D0054228

A Manual of

Laboratory & Diagnostic Tests

Sixth Edition

A Manual of
Laboratory &
Diagnostic Tests

Frances Fischbach, RN, BSN, MSN

Associate Clinical Professor of Nursing
Department of Health Restoration
School of Nursing
University of Wisconsin-Milwaukee
Milwaukee, Wisconsin

Associate Professor of Nursing, Retired
School of Nursing
University of Wisconsin-Milwaukee
Milwaukee, Wisconsin

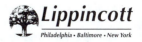

Lippincott

Philadelphia · Baltimore · New York

Editorial Assistant: Dale Thuesen
Project Editor: Nicole Walz
Senior Production Editor: Helen Ewan
Production Coordinator: Pat McCloskey
Art Director: Doug Smock
Indexer: Alexandra Nickerson
Compositor: Peirce Graphic Services, Inc.
Printer: R.R. Donnelly & Sons-Crawfordsville

6th Edition

Copyright © 2000 by Lippincott Williams & Wilkins.
Copyright © 1996, by Lippincott-Raven Publishers. Copyright © 1992, 1988, 1984, 1980, by
J.B. Lippincott Company. All rights reserved. This book is protected by copyright. No part of it may
be reproduced, stored in a retrieval system, or transmitted, in any form or by any means—electronic, mechanical, photocopy, recording, or otherwise—without the prior written permission of
the publisher, except for brief quotations embodied in critical articles and reviews and testing and
evaluation materials provided by publisher to instructors whose schools have adopted its accompanying textbook. Printed in the United States of America. For information write Lippincott
Williams & Wilkins, 530 Walnut Street, Philadelphia, PA, 19106.
Materials appearing in this book prepared by individuals as part of their official duties as U.S. Government employees are not covered by the above-mentioned copyright.

Library of Congress Cataloging in Publication Data

Fischbach, Frances Talaska.
    A manual of laboratory & diagnostic tests / Frances Talaska
Fischbach—6th ed.
      p.   cm.
    Includes bibliographical references and index.
    ISBN 0-7817-1969-0 (alk. paper)
    1. Diagnosis, Laboratory Handbooks, manuals, etc.   1.   Title.
II.   Title: Manual of laboratory and diagnostic tests.
        [DNLM: 1. Laboratory Techniques and Procedures.   QY 25 F528m
    1999]
    RB38.2F27   1999
    616.07′5—dc21
    DNLM/DLC
    for Library of Congress   99-277
                                                                                                      C

Care has been taken to confirm the accuracy of the information presented
and to describe generally accepted practices. However, the author, editors,
and publisher are not responsible for errors or omissions or for any consequences from application of the information in this book and make no warranty, express or implied, with respect to the content of the publication.

The authors, editors, and publisher have exerted every effort to ensure that
drug selection and dosage set forth in this text are in accordance with current
recommendations and practice at the time of publication. However, in view of
ongoing research, changes in government regulations, and the constant flow of
information relating to drug therapy and drug reactions, the reader is urged to
check the package insert for each drug for any change in indications
and dosage and for added warnings and precautions. This is particularly important when the recommended agent is a new or infrequently employed drug.

Some drugs and medical devices presented in this publication have Food
and Drug Administration (FDA) clearance for limited use in restricted research
settings. It is the responsibility of the health care provider to ascertain the FDA
status of each drug or device planned for use in his or her clinical practice.

9 8 7 6 5 4 3 2

To Michael, Mary, Paul, and Margaret

● CONSULTANTS, REVIEWERS, AND RESEARCH ASSISTANTS

Corrinne Strandell, RN, BSN, MSN, PhD
Research and Education Consultant
West Allis, Wisconsin

Marshall B. Dunning, BS, MS, PhD
Associate Professor of Physiology, Department of Critical Care
Pulmonary Medicine
Medical College of Wisconsin
Milwaukee, Wisconsin

Mary Pat Haas Schmidt, BS, MT
Manager, Laboratory Services
OB GYN Associates
Instructor, Medical Technology
Waukesha, Wisconsin

Teresa Friedel Abrams, RN, BSN, MSN
Geriatric Nurse Specialist
Menomonee Falls Health Care Center
Menomonee Falls, Wisconsin

Barbara Barron, MT (ASCP)
Team Immunohematology Department of Pathology
Clement Zablocki VA Medical Center
Milwaukee, Wisconsin

Carol Colasacco, CT (ASCP), CMIAC
Cytotechnologist, Department of Pathology
Fletcher Allen Health Care
Burlington, Vermont

Bernice Gestout DeBoer, RN, BSN, CPAN
Parish Nurse, Covenant Health Care
Milwaukee, Wisconsin

Emma Felder, *RN, BSN, MSN, PhD*
Professor Emeritus, Department of Foundations
University of Wisconsin-Milwaukee
Milwaukee, Wisconsin

Ann Shafranski Fischbach, *RN, BSN*
Occupational Health Nurse
Johnson Controls
Milwaukee, Wisconsin

Cheryl Kaucec, *RN, BSN*
Urologic Nurse
Childrens Hospital of Wisconsin
Milwaukee, Wisconsin

Joan Kizarec, *BS, RTRM*
Director, St. Mary's Hospital
Center for Women's Health
Milwaukee, Wisconsin

Mark S. Lubinsky, *MD*
Associate Professor, Department of Pediatrics
Medical College of Wisconsin
Director, Genetic Services
Children's Hospital of Wisconsin
Milwaukee, Wisconsin

Deborah Martin, *RN, BSN*
Community Health Nurse
Baltimore City Health Department
Maternal and Infant Program Field Office
Baltimore, Maryland

Lyn Mehlberg, *BS, CNMT*
Senior Staff, Nuclear Medicine Technologist
Clinical Instructor, NMT Program
St. Luke's Medical Center
Milwaukee, Wisconsin

Christine Naczek, *MT (ASCP)*
Manager, Blood Banking and Pre-Transfusion Testing
Department of Pathology
United Regional Medical Services, Inc.
Milwaukee, Wisconsin

Anne Witkowiak Nezworski, *RN, BSN*
Maternity and Newborn Specialist
Sacred Heart Hospital
Eau Claire, Wisconsin

Joseph Nezworski, *BS, RN, BSN*
Chief Deputy Medical Examiner
Eau Claire County
Eau Claire, Wisconsin

Richard Nuccio, *MAT, MBA, CNMT (ASCP)*
Global Products
G.E. Medical Systems
Milwaukee, Wisconsin

Patricia Pomahac, *MT (ASCP)*
Supervisor, Diagnostic Immunology
Department of Pathology
United Regional Medical Services, Inc.
Milwaukee, Wisconsin

Tracey Ryan, *RD, CNSD*
Chief Clinical Dietitian
Primary affiliate of the Froedtert Memorial Lutheran Hospital
Medical College of Wisconsin
Milwaukee, Wisconsin

Jean M. Schultz, *BS, RT, RDMS*
Imaging Services
Manager, Metro Region Aurora Health Care
Milwaukee, Wisconsin

Eleanor C. Simms, *RN, BSN*
Specialist, Nursing Student Enrichment Program
Coppin State College
Helene Fuld School of Nursing
Baltimore, Maryland

Rosalie Wilson Steiner, *RN, BSN, MSN, PhD*
Community Health Specialist
Milwaukee, Wisconsin

Keith Templin, *BS, DDS*
Adjunct Instructor, School of Dentistry
Marquette University
Milwaukee, Wisconsin
Private Practice, Germantown, Wisconsin

Jean M. Trione, R.Ph.
Clinical Specialist
Wausau Hospital
Wausau, Wisconsin

Beverly B. Wheeler, RN, MSN, CS
Cardiology/Cardiothoracic Nurse Specialist
National Naval Medical Center
Bethesda, Maryland

● PREFACE

Purpose

The purpose of *A Manual of Laboratory and Diagnostic Tests,* in this Sixth edition, is to promote the delivery of safe, effective, and informed care for patients undergoing diagnostic tests and procedures and also to provide the clinician and student with a unique resource. This comprehensive manual provides a foundation for understanding the relatively simple to the most highly complex diagnostic tests that are delivered to varied populations in varied settings. It describes the clinician's role in providing effective diagnostic services in depth, through affording the necessary information for quality care planning, individualized patient assessment, analysis of patient needs, appropriate interventions, patient education, and timely outcome evaluation.

Potential risks and complications of diagnostic testing mandate that proper tests protocols, interfering factors, follow-up testing, and collaboration among those involved in the testing process be a significant part of the information included in this text.

Organization

This book is organized into 16 chapters and 10 appendices. Chapter 1 outlines the clinician's role in diagnostic testing and includes descriptions of safe, effective, informed pre-, intra-, and posttest care. This chapter has been expanded to include a Patient's Bill of Rights and Responsibilities, a model for the role of the clinical team in providing diagnostic care and services, test environments, reimbursement for diagnostic services, and the importance of communication as key to desired outcomes. The intratest section is new and includes information about collaborative approaches, risk management, the collection, handling, and transport of specimens, controlling pain, comfort measures, and patient monitoring. The reader is referred back to Chapter 1 throughout the text for information about the clinician's role and diagnostic services. Chapters 2 through 16 focus upon specific categories that include:

- Blood Studies
- Urine Studies
- Cerebrospinal Fluid
- Cerebrospinal Fluid Studies

- Cytology, Histology, and Genetic Studies
- Endoscopic Studies
- Ultrasound Studies
- Pulmonary Function and Blood Gas Studies

- Chemistry Studies
- Microbiologic Studies
- Immunodiagnostic Studies
- Nuclear Medicine Studies
- X-ray Studies

- Special Systems, Organ Functions, and Post Mortem Studies
- Prenatal Diagnosis and Tests of Fetal Well-Being

Information about each test includes background rationale, purpose of the test, interfering factors, description of the procedure and test completion, expectations and involvement, and method of specimen collection and handling. Clinical implications with regard to abnormal findings and disease patterns are included. Patient preparation, patient aftercare, and clinical alerts that signal special cautions are integrated into the format. Each test phase has specific guidelines listed. The user-friendly format of the text supports easy information retrieval. Additionally, where possible, age-related reference values are also listed as a component of normal values throughout the text. Numerous examples of test values and clinical considerations for newborn, infant, child, adolescent, and older adult groups have been added where appropriate. A bibliography at the end of each chapter represents a composite of selected references from various disciplines and directs the clinician to information available beyond the scope of this book. The appendices provide the clinician with additional data for everyday practice.

New Information in the Sixth Edition

- The addition of more than 50 new tests and methodologies includes newer procedures for Alzheimer's disease; HIV and hepatitis saliva testing; breast biopsy and prognostic markers; atrial natriuretic factor (ANF) tests for congestive heart failure; fetal well-being tests; ulcer breath test; fertility testing; expanded scope of magnetic resonance imagery (MRI) scans; sleep/sleepiness studies; nuclear tumor detection scans; pediatric considerations for nuclear scans; and bone density scans.

- Appendix J, Drugs Affecting Laboratory Test Values, is new as well as Appendix E, Guidelines for Specimen Transport and/or Storage.

- Revised chapters include changes in the clinician's role and reflect current laboratory and diagnostic practice standards. The appendices are completely revised and contain other additions.

- A greater emphasis is placed upon communication skills and collaboration between health professionals from diverse disciplines, the patients, and their significant others.

Current Developments in Laboratory and Diagnostic Testing

New technologies foster new scientific modalities for patient assessment and clinical interventions. Thus, the clinician is provided a greater understanding of the long chain of events from diagnosis through treatment and outcome. In a brief span of years, new technologies have introduced greatly improved developments in total body and brain scanners; magnetic resonance imagery (MRI); positron emission tomography (PET) scanners; ultrasound and nuclear medicine procedures; genetic studies; new tests for cancer; sleep tests; and postmortem testing after death. Many new technologies are faster, more patient-friendly, more comfortable, and provide an equivalent or higher degree of accuracy (ie, HIV or hepatitis detection, monitoring for drug abuse or therapeutic drug levels). Saliva testing is gaining ground as a mirror of body function, emotional, hormonal, immune, and neurologic status, as well as providing clues about faulty metabolism. Noninvasive testing, which is better suited for testing in environments such as the workplace, private home, and other non-traditional health care settings such as churches, is made possible by better collection methods and standardized collection techniques. Managed care and its drive for control of costs for diagnostic services has a tremendous effect on consumers' access to testing services and the process of care, and results in more access to services in some insurance plans, less in others.

A resurgence in the use of traditional, trusted diagnostic modalities, such as electroencephalogram (EEG), is being seen in certain areas. Diseases such as HIV, antibiotic-resistant strains of pathological organisms, and Type II diabetes are becoming more prevalent. In the workplace, thorough diagnostic testing is more common as applications are made for disability benefits. Also, the number of forensic DNA tests being performed has increased tremendously. Concurrently, consumer perceptions have shifted from implied faith in the health care system to questions about acceptance and trust, related to less independence in choices for health care.

These trends—combined with a shift in diagnostic care from acute care hospital settings to outpatient departments, physicians' offices, clinics, community-based centers, nursing homes, and sometimes even stores and pharmacies—challenge clinicians to provide standards-based, safe, effective, and informed care. Because the health care system is becoming a community-based model, the clinician's role is also changing. Updated knowledge and skills, flexibility, and a heightened awareness of the testing environment are needed to provide diagnostic services in these settings.

Clinicians must also adapt their practice to changes in other areas. This includes developing, coordinating, and following policies and standards set forth by institutions, governmental bodies, and regulatory agencies. Being informed regarding legal implications of informed consent, patient safety, ethical dilemmas about things such as the right to refuse tests, end-of-life decisions, or trends in diagnostic research procedures, add another dimension to the clinician's accountability and responsibility. The consequences of certain types of testing (ie, HIV and genetic) and the implications of confidential versus anonymous testing must also be kept in mind; for example anonymous tests do not require the individual to give his or her name, whereas confidential tests do require the name. This difference has implications in the requirements and process of agency reporting for select groups of infectious diseases such as HIV.

Responding to these trends, the sixth edition of *A Manual of Laboratory and Diagnostic Tests* is a comprehensive, up-to-date diagnostic reference source that includes information about newer technologies, together with the time-honored classic tests that continue to be an important component of diagnostic work. It meets the needs of clinicians, educators, students, and others whose work requires this type of resource or reference manual.

Frances Talaska Fischbach

● ACKNOWLEDGMENTS

I want to give special praise and recognition to my husband, Jack Fischbach, and to my daughters, Mary Fischbach Johnson and Margaret Fischbach, for sharing their expertise and giving their generous help in manuscript preparation, and to my right-hand woman, Kathie Gordon, for carefully arranging and typing the manuscript and for her proficient assistance in all publishing matters.

I would also like to acknowledge and thank all those who provided information and ideas for manuscript revision. This work would not have been complete without the help and information provided by the librarians and staff of the Todd Wehr Library of the Medical College of Wisconsin, the Marquette University Library, and St. Joseph's Hospital Library and the Infection Control Staff at Froedtert Memorial Hospital.

Appreciation and recognition is also due to these persons who encouraged and supported me and assisted with this and previous editions, especially my daughters Mary and Margaret, my daughters-in-law, Ann and Teri, my sons, Michael and Paul, and Gloria Shutte Marolt, Marshall B. Dunning, III, Sheri Watkins, Carolyn Hurst, Timothy Philipp, Theresa Philipp, my cousins, Joe and Anne Nezworski, Jean Pfeiffer Evans, Charles Kerr, Barbara Niemczyski, Randle Pollard, M.D., Richard Kaplon, M.D., Julie Erickson, Rod Doering, Dolaine Genthe, Richard Nuccio, Corrinne Strandell, Sarah Andrus, Mary Pat Schmidt, Bernice DeBoer, and Teri Thode.

As always, many special thanks and compliments to the editorial and production staff at Lippincott Williams & Wilkins, especially the great team of Dale Thuesen and Ilze Rader, who saw the project to completion, to Donna Hilton for her helpful direction, and to Nicole Walz and Helen Ewan for a smooth production. My gratitude to Jay Lippincott, for his personal efforts to foster the author-publisher relationship, for his commitment to excellence in publishing, and for his dedication to the completion of successful projects.

Frances Talaska Fischbach, RN, BSN, MSN

CONTENTS

1

Diagnostic Testing

●————————————————————————————————

Basics of Diagnostic Care

In this era of high technology, health care delivery involves many different disciplines and specialties. Consequently, clinicians must have an understanding and working knowledge of modalities other than their own area of expertise. This includes diagnostic evaluation and diagnostic services. Laboratory and diagnostic tests are tools to gain additional information about the patient. By themselves, these tests are not therapeutic; however, when used in conjunction with a thorough history and physical examination, these tests may confirm a diagnosis or provide valuable information about a patient's status and response to therapy that may not be apparent from the history and physical examination alone. Generally, a tiered approach to selecting tests is used:

1. Basic screening (frequently used with wellness groups and case finding)
2. Establishing (initial) diagnoses
3. Differential diagnosis
4. Evaluation of current medical case management and outcomes
5. Evaluating disease severity
6. Monitoring course of illness and response to treatment
7. Group and panel testing
8. Regularly scheduled screening tests as part of ongoing care
9. Testing related to specific events, certain signs and symptoms, or other exceptional situations (eg, sexual assault, drug screening, pheochromocytoma, postmortem tests)

(See Chart 1-1: Examples of Selecting Tests.)

CHART 1-1 ▶
Examples of Selecting Tests

DIAGNOSTIC TEST	INDICATION
Stool occult blood	Yearly screening after 45 years of age
Serum potassium	Yearly in patients on diuretic agents or potassium supplements
Liver enzyme levels	Yearly if patient is on hepatotoxic drugs; baseline for other patients
Serum amylase	In the presence of abdominal pain
T_4 index or TSH test	Suspicion of hypothyroidism, hyperthyroidism, or thyroid dysfunction, 50 years of age and older
Chlamydia and gonorrhea	In sexually active persons with multiple partners to prevent pelvic inflammatory disease
Hematocrit and hemoglobin	Baseline study; abnormal bleeding; detection of anemia; use CBC results if they are recent
Pap cervical smear	Yearly for all women ≥18 years of age;

(continued)

CHART 1-1 *(continued)*

	more often with high-risk factors (eg, dysplasia, HIV, herpes simplex)
Urine culture	Pyuria
Syphilis serum fluorescent treponemal antibody (FTA) test	Positive VDRL test result
Tuberculosis (TB) skin test	Easiest test to use for TB screening of individuals <35 years of age or those with history of negative TB skin tests
Fasting blood glucose (FBG)	Every 3 years starting at 45 years of age
Urinalysis (UA)	History of recurrent urinary tract disease, pregnant women, men with prostatic hypertrophy
Prothrombin time (PT)	Monitoring anticoagulant treatment
Prostate specific antigen (PSA) and digital rectal examination	Screen men ≥50 years of age for prostate cancer yearly; life expectancy of at least 10 years after detection
Chest x-ray	Follow-up for lung lesions and infiltrates; congestive heart failure; anatomic deformities, posttrauma, before surgery
Mammogram	Screen by 40 years of age in women, then every 12–18 months between 40–49 years of age, annually age ≥50 years of age; follow-up for breast cancer; routine screening when strong family history of breast carcinoma
Colon x-rays and proctosigmoidoscopy	Screen older adults for colon cancer and use after hemoglobin-positive stools, polyps detected, or diverticulosis suspected
Computed tomography (CT) scans	Before and after treatment for certain cancers, injuries, illness (eg, suspected TIA, CVA)
DNA testing of hair, blood, skin tissue or semen samples	To gather postmortem evidence in certain criminal cases; to establish identity and parentage

Some tests are mandated by government agencies or clinical guidelines of professional societies; others are deemed part of necessary care based on the individual practitioner's judgment and expertise or a group practitioner consensus.

T_4, thyroxine; TSH, thyroid-stimulating hormone; PaP, Papanicolaou; HIV, human immunodeficiency virus; VDRL, Venereal Disease Research Laboratory; TIA, transient ischemic attack; CVA, cerebrovascular accident.

As an integral part of their practice, clinicians have long supported patients and their significant others in meeting the demands and challenges incumbent in the simplest to the most complex diagnostic testing. (See Chart 1-2: Basics of Informed Care.) This testing begins before birth and frequently continues

---

CHART 1-2
Basics of Informed Care

- Manage testing environment using collaborative approach
- Communicate effectively and clearly
- Prepare the patient
- Follow standards
- Consider culture, gender, and age diversity
- Measure and evaluate outcomes
- Manage effective diagnostic services using team approach
- Treat, monitor, and counsel about abnormal test outcomes
- Maintain proper test records

---

after death. The clinician who provides diagnostic services must have basic requisite knowledge to plan patient care, make careful judgments, and gather vital information about the patient and the testing process.

The diagnostic testing model incorporates three phases: pretest, intratest,

Test background information	Interfering factors
Normal values	Patient preparation
Explanation of test	Interpreting test results
Indications for testing	Patient aftercare
Actual descriptions of procedures	Clinical alerts
Clinical implications	Special cautions

and posttest (Fig. 1-1). The clinical team actively interacts with the patient and his or her significant others throughout each phase. The following components are included with each laboratory or diagnostic test in this text:

Each phase of testing requires that a specific set of guidelines and standards be followed for accurate and optimal test results. Patient care standards and standards of professional practice are key points in developing a collaborative approach to patient care during diagnostic evaluation. Standards of care provide clinical guidelines and set minimum requirements for professional practice and patient care. They protect the public against less-than-quality care. (See Chart 1-3: Standards for Diagnostic Evaluation.)

If test results are inconclusive or negative and no definitive medical diagnosis can be established, other tests may be ordered. Thus, testing can become an involved and lengthy process (see Fig. 1-1).

Understanding the basics of safe, effective, informed care is important. These basics include assessing risk factors and modifying care accordingly, using a collaborative approach, following proper guidelines for procedures and specimen collection, and delivering appropriate care throughout the process. Providing reassurance and support to the patient and his or her significant oth-

CHART 1-3
Standards For Diagnostic Evaluation

SOURCE OF STANDARDS FOR DIAGNOSTIC SERVICE	STANDARDS FOR DIAGNOSTIC TESTING	EXAMPLES OF APPLIED STANDARDS FOR DIAGNOSTIC TESTING
Professional practice parameters of American Nurses Association (ANA), American Medical Association (AMA), American Society of Clinical Pathologists (ASCP), American College of Radiology, Centers for Disease Control and Prevention (CDC), JCAHO health care practice requirements	Use a decision-making model as a framework for choosing the proper test or procedure and in the interpretation of test results. Use laboratory and diagnostic procedures for screening, differential diagnoses, follow-up, and case management.	Test strategies include single tests or combinations/panels of tests. Panels can be performed in parallel, series, or both.
The guidelines of the major agencies such as American Heart Association, Cancer Society, and American Diabetes Association	Order the correct test, appropriately collect and transport specimens. Properly perform tests in an accredited laboratory or diagnostic facility. Accurately report test results. Communicate and interpret test findings. Treat or monitor the disease and the course of therapy. Provide diagnosis as well as prognosis.	Patients receive diagnostic services based on a documented assessment of need for diagnostic evaluation. Patients have the right to necessary information to enable them to make choices and decisions that reflect their need or wish for diagnostic care.
Individual agency and institution policies and procedures and quality control criteria	Observe standard precautions (formerly known as Universal precautions):use latex allergy protocols and methodology of specimen collection. Use standards and statements for monitoring patients who receive intravenousconscious	The clinician wears protective eye wear and gloves when handling all body fluids and employs proper hand-washing before and after handling specimens and between patient contacts. Labeled biohazard bags are

(continued)

5

CHART 1-3 *(continued)*

procedures. Statements on quality improvement standards. Use standards of professional practice and standards of patient care. Use policy for obtaining informed consent/witnessed consent. Use policies for unusual situations.		sedation for invasive diagnostic used for specimen transport. Vital signs are monitored and recorded at specific times pre- and postprocedure. Patients are monitored for bleeding and respiratory or neurovascular changes. Record data regarding outcomes when defined care criteria are implemented and practiced. Protocols to obtain appropriate consents are employed, and deviations from basic consent policies are documented and reported to the proper individual.
State and federal government communicable disease reporting regulations; Centers for Disease Control and Prevention (CDC), U.S. Department of Health and Human Services, Agency for Health Care Policy and Research (AHCPR), and Clinical Laboratory Improvement Act (CLIA).	Clinical laboratory personnel and other health care providers follow regulations to control the spread of communicable diseases by reporting certain disease conditions, outbreaks, and unusual manifestations and morbidity and mortality data. Findings from research studies provide health care policy makers with guidelines for appropriate selection of tests and procedures.	The clinician reports laboratory evidence of certain disease classes (eg, sexually transmitted diseases, diphtheria, Lyme disease, symptomatic HIV infection; see chap. 7 and 8 for list of reportable diseases.) Persons with hepatitis A may not handle food or care for patients, young children, or the elderly for a specific period of time. Federal government regulates shipment of diagnostic specimens, and MR and CT are used to evaluate persistent low back pain according to AHCPR guidelines.

HIV, human immunodeficiency virus; MR, magnetic resonance; CT, computed tomography.

Diagnostic Testing Process, Care and Services Model **

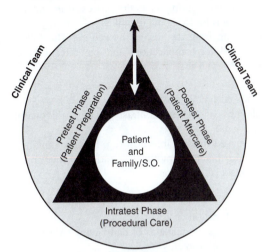

Clinical Team

Pretest
Know test terminology.
Assess for test indications, interferences, contraindictions; identify risk-prone patients and modify care plan and order tests accordingly.
Obtain appropriate consent.
Order tests correctly.
Prepare and educate patient and family.
Consider ethics and law.
Support patient and/or family.
Document and keep proper records.

Posttest
Interpret test results and inform patient.
Know and treat critical values; monitor for post-test complications.
Follow infection control guidelines.

Provide support and counsel for unexpected outcomes.
Order follow-up tests at appropriate intervals and inform patient of same.
Re-educate patient for future testing.
Evaluate the effectiveness of managed care outcomes.
Document and keep proper records.

Intratest
Perform procedure.
Collect and transport specimens.
Observe standard precautions.
Support and reassure patient.
Provide comfort; medicate as necessary.
Monitor appropriately.
Prevent and/or treat complications.
Document and keep proper records.

---

*Components of the Process Model for Diagnostic Care includes: Basic knowledge and skills regarding the following: Test background information, normal reference values, test purpose, indications for testing actual procedures and specimen collection and handling, clinical implications, interfering factors, patient pretest care and preparation, intra-test care, interpreting test results, posttest patient aftercare and clinical alerts for special cautions.

**The role of the Clinical Team is based upon responsibilities, standards, and requisite knowledge addressed in the overview in Chapter One.

***Diagnostic care and services are performed safely, effectively, and in an informed way.
****Services are provided in all 3 phases: Pre-test, Intra-test, and Post-test.

FIGURE 1-1
Model* for the role** of the clinical team in diagnostic care*** and services.****

ers; intervening appropriately; and clearly documenting patient teaching, observations, and outcomes during the entire process is important (see Chart 1-2).

A risk assessment prior to testing identifies risk-prone patients and prevents complications arising from the testing procedure. The following factors increase a patient's risk for complications and may affect outcomes:

Age >70 years
History of falls
History of serious chronic illnesses
History of allergies (eg, latex, contrast iodine, radiopharmaceuticals and other medications)
Infection or increased risk for infection (eg, human immunodeficiency virus [HIV], organ transplant, chemotherapy, radiation therapy)
Aggressive or antisocial behavior
Seizure disorders
Uncontrolled pain
Gastric motility dysfunction
Use of assistive devices for activities of daily living (ADLs)
Unsteady gait, balance problems
Neuromuscular conditions
Weakness, fatigability
Paresthesias
Impaired judgment or illogical thinking
Severe visual problems
Hearing impairment
Use of diuretics, sedatives, analgesics, or other prescription or over-the-counter (OTC) drugs
Alcohol or illegal drug use or addiction

The environments in which diagnostic services are provided; the degree of cultural diversity of the community; and the physical, emotional, social, and spiritual state of the patient all influence the patient's response to the procedure. Including the patient's significant other or others is a vital component of the entire process and must not be taken lightly or casually dismissed.

Testing environments vary. Certain tests (eg, cholesterol screening, blood glucose) can be done "in the field," meaning that the service is brought to the patient's environment. Other tests (eg, electrocardiogram [ECG], hormone levels, and extensive blood chemistry panels) must be done in a physician's office, clinic, or hospital setting. Magnetic resonance (MR) imaging and ultrasound procedures are commonly performed in free-standing diagnostic centers. Complex tests such as endoscopic retrograde cholangiopancreatography (ERCP), cardiac catheterization, or bronchoscopy may require hospital admission or at least outpatient status. As testing equipment becomes more technologically sophisticated and risks associated with testing are reduced, the environment in which diagnostic procedures take place will also shift. Insurance reimbursement for testing influences trends. Managed care and case management, together with collaboration among the diverse health care disciplines and the patient, are key factors in how and to what degree optimal diagnostic services are used.

As societies become more culturally blended, the need to appreciate and work within the realm of cultural diversity becomes imperative. Interacting and directing patients through diagnostic testing can present certain challenges if one is not familiar and sensitive to the health care belief system of the patient and his or her significant others. Something as basic as attempting to communicate in the face of language differences may necessitate arrangements for a relative or translator to be present during all phases of the process. Special attention and communication skills are necessary for these situations as well as when caring for children, and for comatose, confused, or frail patients. Consideration of these issues will significantly influence compliance, outcomes, and positive responses to the procedure. To be most effective, professional care providers must be open to a holistic perspective and attitude that informs their caregiving and communication behaviors.

Preparing patients for diagnostic or therapeutic procedures, collecting specimens, carrying out and assisting with procedures, and providing follow-up care have long been requisite activities of professional practice. This care may continue even after the patient's death. Diagnostic postmortem services include death reporting, possible postmortem investigations, and sensitive communication with grieving families and significant others regarding autopsies and other postmortem testing (see Chap. 15).

Professionals need to work as a team to meet diverse patient needs, to facilitate certain decisions, to develop comprehensive plans of care, and to help patients modify their daily activities to meet test requirements in all three phases. It is a given that institutional protocols are followed.

PRETEST PHASE: ELEMENTS OF SAFE, EFFECTIVE, INFORMED CARE ●

The emphasis of pretest care is on appropriate test selection, proper patient preparation, individualized patient education, and emotional support.

Basic Knowledge and Necessary Skills

Know the test terminology, purpose, process, procedure, and normal test reference values or results. The names of diseases are a convenient way of briefly stating the endpoint of a diagnostic process that begins with assessment of symptoms and signs and ends with knowledge of causation and detection of underlying disorders of structure and function.

The clinical value of a test is related to its *sensitivity,* its *specificity,* and the *incidence of the disease* in the population tested. Sensitivity and specificity do not change with different populations of ill and healthy patients. The *predictive* value of the same test can vary significantly with age, gender, and geographic location.

Specificity refers to the ability of a test to correctly identify those individuals who do not have the disease. The division formula for specificity is as follows:

% of specificity =
$$\frac{\text{persons without disease who test negative}}{\text{divided by the total number of persons without the disease}} \times 100$$

Sensitivity refers to the ability of a test to correctly identify those individuals who truly have the disease. The division formula for sensitivity is as follows:

% of sensitivity =

$$\frac{\text{persons with disease who test positive}}{\text{divided by the total number of persons tested with disease}} \times 100$$

Incidence refers to the prevalence of a disease in a population or community. The predictive value of the same test can be very different when applied to people of differing ages, genders, and geographic locations.

Predicted Values refer to the ability of a screening test result to correctly identify the disease state. *True-positives* correctly identify individuals who actually have the disease, and *true-negatives* correctly identify individuals who do not actually have the disease. *Positive predictive value* equals the percent of positive tests that are true-positives (ie, the individual does have the disease). *Negative predictive value* refers to the percent of negative tests that are true-negatives (ie, the individual does not have the disease).

The following example demonstrates the specificity, sensitivity, and predictive values for a new screening test to identify the cystic fibrosis gene.

Test Result	Have Gene for Cystic Fibrosis	Do Not Have Gene for Cystic Fibrosis	Total
Positive	62	5	67
Negative	15	341	356
Total	77	346	423

$$\% \text{ specificity} = \frac{341}{346} \times 100 = 98.5\%$$

$$\% \text{ sensitivity} = \frac{62}{77} \times 100 = 80.5\%$$

Thus, this new screening test will give a false-negative result about 20% of the time (ie, the person does have the cystic fibrosis gene but his or her test results are negative).

$$\text{positive predictive value} = \frac{62}{67} \times 100 = 92.5\%$$

Thus, there is about an 8% chance that the person will test positive for the cystic fibrosis gene but does not have it.

$$\text{negative predictive value} = \frac{341}{356} \times 100 = 95.7\%$$

Thus, there is about a 5% chance that the person will test negative for the cystic fibrosis gene, but actually does have it.

Look at both current and previous test results and review the most recent laboratory data first, then work sequentially backward to evaluate trends or changes from previous data. The patient's plan of care may need to be modified because of test results and changes in medical management.

Testing Environments

Diagnostic testing occurs in many different environments. Many test sites have shifted into community settings and away from hospitals and clinics.

Point-of-Care Testing refers to tests done in the primary care setting. In acute care settings (eg, critical care units, ambulances), state-of-the-art testing can produce rapid reporting of test results.

Testing in the home care environment requires skill in procedures such as drawing blood samples, collecting samples from retention catheters, proper specimen labeling, documentation, specimen handling, and specimen transporting. Moreover, teaching the patient and his or her significant others how to collect specimens is an important part of the process.

In occupational health environments, testing may be done to reduce or prevent known workplace hazards (eg, exposure to lead) and to monitor identified health problems. This can include preemployment baseline screening, periodic monitoring of exposure to potentially hazardous workplace substances, and drug screening. Skill in drawing blood samples, performing breathing tests, monitoring chain of custody (see page 240 in Chap. 3), and obtaining properly signed and witnessed consent forms for drug testing is required.

More pretest, posttest, and follow-up testing occurs in nursing homes because patients are more frequently taken or transferred to hospitals for more complex procedures (eg, computed tomography [CT] scans, endoscopies), whereas this is not the case with routine testing. Increasing numbers of "full code" (ie, resuscitation) orders leads to greater numbers and varieties of tests. Additionally, confused, combative, or uncooperative behaviors are seen more frequently in these settings. An attitude adopted by nursing home patients of "not wanting to be bothered" or engaging in outright refusal to undergo prescribed tests can make testing difficult. Consequently, understanding patient behaviors and using appropriate communication strategies and interventions for this population is a necessary skill for practicing in this arena.

For those who practice in the realm of public health, diagnostic test responsibilities focus on wellness screenings, preventive services, disease control, counseling, and treatment of individuals with problems. Case finding frequently occurs at health fairs, outreach centers, homeless shelters, neighborhood nurse offices, mobile health vans, and church settings. Responsibilities vary according to setting, and may include providing test information, procuring specimens, and providing referrals to appropriate caregivers. These responsibilities may even extend to transporting and preparing specimens for analysis or actually performing specimen analysis (eg, stool tests for occult blood, tuberculosis [TB] skin testing, procuring blood or saliva samples for HIV/acquired immunodeficiency syndrome [AIDS] testing).

History and Assessment

Obtain a relevant, current health history; perform a physical assessment if indicated. Identify conditions that could influence the actual testing process or test outcomes (eg, pregnancy, diabetes, cultural diversity, language barrier, physical impairment, altered mental state).

1. Perform a risk assessment for potential injury or noncompliance.
2. Identify contraindications to testing such as allergies (eg, iodine, latex, medications, contrast media). Records of previous diagnostic procedures may provide clues.
3. Assess for coping styles and knowledge or teaching needs.
4. Assess fears and phobias (eg, claustrophobia, "panic attacks," fear of needles and blood). Ascertain what strategies the patient uses to deal with these reactions and try to accommodate these.
5. A patient may choose not to disclose drug or alcohol use or HIV and hepatitis risks. Observe universal precautions with every patient (see Appendix A).
6. Document relevant data. Address patient concerns and questions. This information adds to the database for collaborative problem-solving activities among the medical, laboratory/diagnostic, and nursing disciplines.

Reimbursement for Diagnostic Services

Differences in both diagnostic care services and reimbursement may vary between private and government insurance. Nonetheless, quality of care should not be compromised in favor of cost reduction. Advocate for patients regarding insurance coverage for diagnostic services. Inform the patient and his or her family or significant others that it may be necessary to check with their insurance company prior to laboratory and diagnostic testing to make certain that costs are covered.

Many insurance companies employ case managers as gatekeepers for monitoring costs, diagnostic tests ordered, and other care. As a result, the insurance company or third-party payor may reimburse only for certain tests or procedures or may not cover tests considered by them to be preventive care.

Methodology of Testing

Follow testing procedures accurately. Verify orders and document them with complete, accurate, and legible information. Record all drugs the patient is taking because these may influence test outcomes (see Appendix J).

1. Ensure that specimens are correctly obtained, preserved, handled, labeled, and delivered to the appropriate department. For example, it is not generally acceptable to draw blood samples when an intravenous line is infusing proximal to the intended puncture site.
2. Observe precautions for patients in isolation.
3. As much as possible, coordinate patient activities with testing schedules to avoid conflicts with meal times, administration of medications, treatments, or other diagnostic tests.
   a. Maintain NPO (ie, nothing by mouth) status when necessary.
   b. Administer the proper medications in a timely manner. Schedule tests requiring contrast substances in the proper sequence so as to not invalidate succeeding tests.

Interfering Factors

Minimize test outcome deviations by following proper test protocols. Make certain the patient and his or her significant others know what is expected of them. Written instructions are very helpful.

Deviations may include the following:

Incorrect specimen collection, handling, storage, or labeling
Wrong preservative or lack of preservative
Delayed specimen delivery
Incorrect or incomplete patient preparation
Hemolyzed blood samples
Incomplete sample collection, especially of timed samples
Old or deteriorating specimens

Patient factors that can alter test results may include the following:

Incorrect pretest diet
Current drug therapy
Type of illness
Dehydration
Position or activity at time of specimen collection
Postprandial status (ie, time patient last ate)
Time of day
Pregnancy
Age and gender
Level of patient knowledge and understanding of testing process
Stress
Nonadherence or noncompliance with instructions and pretest preparation
Undisclosed drug or alcohol use

Avoiding Errors

To avoid costly mistakes, know what equipment and supplies are needed and how the test is performed. Communication errors account for more incorrect results than do technical errors. Properly identify and label every specimen as soon as it is obtained. Determine the type of sample needed and the collection method to be used. Is the test invasive or noninvasive? Are contrast media injected or swallowed? Is there a need to fast? Are fluids restricted or forced? Are medications administered or withheld? What is the approximate length of the procedure? Are consent forms and conscious sedation, oxygen, or anesthesia required? Report test results as soon as possible. "Critical" or "panic" values must be reported to the proper persons immediately (STAT).

Instruct patients and their significant others regarding their responsibilities. Accurately outline the steps of the testing process and any restrictions that may apply. Conscientious, clear, timely communication among health care departments can reduce errors and inconvenience to both staff and patients.

Proper Preparation

Prepare the patient correctly.

1. Be aware of special needs of those with conditions such as physical limitations or disabilities, ostomies, or diabetes; children; the elderly; and the culturally diverse.
2. Give simple, accurate, precise instructions according to the patient's level of understanding. For example, the patient needs to know when and what to eat and drink or how long they must fast.

3. Encourage dialogue about fears and apprehensions. "Walking" a patient through the procedure using imagery and relaxation techniques may help them to cope with anxieties. Never underestimate the value of a caring presence.
4. Assess for ability to read and understand instructions. Poor eyesight or hearing difficulties may impair understanding and compliance. Speak slowly and clearly. Do not bombard the patient with information. Instruct the patient to use assistive devices such as eyeglasses and hearing aids if necessary. Clear, written instructions can reinforce verbal instructions and should be used whenever possible.
5. Assess for language and cultural barriers. Patients behave according to personal values, perceptions, beliefs, traditions, and cultural and ethnic influences. Take these into consideration and value the patient's uniqueness to the utmost degree possible.
6. Document results accurately in all testing phases.

Patient Education

Educate the patient and family regarding the testing process and what will be expected of them. Record the date, time, type of teaching, and information given, and to whom it was given.

1. Giving sensory and objective information that relates to what the patient will likely physically feel and the equipment that will be used is important so that patients can "see" a realistic representation of what will occur. Avoid technical and medical jargon and adapt information to the patient's level of understanding. Slang terms may be necessary to get a point across.
2. Encourage questions and verbalization of feelings, fears, and concerns. Do not dismiss, minimize, or invalidate the patient's anxiety through remarks such as "Don't worry." Develop "listening ears and eyes" skills. Be aware of nonverbal signals (ie, body language), because these frequently provide a more accurate picture of what the patient really feels than what he or she says. Above all, be nonjudgmental.
3. Emphasize that there is usually a waiting period (ie, "turn-around time") before test results are relayed back to the clinicians and nursing unit. The patient may have to wait several days for results. Offer listening, presence, and support during this time of great concern and anxiety.
4. Record test result information. Include the patient's response. Just because something is taught does not necessarily mean that it is learned or accepted. The possibility that a diagnosis will require a patient to make significant lifestyle changes (eg, diabetes) requires intense support, understanding, education, and motivation. Document specific names of audiovisual and reading materials to be used for audit, reimbursement, and accreditation purposes.

Testing Protocols

Develop consistent protocols for teaching and testing that encompass comprehensive pretest, intratest, and posttest care modalities.

Prepare patients for those aspects of the procedure experienced by the majority of patients. Clinicians can collaborate to collect data and to develop a list of common patient experiences, responses, and reactions.

Patient Independence

Allow the patient to maintain as much control as possible during the diagnostic phases to reduce stress and anxiety. Include the patient and his or her significant others in decision making. Because of factors such as anxiety, language barriers, and physical or emotional impairments, the patient may not fully understand and assimilate instructions and explanations. To validate the patient's understanding of what is presented, ask the patient to repeat instructions given to evaluate assimilation and understanding of presented information.

Include and reinforce information about the diagnostic plan, the procedure, time frames, and the patient's role in the testing.

Test Results

Knowledge of normal or reference values is vital.

1. Normal ranges can vary to some degree from laboratory to laboratory. Theoretically, "normal" can refer to the ideal health state, to average reference values, or to types of statistical distribution. Normal values are those that fall within 2 standard deviations (ie, random variation) from the mean value for the normal population.
2. The reported reference range for a test can vary according to the laboratory used, the method employed, the population tested, and methods of specimen collection and preservation. Laboratories must specify their own normal ranges. Many factors affect laboratory test values and influence ranges. Thus, values may be normal under one set of prevailing conditions but may exhibit different limits in other circumstances. Age, gender, race, environment, posture, diurnal and other cyclic variations, foods, beverages, fasting or postprandial state, drugs, and exercise can affect derived values. Interpretation of laboratory results must always be in the context of the patient's state of being. Circumstances such as hydration, nutrition, fasting state, mental status, or compliance with test protocols are only a few of the situations that can influence test outcomes.
3. The majority of normal blood test values are determined by measuring "fasting" specimens.
4. Be aware of specific influences on test results. Patient posture is important when plasma volume is measured, because this value is 12% to 15% greater in a person who has been supine for several hours. Changing from a supine to standing position can alters values as follows: increased hemoglobin (Hb), red blood cell count (RBC), hematocrit (Hct), calcium, potassium (K), phosphorus (P), aspartate aminotransferase (AST), phosphatases, total protein, albumin, cholesterol, and triglycerides. Going from an upright to a supine position results in decreased Hct, calcium (Ca), total protein, and cholesterol.

A tourniquet applied for >1 minute produces laboratory value increases in protein (5%), iron (6.7%), AST (9.3%), and cholesterol (5%) and decreases in K^+ (6%) and creatinine (2%–3%).

Laboratory Reports

Scientific publications and many professional organizations are changing clinical laboratory data values from conventional units to Système International (SI) units. Currently, much data are reported in both ways.

The SI system uses seven dimensionally independent units of measurement to provide logical and consistent measurements. For example, SI concentrations are written as *amount* per volume (moles or millimoles per liter) rather than as *mass* per volume (grams, milligrams, or milliequivalents per deciliter, 100 milliliters, or liter). Numerical values may differ between systems or may be the same. For example, chloride is the same in both systems: 95 to 105 mEq/L (conventional) and 95 to 105 mmol/L (SI) (see Appendix D).

Margins of Error

Recognize margins of error. For example, if a patient has a battery of chemistry tests, the possibility exists that some tests will be abnormal owing purely to chance. This occurs because a significant margin of error arises from the arbitrary setting of limits. Moreover, if a laboratory test is considered normal up to the 95th percentile, then 5 times out of 100, the test will show an abnormality even though a patient is not ill. A second test performed on the same sample will probably yield the following: 0.95×0.95, or 90.25%. This means that 9.75 times out of 100, a test will show an abnormality even though the person has no underlying health disorder. Each successive testing will produce a higher percentage of abnormal results. If the patient has a group of tests performed on one blood sample, the possibility that some of the tests will "read abnormal" due purely to chance is not uncommon.

Ethics and the Law

Consider legal and ethical implications. These include the patient's right to information, properly signed and witnessed consent forms, and explanations and instructions regarding risks as well as benefits of tests.

1. The patient must demonstrate appropriate cognitive and reasoning faculties to legally sign a valid consent. Conversely, a patient may not legally give consent while under the immediate influence of sedation, anesthetic agents, or certain classes of analgesics and tranquilizers. If the patient cannot validly and legally sign a consent form, an appropriately qualified individual may give consent for the patient.

2. Guidelines and wishes set forth in advance directives or "living will"–type documents must be honored, especially in life-threatening situations. Such directives may prevent more sophisticated invasive procedures from being performed. Some states have legislated that patients can procure "do not resuscitate" (DNR) orders and medical DNR bracelets that indicate their wishes.

3. A collaborative team approach is essential for responsible, lawful, and ethical patient-focused care. The clinician who orders the test has a responsibility to inform the patient about risks and test results and to discuss alternatives for follow-up care. Other caregivers can provide additional information and clarification and can support the patient and family in achieving the best possible outcomes. The duty to maintain confidentiality and provide freedom of choice and the necessity of reporting infectious diseases may result in ethical dilemmas.

Respect for the dignity of the individual reflects basic ethical considerations. Patients and family have a right to consent, to question, to request other opinions, or to refuse diagnostic tests. Conversely, caregivers have the right to know the diagnoses of the patients they care for so they can minimize the risks to themselves.

Patient's Bill of Rights and Patient Responsibilities

Patients have a right to expect that an agency's or institution's policies and procedures will ensure certain rights and responsibilities for them. The patient has the following rights at all times:

1. To considerate, honest, respectful care with consideration given to privacy and maintenance of personal dignity, cultural and personal values and beliefs, and physical and developmental needs, regardless of the setting.

2. To be involved in decision making and to actively participate, if so desired, in the testing process, assuming the patient is competent to make these choices.

3. To participate in the informed consent process prior to testing, and to be told of the benefits, risks, and reasonable alternative approaches to tests ordered.

4. To be informed regarding test costs and reimbursement responsibility.

5. To refuse diagnostic testing.

6. To expect to have the support of family or significant others, if so desired and appropriate during the testing process.

7. To expect that standards of care will be followed by all personnel involved in the testing process.

8. To expect safe, skilled, quality care provided by trained personnel with expertise in their field.

9. To expect patient and family education and instructions regarding all phases of the testing process and procedure, including the nature and purpose of the test, pretest preparation, actual testing, posttest care benefits, risks, side-effects, and complications. Information should be provided in a sensitive and objective manner.

10. To expect to be informed in a timely manner of test results and implications, treatment, and future testing if necessary.

11. To expect to be counseled appropriately regarding abnormal test outcomes as well as alternative options and available treatments.

12. To expect to have acceptable pain control and comfort measures provided throughout the testing process.

13. To expect that all verbal, written, and electronic communication, medical records, and medical record transfers will be accurate and confidential. *Exception: when reporting of situation is required by law* (eg, *certain infectious diseases, child abuse*).

The patient has the following responsibilities:

1. To comply with test requirements (eg, fasting, special preparations, medications, enemas) or to inform the clinician if they are unable to do so.

2. To report active or chronic disease conditions that may alter test outcomes, be adversely affected by the testing process, or pose a risk to health care providers (eg, HIV, hepatitis).

3. To keep appointments for diagnostic procedures and follow-up testing.

4. To disclose drug and alcohol use after being informed that these situations affect test outcome (eg, erroneous test results).

5. To disclose allergies and past history of testing procedures after being informed why this information is important (eg, contrast media).

6. To report any adverse effects attributed to tests and procedures after being advised to watch for possible signs and symptoms.

Cultural Sensitivity

Preserving the cultural well being of any individual or group promotes compliance with testing and easier recovery from routine as well as more invasive and complex procedures. Sensitive questioning and observation may provide information about certain cultural traditions, concerns, and practices related to health. For example, the Hmong people believe the soul resides in the head and that no one should touch an adult's head without permission. Patting a child on the head may violate this belief. Health care personnel should make an effort to understand the cultural differences of populations they serve without passing judgment. Most people of other cultures are willing to share this information if they feel it will be respected. Sometimes a translator is necessary for accurate communication.

Many cultures have diverse beliefs about diagnostic testing that requires blood sampling. For example, alarm about having blood specimens drawn or concerns regarding the disposal of body fluids or tissue may require health care workers to demonstrate the utmost patience, sensitivity, and tact when communicating information about blood tests.

INTRATEST PHASE: ELEMENTS OF SAFE, EFFECTIVE, INFORMED CARE

Basic Knowledge and Required Skills

Intratest care focuses on specimen or tissue collection, performing and/or assisting with procedures, providing emotional and physical comfort and reassurance, administering analgesics and sedatives, and monitoring vital signs and other parameters during testing. The clinician must have basic knowledge about the procedure and test and should have the required skills to perform testing or assist in the process. Safe practice, correct collection of specimens, minimizing delays, providing support to the patient, monitoring as necessary, and being alert to potential side-effects or complications are integral activities of the intratest phase.

Infection Control

Follow accepted infection control protocols. The term *standard precautions* refers to a system of disease control that presupposes each direct contact with body fluids is potentially infectious and that every person exposed to these fluids must protect themselves. Consequently, health care workers must be both informed and conscientious about adhering to standard precautions and strict infection control guidelines. It goes without saying that health care workers must be scrupulous about proper hand washing (see Appendix A). Proper protective clothing and other devices must be worn as necessary.

Procurement and disposal of specimens according to U.S. Occupational Health and Safety Administration (OSHA) standards must be adhered to. Moreover, institutions may have procedures and policies of their own to ensure compliance (eg, specimens are to be placed directly into biohazard bags).

NOTE: *Standard precautions* (formerly known as universal precautions) *prevail in all situations in which risk of exposure to blood, tissue, and other body fluids is even remotely possible.* The terms standard precautions and universal precautions are often used interchangeably.

Collaborative Approaches

A collaborative team approach is necessary for certain procedures. Clinicians must assist and understand each other's role in the procedure. Invasive procedures such as lumbar punctures or cystoscopy place patients at greater risk for complications and usually require closer monitoring during the test. Astute observation of the patient and critical thinking and quick decision-making skills during intense situations is a requisite for clinicians in these settings. Intravenous (IV) sedation and other IV drugs are a frequent part of the scenario in which clinicians from various disciplines work as a team.

Risk Management

Provide a safe environment for the patient at all times. Prevention of complications and management of risk factors is an important part of the intratest phase. As part of risk management, observe standard precautions and infection control precautions as necessary (see Appendices A, B, and C).

Use special care during procedures that include iodine and barium contrasts, radiopharmaceuticals, latex products, and IV conscious sedation. (See Chaps. 9, 10, and 15 for precautions for imaging procedures.) Certain risk factors contribute to a higher incidence of undesirable reactions when contrast agents and radiopharmaceuticals are used.

Classification of Risk Factors	
Preexisting Disorders	*Contributing Elements*
Allergy	Age-related (newborn and older adults)
Asthma	Dehydration
Diabetes	Frequent use of contrast agents
Liver insufficiency	High dosage of contrast and radiopharmaceuticals
Multiple myeloma	Previous reaction to contrast agents
Pheochromocytoma	
Renal failure	
Seizure history	

Assess for a safe environment. Identify patients at risk and environments that may pose a risk. A history of falls, cerebrovascular accident (CVA), neuromuscular disorders, loss of balance, or use of ambulatory assistive devices are contributory risk factors.

Collecting and Transporting Specimens

Procure, process, transport, and store specimens properly for the prescribed test. The community environment and health care setting in which testing takes place dictates protocols for collection, handling, and transporting of specific specimens. Everyone involved in the process must have a thorough understanding of testing principles and protocols to prevent invalid test results and patient injury and to ensure desired outcomes.

Determine specimen type needed and method of sample procurement. Examples may include urine collection, venipuncture, arterial puncture, or bone marrow aspirate. Additionally, special equipment and supplies may be necessary (eg, sterile containers, special kits).

Collection by the patient requires patient cooperation and prior instruction but does not always require direct supervision. Conversely, supervised collection requires participation by trained persons and supervision of the patient during specimen collection. Examples of these two types of collection include a routine urine sample collected by the patient at home (done by patient only) versus a urine sample collection done in a controlled setting (supervised) such as that procured for drug screening.

A third method of collection requires that the clinician perform the entire collection. An example of this type of collection is aspirating a urine sample from an indwelling catheter.

Time of collection is also important. For example, results from a fasting blood glucose test versus results from a 2-hour-postprandial blood glucose test have an entirely different significance from each other as a diagnostic parameter.

Prevent specimen rejection caused by the following errors related to the specimen itself or the collection process.

Specimen Errors	*Collector Errors*
Insufficient volume	Transport delay
Improper type	Improper collection method
Insufficient number of samples	Wrong specimen container
Wrong transport medium or wrong or absent preservative	Wrong time
	Incorrect storage
	Unlabeled or mislabeled specimen and/or wrong patient identification information
	Improperly completed forms or computer data entry
	Discrepancies between test ordered and specimen collected
	Failure to properly transcribe and process orders

Blood collection is normally done by trained persons. (An exception is the self-test for blood glucose using equipment designed specifically for that purpose). The time of collection is an important factor (eg, a sequence of samples for a cardiac panel). For example, a "peak" drug level blood specimen is collected when highest drug concentration in the blood is expected. This type of test is used for therapeutic drug monitoring and dosing. Conversely, a "trough" sample is collected when lowest drug concentration is expected. These types of tests are used for therapeutic drug monitoring and specimens are collected and results reported before the next scheduled dose of medication.

Legal and forensic specimens are collected as evidence in legal proceedings, criminal investigations, and after death. Examples include DNA samples and drug and alcohol levels, and factors such as chain of custody situations and witnessed collections may be involved.

1. Assemble the proper supplies and equipment.

   a. Stool and urine collection requires clean, dry containers and kits. Timed urine collection requires refrigeration and/or containers with special additives. Sterile, dry containers and special kits are needed for midstream clean-catch urine specimens. Oral and sputum specimens require specific techniques and kits and sometimes special preservatives.

   b. Blood collection equipment includes gloves, needles, collection tubes, syringes, tourniquets, needle disposal containers, lancets for skin puncture, cleansing agents or antimicrobial skin preparations, and adhesive bandages. Color-coded stoppers and tubes indicate the type of additive present in the collection tube. Additives preserve the specimen, prevent deterioration and coagulation, and/or block action of certain enzymes in blood cells. Tubes with anticoagulants should be gently and completely inverted (end over end) 7 to 10 times after collection. This process ensures complete mixing of anticoagulants with the blood sample and prevents clot formation.

Blood Specimen Collections

Collection Tube Color and Additives	Use and Precautions
Serum separator tubes (SST): no anticoagulant	For collecting serum samples such as chemistry analysis. SST tubes should be gently inverted (completely, end over end) 5 times after collection to ensure mixing of clot activator with blood and clotting within 30 minutes. After the 30-minute period, centrifuge promptly at designated relative centrifugal force (rct) for 15 ± 5 minutes to separate serum from cells. Serum can be stored in gel separator tubes after centrifugation for up to 48 hours. Do not freeze SST tubes. If frozen specimen is needed, separate serum into a labeled plastic transfer vial. Serum separation tubes must not be used to obtain therapeutic drug levels because the gel may lower values.
Red-topped (plain) tube: no anticoagulant, no additive	For serum chemistry, serology, blood bank, collection of clotted blood specimens.
Plain pink tube: no additive or anticoagulant	For blood bank.
Light green marbled tube: gel separator/lithium, heparin as anticoagulant	For potassium determination.
Black tube: with sodium citrate (binds calcium)	For Westergren sedimentation rate.
Green-topped tube: with anticoagulant heparin (sodium, lithium, and ammonium heparin)	For heparinized plasma specimens, plasma chemistries, arterial blood gases, and special tests such as ammonia levels, hormones, and electrolytes; invert 7–10 times to prevent clot formation.
Gray-topped tube: with oxalate alcohol and fluoride	For glucose levels, glucose tolerance levels.

(continued)

Blood Specimen Collections   *(Continued)*

Collection Tube Color and Additives	*Use and Precautions*
Lavender–topped tube: with ethylene diamine tetraacetic acid (EDTA; removes calcium to prevent clotting)	For whole blood and plasma, for hematology and complete blood counts (CBCs); prevents the filled tube from clotting. If the tube is less than half-filled, the proportion of anti-coagulant to blood may be sufficiently altered to produce unreliable laboratory test results. Invert tube 6–8 times.
Light blue–topped tube: with sodium citrate as anticoagulant (removes calcium to prevent clotting)	For plasma-coagulation studies (eg, prothrombin times [PT], PT/partial thromboplastin time [PTT]) and factor assays. The tube **must** be allowed to fill to its capacity or an improper blood/anticoagulant ratio will invalidate coagulation test results. Invert tube 7–10 times to prevent clotting.
Royal blue–topped tube: no additive, with EDTA or sodium heparin anticoagulant	For toxicology, cadmium and mercury; tube free of trace elements. Invert tube 7–10 times.
Royal blue–topped tube: without EDTA or sodium heparin (no anticoagulant—blood will clot)	For aluminum, arsenic, chromium, copper, nickel, and zinc levels; tube free of trace elements.
Tan/brown–topped tube: with heparin as anticoagulant	For heparinized plasma specimens for testing lead levels (ie, lead-free tube). Invert tube 7–10 times.
Yellow–topped tube: sodium polyethylene sulfonate (SPS)	For collection of blood cultures; aseptic technique for blood draw; invert tube 7–10 times to prevent clot formation.
Gold– or red marbled–topped tube: serum gel separator tube (SST)	For serum, used for most chemistry tests; These tubes should be gently inverted 5 times after collection to ensure mixing of clot activator with blood and clotting within 30 minutes. After 30-minute period, centrifuge promptly at designated rct for 15 ± 5 minutes to separate serum from cells. Serum can be stored in gel separator tubes after centrifugation for up to 48 hours. Do not freeze SST tubes. If frozen specimen is needed, separate serum into a labeled plastic transfer vial. Serum separation tubes must not be used for therapeutic drug levels. The gel may lower values. Not for blood bank use.

2. Store specimens properly after collecting or transport to the laboratory immediately for processing and analysis if possible. Failure to do so may result in specimen deterioration. "STAT" ordered tests should always be hand-delivered to the laboratory and then processed as "STAT." Unacceptable specimens lead to increased costs and time wasted in getting results to the clinician, the patient, the institution, and third-party payor. Exposure to sunlight, air, or other substances and warming or cooling are examples of things that can alter specimen integrity (see Appendix E).

3. As environments for specimen collection become more variable, adapted procedures and protocols require the clinician to keep abreast of the latest information related to these factors (see Appendix E).

Pain Control, Comfort Measures, and Patient Monitoring

Provide proper information, reassurance, and support throughout the entire procedure to allay anxiety and fear. Administer sedatives, pain medication, or antiemetics as ordered. Uphold the dignity of each patient, provide privacy, and minimize any situation that might cause embarrassment or stress. Continue monitoring throughout procedures as well as after completion, if indicated.

1. Do not permit the patient to remain disrobed any longer than necessary. Allow personal clothing and other accessories such as rings or religious medals provided they do not pose a risk or interfere with the procedure. Assure a reasonable degree of privacy.

2. Control pain and provide comfort measures. IV conscious sedation and drugs given to reverse the effects of test medications are part of this scenario. Allow the patient to maintain as much control as possible during all testing phases without compromising safety, the process and procedure, and test integrity. If possible, plan ahead to accommodate persons with special needs such as learning disabilities, visual impairment, ostomy, or diabetes management.

3. Monitor and document vital signs and other relevant parameters (eg, pulse oximetry, ECG) throughout the procedure. Observe for problems and abnormal reactions and take appropriate measures to correct such situations.

4. Document the patient's response to the procedure during all phases. Also document significant events or situations that occur during testing and record disposition of specimens.

POSTTEST PHASE: ELEMENTS OF SAFE, EFFECTIVE, INFORMED CARE

Basic Knowledge and Necessary Skills

The focus of the posttest phase is on patient aftercare and the follow-up activities, observations, and monitoring necessary to prevent or minimize complications. Evaluation of outcomes and effectiveness of care, discharge planning, and appropriate posttest referrals are the major components of this phase.

Abnormal Test Results

Report and interpret test outcomes correctly. Abnormal test patterns or trends can sometimes provide more useful information than single test outcome deviations. Conversely, single test results can be normal in persons with a proven disease or illness.

1. Recognize abnormal test results and consider the implications for the patient in both the acute and the chronic stages of the disease as well as during screening.
2. The greater the degree of test abnormality, the more likely the outcome will be more serious.
3. Consider the role of drugs when tests are abnormal. Use of OTC drugs, vitamins, iron, and other minerals may produce false-positive or false-negative test results. Patients often do not disclose all medications they use, either unintentionally or deliberately. Commonly prescribed drugs that most often affect laboratory test outcomes include anticoagulants, anticonvulsants, antihypertensives, antibiotic or antiviral agents, oral hypoglycemics, hormones, and psychotropic drugs. Consult a pharmacist or Physicians Desk Reference (PDR) source about drugs the patient is taking (eg, current literature search, computerized data, or manufacturer's drug insert sheet) (see Appendix J).
4. Consider biocultural variations when interpreting test results. The table that follows provides examples of some common variations.

Diagnostic Test	*Biocultural Variation*
Orthopedic x-rays	Body proportions and tendencies: African American people exhibit longer arms and legs and shorter trunks than Caucasians. African American women tend to be wider shouldered and more narrow hipped, but with more abdominal adipose tissue than do Caucasian women. Caucasian men tend to exhibit more abdominal adipose tissue than do African American men. Native Americans and Asian Americans have larger trunks and shorter limbs than do African American and Caucasian people. Asian American people tend to be wider hipped and more narrow shouldered than do other peoples.
Bone density measurements	African American men have the densest bones, followed by African American women and Caucasian men, who have similar bone densities. Caucasian women have the least dense bones. Chinese, Japanese, and Inuit bone density is less than that of Caucasian Americans. Additionally, bone density decreases with age.
Test for glucose-6-phosphate dehydrogenase deficiency (G6PD)	G6PD deficiency may be the cause of hemolytic disease of newborns in Asian American and those of Mediterranean descent. Three G6PD variants occur frequently: type A is common in African Americans

(continued)

Diagnostic Test	*Biocultural Variation* *(Continued)*
	(10% of males); the Mediterranean type is common in Iraqis, Kurds, Lebanese, and Sephardic Jews; and the Mahedial type is common in Southeast Asians (22% of males).
Cholesterol levels	African American and Caucasian ethnic groups have similar cholesterol levels at birth. During childhood, African American people develop higher levels than do Caucasian people; however, African American adults have lower cholesterol levels than do Caucasian adults.
Hemoglobin/hematocrit levels	The normal hemoglobin level for African American people is 1 g lower than that for other groups. Given similar socioeconomic conditions, Asian Americans and Mexican Americans have hemoglobin/hematocrit levels higher than those of Caucasian people.
Sickle cell anemia	Sickle cell anemia affects millions of people throughout the world. It is particularly common people whose ancestors come from sub-Sahara Africa; Spanish speaking regions (South America, Cuba, Central America), Saudi Arabia, India, and Mediterranean countries, such as Turkey, Greece, and Italy. In the United States, it affects approximately 72,000 people, most of whose ancestors come from Africa. The disease occures in approximately 1 in every 500 African American births and 1 in every 1,000 to 1,400 Hispanic American births. Approximately 2 million Americans, or 1 in 12 African Americans, carry the sickle cell trait.

Clinical Alert

1. Correct test interpretation also requires knowledge of all medications the patient is taking.
2. Help the patient and his or her significant others to understand and to cope with positive or negative test outcomes.
3. Recognize that "panic values" may pose an immediate threat to the patient's health status. Report these findings to the attending physician or other designated person immediately. Carefully document results and actions taken as soon as possible.
4. Nearly all tests have limitations. Some tests cannot predict future outcomes or events. For example, an ECG cannot predict a future myocardial infarction; it can merely tell what has already occurred. No test is absolute.

(continued)

(Clinical Alert continued)

5. Devastating physical, psychological and social consequences can result from being misdiagnosed with a serious disease because of false-positive or false-negative test results. Major alterations in lifestyles and relationships without just cause can be a consequence of these clinical aberrations (eg, misdiagnosis of HIV or syphilis).

Monitoring for Complications

Observe for complications and take appropriate measures to prevent or deal with them. Provide a safe patient environment.

1. Posttest assessments include evaluation of patient behaviors, complaints, activities, and compliance within the emotional, physical, psychosocial, and spiritual dimensions. Alterations in any of these domains may indicate a need for interventions appropriate to the dimensions affected.

2. Older patients and children may require closer, more lengthy monitoring and observation. For example, invasive procedure sites should be observed and assessed for potential bleeding and circulatory problems in the immediate postprocedure phase and for infection as a later event (possibly several days later).

3. Patients who receive sedation, drugs, contrast media (eg, iodine, barium), or radioactive medications must be evaluated and treated according to established protocols (see Appendix C).

4. Infection control measures with standard precautions and aseptic techniques must be a part of all routine testing regimens.

Test Result Availability

Collaborate with other disciplines to ensure that test results are made available to the clinician, patient, and staff as soon as possible. Time-critical information is of limited value if it is delayed or not received. Even though computerized communication technologies contribute to faster information delivery, clinicians are often left waiting for crucial clinical data. Using facsimile (fax) machines, computers, and wireless networks properly can expedite the reporting of vital patient data to the health care provider so that treatment can begin without delay.

▶ Clinical Alert

The issue of confidentiality demands that access to records and information should be on a strict need-to-know basis with secure and protected access available to select individuals.

Follow-up Care

Follow-up care should be consistent and should provide clearly understood discharge instructions. Emphasize the importance of and protocols for follow-up visits if these are ordered. Have the patient repeat this information back to the person providing the information to ensure that it has been understood. Plan time for listening, support, discussion, and problem-solving according to the patient's needs and requests.

Documentation and Record Keeping

Record information about all phases of the diagnostic testing process in the patient's health care record. Accurately document diagnostic activities and procedures during the pretest, intratest, and posttest phases because of legal, budgetary, reimbursement, and diagnostic related grouping (DRG) implications and constraints.

1. Document that the purpose, side-effects, risks, and expected results and benefits, as well as alternative methods, have been explained to the patient, and note who gave the explanation. Include information about medications, IV conscious sedation, start and end times, and patient responses. Describe allergic or adverse reactions (see Appendix C). Record data regarding disposition of specimens as well as information about follow-up care and discharge instructions.
2. Document the patient's reasons for refusing a test, along with any other pertinent information about the situation and who was given this report.
3. Maintain records of laboratory and diagnostic test data. Frequently, these records are transferred onto compact record storage systems such as microfilm or computer disks. For example, when an individual tests positive for HIV, it is necessary to review donor records at blood donor centers to determine whether the individual ever donated blood. If the infected person donated blood, the recipients of those blood components must be contacted and informed of the situation. This process is called "look back." Because many years may pass between donation and transfusion and the time the donor tests HIV-positive, medical history records of blood donors must be stored indefinitely.

Reporting infectious diseases and outbreaks to state and federal governments is part of record keeping.

Guidelines for Disclosure

Follow agency disclosure guidelines. Ethical standards may be a source of conflict and anxiety when the professional clinician is acting in the role of patient advocate. Recommended guidelines for telling a patient about his or her test results can alleviate some of this frustration. Under normal circumstances, the patient has the right to be informed of his or her test results. Although the clinician who orders the test is responsible for providing initial test result information, other designated individuals may need to facilitate and support the patient's right to know information about their health status.

In certain cases, when the patient brings family and significant others together to inform them about test results, communication becomes open and shared. This prevents the so-called "conspiracy of silence," in which individuals in the scenario withhold information because they feel they are "protecting" the patient or family or because they do not know how to deal with the situation.

Patient Responses to Expected or Unexpected Outcomes

Develop crisis intervention skills to use when communicating with the patient who experiences difficulty dealing with abnormal test results or confirmation of disease or illness.

1. Encourage the patient to take as much control of the situation as possible.
2. Recognize that the different stages of behavioral responses to negative results may last several weeks.

Immediate Response	Secondary Response
Acute emotional turmoil, shock, disbelief about diagnosis, denial	Insomnia, anorexia, difficulty concentrating, depression, difficulty in performing work-related responsibilities and tasks
Anxiety will usually last several days until the person assimilates the information	Depression may last several weeks as the person begins to incorporate the information and to participate realistically in a treatment plan and life style adaptation

3. Monitor changes in patient affect, mood, behaviors, and motivation. Do not assume that a person who initially has a negative perception of their health (eg, denial of diabetes) will not be able to integrate better health behaviors into daily life once they accept the diagnosis.
4. Use the following strategies to lessen the impact of a threatening situation.
   a. Offer appropriate comfort measures.
   b. Allow patients to work through feelings of anxiety and depression. At the appropriate time, reassure them that these feelings and emotions are normal initially. Be more of a therapeutic "listener" than a "talker."
   c. Assist the patient and family in making necessary lifestyle and self-concept adjustments through education, support groups, and other means. Emphasize that risk factors associated with certain diseases can be reduced through lifestyle changes. Be realistic. It is better to introduce change slowly rather than trying to promote adjustments on a grand scale in a short period of time

EXPECTED AND UNEXPECTED OUTCOMES

Evaluate outcomes using the following steps.

1. Learn the normal or reference values and expected outcomes of the test. The patient or his or her significant others should be able to describe the purpose of the test and the testing process and should properly perform expected activities associated with testing. Offer assistance if necessary. If test outcomes are abnormal, the patient should be encouraged to comply

with repeat testing and to introduce appropriate lifestyle changes realistically. Deal with anxiety or fears in a timely manner. Refer the patient to appropriate counseling resources if indicated. Above all, do not dismiss the patient's feelings and concerns casually.

2. Compare normal values with abnormal results and apply these comparisons to the patient's situation. Sometimes desired outcomes cannot be achieved. For example, the patient cannot, for various reasons, fully participate in the teaching/learning process or the actual testing itself. Recommendations for follow-up care and lifestyle changes may not be able to be followed. Verbal and nonverbal cues can sometimes provide reasons (eg, Alzheimer's disease, physical limitations) for this inability. In another instance, the patient might be noncompliant with pretest preparations and posttest activities. Denial of the situation is frequently a reason, although there are many other causes for noncompliance. Patients may refuse diagnostic testing because they feel the results may confirm their worst suspicions and fears.

3. Numerous and varied responses can be related to lack of appropriate problem-solving behaviors, inappropriate behaviors, fears or denial, concern about potential complications, inability to cope or take control of the situation, depression or abnormal emotional patterns of response, and lack of support from significant others and family.

4. Adverse events (eg, perforation, anaphylaxis, death) and health hazards may occur as a result of diagnostic procedures or problems with a medical device or product (eg, reactions to latex gloves or other latex-containing medical devices). Health professionals are asked to monitor and voluntarily report faulty medical devices to the U.S. Food and Drug Administration (FDA) so that action can be taken to protect the public. Reporting does not necessarily constitute an admission that medical personnel or the product caused or contributed to the adverse event.

5. Prompt action is necessary when results are abnormally high or low and are indicative of a serious situation (eg, positive blood culture, abnormally elevated potassium level).

IMPORTANCE OF COMMUNICATION ●

At the heart of informed care is the ability to communicate effectively. Frequently communication must take place within a "compressed" time frame because of time constraints. Thus, the importance of communicating effectively cannot be emphasized enough. Effective communication is the key to achieving desired outcomes and preventing misunderstanding and errors. One must always keep in mind that the human person is an integration of body, mind, and spirit, and that these three entities are intimately bound together to make each of us unique individuals. Skillful assessment of physical, emotional, psychosocial, and spiritual dimensions provides a sound database from which to plan communication and teaching/instruction strategies.

Individuals have different needs and changing capacities for learning as they progress from child to adult to older adult. It is important for the clinician to know the different developmental levels and stages and the ways in which clear communication can be achieved at any level.

For the pediatric patient, teaching tools might include tours of the diagnostic area, play therapy, films or videos, models of equipment that the child can touch or manipulate, and written materials and pictures appropriate to the child's developmental stage. Shorter attention spans and the unpredictable nature of children can make teaching a challenge in this population. Mentally retarded or mentally ill patients may need significant others close by who can guide communication between caretaker and patient. Gentle, simple, nurturing behaviors usually work well with children and developmentally challenged individuals.

Adolescents may be at the stage of developing their own unique identity as they move toward adulthood. Teaching may be more effective without parents present; however, it is important to include parents at some point. Drawings, illustrations, or videos are helpful. Because body image is very important at this stage, honest, supportive behaviors are necessary, especially if some alteration in physical appearance will be necessary (eg, removal of jewelry, no makeup allowed).

The opportunity to actively participate and ask questions is important for adults. They bring to the communication process their lifetime of perceptions and experiences. This can be a proverbial "double-edged sword." Listening well to verbal cues as well as paying attention to nonverbal messages cannot be overemphasized. For example, interacting with patients who have Alzheimer's disease can present special challenges. The presence of a significant other who has experience communicating with this patient can be the key to performing a successful procedure.

Provide an environment that is quiet, private, and free of distractions to promote dialogue and communication. Ask by what name or title the patient wishes to be addressed. Referring to a patient as a room number, a procedure, or a disease is demeaning and inexcusable; it reduces the patient to the level of an object rather than a person.

Nonverbal communication behaviors such as proper eye contact, firm handshake, sense of respect, and *appropriate* humor can reduce anxiety. Do not dismiss the power of touch, the sense of "making time" for the patient, and the use of appropriate and positive verbal cues. The greater part of communication (>70%) is perceived through body language. If words don't match body language and behaviors, the patient will react to the body language they observe as their primary frame of reference.

Every person engaged in the *entire* process of testing is a link in the ongoing communication continuum. This continuum is only as effective as the weakest link that joins all activities and all communication together.

CONCLUSION

As professionals, we need to remember that patients are people just like us. These individuals come to us with their perceptions, worries, and anxieties regarding the diagnostic process and what their illness means to them and their loved ones, what strategies they use for coping, what resources are available for their use, and what other knowledge they have about themselves. As clinicians and patient advocates, we must be willing to "take on the mind" of another—that is, to identify with the patient's point of view as much as possible and to show empathy. Once we reach that point, we can then begin to understand and communicate with each other at the deeper levels necessary for a therapeutic relationship to occur.

BIBLIOGRAPHY ●

AACC Government Affairs Update: House Panel Explores Latext Allergy. April 1999, p5, Washington, DC

Andrews MM, Boyle JS: Competence in trans-cultural nursing care. Am J Nurs 97(8): 16AAA, 16DDD, 1997

Bates DW, Kuperman GJ, Rittenberg E, et al: A radomized trial of a computer-based intervention to reduce utilization of redundant laboratory tests. Am J Med 106:44–150, 1999, February

Beaumont E: Technology scorecard: focus on infection control. Am J Nurs 97(12): 51–54, 1997

Berger JT: The ethics of mandatory HIV testing in newborns. J Clin Ethics 7: 77–84, 1996

Berkowitz CM: Conscious sedation: a primer. RN February: 32–36, 1997

Callahan CM, Kesterson JG, Tierney WM: Association of symptoms of depression with diagnostic test charges among older adults. Ann Intern Med 126(6): 426–432, 1997

Cohen EL, Cesta TG: Nursing Care Management From Concept to Evaluation, 2nd ed. St. Louis, CV Mosby, 1997

Cox M: Wellness guidelines and services. In Hogsted M (ed): Community Resources for Older Adults. St. Louis, CV Mosby, 123–141, 1998

Elixhauser A, Tonantgen M, Andrews R: Agency for health care policy and research: descriptive statistics by insurance status for most frequent hospital diagnoses and procedures. Rockville, MD, U.S. Department of Health and Human Services, AHCPR Pub. No. 97–8009, September, 1997

Escarce JJ, Epstein KR, Colby DC, Schwartz JS: Racial differences in the elderly's use of medical procedures and diagnostic tests. Am J Public Health 83(7): 948–954, 1993

Farrice L: Does a smile cost extra? Lab Med 21(7): 409–410, 1990

Fischbach FT: Quick Reference to Common Laboratory and Diagnostic Tests, 2nd ed. Philadelphia, Lippincott-Raven, 1998

Fischbach FT: Documenting Care—Communication; Nursing Process; Documentation Standards. Philadelphia, FA Davis, 1991

Frizzell J, Credit CE: Avoiding laboratory test pitfalls. Am J Nurs 98(2): 34–38, 1998

Goroll AH, May LH, Mulley AG: Primary Care Medicine: Office Evaluation and Management of the Adult Patient, 3rd ed. Philadelphia, Lippincott-Raven, 1998

Gritter M, Credit CE: The latex threat. Am J Nurs 98(9): 26–32, 1998

Guidelines for Isolation Precautions in Hospitals: Part I Evaluation of Isolation Precautions; Part II Recommendations for Isolation Precautions in Hospitals. Am J Infection Control 24(1):24–52, 1996, February

Hall P: Providing psychosocial support. Am J Nurs 10: 16N–16P, 1996

Hansen M, Fisher JC: Patient-centered teaching from theory to practice. Am J Nurs 98(1): 56–60, 1998

Hanson M: Should we do another test? Decision making in blood banking. Clin Lab Med 16(4): 883–893, 1996

James PA, Cowan TM, Graham RP, Majeroni BA: Family physicians' attitudes about and use of clinical practice guidelines. J Family Pract 45(4), 341–347, 1997

Kravitz RL, Rolph JE, Petersen L: Omission-related malpractice claims and the limits of defensive medicine. Med Care Res Rev 54(4): 456–471, 1997

Kuperman GJ, et al: How promptly are inpatients treated for critical laboratory results? J Am Med Inform Assoc 5: 112–119, 1998

Lehmann CA: Saunders Manual of Clinical Laboratory Science. Philadelphia, WB Saunders, 1998

Long CO, Greenerd DS: Four strategies for keeping patients satisfied. Am J Nurs 94(6): 26–27, 1994

McHugh NG, Christman NJ, Johnson JE: Preparatory information: what helps and why. Am J Nurs 82: 780–782, 1992

National Institute for Occupational Safety and Health: Preventing Allergic Reactions to Natural Rubber Latex in the Work Place. DHHS (N1OSH) Pub. No. 97–135. Cincinnati, OH, U.S. Department of Health and Human Services, 1997

Pasiero CL: Procedural pain management. Am J Nurs 98(7): 18–20, 1998

Research roundup: latex allergy precautions. Am J Nurs 97(10): 16B, 1997

Riordan B, Zana RH: When your patient is a Hmong refugee. Am J Nurs March 92(3): 52–53, 1992

Roberts RR, Zalenski RJ, Mensah EK, et al: Costs of an emergency department-based accelerated diagnostic protocol vs hospitalization in patients with chest pain: a randomized controlled trial. JAMA 278(20): 1670–1676, 1997

Scadding JG: Essentialism and nominalism in medicine: logic of diagnosis in disease terminology. Lancet 348: 594–596, 1996

Sherman LA: Legal issues in blood banking; elements of informed consent. Clin Lab Med 16(4): 931–945, 1996

Slattery M: The epidemic hazards of nursing. Am J Nurs 98(11): 50–53, 1998

Speicher CE: The Right Test: A Physician's Guide to Laboratory Medicine, 3rd ed. Philadelphia, WB Saunders, 1998

Swanson KM: Nursing as informed caring for the well-being of others. J Nurs Scholarship 25(4): 352–357, 1993

Tierney LM, McPhee SJ, Papadakis MA: Current Medical Diagnosis and Treatment, 37th ed. Stanford, CT, Appleton & Lange, 1998

U.S. Department of Health and Human Services: Healthy people 2000: national health promotion and disease prevention objectives. Washington, DC, U.S. Government Printing Office, 1991

U.S. Food and Drug Administration: The F.D.A. Desk Guide for Adverse Event and Product Problem Reporting (form 3500). Rockville, MD, U.S. Food and Drug Administration, 1993

Victoroff MS: The right intentions: errors and accountability [editorial]. J Family Pract 45(1), 8, 1997

Wallach J: Interpretation of Diagnostic Tests, 6th ed. Boston: Little, Brown, 1996

Watson DS: Conscious Sedation/Analgesia. St. Louis: Mosby-Year Book, Inc, 1998

Wilcox W (ed): Health Insurance Sourcebook. Detroit, MI, Omnigraphics, Inc., 1997

Wilfond BS, Rothenberg KH, Thomson ES, et al: Cancer genetic susceptibility testing: ethical and policy implications for future research and clinical practice. J Law Med Ethics 25: 243–251, 1997.

Young DS: Effects of Drugs and Clinical Laboratory Tests, 5th ed. Washington, DC: AACC Press, 1999

2

Blood Studies

●─────────────────────────────────

OVERVIEW OF BASIC BLOOD TESTS ●

Composition of Blood

The average person circulates about 5 L of blood, (1/13 of body weight), of which 3 L is plasma and 2 L is cells. Plasma fluid derives from the intestines and lymphatic systems and provides a vehicle for cell movement. The cells are produced primarily by bone marrow and account for blood "solids." Blood cells are classified as white cells (leukocytes), red cells (erythrocytes), and platelets (thrombocytes). White cells are further categorized as granulocytes, lymphocytes, and monocytes.

Before birth, hematopoiesis occurs in the liver. In midfetal life, the spleen and lymph nodes play a minor role in cell production. Shortly after birth, hematopoiesis in the liver ceases and the bone marrow is the only site of production of erythrocytes, granulocytes, and platelets. B lymphocytes are produced in the marrow and in the secondary lymphoid organs; T lymphocytes are produced in the thymus.

Blood Disorders

Tests in this chapter address disorders of cell production (hematopoiesis), synthesis, and function. Blood and bone marrow examinations constitute the major means of determining certain blood disorders. Specimens are obtained through capillary skin punctures (finger, toe, heel), arterial or venous sampling, or bone marrow aspiration.

● BLOOD SPECIMEN COLLECTION PROCEDURES

Proper specimen collection presumes correct technique and accurate timing where necessary.

CAPILLARY PUNCTURE (SKIN PUNCTURE) ●

Capillary blood is preferred for a peripheral blood smear and can also be used for other hematology studies.

1. Observe standard precautions (Appendix A). Check for latex allergy. If allergy is present, do not use latex-containing products (Appendix B).
2. Obtain capillary blood from fingertips or earlobes (adults) or from the great toe or heel (infants).
3. Disinfect puncture site, dry the site, and puncture skin with sterile disposable lancet no deeper than 2 mm. If povidone-iodine is used, allow to dry thoroughly.
4. Wipe away the initial drop of blood. Collect subsequent drops in a microtube or prepare a smear directly from a drop of blood.

> **Clinical Alert**
>
> 1. Do not squeeze the site to obtain blood because this alters blood composition and invalidates test values.
> 2. Warming the extremity or placing it in a dependent position may facilitate specimen retrieval.

Patient Preparation
Instruct patient about purpose and procedure of test.

Patient Aftercare
Apply small dressing or adhesive strip to site. Evaluate puncture site for bleeding or oozing. Apply compression or pressure to the site if it continues to bleed. Evaluate patient's medication history for anticoagulation or acetylsalicylic acid (ASA)-type drug ingestion.

VENIPUNCTURE

Venipuncture allows procurement of larger quantities of blood for testing. Usually, the antecubital veins are the veins of choice because of ease of access. Blood values remain constant no matter which venipuncture site is selected, so long as it is venous and not arterial blood.

1. Observe standard precautions (Appendix A). If latex allergy is suspected, use latex-free supplies and equipment (Appendix B).
2. Position and tighten a tourniquet on the upper arm to produce venous congestion.

   NOTE: *A blood pressure cuff inflated to a point between systolic and diastolic pressure values can be used.*

3. Ask the patient to close the fist in the designated arm. Select an accessible vein.
4. Cleanse the puncture site and dry it properly with sterile gauze. Povidone-iodine must dry thoroughly.
5. Puncture the vein according to accepted technique. Usually, for an adult, anything smaller than a number 21-gauge needle might make blood withdrawal somewhat more difficult. A Vacutainer system syringe or butterfly system may be used.

   NOTE: *The Vacutainer system consists of vacuum tubes (Vacutainer tubes), a tube holder, and a disposable multisample collecting needle.*

6. Once the vein has been entered by the collecting needle, blood will fill the attached vacuum tubes automatically because of negative pressure within the collection tube.
7. Remove the tourniquet before removing the needle from the puncture site or bruising will occur.
8. Remove needle. Apply pressure and sterile dressing strip to site.
9. The preservative or anticoagulant added to the collection tube depends on the test ordered. In general, most hematology tests use ethylene diamine tetraacetic acid (EDTA) anticoagulant. Even slightly clotted blood invalidates the test and the sample must be redrawn.
10. Take action to prevent these venipuncture errors:

    A. Pretest errors
    (1) Improper patient identification
    (2) Failure to check patient compliance with dietary restrictions
    (3) Failure to calm patient before blood collection
    (4) Using wrong equipment and supplies
    (5) Inappropriate method of blood collection

    B. Procedure errors
    (1) Failure to dry site completely after cleansing with alcohol
    (2) Inserting needle with bevel side down
    (3) Using too small a needle, causing hemolysis of specimen

(4) Venipuncture in unacceptable area (eg, above an intravenous [IV] line)

(5) Prolonged tourniquet application

(6) Wrong order of tube draw

(7) Failure to immediately mix blood collected in additive-containing tubes

(8) Pulling back on syringe plunger too forcefully

(9) Failure to release tourniquet before needle withdrawal

C. Posttest Errors

(1) Failure to apply pressure immediately to venipuncture site

(2) Vigorous shaking of anticoagulated blood specimens

(3) Forcing blood through a syringe needle into tube

(4) Mislabeling of tubes

(5) Failure to label specimens with infectious disease precautions as required

(6) Failure to put date, time, and initials on requisition

(7) Slow transport of specimens to laboratory

Patient Preparation

1. Instruct patient regarding sampling procedure. Assess for circulation or bleeding problems and allergy to latex.

2. Reassure patient that mild discomfort may be felt when the needle is inserted.

3. Place the arm in a fully extended position with palmar surface facing upward (for antecubital access).

> ### Clinical Alert
>
> In patients with leukemia, agranulocytosis, or lowered resistance, fingerstick and earlobe punctures are more likely to cause infection and bleeding than venipunctures. Should a capillary sample be necessary, the cleansing agent should remain in contact with the skin for at least 5 to 10 minutes. Povidone-iodine is the cleansing agent of choice. It should be allowed to dry. It may then be wiped off with alcohol and the site dried with sterile gauze before puncture.

4. If withdrawal of the sample is difficult, warm the extremity with warm towels or blankets. Allow the extremity to remain in a dependent position for several minutes before venipuncture.

Patient Aftercare

1. If oozing or bleeding from the puncture site continues for an unusually long time, elevate the area and apply a pressure dressing. Observe the patient closely. Check for anticoagulant or ASA-type ingestion.

2. Occasionally, a patient becomes dizzy, faint, or nauseated during the venipuncture. The phlebotomist must be constantly aware of the patient's

condition. If a patient feels faint, immediately remove the tourniquet and terminate the procedure. If the patient is sitting, lower the head between the legs and instruct the patient to breathe deeply. A cool, wet towel may be applied to the forehead and back of the neck, and, if necessary, ammonia inhalant may be applied briefly. If the patient remains unconscious, a physician should be notified immediately.

3. Hematomas can be prevented by use of proper technique (not sticking the needle through the vein), release of the tourniquet before the needle is withdrawn, application of sufficient pressure over the puncture site, and maintenance of an extended extremity until bleeding stops.

Clinical Alert

1. Never draw blood from the same extremity being used for IV medications, fluids, or transfusions. If no other site is available, then make sure the venipuncture site is below the IV site. Avoid areas that are edematous, paralyzed, on the same side as a mastectomy, or have infections or skin conditions present. Venipuncture may cause infection, circulatory impairment, or retarded healing.

2. Prolonged tourniquet application causes stasis and hemoconcentration and will alter test results.

BONE MARROW ASPIRATION

Normal Values for Bone Marrow

Formed Cell Elements	Normal Mean (%)	Range (%)
Undifferentiated cells	0.0	0.0–1.0
Reticulum cells	0.4	0.0–1.3
Myeloblasts	2.0	0.3–5.0
Promyelocytes	5.0	1.0–8.0
Myelocytes		
Neutrophilic	12.0	5.0–19.0
Eosinophilic	1.5	0.5–3.0
Basophilic	0.3	0.0–0.5
Metamyelocytes		
Neutrophilic	25.6	17.5–33.7
Eosinophilic	0.4	0.0–1.0
Basophilic	0.0	0.0–0.2
Segmented granulocytes		
Neutrophilic	20.0	11.6–30.0
Eosinophilic	2.0	0.5–4.0
Basophilic	0.2	0.0–3.0
Monocytes	2.0	0–3

(continued)

Normal Values for Bone Marrow *(Continued)*		
Formed Cell Elements	*Normal Mean (%)*	*Range (%)*
Lymphocytes	10.0	8–2
Megakaryocytes	0.4	0.0–3.0
Plasma cells	0.9	0.0–2.0
Erythroid series		
Pronormoblasts	0.5	0.2–4.2
Basophilic normoblasts	1.6	0.25–4.8
Polychromatic normoblasts	10.4	3.5–20.5
Orthochromatic normoblasts	6.4	3.0–25
Promegaloblasts	0	0
Basophilic megaloblasts	0	0
Polychromatic megaloblasts	0	0
Orthochromatic megaloblasts	0	0
Myeloid:erythroid ratio (ratio of WBC, to nucleated RBC)	2:1–4:1	(slightly higher in infants)

*These values are only for adults, and should be used as a guideline. (Each laboratory should establish its own reference range.)

Background

Bone marrow is located within cancellous bone and long bone cavities. It consists of a pattern of vessels and nerves, differentiated and undifferentiated hematopoietic cells, reticuloendothelial cells, and fatty tissue. All of these are encased by endosteum, the membrane lining the bone marrow cavity. After proliferation and maturation have occurred in the marrow, blood cells gain entrance to the blood through or between the endothelial cells of the sinus wall.

Explanation of Test

A bone marrow specimen is obtained through aspiration or biopsy or needle biopsy aspiration. A bone marrow examination is important in the evaluation of a number of hematologic disorders and infectious diseases. The presence or suspicion of a blood disorder is not always an indication for bone marrow studies. A decision to employ this procedure is made on an individual basis.

Sometimes, the aspirate does not contain hematopoietic cells. This "dry tap" occurs when hematopoietic activity is so sparse that there are no cells to be withdrawn or when the marrow contains so many tightly packed cells that they cannot be suctioned out of the marrow. In such cases, a bone marrow biopsy would be advantageous. Before the bone marrow procedure is started, a peripheral blood smear should be obtained from the patient and a differential leukocyte count done.

Procedure

1. Follow standard precautions. Check for latex allergy; if allergy is present, do not use latex-containing products. Position the patient on the back or

side according to site selected. The posterior iliac crest is the preferred site in all patients older than 12 to 18 months. Alternate sites include the anterior iliac crest, sternum, spinous vertebral processes T10 through L4, the ribs, and the tibia in children.

The sternum is not generally used in children because the bone cavity is too shallow, the risk of mediastinal and cardiac perforation is too great, and the child may be uncooperative.

2. Shave, cleanse, and drape the site as for any minor surgical procedure.
3. A local anesthetic (procaine or lidocaine) is injected. This may cause a burning sensation. At this time a skin incision of 3 mm is often made.
4. The physician introduces a short, rigid, sharp-pointed needle with stylet through the periosteum into the marrow cavity.
5. The needle-stylet combination is passed through the incision, subcutaneous tissue, and bone cortex. The stylet is removed and 1.0 to 3.0 ml of marrow fluid is aspirated. When the stylet needle enters the marrow, the patient may experience a feeling of pressure. Moderate discomfort may also be felt as aspiration is done, especially in the iliac crest. The Jamshidi needle is commonly used for biopsy, although the Westerman-Jansen modification of the Vim-Silverman needle may also be used.
6. Once the stylet has been removed, the biopsy needle is advanced with a twisting motion toward the anterior superior iliac spine.
7. After adequate penetration of the base (3 cm), the needle is rotated or "rocked" in several directions several times. This "frees up" the specimen. Once this is done, the needle is then slowly withdrawn.
8. The biopsy specimen is pushed out "backwards" from the needle. It may be used to make touch preparations or may be immediately placed in fixative. Slide smears are made at the bedside.
9. Pressure is applied to the puncture site until bleeding ceases. The site is then dressed.
10. Specimens are placed in biohazard bags, properly labeled, and routed to the appropriate department.

Clinical Implications

1. A specific and diagnostic bone marrow picture provides clues to many diseases. The presence, absence, and ratio of cells are characteristic of the suspected disease.
2. Bone marrow examination may reveal the following abnormal cell patterns:
   A. Multiple myeloma, plasma cell myeloma, macroglobulinemia
   B. Chronic or acute leukemias
   C. Anemia, including megaloblastic, macrocytic, and normocytic anemias
   D. Toxic states that produce bone marrow depression or destruction
   E. Neoplastic diseases in which the marrow is invaded by tumor cells (metastatic carcinoma, myeloproliferative and lymphoproliferative diseases); assists in diagnosis and staging.

F. Agranulocytosis (a decrease in the production of certain types of white cells). This occurs when bone marrow activity is severely depressed, usually as a result of radiation therapy or chemotherapeutic drugs. Implications for the patient focus on the risk of death from overwhelming infection.

G. Platelet dysfunction

H. Some types of infectious diseases, especially histoplasmosis and tuberculosis

I. Deficiency of body iron stores, microcytic anemia

J. Lipid or glycogen storage disease

Patient Preparation

1. Instruct the patient about the test procedure, purpose, benefits, and risks of the test.
2. A legal consent form must be properly signed and witnessed. Bone marrow aspiration is usually contraindicated in the presence of hemophilia and other bleeding dyscrasias. However, risk versus benefit may dictate the choice made.
3. Reassure the patient that analgesics will be available if needed.
4. Bone marrow biopsies or aspirations can be uncomfortable. Squeezing a pillow may be helpful as a distraction technique.
5. Observe standard precautions.

Clinical Alert

1. Complications can include bleeding and sternal fractures. Osteomyelitis or injury to heart or great vessels is rare but can occur if the sternal site is used.
2. Manual and pressure dressings over the puncture site usually control excessive bleeding. Remove dressing in 24 hours. Redress site if necessary.
3. Fever, headache, unusual pain, or redness or pus at biopsy site may indicate infection (later event). Instruct patient to report unusual symptoms to physician immediately.

Patient Aftercare

1. Monitor vital signs until stable and assess site for excess drainage or bleeding.
2. Recommend bed rest for 30 minutes; then normal activities can be resumed.
3. Administer analgesics or sedatives as necessary. Soreness over the puncture site for 3 to 4 days after the procedure is normal. Continued pain may indicate fracture.
4. Interpret test outcomes and monitor appropriately.
5. Follow Chapter 1 guidelines for safe, effective, informed *posttest* care.

● BASIC BLOOD TESTS

HEMOGRAM ●

A hemogram consists of a white blood cell count (WBC), red blood cell count (RBC), hemoglobin (Hb), hematocrit (Hct), red blood cell indices, and a platelet count. A complete blood count consists of a hemogram plus a differential white blood cell count.

COMPLETE BLOOD COUNT (CBC) ●

The CBC is a basic screening test and is one of the most frequently ordered laboratory procedures. The findings in the CBC give valuable diagnostic information about the hematologic and other body systems, prognosis, response to treatment, and recovery. The CBC consists of a series of tests that determine number, variety, percentage, concentrations, and quality of blood cells:

White blood cell count (WBC)
Differential white blood cell count (Diff)
Red blood cell count (RBC)
Hematocrit (Hct)
Hemoglobin (Hb)
Red blood cell indices:
    Mean corpuscular volume (MCV)
    Mean corpuscular hemoglobin concentration (MCHC)
    Mean corpuscular hemoglobin (MCH)
    Stained red cell examination (film or peripheral blood smear)
    Platelet count (often included in CBC)

These tests are described in detail in the following pages.

Normal Values for Hemogram					
Age	*WBC* $(\times 10^3/mm^3)$	*RBC* $(\times 10^6/mm^3)$	*Hb (g/dL)*	*Hct (%)*	*MCV (fL)*
Birth–2 wk	9.0–30.0	4.1–6.1	14.5–24.5	44–64	98–112
2–8 wk	5.0–21.0	4.0–6.0	12.5–20.5	39–59	98–112
2–6 mo	5.0–19.0	3.8–5.6	10.7–17.3	35–49	83–97
6 mo–1 y	5.0–19.0	3.8–5.2	9.9–14.5	29–43	73–87
1–6 y	5.0–19.0	3.9–5.3	9.5–14.1	30–40	70–84
6–16 y	4.8–10.8	4.0–5.2	10.3–14.9	32–42	73–87
16–18 y	4.8–10.8	4.2–5.4	11.1–15.7	34–44	75–89
>18 y males	5.0–10.0	4.5–5.5	14.0–17.4	42–52	84–96
>18 y females	5.0–10.0	4.0–5.0	12.0–16.0	36–48	84–96

(continued)

Normal Values for Hemogram *(Continued)*

Age	MCH (pg)	MCHC (g/dL)	Platelets (× 10³)	RDW (%)	MPV (fL)
Birth–2 wk	34–40	33–37	150–450	—	—
2–8 wk	30–36	32–36	—	—	—
2–6 mo	27–33	31–35	—	—	—
6 mo–1 y	24–30	32–36	—	—	—
1–6 y	23–29	31–35	—	—	—
6–16 y	24–30	32–36	—	—	—
16–18 y	25–31	32–36	—	—	—
>18 y	28–34	32–36	140–400	11.5–14.5	7.4–10.4

Standard Patient Preparation for Hemogram, CBC, and Differential Count (All Components)

1. Explain test procedure. Explain that slight discomfort may be felt the when skin is punctured. Refer to venipuncture procedure for additional information.
2. Avoid stress if possible, because altered physiologic status influences and changes normal hemogram values.
3. Select hemogram components ordered at regular intervals (eg, daily, every other day). These should be drawn consistently at the same time of day for reasons of accurate comparison; natural body rhythms cause fluctuations in laboratory values at certain times of the day.
4. Dehydration or overhydration can dramatically alter values; for example, large volumes of IV fluids can "dilute" the blood and values will appear as lower counts. The presence of either of these states should be communicated to the laboratory.
5. Fasting is not necessary. However, fat-laden meals may alter some test results as a result of lipidemia.

Standard Patient Aftercare for Hemogram, CBC, and Differential Count (All Components)

1. Apply manual pressure and dressings to the puncture site on removal of the needle.
2. Monitor the puncture site for oozing or hematoma formation. Maintain pressure dressings on the site if necessary. Notify physician of unusual problems with bleeding.

Clinical Alert

NEVER apply a total circumferential dressing and wrap *because* this may compromise circulation and nerve function if constriction, from whatever cause, occurs.

3. Resume normal activities and diet.

4. Bruising at the puncture site is not uncommon. Signs of inflammation are unusual and should be reported if the inflamed area appears larger, if "red streaks" develop, or if drainage occurs.

● TESTS OF WHITE BLOOD CELLS

WHITE BLOOD CELL COUNT (WBC; LEUKOCYTE COUNT) ●

Normal Values
Adults: $5.0–10.0 \times 10^3$/cells/mm^3 or $\times 10^9$/L or 5,000–10,000 cells/mm^3
Children:
0–2 wk $9.0–30.0 \times 10^3$/cells/mm^3 or $\times 10^9$/L or 9,000–30,000 cells/mm^3
2–8 wk $5.0–21.0 \times 10^3$/cells/mm^3 or $\times 10^9$/L or 5,000–21,000 cells/mm^3
2 mo–6 y $5.0–19.0 \times 10^3$/cells/mm^3 or $\times 10^9$/L or 5,000–19,000 cells/mm^3
6–18 y $4.8–10.8 \times 10^3$/cells/mm^3 or $\times 10^9$/L or 4,800–10,800 cells/mm^3

Background
White blood cells (WBCs or leukocytes) are divided into two main groups: granulocytes and agranulocytes. The granulocytes receive their name from the distinctive granules that are present in the cytoplasm of neutrophils, basophils, and eosinophils. However, each of these cells also contains a multilobed nucleus, which accounts for their also being called *polymorphonuclear leukocytes*. In laboratory terminology, they are often called "polys" or PMNs. The nongranulocytes, which consist of the lymphocytes and monocytes, do not contain distinctive granules and have nonlobular nuclei that are not necessarily spherical. The term *mononuclear leukocytes* is applied to these cells.

The endocrine system is an important regulator of the number of leukocytes in the blood. Hormones affect the production of leukocytes in the blood-forming organs, their storage and release from the tissue, and their disintegration. A local inflammatory process exerts a definite chemical effect on the mobilization of leukocytes. The life span of leukocytes varies from 13 to 20 days, after which the cells are destroyed in the lymphatic system; many are excreted from the body in fecal matter.

Leukocytes fight infection and defend the body by a process called *phagocytosis,* in which the leukocytes actually encapsulate foreign organisms and destroy them. Leukocytes also produce, transport, and distribute antibodies as part of the immune response to a foreign substance (antigen).

Explanation of Test
The WBC serves as a useful guide to the severity of the disease process. Specific patterns of leukocyte response can be expected in various types of

diseases as determined by the differential count (percentages of the different types of leukocytes). Leukocyte and differential counts, by themselves, are of little value as aids to diagnosis unless the results are related to the clinical condition of the patient; only then is a correct and useful interpretation possible.

Procedure

1. Obtain a venous anticoagulated EDTA blood sample of 5 ml or a finger-stick sample. Place specimen in a biohazard bag.
2. Record the time when specimen was obtained (eg, 7:00 AM).
3. Blood is processed either manually or automatically, using an electronic counting instrument such as the Coulter counter or Abbott Cell-Dyne.

Clinical Implications

1. *Leukocytosis:* WBC >10,000/mm^3 or >10.0 $\times$ 10^3/mm^3 (or >10 $\times$ 10^9/L)
   A. It is usually caused by an increase of only 1 type of leukocyte, and it is given the name of the type of cell that shows the main increase:
      (1) Neutrophilic leukocytosis or neutrophilia
      (2) Lymphocytic leukocytosis or lymphocytosis
      (3) Monocytic leukocytosis or monocytosis
      (4) Basophilic leukocytosis or basophilia
      (5) Eosinophilic leukocytosis or eosinophilia
   B. An increase in circulating leukocytes is rarely caused by a proportional increase in leukocytes of all types. When this does occur, it is usually a result of hemoconcentration.
   C. In certain diseases (eg, measles, pertussis, sepsis), the increase of leukocytes is so great that the blood picture suggests leukemia. *Leukocytosis of a temporary nature* (leukemoid reaction) must be distinguished from leukemia. In leukemia, the leukocytosis is permanent and progressive.
   D. Leukocytosis occurs in acute infections, in which the degree of increase of leukocytes depends on severity of the infection, patient's resistance, patient's age, and marrow efficiency and reserve.
   E. Other causes of leukocytosis include the following:
      (1) Leukemia, myeloproliferative disorders
      (2) Trauma or tissue injury (eg, surgery)
      (3) Malignant neoplasms, especially bronchogenic carcinoma
      (4) Toxins, uremia, coma, eclampsia, thyroid storm
      (5) Drugs—especially ether, chloroform, quinine, epinephrine (Adrenalin), colony-stimulating factors
      (6) Acute hemolysis
      (7) Hemorrhage (acute)
      (8) After splenectomy
      (9) Polycythemia vera
      (10) Tissue necrosis
   F. Occasionally leukocytosis is found when there is no evidence of clinical disease. Such findings suggest the presence of:

(1) Sunlight, ultraviolet irradiation

(2) Physiologic leukocytosis resulting from excitement, stress, exercise, pain, cold or heat, anesthesia

(3) Nausea, vomiting, seizures

G. Steroid therapy modifies the leukocyte response.

(1) When corticotropin (ACTH) is given to a healthy person, leukocytosis occurs.

(2) When ACTH is given to a patient with severe infection, the infection can spread rapidly without producing the expected leukocytosis; therefore, what would normally be an important sign is obscured.

2. *Leukopenia:* WBC <4000/mm^3 or <4.0 × 10^3/mm^3 or 4.0 cells ×10^9/L occurs during and following:

A. Viral infections, some bacterial infections, overwhelming bacterial infections

B. Hypersplenism

C. Bone marrow depression caused by heavy metal intoxication, ionizing radiation, drugs:

(1) Antimetabolites

(2) Barbiturates

(3) Benzine

(4) Antibiotics

(5) Antihistamines

(6) Anticonvulsives

(7) Antithyroid drugs

(8) Arsenicals

(9) Cancer chemotherapy (causes a decrease in leukocytes; leukocyte count is used as a link to disease)

(10) Cardiovascular drugs

(11) Diuretics

(12) Analgesics and antiinflammatory drugs

D. Primary bone marrow disorders:

(1) Leukemia (aleukemic)

(2) Pernicious anemia

(3) Aplastic anemia

(4) Myelodysplastic syndromes

(5) Congenital disorders

(6) Kostmann syndrome

(7) Reticular agenesis

(8) Cartilage-hair hypoplasia

(9) Shwachman-Diamond syndrome

(10) Chédiak-Higashi syndrome

E. Immune-associated neutropenia

F. Marrow-occupying diseases (fungal infection, metastatic tumor)

G. Hypersplenism

H. Iron-deficiency anemia

> **Clinical Alert**
>
> 1. WBC $<500/mm^3$ or $<0.5 \times 10^3/mm^3$ (or $\times 10^9/L$) represents a panic value.
> 2. WBC $>30,000/mm^3$ or 30.0×10^3 (or $\times 10^9/L$) is a panic value.

Interfering Factors

1. Hourly rhythm: There is an early-morning low level and late-afternoon high peak.
2. Age: In newborns and infants, the count is high ($10,000/mm^3$ to $20,000/mm^3$) and gradually decreases in children until the adult values are reached at about age 21 years.
3. Any stressful situation that leads to an increase in endogenous epinephrine production and a rapid rise in the leukocyte count.

Patient Preparation

1. Explain test purpose and procedure.
2. Refer to standard *pretest* care for hemogram, CBC, and differential count on page 44. Also, see Chapter 1 guidelines for safe, effective, informed *pretest* care.

Patient Aftercare

1. Interpret test outcome and monitor appropriately. Refer to standard *posttest* care for hemogram, CBC, and differential count on page • •. Also, follow Chapter 1 guidelines for safe, effective, informed *posttest* care.
2. In prolonged severe granulocytopenia or pancytopenia, give no fresh fruits or vegetables because the kitchen, especially in a hospital, may be a source of food contamination. When the WBC is low, a person can get a pseudomonal or fungal infection from fresh fruits and vegetables. Use a minimal-bacteria or commercially sterile diet. All food must be served from a new or single-serving package. Consider a leukemia diet. See dietary department for restrictions (eg, cooked food only) and careful food preparation. Do not give intramuscular injections. Do not take rectal temperature, give suppositories, or give enemas. Do not use razor blades. Do not give aspirin or nonsteroidal antiinflammatory drugs (NSAIDs), which cause abnormal platelet dysfunction. Watch carefully for any signs or symptoms of infection. Without leukocytes to produce inflammation, serious infections can have very subtle findings. Often patients have only a fever.

DIFFERENTIAL WHITE BLOOD CELL COUNT
(DIFF; DIFFERENTIAL LEUKOCYTE COUNT)

Background

The total count of circulating WBCs is differentiated according to the five types of leukocytes, each of which performs a specific function:

Cell	These Cells Function to Combat
Neutrophils	Pyogenic infections (bacterial)
Eosinophils	Allergic disorders and parasitic infestations
Basophils	Parasitic infections
Lymphocytes	Viral infections (measles, rubella, chickenpox, infectious mononucleosis)
Monocytes	Severe infections, by phagocytosis

Normal Values for Leukocyte Count

Age	Bands/ STAB (%)	Segs/Polys (%)	Eos (%)	Basos (%)	Lymphs (%)	Monos (%)	Metas (%)
Birth–1 wk	10–18	32–62	0–2	0–1	26–36	0–6	—
1–2 wk	8–16	19–49	0–4	0–0	38–46	0–9	—
2–4 wk	7–15	14–34	0–3	0–0	43–53	0–9	—
4–8 wk	7–13	15–35	0–3	0–1	41–71	0–7	—
2–6 mo	5–11	15–35	0–3	0–1	42–72	0–6	—
6 mo–1 y	6–12	13–33	0–3	0–0	46–76	0–5	—
1–6 y	5–11	13–33	0–3	0–0	46–76	0–5	—
6–16 y	5–11	32–54	0–3	0–1	27–57	0–5	—
16–18 y	5–11	34–64	0–3	0–1	25–45	0–5	—
>18 y	3–6	50–62	0–3	0–1	25–40	3–7	0–1

EOS, eosinophils; Basos, basophils; Lymphs, lymphocytes; Monos, monocytes; Metas.

Explanation of Test

The differential count is expressed as a percentage of the total number of leukocytes (WBC). The distribution (number and type) of cells and the degree of increase or decrease are diagnostically significant. The percentages indicate the *relative* number of each type of leukocyte in the blood. The *absolute* count of each type of leukocyte is obtained mathematically by multiplying its relative percentage by the total leukocyte count. The formula is

$$\text{Relative value} \times \text{WBC} = \text{Absolute value}$$
$$(\%) \qquad (\text{cells/mm}^3) \qquad (\text{cells/mm}^3)$$

The differential count alone has limited value; it must always be interpreted in relation to the WBC. If the percentage of 1 type of cell is increased, it can be inferred that cells of that type are relatively more numerous than normal, but it is not known whether this reflects an actual increase in the (absolute) number of cells that are relatively increased or an absolute decrease in cells of another type. On the other hand, if the relative (percentage) values of the differential count and the total WBC are both known, it is possible to calculate absolute values that are not subject to misinterpretation.

SEGMENTED NEUTROPHILS (POLYMORPHONUCLEAR NEUTROPHILS, PMNs, "SEGS," "POLYS") ●

Normal Values
Absolute count: 3000–7000/mm^3
Differential: 50%–60% of total WBC
0%–3% of total PMNs are stab or band cells

Background
Neutrophils, the most numerous and important type of leukocytes in the body's reaction to inflammation, constitute a primary defense against microbial invasion through the process of phagocytosis. These cells can also cause some body tissue damage by their release of enzymes and endogenous pyogenes. In their immature stage of development, neutrophils are referred to as "stab" or "band" cells. The term *band* stems from the appearance of the nucleus, which has not yet assumed the lobed shape of the mature cell.

Explanation of Test
This test determines the presence of neutrophilia or neutropenia. Neutrophilia is an increase in the absolute number of neutrophils in response to invading organisms and tumor cells. Neutropenia occurs when too few neutrophils are produced in the marrow, too many are stored in the blood vessel margin, or too many have been called to action and used up.

Procedure
1. Obtain a 5-ml blood sample in EDTA coagulant and place it in biohazard bag. Count as part of the differential.

Clinical Implications
1. *Neutrophilia* (increased absolute number and relative percentage of neutrophils) >8000/mm^3 or >70% occurs in the following disease states:
   A. Acute, localized and general bacterial infections
   B. Inflammation (eg, acute gout and vasculitis)
   C. Intoxications: metabolic (eg, uremia) and poisoning by chemicals or drugs
   D. Acute hemorrhage
   E. Acute hemolysis of RBCs (hemolytic transfusion reaction)
   F. Myeloproliferative diseases (eg, myelogenous leukemia—often noted in early stages of disease)
   G. Tissue necrosis caused by myocardial infarction, tumors, burns, gangrene, carcinoma, bacterial necrosis
   H. Some viral infections—often noted in early stages of disease
2. *Ratio* of segmented neutrophils to band neutrophils: Normally 1%–3% of PMNs are band forms (immature neutrophils).
   A. Degenerative shift to left: In some overwhelming infections there is an increase in band (immature) forms with no leukocytosis (poor prognosis).

B. Regenerative shift to left: There is an increase in band (immature) forms with leukocytosis (good prognosis) in bacterial infections.

C. Shift to the right: Few band (immature) cells with increased segmented neutrophils can occur in liver disease, megaloblastic anemia, hemolysis, drugs, cancer, and allergies.

D. Hypersegmentation of neutrophils with no band (immature) cells is found in megaloblastic anemias (eg, pernicious anemia) and chronic morphine addiction.

3. *Neutropenia* (decreased neutrophils) $<1800/mm^3$ ($<1000/mm^3$ in African Americans) or $<40\%$ occurs in the following disease states as a result of decreased or ineffective production:

A. Acute, overwhelming bacterial infections (poor prognosis)

B. Viral infections (eg, influenza, infectious hepatitis, mononucleosis)

C. Rickettsial diseases, some parasitical diseases (malaria)

D. Drugs, chemicals, toxic agents, radiation

E. Blood diseases (eg, aplastic anemia, pernicious anemia, aleukemic leukemia, vitamin B_{12} and folate deficiencies)

F. Hormonal disorders (eg, Addison's disease, thyrotoxicosis, acromegaly)

G. Anaphylactic shock, severe renal disease

4. *Neutropenia* resulting from decreased neutrophil survival occurs in:

A. Infections (sepsis due to *Escherichia coli*)

B. Drug-induced

C. Autoimmune-mediated

D. Splenic sequestration

E. Systemic lupus erythematosus (SLE)

5. *Neutropenia* in neonates ($<5000/mm^3$) or in infants ($<1000/mm^3$):

A. Maternal neutropenia, maternal drug ingestion, maternal isoimmunization to fetal leukocytes

B. Inborn errors of metabolism (eg, maple syrup urine disease)

C. Immune deficits

D. Deficits and disorders of myeloid stem cell (eg, leukemia, lymphoma, Kostmann's agranulocytosis, benign chronic granulocytopenia of childhood)

E. Adult-type pernicious anemia, defective intrinsic factor secretion, Imerslund-Graesbeck syndrome

6. Other leukocyte abnormalities and corresponding diseases are listed in the accompanying table.

Leukocyte Abnormalities and Diseases		
Abnormality	*Description*	*Associated Diseases*
Toxic granulation	Coarse, black or purple, cytoplasmic granules	Infections or inflammatory diseases

(continued)

Leukocyte Abnormalities and Diseases   *(Continued)*

Abnormality	Description	Associated Diseases
Döhle bodies	Small (1–2 μm), blue, cytoplasmic inclusions in neutrophils	Infections or inflammatory diseases, burns, myelocytic leukemia, myeloproliferative syndromes, cyclophosphamide therapy
Pelger-Huët anomalies	Neutrophil with bilobed nucleus or no segmentation of nucleus; chromatin is coarse and cytoplasm is pink with normal granulation.	Hereditary, myelocytic leukemias, myeloproliferative syndromes
May-Hegglin anomaly	Basophilic, cytoplasmic inclusions of leukocytes; similar to Döhle bodies.	May-Hegglin syndrome (hereditary), includes thrombocytopenia and giant platelets
Alder's anomaly	Prominent azurophilic granulation in leukocytes; similar to toxic granulation; granulation is seen better with Giemsa stain.	Hereditary, gargoylism
Chédiak-Higashi anomaly	Gray-green, large cytoplasmic inclusions that are fused giant lysomes	Chédiak-Higashi syndrome
LE (lupus erythematosus) cells	Neutrophilic leukocyte with a *homogenous* red-purple inclusion that distends the cell's cytoplasm	Lupus erythematosus and other collagen diseases, chronic hepatitis, drug reactions, serum sickness (not naturally occurring in the body—must be induced to form by mechanical trauma in vitro)
Tart cell	Neutrophilic leukocyte with a phagocytized nucleus of a granulocyte that retains some nuclear structure	Drug reactions (eg, penicillin, procainamide) or actual phagocytosis.

(continued)

Leukocyte Abnormalities and Diseases *(Continued)*

Abnormality	Description	Associated Diseases
Myeloid "shift to left"	Presence of bands, myelocytes, metamyelocytes, or promyelocytes	Infections, intoxications, tissue necrosis, myeloproliferative syndrome, leukemia (chronic myelocytic), leukemoid reaction, pernicious anemia, hyposplenism
Hypersegmented neutrophil	Mature neutrophil with more than 5 distinct lobes	Megaloblastic anemia, hereditary constitutional hypersegmentation of neutrophils; rarely, iron deficiency anemia, malignancy
Leukemic cells (eg, lymphoblasts, myeloblasts)	Presence of lymphoblasts, myeloblasts, monoblasts, myelomonoblasts, promyelocytes (none normally present in peripheral blood)	Leukemia (acute or chronic), leukemoid reaction, severe infectious or inflammatory diseases, myeloproliferative syndrome, intoxications, malignancies, recovery from bone marrow suppression
Auer bodies	Rodlike, 1–6 μm long, red-purple, refractile inclusions in neutrophils	Acute myelocytic leukemia or myelomonocytic leukemia
Smudge cell	Disintegrating nucleus of a ruptured leukocyte	Increased numbers in leukemic blood, particularly in acute lymphocytic leukemia or chronic lymphocytic leukemia when WBC count is greater than 10,000/mm³

Interfering Factors

1. Physiologic conditions such as stress, excitement, fear, anger, joy, and exercise temporarily cause increased neutrophils. Crying babies have neutrophilia.
2. Obstetric labor and delivery cause neutrophilia. Menstruation causes neutrophilia.
3. Steroid administration: Neutrophilia peaks in 4 to 6 hours and returns to normal by 24 hours (in severe infection, expected neutrophilia does not occur).
4. Exposure to extreme heat or cold
5. Age
   A. Children respond to infection with a greater degree of neutrophilic leukocytosis than adults do.

B. Some elderly patients respond weakly or not at all, even when infection is severe.

6. Resistance

   A. People of any age who are weak and debilitated may fail to respond with a significant neutrophilia.

   B. When an infection becomes overwhelming, the patient's resistance is exhausted and, as death approaches, the number of neutrophils decreases greatly.

7. Myelosuppressive chemotherapy

Patient Preparation

1. Explain test purpose and procedure.

2. Refer to standard *pretest* care for hemogram, CBC, and differential count on page 44. Also, see Chapter 1 guidelines for safe, effective, informed *pretest* care.

Patient Aftercare

1. Interpret test outcomes and monitor appropriately for neutrophilia or neutropenia.

> ### Clinical Alert
>
> Agranulocytosis (marked neutropenia and leukopenia) is extremely dangerous and is often fatal because the body is unprotected against invading agents. Patients with agranulocytosis must be protected from infection by means of reverse isolation techniques with strictest emphasis on hand-washing technique.

2. Refer to standard *posttest* care for hemogram, CBC, and differential count on page 44. Also, follow Chapter 1 guidelines for safe, effective, informed *posttest* care.

EOSINOPHILS

Normal Values

Absolute count: 50–250/mm^3 Differential: 1%–4% of total WBC

Background

Eosinophils, capable of phagocytosis, ingest antigen-antibody complexes and become active in the later stages of inflammation. Eosinophils respond to allergic and parasitic diseases. Eosinophilic granules contain histamine (one third of all the histamine in the body).

Explanation of Test

This test is used to diagnose allergic infections, assess severity of infestations with worms and other large parasites, and monitor response to treatment.

Procedure

1. Obtain a 5-ml blood sample in EDTA anticoagulant. Place it in a biohazard bag.
2. Note the time the blood sample is obtained (eg, 3:00 PM).
3. A total WBC is performed, a blood smear is made, 100 cells are counted, and the percentage of eosinophils is reported.
4. An absolute eosinophil count is also available. It is done with a special eosinophil stain and manual counting on a hemacytometer. It must be done within 4 hours after collection or, if refrigerated, within 24 hours.

Clinical Implications

1. *Eosinophilia* (increased circulating eosinophils) >5% or more than 500 cells/mm^3 occurs in:
   A. Allergies, hay fever, asthma
   B. Parasitic disease and trichinosis tapeworm, especially with tissue invasion
   C. Some endocrine disorders, Addison's disease, hypopituitarism
   D. Hodgkin's disease and lymphoma, myeloproliferative disorders, T-cell leukemia
   E. Chronic skin diseases (eg, psoriasis, pemphigus, scabies)
   F. Systemic eosinophilia associated with pulmonary infiltration (PIE)
   G. Some infections (scarlet fever, chlamydia)
   H. Familial eosinophilia (rare), hypereosinophilic syndrome
   I. Polyarteritis nodosa, collagen-vascular diseases (eg, SLE), connective tissue disorders
   J. Eosinophilic gastrointestinal diseases (eg, ulcerative colitis, Crohn's disease)
   K. Immunodeficiency disorders (Wiskott-Aldrich syndrome, immunoglobulin A deficiency)
   L. Many drug reactions, aspirin sensitivity
   M. Löffler's syndrome (related to ascaris infestation)
   N. Tropical eosinophilia (related to filariasis)
   O. Acute renal allograft syndrome
2. *Eosinopenia* (decreased circulating eosinophils) is usually caused by an increased adrenal steroid production that accompanies most conditions of bodily stress and is associated with:
   A. Cushing's syndrome (acute adrenal failure): <50/mm^3
   B. Use of certain drugs such as ACTH, epinephrine, thyroxine, prostaglandins
   C. Acute bacterial infections with a marked shift to the left (increase in immature leukocytes)
3. *Eosinophilic myelocytes* are counted separately because they have a greater significance, being found only in leukemia or leukemoid blood pictures.

Interfering Factors

1. Daily rhythm: The normal eosinophil count is lowest in the morning, then rises from noon until after midnight. For this reason, serial eosinophil counts should be repeated at the same time each day.
2. Stressful situations, such as in burns, postoperative states, electroshock, and labor, cause a decreased count.
3. After administration of corticosteroids, eosinophils disappear.
4. See Appendix J for drugs that affect test outcomes.

Patient Preparation

1. Explain test purpose and procedure.
2. Refer to standard patient care for hemogram, CBC, and differential count on page 44. Also, see Chapter 1 guidelines for safe, effective, informed *pretest* care.

Patient Aftercare

1. Interpret test outcomes and monitor appropriately.
2. Use special precautions if patient is receiving steroid therapy, epinephrine, thyroxine, or prostaglandins. Eosinophilia can be masked by steroid use.
3. Refer to standard *posttest* care for hemogram, CBC, and differential count on page 44. Also, follow Chapter 1 guidelines for safe, effective, informed *posttest* care.

BASOPHILS ●

Normal Values

Absolute count: 15–100/mm^3 Differential: 0.5%–1.0% of total WBC

Background

Basophils, which constitute a small percentage of the total leukocyte count, are considered phagocytic. The basophilic granules contain heparin, histamines, and serotonin. Tissue basophils are called *mast cells* and are similar to blood basophils. Normally, mast cells are not found in peripheral blood and are rarely seen in healthy bone marrow.

Explanation of Test

Basophil counts are used to study chronic inflammation. There is a positive correlation between high basophil counts and high concentrations of blood histamines, although this correlation does not imply cause and effect.

Procedure

1. Obtain a 5-ml blood sample in EDTA and count as part of the differential. Place the sample in a biohazard bag.

Clinical Implications

1. *Basophilia* (increased count) >100/mm^3 is commonly associated with the following:

    A. Granulocytic (myelocytic) leukemia

    B. Acute basophilic leukemia

    C. Myeloid metaplasia

    D. Hodgkin's disease

2. It is less commonly associated with the following:

    A. Inflammation, allergy, or sinusitis

    B. Polycythemia vera

    C. Chronic hemolytic anemia

    D. After splenectomy

    E. After ionizing radiation

    F. Hypothyroidism

    G. Infections, including tuberculosis, smallpox, chickenpox, influenza

    H. Foreign protein ingestion

3. *Basopenia* (decreased count) $<20/mm^3$ associated with the following:

    A. Acute phase of infection

    B. Hyperthyroidism

    C. Stress reactions (eg, pregnancy, myocardial infarction)

    D. After prolonged steroid therapy, chemotherapy, radiation

    E. Hereditary absence of basophils

    F. Acute rheumatic fever in children

4. *Presence of numbers of tissue mast cells* (tissue basophils) is associated with

    A. Rheumatoid arthritis

    B. Urticaria, asthma

    C. Anaphylactic shock

    D. Hypoadrenalism

    E. Lymphoma

    F. Macroglobulinemia

    G. Mast cell leukemia

    H. Lymphoma invading bone marrow

    I. Urticaria pigmentosa

    J. Asthma

    K. Chronic liver or renal disease

    L. Osteoporosis

    M. Systemic mastocytosis

Interfering Factors

1. See Appendix J for drugs that affect test outcomes.

Patient Preparation

1. Explain test purpose and procedure.

2. Refer to standard patient care for hemogram, CBC, and differential count on page 44. Also, see Chapter 1 guidelines for safe, effective, informed *pretest* care.

Patient Aftercare

1. Interpret test outcomes and monitor appropriately.

2. Use special precautions if patient is receiving steroid therapy, epinephrine, thyroxine, or prostaglandins. Eosinophilia can be masked by steroid use.

3. Refer to standard *posttest* care for hemogram, CBC, and differential count on page 44. Also, follow Chapter 1 guidelines for safe, effective, informed *posttest* care.

MONOCYTES (MONOMORPHONUCLEAR MONOCYTES)

Normal Values
Absolute count: 100–500/mm³   Differential: 3%–7% of total WBC

Background
These agranulocytes, the largest cells of normal blood, are the body's second line of defense against infection. Histiocytes, which are large macrophagic phago-cytes, are classified as *monocytes* in a differential leukocyte count. Histiocytes and monocytes are capable of reversible transformation from one to the other.

These phagocytic cells of varying size and mobility remove injured and dead cells, microorganisms, and insoluble particles from the circulating blood. Monocytes escaping from the upper and lower respiratory tracts and the gas-trointestinal and genitourinary organs perform a scavenger function, clearing the body of debris. These phagocytic cells produce the antiviral agent called *interferon*.

Explanation of Test
This test counts monocytes, which circulate in certain specific conditions such as tuberculosis, subacute bacterial endocarditis, and the recovery phase of acute infections.

Procedure
1. Obtain a 5-ml blood sample in EDTA and count as part of the differential.

Clinical Implications
1. In *monocytosis:* A monocyte increase in >500 cells/mm³ or >10%. The most common causes are bacterial infections, tuberculosis, subacute bac-terial endocarditis, and syphilis.
2. Other causes of monocytosis:
   A. Monocytic leukemia and myeloproliferative disorders
   B. Carcinoma of stomach, breast, or ovary
   C. Hodgkin's disease and other lymphomas
   D. Recovery state of neutropenia (favorable sign)
   E. Lipid storage diseases (eg, Gaucher's disease)
   F. Some parasitic mycotic and rickettsial diseases
   G. Surgical trauma
   H. Chronic ulcerative colitis, enteritis, and sprue
   I. Collagen diseases and sarcoidosis
   J. Tetrachloroethane poisoning
3. Phagocytic monocytes (macrophages) may be found in small numbers in the blood in many conditions:

A. Severe infections (sepsis)

B. Lupus erythematosus

C. Hemolytic anemias

4. *Decreased monocyte count* (<100 cells/mm³) is not usually identified with specific diseases:

A. Prednisone treatment

B. Hairy cell leukemia

C. Overwhelming infection that also causes neutropenia

D. Human immunodeficiency virus (HIV) infection

Interfering Factors

1. See Appendix J for drugs that affect test outcomes.

Patient Preparation

1. Explain test purpose and procedure.

2. Refer to standard *pretest* care for hemogram, CBC, and differential count on page 44. Also, see Chapter 1 guidelines for safe, effective, informed *pretest* care.

Patient Aftercare

1. Interpret test outcomes and monitor appropriately for leukemia and infection.

2. Refer to standard *posttest* care for hemogram, CBC, and differential count on page 44. Also, follow Chapter 1 guidelines for safe, effective, informed *posttest* care.

LYMPHOCYTES (MONOMORPHONUCLEAR LYMPHOCYTES); CD4 COUNT; PLASMA CELLS ●

Normal Values

Lymphocytes: 25%–40% of total leukocyte count (relative value) or 1500–4000 cells/mm³

Plasma cells: 0% or none

CD4 count: Mathematical formula (see below)

Background

Lymphocytes are small, mononuclear cells without specific granules. These agranulocytes are motile cells that migrate to areas of inflammation in both early and late stages of the process. These cells are the source of serum immunoglobulins and of cellular immune response and play an important role in immunologic reactions. All lymphocytes are manufactured in the bone marrow. B lymphocytes mature in the bone marrow, and T lymphocytes mature in the thymus gland. B cells control the antigen-antibody response that is specific to the offending antigen and is said to have "memory." The T cells, the master immune cells, include CD4⁺ T-helper cells, killer cells, cytotoxic cells, and CD8⁺ T-suppressor cells (see Chapter 8 for further tests of T cells).

Plasma cells are similar in appearance to lymphocytes. They have abundant blue cytoplasm and an eccentric, round nucleus. Plasma cells are not normally present in blood.

Explanation of Test

This test measures the number of lymphocytes in the peripheral blood. Lymphocytosis is present in various diseases and is especially prominent in viral disorders. Lymphocytes and their derivatives, the plasma cells, operate in the immune defenses of the body.

Procedure

1. Obtain 5 ml of EDTA-anticoagulated blood. Place the specimen in a biohazard bag.
2. Lymphocytes are counted as part of the differential count.

Clinical Implications

1. *Lymphocytosis:* >4000/mm^3 in adults; >7200/mm^3 in children; and >9000/mm^3 in infants occurs in:
    A. Lymphatic leukemia (acute and chronic) lymphoma
    B. Infectious lymphocytosis (occurs mainly in children)
    C. Infectious mononucleosis:
        (1) Caused by Epstein-Barr virus
        (2) Most common in adolescents and young adults
        (3) Characterized by atypical lymphocytes (Downey cells) that are large, deeply indented, with deep blue (basophilic) cytoplasm
        (4) Differential diagnosis—positive heterophil test
    D. Other viral diseases:
        (1) Viral infections of the upper respiratory tract
        (2) Cytomegalovirus
        (3) Measles
        (4) Mumps
        (5) Chicken pox
        (6) Infectious hepatitis
        (7) Toxoplasmosis
    E. Some bacterial diseases such as tuberculosis, brucellosis (undulant fever), and pertussis
    F. Crohn's disease, ulcerative colitis
    G. Serum sickness, drug hypersensitivity
    H. Hypoadrenalism, Addison's disease
    I. Thyrotoxicosis
    J. Neutropenia with relative lymphocytosis
2. *Lymphopenia:* <1000 cells/mm^3 in adults; <2500 cells/mm^3 in children occurs in:
    A. Chemotherapy, radiation treatment (immunosuppressive medications)
    B. After administration of ACTH or cortisone (steroids); with ACTH-producing pituitary tumors
    C. Increased loss via gastrointestinal tract owing to obstruction of lymphatic drainage (eg, tumor, Whipple's disease, intestinal lymphectasia)
    D. Aplastic anemia
    E. Hodgkin's disease and other malignancies
    F. Inherited immune disorders, acquired immunodeficiency syndrome (AIDS), and AIDS-immune dysfunction

G. Advanced tuberculosis

H. Severe debilitating illness of any kind

I. Congestive heart failure

J. Renal failure, SLE

3. *CD4 count:* The number of CD4$^+$ lymphocytes is equal to the absolute number of lymphocytes (total WBC × differential % of lymphocytes) times the percentage of lymphocytes staining positively for CD4. A severely depressed CD4 count is the single best indicator of imminent opportunistic infection.

   A. *Decreased* CD4 lymphocytes

      (1) Immune dysfunction, especially AIDS

      (2) Acute minor viral infections

   B. *Increased* CD4 lymphocytes

      (1) Therapeutic effect of drugs

      (2) Diurnal variation: Peak evening values may be 2 times morning values.

4. *Plasma cells* (not normally present in blood) are *increased* in:

   A. Plasma cell leukemia

   B. Multiple myeloma

   C. Hodgkin's disease

   D. Chronic lymphatic leukemia

   E. Cancer of liver, breast, prostate

   F. Cirrhosis

   G. Rheumatoid arthritis, SLE

   H. Serum reaction

   I. Some bacterial, viral, and parasitic infections

Interfering Factors

1. Physiologic pediatric lymphocytosis is a condition in newborns that includes an elevated WBC and abnormal-appearing lymphocytes that can be mistaken for malignant cells

2. Exercise, emotional stress, and menstruation can cause an increase in lymphocytes.

3. African Americans normally have a relative (not absolute) increase in lymphocytes.

4. See Appendix J for drugs that affect outcomes.

Abnormal Lymphocytes

Abnormality	Description	Associated Diseases
Atypical lymphocytes Reactive lymphocytes "Downey" cells "Turk" cells	Lymphocytes, some with vacuolated cytoplasm, irregularly shaped nucleus, increased numbers of cytoplasmic azurophilic granules, peripheral basophilia, or some with more abundant basophilic cytoplasm, grossly indented cytoplasm	Infectious mononucleosis, viral hepatitis, other viral infections, tuberculosis, drug (eg, penicillin) sensitivity, posttransfusion syndrome

Patient Preparation

1. Explain test purpose and procedure.
2. Refer to standard *pretest* care for hemogram, CBC, and differential count on page 44. Also, see Chapter 1 guidelines for safe, effective, informed *pretest* care.

Patient Aftercare

Clinical Alert

A decreased lymphocyte count <500/mm³ means that a patient is dangerously susceptible to infection, especially viral infections. *Institute measures to protect patient from infection.*

1. Interpret test outcomes and monitor appropriately for lymphocytosis or lymphopenia.
2. Refer to standard *posttest* care for hemogram, CBC, and differential count on page 44. Also, follow Chapter 1 guidelines for safe, effective, informed *posttest* care.

LYMPHOCYTE IMMUNOPHENOTYPING (T AND B CELLS) ●

Normal Values for Adult Peripheral Blood by Flow Cytometry

T and B Surface Markers

Total T cells (CD3⁺)	53%–88%
T-helper cells (CD3⁺ CD4⁺)	32%–61%
T-suppressor cells (CD3⁺ CD8⁺)	18%–42%
B cells (CD19⁺)	5%–20%
Natural killer cells (CD16⁺)	4%–32%

Absolute Counts (based on pathologist's interpretation)

Total lymphocytes	660–4600/mm³
Total T cells (CD3⁺)	812–2318/mm³
T-helper cells (CD3⁺ CD4⁺)	589–1505/mm³
T-suppressor cells (CD3⁺ CD8⁺)	325–997/mm³
B cells (CD19⁺)	92–426/mm³
Natural killer cells (CD16⁺)	78–602/mm³

Lymphocyte Ratio

T-helper/T-suppressor ratio	>1.0

Background

Lymphocytes are divided into two categories, T and B cells, according to their primary function within the immune system. In the body, T and B cells work together to help provide protection against infections, oncogenic agents, and foreign tissue, and they play a vital role in regulating self-destruction or autoimmunity.

The majority of circulating lymphocytes are T cells with a life span of months to years. The life span of B cells is measured in days. *B cells (antibody)* are considered "bursa or bone marrow dependent" and are responsible for humoral immunity (in which antibodies are present in the serum). *T cells (cellular)* are thymus-derived and are responsible for cellular immunity. T cells are further divided into T-helper ($CD3^+$ $CD4^+$) cells and T-suppressor ($CD3^+$ $CD8^+$) cells.

Explanation of Test

Evaluation of lymphocytes in the clinical laboratory is performed by quantitation of the lymphocytes and their subpopulations and by assessment of their functional activity. These laboratory analyses have become an essential component of the clinical assessment of two major disease states: *lymphoproliferative* states (eg, leukemia, lymphoma), in which characterization of the malignant cell in terms of lineage and stage of differentiation provides valuable information to the oncologist to guide prognosis and appropriate therapy, and *immunodeficient* states (eg, HIV infection, organ transplantation), in which the alterations in the immune system that occur secondary to infection are evaluated.

The method of lymphocyte quantitation and characterization is based on the detection of cell surface markers by very specific monoclonal antibodies. For cell surface immunophenotyping, flow cytometry has become the method of choice. Cell surface phenotyping is accomplished by reacting cells from an appropriate specimen with one or more labeled monoclonal antibodies and passing them through a flow cytometer, which counts the proportion of labeled cells.

Procedure

1. A 7-ml EDTA-anticoagulated blood sample (lavender-top tube) is obtained. The sample must not be refrigerated or frozen; it should remain at room temperature until testing is performed. A separate 7-ml venous EDTA-anticoagulated blood sample for hematology should be collected at the same time. Because the interpretation of data is based on absolute values, it is imperative that a WBC and differential count also be performed so that the appropriate data can be obtained.

Clinical Implications

1. Standard immunosuppressive drug therapy usually *decreases* lymphocyte totals.
2. Patients with an absolute T-helper lymphocyte count $<200/mm^3$ are at greatest risk for developing clinical AIDS.
3. *Decreased* T cells occur in congenital immunodeficiency diseases (eg, DiGeorge syndrome, thymic hypoplasia).
4. *Decreased* T cells occur in kidney and heart transplant patients receiving OKT-3, an immunomodulatory drug used to prevent rejection.
5. A marked *increase* in B cells occurs in lymphoproliferative disorders (eg, chronic lymphocytic leukemia). In the typical case of chronic lymphocytic

leukemia, the B cells would be positive for either κ or λ light chains (indicating monoclonality) and would express CD19 (a B-cell antigen).

Patient Preparation

1. Explain purpose and specimen collection procedure. A recent viral cold can cause a decrease in total T cells, as can medications such as corticosteroids. Nicotine and strenuous exercise have also been shown to decrease lymphocyte counts.
2. Follow guidelines in Chapter 1 for safe, effective, informed *pretest* care.

Patient Aftercare

1. Interpret test outcomes and possible need for repeat testing. Lymphocyte immunophenotyping is performed to monitor patients who are HIV⁺ and have begun medication treatment. Transplantation patients are also retested at regular intervals to assess the threat of organ rejection or host infection.
2. See guidelines in Chapter 1 for safe, effective, informed *posttest* care.

● STAINS FOR LEUKEMIAS

Several special WBC staining methods are used to diagnose leukemia, amyloid disease, lymphoma, and erythroleukemia; to differentiate erythema myelosis from sideroblastic anemia; to monitor progress and response to therapy; and to detect early relapse. *Amyloid* refers to starch-like substances deposited in certain diseases (eg, tuberculosis, osteomyelitis, leprosy, Hodgkin's disease, and carcinoma).

SUDAN BLACK B (SBB) STAIN ●

Normal Values

Acute myeloblastic leukemia	Stain (positive)
Granulocytes and monocytes	Stain (positive in characteristic patterns)
Lymphoblasts and lymphocytes	Do not stain (negative)
Monoblasts	Do not stain (negative)
Erythroblasts (erythroleukemia)	Do not stain (negative)
Plasma cells	Do not stain (negative)

Background

This stain aids in differentiation of the immature cells of acute leukemias, especially acute myeloblastic leukemia. The SBB stains a variety of fats and lipids that are present in myeloid leukemias but not present in the lymphoid leukemias.

Procedure

1. Obtain bone marrow aspirate. Prepare slide, stain with SBB, and scan microscopically. Use normal smear control.

Clinical Implications

1. Positive staining of primitive (blast) cells indicates myelogenous origin of cells. SBB is positive in acute granulocytic leukemia.
2. SBB is negative in acute lymphocytic leukemia, monocytic leukemia, and plasma cell leukemia.
3. SBB is weakly positive for monocytes.

Interfering Factors

There are cases of acute leukemia in which the cytochemical stains are not useful and fail to reveal the differentiating features of any specific cell line.

Patient Preparation

1. Explain test purposes and procedures. If bone marrow aspiration is done, see pages 39 for special care.
2. See Chapter 1 guidelines for safe, effective, informed *pretest* care.

Patient Aftercare

1. Interpret test outcomes; counsel and monitor appropriately for leukemia, amyloid disease, anemia, and infection.
2. Follow Chapter 1 guidelines for safe, effective, informed *posttest* care.

PERIODIC ACID–SCHIFF (PAS) STAIN   ●

Normal Values

Lymphoblasts	Stain (positive)
Myeloblasts	Do not stain (negative)

Background

PAS stain aids in the diagnosis of acute lymphoblastic leukemia (ALL). Early myeloid precursors and erythrocyte precursors are negative. As granulocytes mature, they increase in PAS positivity, whereas mature RBCs stay negative.

Procedure

1. Obtain bone marrow aspirate. Prepare slide, stain with PAS, and scan microscopically.

Clinical Implications

1. Blasts in acute lymphoblastic leukemia (ALL) in childhood often have coarse clumps or masses of PAS-positive material within their scent cytoplasm. The staining pattern is usually heterogeneous, with some cells containing PAS-positive clumps and others virtually unstained.

2. In acute granulocytic leukemia, the blasts display either a negative or weakly positive, finely granular pattern.

3. Conspicuous PAS positivity in the erythroid precursors is strongly suggestive of erythroleukemia (M_6).

4. In some cases of thalassemia and in anemias with blocked or deficient iron, the red blood cell precursors also contain PAS-positive material.

TERMINAL DEOXYNUCLEOTIDYL TRANSFERASE (TDT) STAIN

Normal Values
Negative in nonlymphoblastic leukemia
Negative in peripheral blood
0% to 2% positive in bone marrow

Background
The thymus is the primary site of TDT-positive cells, and TDT is found in the nucleus of the more primitive T cells. A thymus-related population of TDT-positive cells resides in the bone marrow (normally a minor population, 0% to 2%). TDT is increased in >90% of cases of ALL of childhood. A minor (5% to 10%) population of patients with acute nonlymphoblastic leukemia have TDT-positive blasts. TDT-positive blasts are prominent in some cases of chronic myelogenous leukemia (CML), relating to the development of an acute blast phase. TDT has been reported to assist in establishing the diagnosis of ALL. TDT-positive cases of blast-phase CML correlate with a positive response to chemotherapy (vincristine and prednisone).

Procedure
1. Obtain a 5-ml EDTA-anticoagulated peripheral blood sample or a 2-ml EDTA-anticoagulated bone marrow aspirate.

2. Slides are dried (stored at room temperature for up to 5 days), processed, and stained, then examined under the microscope for positive cells.

Clinical Implications
TDT is positive in ALL, lymphoblastic lymphoma, and CML (blast crisis).

LEUKOCYTE ALKALINE PHOSPHATASE (LAP) STAIN

Normal Values
24–180 LAP units

Background
Neutrophils are the only leukocytes to contain various amounts of alkaline phosphatase.

Explanation of Test
The LAP stain is used as an aid to distinguish chronic granulocytic leukemia from a leukemoid reaction. A leukemoid reaction is a high WBC count that may look like leukemia but is not.

Procedure
1. Obtain specimen by capillary puncture, venous blood (EDTA), or bone marrow aspirate. Prepare smear and air-dry; stain with LAP.
2. A count of 100 granulocytes is made and scored (from 0 to 4+) as to the degree of LAP units.

Clinical Implications
1. *Decreased* values (0–13 LAP units):
   - **A.** Chronic myelogenous leukemia (CML)
   - **B.** Paroxysmal nocturnal hemoglobinuria (PNH)
   - **C.** Idiopathic thrombocytopenic purpura
   - **D.** Hereditary hypophosphatasia
   - **E.** Sideroblastic anemia
   - **F.** Nephrotic syndrome
   - **G.** Sickle cell anemia
   - **H.** Nephrotic syndrome
2. *Increased* values:
   - **A.** Leukemoid reactions, all kinds of neutrophilia with elevated WBC
   - **B.** Polycythemia vera
   - **C.** Thrombocytopenia
   - **D.** Down syndrome
   - **E.** Multiple myeloma
   - **F.** Hodgkin's disease, lymphoma
   - **G.** Hairy cell leukemia
   - **H.** Aplastic leukemia, acute and chronic lymphatic leukemia
   - **I.** Myelofibrosis
3. Serial LAP tests can be a useful adjunct in evaluating the activity of Hodgkin's disease and the response to therapy.

Interfering Factors
1. Any physiologic stress such as third-trimester pregnancy, labor, or severe exercise cause an *increased* LAP score.
2. Steroid therapy *increases* the LAP score.
3. CML with infection *increase* the LAP score.

TARTRATE-RESISTANT ACID PHOSPHATASE (TRAP) STAIN ●

Normal Values
No TRAP activity

Background
The malignant mononuclear cells of leukemic reticuloendotheliosis (hairy cell leukemia) are resistant to inhibition by tartaric acid. There is evidence the re-

action is not entirely specific, because TRAP reactions have been reported in prolymphocytic leukemia and malignant lymphoma and in some cases of infectious mononucleosis.

Procedure
1. Obtain venous blood sample (5 ml) or bone marrow smear. Blood smear is incubated with TRAP, counterstained, and examined microscopically.

Clinical Implications
1. TRAP is present in the leukemic cells of most patients with hairy cell leukemia; 5% of patients with otherwise typical hairy cell leukemia lack the enzyme.
2. TRAP occasionally occurs in malignant cells of patients with lymphoproliferative disorders other than hairy cell leukemia.
3. Histocytes have weakly positive reactions.

●TESTS OF RED BLOOD CELLS

Many tests look at the red blood cells: their number and size, amount of hemoglobin, rate of production, and percent composition of the blood. The red blood cell count (RBC), hematocrit (Hct), and hemoglobin (Hb) are closely related but different ways to look at the adequacy of erythrocyte production. The same conditions cause an increase (or a decrease) in each of these indicators.

RED BLOOD CELL COUNT (RBC; ERYTHROCYTE COUNT)
Normal Values

Normal Values for RBC	
Men: 4.2–5.4 × 10^6/mm^3 or × 10^{12}/L (average, 4.8)	
Women: 3.6–5.0 × 10^6/mm^3 or × 10^{12}/L (average 4.3)	
Children:	
Birth–2 wk	4.1–6.1 × 10^6/mm^3
2–8 wk	4.0–6.0 × 10^6/mm^3
2–6 mo	3.8–5.6 × 10^6/mm^3
6 mo–1 y	3.8–5.2 × 10^6/mm^3
1–6 y	3.9–5.3 × 10^6/mm^3
6–16 y	4.0–5.2 × 10^6/mm^3
16–18 y	4.2–5.4 × 10^6/mm^3
>18 y males	4.5–5.5 × 10^6/mm^3
>18 y females	4.0–5.0 × 10^6/mm^3

Background
The main function of the red blood cell (RBC or erythrocyte) is to carry oxygen from the lungs to the body tissues and to transfer carbon dioxide from the tissues to the lungs. This process is achieved by means of the *hemoglobin* (Hb)

in the RBCs, which combines easily with oxygen and carbon dioxide and gives arterial blood a bright red appearance. To enable utilization of the maximal amount of Hb, the RBC is shaped like a biconcave disk; this affords more surface area for the Hb to combine with oxygen. The cell is also able to change its shape when necessary to allow for passage through the smaller capillaries.

Explanation of Test

The RBC test, an important measurement in the evaluation of anemia or polycythemia, determines the total number of erythrocytes in a microliter (cubic millimeter) of blood.

Procedure

1. Obtain 5 ml of EDTA-anticoagulated venous blood. Place the specimen in a biohazard bag.
2. Automated electronic devices are generally used to determine the number of RBCs.
3. Note patient age and time of day on the laboratory slip.

Clinical Implications

1. *Decreased RBC values* occur in
   A. Anemia, a condition in which there is a reduction in the number of circulating erythrocytes, the amount of Hb, or the volume of packed cells (Hct). Anemia is associated with cell destruction, blood loss, or dietary insufficiency of iron or of certain vitamins that are essential in the production of RBCs. See the table on page 78 for a classification of anemias based on their underlying mechanisms and pages 88 and 89 for a discussion of the purpose and clinical implications of the reticulocyte count.
   B. Disorders such as
      (1) Hodgkin's disease and other lymphomas
      (2) Multiple myeloma, myeloproliferative disorders, leukemia
      (3) Acute and chronic hemorrhage
      (4) Lupus erythematosus
      (5) Addison's disease
      (6) Rheumatic fever
      (7) Subacute endocarditis, chronic infection
      (8) This list is not meant to be all-inclusive.

Clinical Alert

Refer to page 78 for a discussion of the combined clinical implications of *decreased* RBC, Hct, and Hb values. The same underlying conditions cause a *decrease* in each of these three tests of erythrocyte production.

2. *Erythrocytosis* (increased RBC) occurs in
  A. Primary erythrocytosis
    (1) Polycythemia vera (myeloproliferative disorder)
    (2) Erythremic erythrocytosis (increased RBC production in bone marrow)
  B. Secondary erythrocytosis
    (1) Renal disease
    (2) Extrarenal tumors
    (3) High altitude
    (4) Pulmonary disease
    (5) Cardiovascular disease
    (6) Alveolar hypoventilation
    (7) Hemoglobinopathy
    (8) Tobacco/carboxyhemoglobin
  C. Relative erythrocytosis (decrease in plasma volume)
    (1) Dehydration (vomiting, diarrhea)
    (2) Gaisböck's syndrome

> **Clinical Alert**
>
> Please refer to page 77 for a discussion of the combined clinical impli-
> cations of *increased* RBC, Hct, and Hb values. The same underlying
> conditions cause an *increase* in each of these three tests of erythrocyte
> production.

Interfering Factors

1. Posture: When a blood sample is obtained from a healthy person in a recumbent position, the RBC is 5% lower. (If the patient is anemic, the count
will be lower still.)
2. Dehydration: Hemoconcentration in dehydrated adults (caused by severe
burns, untreated intestinal obstruction, severe persistent vomiting, or diuretic abuse) may obscure significant anemia.
3. Age: The normal RBC of a newborn is higher than that of an adult, with a
rapid drop to the lowest point in life at 2 to 4 months. The normal adult
level is reached at age 14 years and is maintained until old age, when there
is a gradual drop (see Normal Values).
4. Falsely high counts may occur because of prolonged venous stasis during
venipuncture.
5. Stress can cause a higher RBC.
6. Altitude: The higher the altitude, the greater the increase in RBC. Decreased
oxygen content of the air stimulates the RBC to rise (erythrocytosis).
7. Pregnancy: There is a relative decrease in RBC when the body fluid increases in pregnancy, with the normal number of erythrocytes becoming
more diluted.
8. There are many drugs that may cause *decreased* or increased RBCs. See Appendix J for drugs that affect test outcomes.

9. The EDTA blood sample tube must be at least three-fourths filled or values will be invalid because of cell shrinkage.
10. The blood sample must not be clotted (even slightly) or the values will be invalid.

Patient Preparation

1. Explain test purpose and procedure.
2. Refer to standard *pretest* care for hemogram, CBC, and differential count on page 44.
3. Have the patient avoid extensive exercise, stress, or excitement before the test. These cause elevated counts of doubtful clinical value.
4. Avoid overhydration or dehydration, if possible; either causes invalid results. If patient is receiving IV fluids or therapy, note on requisition.
5. Note any medications patient is taking.
6. See Chapter 1 guidelines for safe, effective, informed *pretest* care.

Patient Aftercare

1. Interpret test outcomes and monitor appropriately for anemia and erythrocytosis.
2. Refer to standard *posttest* care for hemogram, CBC, and differential count on page 44.
3. See Chapter 1 guidelines for safe, effective, informed *posttest* care.
4. Resume normal activities and diet.

HEMATOCRIT (HCT); PACKED CELL VOLUME (PCV)

Normal Values for Hematocrit			
Women:	36%–48%	Children:	
Men:	42%–52%	0–2 wk	44%–64%
		2–8 wk	39%–59%
		2–6 mo	35%–49%
		6 mo–1 y	29%–43%
		1–6 y	30%–40%
		6–16 y	32%–42%
		16–18 y	34%–44%

NOTE: *If blood is drawn from a capillary puncture and a microhematocrit is done, values are slightly higher.*

Background

The word *hematocrit* means "to separate blood," which underscores the mechanism of the test, because the plasma and blood cells are separated by centrifugation.

Explanation of Test

The Hct test is part of the CBC. This test indirectly measures the RBC mass. The results are expressed as the percentage by volume of packed RBCs in whole blood (PCV). It is an important measurement in the determination of anemia or polycythemia.

Procedure

1. Observe standard precautions. When doing a capillary puncture (finger puncture), the microcapillary tube is filled three-fourths full with blood, directly from puncture site. These tubes are coated with an anticoagulative.
2. The tubes are centrifuged in a microcentrifuge and the height of packed cells in the tube is measured.
3. The measurement is recorded as a percentage of the total amount of blood in the capillary tube.
4. An Hct can be done on automated hematology instruments, in which case a 5-ml EDTA-anticoagulated venous blood sample is obtained.

Clinical Implications

1. *Decreased Hct values* are an indicator of anemia, a condition in which there is a reduction in the PCV. An Hct ≤30% means that the patient is moderately to severely anemic. Decreased values also occur in the following conditions:
   A. Leukemias, lymphomas, Hodgkin's disease, myeloproliferative disorders
   B. Adrenal insufficiency
   C. Chronic disease
   D. Acute and chronic blood loss
   E. Hemolytic reaction: This condition may be found in transfusion of incompatible blood or as a reaction to chemicals or drugs, infectious agents, or physical agents (eg, severe burns, prosthetic heart valves).
2. The Hct may or may not be reliable immediately after even a moderate loss of blood or immediately after transfusion.
3. The Hct may be normal after acute hemorrhage. During the recovery phase, both the Hct and the RBC drop markedly.
4. Usually, the Hct parallels the RBC when the cells are of normal size. As the number of normal-sized erythrocytes increases, so does the Hct.
   A. However, for the patient with microcytic or macrocytic anemia, this relationship does not hold true.
   B. If a patient has an iron-deficiency anemia with small RBCs, the Hct decreases because the microcytic cells pack to a smaller volume. The RBC, however, may be normal or higher than normal.

▶ **Clinical Alert**

Please refer to page 78 for a discussion of the combined clinical implications of *decreased* Hct, Hb, and RBC values. The same underlying conditions cause a *decrease* in each of these three tests of erythrocyte production.

5. *Increased Hct values* occur in
   A. Erythrocytosis
   B. Polycythemia vera
   C. Shock, when hemoconcentration rise considerably

> **Clinical Alert**
>
> Please refer to page 77 for a discussion of the combined clinical impli-
> cations of *increased* Hct, Hb, and RBC values. The same underlying
> conditions cause an *increase* in each of these three tests of erythrocyte
> production.

Interfering Factors

1. People living at high altitudes have high Hct values, as well as high Hb and
   RBC.
2. Normally, the Hct slightly decreases in the physiologic hydremia of pregnancy.
3. The normal values for Hct vary with age and gender. The normal value for
   infants is higher because the newborn has many macrocytic red cells. Hct
   values in females are usually slightly lower than in males.
4. There is also a tendency toward lower Hct values in men and women older
   than 60 years of age, corresponding to lower RBC values in this age group.
5. Severe dehydration from any cause falsely raises the Hct.

Patient Preparation

1. Explain test purpose and procedure.
2. Refer to standard *pretest* care for hemogram, CBC, and differential count on
   page 44. Also, see Chapter 1 guidelines for safe, effective, informed *pretest* care.

> **Clinical Alert**
>
> An Hct <20% can lead to cardiac failure and death; an Hct >60% is as-
> sociated with spontaneous clotting of blood.

Patient Aftercare

1. Interpret test results and monitor for anemia or polycythemia.
2. Refer to standard *posttest* care for hemogram, CBC, and differential count
   on page 44. Also, follow Chapter 1 guidelines for safe, effective, informed
   posttest care.

HEMOGLOBIN (HB) ●

Background

Hemoglobin (Hb), the main component of erythrocytes, serves as the vehicle
for the transportation of oxygen and carbon dioxide. It is composed of amino

Normal Values for Hemoglobin	
Women:	12.0–16.0 g/dl or 120–160 g/L
Men:	14.0–17.4 g/dl or 140–174 g/L
Children:	
0–2 wk	14.5–24.5 g/dl or 145–245 g/L
2–8 wk	12.5–20.5 g/dl or 125–205 g/L
2–6 mo	10.7–17.3 g/dl or 107–173 g/L
6 mo–1 y	9.9–14.5 g/dl or 99–145 g/L
1–6 y	9.5–14.1 g/dl or 95–141 g/L
6–16 y	10.3–14.9 g/dl or 103–149 g/L
16–18y	11.1–15.7 g/dl or 111–157 g/L

acids that form a single protein, called *globin,* and a compound called *heme,* which contains iron atoms and the red pigment porphyrin. It is the iron pigment that combines readily with oxygen and gives blood its characteristic red color. Each gram of Hb can carry 1.34 ml of oxygen. The oxygen-combining capacity of the blood is directly proportional to the Hb concentration rather than to the RBC, because some RBCs contain more Hb than others. This is why Hb determinations are important in the evaluation of anemia.

Hb also serves as an important buffer in the extracellular fluid. In tissue, the oxygen concentration is lower and the carbon dioxide level and hydrogen ion concentration are higher. At a lower pH, more oxygen dissociates from Hb. The unoxygenated Hb binds to hydrogen ion, thereby raising the pH. As carbon dioxide diffuses into the RBC, carbonic anhydrase converts carbon dioxide to bicarbonate and protons. As the protons are bound to Hb, the bicarbonate ions leave the cell. For every bicarbonate ion leaving the cell, a chloride ion enters. The efficiency of this buffer system depends on the ability of the lungs and kidneys to eliminate, respectively, carbon dioxide and bicarbonate. Refer to the discussion of arterial blood gases in Chapter 14.

Explanation of Test
The Hb determination is part of a CBC. It is used to screen for disease associated with anemia, to determine the severity of anemia, to monitor the response to treatment for anemia, and to evaluate polycythemia.

Procedure
1. A venous blood EDTA-anticoagulated sample of 5 ml is obtained. The Vacutainer tube must be filled at least three-fourths full. Automated electronic devices are generally used to determine the Hb; however, a manual colorimetric procedure is also widely used.
2. The blood sample must not be clotted or the results will be invalid. Place the specimen in a biohazard bag.

Clinical Implications
1. *Decreased Hb levels* are found in anemia states (a condition in which there

is a reduction of Hb, Hct, and/or RBC values). The Hb must be evaluated along with the RBC and Hct.

A. Iron deficiency, thalassemia, pernicious anemia, hemoglobinopathies
B. Liver disease, hypothyroidism
C. Hemorrhage (chronic or acute)
D. Hemolytic anemia caused by

  (1) Transfusions of incompatible blood
  (2) Reactions to chemicals or drugs
  (3) Reactions to infectious agents
  (4) Reactions to physical agents (eg, severe burns, artificial heart valves)
  (5) Various systemic diseases:

    (a) Hodgkin's disease
    (b) Leukemia
    (c) Lymphoma
    (d) SLE
    (e) Carcinomatosis
    (f) Sarcoidosis
    (g) Renal cortical necrosis
    (h) This list is not meant to be all-inclusive.

Clinical Alert

Please refer to page 77 for a discussion of the combined clinical implications of *decreased* Hb, Hct, and RBC values. The same underlying conditions cause a *decrease* in each of these three tests of erythrocyte production.

---

2. *Increased Hb levels* are found in

  A. Polycythemia vera
  B. Congestive heart failure
  C. Chronic obstructive pulmonary disease

3. *Variation* in Hb levels

  A. Occurs after transfusions, hemorrhages, burns. (Hb and Hct are both high during and immediately after hemorrhage.)
  B. The Hb and Hct provide valuable information in an emergency situation

---

Clinical Alert

Please refer to page 78 for a discussion of the combined clinical implications of *increased* Hb, Hct, and RBC values. The same underlying conditions cause an *increase* in each of these three tests of erythrocyte production.

if they are interpreted not in an isolated fashion but in conjunction with other pertinent laboratory data.

Interfering Factors
1. People living at high altitudes have increased Hb values, as well as increased Hct and RBC.
2. Excessive fluid intake cause a decreased Hb.
3. Normally, the Hb is higher in infants (before active erythropoiesis begins).
4. Hb is normally decreased in pregnancy as a result of increased plasma volume.
5. There are many drugs that may cause a *decreased* Hb. Drugs that may cause an *increased* Hb include gentamicin and methyldopa.
6. Extreme physical exercise causes increased Hb.

Patient Preparation
1. Explain test purpose and procedure. Assess medication history.
2. Refer to standard *pretest* care for hemogram, CBC, and differential count on page 44. Also, see Chapter 1 guidelines for safe, effective, informed *pretest* care.

Patient Aftercare
1. Interpret test results and monitor appropriately for anemia or polycythemia.

> ### Clinical Alert
>
> The panic Hb value is <5.0 g/dl, a condition that leads to heart failure and death. A value >20 g/dl leads to clogging of the capillaries as a result of hemoconcentration.

2. Refer to standard *posttest* care for hemogram, CBC, and differential count on page 44. Also, follow Chapter 1 guidelines for safe, effective, informed *posttest* care.

Clinical Implications of Polycythemia: Increased RBC, Hct, and/or Hb
Polycythemia is the term used to describe an abnormal increase in the number of RBCs. Although there are several tests to directly determine the RBC mass, these tests are expensive and somewhat cumbersome. For screening purposes, we rely on the Hct and Hb to indirectly evaluate polycythemia. Polycythemias are classified as follows:
1. *Relative* polycythemia: an increase in Hb, Hct, or RBC caused by a decrease in the plasma volume (eg, dehydration, spurious erythrocytosis from stress or smoking)
2. *Absolute* or *true* polycythemia:
   A. Primary (eg, polycythemia vera, erythremic erythrocytosis)
   B. Secondary
      (1) Appropriate (an appropriate bone marrow response to physiologic conditions)
         (a) Altitude

(b) Cardiopulmonary disorder
(c) Increased affinity for oxygen
(2) Inappropriate (an overproduction of RBCs not necessary to deliver oxygen to the tissues)
  (a) Renal tumor or cyst
  (b) Hepatoma
  (c) Cerebellar hemangioblastoma

Clinical Implications of Anemia: Decreased RBC, Hct, and/or Decreased Hb

Anemia is the term used to describe a condition in which there is a reduction in the number of circulating RBCs, the amount of Hb, and/or the volume of packed cells (Hct). A pathophysiologic classification of anemias based on their underlying mechanisms follows. Anemias are further explained in the table on page 80. Anemias are classified as follows:

1. *Hypoproliferative* anemias (inadequate production of RBCs):
  A. Marrow aplasias
  B. Myelophthisic anemia
  C. Anemia with blood dyscrasias
  D. Anemia of chronic disease
  E. Anemia with organ failure
2. *Maturation defect* anemias:
  A. Cytoplasmic: hypochromic anemias
  B. Nuclear: megaloblastic anemias
  C. Combined: myelodysplastic syndromes
3. *Hyperproliferative* anemias (decreased Hb or Hct despite an increased production of RBCs):
  A. Hemorrhagic: acute blood loss
  B. Hemolytic: a premature, accelerated destruction of RBCs
    (1) Immune hemolysis
    (2) Primary membrane
    (3) Hemoglobinopathies
    (4) Toxic hemolysis (physical-chemical)
    (5) Traumatic or microangiopathic hemolysis
    (6) Hypersplenism
    (7) Enzymopathies
    (8) Parasitic infections
4. *Dilutional* anemias:
  A. Pregnancy
  B. Splenomegaly

RED BLOOD CELL INDICES ●

Background

These indices define the size and Hb content of the RBC and consist of the mean corpuscular volume (MCV), the mean corpuscular hemoglobin concentration (MCHC), and the mean corpuscular hemoglobin (MCH).

Explanation of Tests

The RBC indices are used in differentiating anemias. When they are used together with an examination of the erythrocytes on the stained smear, a clear picture of RBC morphology may be ascertained. On the basis of the RBC indices, the erythrocytes can be characterized as normal in every respect or as abnormal in volume or hemoglobin content. In deficient states, the anemias can be classified by cell size as macrocytic, normocytic, or simple microcytic, or by cell size and color as microcytic hypochromic.

Procedure

1. These are calculated values. An explanation of each measurement is given after the descriptions of general patient pretest and posttest care.

Patient Preparation for MCV, MCHC, and MCH

1. Explain the purpose and procedure for testing. Assess for possible causes of anemia. No fasting is required.
2. See Chapter 1 guidelines for safe, effective, informed *pretest* care.

Patient Aftercare for MCV, MCHC, and MCH

1. Interpret test results and monitor appropriately for anemia. Counsel appropriately for proper diet, medication, related hormone and enzyme problems, and genetically linked disorders.
2. Follow Chapter 1 guidelines for safe, effective, informed *posttest* care.

MEAN CORPUSCULAR VOLUME (MCV)   ●

Normal Values

82–98 fl μm³ or fl (higher values in infants and newborns)

Explanation of Test

Individual cell size is the best index for classifying anemias. This index expresses the volume occupied by a single erythrocyte and is a measure in cubic micrometers (femtoliters) of the mean volume. The MCV indicates whether the RBC size appears normal (normocytic), smaller than normal (<82 μm³, microcytic), or larger than normal (>100 μm³, macrocytic).

Procedure

1. The MCV is calculated from the RBC count (the number of cells per cubic millimeter of blood) and the Hct (the proportion of the blood occupied by the RBCs). The formula is

$$\frac{MCV}{(fl)} = \frac{Hct\ (\%) \times 10}{RBC\ (10^{12}/L)}$$

Clinical Implications

The MCV results are the basis of the classification system used to evaluate an anemia. The categorizations shown in the following table aid in orderly investigation.

Anemias Characterized by Deficient Hemoglobin Synthesis

Microcytic Anemias (MCV 50–82 fl)

DISORDERS OF IRON METABOLISM
Iron-deficiency anemia: the most prevalent worldwide cause of anemia; the major causes are dietary inadequacy, malabsorption, increased iron loss, and increased iron requirements.
Anemia of chronic disease, hereditary atransferrinemia
Congenital hypochromic-microcytic anemia with iron overload (Shahidi-Nathan-Diamond syndrome)

DISORDERS OF PORPHYRIN AND HEME SYNTHESIS
Acquired sideroblastic anemias
Idiopathic refractory sideroblastic anemia, complicating other diseases associated with drugs or toxin (ethanol, isoniazid, lead)
Hereditary sideroblastic anemias
X chromosome–linked, autosomal

DISORDERS OF GLOBIN SYNTHESIS
Thalassemias, hemoglobinopathies, characterized by unstable hemoglobins

Normocytic Normochromic Anemias (MCV 82–98 fl)

ANEMIA WITH APPROPRIATE BONE MARROW RESPONSE
Acute posthemorrhagic anemia
Hemolytic anemia (may be macrocytic when there is pronounced reticulocytosis)

ANEMIA WITH IMPAIRED MARROW RESPONSE
Marrow Hypoplasia
Aplastic anemia, pure red cell aplasia

Marrow Infiltration
Infiltration by malignant cells, myelofibrosis, inherited storage diseases

Decreased Erythropoietin Production
Kidney and liver disease, endocrine deficiencies, malnutrition, anemia of chronic disease

Macrocytic Anemias (MCV 100–150 fl)

COBALAMIN (B_{12}) DEFICIENCY
Decreased Ingestion
Lack of animal products, strict vegetarianism

(continued)

Anemias Characterized by Deficient Hemoglobin Synthesis *(Continued)*

Impaired Absorption
Intrinsic factor deficiency, pernicious anemia, gastrectomy (total or partial), destruction of gastric mucosa by caustics, anti–intrinsic factor antibody in gastric juice, abnormal intrinsic factor molecule, intrinsic intestinal disease, familial selective malabsorption (Imerslund's syndrome), ileal resection, ileitis, sprue, celiac disease, infiltrative intestinal disease (eg, lymphoma, scleroderma) drug-induced malabsorption

Competitive Parasites
Fish tapeworm infestations (*Diphyllobothrium latum*); bacteria in diverticulum of bowel, blind loops

Increased Requirements
Chronic pancreatic disease, pregnancy, neoplastic disease, hyperthyroidism

Impaired Utilization
Enzyme deficiencies, abnormal serum cobalamin binding protein, lack of transcobalamin II, nitrous oxide administration

FOLATE DEFICIENCY
Decreased Ingestion
Lack of vegetables, alcoholism, infancy

Impaired Absorption
Intestinal short circuits, steatorrhea, sprue, celiac disease, intrinsic intestinal disease, anticonvulsants, oral contraceptives, other drugs

Increased Requirement
Pregnancy, infancy, hypothyroidism, hyperactive hematopoiesis, neoplastic disease, exfoliative skin disease

Impaired Utilization
Folic acid antagonists: methotrexate, triamterene, trimethoprim, enzyme deficiencies

Increased Loss
Hemodialysis

UNRESPONSIVE TO COBALAMIN OR FOLATE
Metabolic Inhibitors
Purine synthesis: 6-mercaptopurine, 6-thioguanine, azathioprine
Pyrimidine synthesis: 6-azauridine
Thymidylate synthesis: methotrexate, 5-fluorouracil
Deoxybonucleotide synthesis: hydroxyurea, cytarabine, severe iron deficiency

Inborn Errors
Lesch-Nyhan syndrome, hereditary orotic aciduria, deficiency of formiminotransferase, methyltransferase, others

Interfering Factors

1. Mixed (bimorphic) population of macrocytes and microcytes can result in a normal MCV. Examination of the blood film confirms this.
2. Increased reticulocytes can increase the MCV.
3. Marked leukocytosis increases the MCV.

MEAN CORPUSCULAR HEMOGLOBIN CONCENTRATION (MCHC) ●

Normal Values
31–37 g/dl

Explanation of Test
This test measures the average concentration of Hb in the RBCs. The MCHC is most valuable in monitoring therapy for anemia because the 2 most accurate hematologic determinations (Hb and Hct) are used in its calculation.

Procedure
1. The MCHC is a calculated value. It is an expression of the average concentration of Hb in the RBCs and, as such, it represents the ratio of the weight of Hb to the volume of the erythrocyte. The formula is

$$\frac{MCHC}{(g/dl)} = \frac{Hb\ (g/dl) \times 100}{Hct\ (\%)}$$

Clinical Implications
1. *Decreased MCHC values* signify that a unit volume of packed RBCs contains less Hb than normal. Hypochromic anemia (MCHC <30) occurs in
   A. Iron deficiency
   B. Microcytic anemias, chronic blood loss anemia
   C. Some thalassemias
2. *Increased MCHC values* (RBCs cannot accommodate more than 37 g/dl Hb) occurs in
   A. Spherocytosis
   B. Newborns and infants

Interfering Factors
1. The MCHC may be falsely high in the presence of lipemia, cold agglutinins, or rouleaux and with high heparin concentrations.
2. The MCHC cannot be greater than 37 g/dl because the RBC cannot accommodate more than 37 g/dl Hb. (Check for errors in calculation or in Hb determination.)

MEAN CORPUSCULAR HEMOGLOBIN (MCH) ●

Normal Values
26–34 pg/cell or 0.40–0.53 fmol/cell (normally higher in newborns and infants)

Explanation of Test

The MCH is a measure of the average weight of hemoglobin per RBC. This index is of value in diagnosing severely anemic patients.

Procedure

1. The MCH is a calculated value. The average weight of hemoglobin in the RBC is expressed as picograms of Hb per RBC. The formula is

$$\frac{MCH}{(pg)} = \frac{Hb\ (g/dl) \times 10}{RBC\ (10^{12}/L)}$$

Clinical Implications

1. An increase of the MCH is associated with macrocytic anemia.
2. A decrease of the MCH is associated with microcytic anemia.

Interfering Factors

1. Hyperlipidemia falsely elevates the MCH.
2. WBC counts $>50,000/mm^3$ falsely raise the Hb value and therefore falsely elevates the MCH.
3. High heparin concentrations falsely elevate the MCH.

RED CELL SIZE DISTRIBUTION WIDTH (RDW)   ●

Normal Values

11.5–14.5 coefficient of variation of red cell size (CV)

Explanation of Test

This automated method of measurement is helpful in the investigation of some hematologic disorders and in monitoring response to therapy. The RDW is essentially an indication of the degree of anisocytosis (abnormal variation in size of RBCs). Normal RBCs have a slight degree of variation.

Procedure

1. The CV of RDW is determined and calculated by the analyzer.
2. The CV of RDW should be used with caution and should not replace other diagnostic tests.
3. Calculation:

$$\frac{RDW}{(CV\%)} = \frac{Standard\ deviation\ of\ RBC\ size \times 100}{MCV}$$

Clinical Implications

1. The RDW can be helpful in distinguishing uncomplicated heterozygous thalassemia (low MCV, normal RDW) from iron-deficiency anemia (low MCV, high RDW).

2. The RDW can be helpful in distinguishing anemia of chronic disease (low-normal MCV, normal RDW) from early iron-deficiency anemia (low-normal MCV, elevated RDW).

3. *Increased* RDW occurs in

   A. Iron deficiency
   B. Vitamin B_{12} or folate deficiency (pernicious anemia)
   C. Abnormal hemoglobin: S, S-C, or H
   D. S-β-Thalassemia
   E. Immune hemolytic anemia
   F. Marked reticulocytosis
   G. Posthemorrhagic anemia

Interfering Factors
This test is not helpful for persons who do not have anemia.

Patient Care
Patient preparation and patient aftercare are the same as for the Red Blood Cell Indices on page 79.

STAINED RED CELL EXAMINATION (FILM; STAINED ERYTHROCYTE EXAMINATION) ●

Normal Values
Size: Normocytic (normal size, 7–8 μm)
Color: Normochromic (normal)
Shape: Normocyte (biconcave disk)
Structure: Normocytes or erythrocytes (anucleated cells)

Explanation of Test
The stained film examination determines variations and abnormalities in erythrocyte size, shape, structure, Hb content, and staining properties. It is useful in diagnosing blood disorders such as anemia, thalassemia, and other hemoglobinopathies. This examination also serves as a guide to therapy and as an indicator of harmful effects of chemotherapy and radiation therapy. The leukocytes are also examined at this time.

Procedure
1. A 5-ml blood sample in EDTA is collected. A stained blood smear is studied under a microscope to determine size, shape, and other characteristics of the RBCs.
2. A capillary smear may also be used and may be preferred for detection of some abnormalities.

Clinical Implications
1. *Variations* in staining, color, shape, and RBC inclusions are indicative of RBC abnormalities.

> ### Clinical Alert
>
> Marked abnormalities in size and shape of RBCs without a known cause are an indication for more complete blood studies.

Patient Care

Patient preparation and patient aftercare are the same as for the Red Blood Cell Indices on page 79.

Peripheral Blood Red Cell Abnormalities

Abnormality	*Description*	*Associated Diseases*
Anisocytosis (diameter)	Abnormal variation in size (normal diameter = 6–8 μm)	Any severe anemia (eg, iron-deficiency, hemolytic hypersplenism)
Microcytes	Small cells, <6 μm (MCV <80 fl)	Iron-deficiency and iron-loading (sideroblastic) anemia, thalassemia, lead poisoning, vitamin B_6 deficiency
Macrocytes	Large cells, > 8 μm (MCV >100 fl), MCV >94 fl male, >97 fl female	Megaloblastic anemia, liver disease, hemolytic anemia (reticulocytes), physiologic macrocytosis of newborn, myelophthisis, hypothyroidism
Megalocytes	Large (>8 μm) oval cells	Megaloblastic anemia, pernicious anemia
Hypochromia	Pale cells with decreased concentration of hemoglobin (MCHC <31 g/dl)	Severe iron-deficiency and iron-loading (sideroblastic) anemia, thalassemia, lead poisoning, transferrin deficiency
Poikilocytes	Abnormal variation in shape	Any severe anemia (eg, megaloblastic iron-deficiency, myeloproliferative syndrome, hemolytic); certain shapes are diagnostically helpful (see entries for Spherocytes through Teardrop cells)

(continued)

Peripheral Blood Red Cell Abnormalities   *(Continued)*

Abnormality	*Description*	*Associated Diseases*
Spherocytes	Spherical cells without pale centers; often small (ie, microspherocytosis)	Hereditary spherocytosis, Coombs'-positive hemolytic anemia; small numbers are seen in any hemolytic anemia and after transfusion of stored blood
Ovalocytes	Oval cells	Hereditary elliptocytosis, iron deficiency
Stomatocytosis	Red cells with slit-like (instead of circular) areas of central pallor	Congenital hemolytic anemia, thalassemia, burns, lupus erythematosus, lead poisoning, liver disease, artifact
Sickle cells	Crescent-shaped cells	Sickle cell hemoglobinopathies
Target cells	Cells with a dark center and periphery and a clear ring in between	Liver disease, thalassemia, hemoglobinopathies (S, C, S-C, S-thalassemia)
Schistocytes	Irregularly contracted cells (severe poikilocytosis), fragmented cells	Uremia, carcinoma, hemolytic-uremic syndrome, disseminated intravascular coagulation, microangiopathic hemolytic anemia, toxins (lead, phenylhydrazine); burns, thrombotic thrombocytopenic purpura
"Burr" cells	Burr-like cells, spinous processes	Hemolytic anemias, liver disease ("spur cell" anemia), uremia, microangiopathic hemolytic anemia, disseminated intravascular coagulation
Acanthocytes	Small cells with thorny projections	Abetalipoproteinemia (hereditary acanthocytosis or Bassen-Kornzweig disease), after splenectomy

(continued)

Peripheral Blood Red Cell Abnormalities   *(Continued)*

Abnormality	Description	Associated Diseases
Teardrop cells	Cells shaped like teardrops	Myeloproliferative syndrome, myelophthisic anemia (neoplastic, granulomatous, or fibrotic marrow infiltration), thalassemia
Nucleated red cells	Erythrocytes with nuclei still present, normoblastic or megaloblastic	Hemolytic anemias, leukemias, myeloproliferative syndrome, polycythemia vera, myelophthisic anemia (neoplastic, granulomatous, or fibrotic marrow infiltration), multiple myeloma, extramedullary hematopoiesis, megaloblastic anemias, any severe anemia
Howell-Jolly bodies	Spherical purple bodies (Wright stain) within or on erythrocytes, nuclear debris	Hyposplenism, pernicious anemia, thalassemia
Heinz inclusion bodies	Small round inclusions of denatured hemoglobin seen under phase microscopy or with supravital staining	Congenital hemolytic anemias (eg, glucose-6-phosphate dehydrogenase deficiency), hemolytic anemia secondary to drugs (dapsone, phenacetin), thalassemia (Hb H), hemoglobinopathies (Hb Zurich, Koln, Ube, I, and so on)
Pappenheimer bodies (siderocytes)	Siderotic granules, staining blue with Wright or Prussian blue stain	Iron-loading anemias, hyposplenism
Cabot's rings	Purple, fine, ring-like, intraerythrocytic structure	Pernicious anemia, lead poisoning
Basophilic stippling	Punctate stippling when Wright-stained	Hemolytic anemia, punctate stippling seen in lead poisoning (mitochondrial RNA and iron), thalassemia

(continued)

Peripheral Blood Red Cell Abnormalities *(Continued)*		
Abnormality	*Description*	*Associated Diseases*
Rouleaux	Aggregated erythrocytes regularly stacked on one another	Multiple myeloma, Waldenström's macroglobulinemia, cord blood, pregnancy, hypergammaglobulinemia, hyperfibrinogenemia
Polychromatophilia	RBCs containing RNA, staining a pinkish-blue color; stains supravitally as reticular network with new methylene blue	Hemolytic anemia, blood loss, uremia, after treatment of iron-deficiency or megaloblastic anemia

RETICULOCYTE COUNT ●

Normal Values

Men:	0.5%–1.5% of total erythrocytes
Women:	0.5%–2.5% of total erythrocytes
Children:	0.4%–4% of total erythrocytes
Infants:	2%–5% of total erythrocytes
Absolute count:	25–85 × 10^3/mm^3 or × 10^9 cells/L
Reticulocyte index (RI):	1% increase in RBC production above normal in anemia or corrected reticulocyte count (CRC) or hematocrit correction

Background

A *reticulocyte*—a young, immature, nonnucleated RBC—contains reticular material (RNA) that stains a gray-blue. Reticulum is present in newly released blood cells for 1 to 2 days before the cell reaches its full mature state. Normally a small number of these cells are found in circulating blood. For the reticulocyte count to be meaningful, it must be viewed in relation to the total number of erythrocytes (absolute reticulocyte count = % reticulocytes × erythrocyte count).

Explanation of Test

The reticulocyte count is used to differentiate anemias caused by bone marrow failure from those caused by hemorrhage or hemolysis (destruction of RBCs), to check the effectiveness of treatment in pernicious anemia, to assess the recovery of bone marrow function in aplastic anemia, and to determine the effects of radioactive substances on exposed workers.

Procedure

1. Obtain an EDTA-anticoagulated venous blood sample. Place the specimen in a biohazard bag.

2. The blood sample is mixed with a supravital stain such as brilliant cresyl blue. After the stain is allowed to react with the blood, a smear is prepared with this mixture and scanned under a microscope. The reticulocytes are counted and calculated.
3. Calculation: RI or CRC = Reticulocytes (%) $\times \dfrac{\text{HCT (L/L)}}{0.45 \text{ L/L}}$

Clinical Implications

1. *Increased reticulocyte count* (reticulocytosis) means that increased RBC production is occurring as the bone marrow replaces cells lost or prematurely destroyed. Identification of reticulocytosis may lead to the recognition of an otherwise occult disease, such as hidden chronic hemorrhage or unrecognized hemolysis (eg, sickle cell anemia, thalassemia). Increased levels are observed in the following:
   A. Hemolytic anemia
      (1) Immune hemolytic anemia
      (2) Primary RBC membrane problems
      (3) Hemoglobinopathic and sickle cell disease
      (4) RBC enzyme deficits
      (5) Malaria
   B. After hemorrhage (3 to 4 days)
   C. After treatment of anemias
      (1) An increased reticulocyte count may be used as an index of the effectiveness of treatment.
      (2) After adequate doses of iron in iron-deficiency anemia, the rise in reticulocytes may exceed 20%.
      (3) There is a proportional increase when pernicious anemia is treated by transfusion or vitamin B_{12} therapy.
2. *Decreased reticulocyte count* means that bone marrow is not producing enough erythrocytes; this occurs in
   A. Untreated iron-deficiency anemia
   B. Aplastic anemia (a persistent deficiency of reticulocytes suggests a poor prognosis)
   C. Untreated pernicious anemia
   D. Anemia of chronic disease
   E. Radiation therapy
   F. Endocrine problems
   G. Tumor in marrow (bone marrow failure)
   H. Myelodysplastic syndromes
   I. Alcoholism

Interfering Factors

1. Reticulocytes are normally increased in infants and during pregnancy.
2. Recently transfused patients have a lower count because of the dilutional effect.
3. The presence of Howell-Jolly bodies falsely elevates the reticulocyte count when automated methods are used.

Patient Preparation

1. Explain test purpose and procedure. *Pretest* and *posttest* care are the same as for the hemogram (page 44). Also, see Chapter 1 guidelines for safe, effective, informed *pretest* care.
2. Note medications. Some drugs cause aplastic anemia.

Patient Aftercare

1. Interpret test outcome and monitor appropriately for anemias.
2. Follow Chapter 1 guidelines for safe, effective, informed *posttest* care.

SEDIMENTATION RATE (SED RATE); ERYTHROCYTE SEDIMENTATION RATE (ESR) ●

Normal Values by Westergren's Method
Men: 0–15 mm/h
Women: 0–20 mm/h
Children: 0–10 mm/h

Background
Sedimentation occurs when the erythrocytes clump or aggregate together in a column-like manner (rouleau formation). These changes are related to alterations in the plasma proteins.

Explanation of Test
The ESR is the rate at which erythrocytes settle out of anticoagulated blood in 1 hour. This test is based on the fact that inflammatory and necrotic processes cause an alteration in blood proteins, resulting in aggregation of RBCs, which makes them heavier and more likely to fall rapidly when placed in a special vertical test tube. The faster the settling of cells, the higher the ESR. The ESR should not be used to screen asymptomatic patients for disease. It is most useful for diagnosis of temporal arteritis, rheumatoid arthritis, and polymyalgia rheumatica. The sedimentation rate is not diagnostic of any particular disease but rather is an indication that a disease process is ongoing and must be investigated. It is also quite useful in monitoring the progression of inflammatory diseases; if the patient is being treated with steroids, the ESR will decrease with clinical improvement.

Procedure
1. Obtain an EDTA-anticoagulated venous sample of 5 ml. Place the specimen in a biohazard bag.
2. The specimen is suctioned into a graduated sedimentation tube and allowed to settle for exactly 1 hour. The amount of settling is the patient's ESR.

Clinical Implications
1. *Increased* ESR is found in
   A. All collagen diseases, SLE
   B. Infections, pneumonia, syphilis
   C. Inflammatory diseases
   D. Carcinoma, lymphoma, neoplasms

    E. Acute heavy metal poisoning

    F. Cell or tissue destruction

    G. Toxemia

    H. Waldenström's macroglobulinemia

    I. Nephritis, nephrosis

    J. Subacute bacterial endocarditis

    K. Anemia

    L. Rheumatoid arthritis, gout, arthritis

2. *Normal* ESR (no increase) is found in

    A. Polycythemia vera, erythrocytosis

    B. Sickle cell anemia, hemoglobin C disease

    C. Congestive heart failure

    D. Hypofibrinogenemia (from any cause)

    E. Pyruvate kinase deficiency

    F. Hereditary spherocytosis

3. *Normal or varied* ESR is found in

    A. Acute disease: The change in ESR may lag behind the temperature elevation and leukocytosis for 6 to 24 hours, reaching a peak after several days.

    B. Convalescence: The increased ESR tends to persist longer than the fever or the leukocytosis.

    C. Unruptured acute appendicitis (early): Even when appendicitis is suppurative or gangrenous, the ESR is normal, but if abscess or peritonitis develops, the rate increases rapidly.

    D. Musculoskeletal conditions:

        (1) In rheumatic, gonorrheal, and acute gouty arthritis, the ESR is significantly increased.

        (2) In osteoarthritis, the ESR is slightly increased.

        (3) In neuritis, myositis, and lumbago, the ESR is within the normal range.

    E. Cardiovascular conditions:

        (1) In myocardial infarction, the ESR is increased.

        (2) In angina pectoris, the ESR is not increased.

    F. Malignant diseases:

        (1) In multiple myeloma, lymphoma, and metastatic cancer, the ESR is very high.

        (2) However, there is little correlation between the degree of elevation of the ESR and the prognosis in any one case.

    G. Uncomplicated viral disease and infectious mononucleosis

    H. Active renal failure with heart failure

    I. Acute allergy

    J. Peptic ulcer

Clinical Alert

Extreme elevation of the ESR is found with malignant lymphocarcinoma of colon or breast, myeloma, and rheumatoid arthritis.

Interfering Factors

1. Allowing the blood sample to stand >24 hours before the test is started causes the ESR to decrease.
2. In refrigerated blood, the ESR is increased. Refrigerated blood should be allowed to return to room temperature before the test is performed.
3. Factors leading to an increased ESR include
   A. The presence of fibrinogen, globulins, C-reactive protein
   B. Pregnancy after 12 weeks until about the fourth postpartum week
   C. Young children
   D. Menstruation
   E. Certain drugs (eg, heparin, oral contraceptives) (see Appendix J)
   F. Anemia (low Hct)
4. The ESR may be very high (up to 60 mm/h) in apparently healthy women age 70 to 89 years.
5. Factors leading to reduced ESR include
   A. High blood sugar, high albumin level, high phospholipids
   B. Decreased fibrinogen level in the blood in newborns
   C. Certain drugs (eg, steroids, high-dose aspirin) (see Appendix J)
   D. High Hb and RBC count.

Patient Preparation

1. Explain test purpose and procedure. Obtain appropriate medication history. Fasting is not necessary, but a fatty meal can cause plasma alterations.
2. See Chapter 1 guidelines for safe, effective, informed *pretest* care.

Patient Aftercare

1. Resume normal activities and diet.
2. Interpret test outcome, counsel and monitor appropriately for rheumatic disorders and inflammatory conditions.
3. See Chapter 1 guidelines for safe, effective, informed *posttest* care.

●TESTS FOR PORPHYRIA

Tests of blood, urine, and stool are done to diagnose porphyria, an abnormal accumulation of porphyrins in body fluids. *Porphyrias* are a group of diseases caused by a deficit in the enzymes involved in porphyrin metabolism and abnormalities in the production of the metalloporphyrin heme. These tests are indicated in persons who have unexplained neurologic manifestations, unexplained abdominal pain, cutaneous blisters, and/or the presence of a relevant family history. Test results may identify clinical conditions associated with abnormal heme production, including anemia and porphyria (abnormal accumulation of the porphyrins) associated with enzyme disorders that may be genetic (hereditary) or acquired (eg, lead poisoning, alcohol). Accumulation of porphyrins occurs in blood plasma, serum, erythrocytes, urine, and feces. A discussion of erythrocyte totals and fractionation of erythrocytes and plasma follows. For details of urine, serum, and stool testing for porphyrias, see Chapters 3, 6, and 5, respectively.

ERYTHROPOIETIC PORPHYRINS; FREE ERYTHROCYTE PROTOPORPHYRIN (FEP) ●

Normal Values
<100 μg/dl of packed RBCs

Background
Normally there is a small amount of excess porphyrin at the completion of heme synthesis. This excess is cell-free erythrocyte protoporphyrin (FEP). The amount of FEP in the erythrocyte is elevated when the iron supply is diminished.

Explanation of Test
This test is useful in diagnosing RBC disorders such as iron deficiency and erythropoietic protoporphyria. It is also used to support the diagnosis of lead poisoning, especially in children 6 months to 5 years of age.

Procedure
1. Obtain a 5-ml sample of anticoagulated venous blood. EDTA, heparin, or another anticoagulant may be used. Place the specimen in a biohazard bag.
2. Protect the blood sample from light.
3. The cells are washed and then tested for porphyrins.
4. The Hct must be known for test interpretation.

Clinical Implications
1. *Increased* FEP is associated with
   A. Iron-deficiency anemias (elevated before anemia)
   B. Lead poisoning (chronic)
   C. Halogenated solvents and many drugs (see Appendix J)
   D. Anemia of chronic disease
   E. Acquired idiopathic sideroblastic anemia (some cases)
   F. Erythropoietic prophyria
2. FEP is *normal* in
   A. Thalassemia minor (and therefore can be used to differentiate this from iron deficiency and other disorders of globin synthesis)
   B. Pyridoxine-responsive anemia
   C. Certain forms of sideroblastic anemia

Patient Preparation

1. Explain test purpose and sampling procedure.
2. Note on laboratory slip or computer any medications the patient is taking that cause intermittent porphyria. Discontinue such medications before testing (after checking with physician).
3. See Chapter 1 guidelines for safe, effective, informed *pretest* care.

Patient Aftercare

1. Resume normal activities and diet.
2. Interpret test outcome and monitor appropriately for porphyria or lead poisoning. See page 92 for explanation of porphyrins.
3. See Chapter 1 guidelines for safe, effective, informed *pretest* care.

Clinical Alert

The critical value is FEP >300 μg/dl.

PORPHYRINS; FRACTIONATION OF ERYTHROCYTES AND OF PLASMA

Normal Values

The value is reported in micrograms per deciliter (μg/dl). Check with your laboratory for reference values.

Background

The primary porphyrins of erythrocytes (RBCs) are protoporphyrin, uroporphyrin, and coproporphyrin.

Explanation of Test

Fractionation of erythrocytes is used to differentiate congenital erythropoietic coproporphyria from erythropoietic protoporphyria and to confirm a diagnosis of protoporphyria. This test establishes a specific type of porphyria by naming the specific porphyrin in *plasma*. In persons with renal failure, plasma fractionation can help to determine whether the porphyria is caused by a deficiency of uroporphyrinogenic decarboxylase or by failure of the renal system to excrete porphyrinogens.

Procedure

1. A 5-ml sample of anticoagulated blood is drawn. EDTA or heparin can be used as an anticoagulant. Place the specimen in a biohazard bag.
2. Protect the specimen from light.

Clinical Implications

1. *Increased erythrocyte porphyrins* are associated with primary porphyrias:
   A. Congenital erythropoietic protoporphyria

B. Protoporphyria (autosomal dominant deficiency of heme synthetase)
C. Hereditary porphobilinogen synthase deficiency
2. *Increased plasma porphyrins* are associated with
A. Congenital erythropoietic protoporphyria
B. Coproporphyria
C. Porphyria cutanea tarda

Patient Preparation
1. Advise patient of test purpose.
2. Note on the requisition any drugs the patient is taking.
3. Before testing, drugs that are known to cause intermittent porphyria should be discontinued (after checking with physician).
4. See Chapter 1 guidelines for safe, effective, informed *pretest* care.

Patient Aftercare
1. Resume medications.
2. Interpret test outcome and monitor appropriately for porphyria or lead poisoning.
3. Caution persons diagnosed with porphyria (with cutaneous manifestations) to avoid sun exposure.
4. Advise persons diagnosed with porphyria (with neurologic symptoms) that attacks can be precipitated by infections, various phases of the menstrual cycle, fasting states, and certain drugs. A listing of drugs (not all inclusive) that may precipitate acute attacks follows:
   Barbiturates
   Chlordiazepoxide
   Chloroquine
   Chlorpropamide
   Dichloralphenazone
   Ergot preparations
   Estrogens
   Ethanol
   Glutethimide
   Griseofulvin
   Hydantoins
   Imipramine
   Meprobamate
   Methsuximide
   Methyldopa
   Sulfonamides
5. Follow Chapter 1 guidelines for safe, effective, informed *posttest* care.

> ### Clinical Alert
>
> 1. A blood test for uroporphyrinogen I synthase can be done to iden-
>   tify persons at risk for acute intermittent porphyria, to detect latent-
>   phase intermittent porphyria, and to confirm the diagnosis during an
>   acute episode.
> 2. The normal value is 8–16.8 nmol/L (or 1.27–200 ml per gram of he-
>   moglobin) in women; 7–14.7 nmol/L in men. A value of <6 nmol/L
>   is diagnostic of acute intermittent porphyria.

●ADDITIONAL TESTS FOR HEMOLYTIC ANEMIA

Several RBC enzyme and fragility tests can be done to screen, detect, and confirm the cause of chronic hemolytic anemia. Many persons with hemolytic anemia have no clinical signs or symptoms. Abnormal test outcomes are associated with inherited deficiencies, abnormal hemoglobins, and exposure to
chemicals and drugs. Definitive test results indicate some type of injury to the
RBC, oxidated activity that interferes with normal hemoglobin function, and/or
increased RBC fragility.

PYRUVATE KINASE (PK) ●

Normal Values:
1.5–2.5 U/ml of packed RBCs or 1.1–8.8 U/g Hb

Background
PK deficiency is a genetic disorder characterized by a lowered concentration
of adenosine triphosphate in the RBC and consequential membrane defect.
The result is a nonspherocytic, chronic hemolytic anemia. PK deficiency is the
most common and most important form of hemolytic anemia resulting from a
deficiency of glycolytic enzymes in the RBC.

Procedure
1. Obtain a venous blood sample of at least 5 ml with EDTA or heparin anticoagulant; refrigerate immediately.

Clinical Implications
PK is *increased* in
1. Congenital PK deficiency: recessive, nonspherocytic hemolytic anemia. Patients tolerate anemia well because of increased 2,3-diphosphoglycerate
   (2,3-DPG).
2. Acquired PK deficiency caused by
   A. Myelodysplastic disorders
   B. Leukemias

Patient Preparation

1. Explain test purpose and procedure. There should be no exercising before tests.
2. Withhold transfusion until after blood samples are drawn (especially with osmotic fragility).
3. See Chapter 1 guidelines for safe, effective, informed *pretest* care.

Patient Aftercare

1. Interpret test results and monitor appropriately for hemolytic anemia, hypoxia, or polycythemia.
2. Splenectomy is indicated when anemia is severe enough to require transfusions.
3. Follow Chapter 1 guidelines for safe, effective, informed *posttest* care.

> ### Clinical Alert
>
> Many prescribed drugs interfere with the normal functioning of hemoglobin in susceptible persons, especially sulfonamides, antipyretics, analgesics, large doses of vitamin K, and nitrofurans.

ERYTHROCYTE FRAGILITY (OSMOTIC FRAGILITY AND AUTOHEMOLYSIS)

Normal Values

Immediate Test
Hemolysis begins at 0.50 NaCl; complete at 0.30 NaCl

24-Hour Incubation
Hemolysis begins at 0.70 NaCl; complete at 0.40–0.15 NaCl

Background

Spherocytes of any origin (including conditions other than hereditary spherocytosis) are more susceptible than normal RBCs to hemolysis in dilute (hypotonic) saline and show increased osmotic fragility. Generally, fully expanded cells (spheroidal cells or spherocytes) have increased osmotic fragility, whereas cells with higher surface area-to-volume ratios (eg, thin cells, hypochromic cells, tart cells) have decreased osmotic fragility.

Procedure

1. Obtain a 7-ml venous blood sample using heparin as anticoagulant. Place the specimen in a biohazard bag.
2. Erythrocytes are exposed to varying dilutions of sodium chloride. Hemolysis is read on a spectrophotometer (optical density measurement). Studies are performed and measured both before and after 24-hour incubation of the RBCs.

Clinical Implications

1. *Increased* osmotic fragility is found in
   A. Hemolytic anemia (acquired immune)
   B. Hereditary spherocytosis (stomatocytosis)
   C. Hemolytic disease of the newborn
   D. Malaria
   E. Severe pyruvate kinase deficiency
2. *Decreased* osmotic fragility occurs in
   A. Iron deficiency anemia (macrocytic hypochromic)
   B. Thalassemias
   C. Asplenia (postsplenectomy)
   D. Liver disease
   E. Reticulocytosis
   F. Hemoglobinopathies, especially Hb C, Hb S

Patient Preparation

1. Explain test purpose and procedure. There should be no exercising before tests.
2. Withhold transfusion until after blood samples are drawn (especially with osmotic fragility).
3. See Chapter 1 guidelines for safe, effective, informed *pretest* care.

Patient Aftercare

1. Follow Chapter 1 guidelines for safe, effective, informed *posttest* care.

GLUCOSE-6-PHOSPHATE DEHYDROGENASE (G6PD) ●

Normal Values

Adults: 2.4–5.1 U/ml of RBCs
Infants: 1.5–2.2 U/ml of RBCs
If done as a screening test, G6PD activity is reported as within normal limits.

Background

G6PD is a sex-linked disorder. The major variants occur in specific ethnic groups. In a large group of African American men the incidence of type A G6PD deficiency was found to be 11%. Approximately 20% of African American women are heterozygous. With some variants there is chronic lifelong hemolysis, but more commonly the condition is asymptomatic and results only in susceptibility to acute hemolytic episodes, which may be triggered by certain drugs, ingestion of fava beans, or viral or bacterial infection. G6PD hemolysis is associated with formation of Heinz bodies in peripheral RBCs.

The other two most common types are Mediterranean, which is common in Iraqis, Kurds, Sephardic Jews, and Lebanese and less common in Greeks, Italians, Turks, and North Africans, and the MAHIDOL variant, which is common in Southeast Asians.

Procedure

1. Obtain a blood sample of at least 5 ml, using EDTA anticoagulant. Place the specimen in a biohazard bag.

Clinical Implications

1. G6PD is *decreased* in
   A. G6PD deficiency (causes hemolytic episodes after exposure to certain drugs and fava beans)
   B. Congenital nonspherocytic anemia
   C. Nonimmunologic hemolytic disease of the newborn
2. G6PD is *increased* in
   A. Untreated megaloblastic anemia (pernicious anemia)
   B. Thrombocytopenia purpura
   C. Hyperthyroidism
   D. Viral hepatitis
   E. Myocardial infarction

Interfering Factors

1. Marked reticulocytosis may give a falsely high G6PD.
2. G6PD may be falsely normal for 6 to 8 weeks after a hemolytic episode, especially in black persons with the type A variant.

> **Clinical Alert**
>
> In G6PD-Mediterranean, G6PD levels are grossly deficient in all RBCs. Patients with this variant commonly experience hemolysis induced by diabetic acidosis, infections, and oxidant drugs and potentially fatal hemolytic crises after ingestion of fava beans.

Patient Preparation

1. Explain test purpose and procedure. There should be no exercising before tests.
2. Withhold transfusion until after blood samples are drawn (especially with osmotic fragility).
3. See Chapter 1 guidelines for safe, effective, informed *pretest* care.

Patient Aftercare

1. Follow Chapter 1 guidelines for safe, effective, informed *posttest* care.

HEINZ BODIES; HEINZ STAIN; GLUTATHIONE INSTABILITY ●

Normal Values

<30% Heinz bodies present

Background

Heinz bodies are insoluble intracellular inclusions of hemoglobin attached to the RBC membrane. Heinz bodies are uncommon except with G6PD deficiency immediately after hemolysis and in patients with unstable Hb variants.

Oxidative denaturation of the Hb molecule leads to Heinz body formation and is probably the mechanism for the precipitation of unstable Hb. Heinz bodies are usually removed by the spleen; after splenectomy they increase in the peripheral blood and may appear in >50% of RBCs.

Procedure

1. Obtain a venous blood sample, anticoagulated with heparin. Place the specimen in a biohazard bag.
2. Cells are mixed with a supravital stain and examined microscopically.

Clinical Implications

1. *Increased* Heinz bodies are found in
   A. G6PD deficiency, especially after hemolysis
   B. Congenital Heinz body hemolytic anemia
   C. Unstable Hb variants (eg, Hb Zurich, Hb Philly)
   D. Glutathione deficiency
2. Heinz bodies are found in blood of normal persons who have been poisoned by certain drugs used in treatment protocols (eg, chlorates, phenylhydrazine, primaquine).

Interfering Factors

1. See Appendix J for drugs that affect test outcomes.

2,3-DIPHOSPHOGLYCERATE (2,3-DPG) ●

Normal Values

Males: 4.5–5.1 μmol/ml of packed RBCs or 10.4–14.2 μmol/g Hb
Females: 4.9–5.7 μmol/ml of packed RBCs or 10.4–14.2 μmol/g Hb

Procedure

1. Obtain a venous blood sample of at least 3 ml, anticoagulated with heparin. Place on ice immediately (2.3-DPG is stable for only 2 hours) and transport to laboratory as soon as possible in a biohazard bag.

Clinical Implications

1. *Increased* 2,3-DPG occurs in
   A. Emphysema, cystic fibrosis with pulmonary involvement
   B. Acute leukemia
   C. Pulmonary vascular disease
   D. Sickle cell anemia, iron-deficiency anemia
   E. Pyruvate kinase deficiency
   F. Hyperthyroidism

2. *Decreased* 2,3-DPG
   A. Polycythemia vera
   B. Respiratory distress syndrome
   C. 2,3-DPG deficiency
   D. Hexokinase deficiency

Interfering Factors
1. High altitude *increases* 2,3-DPG.
2. Exercise *increases* 2,3-DPG.

> **Clinical Alert**
>
> If blood with decreased 2,3-DPG is used for transfusion, the Hb may not release O_2 when needed.

Patient Preparation for Tests for Hemolytic Anemia
1. Explain test purpose and procedure. There should be no exercising before tests.
2. Withhold transfusion until after blood samples are drawn (especially with osmotic fragility).
3. See Chapter 1 guidelines for safe, effective, informed *pretest* care.

Patient Aftercare for Tests for Hemolytic Anemia
1. Interpret test results and monitor appropriately for hemolytic anemia, hypoxia, or polycythemia.
2. Follow Chapter 1 guidelines for safe, effective, informed *posttest* care.

● IRON TESTS

IRON, TOTAL IRON-BINDING CAPACITY (TIBC), AND TRANSFERRIN TESTS ●

Normal Values

Iron
Adult Men: 75–175 μg/dl
Adult Women: 65–165 μg/dl
Newborns: 100–250 μg/dl
Children: 50–120 μg/dl

Total Iron-Binding Capacity (TIBC)
240–450 μg/dl

Transferrin
Adults: 250–425 mg/dl

Newborns: 130–275 mg/dl
Children: 203–360 mg/dl

Transferrin (Iron) Saturation
Men: 10%–50%
Women: 15%–50%

Background

Iron is necessary for the production of hemoglobin. Iron is contained in several components. Transferrin (also called *siderophilin*), a transport protein largely synthesized by the liver, regulates iron absorption. High levels of transferrin relate to the ability of the body to deal with infections. Total iron binding capacity (TIBC) correlates with serum transferrin, but the relation is not linear. A serum iron test without a TIBC and transferrin determination has very limited value except in cases of iron poisoning. Transferrin saturation is a better index of iron saturation; it is evaluated as follows:

$$\text{Transferrin saturation (\%)} = \frac{\text{Serum iron} \times 100}{\text{TIBC}}$$

Explanation of Test

The combined results of transferrin, iron, and TIBC tests are helpful in the differential diagnosis of anemia, in assessment of iron-deficiency anemia, and in the evaluation of thalassemia, sideroblastic anemia, and hemochromatosis.

Procedure

1. Obtain a venous blood sample of 10 ml. Place the specimen in a biohazard bag.

Clinical Implications

1. *Increased transferrin* is observed in
   A. Iron-deficiency anemia
   B. Pregnancy
   C. Estrogen therapy
2. *Decreased transferrin* is found in
   A. Microcytic anemia of chronic disease
   B. Protein deficiency or loss from burns or malnutrition
   C. Chronic infection
   D. Acquired liver disease
   E. Renal disease (nephrosis)
   F. Genetic deficiency, hereditary atransferrinemia
   G. Iron-overload states
3. *Decreased iron* occurs in
   A. Iron-deficiency anemia
   B. Chronic blood loss

    C. Chronic diseases (eg, lupus, rheumatoid arthritis, chronic infections)

    D. Third-trimester pregnancy

    E. Remission of pernicious anemia

    F. Inadequate absorption of iron

    G. Hemolytic anemia (PNH)

4. *Increased iron* occurs in

    A. Hemolytic anemias, especially thalassemia and pernicious anemia in relapse

    B. Acute iron poisoning (children)

    C. Iron-overload syndromes

    D. Hemochromatosis

    E. Transfusions (multiple), intramuscular iron

    F. Acute hepatitis, liver damage

    G. Inappropriate iron therapy

    H. Lead poisoning

    I. Acute leukemia

    J. Nephritis

5. *Increased TIBC* is found in

    A. Iron deficiency

    B. Pregnancy (late)

    C. Acute and chronic blood loss

    D. Acute hepatitis

6. *Decreased TIBC* is observed in

    A. Hypoproteinemia (malnutrition and burns)

    B. Hemochromatosis

    C. Non-iron anemia (infection and chronic disease)

    D. Cirrhosis of liver

    E. Nephroses and other renal diseases

    F. Thalassemia

7. The iron saturation index is *increased* in

    A. Hemochromatosis

    B. Increased iron intake

    C. Thalassemia

    D. Hemosiderosis

8. The iron saturation index is *decreased* in

    A. Iron-deficiency anemias

    B. Malignancy (standard and small intestine)

    C. Anemia of infection and chronic disease

    D. Iron neoplasms

Interfering Factors

1. Many drugs affect test outcomes (see Appendix J).

2. Drugs that may cause increased iron include ethanol, estrogens, and oral contraceptives.

3. Drugs that may cause decreased iron include some antibiotics, aspirin, and testosterone.
4. Hemolysis of the blood sample interferes with testing.
5. Iron contamination of glassware used in testing can give high values.
6. Menstruation causes decreased iron; iron is elevated in the premenstrual period.
7. There is a diurnal variation in iron: normal values in the morning, lower in midafternoon, very low in the evening.

Patient Preparation
1. Explain test purpose and procedure.
2. Draw fasting blood in the morning, when levels are higher.
3. Draw iron sample before iron therapy is initiated or blood is transfused.
4. If the patient has received a transfusion, delay iron testing for 4 days.
5. Any iron-chelating drug (eg, Desferal) must be avoided.
6. Avoid sleep deprivation or extreme stress, which cause lower iron levels.
7. Note on laboratory slip or computer screen whether the patient is taking oral contraceptives or estrogen therapy or is pregnant.
8. See Chapter 1 guidelines for safe, effective, informed *pretest* care.

Patient Aftercare
1. Resume normal activities.
2. Interpret test outcome and monitor appropriately. The combination of low serum iron, high TIBC, and high transferrin levels indicates iron deficiency. Diagnosis of iron deficiency may lead further to detection of adenocarcinoma of the gastrointestinal tract, a point that cannot be overemphasized. A significant minority of patients with megaloblastic anemias (20%–40%) have coexisting iron deficiency. Megaloblastic anemia can interfere with the interpretation of iron studies; repeat iron studies 1 to 3 months after folate or B_{12} replacement.
3. Use Chapter 1 guidelines for safe, effective, informed *posttest* care.

▶ Clinical Alert
1. Critical iron values: intoxicated child, 280–2550 µg/dl; fatally poisoned child, >1800 µg/dl.
2. Symptoms of iron poisoning include abdominal pain, vomiting, bloody diarrhea, cyanosis, and convulsions.

FERRITIN

Normal Values
Men: 18–270 ng/ml or μg/L
Women: 18–160 ng/ml or μg/L
Children: 7–140 ng/ml or μg/L
Newborns: 25–200 ng/ml or μg/L
1 month: 50–200 ng/ml or μg/L
2–5 months: 50–200 ng/ml or μg/L

Background
Ferritin, a complex of ferric (Fe^{2+}) hydroxide and a protein, apoferritin, originates in the reticuloendothelial system. Ferritin reflects the body iron stores and is the most reliable indicator of total body iron status. A bone marrow examination is the only better test. Bone marrow aspiration may be necessary in some cases, such as low-normal ferritin and low serum iron in the anemia of chronic disease.

Explanation of Test
The ferritin test is more specific and more sensitive than iron concentration or TIBC for diagnosing iron deficiency. Ferritin decreases before anemia and other changes occur.

Procedure
1. Obtain a venous sample of 6 ml. Place the specimen in a biohazard bag.

Ferritin, Iron, and Iron Saturation Changes in Anemias*			
Anemia	*Ferritin*	*Iron*	*Iron Saturation*
Hemorrhage, acute	N	D	D
Hemorrhage, chronic	D	D	D
Iron-deficiency	D	D	D
Aplastic	D	I	I
Megaloblastic	I	D	D
Hemolytic	I	I	I
Sideroblastic	I	I	I
Thalassemia, major	I	I	I
Thalassemia, minor	I	N/I	N/I
Bone marrow neoplasia	N/I	I	I
Uremia, nephrosis, or nephrotic syndrome	N/I	D/I	D
Liver disease	N/I	N/I	N/I
Chronic disorders	I	D	D

*N, no change; D, decrease; I, increase.

Clinical Implications

1. *Decreased ferritin* (<10 ng/ml) usually indicates iron-deficiency anemia.
2. *Increased ferritin* (>400 ng/ml) occurs in iron excess and in the following:
   A. Iron overload from hemochromatosis or hemosiderosis
   B. Oral or parenteral iron administration
   C. Inflammatory diseases
   D. Acute or chronic liver disease involving alcoholism
   E. Acute myoblastic or lymphoblastic leukemia
   F. Other malignancies (Hodgkin's disease, breast carcinoma, malignant lymphoma)
   G. Hyperthyroidism
   H. Hemolytic anemia, megaloblastic anemia
   I. Thalassemia (normal or sometimes higher)

Interfering Factors

1. Recently administered radioactive medications cause spurious results.
2. Oral contraceptives and antithyroid therapy interfere with testing (see Appendix J).
3. Hemolyzed blood may cause high results.

Patient Preparation

1. Explain test purpose and procedure. Fasting is not necessary.
2. Radioactive medications may not be given for 3 to 4 days before testing.
3. Refrain from alcohol (higher levels of ferritin occur in alcoholism).
4. See Chapter 1 guidelines for safe, effective, informed *pretest* care.

Patient Aftercare

1. Resume normal activities.
2. Interpret test results and monitor appropriately for iron-deficiency anemia and/or ferritin increases. When iron and TIBC tests are used together with ferritin, they can better distinguish between iron-deficiency anemia and the anemia of chronic disease.
3. See Chapter 1 guidelines for safe, effective, informed *posttest* care.

IRON STAIN (STAINABLE IRON IN BONE MARROW; PRUSSIAN BLUE STAIN) ●

Normal Values

Bone marrow: 33% sideroblasts present
Peripheral blood: no siderocytes present

Background

In the bone marrow, normoblasts containing iron granules (stainable) are known as *sideroblasts*. Erythrocytes (RBCs that contain stainable iron) are called *siderocytes*. Normally, about 33% of the normoblasts are sideroblasts. Other storage iron is readily identifiable in monophages in bone marrow particles on the marrow slides.

Explanation of Test

The bone marrow iron stain is the most reliable index of iron deficiency: the presence of iron rules out iron deficiency. Marrow iron disappears before peripheral blood changes occur in iron-deficiency anemia.

Procedure

1. Bone marrow slides are made (or bone marrow biopsy material can be used), stained, and examined under the microscope for the presence of iron. This test may also be done on peripheral blood for the detection of sideroblastic anemias.

Clinical Implications

1. Bone marrow iron is *decreased* in
   A. Iron deficiency from all causes of chronic bleeding, hemorrhage, malignancy.
   B. Polycythemia vera
   C. Pernicious anemia
   D. Collagen diseases (eg, rheumatoid arthritis, SLE)
   E. Infiltration of marrow by malignant lymphomas, carcinoma
   F. Chronic infection
   G. Myeloproliferative diseases
2. Bone marrow iron is *increased* in
   A. Hemochromatosis (primary and secondary)
   B. Anemia—especially thalassemia major and minor, PNH, and other hemolytic anemias
   C. Myeloblastic anemia in relapse

Interfering Factors

Ingestion of iron dextran will bring values to normal despite other evidence of iron-deficiency anemia.

Patient Preparation

1. Preparation is the same as for bone marrow aspiration (see page 42).
2. See Chapter 1 guidelines for safe, effective, informed *pretest* care.

Patient Aftercare

1. Aftercare is the same as for bone marrow aspiration (see page 42).
2. See Chapter 1 guidelines for safe, effective, informed *posttest* care.

● TESTS FOR HEMOGLOBIN DISORDERS

HEMOGLOBIN ELECTROPHORESIS   ●

Normal Values

Hemoglobin A_1: 96.5%–98.5%
Hemoglobin A_2: 1.5%–3.5%
Hemoglobin F: 0%–1%

Background

Normal and abnormal Hbs can be detected by electrophoresis, which matches hemolyzed RBC material against standard bands for the various Hbs known. The most common forms of normal adult Hb are Hb A_1, Hb A_2, and Hb F (fetal hemoglobin). Of the various types of abnormal Hb (hemoglobinopathies), the best known are Hb S (responsible for sickle cell anemia) and Hb C (results in a mild hemolytic anemia). The most common abnormality is a significant increase in Hb A_2, which is diagnostic of the thalassemias, especially β-thalassemia trait. More than 350 variants of Hb have been recognized and identified.

◗ Clinical Alert

The results may be questionable if a blood transfusion has been given in the months preceding testing.

FETAL HEMOGLOBIN (HEMOGLOBIN F; ALKALI-RESISTANT HEMOGLOBIN)   ●

Normal Values

Adults: 0%–2%
Newborns: 60%–90%
By 6 months of age: 2%

Background

Fetal hemoglobin (Hb F) is a normal Hb manufactured in the RBCs of the fetus and infant; it makes up 50% to 90% of the Hb in the newborn. The remaining portion of the Hb in the newborn is made up of Hb A_1 and Hb A_2, the adult types.

Under normal conditions, the manufacture of Hb F is replaced by the manufacture of adult Hb types during the first year of life. But if Hb F persists and constitutes more than 5% of the Hb after 6 months of age, an abnormality should be expected.

Explanation of Test
Determination of Hb F is used to diagnose thalassemia, an inherited abnormality in the manufacture of hemoglobin.

Procedure
1. A 7-ml venous blood EDTA-anticoagulated sample is used for hemoglobin electrophoresis.
2. A blood smear stain may also be done to identify cells containing Hb F (Kleihauer-Betke stain).

Clinical Implications
1. *Increased Hb F* is found in
   A. Thalassemias (major and minor)
   B. Hereditary familial fetal hemoglobinemia (persistence of Hb F)
   C. Hyperthyroidism
   D. Sickle cell disease
   E. Hemoglobin H disease
   F. Anemia, as a compensatory mechanism (pernicious anemia, PNH, sideroblastic anemia)
   G. Leakage of fetal blood into the maternal bloodstream
   H. Aplastic anemia (acquired)
   I. Acute or chronic leukemia
   J. Myeloproliferative disorders, multiple myeloma, lymphoma
   K. Metastatic carcinoma to the bone marrow
   L. Juvenile myeloid leukemia with absence of Philadelphia chromosome

> ### Clinical Alert
>
> In *thalassemia minor,* continued production of Hb F may occur on a minor scale (5% to 10%), and the patient usually lives. In *thalassemia major,* the values may reach 40% to 90%. This continued production of Hb F leads to a severe anemia, and death usually ensues.

Interfering Factors
1. If analysis of the specimen is delayed for more than 2 to 3 hours, the level of Hb F may be falsely increased.
2. Infants small for gestational age or with chronic intrauterine anoxia have persistently elevated Hg F.
3. Hg F is increased during anticonvulsant drug therapy.

Patient Preparation

1. Explain test purpose and procedure.
2. The test should be done before transfusion.
3. See Chapter 1 guidelines for safe, effective, informed *pretest* care.

Patient Aftercare

1. Interpret test outcome, counsel and monitor appropriately for thalassemia and anemia.
2. Follow Chapter 1 guidelines for safe, effective, informed *posttest* care.

HEMOGLOBIN A₂ (Hb A₂) ●

Normal Values

Newborn: 0%–1.8%
Adult: 1.5%–3.0%

Background

Hb A_2 levels have special application to the diagnosis of β-thalassemia trait, which may be present even though the peripheral blood smear is normal. The microcytosis and other morphologic changes of β-thalassemia trait must be differentiated from iron deficiency. Low mean corpuscular volume (MCV) may include the majority of patients with β-thalassemia trait, but it does not differentiate iron-deficient patients.

Explanation of Test

This measurement is used in the investigation of hemolytic anemias for hemoglobinopathies, especially thalassemia and β-thalassemia.

Procedure

1. Draw a venous sample of blood with EDTA anticoagulant.
2. Electrophoresis is then performed.

Clinical Implications

1. *Increased* Hb A_2 occurs in
   A. β-Thalassemia major (3–11%)
   B. Thalassemia minor (3.5–7.5%)
   C. Thalassemia intermedia (6–8%)
   D. Hb A/S (sickle cell trait) (15–45%)
   E. Hb S/S (sickle cell disease) (2–6%)
   F. S-β-thalassemia (3.0–8.5%)
   G. Megaloblastic anemia

2. *Decreased* Hb A_2 occurs in
  A. Untreated iron-deficiency anemia
  B. Sideroblastic anemia
  C. Hb H disease
  D. Erythroleukemia

Patient Preparation
1. Explain test purpose and procedure.
2. Provide genetic counseling.
3. Follow Chapter 1 guidelines for safe, effective, informed *pretest* care.

Patient Aftercare
1. Interpret test outcome, counsel and monitor appropriately.
2. A positive diagnosis of sickle cell disorder has genetic implications, including the need for genetic counseling.
3. A person with sickle cell disease should avoid situations in which hypoxia may occur, such as very strenuous exercise, traveling to high-altitude regions, or traveling in an unpressurized aircraft.
4. Because of the hypoxia created by general anesthetics and a state of shock, surgical and maternity patients with sickle cell disease need very close observation.
5. See Chapter 1 guidelines for safe, effective, informed *posttest* care.

HEMOGLOBIN S (SICKLE CELL TEST; SICKLEDEX) ●

Normal Values
Adult: None present

Background
Sickle cell disease is a term for a group of hereditary blood disorders. Sickle cell anemia is caused by an abnormality of hemoglobin, the red protein in red blood cells that carries oxygen from the lungs to the tissues. People with sickle cell disease make an abnormal hemoglobin, *hemoglobin S* (Hb S). The red blood cells of a person with sickle cell disease don't last as long as "normal" red blood cells. This result is chronic anemia. Also, these red blood cells lose their normal disc shape. They become rigid and deformed and take on a "sickle" or crescent shape. These odd shaped cells are not flexible enough to squeeze through small blood vessels. This may result in blood vessels being blocked. The areas of the body served by those blood vessels will then be deprived of their blood circulation. This damages tissues and organs and causes pain.

Explanation of Test
This blood measurement is routinely done as a screening test for sickle cell anemia or trait and to confirm these disorders. This test detects hemoglobin S, an inherited, recessive gene. An examination is made of erythrocytes for the sickle-

shaped forms characteristic of sickle cell anemia or trait. This is done by removing oxygen from the erythrocyte. In erythrocytes with normal hemoglobin the shape is retained, but erythrocytes containing hemoglobin S will assume a sickle shape. However, the distinction between sickle cell trait and sickle cell disease is done by electrophoresis, which identifies a hemoglobin pattern.

Procedure

1. A venous blood sample of 5 ml with EDTA is obtained. Place the specimen in a biohazard bag.
2. The Sickledex test or hemoglobin electrophoresis is performed. Electrophoresis is more accurate and should be done in all positive Sickledex screens.

Clinical Implications

A *positive test* (Hb S present) means that great numbers of erythrocytes have assumed the typical sickle cell (crescent) shape. Positive tests are 99% accurate.

1. *Sickle cell trait*
   A. Definite confirmation of sickle cell trait by hemoglobin electrophoresis reveals the following heterozygous (A/S) pattern: Hb S, 20%–40%; Hb A_1, 60%–80%; Hb F, small amount. This means that the patient has inherited a normal Hb gene from one parent and an Hb S gene from the other (heterozygous pattern). This patient does not have any clinical manifestations of the disease, but some of the children of this patient may inherit the disease if the patient's mate also has the recessive gene pattern.
   B. The diagnosis of sickle cell trait does not affect longevity and is not accompanied by signs and symptoms of sickle cell anemia.
   C. Sickle cell trait can lead to renal papillary necrosis, hematuria, and an increased risk of pulmonary embolus.
2. *Sickle cell anemia*
   A. Definite confirmation of sickle cell anemia by hemoglobin electrophoresis reveals the following homozygous (S/S) pattern: Hb S, 80%–100%; Hb F, most of the rest, Hb A_1, 0% or small amount. This means that an abnormal Hb S gene has been inherited from both parents (homozygous pattern). Such a patient has all the clinical manifestations of the disease.
3. Hb C-Harlem (rare)
4. Hb S in combination with other disorders, such as thalassemia or Hb S-C.

Interfering Factors

1. False-negative results occur in
   A. Infants before the age of 3 months
   B. Coexisting thalassemias or iron deficiency
   C. The solubility test is unreliable in pernicious anemia and polycythemia.

2. False-positive results occur up to 4 months after transfusion with RBCs having sickle cell trait.

3. Hb D and Hb G migrate to same place as Hb F in electrophoresis.

> **Clinical Alert**
>
> A positive Sickledex test must be confirmed by electrophoresis.

Patient Preparation

1. Explain test purpose and procedure.

2. Provide genetic counseling.

3. Follow Chapter 1 guidelines for safe, effective, informed *pretest* care.

Patient Aftercare

1. Interpret test outcome, counsel and monitor appropriately.

2. A positive diagnosis of sickle cell disorder has genetic implications, including the need for genetic counseling.

3. A person with sickle cell disease should avoid situations in which hypoxia may occur, such as very strenuous exercise, traveling to high-altitude regions, or traveling in an unpressurized aircraft.

4. Because of the hypoxia created by general anesthetics and a state of shock, surgical and maternity patients with sickle cell disease need very close observation.

5. See Chapter 1 guidelines for safe, effective, informed *posttest* care.

METHEMOGLOBIN (HEMOGLOBIN M)

Normal Values

0.4%–1.5% of total hemoglobin

A value of >10% is a critical value.

Background

Methemoglobin is formed when the iron in the heme portion of deoxygenated Hb is oxidized to a ferric form rather than a ferrous form. In the ferric form, oxygen and iron cannot combine. The formation of methemoglobin is a normal process and is kept within bounds by the reduction of methemoglobin to Hb. Methemoglobin causes a shift to the left of the oxyhemoglobin dissociation curve. When a high concentration of methemoglobin is produced in the RBCs, it reduces their capacity to combine with oxygen; anoxia and cyanosis result.

Explanation of Test

This test is used to diagnose hereditary or acquired methemoglobinemia in patients with symptoms of anoxia or cyanosis and no evidence of cardiovascular or pulmonary disease. Hemoglobin M is an inherited disorder of the hemoglobin that produces cyanosis.

Procedure
1. A venous or arterial blood sample, anticoagulated with heparin, is obtained. Place on ice immediately and transport to laboratory in a biohazard bag.

Clinical Implications
1. *Hereditary methemoglobinemia* (uncommon) is associated with
   A. A hemoglobinopathy, Hb M (40% of the total Hb)
   B. Deficiency of methemoglobin reductase (autosomal recessive)
   C. Glutathione deficiency (dominant mode of transmission)
2. *Acquired methemoglobinemia* is associated with
   A. Black water fever
   B. Paroxysmal hemoglobinuria
   C. Clostridial infection
3. Toxic effect of drugs or chemicals (most common cause):
   A. Analgesics
   B. Sulfonamide derivatives
   C. Nitrates and nitrites; nitroglycerin
   D. Antimalarials
   E. Isoniazid
   F. Quinones
   G. Potassium chloride
   H. Benzocaine, lidocaine
   I. Dapsone (most common drug causing methemoglobinemia)

Interfering Factors
1. Consumption of sausage, processed meats, or other foods rich in nitrite and nitrate
2. Absorption of silver nitrate used to treat extensive burns
3. Excessive intake of Bromo-Seltzer is a common cause of methemoglobinemia. (The patient appears cyanotic but otherwise feels well.)
4. Smoking
5. Use of bismuth preparations for diarrhea (see Appendix J)

Patient Preparation
1. Advise patient of purpose of test. Assess for history of Bromo-Seltzer or toxic drugs or chemicals.
2. See Chapter 1 guidelines for safe, effective, informed *pretest* care.

Patient Aftercare
1. Interpret test outcome, counsel for cause of cyanosis and monitor appropriately for anoxia.
2. Treatment includes intravenous methylene blue and oral ascorbic acid.
3. Follow Chapter 1 guidelines for safe, effective, informed *posttest* care.

> **Clinical Alert**
>
> Because fetal hemoglobin is more easily converted to methemoglobin than to adult hemoglobin, infants are more susceptible than adults to methemoglobinemia, which may be caused by drinking well water containing nitrites. Bismuth preparations for diarrhea may also be reduced to nitrites by bowel action.

SULFHEMOGLOBIN

Normal Values
None present or 0–1.0% of total hemoglobin

Background
Sulfhemoglobin is an abnormal hemoglobin pigment produced by the combination of inorganic sulfides with hemoglobin. Sulfhemoglobinemia manifests as a cyanosis.

Explanation of Test
This test is indicated in persons with cyanosis. Sulfhemoglobinemia may occur in association with the administration of various drugs and toxins. The symptoms are few, but cyanosis is intense even though the concentration of sulfhemoglobin seldom exceeds 10%.

Procedure
1. Draw a 5-ml venous blood sample, anticoagulated with EDTA. Place the specimen in a biohazard bag.

Clinical Implications
1. Sulfhemoglobin is observed in patients who take oxidant drugs such as phenacetin, excessive intake of Bromo-Seltzer, sulfonamides, and acetanilid. See Appendix J.
2. Sulfhemoglobin is formed rarely without exposure to drugs or toxins, as in chronic constipation and purging.

Patient Preparation
1. Explain test purpose and procedure. Assess for exposure to drugs and toxins.
2. See Chapter 1 guidelines for safe, effective, informed *pretest* care.

Patient Aftercare
1. Interpret test outcome, counsel for cause of cyanosis and use of certain medications.
2. See Chapter 1 guidelines for safe, effective, informed *posttest* care.

CARBOXYHEMOGLOBIN; CARBON MONOXIDE (CO) ●

Normal Values
0%–2.0% of total hemoglobin (as a proportion, 0–0.02)
In heavy smokers: 6.0%–8.0% (0.06–0.08)
In light smokers: 4.0%–5.0% (0.04–0.05)

Background
Carboxyhemoglobin is formed when Hb is exposed to carbon monoxide (CO). The affinity of Hb for CO is 218 times greater than for oxygen. CO poisoning causes anoxia because the carboxyhemoglobin formed does not permit Hb to combine with oxygen.

Explanation of Test
This test is done to detect CO poisoning. Because carboxyhemoglobin is not capable of transporting oxygen, hypoxia results, causing headache, nausea, vomiting, vertigo, collapse, or convulsions. Death may result from anoxia and irreversible tissue changes. Carboxyhemoglobin produces a cherry-red or violet color of the blood and skin, but this may not be present in chronic exposure. The most common causes of CO toxicity are automobile exhaust fumes, coal gas, water gas, and smoke inhalation from fires. Smoking is a minor cause.

Procedure
1. A heparinized venous blood sample of 5 ml is drawn and put on ice. Keep sample tightly capped and transport to laboratory immediately in a biohazard bag.

Clinical Implications
1. Carboxyhemoglobin is *increased* in
   A. CO poisoning from many sources, including smoking, exhaust fumes, fires
   B. Hemolytic disease
   C. Blood in intestines
2. A direct correlation has been found between CO and symptoms of heart disease, angina, and myocardial infarction.

Patient Preparation
1. Advise patient of purpose of test.
2. Draw blood sample before oxygen therapy has started.
3. See Chapter 1 guidelines for safe, effective, informed *pretest* care.

Patient Aftercare
1. Interpret test outcome and counsel for cause of headache, dizziness, vomiting, convulsions, or coma.
2. Treatment consists of removal of the patient from the source of CO.
3. Oxygen therapy is initiated either by supplemental oxygen at atmospheric pressure or by hyperbaric oxygen.
4. See Chapter 1 guidelines for safe, effective, informed *posttest* care.

Clinical Alert

1. With values of 10%–20%, the patient may be asymptomatic.
2. With 20%–30%, headache, nausea, vomiting, and loss of judgment occur.
3. With 30%–40%, tachycardia, hyperpnea, hypotension, and confusion occur.
4. With 50%–60%, there is loss of consciousness.
5. Values of 60% or higher cause convulsions, respiratory arrest, and death.

MYOGLOBIN (MB)

Normal Values
<70 ng/ml or μg/L

Background
Myoglobin is the oxygen-binding protein of striated muscle. It resembles Hb but is unable to release oxygen except at extremely low tension. Injury to skeletal muscle results in release of myoglobin.

Explanation of Test
The myoglobin test is used as an early marker of muscle damage in myocardial infarction and to detect polymyositis and muscle injuries.

Procedure
1. A venous blood sample of at least 5 ml is drawn; serum is used. Lipemic or grossly hemolyzed specimens are not acceptable.

Clinical Implications
1. *Increased myoglobin values* are associated with
   A. Myocardial infarction (elevates 1 to 3 hours after pain onset, earlier than creatine kinase)
   B. Other muscle injury (trauma, exercise, open heart surgery)
   C. Polymyositis and progressive muscular dystrophy
   D. Myocarditis
   E. Metabolic stress (eg, carbon dioxide poisoning, hypoglycemia, hypokalemia, water intoxication)
   F. Inflammatory myopathy (eg, SLE)
   G. Toxin exposure: narcotics, Malayan sea snake toxin
   H. Malignant hyperthermia
   I. Acute infectious disease
2. *Decreased myoglobin values* are found in
   A. Circulating antibodies to myoglobin (many patients with polymyositis)
   B. Rheumatoid arthritis

C. Myasthenia gravis

D. Kidney insufficiency or renal failure

Interfering Factors

1. See Appendix J for drugs that affect test outcomes.

Patient Preparation

1. Advise patient of test purpose.

2. Radioisotopes must be avoided until after blood is drawn.

3. Avoid vigorous exercise before the test because it may elevate myoglobin.

4. See Chapter 1 guidelines for safe, effective, informed *pretest* care.

Patient Aftercare

1. Resume normal activities.

2. Interpret test outcomes, counsel and monitor appropriately for myocardial infarction, muscle inflammation, and metabolic stress.

3. See Chapter 1 guidelines for safe, effective, informed *posttest* care.

> **Clinical Alert**
>
> Myoglobin is currently the earliest biologic marker of myocardial necrosis. It appears in the peripheral blood 2 to 3 hours after pain onset and reaches peak levels at 6 to 9 hours. Myoglobin is a sensitive indicator of acute myocardial infarction but is not specific for cardiac muscle.

HAPTOGLOBIN (HP)

Normal Values

Newborns: absent in 90%

Infants: 5–48 mg/dl

Children: 25–138 mg/dl

Adults: 40–240 mg/dl

Background

Haptoglobin (Hp) is a transport glycoprotein synthesized solely in the liver. It is a carrier for free Hb in plasma; its primary physiologic function is the preservation of iron.

Explanation of Test

A decrease in Hp (with normal liver function) is most likely to occur with increased consumption of Hp due to intravascular hemolysis. The concentration of Hp is inversely related to the degree of hemolysis and to the duration of the hemolytic episode.

Procedure

1. A venous blood sample of at least 2 ml is obtained. Place the specimen in a biohazard bag.

2. The serum is measured for Hp by a radial immunodiffusion method. A single determination is of limited value.

Clinical Implications

1. *Hp is decreased in acquired disorders* such as
   A. Transfusion reactions
   B. Erythroblastosis fetalis
   C. SLE
   D. Autoimmune hemolytic anemia
   E. Other hemoglobinemias caused by intravascular hemorrhages, especially artificial heart valves, acute bacterial endocarditis
   F. Malarial infestation
   G. PNH
   H. Hematoma, tissue hemorrhage
   I. Thrombotic thrombocytopenic purpura
   J. Drug-induced hemolytic anemia (methyldopa)
   K. Acute or chronic liver disease
2. *Hp is decreased in some inherited disorders,* such as
   A. Sickle cell disease
   B. G6PD and pyruvate kinase deficiency
   C. Hereditary spherocytosis
   D. Thalassemia and megaloblastic anemias
   E. Congenital absence is observed in 1% of black and Asian populations.
3. *Hp is increased* in
   A. Infection and inflammation (acute or chronic)
   B. Neoplasias, lymphomas (advanced)
   C. Biliary obstruction
   D. Acute rheumatic disease and other collagen diseases
   E. Tissue destruction

Interfering Factors

1. Estrogen and oral contraceptives lower Hp.
2. Steroid therapy raises Hp.
3. Androgens increase Hp.

> ### Clinical Alert
>
> Normal Hp results measured during inflammatory episodes or during steroid treatment do not rule out hemolysis.

Patient Preparation

1. Advise patient of test purpose.
2. Avoid use of oral contraceptives and androgens before blood is drawn. (Check with physician.)
3. Avoid exercise before test.
4. Follow Chapter 1 guidelines for safe, effective, informed *pretest* care.

Patient Aftercare
1. Resume normal activities and medications.
2. Interpret test results. Repeat testing may be necessary. Monitor appropriately for abnormal bleeding.
3. See Chapter 1 guidelines for safe, effective, informed *posttest* care.

BART'S HEMOGLOBIN　●

Normal Values
Adults: none
Children: none
Newborns: <0.5%

Background
Bart's hemoglobin is an unstable Hb with high oxygen affinity. When there is complete absence of production of the chain of Hb and deletion of all 4 globin genes, the disorder is known as Bart's hydrops fetalis. Both parents of the affected infant have heterozygous thalassemia; they are almost all Southeast Asians. Affected infants are either stillborn or die shortly after birth.

Explanation of Test
This test determines the percentage of the abnormal Bart's Hb in cord blood and identifies α-thalassemia hemoglobinopathies.

Procedure
1. A sample of cord blood is obtained, and hemoglobin electrophoresis is performed. Venous blood anticoagulated with EDTA or heparin can be used.

Clinical Implications
Increased levels are associated with

1. Homozygous α-thalassemia (hydrops fetalis syndrome, which causes stillbirth)
2. Hb H disease
3. α-Thalassemia minor

Patient Preparation
1. Explain test purpose and procedure to parents.
2. Obstetric complications may lead to significant morbidity and mortality for the mothers of these infants.
3. Provide genetic counseling in a sensitive manner.
4. See Chapter 1 guidelines for safe, effective, informed *pretest* care.

Patient Aftercare
1. Interpret test outcome and counsel parents.
2. See Chapter 1 guidelines for safe, effective, informed *posttest* care.

PAROXYSMAL NOCTURNAL HEMOGLOBINURIA (PNH) TEST; ACID HEMOLYSIS TEST; HAM'S TEST ●

Normal Values
Negative or <1% hemolysis

Background
PNH was first described by a patient who noted hemoglobinuria after sleep. In many patients, the hemolysis is irregular or occult. PNH is a hemolytic anemia in which there is also production of defective platelets and granulocytes. The diagnostic feature of PNH is an increased sensitivity of the erythrocytes to complement-mediated lysis. Although patients with PNH can present with hemoglobinuria or a hemolytic anemia, they may also present with iron deficiency (because of urinary loss of blood), bleeding secondary to thrombocytopenia, thrombosis, renal abnormalities, or neurologic abnormalities.

Explanation of Test
These tests are carried out to make a definitive diagnosis of PNH. The basis of these tests is that the cells peculiar to PNH have membrane defects, making them extrasensitive to complement in the plasma. Cells from patients with PNH undergo marked hemolysis after 15 minutes in the laboratory test. The tests are performed for patients who have hemoglobinuria, bone marrow aplasia (hypoplasia), or undiagnosed hemolytic anemia; they may be useful in the evaluation of patients with unexplained thrombosis or acute leukemia.

Procedure
1. Obtain a venous blood sample of 5 ml anticoagulated with EDTA. Place the specimen in a biohazard bag.
2. The patient's RBCs are mixed with normal serum and also with the patient's own serum, acidified, incubated at 37°C, and examined for hemolysis. Normally, there should be no lysis of the RBCs in this test (also called Ham's test).
3. A separate test called the sugar water test or sucrose hemolysis test may also be done at this time.

Clinical Implications
A *positive test* (hemolysis) is found in

1. PNH: A positive test (10%–50% lysis) is needed for diagnosis. The sucrose hemolysis test is also positive in PNH.
2. Hereditary erythroblastic multinuclearity associated with a positive acidified serum test (HEMPAS): The sucrose hemolysis test is negative.

Interfering Factors
1. False-positive results may be obtained with the following:
   A. Blood containing large numbers of spherocytes (hereditary or acquired)
   B. Dyserythropoietic anemia
   C. Specimen >8 hours old, specimen hemolyzed

D. Aplastic anemia
E. Leukemia and myeloproliferative syndromes

2. These conditions can be distinguished from PNH by the fact that hemolysis occurs in both acidified serum and complement. In PNH, hemolysis occurs only in complement (complement dependent).

Patient Preparation

1. Explain test purpose.
2. See Chapter 1 guidelines for safe, effective, informed *pretest* care.

Patient Aftercare

1. Interpret test results, counsel and monitor appropriately for anemia.
2. See Chapter 1 guidelines for safe, effective, informed *posttest* care.

●OTHER BLOOD TESTS

VITAMIN B$_{12}$ (VB$_{12}$) ●

Normal Values
Adults: 100–700 pg/ml or 74–517 pmol/L
Newborn: 160–1300 pg/ml
Unsaturated vitamin B$_{12}$ binding capacity: 743–1632 pg/ml

Background
Vitamin B$_{12}$ (VB$_{12}$), also known as the antipernicious anemia factor, is necessary for the production of RBCs. It is obtained only from ingestion of animal protein and requires an intrinsic factor for absorption. Both VB$_{12}$ and folic acid depend on a normally functioning intestinal mucosa for their absorption and are important for the production of RBCs. Levels of VB$_{12}$ and folate are usually tested in conjunction with one another because the diagnosis of macrocytic anemia requires measurement of both.

Explanation of Test
This determination is used in the differential diagnosis of anemia and conditions marked by high turnover of myeloid cells, as in the leukemias. When binding capacity is measured, it is the unsaturated fraction that is determined. The measurement of unsaturated vitamin B$_{12}$ binding capacity (UBBC) is valuable in distinguishing between untreated polycythemia vera and other conditions in which there is an elevated Hct.

Procedure
1. A fasting venous blood sample of at least 5 ml is obtained.
2. The specimen must be obtained before an injection of vitamin B$_{12}$ is administered and before a Schilling test is done. Place the specimen in a biohazard bag.

Clinical Implications

1. *Decreased VB_{12} (<100 pg/ml) is associated with*
   A. Pernicious anemia (megaloblastic anemia)
   B. Malabsorption syndromes and inflammatory bowel disease
   C. Fish tapeworm infestation
   D. Primary hypothyroidism
   E. Loss of gastric mucosa, as in gastrectomy and resection
   F. Zollinger-Ellison syndrome
   G. Blind loop syndromes (bacterial overgrowth)
   H. Vegetarian diets
   I. Folic acid deficiency
   J. Iron deficiency may be present in some patients (eg, gastrectomy)
2. *Increased VB_{12} (>700 pg/ml) is associated with*
   A. Chronic granulocytic leukemia, lymphatic and monocytic leukemia
   B. Chronic renal failure
   C. Liver disease (hepatitis, cirrhosis)
   D. Some cases of cancer, especially with liver metastasis
   E. Polycythemia vera
   F. Congestive heart failure
   G. Diabetes
   H. Obesity
3. Increased UBBC is found in
   A. Sixty percent of cases of polycythemia vera. (This test is normal in secondary relative polycythemia, aiding in the differential diagnosis of these 2 states).
   B. Reactive leukocytosis (leukemoid reaction).
   C. Chronic myelogenous leukemia.

Interfering Factors

1. The following result in increased VB_{12} values:
   A. Pregnancy
   B. Blood transfusion
   C. Aged persons
   D. High vitamin C and A doses
   E. Smoking
   F. Drugs capable of interfering with VB_{12} absorption (see Appendix J)

Patient Preparation

1. Explain test purpose and procedure.
2. Overnight fasting from food is necessary. Water is permitted.
3. Withhold VB_{12} injection before the blood is drawn.
4. Follow Chapter 1 guidelines for safe, effective, informed *pretest* care.

Patient Aftercare

1. Resume normal activities and diet.
2. Interpret test results, counsel and monitor appropriately for anemia, leukemia, or polycythemia.

3. See Chapter 1 guidelines for safe, effective, informed *posttest* care. See Appendix F for more information on vitamin testing.

> **Clinical Alert**
>
> **1.** Persons who have recently received therapeutic or diagnostic doses of radionuclides will have unreliable results.
> **2.** See Appendix F for more information on nutritional status of vitamin B_{12}.

> **Clinical Alert**
>
> The Schilling test is used to confirm pernicious anemia and to determine whether vitamin B_{12} deficiency is caused by malabsorption.

FOLIC ACID (FOLATE)

Normal Values

Adult: 2–20 ng/ml (serum)
Child: 5–21 ng/ml (serum)
Red blood cell folate: 110–700 ng/ml

Background

Folic acid is needed for normal RBC and WBC function and for the production of cellular genes. Folic acid is a more potent growth promoter than VB_{12}, although both depend on the normal functioning of intestinal mucosa for their absorption. Folic acid, like VB_{12}, is required for DNA production. Folic acid is formed by bacteria in the intestines, is stored in the liver, and is present in eggs, milk, leafy vegetables, yeast, liver, fruits, and other elements of a well-balanced diet.

Explanation of Test

This test is indicated for the differential diagnosis of megaloblastic anemia and in the investigation of folic acid deficiency, iron deficiency, and hypersegmental granulocytes. Measurement of both serum and RBC folate levels constitutes a reliable means of determining the existence of folate deficiency. The finding of low serum folate means that the patient's recent diet was subnormal in folate content, or that the patient's recent absorption of folate was subnormal, or both. Low RBC folate can mean either that there is tissue folate depletion due to folate deficiency requiring folate therapy or, alternatively, that the patient has primary VB_{12} deficiency that is blocking the ability of cells to take up folate. Serum levels are commonly high in patients with VB_{12} deficiency, because this vitamin is needed to allow incorporation of folate into tissue cells. For thoroughness, the serum VB_{12} should also be determined, because >50%

of all patients with significant megaloblastic anemia have VB_{12} deficiency rather than folate deficiency.

Procedure

1. Obtain a fasting venous sample of 10 ml. Protect the sample from light. Place the specimen in a biohazard bag. If RBC folate is ordered, 5 ml of venous blood is drawn with EDTA anticoagulant. An Hct determination is also required.

Clinical Implications

1. *Decreased* folic acid levels are associated with
   A. Inadequate intake owing to alcoholism, chronic disease, malnutrition, diet devoid of fresh vegetables, or anorexia
   B. Malabsorption of folic acid (eg, small-bowel disease)
   C. Excessive use of folic acid by the body (eg, pregnancy, hypothyroidism)
   D. Megaloblastic (macrocytic) anemia
   E. Hemolytic anemia (sickle cell, phenocytosis, PNH)
   F. Liver disease associated with cirrhosis, alcoholism, hepatoma
   G. Adult celiac disease, sprue
   H. Exfoliative dermatitis
   I. Carcinomas (mainly metastatic), acute leukemia
   J. Crohn's disease, ulcerative colitis
   K. Infantile hyperthyroidism
   L. Myelofibrosis
   M. Drugs that are folic antagonists (interfere with nucleic acid synthesis):
      (1) Anticonvulsants (phenytoin)
      (2) Aminopterin and methotrexate used in leukemia treatment
      (3) Antimalarials
      (4) Alcohol (ethanol)
      (5) Oral contraceptives
2. *Increased* folic acid levels are associated with
   A. Blind loop syndrome
   B. Vegetarian diet
   C. Pernicious anemia, VB_{12} deficiency

Interfering Factors

1. Drugs that are folic acid antagonists, among others (see Appendix J)
2. Hemolyzed specimens (false elevation)
3. Iron-deficiency anemia (false increase)

Clinical Alert

Elderly persons and those with inadequate diets develop folate-deficient megaloblastic anemia.

Patient Preparation
1. Explain test purpose and procedure. Obtain pertinent medication history.
2. Fasting from food for 8 hours before testing is required; water is permitted.
3. Blood must be drawn before VB_{12} injection.
4. No radioisotopes can be administered for 24 hours before the specimen is drawn.
5. See Chapter 1 guidelines for safe, effective, informed *pretest* care.

Patient Aftercare
1. Resume normal activities and medications.
2. Interpret test results, counsel and monitor appropriately for anemia.
3. See Chapter 1 guidelines for safe, effective, informed *posttest* care. See Appendix F for more information on vitamin testing.

ERYTHROPOIETIN (EP)   ●

Normal Values
4–20 U/L

Background
Erythropoietin (Ep) is a glycoprotein hormone that regulates erythropoiesis. The levels of Ep in anemia are primarily determined by the degree of anemia; Ep is inversely related to RBC volume and Hct.

Explanation of Test
This test is useful in differentiating primary from secondary polycythemia and in detecting the recurrence of Ep-producing tumors. It is also used as an indicator of need for Ep therapy in patients with renal failure.

Procedure
1. Obtain a venous blood serum sample of 5 ml. Place the specimen in biohazard bag. Separate serum from cells as soon as possible and place in polypropylene tube (*not* clear plastic-polystyrene). Freeze.

Clinical Implications
1. Ep is *increased appropriately* in
   A. Anemias with very low Hb (eg, aplastic anemia, hemolytic anemia); hematologic cancers have very high levels.
   B. Patients with any kind of moderate anemia have moderately high levels.
   C. Myelodysplasia, chemotherapy, AIDS
   D. Secondary polycythemia vera caused by tissue hypoxia (eg, high altitude, chronic obstructive pulmonary disease)
   E. Pregnancy (very high values)

2. Ep is *increased inappropriately* in erythropoietin-producing tumors:
   A. Renal cysts, renal transplant
   B. Renal adenocarcinoma
   C. Pheochromocytomas
   D. Cerebellar hemangioblastomas
   E. Uterine fibroids
   F. Occasionally, adrenal, ovarian, testicular, breast, and hepatic carcinoma
3. Ep is *decreased appropriately* in
   A. Renal failure
   B. Rheumatoid arthritis
   C. Multiple myeloma
   D. Cancer
4. Ep is *decreased inappropriately* in
   A. Polycythemia vera
   B. After bone marrow transplantation (weeks 3 and 4)
   C. AIDS before initiating therapy
   D. Autonomic neuropathy

Interfering Factors

1. Ep is *increased* in
   A. Pregnancy
   B. Use of anabolic steroids
   C. Administration of thyroid-stimulating hormone, ACTH, epinephrine
   D. Growth hormone (see Appendix J)
2. Ep is *decreased* in
   A. Transfusions
   B. Use of some prescribed drugs (see Appendix J)
   C. Drugs that increase renal blood flow (eg, enalapril)
   D. High plasma viscosity

Patient Preparation

1. Explain test purpose and procedure.
2. Draw blood at the same time for serial determinations: Circadian rhythm is lowest in the morning and 40% higher in late evening.
3. Fasting is not necessary, but a morning specimen is needed.
4. Note use of any drugs.
5. See Chapter 1 guidelines for safe, effective, informed *pretest* care.

Patient Aftercare

1. Resume normal activities and medications.
2. Interpret test results, counsel and monitor appropriately for anemia.
3. See Chapter 1 guidelines for safe, effective, informed *posttest* care. See Appendix F for more information on vitamin testing.

●TESTS OF HEMOSTASIS AND COAGULATION

OVERVIEW OF TESTING FOR ABNORMAL BLEEDING AND CLOTTING ●

Hemostasis and coagulation tests are generally done for patients with bleeding disorders, vascular injury or trauma, or coagulopathies. Reflex vasoconstriction is the normal response to vascular insult once the first-line defenses (skin and tissue) are breached. In larger vessels, vasoconstriction may be the primary mechanism for hemostasis. With smaller vessels, vasoconstriction reduces the size of the area that must be occluded by the hemostatic plug. Part of this cascade of sequential clotting events relates to the fact that platelets adhere to the injured and exposed subendothelial tissues. This phenomenon initiates the complex clotting mechanism whereby thrombin and fibrin are formed and deposited to aid in intravascular clotting (Table 2-1).

The entire mechanism of coagulation and fibrinolysis (removal of fibrin clot) is one of balance. It may best be understood by referring to the diagrams in this section. Abnormal bleeding does not always indicate coagulopathy, in much the same way that lack of bleeding does not necessarily indicate absence of a bleeding disorder.

The most common causes of hemorrhage are thrombocytopenia (platelet deficiency) and other acquired coagulation disorders, including liver disease, uremia, disseminated intravascular coagulation (DIC), and anticoagulant administration. Together they account for most hemorrhagic problems. Hemophilia and other inherited factor deficiencies are seen less frequently. Bleeding tendencies are associated with delays in clot formation or premature clot lysis. Thrombosis is associated with inappropriate clot activation or localization of the blood coagulation process. Finally, clotting disorders are divided into two classes: those caused by impaired coagulation and those caused by hypercoagulability.

HYPERCOAGULABILITY STATES ●

Two general forms of hypercoagulability exist: hyperreactivity of the platelet system, which results in arterial thrombosis, and accelerated activity of the clotting system, which results in venous thrombosis. Hypercoagulability refers to an unnatural tendency toward thrombosis. The thrombus is the actual insoluble mass (fibrin or platelets) present in the bloodstream or chambers of the heart.

Conditions and classifications associated with hypercoagulability include the following:

PLATELET ABNORMALITIES. These conditions are associated with arteriosclerosis, diabetes mellitus, increased blood lipids or cholesterol levels, increased platelet levels, and smoking. Arterial thrombosis may be related to blood flow

TABLE 2-1
The Complex Chain of Coagulation Reactions

A balance normally exists between the factors that stimulate formation of thrombin and forces acting to delay thrombin formation. This balance maintains circulating blood as a fluid. When injury occurs or blood is removed from a vessel, this balance is upset and coagulation occurs. Blood clotting involves 4 progressive stages. The Roman numerals assigned to the coagulation factors identify their order of discovery rather than their involvement in the stages of clot formation.

Stage	*Components of Stages*
STAGE I (3–5 MIN)	
Phase I—Platelet activity. Platelets serve as a source of thromboplastin.	90% of all coagulation disorders are caused by defects in phase I. Platelet counts $<1 \times 10^6/mm^3$ indicate moderate interference with phase I activity.
Phase II—Thromboplastin. Factor III, an enzyme thought to be liberated by damaged cells, is formed by 6 different factors plus calcium.	Calcium Factor V Factor VIII Factor IX } are involved in the formation of tissue thromboplastin (intrinsic prothrombin activation) Factor X Factor XI Factor XII
STAGE II (8–15 SEC)	
Prothrombin factor II is converted to thrombin in the presence of calcium.	Factor II Factor X } are involved in the conversion of fibrinogen to fibrin Factor VII Factor V
STAGE III (1 SEC)	
Thrombin interacts with fibrinogen (factor I) to form the framework of the clot.	At the end of stage III, factor XIII functions in the stabilization of the clot.
STAGE IV	
Fibrinolytic system (antagonistic check-and-balance to the clotting mechanism) is activated.	Removal of fibrin clot through fibrinolysis. Plasminogen is converted to plasmin, which breaks clot into fibrin split products.

disturbances, vessel wall changes, and increased platelet sensitivity to factors causing platelet adherence and aggregation.

CLOTTING SYSTEM ABNORMALITIES. These are associated with congestive heart failure, immobility, artificial surfaces (eg, artificial heart valves), damaged vasculature, use of oral contraceptives or estrogen, pregnancy and the postpartum state, and the postsurgical state. Other influences include malignancy, myeloproliferative (bone marrow) disorders, obesity, lupus disorders, and genetic predisposition.

VENOUS THROMBOSIS. This can be related to stasis of blood flow, to coagulation alterations, or to increases in procoagulation factors or decreases in anticoagulation factors (Table 2-2).

DISORDERS OF HEMOSTASIS ●

CONGENITAL VASCULAR ABNORMALITIES (VESSEL WALL STRUCTURE DEFECTS). Defects of the actual blood vessel are poorly defined and difficult to test for. Hereditary telangiectasia is the most commonly recognized vascular abnormality. Laboratory studies are normal, so the diagnosis must be made from clinical signs and symptoms. Patients frequently report epistaxis and symptoms of anemia. Another abnormality is congenital hemangiomata (Kasabach-Merritt syndrome).

ACQUIRED ABNORMALITIES OF THE VESSEL WALL STRUCTURE. Causes include Schönlein-Henoch purpura as an allergic response to infection or drugs, diabetes mellitus, rickettsial diseases, septicemia, and amyloidosis present with some degree of vascular abnormalities. Purpura can also be associated with steroid therapy and easy bruising in females (infectious purpura), or it can be a result of drug use.

HEREDITARY CONNECTIVE TISSUE DISORDERS. These include Ehlers-Danlos syndrome (hyperplastic skin and hyperflexible joints) and pseudoxanthoma elasticum (rare connective tissue disorder).

ACQUIRED CONNECTIVE TISSUE DEFECTS. These can be caused by scurvy (vitamin C deficiency) or senile purpura.

QUALITATIVE PLATELET ABNORMALITIES. These disorders can be divided into subclasses:

1. *Thrombocytopenia* (platelet count $<150 \times 10^3/mm^3$) is caused by decreased production of platelets, increased use or destruction of platelets, or hypersplenism. Contributing factors include bone marrow disease, autoimmune diseases, DIC, bacterial or viral infection, chemotherapy, therapy radiation, multiple transfusions, and certain drugs (eg, NSAIDs, thiazides, estrogens).
2. *Thrombocytosis* (elevated platelet count) is caused by hemorrhage, iron-deficiency anemia, inflammation, or splenectomy.

> ### ▶ Clinical Alert
>
> An increased platelet count predisposes the patient to arterial thrombosis.

TABLE 2-2
Proteins Involved in Blood Coagulation

Protein	Synonym	Plasma Concentration (mg/dl)	Function
Fibrinogen	Factor I	200–400	Converted to fibrin along with platelets to form clot
Factor II	Prothrombin (Prethrombin)	10–15	Is converted to thrombin (IIa) which splits fibrinogen into fibrin
Factor V	Proaccelerin, Labile factor	0.5–1.0	Supports Xa activation of II to IIa
Factor VII	Stable factor Proconvertin	0.2	Activates X
Factor VIII;c	Antihemophlic factor (AHF) Platelet Co-factor I	1.0–2.0	Supports IXa activation of X
Factor IX	Christmas factor Plasmas thrombo-plastin component (PTC)	0.3–0.4	Activates X
Factor X	Stuart-Prower factor (AVTD Prothrombin III)	0.6–0.8	Activates II
Factor XI	Plasmas thrombo-plastin antecedent (Antihemophlic factor C)	0.4	Actives XII and Prekallikrein
Factor XII	Hageman factor	2.9	Activates XI and prekallikrein
Factor XIII	Fibrin-stabilizing factor Laki-Lorand factor	2.5	Crosslinks fibrin and other proteins
von Willebrand's factor	Factor VIII-related antigen VIII:VWD	1.0	Stabilizes VIII, mediates platelet adhesion
Prekallikrein	Fletcher factor	5.0	Activates XII and prekallikrein, cleaves HMWK
High molecular weight, kinin-ogen (HMWK)	Fitzgerald factor	4.7–12.2	Supports reciprocal activation of XII, XI and prekallikrein

(continued)

TABLE 2-2 *(Continued)*
Proteins Involved in Blood Coagulation

Protein	*Synonym*	*Plasma Concentration (mg/dl)*	*Function*
Fibronectin	Cold insoluble globulin	20–40	Mediates cell adhesion
Major anti-thrombin	Antithrombin III	20–40	Inhibits IIa, Xa, and XIa, XIIa, and Kallikrein
Protein C	—	0.5	Complexed with Protein S, Inactivates V and VIII
Protein S	—	1.5	Protein S and C work together
Plasminogen	—	20	Forms plasmin which lyses the fibrin clot and inhibits other factors
a2 Antiplasmin	—	9.6–13.5	Inhibits plasmin
a1 Antitrypsin	—	245–335	Week inhibitor of thrombin, potent inhibitor of XIa
Tissue plasminogen	—	—	Activates plasminogen
Plasminogen activator inhibitor I	—		Inactivates tPA
Plasminogen activator inhibitor II	—		Inactivates urokinase

The clotting factors of the blood are proteins; they are present in the blood plasma in an inactive form.

3. *Thrombocythemia* (platelet count $>1000 \times 10^3/mm^3$) is caused by granulocytic leukemia, polycythemia vera, or myeloid metaplasia.

Clinical Alert

When the platelet count is substantially increased, bleeding can occur in the nose, gastrointestinal tract, skin, and gums.

QUANTITATIVE PLATELET ABNORMALITIES. These are associated with Glanz-mann's thrombasthenia, a hereditary autosomal-recessive disorder that can produce severe bleeding, especially with trauma and surgical procedures. Platelet factor 3 differences associated with aggregation, adhesion, or release defects may be manifested in storage-pool disease, May-Hegglin anomaly, Bernard-Soulier syndrome, and Wiskott-Aldrich syndrome. Dialysis and use of drugs such as aspirin, other antiinflammatory agents, dipyridamole, and prostaglandin E also can be tied to platelet abnormalities.

CONGENITAL COAGULATION ABNORMALITIES. These include hemophilia A and B (deficiencies of factors VIII and IX, respectively), rare autosomal recessive traits (hemophilia C), and autosomal dominant traits (eg, von Willebrand's disease).

ACQUIRED COAGULATION ABNORMALITIES. These are associated with several disease states and are much more common than inherited deficiencies.

1. Circulatory anticoagulant activity may be evident in the presence of anti-factor VIII, rheumatoid arthritis, immediate postpartum period, SLE, or multiple myeloma.
2. Vitamin D deficiency may be caused by oral anticoagulants, biliary obstruction and malabsorption syndrome, or intestinal sterilization by antibiotic therapy. Newborns are prone to vitamin D deficiency.
3. DIC causes continuous production of thrombin which, in turn, consumes the other clotting factors and results in uncontrolled bleeding.
4. Primary fibrinolysis is the situation whereby isolated activation of the fibrinolytic mechanism occurs without prior coagulation activity, as in streptokinase therapy, severe liver disease, prostate cancer, or, more rarely, electroshock.
5. Most coagulation factors are manufactured in liver. Consequently, in liver disease the extent of coagulation abnormalities is directly proportional to the severity of the liver disease.

TESTS FOR DISSEMINATED INTRAVASCULAR COAGULATION (DIC) ●

DIC is an acquired hemorrhagic syndrome characterized by uncontrolled formation and deposition of fibrin thrombi. Continuous generation of thrombin causes depletion (consumption) of the coagulation factors and results in uncontrolled bleeding. Also, fibrinolysis is activated in DIC. This further adds to the hemostasis defect caused by the consumption of clotting factors. The many coagulation test abnormalities found in acute DIC include the following:

Prothrombin time (PT):	Prolonged
Partial thromboplastin time (PTT) or APTT:	Prolonged
Bleeding time:	Prolonged

Fibrinogen:	Decreased
Platelet count:	Decreased
Fibrinolysin test:	Increased
Fibrin split products:	Positive
Thrombin time (TT):	Prolonged
Clotting factors II, V, VIII, and X:	Decreased
Fibrinopeptide A:	Increased
D-dimer:	Positive
Antithrombin III:	Decreased

In chronic DIC the results are variable, especially the PT, PTT, TT, and fibrinogen, making the diagnosis much more difficult. No single test or group of tests is diagnostic, and diagnosis usually depends on a combination of findings. Normal levels do not rule out DIC, and a repeat profile should be done a few hours later to look for changes in platelet count and fibrinogen.

Causes of DIC include septicemia, malignancies and cancer, obstetric emergencies, cirrhosis of liver, sickle cell disease, trauma or crushing injuries, malaria, incompatible blood transfusion, cold hemoglobinuria or PNH, connective tissue diseases, snake bites, and brown recluse spider bites.

Paradoxically, the treatment for uncontrolled bleeding in DIC is heparin administration. The heparin blocks thrombin formation, which blocks consumption of the other clotting factors and allows hemostasis to occur.

Laboratory Investigation of Hemostasis

Usually, a blood sample of at least 20 ml is obtained by the 2-tube technique. In the first tube, a 5-ml blood sample is obtained and discarded. Then 15 to 20 ml of blood is drawn into Vacutainer tubes with sodium citrate as the anticoagulant. A butterfly needle may be used to prevent backflow or to make sampling easier in the case of a "difficult draw." Coagulation studies (*coagulation profiles, coag panels, coagulograms*) are used for screening or as diagnostic tools for evaluation of symptoms such as easy or spontaneous bruising, petechiae, prolonged bleeding (eg, from cuts), abnormal nosebleeds, heavy menstrual flow, family history of coagulopathies, or gastrointestinal bleeding (Table 2-3).

1. These five primary screening tests are initially performed to diagnose suspected coagulation disorders:
   A. Platelet count, size, and shape
   B. Bleeding time—reflects data about the ability of platelets to function normally and the ability of the capillaries to constrict their walls
   C. PTT—determines the overall ability of the blood to clot
   D. PT—measures the function of second-stage clotting factors
   E. Fibrinogen level
2. Factor assays are definitive coagulation studies of a specific clotting factor (eg, factor VIII for hemophilia). These are done if the screening test indicates a problem with a specific factor or factors.
3. Fibrinolysis is used to address problems of the fibrinolytic system. This includes the following studies:

TABLE 2-3
Laboratory Tests to Measure Hemostasis*

Name of Test	Vascular Function	Platelet Function	Stage I	Stage II	Stage III	Stage IV
Bleeding time	X	X				
Platelet count		X				
Platelet adhesiveness		X				
Platelet aggregation		X				
Aspirin tolerance		X				
Platelet factor 3 assay		X				
Activated clotting		X	X	X	X	
Activated recalcification time			X	X		
Activated partial thromboplastin			X	X		
Prothrombin time				X		
Stypven time				X		
Circulating anticoagulant factor I.D. substitution			X	X	X	
Factor assay			X	X	X	
Thrombin time				X	X	X
Reptilase time				X		
Fibrinogen assay					X	
Factor XIII assay				X		
Euglobulin lysis time						X
Thrombin time-diluted					X	X
Plasminogen assay						X
Protamine sulfate (ethanal gelation)					X	X
D-dimer						X
Fibrin monomer						X
Fibrinopeptide-A						X
Latex agglutination for fibrin split products						X

*These tests measure all facets of hemostasis: vascular function, platelets, and clotting factors.

A. Euglobulin clot lysis—identifies increased plasminogen activator activity. (Plasmin is *not* usually present in the blood plasma.)

B. Factor XIII (fibrin stabilizing factor)

C. Fibrin split products (eg, protamine sulfate test)

4. The investigation of hypercoagulable status (thrombotic tendency, thromboembolic disorders) covers both primary causes (deficiencies of antithrombin III, protein C, protein S, and factor XII; fibrinolytic mechanisms) and secondary causes (acquired platelet disorders and acquired diseases of coagulation and fibrinolytic impairment). These include the following tests:

A. PT

B. PTT

C. Fibrinogen test

D. Antiplatelet factors (eg, prostacyclin)

E. Anticoagulant factors (eg, antithrombin III, protein C, protein S, lupus anticoagulant)

F. Fibrinolysis tests (eg, fibrin degradation products [FDPs], euglobulin lysis time, fibrin monomers)

G. TT

NOTE: *The lupus inhibitor (lupus anticoagulant) is an antibody (against the phospholipid used in the PT and PTT tests) that is responsible for inhibition of the PT, PTT, Russell viper venom time (dRVVT), and Kaolen clotting time (KCT). To demonstrate its presence, 1 ml of the patient's plasma is mixed with 1 ml of normal plasma and a PTT test of the mixture is done. When an inhibitor of any sort is present, the PTT will not return to normal range. An inhibitor of the lupus type can be shown by correcting the PTT through use of platelets as a phospholipid source or by demonstrating a characteristic pattern in the PTT that results from sequential dilution of the phospholipid reagent. Lupus anticoagulants may be associated with false-positive Venereal Disease Research Laboratory (VDRL) test reports and with another antiphospholipid— the anticardiolipin antibody (B2-glycoprotein I).*

Clinical Alert

Conditions associated with the presence of the lupus anticoagulant include

1. SLE (one fifth of patients)

2. Other autoimmune diseases (rheumatoid arthritis, Raynaud's syndrome)

3. Spontaneous abortions (associated with presence of anticardiolipin autoantibody).

4. Lupus anticoagulant is more often associated with thromboembolism than with bleeding problems.

5. Most lupus anticoagulant antibodies are directed against prothrombin or B2-glycoprotein I.

> ### Clinical Alert
>
> 1. All patients with hemorrhagic or thrombotic tendencies, or undergoing coagulation studies, should be observed closely for possible bleeding emergencies. A comprehensive history and physical examination should be done.
> 2. Blood samples for coagulation studies should be drawn last if other blood studies are indicated.
> 3. Procedure alert: When a blood sample is obtained for PT, PTT, and TT, sodium citrate is used as the anticoagulant in the sampling tubes.

Patient Assessment for Bleeding Tendency

1. Examine all skin for bruising.
2. Record petechiae associated with use of blood pressure cuffs or tourniquets.
3. Note bleeding from the nose or gums for no apparent cause.
4. Estimate blood quantity in vomitus, expectorated mucus, urine, stools, and menstrual flow.
5. Note prolonged bleeding from injection sites.
6. Watch for symptoms, especially changes in levels of consciousness or neurologic checks that may signal an "intracranial bleed."
7. Determine whether the patient is taking anticoagulants or aspirin.

BLEEDING TIME (IVY METHOD; TEMPLATE BLEEDING TIME)

Normal Values
3–10 minutes in most laboratories
Ivy method (forearm with template): 2–9.5 minutes

Background
Bleeding time measures the primary phase of hemostasis: the interaction of the platelet with the blood vessel wall and the formation of a hemostatic plug. Bleeding time is the best single screening test for platelet function disorders and is one of the primary screening tests for coagulation disorders.

Explanation of Test
This test is of value in detecting vascular abnormalities and platelet abnormalities or deficiencies. It is not recommended for routine presurgical workup.

A small stab wound is made in either the earlobe or the forearm; the bleeding time (the amount of time it takes to form a clot) is recorded. The duration of bleeding from a punctured capillary depends on the quantity and quality of platelets and the ability of the blood vessel wall to constrict.

The principal use of this test today is in the diagnosis of von Willebrand's disease, an inherited defective molecule of factor VIII, and a type of pseudo-hemophilia. It has been established that aspirin may cause abnormal bleeding in some normal persons, but the bleeding time test has not proved consistently valuable in identifying such persons.

Procedure (Ivy Method)

1. The area three finger-widths below the antecubital space is cleansed with alcohol and allowed to dry.
2. A blood pressure cuff is placed on the arm above the elbow and inflated to 40 mm Hg.
3. A cleansed area of the forearm without superficial veins is selected. The skin is stretched laterally and tautly between the thumb and forefinger.
3. The skin is punctured with a sterile disposable template to a uniform depth of 3 mm and width of 5 mm.
4. A stopwatch is started. The edge of a 4 × 4-inch filter paper is used to blot the blood through capillary action by gently touching the drop every 30 seconds. The wound itself is not disturbed. The blood pressure gauge is removed when bleeding stops and a clot has formed. A sterile dressing is applied when the test is completed.
5. The end point (by this or the earlobe method) is reached when blood is no longer blotted from the forearm puncture. It is reported in minutes and half minutes (eg, 5 minutes 30 seconds).

Clinical Implications

1. Bleeding time is *prolonged* when the level of platelets is decreased or when platelets are qualitatively abnormal:
   A. Thrombocytopenia (platelet count $<80 \times 10^3/mm^3$)
   B. Platelet dysfunction syndromes
   C. Decrease or abnormality in plasma factors (eg, von Willebrand's factor, fibrinogen)
   D. Abnormalities in the walls of the small blood vessels, vascular disease
   E. Advanced renal failure
   F. Severe liver disease
   G. Leukemia, other myeloproliferative diseases
   H. Scurvy
   I. DIC disease (owing to the presence of FDPs)
2. In von Willebrand's disease, bleeding time can be variable; it will definitely be prolonged if aspirin is taken before testing (aspirin tolerance test).
3. A single prolonged bleeding time does not prove the existence of hemorrhagic disease. Because a larger vessel can be punctured, the puncture should be repeated on an alternate body site, and the 2 values obtained should be averaged.
4. Bleeding time is normal in the presence of coagulation disorders other than platelet dysfunction, vascular disease, or von Willebrand's disease.

5. Aspirin therapy (anti-platelet function therapy): When thrombus formation is thought to be mediated by platelet activation, the patient frequently is given agents to interrupt normal platelet function, which may be monitored by bleeding times or platelet aggregation studies. Aspirin is the most commonly used inhibitor; it inhibits platelet adhesion or "stickiness."

Interfering Factors
1. Normal values for bleeding time vary when the puncture site is not of uniform depth and width.
2. Touching the puncture site during this test will break off fibrin particles and prolong the bleeding time.
3. Excessive alcohol consumption (as in alcoholics) may cause increased bleeding time.
4. Prolonged bleeding time can reflect ingestion of 10 g of aspirin as long as 5 days before the test.
5. Other drugs that may cause increased bleeding times include dextran, streptokinase-streptodornase (fibrinolytic agents), mithramycin, pantothenyl alcohol. See Appendix J.
6. Extreme hot or cold conditions can alter the results.
7. Edema of patient's hands or cyanotic hands will invalidate the test.

Patient Preparation
1. Explain test purpose and procedure. See Patient Assessment for Bleeding Tendency on page 136.
2. Instruct patient to abstain from aspirin and aspirin-like drugs for at least 7 days before the test.
3. Advise the patient to abstain from alcohol before the test.
4. Inform the patient that scar tissue may form at the puncture site (keloid formation).
5. If the patient has an infectious skin disease, the test should be postponed.
6. See Chapter 1 guidelines for safe, effective, informed *pretest* care.

Patient Aftercare
1. Interpret test outcome and monitor appropriately for prolonged bleeding. See Patient Assessment for Bleeding Tendency on page 136.
2. See Chapter 1 guidelines for safe, effective, informed *posttest* care.

Clinical Alert
1. The critical value for bleeding time is >15 minutes.
2. If the puncture site is still bleeding after 15 minutes, discontinue the test and apply pressure to the site. Document and report the results to the clinician.

PLATELET COUNT; MEAN PLATELET VOLUME (MPV) ●

Normal Values

Platelet Count
Adults: 140–400 × 10³/mm³
Children: 150–450 × 10³/mm³

Mean Platelet Volume
7.4–10.4 μm³ or fl

Background

Platelets (thrombocytes) are the smallest of the formed elements in the blood. These cells are nonnucleated, round or oval, flattened, disk-shaped structures. Platelet activity is necessary for blood clotting, vascular integrity and vasoconstriction, and the adhesion and aggregation activity that occurs during the formation of platelet plugs that occlude (plug) breaks in small vessels. Thrombocyte development takes place primarily in the bone marrow. The life span of a platelet is about 7.5 days. Normally, two thirds of all the body platelets are found in the circulating blood and one third in the spleen.

Explanation of Test

The platelet count is of value for assessing bleeding disorders that occur with thrombocytopenia, uremia, liver disease, or malignancies and for monitoring the course of disease associated with bone marrow failure. This test is indicated when the estimated platelet count (on a blood smear) appears abnormal. It is also part of a coagulation profile or workup.

The mean platelet volume (MPV) is sometimes ordered in conjunction with a platelet count. The MPV indicates the uniformity of size of the platelet population. It is used for the differential diagnosis of thrombocytopenia.

Procedure

1. A 7-ml venous blood sample is mixed with an EDTA anticoagulant tube. The platelets are counted by phase microscopy or by an automated counting instrument. The MPV is also calculated by many instruments at the time of the platelet count. A blood smear is also made, and the size, shape, and clumping of the platelets are noted. Place the specimen in a biohazard bag.

Clinical Implications

1. *Abnormally increased* numbers of platelets (thrombocythemia, thrombocytosis) occur in
   A. Essential thrombocythemia
   B. Chronic myelogenous and granulocytic leukemia, myeloproliferative diseases
   C. Polycythemia vera and primary thrombocytosis
   D. Splenectomy

E. Iron-deficiency anemia
F. Asphyxiation
G. Rheumatoid arthritis and other collagen diseases, SLE
H. Rapid blood regeneration caused by acute blood loss, hemolytic anemia
I. Acute infections, inflammatory diseases
J. Hodgkin's disease, lymphomas, malignancies
K. Chronic pancreatitis, tuberculosis, inflammatory bowel disease
L. Renal failure
M. Recovery from bone marrow suppression (thrombocytopenia)

> **Clinical Alert**
>
> 1. In 50% of patients who exhibit unexpected platelet increases, a malignancy is found.
> 2. In patients with an extremely elevated platelet count ($>1000 \times 10^3/mm^3$) as a result of a myeloproliferative disorder, assess for bleeding caused by abnormal platelet function.

---

2. *Abnormally decreased* numbers of platelets (thrombocytopenia) occur in
   A. Idiopathic thrombocytopenic purpura, neonatal purpura
   B. Pernicious, aplastic, and hemolytic anemias
   C. After massive blood transfusion (dilution effect)
   D. Viral, bacterial, and rickettsial infections
   E. Congestive heart failure
   F. Thrombopoietin deficiency
   G. During cancer chemotherapy and radiation, exposure to dichloro-diphenyltrichloroethane (DDT) and other chemicals
   H. HIV infection
   I. Lesions involving the bone marrow (eg, leukemias, carcinomas, myelofibrosis)
   K. DIC and thrombotic thrombocytopenic purpura
   L. Inherited syndromes as Bernard-Soulier syndrome, May-Hegglin anomaly, Wiskott-Aldrich syndrome, Fanconi syndrome
   M. Toxemia of pregnancy, eclampsia
   N. Alcohol toxicity, ethanol abuse
   O. Hypersplenism
   P. Renal insufficiency

NOTE: *Many drugs have toxic effects. The dosage does not have to be high to be toxic. Toxic thrombocytopenia depends on the inability of the body to metabolize and secrete the toxic substance.*

3. *Increased MPV* is observed in
   A. Idiopathic thrombocytopenic purpura (autoimmune)
   B. Thrombocytopenia caused by sepsis

C. Prosthetic heart valve
D. Massive hemorrhage
E. Myeloproliferative disorders
F. Acute and chronic myelogenous leukemia
G. Splenectomy
H. Vasculitis
I. Megaloblastic anemia
4. *Decreased MPV* occurs in Wiskott-Aldrich syndrome.

Clinical Alert

1. Panic values: A decrease in platelets to $<20 \times 10^3/mm^3$ is associated with a tendency for spontaneous bleeding, prolonged bleeding time, petechiae, and ecchymosis.
2. Platelet counts $>50 \times 10^3/mm^3$ are not generally associated with spontaneous bleeding.

Interfering Factors

1. Platelet counts normally increase at high altitudes; after strenuous exercise, trauma, or excitement; and in winter.
2. Platelet counts normally decrease before menstruation and during pregnancy.
3. Clumping of platelets may cause falsely lowered results.
4. Oral contraceptives cause a slight increase.
5. See Appendix J for drugs that affect test outcomes.

Patient Preparation

1. Explain test purpose and procedure.
2. Avoid strenuous exercise before blood is drawn.
3. Note what medications and what treatments the patient is receiving.
4. See Chapter 1 guidelines for safe, effective, informed *pretest* care.

Patient Aftercare

1. Interpret test outcomes and monitor appropriately. Observe for signs and symptoms of gastrointestinal bleeding, hemolysis, hematuria, petechiae, vaginal bleeding, epistasis, and bleeding from the gums. When hemorrhage is apparent, use emergency measures to control bleeding and notify the attending physician.
2. Platelet transfusions are used if the platelet count is $<20 \times 10^3/mm^3$ or if there is a specific bleeding lesion. One unit of platelet concentrate raises the count by $15 \times 10^3/mm^3$.
3. See Chapter 1 guidelines for safe, effective, informed *posttest* care.

PLATELET AGGREGATION ●

Normal Values
Full platelet aggregation in response to adenosine diphosphate, collagen, epinephrine, thrombin, and ristocetin.

Explanation of Test
Platelet aggregation is used in the classification of congenital qualitative functional disorders of adhesion, release, or aggregation. It is rarely used to evaluate acquired bleeding disorders.

Procedure
1. Obtain a 5-ml venous blood sample (anticoagulated in a tube containing sodium citrate). Place it in biohazard bag. The sample is kept at room temperature (*never refrigerate*) and must be run within 30 minutes after the blood is drawn. When platelets aggregate, the transmission of light through a sample of platelet-rich plasma is increased. This increase in light transmission can be used as an index to the aggregation in response to various agonists.

Clinical Implications
1. Decreased platelet aggregation occurs in *congenital diseases:*
   A. Bernard-Soulier syndrome
   B. Glanzmann's thrombasthenia
   C. Storage pool diseases (eg, Chédiak Higashi syndrome, gray platelet disease)
   D. Cyclooxygenase deficiency
   E. Wiskott-Aldrich syndrome
   F. Albinism
   G. β-Thalassemia major
   H. May-Hegglin anomaly
   I. Various connective tissue disorders (eg, Marfan's syndrome)
   J. von Willebrand's disease
2. Decreased platelet aggregation also occurs in *acquired disorders:*
   A. Uremia
   B. Antiplatelet antibodies
   C. Cardiopulmonary bypass
   D. Myeloproliferative disorders
   E. Dysproteinemias (macroglobulinemia)
   F. Idiopathic thrombocytopenic purpura
   G. Polycythemia vera
   H. Use of drugs and aspirin, some antibiotics, antiinflammatory drugs, psychotropic drugs, and others (see Appendix J)
   I. DIC
3. *Increased* aggregation occurs in primary and secondary Raynaud's syndrome.

Patient Preparation

1. Explain test purpose and procedure.
2. For 10 days before the test, drugs that inhibit platelet aggregation are contraindicated. These include aspirin, antihistamines, steroids, cocaine, antiinflammatories, and theophylline.
3. On the day of the test, avoid caffeine.
4. Avoid Coumadin for 2 weeks and heparin therapy for 1 week before testing.
5. See Chapter 1 guidelines for safe, effective, informed *pretest* care.

Patient Aftercare

1. Interpret test outcome and counsel appropriately for congenital disorders.
2. Resume medications and normal diet.
3. See Chapter 1 guidelines for safe, effective, informed *posttest* care.

THROMBIN TIME (TT); THROMBIN CLOTTING TIME (TCT)

Normal Values

7.0–12.0 seconds (varies widely by laboratory)
Check with your laboratory for reference values.

Explanation of Test

Stage III fibrinogen defects can be detected by the TT test. It can detect DIC and hypofibrinogenemia and may also be used for monitoring streptokinase therapy. The test actually measures the time needed for plasma to clot when thrombin is added. Normally, a clot forms rapidly; if it does not, a stage III deficiency is present (Fig. 2-1). A TT test is often included as part of a panel for coagulation defects.

Procedure

1. With the procedure for 2-tube specimen collection, a 7-ml venous blood sample is anticoagulated with sodium citrate and put on ice. Care must be taken not to contaminate the specimen with heparin from IV apparatus or other sources.

Clinical Implications

1. *Prolonged TT* occurs in
   A. Hypofibrinogenemia
   B. Therapy with heparin or heparin-like anticoagulants
   C. DIC
   D. Fibrinolysis
   E. Multiple myeloma
   F. Presence of large amounts of FSPs/FDPs, as in DIC
   G. Uremia
   H. Severe liver diseases

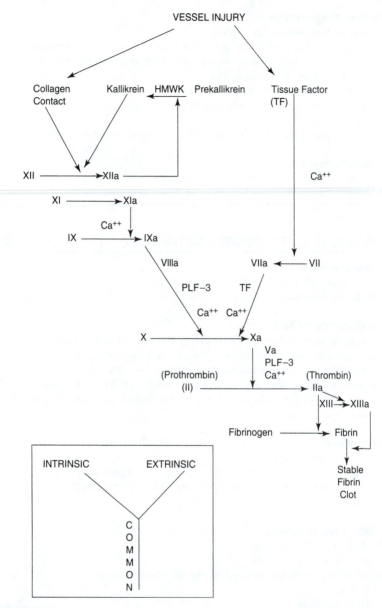

FIGURE 2-1

Intrinsic, extrinsic, and common pathways of coagulation. Vessel injury initiates intrinsic pathway through contact activation by exposed collagen. Extrinsic pathway is initiated by endothelial release of tissue factor (i.e., tissue thromboplastin). Extrinsic and intrinsic pathway each initiate common pathway to create stable fibrin clot. (Lotspeich-Steininger, C. A., et al. (1992) *Clinical Hematology*, Philadelphia: JB Lippincott Co.)

2. *Shortened TT* occurs in
   A. Hyperfibrinogenemia
   B. Elevated Hct (>55%)
3. Therapy with plasminogen activators—streptokinase, urokinase, or tissue plasminogen activator (tPA): Anticoagulant therapy is an attempt either to prevent thrombus formation or to promote thrombus lysis. The type and location of the thrombus usually determine the type of anticoagulant to be administered and the treatment protocol. The newest treatment for life-threatening thrombus formation uses plasminogen activators to accelerate fibrinolysis, which is the enzymatic dissolution of already organized clots (Fig. 2-2). The action of some of these agents produces a lytic state that can be monitored by the TT.

Although several tests are sensitive to the effects of thrombolytic drugs, many require lengthy assay procedures or special techniques. Of the laboratory procedures that have been recommended (PT, TT, APTT, quantitative fibrinogen, euglobulin clot lysis, and plasminogen levels), the TT has become widely accepted because it is fast and practical, does not require special equipment, and can detect the decrease in fibrinogen levels as well as the presence of fibrin and FDPs.

The half-life for these activators is relatively short (10–90 minutes); therefore, the antidote for overdose is to hold giving the next dose.

> ### Clinical Alert
>
> TT is *severely* prolonged in the presence of afibrinogenemia (<80 mg/dl of fibrinogen). Critical value: >60 seconds.

Interfering Factors

1. Heparin prolongs thrombin time. Interpret test results within this context.
2. Plasminogen activator therapy prolongs thrombin clotting time.
3. See Appendix J for drugs that affect test outcomes.

Patient Preparation

1. Explain test purpose and procedure.
2. If possible, no heparin should be taken for 2 days before testing.
3. See Chapter 1 guidelines for safe, effective, informed *pretest* care.

Patient Aftercare

1. Resume normal activities and medications as ordered.
2. Interpret test outcomes and monitor appropriately. Check for excess bleeding. If plasminogen activator is being monitored, see Patient Aftercare for APTT, page 149.
3. See Chapter 1 guidelines for safe, effective, informed *posttest* care.

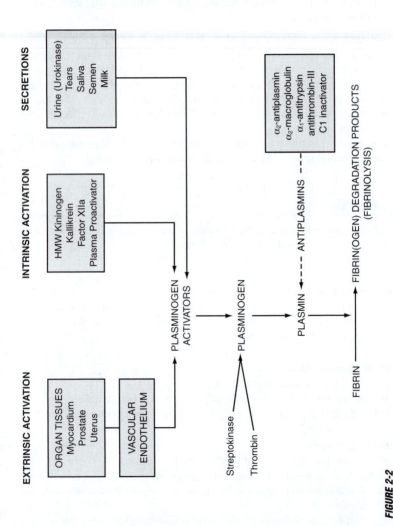

Fibrinolytic system may be activated by plasminogen activators from extrinsic sources such as vascular endothelium or by intrinsic sources such as factor XIIa and others as shown. These plasminogen activators convert plasminogen to plasmin. Thrombin also activates plasminogen; streptokinase, administered therapeutically in thrombotic disorders, acts in the same way. Plasmin promotes fibrinolysis. Antiplasmins control (inhibit and neutralize) excess plasmin, thus preventing excessive and premature fibrinolysis.

EXTRINSIC ACTIVATION

ORGAN TISSUES
Myocardium
Prostate
Uterus

VASCULAR
ENDOTHELIUM

INTRINSIC ACTIVATION

HMW Kininogen
Kallikrein
Factor XIIa
Plasma Proactivator

SECRETIONS

Urine (Urokinase)
Tears
Saliva
Semen
Milk

PLASMINOGEN
ACTIVATORS

Streptokinase

Thrombin

PLASMINOGEN

PLASMIN - - - - > ANTIPLASMINS - - - - α_2-antiplasmin
α_2-macroglobulin
α_1-antitrypsin
antithrombin-III
C1 inactivator

FIBRIN ⟶ FIBRIN(OGEN) DEGRADATION PRODUCTS
(FIBRINOLYSIS)

FIGURE 2-2

Stage Four Activation of the Fibrinolytic System

PARTIAL THROMBOPLASTIN TIME (PTT); ACTIVATED PARTIAL THROMBOPLASTIN TIME (APTT) ●

Normal Values
APTT: 21–35 seconds
Check with your laboratory for therapeutic range values during heparin therapy.

Background
The PTT, a one-stage clotting test, screens for coagulation disorders. Specifically, it can detect deficiencies of the intrinsic thromboplastin system and also reveals defects in the extrinsic coagulation mechanism pathway.

NOTE: *The PTT and APTT test for the same functions. APTT is a more sensitive version of PTT that is used to monitor heparin therapy.*

Explanation of Test
The APTT is used to detect deficiencies in the intrinsic coagulation system, to detect incubating anticoagulants, and to monitor heparin therapy. It is part of a coagulation panel workup.

Procedure
1. A 7-ml venous blood sample is obtained and anticoagulated with sodium citrate. Use the 2-tube method. Place the specimen in a biohazard bag.
2. Do not draw blood samples from a heparin lock or heparinized catheter.
3. The sample may be transported at room temperature, but the vacuum must be intact (do not remove stopper). It is stable for 12 hours.

Clinical Implications
1. *Prolonged APTT* occurs in
   A. All congenital deficiencies of intrinsic system coagulation factors, including hemophilia A and hemophilia B
   B. Congenital deficiency of Fitzgerald's factor, Fletcher's factor (prekallikrein)
   C. Heparin therapy, streptokinase, urokinase
   D. Warfarin (Coumadin)-like therapy
   E. Vitamin K deficiency
   F. Hypofibrinogenemia
   G. Liver disease
   H. DIC (chronic or acute)
   I. Fibrin breakdown products
2. When APTT is performed in conjunction with a PT, a further clarification of coagulation defects is possible. For example, a normal PT with an abnormal APTT means that the defect lies within the first stage of the clotting cascade (factors VIII, IX, X, XI, and/or XII). The pattern of a normal PTT with an abnormal PT suggests a possible factor VII deficiency. If both PT and APTT are prolonged, a deficiency of factor I, II, V, or X is suggested.

Used together, APTT and PT will detect approximately 95% of coagulation defects.

3. *Shortened APTT* occurs in
   A. Extensive cancer, except when the liver is involved
   B. Immediately after acute hemorrhage
   C. Very early stages of DIC

4. *Circulating anticoagulants* (inhibitors) usually occur as inhibitors of a specific factor (eg, factor VIII). These are most commonly seen in the development of anti-factor VIII or anti-factor IX in 5% to 10% of hemophiliac patients. Anticoagulants that develop in the treated hemophiliac are detected through prolonged APTT. Circulating anticoagulants are also associated with other conditions:
   A. After many plasma transfusions
   B. Drug reactions
   C. Tuberculosis
   D. Chronic glomerulonephritis
   E. SLE
   F. Rheumatoid arthritis

NOTE: *Mixing equal parts of patient plasma and normal plasma corrects the APTT if it is caused by a coagulation factor defect but does not correct the APTT to normal if it caused by a circulating inhibitor. A more sensitive test is the Russell viper venom test, which demonstrates the presence of the lupus anticoagulant. This test is unaffected by inhibitors of factor VIII or deficiencies of factors VIII, IX, XI, or XII; it is affected by deficiencies of factors II, V, or X and by the use of sodium, warfarin, or heparin. Because lupus-type anticoagulants vary greatly in their reactivity in various test systems, it is recommended that this test be done in conjunction with the APTT and the anticardiolipin antibody assay. The reference range is 33.5–41.5 seconds.*

> ### Clinical Alert
>
> APTT >100 seconds signifies spontaneous bleeding.

5. *Heparin therapy:* In deep vein thrombosis or acute myocardial infarction, the usual protocol requires injection of heparin (monitored by the APTT), followed by long-term therapy with oral anticoagulants (monitored by the PT, APTT, or both).
   A. In the blood, heparin combines with an α-globulin (heparin cofactor) to form a potent antithrombin. It is a direct anticoagulant.
   B. Intravenous heparin injection produces an immediate anticoagulant effect; it is chosen when rapid anticoagulant effects are desired.
   C. Because the half-life of heparin is 3 hours, the APTT is measured 3 hours after heparin administration.

D. Therapeutic APTT levels are ordinarily maintained at 2 to 2.5 times the normal values.

E. To evaluate heparin effects, blood is tested:

(1) For baseline values before therapy is initiated

(2) One hour before the next dose is due (when a 4-hour administration cycle is ordered)

(3) According to the patient's status (eg, bleeding)

Interfering Factors

1. See Appendix J for drugs that affect test outcomes.

Patient Preparation

1. Explain test purpose, procedure, benefits, and risks.

2. See Chapter 1 guidelines for safe, effective, informed, *pretest* care.

3. Draw blood sample 1 hour before next dose of heparin. The heparin dose given relates to the APTT result.

Patient Aftercare for APTT

1. Interpret test outcome and monitor appropriately. Protamine sulfate is the antidote for heparin overdose or for reversal of heparin anticoagulation therapy.

2. Follow Chapter 1 guidelines for safe, effective, informed *posttest* care.

3. Watch for signs of spontaneous bleeding, notify physician immediately and treat accordingly.

4. Alert the patient to watch for bleeding gums, hematuria, oozing from wounds, and excessive bruising.

5. Instruct the patient to use an electric shaver instead of a blade and to exercise caution in all activities.

6. Avoid use of aspirin or ASA-like drugs (unless specifically prescribed) because they contribute to bleeding tendencies.

ACTIVATED COAGULATION TIME (ACT) ●

Normal Values

ACT: 150–180 seconds
Therapeutic range: 75–120 seconds

Background and Explanation of Test

This test evaluates coagulation status. The ACT responds linearly to heparin level changes and responds to wider ranges of heparin concentrations than does the APTT.

The ACT can be a bedside procedure and requires only 0.4 ml of blood. Heparin infusion or reversal with protamine can then be titrated almost immediately according to the ACT results. ACT also is routinely used during dialysis, coronary artery bypass procedures, arteriograms, and percutaneous transluminal coronary arteriography. This test is hard to standardize, and no controls are available; therefore, it is not in widespread use.

PROTHROMBIN TIME (PRO TIME; PT) ●

Normal Values
PT: 11.0–13.0 seconds (can vary by laboratory)
Therapeutic levels are at a P/C ratio of 2.0–2.5. Recommended therapeutic ranges are shown in the following table:

Therapeutic Context	INR	Target
Preoperative oral anticoagulant started 2 wk before surgery		
Non–hip surgery	1.5–2.5	2.0
Hip surgery	2.0–3.0	2.5
Primary and secondary prevention of deep vein thrombosis	2.0–3.0	2.5
Prevention of systemic embolism in patients with atrial fibrillation	2.0–3.0	2.5
Recurrent systemic embolism	3.0–4.5	3.5
Prevention of recurrent deep vein thrombosis (≥2 episodes)	2.5–4.0	3.0
Cardiac stents	3.0–4.5	3.5
Prevention of arterial thrombosis, including patients with mechanical heart valves	3.0–4.5	3.5

DEFINITIONS

- *P/C ratio (prothrombin time ratio):* the observed patient PT divided by the laboratory PT mean normal value
- *INR (International Normalized Ratio):* a comparative rating of PT ratios (representing the observed PT ratio adjusted by the International Reference Thromboplastin)
- *ISI (International Sensitivity Index):* a comparative rating of thromboplastin (supplied by the manufacturer of the reagent)

Background
Prothrombin is a protein produced by the liver for clotting of blood. Prothrombin production depends on adequate vitamin K intake and absorption. During the clotting process, prothrombin is converted to thrombin. The prothrombin content of the blood is reduced in patients with liver disease.

Explanation of Test
The PT is 1 of the 4 most important screening tests used in diagnostic coagulation studies. It directly measures a potential defect in stage II of the clotting mechanism through analysis of the clotting ability of 5 plasma coagulation factors (prothrombin, fibrinogen, factor V, factor VII, and factor X). This is known as the pro time, and it is commonly ordered during management of oral anticoagulant (Coumadin) therapy.

Procedure

1. A 5-ml venous blood sample is drawn (by the 2-tube technique) into a tube containing a calcium-binding anticoagulant (sodium citrate). The ratio of sodium citrate to blood is critical.
2. Blue-top vacuum tubes keep prothrombin levels stable at room temperature for 12 hours if left capped (vacuum intact). Place the specimen in biohazard bag.

Oral Anticoagulant Therapy

Oral anticoagulant drugs (eg, Coumadin, dicumarol) are commonly prescribed to treat blood clots. These are *indirect* anticoagulants (compared with heparin, which is a direct anticoagulant). However, if necessary, heparin is the anticoagulant of choice for initiating treatment because it acts rapidly and also partially lyses the clot.

1. These drugs act via the liver to delay coagulation by interfering with the action of the vitamin K–related factors (II, VII, IX, and X), which promote clotting.
2. Oral anticoagulants delay vitamin K formation and cause the PT to increase as a result of decreased factors II, VII, IX, and X.
3. The usual procedure is to run a PT test every day when beginning therapy. The anticoagulant dose is adjusted until the therapeutic range is reached. Then, weekly to monthly PT testing continues for the duration of therapy.
4. Coumadin takes 48 to 72 hours to cause a measurable change in the PT (3 to 4 days of drug therapy).

Drug Therapy and PT Protocols

1. Patients with cardiac problems are usually maintained at a PT level 2 to 2.5 times the normal (baseline) values.
2. Use of the INR values allows more sensitive control. A reasonable INR target for virtually all thromboembolic problems is 2.0 to 3.0. See the table for more specific guidelines.
3. For treatment of blood clots, the PT is maintained within 2 to 2.5 times normal. If the PT drops below this range, treatment may be ineffective and old clots may expand or new clots may form. Conversely, if the PT rises above 30 seconds, bleeding or hemorrhage may occur.

Clinical Implications

1. Conditions that cause *increased PT* include
   A. Deficiency of factors II (prothrombin), V, VII, or X
   B. Vitamin K deficiency
   C. Hemorrhagic disease of the newborn
   D. Liver disease (eg, alcoholic hepatitis), liver damage
   E. Current anticoagulant therapy with Coumadin
   F. Biliary obstruction
   G. Poor fat absorption (eg, sprue, celiac disease, chronic diarrhea)

H. Hypervitaminosis
I. DIC
J. Zollinger-Ellison syndrome
K. Hypofibrinogenemia (factor I deficiency)
L. SLE (circulating anticoagulants)
2. Conditions that cause *decreased PT* include
   A. Ovarian hyperfunction
   B. Regional enteritis or ileitis
3. Conditions that *do not affect the PT* include
   A. Polycythemia vera
   B. Tannin disease
   C. Christmas disease (factor IX deficiency)
   D. Hemophilia A (factor VIII deficiency)
   E. von Willebrand's disease
   F. Platelet disorders (idiopathic thrombocytopenic purpura)

Interfering Factors
1. Diet: Ingestion of excessive green, leafy vegetables increases the body's absorption of vitamin K, which promotes blood clotting.
2. Alcoholism or excessive alcohol ingestion raises PT levels.
3. Diarrhea and vomiting decrease PT because of dehydration.
4. Quality of venipuncture: PT can be shortened if technique is traumatic and tissue thromboplastin is introduced to the sample.
5. Influence of prescribed medications: antibiotics, aspirin, cimetidine, isoniazid, phenothiazines, cephalosporins, cholestyramines, phenylbutazone, metronidazole, oral hypoglycemics, phenytoin.

Patient Preparation
1. Explain the purpose, procedure, and need for frequent testing. Emphasize the need for regular monitoring through frequent blood testing if long-term therapy is prescribed. *Do not refer to anticoagulants as "blood thinners."* One explanation might be, "Your blood will be tested periodically to determine the pro time, which is an indication of how the blood clots." The anticoagulant dose will be adjusted according to PT results.
2. Caution against self-medication. Ascertain what drugs the patient has been taking. Many drugs, including over-the-counter medications, alter the effects of anticoagulants and the PT value. Aspirin, acetaminophen, and laxative products should be avoided unless specifically ordered by the physician.
3. Instruct the patient never to start or discontinue any drug without the doctor's permission. This will affect PT values and may also interfere with the healing process.
4. Counsel regarding diet. Excessive amounts of green, leafy vegetables (eg, spinach, broccoli) will increase vitamin K levels and could interfere with anticoagulant metabolism. Caution against using razor blades; electric shavers should be used.
5. These guidelines also apply to aftercare.

Patient Aftercare

1. Interpret test outcomes and monitor appropriately with follow-up testing and observation.

2. Avoid intramuscular injections during anticoagulant therapy, because hematomas may form at the injection site. As the PT increases to upper limits (>30 minutes), assess carefully for bleeding from different areas; this may require neurologic assessment (if cranial bleeding is suspected), lung assessment and auscultation, gastrointestinal and genitourinary assessments, or other assessments as appropriate. Instruct the patient to observe for bleeding from gums, in the urine, or other unusual bleeding. Advise that care should be exercised in all activities to avoid accidental injury.

3. Patients who are being monitored by PT for long-term anticoagulant therapy should not take any other drugs unless they have been specifically prescribed.

4. When unexpected adjustments in anticoagulant doses are required to maintain a stable PT, or when there are erratic changes in PT levels, a drug interaction should be suspected and further investigation should take place.

5. Changes in exercise intensity should be made gradually or avoided. Active sports and contact sports should be avoided because of the potential for injury.

6. See Chapter 1 guidelines for safe, effective, informed *posttest* care.

Clinical Alert

1. *Critical value:* If P/C is >2.5 or >30.0 seconds, notify clinician.
2. If PT is excessively prolonged (>40 seconds), vitamin K may be ordered.
3. Baseline PT levels should be determined before anticoagulant administration.
4. *Critical value:* INR >3.6; notify clinician.

COAGULANT FACTORS (FACTOR ASSAY)   ●

Normal Values

Factor II:	80%–120% of normal
Factor V:	50%–150% of normal
Factor VII:	65%–140% of normal or 65–135 AU
Factor VIII:	55%–145% of normal or 55–145 AU
Factor IX:	60%–140% of normal or 60–140 AU
Factor X:	45%–155% of normal or 45–155 AU
Factor XI:	65%–135% of normal or 65–135 AU
Factor XII:	50%–150% of normal or 50–150 AU
Ristocetin (von Willebrand's factor):	45%–140% of normal or 45–140 AU
Factor VIII antigen:	50–150 mg/dl
Factor VIII–related antigen:	45%–185% of normal or 45–185 AU

Fletcher's factor (prekallikrein):　　80%–120% of normal
Critical value for any　　<10% of normal
　　coagulation factor:

Explanation of Test
This test of specific factors of coagulation is done in the investigation of inherited and acquired bleeding disorders. For example, tests of factor VIII–related antigen are used in the differential diagnosis of classic hemophilia and von Willebrand's disease in cases in which there is no family history of bleeding and bleeding times are borderline or abnormal. A test for ristocetin cofactor is done to help diagnose von Willebrand's disease by determining the degree or rate of platelet aggregation that is taking place.

Procedure
1. A 5-ml venous blood sample is drawn by the 2-tube method and is added to a collection tube containing sodium citrate as the anticoagulant.
2. Samples are capped, put on ice, and sent to the laboratory as soon as possible.

Clinical Implications
1. *Inherited deficiencies:*
   A. Any of the specific factors—I, V, VII, VIII, IX, X, XI, XII, and XIII—may be deficient on a familial basis. Factor VII is decreased in hypoproconvertinemia (autosomal recessive); factor VIII is decreased in classic hemophilia A and von Willebrand's disease (inherited autosomally); factor IX is decreased in Christmas disease or hemophilia B (sex-linked recessive); and factor XI is decreased in hemophilia C (autosomal dominant, occurring predominantly in Jews).
2. *Acquired disorders:*
   A. Factor VII is decreased in
      (1) Liver disease
      (2) Treatment with coumarin-type drugs
      (3) Hemorrhagic disease of the newborn
      (4) Kwashiorkor
   B. Factor VIII is increased in
      (1) Late normal pregnancy
      (2) Thromboembolic conditions
      (3) Coronary artery disease
      (4) Postoperative period
      (5) Rebound activity after sudden cessation of a coumarin-type drug
   C. Factor IX is decreased in
      (1) Uncompensated cirrhosis, liver disease
      (2) Nephrotic syndrome
      (3) Development of circulating anticoagulants against factor IX
      (4) Normal newborn
      (5) Dicumarol and related anticoagulant drugs

(6) DIC

(7) Vitamin K deficiency

D. Factor XI is decreased in

(1) Liver disease

(2) Intestinal malabsorption (vitamin K)

(3) Occasional development of circulatory anticoagulants against factor IX

(4) Congenital heart disease

(5) PNH

(6) DIC

(7) Newborns

E. Factor XII is decreased in the nephrotic syndrome.

F. Factor VIII is decreased in

(1) Presence of factor VIII inhibitors (anticoagulants capable of specifically neutralizing a coagulation factor and thereby disrupting hemostasis), associated with hemophilia A and immunologic reactions

(2) von Willebrand's disease

(3) DIC

G. Factor VIII–related antigen is low in von Willebrand's disease and normal in hemophilia.

H. Ristocetin cofactor is decreased in von Willebrand's disease and in Bernard-Soulier disease, an intrinsic platelet defect.

I. Factor X is increased during normal pregnancy.

J. Factor X is decreased in

(1) Vitamin K deficiency

(2) Liver disease

(3) Oral anticoagulants

K. Factor XII is increased after exercise.

L. Factor XIII is decreased in

(1) Postoperative patients

(2) Liver disease

(3) Persistent increased fibrinogen levels

(4) Obstetric complications with hypofibrinogenemia

(5) Acute myelogenous leukemia

(6) Circulating anticoagulants

PLASMINOGEN (PLASMIN; FIBRINOLYSIN)   ●

Normal Values

Plasminogen Activity
Males: 76%–124% of normal for plasma
Females: 65%–153% of normal for plasma
Infants: 27%–59% of normal for plasma

Background

Plasminogen is a glycoprotein present in plasma. Under normal circumstances, plasminogen is a part of any clot because of the tendency of fibrin to absorb plasminogen from the plasma. When plasminogen activators perform their function, plasmin is formed within the clot; this gradually dissolves the clot while leaving time for tissue repair. Free plasmin also is released to the plasma; however, antiplasmins there immediately destroy any plasmin released from the clot (see Figure 2–2).

Explanation of Test

This test is done to determine plasminogen activity in persons with thrombosis or DIC. When pathologic coagulation processes are involved, excessive free plasmin is released to the plasma. In these situations, the available antiplasmin is depleted, and plasmin begins destroying components other than fibrin, including fibrinogen, factors V and VIII, and other factors. Plasmin acts more quickly to destroy fibrinogen because of fibrinogen's instability.

For therapeutic destruction of thrombi, urokinase, a trypsin-like protease purified from urine, may be administered to a patient to activate plasminogen to plasmin and induce fibrinolysis. Streptokinase is another therapeutic agent used for the same purpose.

Procedure

1. A 5-ml venous blood sample is added to a collection tube containing sodium citrate. The 2-tube method is used. Place the specimen in a biohazard bag.
2. The sample is put on ice and transported to the laboratory immediately.
3. The test must be started within 30 minutes after the blood is drawn.

Clinical Implications

1. *Decreased* plasminogen activity occurs in
    A. Some familial or isolated cases of idiopathic deep vein thrombosis
    B. DIC and systemic fibrinolysis
    C. Liver disease and cirrhosis
    D. Neonatal hyaline membrane disease
    E. Therapy with plasminogen activators
2. Decreased levels of plasminogen or abnormally functioning plasminogen can lead to venous and arterial clotting (thrombosis).
3. *Increased* plasminogen activity occurs in pregnancy (third trimester).

Interfering Factors

1. See Appendix J for drugs that affect test outcomes.

Patient Preparation

1. Explain test purpose and procedure.
2. See Chapter 1 guidelines for safe, effective, informed *pretest* care.

Patient Aftercare

1. Interpret test outcomes and monitor appropriately for thrombotic tendency.
2. See Chapter 1 guidelines for safe, effective, informed *posttest* care.

FIBRINOLYSIS (EUGLOBULIN LYSIS TIME) ●

Normal Values

Euglobulin lysis—no lysis of plasma clot at 37°C in 60–120 minutes. The clot is observed for 24 hours.

Background

Primary fibrinolysis, without any sign of intravascular coagulation, is extremely rare. Secondary fibrinolysis is usually seen and follows or occurs simultaneously with intravascular coagulation. This secondary fibrinolysis is thought to be a protective mechanism against generalized clotting.

Explanation of Test

This test is done to evaluate a fibrinolytic crisis. Shortened time indicates excessive fibrinolytic activity. Lysis is marked and rapid with primary fibrinolysis but is minimal in secondary fibrinolysis.

Procedure

1. A 5-ml venous blood sample is collected in a tube containing sodium citrate using the 2-tube method. Place the specimen in a biohazard bag.
2. The sample is put on ice and transported to the laboratory immediately.
3. The test must be started within 30 minutes after the blood is drawn.

> ### Clinical Alert
>
> A lysis time <1 hour signifies that abnormal fibrinolysis is occurring.

Clinical Implications

1. *Increased* fibrinolysis occurs in the following conditions:
   A. Within 48 hours after surgery
   B. Primary fibrinolysis
   C. Cancer of prostate or pancreas
   D. Circulatory collapse
   E. During lung and cardiac surgery
   F. Obstetric complications (eg, antepartum hemorrhage, amniotic embolism, septic abortion, death of fetus, hydatidiform mole)
   G. Long-term DIC
   H. Liver disease
   I. Administration of plasminogen activators (tPA, streptokinase, urokinase)
2. Heparin does not interfere with this test.

Interfering Factors

1. Increased fibrinolysis occurs with moderate exercise and increasing age.
2. Decreased fibrinolysis occurs in arterial blood, compared with venous blood. This difference is greater in arteriosclerosis (especially in young persons).
3. Decreased fibrinolysis occurs in postmenopausal women and in normal newborns.

4. FDPs interfere with fibrinolysis.
5. Normal results can occur if fibrinolysis is far advanced (plasminogen depleted).
6. Fibrinolysis is increased by very low fibrinogen levels (<80 mg/dl) and decreased by high fibrinogen levels.
7. Increased fibrinolysis can be caused by traumatic venipuncture or a tourniquet that is too tight.
8. See Appendix J for drugs that affect test outcomes.

Patient Preparation
1. Advise patient of test purpose and procedure; no exercise before test.
2. See Chapter 1 guidelines for safe, effective, informed *pretest* care.

Patient Aftercare
1. Interpret test results and monitor appropriately for fibrinolytic crisis.
2. See Chapter 1 guidelines for safe, effective, informed *posttest* care.

FIBRIN SPLIT PRODUCTS (FSP); FIBRIN DEGRADATION PRODUCTS (FDP) ●

Normal Values
Negative at 1:4 dilution or <10 μg/ml

Background
When fibrin is split by plasmin, positive tests for fibrin degradation (split) products, identified by the letters X, Y, D, and E, are produced. These products have an anticoagulant action and inhibit clotting when they are present in excess in the circulation. Increased levels of FDPs may occur with a variety of pathologic processes in which clot formation and lysis occur.

Explanation of Test
This test is done to establish the diagnosis of DIC and other thromboembolic disorders.

Procedure
1. A venous blood sample of at least 4.5 ml is placed in a tube containing thrombin and an inhibitor of fibrinolysis (reptilase, aprotinin, and calcium). Place the specimen in a biohazard bag.
2. Blood must be completely clotted before test is started for the test to be valid.

Clinical Implications
1. *Increased* FSP/FDP is associated with any condition associated with DIC (see pages 133 for examples) and in
   A. Venous thrombosis
   B. Primary fibrinolysis

C. After thoracic and cardiac surgery or renal transplantation
D. Acute myocardial infarction
E. Pulmonary embolism
F. Carcinoma

Interfering Factors

1. Because all of the laboratory methods are sensitive to fibrinogen as well as FDP, it is essential that no unclotted fibrinogen be left in the serum preparation. False-positive reactions can result if any fibrinogen is present.
2. False-positive results occur with heparin therapy.
3. The presence of rheumatoid factor (rheumatoid arthritis) may cause falsely high FSP/FDP values.
4. See Appendix J for drugs that affect test outcomes.

Patient Preparation

1. Explain test purpose and procedure.
2. See Chapter 1 guidelines for safe, effective, informed *pretest* care.

Patient Aftercare

1. Interpret test results and monitor appropriately for DIC and thrombosis.
2. See Chapter 1 guidelines for safe, effective, informed *posttest* care.

Clinical Alert

1. Patients with very high levels of FSP/FDP have blood that does not clot or clots poorly.
2. *Critical Value:* >160 µg/ml

D-DIMER ●

Normal Values

<250 ng/ml or <0.25mg/L
Qualitative: no D-dimer fragments present

Background

D-dimers are produced by the action of plasmin on cross-linked fibrin. They are not produced by the action of plasmin on unclotted fibrinogen or FDPs.

Explanation of Test

This test is used in the diagnosis of DIC disease and to screen for venous thrombosis. The D-dimer test is more specific for DIC than are tests for FSPs. The test verifies in vivo fibrinolysis because D-dimers are produced only by the action of plasmin on cross-linked fibrin, and not by the action of plasmin on unclotted fibrinogen. A positive D-dimer test is presumptive evidence for DIC.

Procedure

1. A venous blood sample of 4.5 ml is collected into a tube containing sodium citrate. It remains stable for 4 hours at room temperature. Place the specimen in biohazard bag.

Clinical Implications

1. *Increased* D-dimer values are associated with
   A. DIC (secondary fibrinolysis)
   B. Arterial or venous thrombosis
   C. Primary fibrinolysis
   D. Pulmonary embolism
   E. Late in pregnancy, postpartum
   F. Sickle cell crisis
   G. Malignancy
2. D-dimer values are increased with tPA anticoagulant therapy.

Interfering Factors

1. False-positive tests are obtained with high titers of rheumatoid factor.
2. False-positive D-dimer levels increase as the tumor marker CA-125 for ovarian cancer increases.
3. The D-dimer test will be positive in all patients after surgery or trauma.

Patient Preparation

1. Explain test purpose and procedure.
2. See Chapter 1 guidelines for safe, effective, informed *pretest* care.

Patient Aftercare

1. Interpret test outcome and monitor appropriately for DIC or thrombin.
2. See Chapter 1 guidelines for safe, effective, informed *posttest* care.

FIBRINOPEPTIDE A (FPA) ●

Normal Values
None present

Explanation of Test
This measurement is the most sensitive assay done to determine thrombin action. FPA reflects the amount of active intravascular blood clotting; this occurs in a subclinical DIC, which is common in patients with leukemia of various types and may be associated with tumor progression. FPA elevations can occur without intravascular thrombosis, decreasing the value of a positive test.

Procedure
1. A venous blood sample of 4.5 ml is collected in blue-top Vacutainer tube containing aprotinin to prevent activation in vitro. Place the specimen in a biohazard bag.

Clinical Implications
1. *Increased* FPA occurs in
   A. DIC
   B. Leukemia of various types
   C. Venous thrombosis and pulmonary embolus
   D. Infections
   E. Postoperative patients
   F. Patients with widespread solid tumors
2. *Decreased* FPA occurs when clinical remission of leukemia is achieved with chemotherapy.

Interfering Factors
1. A traumatic venous puncture may result in falsely increased levels.
2. The biologic half-life (stable for 2 hours or more) imposes limitations on the interpretation of a negative FPA test.

Clinical Alert

DIC occurs commonly in association with death of tumor cells in acute promyelocytic leukemia. For this reason, heparin is used prophylactically and in association with the initiation of chemotherapy for promyelocytic leukemia. DIC occurs less commonly during the treatment of acute myelomonocytic leukemia and acute lymphocyte leukemia. Evidence of DIC should be sought in every patient with leukemia before initiation of treatment.

Patient Preparation
1. Explain test purpose and procedure.
2. Avoid prolonged use of tourniquet.
3. See Chapter 1 guidelines for safe, effective, informed *pretest* care.

Patient Aftercare
1. Interpret test outcome and monitor appropriately for DIC and thrombosis.
2. See Chapter 1 guidelines for safe, effective, informed *posttest* care.
3. Resume normal activities.

PROTHROMBIN F1+2 ASSAY ●

Normal Values
0.5–1.9 nmol/L

Background
The prothrombin F1+2 fragment is liberated from the prothrombin molecule when it is activated by factor Xa to form thrombin. Thrombin may be rapidly inactivated by antithrombin III. The F1+2 fragment, however, has a half-life of about 1.5 hours, making it a useful marker for activated coagulation.

Explanation of Test
Prothrombin F1+2 is used to detect activation of the coagulation system before actual thrombosis occurs. It is used to identify patients with low-grade intravascular coagulation (DIC) and to judge the effectiveness of oral anticoagulant therapy.

Procedure
1. A 4.5-ml sample of venous blood is drawn into a blue-top (sodium citrate anticoagulant) Vacutainer using the 2-tube technique.

Clinical Implications
1. *Increased* prothrombin F1+2 is found in
   A. DIC (early)
   B. Congenital deficiencies of antithrombin III
   C. Congenital deficiencies of protein S and protein C
   D. Patients receiving inadequate amounts of oral anticoagulants (Coumadin).
2. *Decreased* prothrombin F1+2 is found in patients receiving adequate amounts of Coumadin.

NOTE: *Failure to achieve a reduction in prothrombin F1+2 levels during oral anticoagulant therapy, despite an adequately prolonged PT, suggests inadequate anticoagulation.*

Interfering Factors
Levels will be high in the immediate postoperative period.

Patient Preparation
1. Explain test purpose and procedure.
2. Avoid prolonged use of tourniquet.
3. See Chapter 1 guidelines for safe, effective, informed *pretest* care.

Patient Aftercare
1. Interpret test outcome and monitor appropriately for DIC and thrombosis.
2. See Chapter 1 guidelines for safe, effective, informed *posttest* care.
3. Resume normal activities.

FIBRIN MONOMERS (PROTAMINE SULFATE TEST) ●

Normal Values
Negative; no fibrin monomer present

Background
A positive test result reflects the presence of fibrin monomers, indicative of thrombin activity and consistent with a diagnosis of intravascular coagulation. A negative result does not mean that intravascular coagulation is not present. A positive result may also be seen in some cases of severe liver disease and

in inflammatory disorders caused by accumulation of products of coagulation in the circulation.

Explanation of Test

The detection of fibrin monomers and early-stage FSPs in plasma is useful in the diagnosis of DIC. Heparin therapy does not interfere with this test.

Procedure

1. Obtain a 4.5-ml venous blood sample anticoagulated with sodium citrate (blue-top tube). The 2-tube technique is used. Place the specimen on ice and transport to the laboratory. The test must be performed within 1 hour after collection.

Clinical Implications

1. A positive test is indicative of DIC.
2. Patients with deep vein thrombosis occasionally have positive results.
3. The test may be positive in severe liver disease or metastatic cancer.

Interfering Factors

False-positive results may occur in the following situations:

1. Traumatic venipuncture
2. During or immediately before menstruation
3. During streptokinase therapy (thrombolytic therapy)

Patient Preparation

1. Explain test purpose and procedure.
2. Avoid prolonged use of tourniquet.
3. See Chapter 1 guidelines for safe, effective, informed *pretest* care.

Patient Aftercare

1. Interpret test outcome and monitor appropriately for DIC and thrombosis.
2. See Chapter 1 guidelines for safe, effective, informed *posttest* care.
3. Resume normal activities.

FIBRINOGEN

Normal Values

200–400 mg/dl or 2.0–4.0 g/L

Background

Fibrinogen is a complex protein (polypeptide) that, with enzyme action, is converted to fibrin. The fibrin, along with platelets, forms the network for the common blood clot. Although it is of primary importance as a coagulation protein, fibrinogen is also an acute phase protein reactant. It is increased in diseases involving tissue damage or inflammation.

Explanation of Test
This test is done to investigate abnormal PT, APTT, and TT and to screen for DIC and fibrin-fibrinogenolysis. It is part of a coagulation panel.

Procedure
1. A venous blood sample is obtained with a collection tube containing sodium citrate. The 2-tube method is used. Place the specimen in a biohazard bag.

Clinical Implications
1. *Increased* fibrinogen values occur in
   A. Inflammation (rheumatoid arthritis, pneumonia, tuberculosis, streptomycin)
   B. Acute myocardial infarction
   C. Nephrotic syndrome
   D. Cancer, multiple myeloma, Hodgkin's disease
   F. Pregnancy, eclampsia
   G. Various cerebral accidents and diseases
2. *Decreased* fibrinogen occur in
   A. Liver disease
   B. DIC (secondary fibrinolysis)
   C. Cancer
   D. Primary fibrinolysis
   E. Hereditary and congenital hypofibrinogenemia
   F. Dysfibrinogenemia

Interfering Factors
1. High levels of heparin interfere with test results.
2. High levels of FSP/FDP cause low fibrinogen values.
3. Oral contraceptives cause high fibrinogen values.
4. Elevated antithrombin III may cause decreased fibrinogen.
5. See Appendix J for other drugs that affect test outcomes.

> **Clinical Alert**
> _____
>
> 1. Values <50 mg/dl can result in hemorrhage after traumatic surgery.
> 2. Values >700 mg/dl constitute a significant risk for both coronary artery and cerebrovascular disease.

Patient Preparation
1. Explain test purpose and procedure.
2. Aggressive muscular exercise should be avoided before the test.
3. See Chapter 1 guidelines for safe, effective, informed *pretest* care.

Patient Aftercare
1. Interpret test outcome and monitor appropriately for DIC and response to treatment. If fibrinogen is low, cryoprecipitate is the preferred product for therapeutic replacement.
2. See Chapter 1 guidelines for safe, effective, informed *posttest* care.

PROTEIN C (PC ANTIGEN) ●

Normal Values
Qualitative: 71%–142% of increased functional activity
Quantitative: 67%–125% of normal PC antigen

Background
Protein C, a vitamin K–dependent protein that prevents thrombosis, is produced in the liver and circulated in the plasma. It functions as an anticoagulant by inactivating factors V and VIII. Protein C is also a profibrinolytic agent
(ie, it enhances fibrinolysis). The protein C mechanism therefore functions to
prevent extension of intravascular thrombi.

Explanation of Test
This test evaluates patients with severe thrombosis and those with an increased
risk or predisposition to thrombosis. Patients with partial protein C or partial
protein S deficiency (heterozygotes) may experience venous thrombotic
episodes, usually in early adult years. There may be deep vein thromboses,
episodes of thrombophlebitis or pulmonary emboli (or both), and manifestations of a hypercoagulable state. Patients who are heterozygous may have type
I protein C deficiency, with decreased protein C antigen, or type II deficiency,
with normal protein C antigen levels but decreased functional activity.

> **NOTE:** *The protein S level should always be determined when a protein C
> test is ordered.*

Procedure
1. A 45-ml venous blood sample is anticoagulated with sodium citrate (blue-
   top tube). The 2-tube method is used. The specimen should be capped and
   placed on ice.

Clinical Implications
1. *Decreased* protein C is associated with
   A. Severe thrombotic complications in the neonatal period (neonatal purpura fulminans)
   B. Increased risk of venous thrombolic episodes
   C. Warfarin (Coumadin)–induced skin necroses (pathognomonic for protein C deficiency)
   D. DIC, especially when it occurs with cancer (presumably owing to consumption by cofactor thrombin-thrombomodulin catalyst activities)
   E. Thrombophlebitis and pulmonary embolism, especially in early adult years
   F. Other acquired causes of protein C deficiency include
   (1) Liver disease
   (2) Acute respiratory distress syndrome
   (3) L-Asparagine therapy
   (4) Malignancies
2. A deficiency of protein C may also be *congenital* (35%–58%).

> **Clinical Alert**
>
> Homozygous protein C–deficient patients have absent or almost absent protein C antigen and usually succumb in infancy with the picture of purpura fulminans neonatalis, including lower extremity skin ecchymoses, anemia, fever, and shock.

Interfering Factors

1. Decreased protein C is found in the postoperative state.
2. Pregnancy or use of oral contraceptives decreases protein C.
3. A transient drop in protein C occurs with a high loading dose of warfarin.
4. Protein C decreases with age.

NOTE: *This test is not useful in diagnosing DIC.*

Patient Preparation

1. Explain test purpose and procedure.
2. See Chapter 1 guidelines for safe, effective, informed *pretest* care.

Patient Aftercare

1. Interpret test outcome and monitor appropriately for thrombosis. In the case of a protein C deficiency, educate the patient concerning the symptoms and implications of the disease. The risk factors include obesity, oral contraceptives, varicose veins, infection, trauma, surgery, pregnancy, immobility, and congestive heart failure.
2. See Chapter 1 guidelines for safe, effective, informed *posttest* care.

PROTEIN S

Normal Values

Male: 78–130% of normal activity
Female: 70–120% of normal activity

Background

Both protein S and protein C are dependent on vitamin K for their production and function. A deficiency of either one is associated with a tendency toward thrombosis. Protein S serves as a cofactor to enhance the anticoagulant effects of activated protein C. Slightly more than half of protein S is complexed with C4 binding protein and is inactive. Activated protein C in the presence of protein S rapidly inactivates factors V and VIII.

Explanation of Test

This test is done to differentiate acquired from congenital protein S deficiency. Congenital deficiency of protein S is associated with a high risk of thromboembolism. Acquired deficiency of protein S can be seen in various autoimmune disorders and inflammatory states owing to elevation of C4 binding protein. This protein forms an inactive complex with protein S. C4 binding protein levels should be determined in all patients who demonstrate a reduced level of protein S.

Procedure

1. A venous blood sample is anticoagulated with sodium citrate (blue-top tube). The 2-tube method is used. Keep the specimen capped and on ice.

Clinical Implications

1. *Decreased values* are associated with protein S deficiency. Familial protein S deficiency is associated with recurrent thrombosis. Abnormal plasma distribution of protein S occurs in functional protein S deficiency. In type I, free protein S is decreased, although the level of total protein may be normal; in type II, total protein is markedly reduced.
2. Hypercoagulable-state acquired protein S deficiency is found in
   A. Diabetic nephropathy
   B. Chronic renal failure caused by hypertension
   C. Cerebral venous thrombosis
   D. Coumarin-induced skin necrosis
   E. DIC

Interfering Factors

The following factors cause *decreased* protein S:

1. Heparin therapy or specimen contaminated with heparin
2. Patient on unstable warfarin (Coumadin should be discontinued for 30 days for true a protein S determination)
3. Pregnancy
4. Contraceptives (oral)
5. First month of life
6. L-asparaginase therapy

   NOTE: *This test is not useful in diagnosing DIC.*

Patient Preparation

1. Explain test purpose and procedure.
2. See Chapter 1 guidelines for safe, effective, informed *pretest* care.

Patient Aftercare

1. Interpret test outcome and monitor appropriately for thrombotic tendency.
2. See Chapter 1 guidelines for safe, effective, informed *posttest* care.

ANTITHROMBIN III (AT-III; HEPARIN COFACTOR ACTIVITY) ●

Normal Values

Functional Assay
Infants (1–30 days): 26%–61% (premature); 44%–76% (full-term)
Adults and infants older than 6 months: 80%–120%

Immunologic Assay
17–30 mg/dl

Background

AT-III inhibits the activity of activated factors XII, XI, IX, and X as well as factor II. AT-III is the main physiologic inhibitor of activated factor X, on which it appears to exert its most critical effect. AT-III is a "heparin cofactor." Heparin interacts with AT-III and thrombin, increasing the rate of thrombin neutralization (inhibition) but decreasing the total quantity of thrombin inhibited.

Explanation of Test

This test detects a decreased level of antithrombin that is indicative of thrombotic tendency. Only the test of functional activity gives a direct clue to thrombotic tendency. In some families, several members may have a combination of recurrent thromboembolism and reduced plasma antithrombin (30%–60%). A significant number of patients with mesenteric venous thrombosis have AT III deficiency. It has been recommended that patients with such thrombotic disease be screened for AT III levels to identify those patients who may benefit from coumarin anticoagulant prophylaxis.

Procedure

1. A venous blood sample (4.5 ml) is anticoagulated with sodium citrate.
2. The 2-tube method is used.
3. The sample is placed on ice and transported to laboratory immediately.

Clinical Implications

1. *Increased AT-III values* are associated with
  A. Acute hepatitis
  B. Renal transplant
  C. Inflammation
  D. Menstruation
  E. Use of warfarin (Coumadin) anticoagulant
  F. Hyperglobulinemia
2. *Decreased AT-III values* are associated with
  A. Congenital deficiency (hereditary)
  B. Liver transplant and partial liver removal
  C. DIC
  D. Nephrotic syndrome

E. Active thrombotic disease (deep vein thrombosis)
F. Cirrhosis, chronic liver failure
G. Carcinoma
H. Pulmonary embolism
I. Heparin failure
J. Fibrinolytic disorders
K. Gram-negative septicemia

Interfering Factors
1. Antithrombin decreases after 3 days of heparin therapy.
2. Use of oral contraceptives interferes with the test.
3. Results are unreliable in the last trimester of pregnancy and in the early postpartum period.
4. Decreased after surgery.

Patient Preparation
1. Explain test purpose and procedure.
2. See Chapter 1 guidelines for safe, effective, informed *pretest* care.

Patient Aftercare
1. Interpret test outcome and monitor appropriately for thrombotic tendency.
2. If patient has decreased levels of AT-III, coumarin anticoagulant would be used as a prophylaxis.
3. See Chapter 1 guidelines for safe, effective, informed *posttest* care.

BIBLIOGRAPHY

Dahlback B: Resistance to activated protein C as risk factor for thrombosis: Molecular mechanisms, laboratory investigation, and clinical management. Semin Hematol 34(3): 217–234, 1997

Freeman J, Rodgers BA: Lupus: A Patient Care Guide for Nurses and Other Health Professionals. Bethesda, National Institute of Health, National Institute of Arthritis and Musculoskeletal and Skin Diseases, 1999

Goroll AH, May LA, Mulley GA: Primary Care Medicine: Office Evaluation and Management of the Adult Patient, 3rd ed. Philadelphia, JB Lippincott, 1995

Henry J, et al: Clinical Diagnosis and Management by Laboratory Methods, 19th ed. Philadelphia, WB Saunders, 1996

Koepke J: Is ESR useful? Medical Laboratory Observer 29(1): June 1997

Krenzischek DA, Tanseco FV: Comparative study of bedside and laboratory measurements of hemoglobin. Am J Crit Care 5(6): 427, 1996

Looker AC, Dallman PR, Carroll MD, et al: Prevalence of iron deficiency in the United States. JAMA 277: 973, 1997

Lotspeich-Steininger CA, Steine-Martin EA, Koepke JA: Clinical Hematology: Principles, Procedures, Correlations. Philadelphia, JB Lippincott, 1992

Speicher CE: The Right Test: A Physician's Guide to Laboratory Medicine, 3rd ed. Philadelphia, WB Saunders, 1998

Statland B: Tips from clinical experts. Medical Laboratory Observer 29(1): June 1997

3

Urine Studies

OVERVIEW OF URINE STUDIES ●

Urine Formation

Urine is continuously formed by the kidneys. It is actually an ultrafiltrate of plasma from which glucose, amino acids, water, and other substances essential to body metabolism have been reabsorbed. The physiologic process by which approximately 170,000 ml of filtered plasma is converted to the average daily urine output of 1200 ml is complex.

Urine formation takes place in the kidneys, 2 fist-sized organs located outside the peritoneal cavity on each side of the spine, at about the level of the last thoracic and first 2 lumbar vertebrae. The kidneys, together with the skin and the respiratory system, are the chief excretory organs of the body. Each kidney is a highly discriminatory organ that maintains the internal environment of the body by selective secretion or reabsorption of various substances according to specific body needs.

The main functional unit of the kidney is the nephron. There are about 1 to 1.5 million nephrons per kidney, each composed of 2 main parts: a glomerulus, which is essentially a filtering system, and a tubule through which the filtered liquid passes. Each glomerulus consists of a capillary network surrounded by a membrane called *Bowman's capsule,* which continues on to form the beginning of the renal tubule. The kidney's ability to selectively clear waste products from the blood while maintaining the essential water and electrolyte balances in the body is controlled in the nephron by renal blood flow, glomerular filtration, and tubular reabsorption and secretion.

Blood is supplied to the kidney by the renal artery and enters the nephron through the afferent arteriole. It flows through the glomerulus and into the efferent arteriole. The varying size of these arterioles creates the hydrostatic pressure difference necessary for glomerular filtration and serves to maintain glomerular capillary pressure and consistent renal blood flow within the glomerulus. (The smaller size of the efferent arteriole produces an increase in the glomerular capillary pressure, which aids in urine formation.)

As the filtrate passes along the tubule, more solutes are added by excretion from the capillary blood and secretions from the tubular epithelial cells. Essential solutes and water pass back into the blood through the mechanism of tubular reabsorption. Finally, urine concentration and dilution occur in the renal medulla. The kidney has the remarkable ability to dilute or concentrate urine, according to the needs of the individual, and to regulate sodium excretion. Blood chemistry, blood pressure, fluid balance, and nutrient intake, together with the general state of health, are key elements in this entire metabolic process.

Urine Constituents

In general, urine consists of urea and other organic and inorganic chemicals dissolved in water. Considerable variations in the concentrations of these substances can occur as a result of the influence of factors such as dietary intake, physical activity, body metabolism, endocrine function, and even body position. Urea, a metabolic waste product produced in the liver from the breakdown of protein and amino acids, accounts for almost half of the total dissolved solids in urine. Other organic substances include primarily creatinine and uric acid. The major inorganic solid dissolved in urine is chloride, followed by sodium and potassium. Small or trace amounts of many additional inorganic chemicals are also present in urine. The concentrations of these inorganic compounds are greatly influenced by dietary intake, making it difficult to establish normal levels. Other substances found in urine include hormones, vitamins, and medications. Although they are not a part of the original plasma filtrate, the urine may also contain formed elements such as cells, casts, crystals, mucus, and bacteria. Increased amounts of these formed elements are often indicative of disease (Chart 3-1).

Types of Urine Specimens

During the course of 24 hours, the composition and concentration of urine changes continuously. Urine concentration varies according to water intake and pretest activities. To obtain a specimen that is truly representative of a patient's metabolic state, it is often necessary to regulate certain aspects of specimen collection, such as time of collection, length of collection period, patient's dietary and medicinal intake, and method of collection. It is important to instruct patients when special collection procedures must be followed. See Appendix A: Standard Precautions, Appendix B: Latex Precautions, and Appendix E: Guidelines for Specimen Transport for additional guidelines.

URINE TESTING ●

Urinalysis (UA) is an essential procedure for those persons undergoing hospital admission or physical examination. It is a useful indicator of a healthy or diseased state and has remained an integral part of a patient examination. Two unique characteristics of urine specimens can account for this continued popularity:

1. Urine is a readily available and easily collected specimen;
2. Urine contains information about many of the body's major metabolic functions, and this information can be obtained by simple laboratory tests.

These characteristics fit in well with the current trends toward preventive medicine and lower medical costs. By offering an inexpensive way to test large numbers of people, not only for renal disease but also for the asymptomatic beginnings of conditions such as diabetes mellitus and liver disease, the UA can be a valuable metabolic screening procedure.

Should it be necessary to determine whether a particular fluid is actually urine, the specimen can be tested for its urea and creatinine content. Inasmuch

CHART 3–1 ▶
Urinary System and Related Tests

ORGANS AND FUNCTION

The kidneys, ureter, bladder, and urethra compose the urinary system. Kidneys must be able to excrete dietary and waste products (not eliminated by other organs) through the urine. Urine is formed within the functional unit of the kidneys, the nephron, which consists of glomeruli and tubules.

Kidney Glomerulus
Formation of filtrate
Filtration

Kidney Tubule
Secretion of waste products
Reabsorption of waste products needed by the body
Reabsorption of water, sodium chloride, bicarbonates, potassium, and calcium, among others

Kidney: pelvis, ureters, and bladder
Excretion and storage of formed urine
Main urine constituents: water, urea, uric acid, creatinine, sodium, potassium, chloride, calcium, magnesium, phosphates, sulfates, and ammonia

Examples of Selective Filtration, Reabsorption and Excretion by the Urinary System

CONSTITUENT	FILTERED (G/24 H)	REABSORBED (G/24 H)	EXCRETED (G/24 H)
Sodium	540	537	3.3
Chloride	630	625	5.3
Bicarbonate	300	300	0.3
Potassium	28	24	3.9
Glucose	140	140	0.0
Urea	53	28	25
Creatinine	1.4	0.0	1.4
Uric acid	8.5	7.7	0.8

as both of these substances are present in much higher concentrations in urine than in other body fluids, the demonstration of a high urea and creatinine content can identify a fluid as urine.

Laboratory Testing for Routine Urinalysis

First, the physical characteristics of the urine are noted and recorded. Second, a series of chemical tests are run. A chemically impregnated dipstick can be used for many of these tests. Standardized results can be obtained by processing the urine-touched dipstick through special automated instruments. Third, the urine sediment is examined under the microscope.

Dipstick Testing

Although laboratory facilities allow for a wide range of urine tests, some types of tablet, tape, and dipstick tests are available for UA outside the laboratory setting. They can be used and read directly by patients and clinicians.

Similar in appearance to pieces of blotter paper on a plastic strip, dipsticks actually function as miniature laboratories. These chemically impregnated reagent strips provide quick determinations of pH, protein, glucose, ketones, bilirubin, hemoglobin (blood), nitrite, leukocyte esterase, urobilinogen, and specific gravity. The dipstick is impregnated with chemicals that react with specific substances in the urine to produce color-coded visual results. The depth of color produced relates to the concentration of the substance in the urine. Color controls are provided against which the actual color produced by the urine sample can be compared. The reaction times of the impregnated chemicals are standardized for each category of dipstick; it is vital that color changes be matched to the control chart at the correct elapsed time after each stick is dipped into the urine specimen. Instructions that accompany each type of dipstick outline the procedure. When more than 1 type of test is incorporated on a single stick (eg, pH, protein, and glucose), the chemical reagents for each test are separated by a water-impermeable barrier made of plastic so that results do not become altered.

In addition to dipsticks, reagent strips, chemical tablets, and treated slides for special determinations such as bacteria, phenylketonuria (PKU), mucopolysaccharides, salicylate, and cystinuria are available for urine analysis.

Urine Testing by Dipstick/Reagent Strip

| | Possible Reaction Interference | | Correlations with Other Tests |
Measurement	False-Positive	False-Negative	
pH	None	Runover from the protein pad may lower	Nitrite Leukocytes Microscopic examination
Protein	Highly alkaline urine, ammonium compounds (antiseptics), detergents	High salt concentration	Blood Nitrite Leukocytes Microscopic examination
Glucose	Peroxide, oxidizing detergents	Ascorbic acid, 5-HIAA, homogentisic acid, aspirin, levodopa, ketones, high specific gravity with low pH	Ketones

(continued)

Urine Testing by Dipstick/Reagent Strip

| Measurement | Possible Reaction Interference | | Correlations with Other Tests |
	False-Positive	False-Negative	
Ketones	Levodopa, phenylketones	None	Glucose
Blood	Oxidizing agents, vegetable and bacterial peroxidases	Ascorbic acid, nitrite, protein, pH <5.0, high specific gravity, Captopril	Protein Microscopic examination
Bilirubin	Lodine, pigmented urine, indican	Ascorbic acid, nitrite	Urobilinogen
Urobilinogen	Ehrlich-reactive compounds (Multistix), medication color	Nitrite, formalin	Bilirubin
Nitrite	Pigmented urine on automated readers	Ascorbic acid, high specific gravity	Protein Leukocytes Microscopic examination
Leukocytes	Oxidizing detergents	Glucose, protein, high specific gravity, oxalic acid, gentamycin tetracycline, cephalexin, cephalothin	Protein Nitrite Microscopic examination
Specific gravity	Protein	Alkaline urine	None

Procedure

1. Use a fresh urine sample (within 1 hour of collection or a sample that has been refrigerated).
2. Read or review directions for use of the reagent. Periodically check for changes in procedure.
3. Dip a reagent strip into well-mixed urine, then remove it and compare each reagent area on the dipstick with the corresponding color control chart within the established time frame. Correlate color comparisons as closely as possible.

Interfering Factors

1. If the dipstick is kept in the urine sample too long, the impregnated chemicals in the strip may be dissolved and could produce inaccurate readings and values.
2. If the reagent chemicals on the impregnated pad become mixed, the readings will be inaccurate. To avoid this, blot off excess urine after withdrawing the dipstick from the sample.

> **Clinical Alert**
>
> 1. Precise timing is essential. If the test is not timed correctly, color changes may produce invalid or false results.
> 2. When not in use, the container of dipsticks should be kept tightly closed and stored in a cool, dry environment. If the reagents absorb moisture from the air before they are used, they will not produce accurate results. A desiccant comes with the reagents and should be kept in the container.
> 3. Quality control protocols must be followed:
>   **A.** The expiration date must be honored even if there is no detectable deterioration of strips.
>   **B.** Bottles must be discarded 6 months after opening, regardless of expiration date.
>   **C.** Known positive and negative (abnormal and normal) controls must be run for each new bottle of reagent strips when it is opened and whenever there is a question of deterioration.

● COLLECTION OF URINE: SPECIMENS

Standard UA specimens can be collected any time, whereas first morning, fasting, and timed specimens require collection at specific times of day. Patient preparation and education needs vary according to the type of specimen required (Table 3-1) and the patient's ability to cooperate with specimen collection. Clear instructions and assessment of the patient's understanding of the process are key to a successful outcome. Assess the patient's usual urinating patterns and encourage fluid intake (unless contraindicated). Provide verbal and written directions for self-collection of specimens. Assess for presence of interfering factors: failure to follow collection instructions, inadequate fluid intake, certain medications, and patient use of illegal drugs may affect test results. Certain foods, or any type of food consumption in some instances, may also affect test results.

SINGLE, RANDOM URINE SPECIMEN ●

This is the most commonly requested specimen. Because the composition of urine changes over the course of the day, the time of day when the specimen is collected may influence the findings. The first voided morning specimen is particularly valuable, because it is usually more concentrated and therefore more likely to reveal abnormalities as well as the presence of formed substances. It is also relatively free of dietary influences and of changes caused

TABLE 3-1
Collection of Urine Specimens
(Place urine specimens in a biohazard bag).

Type of Specimen	Characteristics
FIRST MORNING SPECIMEN	
Most concentrated	Free of dietary influences
Bladder-incubated	Formed elements may disintegrate if
Best for nitrate, protein, pregnancy tests; microscopic examination; routine screening	pH is high and/or specific gravity is low
RANDOM SPECIMEN	
Most convenient	Most common
Collected any time	
Good for chemical screening, routine screening, microscopic examination	
CLEAN-CATCH (MIDSTREAM)	
Used for random collection and bacterial culture	Minimizes bacterial counts
SECOND (DOUBLE-VOIDED) SPECIMEN	
The first morning specimen is discarded; the second specimen is collected and tested	Diabetic monitoring
	Reflects blood glucose/usually fasting; less concentrated urine.
	Formed elements remain intact.
	Accurately reflect components.
POSTPRANDIAL	
Used for glucose determination, diabetic monitoring	Collected 2 hours after a meal.
TIMED	
Requires collection at certain time	Total specimen must be collected
TIMED 2-HOUR VOLUME	
Used for urobilinogen determination	All urine saved for 2-h period
TIMED 24-HOUR VOLUME	
Necessary for accurate quantitative results	All urine saved for 24-h period
Chemical testing	
CATHETER SPECIMEN	
Clamp catheter 15 to 30 min before collection	Bacterial culture
Cleanse sample port with alcohol	
Insert needle into sample port; after aspirating sample, transfer to specimen container	
ALERT: Unclamp catheter	
SUPRAPUBIC ASPIRATION	
Sterile bladder urine	Bacterial culture cytology

by physical activity, because the specimen is collected after a period of fasting and rest.

Procedure

1. The patient is instructed to void directly into a clean, dry container or bedpan. The specimen is then directly transferred into an appropriate container. Disposable containers are recommended. Women should always have a clean-clatch specimen if a microscopic examination is ordered (see Chap. 7).

2. Specimens from infants and young children can be collected into a disposable collection apparatus consisting of a plastic bag with an adhesive backing around the opening that can be fastened to the perineal area or around the penis to permit voiding directly into the bag. The specimen bag is carefully removed and the urine is transferred to an appropriate specimen container.

3. All specimens should be covered tightly, labeled properly, and sent immediately to the laboratory. The label should be on the cup, not on the lid.

4. If a urine specimen is likely to be contaminated with drainage, vaginal discharge, or menstrual blood, a clean specimen must be obtained using the same procedure as for bacteriologic examination (see Chap. 7).

5. If a urine specimen is obtained from an indwelling catheter, it may be necessary to clamp off the catheter for about 15 to 30 minutes before obtaining the sample. Clean the specimen port (in the tubing) with antiseptic before aspirating the urine sample with a needle and syringe.

6. Observe standard precautions when handling urine specimens (Appendix A).

7. If the specimen cannot be delivered to the laboratory or tested within 1 hour, it should be refrigerated or have an appropriate preservative added.

Interfering Factors

1. Feces, discharges, vaginal secretions, and menstrual blood will contaminate the urine specimen. A clean voided specimen must be obtained.

2. If the specimen is not refrigerated within 1 hour of collection, the following changes in composition may occur:
   A. Increased *pH* from the breakdown of urea to ammonia by urease-producing bacteria
   B. Decreased *glucose* from glycolysis and bacterial utilization
   C. Decreased *ketones* because of volatilization
   D. Decreased *bilirubin* from exposure to light
   E. Decreased *urobilinogen* as a result of its oxidation to urobilin
   F. Increased *nitrite* from bacterial reduction of nitrate
   G. Increased *bacteria* from bacterial reproduction
   H. Increased *turbidity* caused by bacterial growth and possible precipitation of amorphous material

I. Disintegration of *red blood cells* (RBCs) and *casts,* particularly in dilute alkaline urine

J. Changes in *color* caused by oxidation or reduction of metabolites

LONG-TERM, TIMED URINE SPECIMEN (2-HOUR, 24-HOUR) ●

Explanation of Test

Some diseases or conditions require a second morning specimen or a 2-hour or 24-hour urine specimen to evaluate kidney function accurately (see Table 3-1). Substances excreted by the kidney are not excreted at the same rate or in the same amounts during different periods of the day and night; therefore, a random urine specimen might not give an accurate picture of the processes taking place over a 24-hour period. For measurement of total urine protein, creatinine, electrolytes, and so forth, more accurate information is obtained from a long-term specimen. All urine voided in a 24-hour period is collected into a suitable receptacle; depending on the intended test, a preservative is added or the collection is kept refrigerated, or both (Table 3-2).

Procedure

1. At the beginning of a 24-hour timed urine specimen collection (or any other timed specimen collection), the patient is asked to void. This first specimen is *discarded,* and the time is noted.

2. The time the test begins and the time the collection should end are marked on the container. As a reminder, it may be helpful to post a sign above the toilet (eg, "24-Hour Collection in Progress"), with the beginning and ending times noted.

3. All urine voided over the next 24 hours is collected into a large container (usually glass or polyethylene) that is labeled with the patient's name, the time-frame for collection, the test ordered, and other pertinent information. It is not necessary to measure the volume of individual voidings, unless specifically ordered.

4. To conclude the collection, the patient voids 24 hours after the first voiding. Urine from this last voiding must be added to the specimen in the container.

   NOTE: *Because the patient may not always be able to void on request, the last specimen should be obtained as closely as possible to the stated end-time of the test.*

5. Storage

   A. Nonrefrigerated samples may be kept in a specified area or in the patient's bathroom.

   B. If refrigeration is necessary, the collection bottle must either be refrigerated immediately after the patient has voided or be placed into an iced container.

Special Considerations

1. In a health care facility, responsibility for the collection of urine specimens should be specifically assigned.

TABLE 3-2
24-Hour Collection: Standards for Timed Urine Specimen Collection

Test Element and Purpose	Preservative	Specimen Handling and Storage
Acid mucopolysaccharides (inherited enzyme deficiency) in infants with mental retardation or failure to thrive	20 ml toluene (add at start of collection)	Refrigerate during collection; include patient's age
Aldosterone (cause of hypertension)	1 g boric acid per 100 ml urine	Refrigerate
Amino acids, quantitative (aminoaciduria, screen for inborn errors of metabolism and genetic abnormalities)	None	Refrigerate during collection
Aminolevulinic acid (porphyria and lead poisoning)	25 ml of 50% acetic acid; for children <5 y, use 15 ml of 50% acetic acid	Refrigerate or ice; protect from light
Amylase (differentiates acute pancreatitis from other abdominal diseases)	None	Refrigerate during collection
Arsenic (arsenic poisoning—occupational exposure)	20 ml of 6N HNO_3 in a metal-free container	Refrigerate during collection
Cadmium (toxic levels including occupational exposure)	20 ml of 6N HNO_3 in a metal-free container	Refrigerate during collection
Calcium, Quantitative Sulkowitch (hypercalciuria as in hyperparathyroidism, hyperthyroidism, vitamin D toxicity, Paget's disease, osteolytic diseases, and renal tubular acidosis)	30 ml of 6N HCl	Refrigerate during collection
Catecholamine fractions, urinary free catecholamines (measure adrenomedullary function, to diagnose pheochromocytoma)	25 ml of 50% acetic acid; for children <5 y, use 15 ml of 50% acetic acid	Refrigerate or freeze, pH 1–3

(continued)

TABLE 3-2 *(Continued)*
24-Hour Collection: Standards for Timed Urine Specimen Collection

Test Element and Purpose	Preservative	Specimen Handling and Storage
Chloride (electrolyte imbalance, dehydration, metabolic alkalosis)	None	Refrigerate during collection
Chromium (toxic levels, including occupational exposure)	20 ml of 6N HNO_3 in a metal-free container	Refrigerate
Citrate/citric acid (renal disease)	30 ml of 6N HCl	Refrigerate, pH 1–3
Copper (Wilson's disease)	20 ml of 6N HNO_3 in a metal-free container	Refrigerate during collection
Cortisol, free (hydrocortisone levels in adrenal hormone function)	30 ml of 6N HC1	Refrigerate during collection
Creatinine (to evaluate disorders of kidney function)	None	Refrigerate during collection
Creatinine clearance (measures kidney function, primarily glomerular filtration)	None	Refrigerate during collection
Cyclic adenosine monophosphate	None	Refrigerate during collection; freeze a portion after collection
Cystine, quantitative (to diagnose cystinuria, inherited disease characterized by bladder calculi)	None	Refrigerate during collection
Δ-Aminolevulinic acid (porphyria and lead poisoning)	30 ml of 33% glacial acetic acid	Protect from light; refrigerate during collection
Electrolytes, sodium, potassium (electrolyte imbalance)	None, or 1.0 g boric acid	Refrigerate

(continued)

TABLE 3-2 *(Continued)*
24-Hour Collection: Standards for Timed Urine Specimen Collection

Test Element and Purpose	Preservative	Specimen Handling and Storage
Estriol, estradiol (menstrual and fertility problems, male feminization characteristics, estrogen-producing tumors, and pregnancy)	1.0 g boric acid	Refrigerate during collection
Estrogens, total, nonpregnancy or third trimester (estrogen levels for menstrual and fertility problems, pregnancy and estrogen-producing tumors)	1.0 g boric acid	Refrigerate during collection
Follicle-stimulating/ luteinizing hormone (gonadotropic hormones, FSH and LH to determine cause of gonadal deficiency)	1.0 g boric acid or none	Store frozen
Glucose (glucosuria to screen, confirm or monitor diabetes mellitus, rapid intestinal absorption)	1.0 g boric acid	Dark bottle
Histamine (chronic myelogenous leukemia, carcinoids, polycythemia vera)	None	Refrigerate; freeze portion after collection
Homogentisic acid	None	Freeze portion after collection
Homovanillic acid (to diagnose neuroblastoma, pheochromocytoma, ganglioblastoma)	20 ml of 50% acetic acid; for children <5 y, use 15 ml of 50% acetic acid	Refrigerate during collection
17-Hydroxycorticosteroids (adrenal function by measuring urine excretion of steroids to diagnose endocrine disturbances of the adrenal androgens, Cushing's, Addison's, and so forth)	1.0 g boric acid	Refrigerate, pH 5–7; freeze portion after collection

(continued)

TABLE 3-2 *(Continued)*
24-Hour Collection: Standards for Timed Urine Specimen Collection

Test Element and Purpose	Preservative	Specimen Handling and Storage
5-Hydroxyindoleacetic acid, Serotonin (carcinoid tumors)	25 ml of 50% acetic acid; for children <5 y, use 15 ml of 50% acetic acid	Refrigerate during collection; freeze portion after collection
Hydroxyproline, free (measures the free hydroxyproline [less than 10% normally]; rapid growth and increased collagen turnover)	None	Refrigerate during collection; store frozen
Hydroxyproline, total, 24-hour collection (bone collagen reabsorption and the degree of bone destruction from bone tumors)	None	Refrigerate during collection; use gelatin-free and low-collagen diet
Immunofixation electrophoresis (measures immune status and competence by identifying monoclonal and particle protein band immunoglobulins)	None	Refrigerate
κ and λ chains, quantitative, also in serum (monoclonal gammopathies, myeloma tumor burden)	None	Refrigerate
17-Ketogenic steroids, (Porter-Silber and Cushing's syndrome, adrenogenital syndrome)	1.0 g boric acid	Do not refrigerate
17-Ketosteroid, fractions (adrenal and gonadal abnormalities)	1.0 g boric acid	Do not refrigerate
Lead (lead poisoning and chelation therapy)	20 ml of 6N HNO_3 in a metal-free container	Refrigerate

(continued)

TABLE 3-2 *(Continued)*
24-Hour Collection: Standards for Timed Urine Specimen Collection

Test Element and Purpose	Preservative	Specimen Handling and Storage
Lipase (acute pancreatitis and to differentiate pancreatitis from other abdominal disorders)	None	Refrigerate
Lysozyme, muramidase (to differentiate acute myelogenous or monocytic leukemia from acute lymphatic leukemia)	None	Refrigerate
Magnesium (magnesium metabolism, electrolyte status, and nephrolithiasis)	20 ml of 6N HCl in a metal-free container	Refrigerate
Manganese (toxicity, parenteral nutrition)	None	Refrigerate during collection
Mercury (toxicity, industrial and dental overexposure; inorganic mercury)	20 ml of 6N HNO_3 in a metal-free container	Refrigerate; pH 2 with nitric acid
Metanephrine, total (assays of catecholamines and vanillylmandelic acid; frequently to diagnose pheochromocytoma)	30 ml of 6N HCl	pH 1–3
Metanephrine, fractions (to diagnose and monitor pheochromocytoma and ganglioneuroblastoma)	30 ml of 6N HCl, final pH <3	Refrigerate; no caffeine before or during testing
Metanephrine, total (pheochromocytoma, children with neuroblastoma, ganglioneuroma)	25 ml of 50% acetic acid; for children <5 y, use of 15 ml of 50% acetic acid; or 30 ml of 6NHCl.	Refrigerate; no caffeine before or during testing
MHPG (3-Methoxy-4-hydroxyphenylglycol) (to classify bipolar manic depression for drug therapy)	None	Refrigerate
Microalbumin, 24-hour (diabetic nephropathy)	None	Refrigerate

(continued)

TABLE 3-2 *(Continued)*
24-Hour Collection: Standards for Timed Urine Specimen Collection

Test Element and Purpose	Preservative	Specimen Handling and Storage
Osmolality, 24-hour (diabetes insipidus, primary polypepsia)	None	Refrigerate
Oxalate (nephrolithiasis and inflammatory bowel diseases)	20 ml of 6N HCl	Refrigerate, pH 2–3
Phosphorous, 24-hour (renal losses; hyperparathyroidism and hypoparathyroidism)	Acid washed, detergent-free container	Refrigerate during collection; acidify after collection
Porphobilinogens	None	Refrigerate during collection; freeze a portion; protect from light
Porphyrins, quantitative (to diagnose porphyrias and lead poisoning).	5 g sodium carbonate (do not use sodium bicarbonate)	Refrigerate; protect specimen from light
Porphyrins (to diagnose porphyrias and lead poisoning).	None (preservative is added on receipt in laboratory)	Refrigerate; protect specimen from light
Potassium, 24-hour (electrolyte imbalance, renal and adrenal disorders)	None	Refrigerate during collection
Pregnanediol, 24-hour (measures ovarian and placental function)	Boric acid	Refrigerate during collection
Pregnanetriol (adrenogenital syndrome)	25 ml of 50% acetic acid; for children <5 y, use 15 ml of 50% acetic acid	Refrigerate during collection; pH 4–4.5 after receipt in laboratory
Protein electrophoresis, 24-hour (average 35 in amyloidosis and myeloma)	None	Refrigerate
Protein, total (proteinuria, differential diagnosis of renal disease)	None	Refrigerate during collection

(continued)

TABLE 3-2 *(Continued)*
24-Hour Collection: Standards for Timed Urine Specimen Collection

Test Element and Purpose	Preservative	Specimen Handling and Storage
Schilling test (vitamin B-12 deficiency, pernicious anemia)	None	Refrigerate during collection; transport entire specimen to laboratory
Selenium (nutritional deficiency, industrial exposure)	20 ml of 6N HNO_3 in a metal-free container	Refrigerate; transport entire specimen to laboratory
Sodium, 24-hour (electrolyte imbalance, acute renal failure, oliguria and hyponatremia, sodium excreted for diagnosis of renal and adrenal imbalances)	None	Refrigerate during collection
Substance abuse screen (specific drugs and alcohol involved in substance abuse)	None	Refrigerate or freeze
Thallium (thallium toxicity, occupational exposure)	20 ml of 6N HNO_3 in a metal-free container	Refrigerate
Thiocyanate (short-term nitroprusside therapy, cyanide poisoning)	None	Refrigerate during collection
Total protein (renal disease)	None	Refrigerate during collection
Urea nitrogen, 24-hour (kidney function, hyperalimentation)	None	Refrigerate; adjust pH <5 with concentrated HCl after receipt in laboratory
Uric acid, 24-hour (uric acid metabolism in gout and renal calculus formation)	None	Refrigerate during collection
Urobilinogen (liver function and liver cell damage)	5 g sodium carbonate and 100 ml petroleum ether (do not use sodium bicarbonate)	Refrigerate during collection; protect specimen from light; check with laboratory

(continued)

TABLE 3-2 *(Continued)*
24-Hour Collection: Standards for Timed Urine Specimen Collection

Test Element and Purpose	Preservative	Specimen Handling and Storage
Vanillylmandelic acid, quantitative (adrenomedular pheochromocytoma, hypertension)	25 ml 50% of acetic acid; for children <5 y use 15 ml 50% acetic acid	Refrigerate, pH 1–3; protect from light
Zinc (industrial exposure, toxicity, nutritional, acrodermatitis enteropathies)	20 ml 6N HNO_3 in a metal-free container	Refrigerate

2. When instructing a patient about 24-hour urine collections, make certain the patient understands that the bladder must be emptied just before the 24-hour collection starts and that this preliminary specimen must be discarded; then, all urine voided until the ending time is saved.

3. Do not predate and pretime requisitions for serial collections. It is difficult for some patients to void at specific times. Instead, mark the actual times of collection on containers.

4. Documentation of the exact times at which the specimens are obtained is crucial to many urine tests.

5. Instruct the patient to urinate as near to the end of the collection period as possible.

6. When a preservative is added to the collection container (eg, acetic acid preservative in 24-hour urine collection for vanillylmandelic acid [VMA]), the patient must take precautions against spilling the contents. Instructions regarding spillage need to be provided before the test begins.

7. The preservative used is determined by the urine substance to be tested for. The laboratory usually provides the container and the proper preservative when the test is ordered. If in doubt, verify this with the laboratory personnel.

Interfering Factors

1. Failure of patient or attending personnel to follow the procedure is the most common source of error.

   A. The patient should be given both verbal and written instructions. If the patient is unable to comprehend these directions, a significant other should be instructed in the process.

   B. If required, the proper preservative must be used.

2. Instruct the patient to use toilet paper *after* transferring the urine to the 24-hour collection container. Toilet paper placed in the specimen decreases the actual amount of urine available and contaminates the specimen.

3. The presence of feces contaminates the specimen. Patients should void first and transfer the urine to the collection receptacle before defecating.
4. If heavy menstrual flow or other discharges or secretions are present, the test may have to be postponed or an indwelling catheter may need to be inserted to keep the specimen free of contamination. In some cases, thorough cleansing of the perineal or urethral area before voiding may be sufficient. If in doubt, communicate with laboratory personnel and the patient's physician.

Patient Preparation

Most 24-hour urine specimen collections start in the early morning at about 7:00 AM (0700). Instruct the patient to do the following:

1. Empty the bladder completely on awakening and then discard that urine specimen. Record the time the voided specimen is discarded and the time the test is begun.
2. Save all urine voided during the next 24 hours, including the first specimen voided the next morning.
3. The urine voided the next morning (as close to the ending time as possible) is added to the collection container. The 24-hour test is then terminated, and the ending time is recorded.
4. A urinal, wide-mouth container, special toilet device, bedpan, or the collection container itself can be used to catch urine. It is probably easier for women to void into another wide-mouth receptacle first and then to *carefully* transfer the entire specimen to the collection bottle. Men may find it simpler to void directly into the 24-hour collection container.
5. It is most important that *all* urine be saved in the 24-hour container. Ideally, the container should be refrigerated or placed on ice.
6. Test results are calculated on the basis of a 24-hour output. Unless *all* urine is saved, results will not be accurate. Moreover, these tests are usually expensive, complicated, and necessary for the evaluation and treatment of the patient's condition.

● ROUTINE URINALYSIS (UA) AND RELATED TESTS

Normal Values in Urinalysis		
General Characteristics and Measurements	**Chemical Determinations**	**Microscopic Examination of Sediment**
Color: pale yellow to amber	Glucose: negative	Casts negative: occasional hyaline casts
Appearance: clear to slightly hazy	Ketones: negative	Red blood cells: negative or rare

(continued)

Normal Values in Urinalysis   *(Continued)*

General Characteristics and Measurements	Chemical Determinations	Microscopic Examination of Sediment
Specific gravity: 1.005–1.025 with a normal fluid intake	Blood: negative	Crystals: negative (none)
pH: 4.5–8.0; average person has a pH of about 5 to 6	Protein: negative	White blood cells: negative or rare
Volume: 600–2500 ml/24 h; average 1200 ml/24 h	Bilirubin: negative	Epithelial cells: few; hyaline casts 0–1/lpf
	Urobilinogen: 0.2–1.0	
	Nitrate for bacteria: negative	
	Leukocyte esterase: negative	

Explanation of Test

The process of urinalysis (UA) determines the following properties of urine: color, odor, turbidity, specific gravity, pH, glucose, ketones, blood, protein, bilirubin, urobilinogen, nitrite, leukocyte esterase, and other abnormal constituents revealed by microscopic examination of the urine sediment. A 10-ml urine specimen is usually sufficient for conducting these tests.

URINE VOLUME

Normal Values

600–2500 ml in 24 h

Background

Urine volume measurements are part of the assessment for fluid balance and kidney function. The normal volume of urine voided by the average adult in a 24-hour period ranges from 600 to 2500 ml; the typical amount is about 1200 ml. The amount voided over any period is directly related to the individual's fluid intake, the temperature and climate, and the amount of perspiration that occurs. Children void smaller quantities than adults, but the total volume voided is greater in proportion to their body size.

The volume of urine produced at night is <700 ml, making the day/night ratio approximately 2:1 to 4:1.

Explanation of Test

Urine volume depends on the amount of water excreted by the kidneys. Water is a major body constituent; therefore, the amount excreted is usually determined by the body's state of hydration. Factors that influence urine volume include fluid intake, fluid loss from nonrenal sources, variations in the secretion of antidiuretic hormone (ADH), and the necessity to excrete increased amount of solutes such as glucose or salts. *Polyuria* is a marked increase of urine production. *Oliguria* is decreased urinary output. The extreme form of this process is *anuria,* a total lack of urine production.

Procedure

1. Collect a 24-hour urine specimen and keep it refrigerated or on ice.
2. Record the exact collection starting time and collection ending time on the specimen container and in the patient's health care record.
3. When the collection is completed, transfer the specimen container to the laboratory refrigerator. Make out the proper forms and document accordingly.
4. Volume is ascertained by measuring the entire urine amount in a graduated and appropriately calibrated pitcher or other receptacle. The total volume is recorded as urine volume in milliliters (cubic centimeters) per 24 hours.

Clinical Implications

1. *Polyuria* (increased urine output) with elevated urea nitrogen (BUN) and creatinine levels
   A. Diabetic ketoacidosis
   B. Partial obstruction of urinary tract
   C. Some types of tubular necrosis (aminoglycoside)
2. *Polyuria* with normal BUN and creatinine
   A. Diabetes mellitus and diabetes insipidus
   B. Neurotic states (compulsive water drinking)
   C. Certain tumors of brain and spinal cord
3. *Oliguria* (<200 ml in adults, or <15 to 20 ml/kg in children, per 24 hours)
   A. Renal causes
      (1) Renal ischemia
      (2) Renal disease due to toxic agents (certain drugs are toxic to the renal system)
      (3) Glomerulonephritis
   B. Dehydration caused by prolonged vomiting, diarrhea, excessive diaphoresis, or burns
   C. Obstruction (mechanical) of some area of the urinary tract or system
   D. Cardiac insufficiency
4. *Anuria* (<100 ml in 24 h)
   A. Complete urinary tract obstruction
   B. Acute cortical necrosis (cortex of the kidney)
   C. Glomerulonephritis (acute, necrotizing)
   D. Acute tubular necrosis
   E. Hemolytic transfusion reaction

Interfering Factors

1. Polyuria
   A. Intravenous glucose or saline
   B. Pharmacologic agents such as thiazides and other diuretics
   C. Coffee, alcohol, tea, caffeine

2. Oliguria
   A. Water deprivation, dehydration
   B. Excessive salt intake

Patient Preparation
1. Explain the purpose and procedure of the test.
2. Withhold diuretics for 3 days before the test. Check with clinician.
3. Avoid excessive water (liquid) intake and excessive salt intake. Advise patients to avoid salty foods and added salt in the diet. Eliminate caffeine and alcohol. Determine the patient's usual liquid intake and request that intake not be increased beyond this daily amount during testing.
4. Follow guidelines in Chapter 1 for safe, effective, *pretest* care.

Patient Aftercare
1. Patient can resume normal fluid and dietary intake and medications, unless specifically ordered otherwise.
2. Interpret test outcomes and counsel appropriately.
3. Follow guidelines in Chapter 1 for safe, effective, *posttest* care.

URINE SPECIFIC GRAVITY (SG)   ●

Normal Values
Normal hydration and volume: 1.005–1.030 (usually between 1.010 and 1.025)
Concentrated urine: 1.025–1.030+
Dilute urine: 1.001–1.010
Infant <2 y: 1.001–1.018

Explanation of Test
Specific gravity (SG) is a measurement of the kidneys' ability to concentrate urine. The test compares the density of urine against the density of distilled water, which has an SG of 1.000. Because urine is a solution of minerals, salts, and compounds dissolved in water, the SG is a measure of the density of the dissolved chemicals in the specimen. As a measurement of specimen density, SG is influenced by both the number of particles present and the size of the particles. Osmolality is a more exact measurement and may be needed in certain circumstances.

The range of urine SG depends on the state of hydration and varies with urine volume and the load of solids to be excreted under standardized conditions; when fluid intake is restricted or increased, SG measures the concentrating and diluting functions of the kidney. Loss of these functions is an indication of renal dysfunction.

Procedure
1. SG can be tested with the use of a multiple-test *dipstick* that has a separate reagent area for SG. An indicator changes color in relation to ionic concentration, and this result is translated into a value for SG.
2. SG can be determined with a *refractometer* or total solids meter. The refractive index is the ratio of the velocity of light in air to the velocity of light

in the test solution. A drop of urine is placed on a clear glass plate of the urinometer and another "plate" is pressed on top of the urine sample. The path of light is deviated when it enters the solution, and the degree of deviation (refraction) is proportional to the density of the solution.

3. The *urinometer* (hydrometer) is the most widely known but least accurate method. It has been used for many years and consists of a bulb-shaped instrument that contains a scale calibrated in SG readings. Urine (10 to 20 ml) is transferred into a small test tube–like cylinder, and the urinometer is floated in the urine. The SG is read off the urinometer at the meniscus level of the urine.

4. Specimen collection
   A. For regular UA testing, about 20 ml of a random sample is needed for urinometer testing.
   B. When a special evaluation of SG is ordered separately from the UA, the patient should fast for 12 hours before specimen collection.

Clinical Implications

1. *Normal SG:* SG values usually vary inversely with the amount of urine excreted (decreased urine volume = increased SG). However, this relationship is not valid in certain conditions, including
   A. Diabetes—increased urine volume, increased SG
   B. Hypertension—normal volume, decreased SG
   C. Early chronic renal disease—increased volume, decreased SG
2. *Hyposthenuria* (low SG, 1.001 to 1.010) occurs in the following conditions:
   A. Diabetes insipidus (low SG with large urine volume). It is caused by absence or decrease of ADH, a hormone that triggers kidney absorption of water. Without ADH, the kidneys produce excessive amounts of urine that are not reabsorbed (sometimes 15 to 20 L/day).
   B. Glomerulonephritis (kidney inflammation without infection) and pyelonephritis (kidney inflammation with bacterial infection, but not in the acute type of this disease). SG can be low in glomerulonephritis, with decreased urine volume. Tubular damage affects kidneys' ability to concentrate urine.
   C. Severe renal damage with disturbance of both concentrating and diluting abilities of urine. The SG is low (1.010) and fixed (varying little from specimen to specimen); this is termed *isosthenuria.*
3. *Hypersthenuria* (increased SG, 1.025 to 1.035) occurs in the following conditions:
   A. Diabetes mellitus
   B. Nephrosis
   C. Excessive water loss (dehydration, fever, vomiting, diarrhea)
   D. Increased secretion of ADH and diuretic effects related to the stress of a surgical procedure
   E. Congestive heart failure
   F. Toxemia of pregnancy

Interfering Factors
1. Radiopaque x-ray contrast media, minerals, and dextran may cause falsely high SG readings. The reagent dipstick method is not affected by high-molecular-weight substances.
2. Temperature of urine specimens affects SG; cold specimens produce falsely high values.
3. Highly buffered alkaline urine may also cause low readings (with dipsticks only).
4. Elevated readings may occur in the presence of moderate amounts of protein (100 to 750 mg/dl).
5. Detergent residue (on specimen containers) can produce elevated SG results.
6. Diuretics and antibiotics cause high readings.
7. See Appendix J for drugs that affect test outcomes.

Patient Preparation
1. Explain the purpose and procedure for urine collection.
2. Follow guidelines in Chapter 1 for safe, effective, informed *pretest* care.

Patient Aftercare
1. Interpret test outcomes, counsel, and monitor appropriately for conditions associated with altered SG.
2. Follow Chapter 1 guidelines for safe, effective, informed *posttest* care.

URINE OSMOLALITY

Normal Values
24-h specimen: 300–900 mOsm/kg of water
Random specimen: 50–1200 mOsm/kg of water
Urine/serum ratio: 1:1 to 3:1

Background
Osmolality, a more exact measurement of urine concentration than SG, depends on the number of particles of solute in a unit of solution. More information concerning renal function can be obtained if serum and urine osmolality tests are run at the same time. The normal ratio between urine and serum osmolality is 3:1. A high urine/serum ratio is seen with concentrated urine. With poor concentrating ability, the ratio is low.

Explanation of Test
Whenever a precise measurement is indicated to evaluate the concentrating and diluting ability of the kidney, this test is done. Urine osmolality during water restriction is an accurate test of decreased kidney function. It is also used to monitor the course of renal disease; to monitor fluid and electrolyte therapy; to establish the differential diagnosis of hypernatremia, hyponatremia, and polyuria; and to evaluate the renal response to ADH.

Procedure

1. This is a 24-hour urine collection test.
2. For the 24-hour test, the patient voids at approximately 7:00 AM (0700). All of the urine voided is saved in a special 24-hour collection container kept on ice or refrigerated (see Patient Preparation on p. 188). A high-protein diet may be ordered.
3. At the end of the test, the specimen is labeled and sent to the laboratory.
4. Simultaneous determination of serum osmolality may be done. A high urine/serum ratio is seen with concentrated urine.

Clinical Implications

1. Osmolality is *increased* in
   A. Prerenal azotemia
   B. Congestive heart failure
   C. Addison's disease
   D. Inappropriate ADH secretion (SIADH)
   E. Dehydration
   F. Amyloidosis
   G. Hyponatremia
2. Osmolality is *decreased* in
   A. Acute renal failure
   B. Diabetes insipidus
   C. Hypokalemia
   D. Hypernatremia
   E. Primary polydipsia
   F. Compulsive water drinking
3. Urine/serum ratio is
   A. *Increased* in prerenal azotemia.
   B. *Decreased* in acute tubular necrosis.

Interfering Factors

1. Intravenous sodium administration.
2. Intravenous dextrose and water administration.

Patient Preparation

1. Explain purpose and procedure of the test to the patient.
2. A normal diet is prescribed for 3 days before testing.
3. To increase sensitivity of the osmolality test, a high-protein diet may be ordered for 3 days before the test. No liquids with the evening meal and no food or liquids should be taken after the evening meal until collection. Check with your laboratory if the patient has diabetes.
4. Follow guidelines in Chapter 1 for safe, effective, informed *pretest* care.

Patient Aftercare

1. Provide the patient with foods and fluids as soon as the last urine sample is obtained.

2. Interpret test outcomes and monitor appropriately.

3. Follow guidelines in Chapter 1 for safe, effective, *posttest* care.

URINE APPEARANCE   ●

Normal Values
Fresh urine is clear to slightly hazy.

Background
The first observation made about a urine specimen is usually its appearance, which generally refers to the clarity of the specimen.

Explanation of Test
Cloudy urine signals a possible abnormal constituent, such as white blood cells (WBCs), RBCs, or bacteria. On the other hand, excretion of cloudy urine may not be abnormal, because a change in urine pH can cause precipitation, within the bladder, of normal urinary components. Alkaline urine may appear cloudy because of phosphates; acid urine may appear cloudy because of urates.

Procedure
1. Observe the clarity of a fresh urine sample by visually examining a well-mixed specimen in front of a light source.

2. Common terms used to report appearance include the following: clear, hazy, slightly cloudy, cloudy, turbid, and milky.

3. The degree of turbidity should correspond to the amount of material observed under the microscope.

4. Document results.

Clinical Implications
1. Pathologic urines are often turbid or cloudy; however, many normal urines can also appear cloudy.

2. Urine turbidity may result from urinary tract infections (UTIs).

3. Urines may be cloudy because of the presence of RBCs, WBCs, epithelial cells, or bacteria.

Interfering Factors
1. After ingestion of food, urates, carbonates, or phosphates may produce cloudiness in normal urine on standing.

2. Semen or vaginal discharges mixed with urine are common causes of turbidity.

3. Fecal contamination causes turbidity.

4. Extraneous contamination (eg, talcum, vaginal creams, radiographic contrast media) can cause turbidity.

5. "Greasy" cloudiness may be caused by large amounts of fat.

6. Often normal urine develops a haze or turbidity after refrigeration or standing at room temperature because of precipitation of crystals of calcium oxalate or uric acid.

URINE COLOR ●

Normal Values

The normal color of urine is pale yellow to amber.

Straw-colored urine is normal and indicates a low SG, usually <1.010. (The exception may be a patient with an elevated blood glucose concentration, whose urine is very pale yellow but has a high SG.)

Amber-colored urine is normal and indicates a high SG and a small output of urine.

Background

The yellow color of urine is caused by the presence of the pigment urochrome, a product of metabolism that under normal conditions is produced at a constant rate. The actual amount of urochrome produced depends on the body's metabolic state, with increased amounts being produced in thyroid conditions and fasting states.

Explanation of Test

Urine specimens may vary in color from pale yellow to dark amber. Variations in the yellow color are related to the body's state of hydration. The darker amber color may be directly related to the urine concentration or SG.

Procedure

Observe and record the color of freshly voided urine.

Clinical Implications

1. Almost *colorless* (straw-colored) urine:
   A. Large fluid intake
   B. Chronic interstitial nephritis
   C. Untreated diabetes mellitus
   D. Diabetes insipidus
   E. Alcohol and caffeine ingestion
   F. Diuretic therapy
   G. Nervousness
2. *Orange-colored* (amber) urine:
   A. Concentrated urine caused by fever, sweating, reduced fluid intake, or first morning specimen
   B. Bilirubin (yellow foam when shaken)
   C. Carrots or vitamin A ingestion
   D. Certain urinary tract medications (eg, phenazopyridine [Pyridium], nitrofurantoin)
3. *Brownish-yellow or greenish-yellow* urine may indicate bilirubin in the urine that has been oxidized to biliverdin (greenish foam when shaken).
4. *Green* urine:
   A. Pseudomonal infection
   B. Indican

5. *Pink to red* urine:
   A. RBCs
   B. Hemoglobin, methemoglobin, oxyhemoglobin
   C. Myoglobin
   D. Porphyrins
6. *Brown-black* urine:
   A. RBCs oxidized to methemoglobin
   B. Methemoglobin
   C. Homogentisic acid (alkaptonuria)
   D. Melanin or melanogen
   E. Phenol poisoning (Lysol)
7. *Smoky* urine may be caused by RBCs.
8. *Milky* urine is associated with fat, cystinuria, many WBCs, or phosphates (not pathologic).

Interfering Factors

1. Normal urine color darkens on standing because of the oxidation of urobilinogen to urobilin. This decomposition process starts about 30 minutes after voiding.
2. Some foods cause changes in urine color:
   A. Beets turn the urine *red*.
   B. Rhubarb can cause *brown* urine.
3. Many drugs alter the color of urine:
   A. Cascara and senna laxatives in the presence of acid urine turn the urine *reddish-brown;* in the presence of alkaline urine, they turn the urine *red*.
   B. *Bright yellow* color in alkaline urine may be a result of riboflavin or phenazopyridine.
   C. Urine that *darkens* on standing may indicate antiparkinsonian agents such as levodopa (Sinemet).
   D. *Black* urine may be caused by cascara, chloroquine, iron salts (ferrous sulfate, ferrous fumarate, ferrous gluconate), metronidazole, nitrofurantoin, quinine, or senna.
   E. *Blue* urine may be caused by triamterene.
   F. *Blue-green* urine may be caused by amitriptyline, methylene blue, or mitoxantrone.
   G. *Orange* urine may be caused by heparin, phenazopyridine, rifampin, sulfasalazine, or warfarin.
   H. *Red-pink* urine may be caused by chloroxazone, daunorubicin, doxorubicin, heparin, ibuprofen, methyldopa, phenytoin, rifampin, or senna.
   I. *Pink to brown* urine may be caused by laxatives.
   J. *Brown* urine may be caused by chloroquine, furazolidone, or primaquine.
   K. *Green* urine may be caused by indomethacin.

Patient Preparation

Assess color of urine; instruct patient to monitor and to report abnormal urine colors.

> **Clinical Alert**
>
> 1. If the urine is a red color, do not assume drug causation. Check the urine for hemoglobin. Question the patient regarding hematuria and recent activity, injury, or infection. Sometimes vigorous exercise can bring on hematuria.
> 2. Red urine that is negative for occult blood is an indication that porphyria may be present. Report at once and document test results.
> 3. Other grossly abnormal colors (eg, black, brown) should be documented and reported.

Patient Aftercare
1. Interpret abnormal urine colors and counsel appropriately.
2. Explain that follow-up testing may be needed.

URINE ODOR

Normal, freshly voided urine has a faint odor owing to the presence of volatile acids. It is not generally offensive. Although not part of the routine UA, abnormal odors should be noted.

Normal Values
Fresh urine from most healthy persons has a characteristic aromatic odor.

Procedure
Smell the urine and record perceptions.

Clinical Implications
1. The urine of patients with diabetes mellitus may have a fruity (acetone) odor because of ketosis.
2. UTIs result in a foul-smelling urine because of the presence of bacteria, which split urea to form ammonia.
3. The urine of infants with an inherited disorder of amino acid metabolism known as "maple syrup urine disease" smells like maple or burnt sugar.
4. Cystinuria and homocystinuria result in a sulfurous odor.
5. Oasthouse urine disease caused a smell associated with the smell of a brewery (yeasts, hops).
6. In phenylketonuria, a musty, mousy smell may be evident.
7. Tyrosinemia is characterized by a cabbage-like or "fishy" urine odor.
8. Butyric/hexanoic acidemia produces a urine odor resembling that of sweaty feet.

Interfering Factors

1. Some foods, such as asparagus, produce characteristic urine odors.
2. Bacterial activity produces ammonia from the decomposition of urea, with its characteristic pungent odor.

URINE PH   ●

Normal Values
The pH of normal urine can vary widely, from 4.6 to 8.0.
The average pH value is about 6.0 (acid).

Background
The symbol *pH* expresses the urine as a dilute acid or base solution and measures the free hydrogen ion (H^+) concentration in the urine; "7.0" is the point of neutrality on the pH scale. The lower the pH, the greater the acidity; the higher the pH, the greater the alkalinity. The pH is an indicator of the renal tubules' ability to maintain normal hydrogen ion concentration in the plasma and extracellular fluid. The kidneys maintain normal acid-base balance primarily through reabsorption of sodium and tubular secretion of hydrogen and ammonium ions. Secretion of an acid or alkaline urine by the kidneys is 1 of the most important mechanisms the body has for maintaining a constant body pH.

Urine becomes increasingly acidic as the amount of sodium and excess acid retained by the body increases. Alkaline urine, usually containing bicarbonate–carbonic acid buffer, is normally excreted when there is an excess of base or alkali in the body.

Control of Urine pH
Control of urinary pH is important in the management of several diseases, including bacteriuria, renal calculi, and drug therapy in which streptomycin or methenamine mandelate is being administered.

1. *Renal calculi:* Renal stone formation partially depends on the pH of urine. Patients being treated for renal calculi are frequently given diets or medication to change the pH of the urine so that kidney stones will not form.
   A. Calcium phosphate, calcium carbonate, and magnesium phosphate stones develop in alkaline urine. In such instances the urine must be kept acid (see Diet).
   B. Uric acid, cystine, and calcium oxalate stones precipitate in acid urines. Therefore, as part of treatment, the urine should be kept alkaline (see Diet).
2. *Drug treatment*
   A. Streptomycin, neomycin, and kanamycin are effective for treating genitourinary tract infections, provided the urine is alkaline.
   B. During sulfa therapy, an alkaline urine should help prevent formation of sulfonamide crystals.

    C. Urine should also be kept persistently alkaline in the presence of salicylate intoxication (to enhance excretion) and during blood transfusions.

3. *Clinical conditions*

    A. The urine should be kept acid during treatment of UTI or persistent bacteriuria and during management of urinary calculi that develop in alkaline urine.

    B. An accurate measurement of urinary pH can be made only on a freshly voided specimen. If the urine must be kept for any length of time before analysis, it must be refrigerated.

    C. Highly concentrated urine, such as that formed in hot, dry environments, is strongly acidic and may produce irritation.

    D. During sleep, decreased pulmonary ventilation causes respiratory acidosis; as a result, urine becomes highly acid.

    E. Chlorothiazide diuretic administration causes acid urine to be excreted.

    F. Bacteria from a UTI or from bacterial contamination of the specimen produce alkaline urine. Urea is converted to ammonia.

4. *Diet*

    A. A vegetarian diet that emphasizes citrus fruits and most vegetables, particularly legumes, helps keep the urine alkaline. Alkaline urine after meals is a normal response to the secretions of hydrochloric acid in gastric juice.

    B. A diet high in meat and protein keeps the urine acid.

    C. Cranberry juice is the 1 fruit that will maintain an acid urine, and it has long been used as a remedy for minor UTIs.

Explanation of Test

The importance of urinary pH lies primarily in determining the existence of systemic acid-base disorders of metabolic or respiratory origin and in the management of urinary conditions that require the urine to be maintained at a specific pH.

Procedure

1. *Dipstick measurement:* Reagent strips produce a spectrum of color changes from orange to green-blue to identify pH ranges from 5 to 9.

2. The reagent strip is dipped into a freshly voided urine specimen, and the color change is compared with a standardized color chart on the bottle that correlates color results with pH values.

3. Maintenance of the urine at a consistent pH requires frequent urine pH testing.

Clinical Implications

1. *To be useful, the urine pH measurement must be used in conjunction with other diagnostic information.* For example, in renal tubular necrosis, the kidney is not able to excrete a urine that is strongly acid. Therefore, if the urine pH is 5, renal tubular necrosis is eliminated as a possible diagnosis.

A. *Acidic urine* (pH <7.0) occurs in

(1) Metabolic acidosis, diabetic ketosis, diarrhea, starvation, uremia

(2) UTIs caused by *Escherichia coli*

(3) Respiratory acidosis (carbon dioxide retention)

(4) Deficiency of potassium (patient may be in metabolic alkalosis)

B. *Alkaline urine* (pH >7.0) occurs in

(1) UTIs caused by urea-splitting bacteria (*Proteus* and *Pseudomonas*)

(2) Renal tubular acidosis, chronic renal failure

(3) Metabolic acidosis (vomiting)

(4) Respiratory alkalosis involving hyperventilation ("blowing off" carbon dioxide)

Interfering Factors

1. With prolonged standing, the pH of a urine specimen becomes alkaline because bacteria split urea and produce ammonia.

2. Ammonium chloride and mandelic acid may produce acid urines.

3. "Runover" between the pH testing area and the highly acidic protein area on the dipsticks may cause alkaline urine to give an acidic reading.

4. Sodium bicarbonate, potassium citrate, and acetazolamide may produce alkaline urine.

5. Urine becomes alkaline after eating because of excretion of stomach acid; this is known as the "alkaline tide."

Clinical Alert

The pH of urine never reaches 9, either in normal or abnormal conditions. Therefore, a pH finding of 9 indicates that a fresh specimen should be obtained to ensure the validity of the UA.

Patient Preparation

1. Explain test purpose and specimen collection procedure.

2. Follow guidelines in Chapter 1 for safe, effective, informed *pretest* care.

Patient Aftercare

1. Interpret test outcomes and monitor patient appropriately (see Control of Urine pH).

2. Follow guidelines in Chapter 1 for safe, effective, informed *posttest* care.

URINE BLOOD OR HEMOGLOBIN (HEME) ●

Normal Values
Negative/none

Background
The presence of free hemoglobin in the urine is referred to as *hemoglobin-uria*. Hemoglobinuria can be related to conditions outside the urinary tract and occurs when there is such extensive or rapid destruction (intravascular he-molysis) of circulating erythrocytes that the reticuloendothelial system cannot metabolize or store the excess free hemoglobin. The hemoglobin is then fil-tered through the glomerulus. Hemoglobinuria may also occur as a result of lysis of RBCs in the urinary tract.

When intact RBCs are present in the urine, the term *hematuria* is used. Hema-turia is most closely related to disorders of the renal or genitourinary systems in which bleeding is the result of trauma or damage to these organs or systems.

Explanation of Test
This test detects RBCs, hemoglobin, and myoglobin in urine. Blood in urine is *always* an indicator of damage to the kidney or urinary tract.

The use of both a urine dipstick measurement and microscopic examina-tion of urine provides a complete clinical evaluation of hemoglobinuria and hematuria. Newer forms of dipsticks contain a lysing reagent that reacts with occult blood and detects intact as well as lysed RBCs.

When urine sediment is positive for occult blood but no RBCs are seen mi-croscopically, *myoglobinuria* can be suspected. Myoglobinuria is caused by excretion of myoglobin, a muscle protein, into the urine as a result of (1) trau-matic muscle injury, such as may occur in automobile accidents, football in-juries, or electric shock; (2) a muscle disorder, such as an arterial occlusion to a muscle or muscular dystrophy; (3) certain kinds of poisoning, such as car-bon monoxide or fish poisoning; or (4) malignant hyperthermia related to ad-ministration of certain anesthetic agents. Myoglobin can be distinguished from free hemoglobin in the urine by chemical tests.

Procedure
1. Collect a fresh, random urine specimen.
   - **A.** *Hemoglobinuria* (hemoglobin in urine)
     - **(1)** Reagent sticks are dipped into the urine, and the color change on the dipstick is correlated with a standardized color chart specifically used with that particular type of dipstick.
     - **(2)** The color chart indicates color gradients for negative, moderate, and large amounts of hemoglobin.
   - **B.** *Hematuria* (RBCs in urine)
     - **(1)** This dipstick method allows detection of intact RBCs when the num-ber is greater than 10 cells/μl of urine. The color change appears stippled on the dipstick.

(2) The degree of hematuria can be estimated by the intensity of the speckled pattern.
2. To verify the presence of RBCs, the urine sample is centrifuged and the sediment is examined microscopically (see page 222).
   A. Hemoglobinuria is suspected when no RBCs are seen or the number seen does not correspond to the degree of color on the dipstick.
   B. Myoglobinemia may be suspected if the urine is cherry-red, no RBCs are seen, and blood serum enzymes for muscle destruction are elevated.

Clinical Implications
1. *Hematuria* is found in
   A. Acute UTI (cystitis)
   B. Lupus nephritis
   C. Urinary tract or renal tumors
   D. Urinary calculi (intermittent hematuria)
   E. Malignant hypertension
   F. Glomerulonephritis (acute or chronic)
   G. Pyelonephritis
   H. Trauma to kidneys
   I. Polycystic kidney disease
   J. Leukemia
   K. Thrombocytopenia
   L. Strenuous exercise
   M. Benign familial or recurrent hematuria (asymptomatic hematuria without proteinuria; other clinical and laboratory data are normal)
   N. Heavy smokers
2. *Hemoglobinuria* is found in
   A. Extensive burns
   B. Transfusion reactions (incompatible blood products)
   C. Febrile intoxication
   D. Certain chemical agents and alkaloids (poisonous mushrooms, snake venom)
   E. Malaria
   F. Bleeding resulting from operative procedures on the prostate (can be difficult to control, especially in the presence of malignancies)
   G. Hemolytic disorders such as sickle cell anemia, thalassemia, and glucose-6-phosphate dehydrogenase deficiency
   H. Paroxysmal hemoglobinuria (large quantities of hemoglobin appear in urine at irregular intervals)
   I. Kidney infarction
   J. Hemolysis occurring while the urine is in the urinary tract (RBC lysis from hypotonic urine or alkaline urine)
   K. Fava bean sensitivity (causes severe hemolytic anemia)
   L. Disseminated intravascular coagulation
   M. Strenuous exercise ("march hemoglobinuria")

> ### Clinical Alert
>
> One of the early indicators of possible renal or urinary tract disease is the appearance of blood in the urine. This does not mean that blood will be present in every voided specimen, but in most cases of renal or urinary tract disease, occult blood will appear in the urine with a reasonable degree of frequency. Any positive test for blood should be rechecked on a new urine specimen. If blood still appears, the patient should be further evaluated.

Interfering Factors

1. Drugs causing a positive result for blood or hemoglobin include
   A. Drugs toxic to the kidneys (eg, bacitracin, amphotericin)
   B. Drugs that alter blood clotting (coumarin)
   C. Drugs that cause hemolysis of RBCs (aspirin)
   D. Drugs that may give a false-positive result (eg, bromides, copper, iodides, oxidizing agents)
2. High doses of ascorbic acid or vitamin C may cause a false-negative result.
3. High SG or elevated protein reduces sensitivity (see Chap. 1).
4. Myoglobin produces a false-positive result.
5. Hypochlorites or bleach used to clean urine containers causes false-positive results.
6. Menstrual blood may contaminate the specimen and alter results.
7. Prostatic infections may cause false-positive results.
8. See Appendix J for a complete list of drugs that affect test outcomes.

Patient Preparation

1. Explain test purpose and procedure for urine specimen collection.
2. Follow guidelines in Chapter 1 for safe, effective, informed *pretest* care.

Patient Aftercare

1. Interpret test outcomes and explain possible need for follow-up testing.
2. Follow guidelines in Chapter 1 for safe, effective, informed *posttest* care.

URINE PROTEIN (ALBUMIN), QUALITATIVE AND 24-HOUR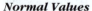

Normal Values
Adult: 10–140 mg/L or 1–14 mg/dl in 24 h
Child <10 y: 10–100 mg/L or 1–10 mg/dl in 24 h

Background
The presence of increased amounts of protein in the urine can be an important indicator of renal disease. It may be the first sign of a serious problem and may appear before any other clinical symptoms. However, there are other physiologic conditions (eg, exercise, fever) that can lead to increased protein excretion in urine. Also, there are some renal disorders in which proteinuria is absent.

Explanation of Test

In a healthy renal and urinary tract system, the urine contains no protein or only trace amounts. These consist of albumin (one-third of normal urine protein is albumin) and globulins from the plasma. Because albumin is filtered more readily than the globulins, it is usually abundant in pathologic conditions. Therefore, the term *albuminuria* is often used synonymously with *proteinuria*.

Normally, the glomeruli prevent passage of protein from the blood to the glomerular filtrate. Therefore, the presence of protein in the urine is the *single most important indication* of renal disease. If more than a trace of protein is found persistently in the urine, a quantitative 24-hour evaluation of protein excretion is necessary.

Procedure

QUALITATIVE PROTEIN COLLECTION

1. Collect a random urine sample in a clean container and test it as soon as possible.
2. Use a protein reagent dipstick, and compare the test result color with the color comparison chart provided on the reagent strip bottle. Protein can also be detected by turbidimetric methods using sulfosalicylic acid.
3. If 1 of these methods produces positive results, a new second specimen should be tested and any interfering factors investigated. Then a 24-hour urine test may be ordered for a quantitative measurement of protein.

24-HOUR URINE PROTEIN COLLECTION

1. Label a 24-hour urine container with the name of the patient, the test, and the date and time the test is started.
2. Refrigerate the specimen as it is being collected.
3. See general instructions for 24-hour urine collection listed (page 179).
4. Record the exact starting and ending times for the 24-hour collection on the specimen container and on the patient's record. (The usual starting and ending times are 0700 to 0700).

Clinical Implications

1. Proteinuria occurs by 2 main mechanisms: damage to the glomeruli or a defect in the reabsorption process that occurs in the tubules.
   - **A.** *Glomerular damage*
     - **(1)** Glomerulonephritis
     - **(2)** Systemic lupus erythematosus (SLE)
     - **(3)** Malignant hypertension
     - **(4)** Amyloidosis
     - **(5)** Diabetes mellitus
     - **(6)** Lipoid nephrosis
   - **B.** *Diminished tubular reabsorption*
     - **(1)** Renal tubular acidosis
     - **(2)** Pyelonephritis
     - **(3)** Cystinosis
     - **(4)** Wilson's disease

     (5) Fanconi's syndrome
     (6) Interstitial nephritis

2. In pathologic states, the level of proteinuria is rarely constant, so not every sample of urine is abnormal in patients with renal disease, and the concentration of protein in the urine is not necessarily indicative of the severity of renal disease.

3. Proteinuria may result from glomerular blood flow changes without the presence of a structural abnormality, as in congestive heart failure.

4. Proteinuria may be caused by increased serum protein levels
   A. Multiple myeloma (Bence Jones protein)
   B. Waldenström's macroglobulinemia
   C. Malignant lymphoma

5. Proteinuria can occur in other nonrenal diseases
   A. Acute infection
   B. Trauma
   C. Leukemia
   D. Toxemia, preeclampsia of pregnancy
   E. Malaria
   F. Vascular disease (hypertension)
   G. Renal transport rejection
   H. Sickle cell disease
   I. Poisoning from turpentine, phosphorus, mercury, gold, lead, phenol, opiates, or other drugs

6. Large numbers of leukocytes accompanying proteinuria usually indicate infection at some level in the urinary tract. Large numbers of both leukocytes and erythrocytes indicate a noninfectious inflammatory disease of the glomerulus. Proteinuria associated with pyelonephritis may have as many RBCs as WBCs.

7. Proteinuria does not always accompany renal disease
   A. Pyelonephritis
   B. Urinary tract obstructions
   C. Nephrolithiasis
   D. Tumors
   E. Congenital malformations
   F. Renal artery stenosis

8. Proteinuria is often associated with the finding of casts on sediment examination because protein is necessary for cast formation.

9. Postural proteinuria results from the excretion of protein by some patients when they stand or move about. This type of proteinuria is intermittent and disappears when the patient lies down. Postural proteinuria occurs in 3% to 15% of healthy young adults. It is also known as *orthostatic proteinuria*.

COLLECTING THE SPECIMEN FOR ORTHOSTATIC PROTEINURIA

1. The patient is instructed to void at bedtime and to discard this urine.

2. The next morning, a urine specimen is collected immediately after the patient awakens and before the patient has been in an upright position for longer than 1 minute. This may involve the use of a bedpan or urinal.

3. A second specimen is collected after the patient has been standing or walking for at least 2 hours.
4. With postural proteinuria, the first specimen contains no protein but the second one is positive for protein.
5. The urine looks microscopically normal; no RBCs or WBCs are apparent. Orthostatic proteinuria is considered a benign condition and slowly disappears with time. Progressive renal impairment usually does not occur.

Clinical Alert

1. Proteinuria of >2000 mg/24 hours in an adult or ≥40 mg/24 hours in a child usually indicates a glomerular cause.
2. Proteinuria of >3500 mg/24 hours points to a nephrotic syndrome.

Interfering Factors for Qualitative Protein Test

1. Because of renal vasoconstriction, the presence of a functional, mild, and transitory proteinuria is associated with
   A. Strenuous exercise
   B. Severe emotional stress, seizures
   C. Cold baths, exposure to very cold temperatures
2. Increased protein in urine occurs in these benign states:
   A. Fever and dehydration
   B. Non–immunoglobulin E food allergies
   C. Salicylate therapy
   D. In the premenstrual period and immediately after delivery
3. False or accidental proteinuria may occur because of a mixture of pus and RBCs in the urinary tract related to infections, menstrual or vaginal discharge, mucus, or semen.
4. False-positive results can occur from incorrect use and interpretation of the color reagent strip test.
5. Alkaline, highly buffered urine can produce false-positive results on the dipstick test.
6. Very dilute urine may give a falsely low protein value.
7. Certain drugs may cause false-positive or false-negative urine protein tests (see Appendix J).
8. Radiographic contrast agents may produce false-positive results with turbidimetric measurements.

Patient Preparation

1. Instruct the patient about the purpose and procedure for collection of the 24-hour urine specimen. Emphasize the importance of compliance with the procedure.
2. Food and fluids are permitted; however, fluids should not be forced, because very dilute urine can produce false-negative values.
3. Follow guidelines in Chapter 1 for safe, effective, informed *pretest* care.

Patient Aftercare

1. Interpret test outcomes and explain the possible need for follow-up testing and treatment.

2. See guidelines in Chapter 1 for safe, effective, informed *posttest* care.

URINE BENCE JONES PROTEIN

Normal Values

Negative

Background

Bence Jones proteins are monoclonal immunoglobulin light chains that may be present in either serum or urine. The molecular weights of these proteins are low, so they are easily filtered through the glomeruli and excreted in the urine. They are also referred to as "free" light chains, because they are not attached to other immunoglobulins.

Explanation of Test

This test is helpful in the diagnosis of multiple myeloma, lymphoma, macroglobulinemia, leukemia, osteogenic sarcoma, amyloidosis, and other malignancies.

Screening for Bence Jones protein can be done by a turbidimetric test such as the sulfosalicylic acid test or by the heat precipitation test. Bence Jones protein precipitates on heating between 45°C and 60°C and then redissolves with further heating to the boiling point. When a screening test is positive, confirmatory testing must be done, because the screening tests in themselves are not diagnostic. The best confirmatory tests are urine protein electrophoresis and immunoelectrophoresis of the urine (see Chap. 8).

Procedure

1. Collect a random urine specimen.

2. Refrigerate the specimen or take it to the laboratory as soon as possible.

3. If screening is positive, a urine and blood serum electrophoresis should be done to confirm.

Clinical Implications

A positive Bence Jones protein test (free light chains) is found in

1. Fifty percent to 80% of multiple myeloma cases (malignant proliferation of plasma cells)

2. Waldenström's macroglobulinemia

3. Cryoglobulinemia

4. Primary amyloidosis

5. Adult Fanconi's syndrome

6. Benign monoclonal gammopathy

7. Other malignant B-cell diseases

8. Light chain disease

Interfering Factors

Conditions that may produce a false-positive result include

1. Connective tissue disorders, (eg, SLE, rheumatoid arthritis)
2. Chronic renal insufficiency
3. Metastatic carcinoma of lung, gastrointestinal tract, or genitourinary tract
4. High doses of penicillin or aspirin
5. Radiographic contrast media
6. Blood in urine
7. Lymphoma and leukemia

Clinical Alert

1. The dipstick method for detecting protein will give a false-negative result for Bence Jones protein—the protein dipstick reacts mainly with albumin. Bence Jones is a globulin; therefore, this method cannot be used for screening.
2. When significant amounts of free κ and λ light chains are detected by electrophoresis, they should be confirmed by urine immunofixation for early diagnosis and assessment of this type of light chain disease.

Patient Preparation

1. Explain test purpose and specimen collection procedure.
2. See Chapter 1 guidelines for safe, effective, informed *pretest* care.

Patient Aftercare

1. Interpret test outcomes and monitor appropriately.
2. Follow Chapter 1 guidelines for safe, effective, informed *posttest* care.

URINE β₂-MICROGLOBULIN ●

Normal Values

24-h specimen: <1 mg
Blood serum specimen: <2.7 μg/ml

Background

β₂-Microglobulin is a small membrane associated with amino acid peptide, a component of the lymphatic human lymphocyte antibody (HLA) complex. It is structurally related to the immunoglobulins.

Explanation of Test

This test measures β₂-microglobulin, which is nonspecifically increased in inflammatory conditions and in active chronic lymphatic leukemia. It may be used to differentiate glomerular from tubular dysfunction. In glomerular disease, β₂-microglobulin is increased in serum and decreased in urine, whereas in tubular disorders it is decreased in serum and increased in urine. In aminoglycoside toxicity, β_2-microglobulin levels become abnormal before creatinine levels begin to show abnormal values. Serum is also used to evaluate the prognosis of multiple myeloma.

Procedure

1. Collect a 10-ml random fresh urine sample, a 24-hour specimen, or a serum sample.
2. Keep the pH neutral.
3. Either specimen must be frozen if not analyzed immediately.

Clinical Implications

1. Increased urine β_2-microglobulin occurs in
   a. Renal tubular disorders (>50 mg/day)
   b. Heavy metal poisoning (mercury, cadmium)
   c. Drug toxicity (aminoglycosides, cyclosporine)
   d. Fanconi's syndrome
   e. Pyelonephritis
   f. Renal allograft rejection
   g. Lymphoid malignancies
   h. Acquired immunodeficiency syndrome (AIDS)—progressive disease
2. Serum β_2-microglobulin <4μg/ml is associated with a poor survival prognosis in multiple myeloma.

Interfering Factors

1. Highly acid urine
2. Certain antibiotics (eg, gentamicin, tobramycin)
3. Recent nuclear medicine scan
4. Increased synthesis in certain diseases (eg, Crohn's disease, hepatitis, sarcoidosis) decreases the usefulness of the blood serum test.

Patient Preparation

1. Instruct patient regarding the purpose and procedure of test.
2. See instructions for 24-hour urine collection, page 179.
3. See Chapter 1 for guidelines for safe, effective, informed *pretest* care.

Patient Aftercare

1. Interpret test outcomes and monitor appropriately.
2. See Chapter 1 guidelines for safe, effective, informed *posttest* care.

URINE GLUCOSE (SUGAR) ●

Normal Values

Random specimen: Negative
24-h specimen: <0.3 g

Background

Glucose is present in glomerular filtrate and is reabsorbed by the proximal convoluted tubule. If the blood glucose level exceeds the reabsorption capacity of the tubules, glucose will appear in the urine. Tubular reabsorption of glucose is by active transport in response to the body's need to maintain an adequate concentration of glucose. The blood level at which tubular reabsorption stops is termed the *renal threshold,* which for glucose is between 160 and 180 mg/dl.

Explanation of Test
Urine glucose tests are used to screen for diabetes, to confirm a diagnosis of diabetes, and to monitor the degree of diabetic control. Diabetes mellitus is the main cause of glycosuria. In diabetes, the blood glucose levels are high. Glycosuria that is not accompanied by high glucose levels is seen in conditions that affect tubular reabsorption, in central nervous system damage, and in thyroid disorders.

Types of Glucose Tests
1. *Reduction tests* (Clinitest)
   A. These are based on reduction of cupric ions by glucose. When the compounds are added to urine, a heat reaction takes place. This results in precipitation and a change in the color of the urine if glucose is present.
   B. These tests are nonspecific for glucose because the reaction can also be caused by other reducing substances in the urine, including
   (1) Creatinine, uric acid, ascorbic acid
   (2) Other sugars, such as galactose, lactose, fructose, pentose, and maltose
2. *Enzyme tests* (Clinistix, Diastix, Tes-Tape)
   A. These tests are based on interaction between glucose oxidase (an enzyme) and glucose. When dipped into urine, the enzyme-impregnated strip changes color according to the amount of glucose in the urine. The manufacturer's color chart provides a basis for comparison of colors between the sample and the manufacturer's control.
   B. These tests are specific for glucose only.

Procedure
1. Use a freshly voided specimen.
2. Follow directions on the test container exactly. Timing must be exact; the color reaction must be compared with the closest matching control color on the manufacturer's color chart to ascertain accurate results.
3. Record the results on the patient's record.
4. If a 24-hour urine specimen is also ordered, the entire urine sample must be refrigerated or iced during collection. See Table 3-2 for proper preservative.

Clinical Alert

1. Urine glucose >1000 mg (4+) is a critical value.
2. Determine exactly what drugs the patient is taking and whether the metabolites of these drugs can affect the urine glucose results. Frequent updating in regard to the effects of drugs on blood glucose levels is necessary in light of the many new drugs introduced and prescribed.

(continued)

(Clinical Alert continued)
3. Test results may be reported as "plus" (+) or as percentages. Percentages are more accurate.
4. When screening for galactose (galactosuria) in infants, the reduction test must be used. The enzyme tests do not react with galactose.

Clinical Implications

1. *Increased glucose* occurs in
   A. Diabetes mellitus
   B. Thyroid disorders (thyrotoxicosis)
   C. Cushing's syndrome, acromegaly
   D. Central nervous system disorders (brain injury)
   E. Impaired tubular reabsorption
      (1) Fanconi's syndrome
      (2) Advanced renal tubular disease
   F. Pregnancy with possible latent diabetes
2. *Increase of other sugars* (react only with reduction tests, not dipstick tests):
   A. Lactose—pregnancy, lactation, lactose intolerance
   B. Galactose—hereditary galactosuria (severe enzyme deficiency in infants; must be treated promptly)
   C. Xylose—excessive ingestion of fruit
   D. Fructose—hereditary fructose intolerance, hepatic disorders
   E. Pentose—certain drug therapies and rare hereditary conditions

Interfering Factors

1. Interfering factors for reduction test (false-positive results):
   A. Presence of non–sugar-reducing substances such as ascorbic acid, homogentisic acid, creatinine
   B. Tyrosine
   C. Nalidixic acid, cephalosporins, probenecid, and penicillin
   D. Large amounts of urine protein (slows reaction)
2. Interfering factors for dipstick enzyme tests
   A. Ascorbic acid (in large amounts) may cause a false-negative result
   B. Large amount of ketones may cause a false-negative result
   C. Peroxide or strong oxidizing agents may cause a false-positive result
3. Stress, excitement, myocardial infarction, testing after a heavy meal, and testing soon after the administration of intravenous glucose may all cause false-positive results, most frequently trace reactions
4. Contamination of the urine sample with bleach or hydrogen peroxide may invalidate results.
5. False-negative results may occur if urine is left to sit at room temperature for an extended period, owing to the rapid glycolysis of glucose.
6. See Appendix J for other drugs that affect test outcomes.

Patient Preparation

1. Instruct the patient about the test purpose, the procedure, and the double-voiding technique.

A. Discard the first voided morning specimen, then void 30 to 45 minutes later for the test specimen. This second specimen reflects the immediate state of glucosuria more accurately, because the first morning specimen consists of urine that has been present in the bladder for several hours.

B. Advise the patient not to drink liquids between the first and second voiding so as not to dilute the glucose present in the specimen.

C. A urine glucose test combined with a blood glucose test gives a more complete assessment of diabetes.

2. Instruct the patient about the 24-hour urine collection procedure when applicable (see page 179).

3. Follow Chapter 1 guidelines for safe, effective, informed *pretest* care.

Patient Aftercare

1. Interpret test outcomes and counsel appropriately.

2. See Chapter 1 guidelines for safe, effective, informed *posttest* care.

URINE KETONES (ACETONE; KETONE BODIES) ●

Normal Values

Negative

Background

Ketones, which result from the metabolism of fatty acid and fat, consist mainly of 3 substances: acetone, β-hydroxybutyric acid, and acetoacetic acid. The last 2 substances readily convert to acetone, in essence making acetone the main substance being tested. However, some testing products measure only acetoacetic acid.

In healthy persons, ketones are formed in the liver and are completely metabolized so that only negligible amounts appear in the urine. However, when carbohydrate metabolism is altered, an excessive amount of ketones is formed (acidosis) because fat becomes the predominant body fuel instead of carbohydrates. When the metabolic pathways of carbohydrates are disturbed, carbon fragments from fat and protein are diverted to form abnormal amounts of ketone bodies. Increased ketones in the blood lead to electrolyte imbalance, dehydration, and, if not corrected, acidosis and eventual coma.

Explanation of Test

The excess presence of ketones in the urine (ketonuria) is associated with diabetes or altered carbohydrate metabolism. Some "fad" diets that are low in carbohydrates and high in fat and protein also produce ketones in the urine. Testing for urine ketones by patients with diabetes may provide the clue to early diagnosis of ketoacidosis and diabetic coma.

Indications for Ketone Testing

1. *General:* Screening for ketonuria is frequently done for hospitalized patients, presurgical patients, pregnant women, children, and persons with diabetes.

2. *Glycosuria* (diabetes):
   A. Testing for ketones is indicated for any patient showing elevated urine and blood sugars.
   B. When treatment is being switched from insulin to oral hypoglycemic agents, the development of ketonuria within 24 hours after withdrawal of insulin usually indicates a poor response to the oral hypoglycemic agents.
   C. The urine of diabetic patients treated with oral hypoglycemic agents should be tested regularly for glucose and ketones, because oral hypoglycemic agents, unlike insulin, do not control diabetes when acute complications such as infection develop.
   D. Ketone testing is done to differentiate between diabetic coma and insulin shock.
3. *Acidosis:*
   A. Ketone testing is used to judge the severity of acidosis and to monitor the response to treatment.
   B. Urine ketone measurement frequently provides a more reliable indicator of acidosis than blood testing (it is especially useful in emergency situations).
   C. Ketones appear in the urine before there is any significant increase of ketones in the blood.
4. *Pregnancy:* During pregnancy, the early detection of ketones is essential because ketoacidosis is a prominent factor that contributes to intrauterine death.

Procedure

1. Dip the ketone reagent strip in fresh urine, tap off excess urine, time the reaction accurately, and then compare the strip with the control color chart on the container.
2. If procedure differs from the technique just described, follow the manufacturer's directions exactly.
3. Do not use dipsticks to test for ketones in blood. Special testing products are designed for blood.

Clinical Implications

1. Ketosis and ketonuria may occur whenever increased amounts of fat are metabolized, carbohydrate intake is restricted, or the diet is rich in fats (either "hidden" or obvious). This state can occur in the following situations:
   A. Metabolic conditions
      (1) Diabetes mellitus (diabetic acidosis)
      (2) Renal glycosuria
      (3) Glycogen storage disease (von Gierke's disease)
   B. Dietary conditions
      (1) Starvation, fasting
      (2) High-fat diets
      (3) Prolonged vomiting

(**4**) Anorexia

(**5**) Low-carbohydrate diet

(**6**) Eclampsia

C. Increased metabolic states caused by

(**1**) Hyperthyroidism

(**2**) Fever

(**3**) Pregnancy or lactation

2. In nondiabetic persons, ketonuria occurs frequently during acute illness, severe stress, or strenuous exercise. Approximately 15% of hospitalized patients have ketones in their urine even though they do not have diabetes.

3. Children are particularly prone to developing ketonuria and ketosis.

4. Ketonuria occurs after anesthesia (ether or chloroform).

Interfering Factors

1. Drugs that may cause a false-positive result include

A. Levodopa

B. Phenothiazines

C. Ether

D. Insulin

E. Aspirin

F. Metformin

G. Penicilliamine

H. Phenazopyridine (Pyridium)

I. Captopril

2. False-negative results occur if urine stands too long, owing to loss of ketones into the air.

3. See Appendix J for other drugs that affect test outcomes.

> ### Clinical Alert
>
> Ketonuria signals a need for caution, rather than crisis intervention, in either a diabetic or a nondiabetic patient. However, this condition should not be taken lightly.

1. In the diabetic patient, ketone bodies in the urine suggest that the diabetes is not adequately controlled and that adjustments of either the medication or the diet should be made promptly.

2. In the nondiabetic patient, ketone bodies indicate a reduced carbohydrate metabolism and excessive fat metabolism.

3. Positive urine ketones in a child younger than 2 years of age is a critical alert.

Patient Preparation

1. Explain test purpose and procedure.

2. Follow guidelines in Chapter 1 for safe, effective, informed *pretest* care.

Patient Aftercare
1. Interpret test outcomes and monitor appropriately.
2. See Chapter 1 guidelines for safe, effective, informed *posttest* care.

URINE NITRITE (BACTERIA) ●

Normal Values
Negative for bacteria

Background
This test is a rapid, indirect method for detecting bacteria in the urine. Significant UTI may be present in a patient who does not experience any symptoms. Common gram-negative organisms contain enzymes that reduce the nitrate in the urine to nitrite.

Explanation of Test
Clinicians frequently request the urine nitrate test to screen high-risk patients: pregnant women, school-age children (especially girls), diabetic patients, elderly patients, patients with a history of recurrent infections.

The majority of UTIs are believed to start in the bladder as a result of extreme contamination; if left untreated, they can progress upward all the way to the kidneys. Pyelonephritis is a frequent complication of untreated cystitis and can lead to renal damage. Detection of bacteria using the nitrate test and subsequent antibiotic therapy can prevent these serious complications. The nitrate test can also be used to evaluate the success of antibiotic therapy.

Procedure
1. A first morning specimen is preferred, because urine that has been in the bladder for several hours is more likely to yield a positive nitrate test than a random urine sample that may have been in the bladder for only a short time. A clean-catch (midstream) urine specimen is needed to minimize bacterial contamination from adjacent areas.
2. Follow the exact testing procedure according to prescribed guidelines for reliable test results. Any shade of pink is positive for nitrite-producing bacteria.
3. Comparison of the reacted reagent area on the dipstick with a white background may aid in the detection of a faint pink hue that might otherwise be missed.
4. A microscopic examination should be done to verify results, if at all possible.

Clinical Implications
1. Under the light microscope, the presence of ≥20 bacteria per high-power field (hpf) may indicate a UTI. Untreated bacteriuria can lead to serious kidney disease.
2. The presence of a few bacteria suggests a UTI that cannot be confirmed or excluded until more definitive studies, such as culture and sensitivity tests, are performed. Again, this finding merits serious consideration for treatment.

3. A positive nitrate test is a reliable indicator of significant bacteriuria and is a cue for performing urine culture.

4. A negative result should *never* be interpreted as indicating absence of bacteriuria, for the following reasons:

    A. If an overnight urine sample is not used, there may not have been enough time for the nitrate to convert to nitrite in the bladder.

    B. Some UTIs are caused by organisms that do not convert nitrate to nitrite (eg, staphylococci, streptococci).

    C. Sufficient dietary nitrate may not be present for the nitrate-to-nitrite reaction to occur.

Interfering Factors

1. Azo dye metabolites and bilirubin can produce false-positive results.

2. Ascorbic acid can produce false-negative results.

3. False-positive results can be obtained if the urine sits too long at room temperature, allowing contaminant bacteria to multiply.

Clinical Alert

A negative urine nitrate test should never be interpreted as indicating the absence of bacteria.

Patient Preparation

1. Explain the test purpose and urine specimen collection procedure. Instruct the patient in the procedure necessary for a clean-catch (midstream) specimen.

2. Follow guidelines in Chapter 1 for safe, effective, informed *pretest* care.

Patient Aftercare

1. Interpret test outcomes and monitor appropriately.

2. See Chapter 1 guidelines for safe, effective, informed *posttest* care.

URINE LEUKOCYTE ESTERASE

Normal Values
Negative

Background
Usually, the presence of leukocytes (WBCs) in the urine indicates a UTI. The leukocyte esterase test detects esterase released by the leukocytes into the urine. This is a standardized means for the detection of WBCs.

Explanation of Test
Microscopic examination and chemical testing are used to determine the presence of leukocytes in the urine. The chemical test is done with a leukocyte esterase dipstick. This test can also detect intact leukocytes, lysed leukocytes, and WBC casts.

Procedure

1. Collect a fresh, random urine specimen with a clean-catch or midstream technique.
2. Directions for dipstick use must be followed exactly. Timing is critical for accurate results.
3. A positive result causes a purple color on the dipstick. The test is not designed to measure the amount of leukocytes.

Clinical Implications

1. Positive results are clinically significant and indicate pyuria (UTI).
2. Urine with positive results from the dipstick should be examined microscopically for WBCs and bacteria.

Interfering Factors

1. Vaginal discharge, *Trichomonas,* parasites, and histocytes can cause false-positive results.
2. False-negative results may occur with large amounts of glucose or protein.

> ### Clinical Alert
>
> A urine sample that tests positive for both nitrite and leukocyte esterase should be cultured for pathogenic bacteria.

Patient Preparation

1. Explain test purpose and procedure.
2. See Chapter 1 guidelines for safe, effective, informed *pretest* care.

Patient Aftercare

1. Interpret test outcomes and monitor appropriately.
2. Follow Chapter 1 guidelines for safe, effective, informed *posttest* care.

URINE BILIRUBIN ●

Normal Values

Negative (0–0.02 mg/dl)

Background

Bilirubin is formed in the reticuloendothelial cells of the spleen and bone marrow as a result of the breakdown of hemoglobin; it is then transported to the liver. Urinary bilirubin levels are increased to significant levels in the presence of any disease process that increases the amount of conjugated bilirubin in the bloodstream (see Chap. 6). Elevated amounts appear when the normal degradation cycle is disrupted by obstruction of the bile duct or when the integrity of the liver is damaged.

Explanation of Test
Urine bilirubin aids in the diagnosis and monitoring of treatment for hepatitis and liver damage.

Urine bilirubin is an early sign of hepatocellular disease or intrahepatic or extrahepatic biliary obstruction. It should be a part of every UA, because bilirubin often appears in the urine before other signs of liver dysfunction (eg, jaundice, weakness) become apparent. Not only does the detection of urinary bilirubin provide an early indication of liver disease, but its presence or absence can be used in determining the cause of clinical jaundice.

Procedure
1. Examine the urine within 1 hour of collection, because urine bilirubin is unstable, especially when exposed to light. If the urine is yellowish-greenish to brownish, shake the urine. If a yellowish-greenish foam develops, bilirubin is probably present. Bilirubin alters the surface tension and allows foam to form. The yellow color is the bilirubin.
2. Chemical strip testing:
   A. Dip a chemically reactive dipstick into the urine sample according to manufacturer's directions.
   B. Close comparison of color changes on the dipstick with control colors on the color chart is an absolute necessity. Failure to make a close approximation of color may result in failure to recognize urine bilirubin. Good lighting is required.
   C. Interpret results as "negative" to "3+" or as "small," "moderate," or "large" amounts of bilirubin.
3. When it is crucial to detect even very small amounts of bilirubin in the urine, as in the earliest phase of viral hepatitis, Icotest tablets are preferred for testing because they are more sensitive to urine bilirubin. When elevated amounts of urine bilirubin are present, a blue to purplish color forms on the absorptive mat. The the intensity of the color and the rapidity of its development are directly proportional to the amount of bilirubin in the urine.

Clinical Implications
1. Even trace amounts of bilirubin are abnormal and warrant further investigation. Normally, there is no detectable bilirubin in the urine.
2. Increased bilirubin occurs in
   A. Hepatitis and liver diseases caused by infections or exposure to toxic agents
   B. Obstructive biliary tract disease

   NOTE: *Urine bilirubin is negative in hemolytic disease.*

Interfering Factors
1. Drugs may cause false-positive or false-negative results. See Appendix J.
2. Bilirubin rapidly decomposes when exposed to light; therefore, urine should be tested immediately.
3. High concentrations of ascorbic acid or nitrate cause decreased sensitivity.

> ### Clinical Alert
>
> Pyridium-like drugs or urochromes may give the urine an amber or reddish color and can mask the bilirubin reaction.

Patient Preparation
1. Explain test purpose and procedure.
2. See Chapter 1 guidelines for safe, effective, informed *pretest* care.

Patient Aftercare
1. Interpret test outcomes and monitor appropriately for liver disease.
2. Follow Chapter 1 guidelines for safe, effective, informed *posttest* care.

URINE UROBILINOGEN, RANDOM AND TIMED ●

Normal Values
Random specimen: 0.1–1 Ehrlich U/dl or < 1mg
2-h specimen: 0.1–1.0 Ehrlich U or < 1mg
24-h specimen: 0.5–4.0 Ehrlich U or 0.5–4.0 mg/d

Background
Bilirubin, which is formed from the degradation of hemoglobin, is transformed through the action of bacterial enzymes into *urobilinogen* after it enters the intestines. Some of the urobilinogen formed in the intestine is excreted as part of the feces, where it is oxidized to urobilin; another portion is absorbed into the portal bloodstream and carried to the liver, where it is metabolized and excreted in the bile. Traces of urobilinogen in the blood that escape removal by the liver are carried to the kidneys and excreted in the urine. This is the basis of the urine urobilinogen test. Unlike bilirubin, urobilinogen is *colorless*.

Explanation of Test
Urine urobilinogen is one of the most sensitive tests available to determine impaired liver function. Urinary urobilinogen is increased by any condition that causes an increase in the production of bilirubin and by any disease that prevents the liver from normally removing the reabsorbed urobilinogen from the portal circulation. An increased urobilinogen level is one of the earliest signs of liver disease and hemolytic disorders.

Although it cannot be determined by reagent strip, the absence of urobilinogen is also diagnostically significant and represents an obstruction of the bile duct.

Procedure
1. Follow instructions for collecting a timed 24-hour, 2-hour, or random specimen. Check with the laboratory for specific protocols.
2. The 2-hour timed collection is best done from 1:00 PM to 3:00 PM (1300 to

1500) or from 2:00 PM to 4:00 PM (1400 to 1600), because peak excretion occurs during this time. No preservatives are necessary. Record the total amount of urine voided. Protect the collection receptacle from light. Test immediately after specimen collection is completed.

Clinical Implications

1. Urine urobilinogen is *increased* when there is
   A. Increased destruction of RBCs
      (1) Hemolytic anemias
      (2) Pernicious anemia (megaloblastic)
      (3) Malaria
   B. Hemorrhage into tissues
      (1) Pulmonary infarction
      (2) Excessive bruising
   C. Hepatic damage
      (1) Biliary disease
      (2) Cirrhosis (viral and chemical)
      (3) Acute hepatitis
   D. Cholangitis
2. Urine urobilinogen is *decreased* or absent when normal amounts of bilirubin are not excreted into the intestinal tract. This usually indicates partial or complete obstruction of the bile ducts. The stool is pale in color. Decreased urinary urobilinogen is associated with
   A. Cholelithiasis
   B. Severe inflammation of the biliary ducts
   C. Cancer of the head of the pancreas
3. During antibiotic therapy, suppression of normal gut flora may prevent the breakdown of bilirubin to urobilinogen; therefore urine levels will be decreased or absent.
4. More comprehensive information is obtained when the tests for urobilinogen and bilirubin are correlated (see the following comparisons).

Comparison of Urine Urobilinogen and Urine Bilirubin Values

Test	In Health	In Hemolytic Disease	In Hepatic Disease	In Biliary Obstruction
Urine urobilinogen	Normal	Increased	Increased	Low or absent
Urine bilirubin	Negative	Negative	Positive or negative	Positive

Clinical Alert

Urine urobilinogen rapidly decomposes at room temperature or when exposed to light.

Interfering Factors

1. Drugs that may affect urobilinogen levels include those that cause cholestasis and those that reduce the bacterial flora in the gastrointestinal tract. Check with pharmacist for specific drugs patient is taking.
2. Peak excretion is known to occur from noon to 4:00 PM. The amount of urobilinogen in the urine is subject to diurnal variation.
3. Strongly alkaline urine shows a higher urobilinogen level, and strongly acid urine shows a lower urobilinogen level.
4. Drugs that may cause *increased* urobilinogen include drugs that cause hemolysis. Check with pharmacist for specific drugs patient is taking.
5. If the urine is highly colored, the strip will be difficult to read.

Patient Preparation

1. Explain test purpose and urine collection procedures.
2. See Chapter 1 guidelines for safe, effective, informed *pretest* care.

Patient Aftercare

1. Interpret test outcomes and monitor appropriately for anemia and gastrointestinal disorders. Advise concerning need for follow-up testing.
2. Follow Chapter 1 guidelines for safe, effective, informed *posttest* care.

●MICROSCOPIC EXAMINATION OF URINE SEDIMENT

In health, the urine contains small numbers of cells and other formed elements from the entire genitourinary tract: casts and epithelial cells from the nephron; epithelial cells from the kidney, pelvis, ureters, bladder, and urethra; mucous threads and spermatozoa from the prostate; possibly RBCs or WBCs and an occasional cast. In renal parenchymal disease, the urine usually contains increased numbers of cells and casts discharged from an organ that is otherwise accessible only by biopsy or surgery (see the following list of elements and their significance). Urinary sediment provides information useful for both diagnosis and prognosis. It provides a direct sampling of urinary tract morphology.

The urinary sediment is obtained by pouring 10 ml of fresh, well-mixed urine into a conical tube and centrifuging the sample at a specific speed for 10 minutes. The supernatant is poured off, and 1 ml of the sediment is mixed under a coverslip on a slide and examined microscopically.

The urine sediment can be broken down into cellular elements (RBCs, WBCs, and epithelial cells), casts, crystals, and bacteria. These may originate anywhere in the urinary tract. When casts do occur in the urine, they may indicate tubular or glomerular disorders.

Casts are the only elements found in urinary sediment that are unique to

Microscopic Examination of Urine Sediment

Urine Sediment Component	Clinical Significance
Bacteria	Urinary tract infection
Casts	Tubular or glomerular disorders
Broad casts	Formation occurs in collecting tubules; serious kidney disorder
Epithelial (renal) casts	Tubular degeneration
Fatty casts	Nephrotic syndrome
Granular or waxy casts	Renal parenchymal disease
Hyaline casts	Acid urine, high salt content
Red blood cell casts	Acute glomerulonephritis
White blood cell casts	Pyelonephritis
Epithelial cells	Damage to various parts of urinary tract
Renal cells	Tubular damage
Squamous cells	Normal or contamination
Erythrocytes	st renal disorders; menstruation; strenuous exercise
Fat bodies (oval)	Nephrotic syndrome
Leukocytes	Most renal disorders; urinary tract infection; pyelonephritis

the kidneys. They are formed primarily within the lumen of the distal convoluted tubule and collecting duct, providing a microscopic view of conditions within the nephron. Their shapes are representative of the tubular lumen.

Cast width is significant in determining the site of origin and may indicate the extent of renal damage. The width of the cast indicates the diameter of the tubule responsible for its formation. Cast width is described as *narrow* (as wide as 1 to 2 RBCs), *medium-broad* (3 to 4 RBCs), or *broad* (5 RBCs). The broad casts form in the collecting tubule and may be of any composition. Their presence usually indicates a marked reduction in the functional capacity of the nephron and suggests severe renal damage or end-stage renal disease.

The major constituent of casts is Tamm-Horsfall protein, a glycoprotein excreted by the renal tubular cells. It is found in normal and abnormal urine and is not detected by the urine dipstick method.

Clinical Alert

Microscopic examination of urine sediment can provide the following information:

1. Evidence of renal disease as opposed to infection of the lower urinary tract.
2. Type and status of a renal lesion or disease.

URINE RED BLOOD CELLS AND RED BLOOD CELL CASTS ●

Normal Values

RBCs: 0–3/hpf
RBC casts: 0/lpf

Explanation of Test

In health, erythrocytes (RBCs) occasionally appear in the urine. However, *persistent* findings of even small numbers of RBCs should be thoroughly investigated, because these cells come from the kidney and may signal serious renal disease. They are usually diagnostic of glomerular disease.

Procedure for Microscopic Urine Examination

1. Collect a random urine specimen. Transport the specimen to the laboratory as soon as possible.
2. Urinary sediment is microscopically examined under both the low-power field (lpf) and the high-power field (hpf). Low power is used to find and count casts; RBCs, WBCs and bacteria show up and are counted under high power. Amounts present are defined in the following terms: few, moderate, packed, and packed solid; or 1+, 2+, 3+, and 4+. Crystals and other elements are also noted.
3. Microscopic results should be correlated with the physical and chemical findings to ensure the accuracy of the report.

Common Correlations in Urinalysis

Microscopic Elements	Physical Examination	Dipstick Measurement*
Red blood cells	Turbidity, red color	Blood
White blood cells	Turbidity	Protein
		Nitrite
		Leukocytes
Epithelial cast cells	Turbidity	Protein
Bacteria	Turbidity	pH
		Nitrite
		Leukocytes
Crystals	Turbidity, color	pH

* positive result.

Clinical Implications

1. *RBC casts* indicate hemorrhage in the nephron.
   A. RBC casts are found in 3 forms
      (1) Intact RBCs
      (2) Degenerating cells within a protein matrix
      (3) Homogenous blood casts ("hemoglobin casts")

B. RBC casts indicate acute inflammatory or vascular disorders in the glomerulus and are found in
  (1) Glomerulonephritis (acute and chronic)
  (2) Renal infarction
  (3) Lupus nephritis
  (4) Goodpasture's syndrome
  (5) Severe pyelonephritis
  (6) Congestive heart failure
  (7) Renal vein thrombosis
  (8) Kidney involvement in subacute bacterial endocarditis
  (9) Malignant hypertension
  (10) Periarteritis nodosa
C. RBCs and epithelial cell casts are usually associated with SLE and glomerulonephritis.
D. RBCs *should be present* if RBC casts are in the sediment.

2. *Red blood cells*
  A. The finding of more than 1 or 2 RBCs/hpf is abnormal and can indicate
    (1) Renal or systemic disease (glomerulonephritis)
    (2) Trauma to the kidney (vascular injury)
  B. Increased numbers of RBCs occur in
    (1) Pyelonephritis
    (2) SLE
    (3) Renal stones
    (4) Cystitis (acute or chronic)
    (5) Prostatitis
    (6) Tuberculosis (renal)
    (7) Genitourinary tract malignancies
    (8) Hemophilia, coagulation disorders
    (9) Malaria
    (10) Polyarteritis nodosa
    (11) Malignant hypertension
    (12) Acute febrile episodes
  C. Greater numbers of RBCs than WBCs indicates bleeding into the urinary tract, as may occur with
    (1) Trauma
    (2) Tumors of rectum, colon, pelvis
    (3) Aspirin overdose or other toxic drugs
    (4) Anticoagulant therapy overdose
    (5) Thrombocytopenia

Clinical Alert

1. In health, RBCs are occasionally found in the urine. However, persistent findings of even small numbers of RBCs should be thoroughly
(continued)

(Clinical Alert continued)

investigated, the first step being to request a fresh urine specimen for repeat testing.

2. Rule out the possible presence of menstrual blood, vaginal bleeding, or trauma to the perineal area in a female patient.

Interfering Factors

1. Increased numbers of RBCs may be found after a traumatic catheterization and after passage of urinary tract or kidney stones.
2. Alkaline urine hemolyzes RBCs and dissolves casts ("ghosts").
3. Some drugs can cause increased numbers of RBCs in the urine. See Appendix J.
4. RBC casts and RBCs may appear after very strenuous physical activity or participation in contact sports.
5. Heavy smokers show small numbers of RBCs in the urine.
6. Yeast or oil droplets may be mistaken for RBCs.

Patient Preparation

1. Explain test purpose and procedure for random urine sample collection.
2. See Chapter 1 guidelines for safe, effective, informed *pretest* care.

Patient Aftercare

1. Interpret test outcomes and counsel appropriately.
2. Follow Chapter 1 guidelines for safe, effective, informed *posttest* care.

URINE WHITE BLOOD CELLS AND WHITE BLOOD CELL CASTS

Normal Values

WBCs: 0–4/hpf
Normal women may have slightly more WBCs.
WBC casts: 0/lpf

Background

Leukocytes (WBCs) may originate from anywhere in the genitourinary tract. They are also capable of amoeboid migration through the tissues to sites of infection or inflammation. An increase in urinary WBCs is called pyuria and indicates the presence of an infection or inflammation in the genitourinary system. However, WBC casts always come from the kidney tubules.

Procedure

1. Collect a random urine specimen and transport it to laboratory as soon as possible.
2. Urinary sediment is microscopically examined under high power for cells and under low power for casts.

Clinical Implications

1. *White blood cells*
   A. Large numbers of WBCs (≥30 cells/hpf) usually indicate acute bacterial infection within the urinary tract.

B. Increased WBCs are seen in
  (1) All renal disease
  (2) Urinary tract disease (eg, cystitis, prostatitis)
  (3) Viral infection
  (4) Strenuous exercise
  (5) Chronic pyelonephritis
  (6) Bladder tumors
  (7) Tuberculosis
  (8) Lupus erythematosus
  (9) Interstitial nephritis
  (10) Glomerulonephritis
C. In bladder infections, WBCs tend to be associated with bacteria, epithelial cells, and relatively few RBCs.
D. Large numbers of lymphocytes and plasma cells in the presence of a kidney transplant may indicate early tissue rejection (acute renal allograft rejection).
E. Eosinophils are associated with tubulointerstitial disease and hypersensitivity to penicillin.

Clinical Alert

A urine culture (see Chap. 7) should be done if elevated urine WBCs are found.

---

2. *WBC casts*
  A. WBC casts indicate renal parenchymal infection and may occur in
    (1) Pyelonephritis (most common cause)
    (2) Acute glomerulonephritis
    (3) Interstitial nephritis
    (4) Lupus nephritis
  B. It can be very difficult to differentiate between WBC casts and epithelial cell casts.

Interfering Factors
Vaginal discharge can contaminate a specimen with WBCs. Either a clean-catch urine specimen or a catheterized urine specimen should be obtained to rule out contamination as the cause for WBCs in the urine.

Clinical Alert

Pyelonephritis may remain completely asymptomatic even though renal tissue is being progressively destroyed. Therefore, careful examination (using low power) of urinary sediment for leukocyte casts is vital.

Patient Preparation
The *pretest* care is the same as for the urine RBC test.

Patient Aftercare
The *posttest* care is the same as for the urine RBC test.

URINE EPITHELIAL CELLS AND EPITHELIAL CASTS   ●

Normal Values
Renal tubule epithelial cells: 0–3/hpf
Squamous epithelial cells are common in normal urine sample.
Renal tubule epithelial casts: 0 (not seen)

Background
Renal epithelial cell casts are formed from cast-off tubule cells that slowly degenerate, first into coarse and then into fine granular material. Epithelial casts are the rarest of casts.

Urine epithelial cells are of 3 kinds:

1. *Renal tubule epithelial cells* are round and slightly larger than WBCs. Each cell contains a single large nucleus. These are the types of epithelial cells associated with renal disease. However, the presence of an occasional renal epithelial cell is not unusual, because the renal tubules are continually sloughing old cells. In cases of acute tubular necrosis, renal tubular epithelial cells containing large nonlipid vacuoles may be seen. These are referred to as *bubble cells*. When lipids cross the glomerular membrane, the renal epithelial cells absorb the lipids and become highly refractive. These are called *oval fat bodies*. Both of these findings are significant and should be reported.

2. *Bladder epithelial cells* are larger than renal epithelial cells. They range from round to pear-shaped to columnar. Also known as "transitional" epithelial cells, they line the urinary tract from the renal pelvis to the proximal two thirds of the urethra.

3. *Squamous epithelial cells* are large, flat cells with irregular borders, a single small nucleus, and abundant cytoplasm. Most of these cells are urethral and vaginal in origin and do not have much diagnostic importance.

Procedure
1. Collect a random urine specimen.
2. Examine the urine sediment microscopically.

Clinical Implications
1. Greater numbers of epithelial cell casts are found when the following diseases have damaged tubule epithelium:
   A. Nephrosis
   B. Amyloidosis
   C. Poisoning from heavy metals or other toxins
   D. Glomerulonephritis
   E. Acute tubular necrosis
   F. Pyelonephritis

2. Renal tubular epithelial cells are found in
   A. Acute tubular necrosis
   B. Acute glomerulonephritis (secondary effects)
   C. Pyelonephritis
   D. Salicylate overdose (toxic reaction)
   E. Impending allograft rejection
   F. Viral infections

URINE HYALINE CASTS ●

Normal Values
Occasional (0–2/lpf)

Background
Hyaline casts are clear, colorless casts that are formed when a renal protein within the tubules (Tamm-Horsfall protein) precipitates and gels. Tamm-Horsfall protein is excreted at a fairly constant rate by the tubule cells and provides immunologic protection from infection. Hyaline casts form under conditions of urine stasis and in the presence of sodium and calcium.

Procedure
1. Obtain a fresh urine sample.
2. Urinary sediment is microscopically examined for casts under low power.
3. Casts are best seen when the light intensity is reduced.
4. Wrinkling and convoluting of the cast occurs as it ages.

Clinical Implications
1. Hyaline casts indicate possible damage to the glomerular capillary membrane. These casts appear in
   A. Glomerulonephritis, pyelonephritis
   B. Malignant hypertension
   C. Chronic renal disease
   D. Congestive heart failure
   E. Diabetic nephropathy
2. Hyaline casts may be a temporary phenomenon in the presence of
   A. Fever (dehydration)
   B. Postural orthostatic lordotic strain
   C. Emotional stress
   D. Strenuous exercise
   E. Heat exposure
3. Nephrotic syndrome may be suspected when large numbers of hyaline casts appear in the urine together with significant proteinuria, fine granular casts, fatty casts, oval fat bodies, or fat droplets.
4. In cylindruria, large numbers of hyaline casts may be present but protein in the urine is absent.

> ### Clinical Alert
>
> Casts may not be found even when proteinuria is significant if the urine is dilute (1.010 SG) or alkaline. In these cases, the casts are dissolved as soon as they are formed.

Patient Preparation and Aftercare

The *pretest* and *posttest* care are the same as for the urine RBC test.

URINE GRANULAR CASTS

Normal Values

Occasional (0–2/lpf)

Background

Granular casts appear homogeneous, coarsely granular, colorless, and very dense. They then further degenerate into finely granular casts. It is not necessary to distinguish the different granular casts. Granular casts may result from degradation of cellular casts, or they may represent direct aggregation of serum proteins into a matrix of Tamm-Horsfall microprotein.

Procedure

1. Collect a random urine specimen and transport it to laboratory as soon as possible.
2. Examine urinary sediment microscopically under low power.

Clinical Implications

1. Granular casts are found in
   A. Acute tubular necrosis
   B. Advanced glomerulonephritis
   C. Pyelonephritis
   D. Malignant nephrosclerosis
2. Granular casts are found with hyaline casts after strenuous exercise or severe stress.

Patient Preparation and Aftercare

The *pretest* and *posttest* care are the same as for the urine RBC test.

URINE WAXY CASTS OR BROAD CASTS (RENAL FAILURE CASTS) AND FATTY CASTS

Normal Values

Negative (not seen)

Background

Casts are formed in the collecting tubules under conditions of extreme renal stasis. Waxy casts form from the degeneration of granular casts.

Broad, waxy casts are 2 to 6 times the width of ordinary casts and appear waxy and granular. Casts may vary in size as disease distorts the tubular structure (they get wider because they are a mold of the tubules). Also, as urine flow from the tubules becomes compromised, casts are more likely to form. The finding of broad, waxy casts suggests a serious prognosis—hence, the term *renal failure casts*.

Fatty casts are formed from the attachment of fat droplets and degenerating oval fat bodies into a protein matrix. Fatty casts are highly refractile and contain yellow-brown fat droplets.

Procedure
Urine sediment is microscopically examined under low power.

Clinical Implications
1. Broad and waxy casts occur in
   A. Chronic renal disease
   B. Tubular inflammation and degeneration (nephrotic syndrome)
   C. Localized nephron obstruction (extreme stasis of urine flow)
2. Fatty casts are found in disorders causing lipiduria, such as nephrotic syndrome.

> ### Clinical Alert
> The presence of broad, waxy casts signals very serious renal disease.

Patient Preparation and Aftercare
The *pretest* and *posttest* care are the same as for the urine RBC test.

URINE CRYSTALS

Background
A variety of crystals may appear in the urine. They can be identified by their specific appearance and solubility characteristics. Crystals in the urine may present no symptoms, or they may be associated with the formation of urinary tract calculi and give rise to clinical manifestations associated with partial or complete obstruction of urine flow.

Explanation of Test
The type and quantity of crystalline precipitate varies with the pH of the urine. Amorphous crystalline material has no significance and forms as normal urine cools.

Procedure
1. Collect a random urine specimen.
2. Examine the urinary sediment microscopically under high power.
3. The pH of the urine is an important aid to identification of crystals.

Clinical Implications

The following table describes the meaning of urine crystal findings.

Urine Crystals			
Type of Crystal	*Color*	*Shape*	*Clinical Implications*
ACID URINE			
Amorphous urates	Pink to brick red	Granules	Normal
Uric acid	Yellow-brown	Polymorphous—whetstones, rosettes or prisms, rhombohedral prisms, hexagonal plate	Normal or increased purine metabolism, gout
Sodium urate	Colorless to yellow	Fan of slender prisms	
Cystine (rare)	Colorless, highly refractile	Flat hexagonal plates with well-defined edges, singly or in clusters	Cystinuria—cystine stones in kidney, crystals also in spleen and eyes
Cholesterol (rare)	Colorless	"Broken window panes" with notched corners	Elevated cholesterol, chyluria
Leucine (rare)	Yellow or brown, highly refractile	Spheroids with striations; pure form hexagonal	Protein breakdown, severe liver disease
Tyrosine (rare)	Colorless or yellow	Fine, silky needles in sheaves or rosettes	Protein breakdown, severe liver disease
Bilirubin	Reddish-brown	Cubes, rhombic plates, amorphous needles	Elevated bilirubin
ACID, NEUTRAL, OR SLIGHTLY ALKALINE URINE			
Calcium oxalate	Colorless	Octahedral dumbbells, often small—use high power	Normal; large amounts in fresh urine may indicate severe chronic renal disease

(continued)

Urine Crystals   *(Continued)*

Type of Crystal	Color	Shape	Clinical Implications
Hippuric acid (rare)	Colorless	Rhombic plates, four-sided prisms	No significance
ALKALINE, NEUTRAL, OR SLIGHTLY ACID URINE			
Triple phosphate	Colorless	"Coffin lids," 3–6 sided prism; occasionally fern-leaf	Urine stasis and chronic infection
ALKALINE URINE			
Calcium carbonate	Colorless	Needles, spheres, dumbbells	Normal
Ammonium biurate	Yellow opaque brown	"Thorn apple" spheres, dumbbells, sheaves of needles	Normal
Calcium phosphate	Colorless	Prisms, plates, needles	Normal; large amounts in chronic cystitis or prostatic hypertrophy
Amorphous phosphates	White	Granules	Normal

Clinical Alert

Specific drugs may cause increased levels of their own crystals. Unless toxicity is suspected, they are of little clinical significance.

Patient Preparation and Aftercare
The *pretest* and *posttest* care are the same as for the urine RBC test.

URINE SHREDS

Background
Shreds consist of a mixture of mucus, pus, and epithelial (squamous) cells. They can be seen on gross examination.

Procedure
1. Examine a fresh urine specimen by visually checking for a hazy mass.
2. Centrifuge the specimen and examine the sediment microscopically to verify the presence of formed elements.

Clinical Implications

1. When mucus predominates, the shreds float on the surface.
2. When epithelial cells predominate, the shreds occupy the middle zone.
3. When pus (WBCs) predominates, the shreds are drawn to the bottom of the specimen.
4. Other findings in urine caused by specimen contamination include microscopic yeast, *Trichomonas,* spermatozoa, vegetable fibers, parasites, and meat fibers. These should be reported because they have clinical significance.
    A. Yeast—may indicate urinary moniliasis or vaginal moniliasis (*Candida albicans*)
    B. Parasites—usually from fecal or vaginal contamination
    C. Spermatozoa—seen after sexual intercourse, after nocturnal emissions, or in the presence of prostatic disease

URINE PREGNANCY TEST; HUMAN CHORIONIC GONADOTROPIN (HCG) TEST ●

Normal Values

Positive: pregnancy exists
Negative: nonpregnant state

Background

From the earliest stage of development, the placenta produces hormones, either on its own or in conjunction with the fetus. The very young placental trophoblast produces appreciable amounts of the hormone human chorionic gonadotropin (hCG), which is excreted in the urine. This hormone is not found in the urine of men or of normal, young, nonpregnant women.

Explanation of Test

Increased urinary hCG levels form the basis of the tests for pregnancy; hCG is present in blood and urine whenever there is living chorionic/placental tissue. hCG is made up of α- and β-subunits. hCG can be detected in the urine of pregnant women 26 to 36 days after the first day of the last menstrual period (ie, 8 to 10 days after conception). Pregnancy tests should return to negative 3 to 4 days after delivery.

Procedure

1. Collect an early morning urine specimen. The first morning specimen generally contains the greatest concentration of hCG. A random specimen may be used, but the SG must be at least 1.005.
2. Do not use grossly bloody specimens. If necessary, a catheterized specimen should be used.

Clinical Implications

1. A *positive* result usually indicates pregnancy.
2. *Positive* results also occur in
    A. Choriocarcinoma
    B. Hydatidiform mole
    C. Testicular tumors

D. Chorioepithelioma
E. Chorioadenoma destruens
F. About 65% of ectopic pregnancies
3. *Negative or decreased* results occur in
   A. Fetal death
   B. Abortion (test remains positive for 1 week after procedure)

Interfering Factors

1. False-negative tests and falsely low levels of hCG may be caused by very dilute urine (low SG) or by using a specimen obtained too early in pregnancy.
2. False-positive tests are associated with
   A. Proteinuria
   B. Hematuria
   C. The presence of excess pituitary gonadotropin

URINE ESTROGEN, TOTAL AND FRACTIONS (ESTRADIOL [E_2] AND ESTRIOL [E_3]), 24-HOUR URINE AND BLOOD   ●

Normal Values

Normal values vary widely between women and men and in the presence of pregnancy, the menopausal state, or the follicular, ovulatory, or luteal stage of the menstrual cycle.

Urine Estradiol (E_2)
Men: 0–6 µg/24 h
Women: Follicular phase, 0–3 µg/24 h
              Ovulatory peak, 4–14 µg/24 h
              Luteal phase, 4–10 µg/24 h
              Postmenopausal, 0–4 µg/24 h

Urine Estriol (E_3) (wide range of normal)
Men: 1–11 µg/24 h
Women: Follicular phase, 0–14 µg/24 h
              Ovulatory phase, 13–54 µg/24 h
              Luteal phase, 8–60 µg/24 h
              Postmenopausal, 0–11 µg/24 h
Pregnancy: 1st trimester, 0–800 µg/24 h
              2nd trimester, 800–12,000 µg/24 h
              3rd trimester, 5000–50,000 µg/24 h

Urine Total Estrogens
Men: 15–40 µg/24 h or 52–139 µml/d
Women: Menstruating, 15–80 µg/24 h or 52–277 µmol/d
Postmeno-
  pausal: < 20µg/24h or < 69µmol/d
Pregnancy: 1st trimester, 0–800 µg/24 h
              2nd trimester, 800–5,000 µg/24 h
              3rd trimester, 5000–50,000 µg/24 h

Background

Estradiol is the most active of the endogenous estrogens. The test evaluates female menstrual and fertility problems. In men, estradiol is useful for evaluating estrogen-producing tumors. *Estriol* is the prominent urinary estrogen in pregnancy. Serial measurements reflect the integrity of the fetal-placental complex.

Total estrogens evaluate ovarian estrogen-producing tumors in premenarchal or postmenopausal females.

Explanation of Test

These measurements, together with the gonadotropin (FSH) level (see Chapter 6), are useful in evaluating menstrual and fertility problems, male feminization characteristics, estrogen-producing tumors, and pregnancy. Estradiol (E_2) is the most active of the endogenous estrogens. Estriol (E_3) levels in both plasma and urine rise as pregnancy advances; significant amounts are produced in the third trimester. E_3 is no longer considered useful for detection of fetal distress. Total estrogens may be helpful to establish time of ovulation and the optimum time for conception.

Procedure

1. Obtain a venous blood sample.
2. Collect a 24-hour urine specimen and use boric acid preservative for all estrogen tests. Keep the container refrigerated or on ice during collection.
3. Follow general collection procedures for a 24-hour urine specimen (page 179).
4. Record the age and sex of the patient.
5. The number of gestation weeks must be communicated if patient is pregnant.
6. The number of days into the menstrual cycle must be documented for the nonpregnant woman.

Clinical Implications

1. *Increased urine E_2* is found in the following conditions:
   A. Feminization in children (testicular feminization syndrome)
   B. Estrogen-producing tumors
   C. Precocious puberty related to adrenal tumors
   D. Hepatic cirrhosis
   E. Hyperthyroidism
   F. In women, estradiol increases during menstruation, before ovulation, and during the 23rd to 41st weeks of pregnancy.
2. *Decreased urine E_2* occurs in
   A. Primary and secondary hypogonadism
   B. Kallmann's syndrome
   C. Hypofunction or dysfunction of the pituitary or adrenal glands
   D. Menopause

> **Clinical Alert**
>
> Estradiol may be used for Pergonal monitoring. Serial measurements of E_2 during ovulation induction enable the physician to minimize high E_2 levels caused by ovarian overstimulation and thereby decrease side effects.

3. *Increased urine E_3* occurs in pregnancy; there is a sharp rise when delivery is imminent.

4. *Decreased urine E_3* is found in cases of placental insufficiency or fetal distress (abrupt drop of $\geq 40\%$ on 2 consecutive days). Serial monitoring of estriol for 4 consecutive days is recommended to evaluate fetal distress.

> **Clinical Alert**
>
> Normal values are guidelines and must be interpreted in conjunction with clinical findings.

6. Urine total estrogens are *increased* in
  A. Malignant neoplasm of adrenal gland
  B. Malignant neoplasm of cell tumor of ovary
  C. Benign neoplasm of ovary
  D. Granulosa cell tumor of ovary
  E. Lutein cell tumor of ovary
  F. Theca cell tumor of ovary
  G. Benign neoplasm of testis

7. Urine total estrogens are *decreased* in
  A. Ovarian hypofunction (ovarian agenesis, primary ovarian malfunction)
  B. Intrauterine death
  C. Preeclampsia
  D. Hypopituitarism
  E. Hypofunction of adrenal cortex
  F. Menopause
  G. Anorexia nervosa

Interfering Factors

1. Total estrogens
  A. Oral contraceptives
  B. Estrogen
  C. Progesterone therapy
  D. Pregnancy and after administration of acetazolamide during pregnancy

2. Estradiol
  A. Radioactive pharmaceuticals
  B. Oral contraceptives

3. Estriol

    A. Glucose and protein interfere with outcome.

    B. Day-to-day physiologic variation can be as much as 30%; therefore, single determinations are of limited use.

    C. Renal disease—in which case a serum assay would be more accurate.

Patient Preparation

1. Explain the test purpose and procedure.

2. Stress test compliance. The patient must be able to adjust daily activities to accommodate urine collection protocols.

3. Do not administer radioisotopes for 48 hours before specimen collection.

4. Discontinue all medications for 48 hours before specimen collection (with physician's approval). Drugs deemed necessary must be documented and communicated.

5. See Chapter 1 guidelines for safe, effective, informed *pretest* care.

Patient Aftercare

1. Resume medications and activity.

2. Interpret test outcomes, monitor, and counsel appropriately.

3. Follow Chapter 1 guidelines for safe, effective, informed *posttest* care.

●URINE DRUG INVESTIGATION SPECIMENS

When screening for unknown drugs, the most valuable samples are obtained from urine, gastric contents, and blood. Urine drug screening is preferred for several reasons:

1. Specimens are easily procured.

2. It is not an invasive procedure (unless bladder catheterization is involved).

3. Drug concentrations are more elevated in urine or may not be detectable in blood (Table 3-3).

4. Drug metabolites are excreted for a longer period (days or weeks) through urine, indicating past drug use.

5. Urine test procedures are more easily done and are more economical.

    NOTE: *Blood is the preferred medium for ethyl alcohol testing because the alcohol concentration is more elevated and therefore more reliably measured in a blood sample (see Chap. 6).*

Indications for Toxicology Screening

1. To confirm clinical or postmortem diagnosis

2. To differentiate drug-induced disease from other causes, such as trauma or metabolic or infectious disease processes

3. To identify contributing diagnoses, such as ethanol abuse, trauma, presence of other drugs, or underlying psychosis

TABLE 3-3
Common Urine Drug Tests*

Amphetamines	Phencyclidine (PCP)
Alcohol	Lysergic acid diethylamide (LSD)
Barbiturates	Analgesics
Benzodiazepines	Sedatives
Cocaine, "crack"	Major tranquilizers[†]
Cyanide	Stimulants
Opiates	Sympathomimetics
Marijuana	

*Many of these drugs are detectable in urine but are not detectable in blood serum. However, all drugs detectable in blood serum are also detectable in urine, except for glutethimide.
[†]Because minor tranquilizers are almost completely metabolized, they are not likely to be detected in urine unless an overdose is taken.

4. To seek a basis for high-risk interventions such as hemodialysis
5. To test for drug abuse in the workplace, especially where public safety is at risk or concern
6. As part of preemployment screening for drug use or abuse
7. To randomly test prisoners and parolees to deter or detect drug use

Clinical Alert

When reporting drug test results for substance abuse, health care workers and patients need to be aware of the psychological, social, economic, and legal implications and the potential liabilities associated with mismanaged or incorrectly reported results. Documented procedures should be established and followed to ensure that before a result is reported corroborating evidence exists to support that result. Confirmation of all positive results must be done through an equally sensitive and specific method that uses a different chemical principle to cross-check the initial results. Keep in mind that problems associated with incorrect test results are directly proportional to the volume of drug abuse testing being done.

Urine screening is not a cure-all for preventing substance abuse in the workplace. When properly implemented, however, it can support a well thought-out substance abuse rehabilitation program. Screening can detect a problem that the employee may not admit to having. Sure knowledge that an employee abuses drugs allows an employer to move with confidence toward handling the problem.

WITNESSED URINE SAMPLING FOR SUSPECTED SUBSTANCE ABUSE ●

Procedure

1. A trained individual must witness the actual procurement or delivery of a 50-ml random urine sample. After collection, tag the sample with a numerical code. (Check institutional protocols.)
2. A signed consent form must be obtained from the testee (patient).
3. Place the sample in a plastic, sealed sack and mark it with a notary-style seal or with tamper-proof tape to protect against tampering.
4. Originate a "chain-of-custody" document at the time of the sample collection. The person who provides the urine specimen must sign the document, as does every other person who handles the sample.
5. After both initial and confirmatory testing, mark the sample, reseal it, marked, and securely store it for a minimum of 30 days.
6. Records of all tests done must be carefully maintained, together with the chain-of-custody report.
7. Confirm all positive test results by a second, different test method, because a false-negative result can misrepresent the danger a drug abuser poses; a false-positive result can seriously violate the civil and occupational rights of the testee, for which the testing laboratory can be held accountable.
8. Release the results of the test only to predesignated, authorized persons; this lessens the risk of false or speculative information being disseminated.

Clinical Implications

Certain drugs can be detected in the urine for hours to several days after ingestion, including (Check with agency laboratory for specific drugs and specific time intervals.)

1. Amphetamines, 30-mg dose (1–12 hours)
2. Barbiturates, 30-mg dose (4.5 to 7 days)
3. Benzodiazepines, 10-mg dose of diazepam (7 days)
4. Cannabinoids, weekly use (7–34 days)
5. Cocaine as metabolites (2–3 days)
6. Codeine (4 hours)
7. Methadone, 40-mg dose (7.5–56 hours)
8. Methaqualone, 150-mg dose (7 days)
9. Morphine, 10-mg intravenous dose (84 hours)
10. Phencyclidine (7 days)
11. Propoxyphene (6 hours)

Interfering Factors

Factors associated with incorrect test results for urine drug screens include the presence of

1. Detergents
2. Sodium chloride (table salt)
3. Low SG (dilute urine)

4. High pH (acid urine)
5. Low pH (alkaline urine)
6. Blood in the urine

Patient Preparation
1. Explain the test purpose and the procedure for specimen collection.
2. Follow Chapter 1 guidelines for safe, effective, informed *pretest* care.

Patient Aftercare
1. Interpret test outcomes and counsel appropriately regarding results and possible retesting.
2. See Chapter 1 guidelines for safe, effective, informed *posttest* care.

●TIMED URINE TESTS

URINE CHLORIDES (CL), QUANTITATIVE (24-HOUR) ●

Normal Values
Adult: 140–250 mEq/24 h or 140–250 mmol/d
Child >6 y: 15–40 mEq/24 h or 15–40 mmol/d
Child 10–14 y: 64–176 mEq/24 h or 64–176 mmol/d
Children's values are much lower than adult values.
Values vary greatly with salt intake and perspiration.

It is difficult to talk about normal and abnormal ranges, because the test findings have meaning only in relation to salt intake and output.

Background
The amount of chloride excreted in the urine in a 24-hour period is an indication of the state of the electrolyte balance. Chloride is most often associated with sodium balance and fluid change.

Explanation of Test
The urine chloride measurement may be used to diagnose dehydration or as a guide in adjusting fluid and electrolyte balance in postoperative patients. It also serves as a means of monitoring the effects of reduced-salt diets, which are of great therapeutic importance in patients with cardiovascular disease, hypertension, liver disease, and kidney ailments.

Urine chloride is often ordered along with sodium and potassium as a 24-hour urine test. The urinary anion gap (Na + K) − Cl is useful for initial evaluation of hyperchloremic metabolic acidosis. It is also used to determine whether a case of metabolic alkalosis is salt responsive.

Procedure
1. Collect a 24-hour urine specimen.
2. Record the exact starting and ending times on the specimen container and in the patient's health care record.

3. The complete specimen should be sent to the laboratory for refrigeration until it can be analyzed.

> ### Clinical Alert
>
> Because electrolytes and water balance are so closely related, evaluate the patient's state of hydration by checking daily weight, by recording accurate intake and output, and by observing and recording skin turgor, the appearance of the tongue, and the appearance of the urine sample.

Clinical Implications

1. *Decreased* urine chloride occurs in
   A. Chloride-depleted patients (<10 mEq/L); these patients have low serum chloride and are chloride responsive (they respond to chloride therapy so that serum and urine levels return to normal).
      (1) Inappropriate secretion of antidiuretic hormone (SIADH)
      (2) Vomiting, diarrhea
      (3) Gastric suction
      (4) Addison's disease
      (5) Metabolic alkalosis
      (6) Diuretic therapy
      (7) Villous tumors of the colon
   B. Chloride is decreased by endogenous or exogenous corticosteroids (>20 mEq/L); this condition is not responsive to the chloride administration. Diagnosis of a chloride-resistant metabolic alkalosis helps identify a corticotropin (ACTH)—or aldosterone-producing neoplasm, such as
      (1) Cushing's syndrome
      (2) Conn's syndrome
      (3) Mineralocorticoid therapy
      (4) Bartter's syndrome
2. *Increased* urine chloride occurs in
   A. Dehydration
   B. Renal tubular acidosis
   C. Potassium depletion

Interfering Factors

1. Decreased chloride is associated with
   A. Carbenicillin therapy
   B. Reduced dietary intake of chloride
   C. Ingestion of large amounts of licorice
   D. Alkali ingestion
2. Increased chloride is associated with
   A. Ammonium chloride administration
   B. Excessive infusion of normal saline
   C. Ingestion of sulfides, cyanides, halogens, bromides, and sulfhydryl compounds

Patient Preparation
1. Instruct the patient about the test purpose and the method for collecting a 24-hour specimen.
2. See Chapter 1 guidelines for safe, effective, informed *pretest* care.

Patient Aftercare
1. Interpret test outcomes and monitor appropriately for fluid imbalances.
2. See Chapter 1 guidelines for safe, effective, informed *posttest* care.

URINE SODIUM (NA), QUANTITATIVE (24-HOUR) ●

Normal Values
Adult: 40–220 mEq/24 h or 40–220 mmol/d
Child: 41–115 mEq/24 h or 40–220 mmol/d
Values are diet dependent.

Background
Sodium is a primary regulator for retaining or excreting water and maintaining acid-base balance. The body has a strong tendency to maintain a total base content; on a relative scale, only small shifts are found even under pathologic conditions. As the predominant base substance in the blood, sodium helps to regulate acid-base balance because of its ability to combine with chloride and bicarbonate. Sodium also promotes the normal balance of electrolytes in the intracellular and extracellular fluids by acting in conjunction with potassium under the effect of aldosterone. This hormone promotes the 1:1 exchange of sodium for potassium or the hydrogen ion.

Explanation of Test
This test measures 1 aspect of electrolyte balance by determining the amount of sodium excreted in a 24-hour period. It is done for diagnosis of renal, adrenal, water, and acid-base imbalances.

Procedure
1. Properly label a 24-hour urine container.
2. The urine container must be refrigerated or kept on ice.
3. Follow general instructions for 24-hour urine collections (page 179).
4. Record exact starting and ending times on the specimen container and in the patient's health care record.
5. Transfer the specimen to the laboratory for proper storage when the test is completed.

Clinical Implications
1. *Increased* urine sodium occurs in
   A. Adrenal failure (Addison's disease)
   B. Salt-losing nephritis
   C. Renal tubular acidosis
   D. SIADH

E. Dehydration
F. Aldosterone defect (AIDS-related hypoadrenalism)
G. Hypothyroidism
H. Bartter's syndrome
2. *Decreased* urine sodium occurs in
    A. Excessive sweating, diarrhea
    B. Congestive heart failure
    C. Liver disease
    E. Nephrotic syndromes with acute oliguria
    F. Diabetes insipidus
    G. Prerenal azotemia
    H. Cushing's disease
    I. Overhydration

Interfering Factors

1. Increased sodium levels are associated with caffeine intake, diuretic therapy, dopamine, postmenstrual diuresis, increased sodium intake, and vomiting. See Appendix J.
2. Decreased sodium levels are associated with intake of corticosteroids, and propranolol; low sodium intake; premenstrual sodium and water retention; and stress diuresis. See Appendix J.

Patient Preparation

1. Instruct the patient about the purpose of the test, method of collection, and specimen refrigeration or icing. Written instructions can be helpful.
2. Encourage intake of food and fluids.
3. Follow Chapter 1 guidelines for safe, effective, informed *pretest* care.

> **Clinical Alert**
>
> Because electrolytes and water balance are so closely related, determine the patient's state of hydration by checking and recording daily weights, accurate intake and output of fluids, and observations about skin turgor, the appearance of the tongue, and the appearance of the urine.

Patient Aftercare

1. Interpret test outcomes and monitor as necessary for fluid and electrolyte state.
2. Follow Chapter 1 guidelines for safe, effective, informed *posttest* care.

URINE POTASSIUM (K), QUANTITATIVE (24-HOUR) AND RANDOM

Normal Values

Adult: 25–125 mEq/24 h or 25–125 mmol/d
Child: 22–57 mEq/24 h or 25–125 mmol/d
Values are diet dependent.

Background

Potassium acts as a part of the body's buffer system and serves a vital function in the body's overall electrolyte balance. Because the kidneys cannot completely conserve potassium, this balance is regulated by the excretion of potassium through the urine. It takes the kidney 1 to 3 weeks to effectively conserve potassium.

Explanation of Test

This test provides insight into electrolyte balance by measuring the amount of potassium excreted in 24 hours. This measurement is useful in the study of renal and adrenal disorders and water and acid-base imbalances. An evaluation of urinary potassium can be helpful in determining the origin of abnormal potassium levels. Urine potassium values <20 mmol/L are associated with nonrenal conditions, whereas values >20 mmol/L are associated with renal causes.

Procedure

1. Label a 24-hour urine container properly.
2. Refrigerate the urine container or keep it on ice during the collection.
3. Follow general instructions for 24-hour urine collection (page 179).
4. Record exact starting and ending times on the container and in the patient's health care record.
5. Transfer the specimen to the laboratory for proper storage.
6. A random urine potassium determination may be done.

Clinical Implications

1. *Increased* urine potassium occurs in
   A. Primary renal diseases
   B. Diabetic and renal tubule acidosis
   C. Albright-type renal disease
   D. Starvation (onset)
   E. Primary and secondary aldosteronism
   F. Cushing's syndrome
   G. Onset of alkalosis
   H. Fanconi's syndrome
   I. Bartter's syndrome
2. *Decreased* urine potassium occurs in
   A. Addison's disease
   B. Severe renal disease, (eg, pyelonephritis; glomerulonephritis)
   C. In patients with potassium deficiency, regardless of the cause, the urine pH tends to fall. This occurs because hydrogen ions are released in exchange for sodium ions, given that both potassium and hydrogen are excreted by the same mechanism.

Interfering Factors

1. *Increased* urinary potassium is associated with
   A. Acetazolamide and other diuretics
   B. Cortisone

> **Clinical Alert**
>
> In the presence of excessive vomiting or gastric suctioning, the resulting alkalosis maintains urinary potassium excretion at levels inappropriately high for the degree of actual potassium depletion that occurs.

    C. Sulfates
    D. Ethylenediaminetetraacetic acid (EDTA) anticoagulant
    E. Penicillin, carbenicillin
    F. Thiazides
    G. Licorice
    H. Sulfates (see Appendix J)
2. *Decreased* urinary potassium is associated with
    A. Amiloride
    B. Diazoxide
    C. Intravenous glucose infusion (see Appendix J)

Patient Preparation

1. Instruct the patient about the purpose of the test, the collection procedure, and the need for refrigeration or icing of the 24-hour urine specimen. Written instructions can be helpful.
2. Food and fluids are permitted and encouraged.
3. Follow Chapter 1 guidelines for safe, effective, informed *pretest* care.

> **Clinical Alert**
>
> **1.** Because electrolytes and water balance are so closely related, determine the patient's state of hydration by checking and recording daily weights, accurate intake and output of fluids, and observations about skin turgor, the appearance of the tongue, and the appearance of the urine.
>
> **2.** Observe for signs of muscle weakness, tremors, changes in electro-cardiographic tracings, and dysrhythmias. The degree of hypokalemia or hyperkalemia at which these symptoms occur varies with each person.

Patient Aftercare

1. Interpret test outcomes and monitor appropriately for signs and symptoms of electrolyte imbalances and kidney disorders.
2. See Chapter 1 guidelines for safe, effective, informed *posttest* care.

URINE URIC ACID, QUANTITATIVE (24-HOUR) ●

Normal Values

With normal diet: 250–750 mg/24 h or 1.48–4.43 mmol/d
With purine-free diet: <400 mg/24 h or <2.48 mmol/d
With high-purine diet: <1000 mg/24 h or <5.90 mmol/d

Background

Uric acid is formed from the metabolic breakdown of nucleic acids composed of purines. Excessive uric acid relates to excessive dietary intake of purines or to endogenous uric acid production in certain disorders. Normally, one third of the uric acid formed is degraded by bacteria in the intestines.

Explanation of Test

This test evaluates uric acid metabolism in gout and renal calculus formation. Evaluation of excess uric acid excretion is important to aid in evaluating stone formation and nephrolithiasis. It also reflects the effects of treatment with uricosuric agents by measuring the total amount of uric acid excreted within a 24-hour period.

Procedure

1. Properly label a 24-hour urine container to which the appropriate preservative has been added.
2. Follow general instructions for 24-hour urine collection (page 179).
3. Record exact starting and ending times on the specimen container and in the patient's health care record.
4. When collection is completed, send the specimen to the laboratory.

Clinical Implications

1. *Increased* urine uric acid (uricosuria) occurs in
   A. Nephrolithiasis (primary gout)
   B. Chronic myelogenous leukemia (secondary nephrolithiasis)
   C. Polycythemia vera
   D. Lesch-Nyhan syndrome
   E. Wilson's disease
   F. Viral hepatitis
   G. Sickle cell anemia
   H. High uric acid concentration in urine with low urine pH may produce uric acid stones in the urinary tract. (These patients do not have gout.)
2. *Decreased* urine uric acid is found in
   A. Chronic kidney disease
   B. Xanthinuria
   C. Folic acid deficiency
   D. Lead toxicity

Interfering Factors
1. Many drugs increase uric acid levels, including
   A. Salicylates (aspirin) and other antiinflammatory drugs
   B. Diuretics
   C. Vitamin C (ascorbic acid)
   D. Warfarin
   E. Cytotoxic drugs used to treat lymphoma and leukemia (see Appendix J)
2. Other factors increasing uric acid urine levels include
   A. X-ray contrast media
   B. Strenuous exercise
   C. Diet high in purines (eg, kidney, sweetbreads) (see Chap. 6)
3. Allopurinol decrease, uric acid levels (See Appendix J)

Patient Preparation
1. Instruct the patient about the test purpose, interfering factors, collection process, and refrigeration or icing of the 24-hour urine specimen. A written reminder may be helpful.
2. Encourage food and fluids. In some situations, a diet high or low in purines may be ordered during and before specimen collection.
3. Follow Chapter 1 guidelines for safe, effective, informed *pretest* care.

Patient Aftercare
1. Resume usual diet.
2. Interpret test outcomes and counsel appropriately regarding prescribed treatment and possible need for further testing.
3. See Chapter 1 guidelines for safe, effective, informed *posttest* care.

URINE CALCIUM, QUANTITATIVE (24-HOUR)

Normal Values
Normal diet: 100–300 mg/24 h or 2.50–7.50 mmol/d
Low-calcium diet: 50–150 mg/24 h or 1.25–3.75 mmol/d

Background
Calcium hemostasis is maintained by the parathyroid hormone. The bulk of calcium excreted is eliminated in the stool. However, a small quantity of calcium is normally excreted in the urine. This amount varies with the quantity of dietary calcium ingested. Increased calcium in urine results from an increase in intestinal calcium absorption, a lack of renal tubule reabsorption of calcium, resorption or loss of calcium from bone, or a combination of these mechanisms.

Explanation of Test
The urine calcium test is used for evaluation of calcium intake and/or the rate of intestinal absorption, bone resorption, and renal loss. Urine calcium is high in 30% to 80% of cases of primary hyperparathyroidism but does not reliably diagnose this disease.

Procedure

1. Properly label a 24-hour urine container.
2. Procure an acid-washed bottle. See Table 3-2 beginning on page 180 regarding 24-hour urine collection data.
3. Follow general instructions for 24-hour urine collection (page 179). Refrigerate during collection.
4. Record exact starting and ending times of the collection on the specimen container and in the patient's health care record.
5. Send the specimen to the laboratory when collection is completed.
6. A random (Sulkowitch) test can be done in an emergency. Follow directions for random urine collection in first part of the chapter.

Clinical Implications

1. *Increased* urine calcium is found in
   - **A.** Hyperparathyroidism (30% to 50% of cases)
   - **B.** Sarcoidosis
   - **C.** Primary cancers of breast and bladder
   - **D.** Osteolytic bone metastases
   - **E.** Multiple myeloma
   - **F.** Paget's disease
   - **G.** Renal tubular acidosis
   - **H.** Fanconi's syndrome
   - **I.** Vitamin D intoxication
   - **J.** Idiopathic hypercalcuria
   - **K.** Diabetes mellitus
   - **L.** Crohn's disease and some cases of ulcerative colitis
   - **M.** Thyrotoxicosis
2. Increased urinary calcium almost always accompanies increased blood calcium levels.
3. Calcium excretion levels greater than calcium intake levels are always excessive; urine excretion values >400 to 500 mg/24 hours are reliably abnormal.
4. Increased calcium excretion occurs whenever calcium is mobilized from the bone, as in metastatic cancer or prolonged skeletal immobilization.
5. When calcium is excreted in increasing amounts, the situation creates the potential for nephrolithiasis or nephrocalcinosis, especially with high protein intake.
6. *Decreased* urine calcium is found in
   - **A.** Hypoparathyroidism
   - **B.** Familial hypocalciuria hypercalcemia
   - **C.** Vitamin D deficiency
   - **D.** Preeclampsia
   - **E.** Acute nephrosis, nephritis, renal failure
   - **F.** Renal osteodystrophy
   - **G.** Vitamin D–resistant rickets
   - **H.** Metastatic carcinoma of prostate
   - **I.** Malabsorption syndrome—celiac-sprue disease, steatorrhea
7. Urine calcium decreases in late normal pregnancy.

Interfering Factors

1. Falsely elevated levels may be caused by
   A. Some drugs (eg, calcitonin, vitamins A, K, and C, and corticosteroids—see Appendix J)
   B. Urine procured immediately after meals in which high calcium intake has occurred (eg, milk)
   C. Increased exposure to sunlight
   D. Immobilization (especially in children)
2. Falsely decreased levels may be found with
   A. Increased ingestion of phosphate, bicarbonate, antacids
   B. Alkaline urine
   C. Thiazide diuretics (can be used to lower calcium levels therapeutically)
   D. Oral contraceptives, estrogens
   E. Lithium (see Appendix J)

Patient Preparation

1. Instruct the patient about the test purpose and procedure. Written instructions may be helpful.
2. Encourage food and fluids.
3. If the urine calcium test is done because of a metabolic disorder, the patient should eat a low-calcium diet and calcium medications should be restricted for 1 to 3 days before specimen collection.
4. For a patient with a history of renal stone formation, urinary calcium results will be more meaningful if the patient's usual diet is followed for 3 days before specimen collection. Do *not* stop medications.
5. See Chapter 1 guidelines for safe, effective, informed *pretest* care.

Clinical Alert

1. Observe patients with very low urine calcium levels for signs and symptoms of tetany (muscle spasms, twitching, hyperirritable nervous system).
2. The first sign of calcium imbalance may be a pathologic fracture that can be related to calcium excess.
3. The Sulkowitch test (random urine sample) can be used in an emergency, especially when hypercalcemia is suspected, because hypercalcemia is life-threatening.

Patient Aftercare

1. Interpret test outcomes, monitor and counsel accordingly regarding calcium imbalances.
2. Follow Chapter 1 guidelines regarding safe, effective, informed *posttest* care.

URINE MAGNESIUM, QUANTITATIVE (24-HOUR)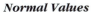

Normal Values
12–199 mg/24 h or 3.0–5.0 mEq/24 h or 3.00–5.00 mmol/d

Background
Magnesium excretion controls serum magnesium balance. Urinary magnesium excretion is diet dependent.

Explanation of Test
This test evaluates magnesium metabolism, investigates electrolyte status, and is a component of a workup for nephrolithiasis.

Procedure
1. Collect a 24-hour urine specimen in a metal-free and acid-rinsed container.
2. Record exact starting and ending times.
3. See page 179 for 24-hour urine collection guidelines.

Clinical Implications
1. *Increased* urine magnesium is associated with
   A. Increased blood alcohol
   B. Bartter's syndrome
2. *Decreased* urine magnesium is associated with
   A. Malabsorption
   B. Long-term chronic alcoholism
   C. Long-term parenteral therapy
   D. Magnesium deficiency
   E. Chronic renal disease

Interfering Factors
1. Increased magnesium levels are associated with
   A. Corticosteroids
   B. Cisplatin therapy
   C. Thiazide diuretics
   D. Amphothericin (see Appendix J)
   E. Blood in urine
2. Decreased magnesium levels are found in hypercalcuria. See Appendix J for drugs that affect test outcomes.

Patient Preparation
1. Explain purpose of test and collection procedures.
2. Instruct that the specimen will be unacceptable if it comes in contact with any type of metal.
3. See Chapter 1 guidelines for safe, effective, informed *pretest*care.

Patient Aftercare

1. Interpret test outcomes and monitor appropriately for abnormal magnesium excretion.
2. Follow Chapter 1 guidelines for safe, effective, informed *posttest* care.

URINE OXALATE, QUANTITATIVE (24-HOUR)

Normal Values
Men: 7–44 mg/24 h or 228–684 μmol/d
Women: 4–31 mg/24 h or 228–627 μmol/d
Children: 13–38 mg/24 h

Background
Normal oxalate is derived from dietary oxalic acid (10%) and from the metabolism of ascorbic acid (35% to 50%) and glycine (40%). Patients who form calcium oxalate kidney stones appear to absorb and excrete a higher proportion of dietary oxalate in the urine.

Explanation of Test
The 24-hour urine collections for oxalate are indicated in patients with surgical loss of distal small intestine, especially those with Crohn's disease. The incidence of nephrolithiasis in patients who have inflammatory bowel disease is 2.6% to 10%. Hyperoxaluria is regularly present after jejunoileal bypass for morbid obesity; such patients may develop nephrolithiasis.

Oxaluria is also a characteristic of ethylene glycol intoxication. Additionally, vitamin C increases oxalate excretion and in some people may be a risk factor for calcium oxalate nephrolithiasis. Such ingestion can usually be determined through the patient's history. If oxalate excretion becomes normal after reduction of vitamin C intake, additional therapy to prevent stones may not be required.

Procedure
1. Collect and refrigerate or place on ice a 24-hour urine specimen according to protocols. Do not acidify.
2. See page 179 for directions for a 24-hour urine collection.

Clinical Implications
1. *Increased* urine oxalate is associated with
  A. Ethylene glycol poisoning (>150 mg/day or >1710 mol/day)
  B. Primary hyperoxaluria, a rare genetic disorder (100–600 mg/day or 1140–6840 mol/day [nephrocalcinosis])
  C. Pancreatic disorders (diabetes, steatorrhea)
  D. Cirrhosis, biliary diversion
  E. Vitamin B_6 deficiency (pyridoxine)

F. Sarcoidosis

G. Crohn's disease (inflammatory bowel disease)

H. Celiac disease (sprue)

I. Jejunoileal bypass for treatment of morbid obesity

2. *Decreased* urine oxalate occurs in

A. Renal failure

B. Hypercalciuria

Interfering Factors

1. Foods such as rhubarb, strawberries, beans, beets, spinach, tomatoes, gelatin, chocolate, cocoa, and tea contain oxalates.
2. Ethylene glycol and methoxyflurane cause increased levels (see Appendix J)
3. Calcium causes decreased levels (see Appendix J)

Patient Preparation

1. Explain test purpose and procedure.
2. Advise the patient to avoid foods that promote oxalate excretion before the test. A list of such foods is helpful. Normal fluid intake should be continued.
3. Vitamin C should not be taken within 24 hours before the of beginning the test nor during the test.
4. The patient should be ambulatory and preferably at home.
5. Follow Chapter 1 guidelines for safe, effective, informed *pretest* care.

Patient Aftercare

1. Resume normal diet and exercise.
2. Interpret test outcomes and counsel appropriately about abnormal levels.
3. See Chapter 1 guidelines for safe, effective, informed *posttest* care.

URINE PREGNANEDIOL (24-HOUR)

Normal Values

This test is difficult to standardize; it varies with age, sex, and length of existing pregnancy.

Men:	0–1 mg/24 h
Women:	Follicular phase, 0.5–1.5 mg/24 h
	Postmenopausal, 0.2–1 mg/24 h
Pregnancy:	1st trimester, 10–30 mg/24 h
	2nd trimester, 35–70 mg/24 h
	3rd trimester, 70–100 mg/24 h

Background

Pregnanediol levels in normally menstruating women are constant during the follicular phase. Levels increase sharply during the luteal phase. During pregnancy, levels gradually increase, falling sharply before the onset of labor and delivery.

Explanation of Test

This test measures ovarian and placental function. Specifically, it measures a part of the hormone progesterone and its principal excreted metabolite, pregnanediol. Progesterone exerts its main effect on the endometrium by causing the endometrium to enter the secretory phase and to become ready for implantation of the blastocyte should fertilization take place.

Pregnanediol excretion is elevated in pregnancy and decreased in luteal deficiency or placental failure.

NOTE: *A serum progesterone test is more informational and is used more frequently.*

Procedure

1. Label a 24-hour urine container properly.
2. Refrigeration of the specimen or use of a boric acid preservative may be required. Check laboratory policy. Protect the specimen from light.
3. Follow general instructions for 24-hour urine collection (page 179).
4. Record exact starting and ending times on the specimen container and in the patient's health care record.
5. Send the completed specimen to the laboratory.

Clinical Implications

1. *Increased* urine pregnanediol is associated with
   A. Luteal cysts of ovary (ovarian cyst)
   B. Arrhenoblastoma of the ovary
   C. Congenital hyperplasia of adrenal gland
   D. Malignant neoplasm of trophoblasts
2. *Decreased* urine pregnanediol is associated with
   A. Amenorrhea (ovarian hypofunction)
   B. Threatened abortion (if <5.0 mg/24 hours, abortion is imminent)
   C. Fetal death, intrauterine death, placental failure
   D. Toxemia, eclampsia
   E. Benign neoplasm of ovary
   F. Granulosa cell tumor of ovary
   G. Lutein cell tumor of ovary
   H. Theca cell tumor of ovary
   I. Hydatidiform mole

Interfering Factors

Decreased values occur with estrogen or progesterone therapy and with the usage of oral contraceptives.

Patient Preparation

1. Instruct the patient about the test purpose and the 24-hour urine specimen collection procedure. A written reminder may be helpful.
2. Allow food and fluids.
3. See Chapter 1 guidelines regarding safe, effective, informed *pretest* care.

Patient Aftercare

1. Interpret test outcomes and counsel appropriately about abnormal ovarian and placental function.
2. Follow Chapter 1 guidelines regarding safe, effective, informed *posttest* care.

URINE PREGNANETRIOL (24-HOUR) ●

Normal Values

Adult: <2.0 mg/24 h
Child: 0.3–1.1 mg/24 h
Infant: <0.2 mg/24 h

Background

Pregnanetriol is a ketogenic steroid reflecting 1 segment of adrenocortical activity. Pregnanetriol should not be confused with pregnanediol, despite the similarity of name.

Explanation of Test

This 24-hour urine test is done to diagnose adrenocortical dysfunction, adrenogenital syndrome, or a defect in 21-hydroxylation. The diagnosis of adrenogenital syndrome is indicated in

1. Adult women who show signs and symptoms of excessive androgen production with or without hypertension
2. Craving for salt
3. Sexual precocity in boys
4. Infants who exhibit signs of failure to thrive
5. Presence of external genitalia in females (pseudohermaphroditism). In males, differentiation must be made between a virilizing tumor of the adrenal gland, neurogenic and constitutional types of sexual precocity, and interstitial cell tumor of the testes.

Procedure

1. Label a 24-hour urine container properly.
2. Refrigerate the specimen if necessary; some laboratories may require a boric acid preservative in the collection receptacle.
3. Follow general instructions for 24-hour urine collection (page 179).
4. Record exact starting and ending times on the specimen container and in the patient's health care record.
5. Send the completed specimen to the laboratory.

Clinical Implications

1. *Elevated* urine pregnanetriol occurs in
   A. Congenital adrenocortical hyperplasia
   B. Stein-Leventhal syndrome
   C. Ovarian and adrenal tumors

2. *Decreased* urine pregnanetriol occurs in
   A. Hydroxylase deficiency
   B. Ovarian failure

Patient Preparation

1. Instruct the patient about the test purpose and procedure for collection of a 24-hour urine specimen. A written reminder may be helpful.
2. Allow food and fluids.
3. Avoid muscular exercise before and during specimen collection.
4. See Chapter 1 guidelines for safe, effective, informed *pretest* care.

Patient Aftercare

1. Interpret test outcomes and counsel appropriately about adrenogenital syndrome.
2. Follow Chapter 1 guidelines for safe, effective, informed *posttest* care.

URINE 5-HYDROXYINDOLEACETIC ACID (5-HIAA), 24-HOUR ●

Normal Values

Qualitative: Negative
Quantitative: 3–15 mg/24 h or 10.4–31.2 μmol/d

Background

Serotonin is a vasoconstricting hormone normally produced by the argentaffin cells of the gastrointestinal tract. The principal function of the cells is to regulate smooth muscle contraction and peristalsis. 5-HIAA (5-hydroxyindoleacetic acid) is the major urinary metabolite of serotonin.

Explanation of Test

This urine test is conducted to diagnose the presence of a functioning carcinoid tumor, which can be shown by significant elevations of 5-HIAA. Excess amounts of 5-HIAA are produced by most carcinoid tumors. Carcinoid tumors produce symptoms of flushing, hepatomegaly, diarrhea, bronchospasm, and heart disease.

Procedure

1. The patient should not eat any bananas, pineapple, tomatoes, eggplants, plums, or avocados for 48 hours before or during the 24-hour test, because these foods contain serotonin.
2. Properly label a 24-hour urine container that contains the preservative (acid).
3. Many drugs must be discontinued 48 hours before sample collection, including acetaminophen, salicylates, phenacetin, naproxen, imipramine, and monoamine oxidase inhibitors.
4. Follow general directions for 24-hour urine collection (page 179).

5. Record exact starting and ending times of the collection on the specimen container and in the patient's health care record.
6. Send the completed specimen to the laboratory.

Clinical Implications

1. Levels >25 mg/24 h indicate large carcinoid tumors, especially when metastatic:
   A. Ileal tumors
   B. Pancreatic tumors
   C. Duodenal tumors
   D. Biliary tumors
2. *Increased* urine 5-HIAA is found in
   A. Cystic fibrosis
   B. Ovarian carcinoid tumor
   C. Tropical sprue
   D. Severe pain of sciatica or skeletal and smooth muscle spasm
   E. Bronchial adenoma (carcinoid type)
   F. Malabsorption
   G. Celiac disease
   H. Whipple's disease
   I. Stasis syndrome
   J. Chronic intestinal obstruction
   K. Oat cell cancer of respiratory system
3. *Decreased* urine 5-HIAA is found in
   A. Depressive illness
   B. Small intestinal resection
   C. Phenylketonuria (PKU)
   D. Hartnup's disease
   E. Mastocytosis

Interfering Factors

1. False-positive results occur with
   A. Ingestion of banana, pineapple, plum, walnut, eggplant, tomato, chocolate, and avocado, because of their serotonin content
   B. Many drugs (see Appendix J)
2. False-negative results can be caused by specific drugs that depress 5-HIAA production.

Patient Preparation

1. Instruct the patient about test purpose and procedure for collection of the 24-hour urine specimen. Written instructions may be helpful.
2. Encourage intake of food and water. Foods high in serotonin content must not be eaten for 48 hours before or during the test.
3. If possible, no drugs should be taken for 72 hours before the test nor during the test (especially aforementioned drugs).
4. See Chapter 1 guidelines for safe, effective, informed *pretest* care.

Patient Aftercare

1. Resume normal diet and medications when test is completed.
2. Interpret test outcome and counsel appropriately about abnormal 5-HIAA levels.
3. Follow Chapter 1 guidelines for safe, effective, informed *posttest* care.

> ### Clinical Alert
>
> A serum serotonin assay may detect some carcinoids missed by the urine 5-HIAA assay.

URINE VANILLYLMANDELIC ACID (VMA); CATECHOLAMINES (24-HOUR)

Normal Values

Adults

VMA: Up to 2–7 mg/24 h or up to 35.4 μmol/d

Catecholamines (total): <100 μg/d or <591 nmol/d

Epinephrine: 0–20 μg/24 h or 0–118 nmol/d

Norepinephrine: 15–80 μg/24d or 89–473 nmol/d

Dopamine: 65–400 μg/24 h or 420–2600 nmol/d

Children's levels are different from those of adults. Check with your laboratory for values in children.

NOTE: *Different laboratories report values in different units—this should be kept in mind when analyzing results.*

Background

The principal substances formed by the adrenal medulla and excreted in urine are VMA, epinephrine, norepinephrine, metanephrine, and normetanephrine. These substances contain a catechol nucleus together with an amine group and therefore are referred to as *catecholamines*. The major portion of these hormones are changed into metabolites, the principal one being 3-methoxy-4-hydroxymandelic acid, known as vanillylmandelic acid or VMA.

VMA is the primary urinary metabolite of the catecholamine group. It has a urine concentration 10 to 100 times greater than those of the other amines. It is also fairly simple to detect; methods used for catecholamine determination are much more complex.

Explanation of Test

This 24-hour urine test of adrenomedullary function is done primarily when pheochromocytoma, a tumor of the chromaffin cells of the adrenal medulla, is suspected in a patient with hypertension.

The assay for pheochromocytoma is most valuable when a urine specimen is collected during a hypertensive episode. Because a 24-hour urine collection represents a longer sampling time than a symptom-directed serum sample, the 24-hour urine test may detect a pheochromocytoma missed by a single blood level determination.

Procedure

1. Properly label a 24-hour urine container with acid preservative and refrigerate the container or keep it on ice.
2. Follow general instructions for 24-hour urine collection (page 179).
3. Record exact starting and ending times of the collection on the specimen container and in the patient's health care record.
4. Send the specimen to the laboratory.

Clinical Implications

1. *Increased urine VMA* occurs as follows:
   A. High levels in pheochromocytoma
   B. Slight to moderate elevations in
      (1) Neuroblastoma
      (2) Ganglioneuroma
      (3) Ganglioblastoma
      (4) Carcinoid tumor (some cases)
2. *Increased urine catecholamines* are found in
   A. Pheochromocytoma
   B. Neuroblastomas
   C. Ganglioneuromas
   D. Myocardial infarction
   E. Hypothyroidism
   F. Diabetic acidosis
   G. Long-term manic depressive states
3. *Decreased urine catecholamines* are found in
   A. Diabetic neuropathy
   B. Parkinson's disease

Interfering Factors

1. Increased urine VMA and catecholamines are caused by
   A. Hypoglycemia—for this reason, the test should *not* be scheduled while the patient is receiving nothing by mouth.
   B. Many foods, such as the following:
      (1) Caffeine-containing products (eg, tea, coffee, cocoa, carbonated drinks)
      (2) Vanilla
      (3) Fruit, especially bananas
      (4) Licorice
   C. Many drugs cause increased VMA levels, especially reserpine, α-methyldopa, levodopa, monoamine oxidase inhibitors, sinus and cough medicines, bronchodilators, and appetite suppressants.

2. Falsely decreased levels of VMA and catecholamines are caused by
   A. Alkaline urine
   B. Uremia (causes toxicity and impaired excretion of VMA)
   C. Radiographic contrast agents—for this reason, an intravenous pyelogram should not be scheduled before a VMA test.
   D. Certain drugs (see Appendix J)

Patient Preparation
1. Instruct the patient about the test purpose and the procedure for collection of the 24-hour urine specimen. A written reminder may be helpful, especially regarding restricted foods.
2. Explain diet and drug restrictions. Diet restrictions vary among laboratories, but coffee, tea, bananas, cocoa products, vanilla products, and aspirin are always excluded for 3 days (2 days before and 1 day during specimen collection).
3. Many laboratories require that all drugs be discontinued for 1 week before testing.
4. Encourage adequate rest, food, and fluids.
5. Stress, strenuous exercise, and smoking should be avoided during the test.
6. See Chapter 1 guidelines for safe, effective, informed *pretest* care.

Patient Aftercare
1. The patient may resume pretest diet, drugs, and activity when the test is completed.
2. Interpret test outcomes and counsel appropriately.
3. Follow Chapter 1 guidelines for safe, effective, informed *posttest* care.

URINE PORPHYRINS AND PORPHOBILINOGENS, 24-HOUR AND RANDOM; Δ-AMINOLEVULINIC ACID (ALA, Δ-ALA) ●

Normal Values

Porphobilinogens
Random specimen: 0–2.0 mg/L or negative
24-h specimen: 0–2.5 mg

Δ-ALA
Random specimen: 0–4.5 mg/L
24-h specimen: 0–7.5 mg

Porphyrins	*Male*	*Female*
Random specimen:	Negative	Negative
24-h specimen (μg):		
Uroporphyrin	8–44	4–22
Coproporphyrin	10–109	3–56
Heptacarboxyporphyrin	0–12	0–9
Pentacarboxyporphyrin	0–4	0–3
Hexacarboxyporphyrin	0–5	0–5
Total porphyrins	8–149	3–78

Background

Porphyrins are cyclic compounds formed from Δ-aminolevulinic acid (Δ-ALA), which plays a role in the formation of hemoglobin and other hemoproteins that function as carriers of oxygen in the blood and tissues. In health, insignificant amounts of porphyrin are excreted in the urine. However, in certain conditions, such as porphyria (disturbance in metabolism of porphyrin), liver disease, lead poisoning, and pellagra, increased levels of porphyrins and Δ-ALA are found in the urine. Disorders in porphyrin metabolism also result in increased amounts of porphobilinogen in urine. The most common signs and symptoms of acute intermittent porphyria are abdominal pain and tachycardia. Patients with the porphyrias may pass urine the color of port wine.

When urine is tested for the presence of porphyrins, porphobilinogen, and/or ALA, it is also given the black light screening test (Wood's light test). Porphyrins are fluorescent when exposed to black or ultraviolet light. See Chapter 2 for other tests for porphyria.

Explanation of Test

This test is used to diagnose porphyrias and lead poisoning. The following is a summary of laboratory findings for various porphyrias.

CONGENITAL ERYTHROPOIETIC PORPHYRIA. Elevations of urine uroporphyrin and coproporphyrin occur, with the former exceeding the latter.

ACUTE INTERMITTENT PORPHYRIA. Porphobilinogen and Δ-ALA are elevated in acute attacks, and small increases of urine uroporphyrin and coproporphyrin may be found.

HEREDITARY COPROPORPHYRIA. Urine coproporphyrin and porphobilinogen are markedly increased during acute attacks; increases of urine uroporphyrin may also be found.

VARIEGATE PORPHYRIA. In acute attacks, results are similar to those seen in acute intermittent porphyria. Porphobilinogen and Δ-ALA usually return to normal between attacks. Urine coproporphyrin exceeds uroporphyrin excretion during acute attacks.

CHEMICAL PORPHYRIAS. Porphyrinogenic chemicals include certain halogenated hydrocarbons, which cause increased uroporphyrin levels in the urine.

LEAD POISONING. Δ-ALA levels exceed those of porphobilinogen, which may remain normal.

Procedure

1. Properly label a 24-hour clean-catch urine container.
2. Provide refrigeration or icing. The specimen must be kept protected from exposure to light. Check with your laboratory regarding the need for preservatives.

3. Follow general instructions for 24-hour urine collection (page 179).
4. Record exact starting and ending times on the specimen container and in the patient's health care record.
5. Send the specimen to the laboratory.
6. For random tests, midmorning or midafternoon specimens are best because it is more likely that the patient will excrete porphyrins at those times. Transport the specimen to the laboratory immediately. Protect the specimen from light.
7. Observe and record the urine color. If porphyrins are present, the urine may appear amber-red or burgundy in color, or it may vary from pale pink to almost black. Some patients excrete urine of normal color that turns dark after standing in the light.

Clinical Implications

1. *Increased urine porphobilinogen* occurs in
   A. Porphyria (acute intermittent type)
   B. Variegate porphyria
   C. Hereditary coproporphyria
   D. See Explanation of Test for others.

> **Clinical Alert**
>
> Porphobilinogen is not increased in lead poisoning.

2. *Increased fractionated porphyrins* occur in
   A. Acute intermittent porphyria
   B. Congenital erythropoietic porphyria
   C. Hereditary coproporphyria
   D. Variegate porphyria
   E. Chemical porphyria caused by heavy metal poisoning or carbon tetrachloride
   F. Lead poisoning
   G. Viral hepatitis
   H. Cirrhosis (alcoholism)
   I. Newborn of mother with porphyria
   J. Congenital hepatic porphyria
3. *Increased urine Δ-ALA* can occur in
   A. Acute intermittent porphyria (acute phase)
   B. Variegate porphyria (during crisis)
   C. Hereditary coproporphyria
   D. Lead poisoning does *not* increase urine Δ-ALA until serum lead levels reach >40 μg/dl; urine Δ-ALA may remain elevated for several months after control of lead exposure.
   E. Congenital hepatic porphyria
   F. Slight increase in pregnancy, diabetic acidosis
4. *Decreased urine Δ-ALA* is found in alcoholic liver disease.

Interfering Factors

1. Oral contraceptives and diazepam can cause acute porphyria attacks in susceptible patients.
2. Alcohol ingestion interferes with the test.
3. Many other drugs, especially phenazopyridine, procaine, sulfamethoxazole, and the tetracyclines, interfere with the test (see Appendix J).

Patient Preparation

1. Instruct the patient about the purpose and procedure of collecting a 24-hour urine specimen. A written reminder may be helpful.
2. Allow food and fluids, but alcohol and excessive fluid intake should be avoided during the 24-hour collection.
3. If possible, discontinue all drugs for 2 to 4 weeks before the test so that results will be accurate.
4. See Chapter 1 guidelines for safe, effective, informed *pretest* care.

Patient Aftercare

1. The patient may resume normal activities and medications.
2. Interpret test outcomes and counsel appropriately.
3. Follow Chapter 1 guidelines for safe, effective, informed *posttest* care.

> **Clinical Alert**
>
> This test should not be ordered for patients receiving Donnatal or other barbiturate preparations. However, if intermittent porphyria is suspected, the patient should take those medications according to prescribed protocols, because these drugs may provoke an attack of porphyria.

URINE AMYLASE EXCRETION AND CLEARANCE
(RANDOM, TIMED URINE, AND BLOOD)

Normal Values

Amylase/creatinine clearance: 1%–4%
This is a ratio calculated as follows:

$$\frac{\text{Urine amylase}}{\text{Serum amylase}} \times \frac{\text{Serum creatinine}}{\text{Urine creatinine}} \times 100$$

Urine Amylase
Random specimen: 70–320 U/g of creatinine
2-h specimen: 2–34 U
24-h specimen: 24–408 U
Values vary according to laboratory methods used.

Background

Amylase is an enzyme that changes starch to sugar. It is produced in the salivary glands, pancreas, liver, and fallopian tubes and is normally excreted in small amounts in the urine. If the pancreas or salivary glands are inflamed, much more of the enzyme enters the blood and, consequently, more amylase is excreted in the urine.

Explanation of Test

This test of blood and urine indicates pancreatic function and is done to differentiate acute pancreatitis from other causes of abdominal pain, epigastric discomfort, or nausea and vomiting.

In patients with acute pancreatitis, the urine often shows a prolonged elevation of amylase, compared with a short-lived peak in the blood. Moreover, urine amylase may be elevated when blood amylase is within normal range, and, conversely, the blood amylase may be elevated when urine amylase is within normal range. The advantage of the amylase/creatinine clearance test is that it can be done on a single random urine specimen and a single serum sample instead of having to wait for a 2- or 24-hour urine collection. The ratio is increased in certain conditions other than acute pancreatitis, such as diabetic acidosis and renal insufficiency.

Procedure

For the amylase clearance test, a venous blood sample of 4 ml must be collected at the same time the random urine specimen is obtained.

1. A random, 2-hour, or 24-hour timed urine specimen will be ordered. A 2-hour specimen is usually collected.
2. Refrigerate the urine specimen.
3. Follow general instructions for the appropriate urine collection.
4. Record exact starting and ending times on the specimen container and on the health care record. This is very important for calculation of results.
5. Send the specimen to the laboratory.

Clinical Implications

1. Amylase/creatinine clearance is *increased* in
   A. Pancreatitis
   B. Diabetic ketoacidosis
   C. Burns
   D. Renal insufficiency
2. Amylase/creatinine clearance is *decreased* in macroamylasia.
3. Urine amylase is *increased* in
   A. Pancreatitis
   B. Parotitis
   C. Intestinal obstruction
   D. Diabetic ketoacidosis
   E. Strangulated bowel

F. Pancreatic cyst
G. Peritonitis
H. Biliary tract disease
4. Urine amylase is *decreased* in
  A. Pancreatic insufficiency
  B. Advanced cystic fibrosis
  C. Severe liver disease
  D. Renal failure
  E. Macroamylasemia

Interfering Factors
1. High levels of glucose (>500 mg/dl) interfere with the amylase excretion test.
2. Some drugs produce increased amylase and possibly pancreatitis.

Patient Preparation
1. Instruct the patient about the test purpose and procedure for urine specimen collection. A written instruction sheet may be helpful.
2. Encourage fluids, if they are not restricted.
3. See Chapter 1 guidelines for safe, effective, informed *pretest* care.

Patient Aftercare
1. Interpret test outcomes and monitor appropriately.
2. Follow Chapter 1 guidelines for safe, effective, informed *posttest* care.

> ### Clinical Alert
>
> Follow-up calcium levels should be checked in fulminating pancreatitis, because extremely low calcium levels can occur.

PHENYLKETONURIA (PKU); URINE PHENYLALANINE (RANDOM URINE AND BLOOD) ●

Normal Values
Blood: <2 mg/dl (2–5 d after birth)
Urine: Negative dipstick (detects phenylalanine in range of 5–10 mg/dl)

Background
Routine blood and urine tests are done on newborns to detect phenylketonuria (PKU), an inherited disease that can lead to mental retardation and brain damage if untreated. This disease is characterized by a lack of the enzyme that converts phenylalanine, an amino acid, to tyrosine, which is necessary for normal metabolic function. Because dietary phenylalanine is not converted to tyrosine, phenylalanine, phenylpyruvic acid, and other metabolites accumulate in

blood and urine. Tyrosine and the derivative catecholamines are deficient, which results in mental retardation. Both sexes are affected equally, with most cases occurring in persons of northern European ancestry.

Explanation of Test

This test is used for newborns to detect the metabolic disorder hyperphenylalaninemia. If untreated, this disorder can lead to mental retardation. Dietary restrictions of phenylalanine have shown good results.

Procedure

COLLECTING THE BLOOD SAMPLE

1. Cleanse the skin with an antiseptic and pierce the infant's heel with a sterile disposable lancet.
2. If bleeding is slow, support the infant so that blood flows by means of gravity while spotting the blood on the filter paper.
3. The circles on the filter paper must be completely filled. This can best be done by placing 1 side of the filter paper against the infant's heel and watching for the blood to appear on the other side of the paper until it completely fills the circle.
4. Do not touch blood circles until they are completely dry. Keep in cool, dry area.
5. Samples must be transported to testing site within 12 to 24 hours.

COLLECTING THE URINE SAMPLE IN NURSERY OR AT HOME

1. Dip the reagent strip into a fresh sample of urine or press it against a wet diaper (phenylalanines and phenylpyruvic acid may not appear in urine until the infant is 2 to 3 weeks of age).
2. After exactly 30 seconds, compare the strip with a color chart according to manufacturer's directions.
3. Salicylates and phenothiazine may cause abnormal color reactions.

Clinical Implications

Increased phenylalanine is found in

1. Hyperphenylalaninemia. In a positive test for PKU, the blood phenylalanine is >15 mg/100 ml. Blood tyrosine is <5 mg/100 ml; it is never increased in PKU.
2. Obesity
3. In low-birth-weight or premature infants, transient hyperphenylalaninemia along with transient hypertyrosinemia may occur.

Interfering Factors

1. Premature infants, those weighing <11 kg (<5 lb), may have elevated phenylalanine and tyrosine levels without having the genetic disease. This is a result of delayed development of appropriate enzyme activity in the liver (liver immaturity).

2. Antibiotics interfere with the blood assay.
3. Cord blood cannot be used for analysis.

Instructions to Mothers

1. Inform the mother about the purpose of the test and the methods of collecting the specimens.
2. Most parents are interested to know that PKU (a genetic disease in which a defective gene is passed on from each parent) was first recognized by a young mother of 2 mentally retarded children. She was aware that the urine of these children had a peculiar odor and, on the basis of this, was able to have a biochemist study the urine and identify phenylpyruvic acid. Her discovery led to the first successful dietary treatment, restriction of phenylalanine (eg, in milk) for those newborn babies identified as having PKU, was started and resulted in normal mental development of these children.
3. Interpret test outcomes and counsel regarding diet if results are positive.

Clinical Alert

1. The blood test must be performed at least 3 days after birth or after the child has ingested protein (milk) for at least 24 to 48 hours.
2. Urine testing is usually done at the 4- or 6-week checkup if a blood test was not done.
3. PKU studies should be done on all infants who weigh ≥11 kg (≥5 pounds) before they leave the hospital.
4. Sick or premature infants should be tested within 7 days after birth regardless of protein intake, weight, or antibiotic therapy.

Clinical Alert

The established standard is that all newborn infants should be tested for PKU and congenital hypothyroidism before discharge.

D-XYLOSE ABSORPTION (TIMED URINE AND BLOOD) ●

Normal Values

60-Minute Serum/Plasma
0–5 mo:	>15 mg/dl
6 mo to 16 y:	>20 mg/dl
17 y and older:	21–57 mg/dl

120-Minute Serum/Plasma

0–5 mo:	>25 mg/dl
6 mo–16 y:	>20 mg/dl
17 y and older:	32–58 mg/dl

Urine Xylose 5-h Reference Range

0–64 y:	>16% of dose or >4.0 g
65 y and older:	>14% of dose or >3.5 g

Background

The D-xylose test is a diagnostic measure for evaluating malabsorptive conditions and intestinal absorption of D-xylose, a pentose not normally present in the blood in significant amounts. It is partially absorbed when ingested and is excreted in the urine. Little is metabolized.

Explanation of Test

This test directly measures intestinal absorption and is used in the differential diagnosis of steatorrhea. The usual problem is differentiating pancreatic from enterogenous steatorrhea. When D-xylose (which is not metabolized by the body) is administered orally, blood and urine levels are checked for absorption rates. Absorption is normal in pancreatic steatorrhea but is impaired in enterogenous steatorrhea.

Procedure

1. The patient should refrain from foods containing pentose for 24 hours before test.
2. Do not allow food or liquids by mouth for at least 8 hours before the start of the test. Pediatric patients should fast only 4 hours.
2. The patient should void at the beginning of the test. Discard this urine.
3. Administer the oral dose of D-xylose after it has been dissolved in water in 100 ml H_2O. Adult dosage is 25 g and for children under 12 years, a 5 g oral dose is recommended. For adults, additional water up to 250 ml should be taken at this time and another 250 ml in 1 hour. Record these times on the patient's health care record. Give no further fluids (except water) or food until the test is completed.
4. Within 60 to 120 minutes later, draw a 3-ml sample of venous blood.
5. The patient must rest quietly in one place until the test is completed.
6. Five hours from the start of the test, the patient should void. Save all urine voided during the test.

Clinical Implications

1. Urine D-xylose is *decreased* in
   A. Tropical and nontropical sprue
   B. Amyloidosis
   C. Small bowel ischemia
   D. Whipple's disease
   E. Viral gastroenteritis

F. Bacterial overgrowth in small intestine

2. The D-xylose test is *normal* in the following conditions:

   A. Malabsorption due to pancreatic insufficiency

   B. Postgastrectomy

   C. Malnutrition

Interfering Factors

1. Many drugs and antibiotics (see Appendix J)
2. Nonfasting state, treatment with hyperalimentation
3. Foods rich in pentose (fruits and preserves)
4. Vomiting of the xylose test meal
5. Impaired renal function

Patient Preparation

1. Explain purpose and procedure of the test and the urine collection process. The entire 5-hour specimen must be collected.
2. The patient must fast at least 8 hours before the start of the test; children younger than 9 years of age should fast for only 4 hours.
3. Water may be taken at any time.
4. Weigh the patient to determine the proper dose of D-xylose.
5. The patient must not ingest contraindicated drugs for 1 week before the test.
6. See Chapter 1 guidelines for safe, effective, informed *pretest* care.

Patient Aftercare

1. Normal food, fluids, and activities can be resumed.
2. See Chapter 1 guidelines for safe, effective, informed *posttest* care.

Clinical Alert

Nausea, vomiting, and diarrhea may result from ingestion of the D-xylose. If vomiting occurs, the test is invalid and must be repeated.

URINE CREATININE; CREATININE CLEARANCE
(TIMED URINE AND BLOOD)

Normal Values

Urine creatinine, men: <0.8–1.8 g/24 h
Urine creatinine, women: 0.6–1.6 g/24 h
Blood creatinine: 0.4–1.5 mg/dl

Creatinine Clearance (ml/min/1.73 m²):

Age (y)	Men	Women
<20	88–146	81–134
20–30	88–146	81–134
30–40	82–140	75–128

40–50	75–133	69–122
50–60	68–126	64–116
60–70	61–120	58–110
70–80	55–113	52–105

Background

Creatinine is a substance that, in health, is easily excreted by the kidney. It is the byproduct of muscle energy metabolism and is produced at a constant rate according to the muscle mass of the individual. Endogenous creatinine production is constant so long as the muscle mass remains constant. Because all creatinine filtered by the kidneys in a given time interval is excreted into the urine, creatinine levels are equivalent to the glomerular filtration rate (GFR). Disorders of kidney function prevent maximum excretion of creatinine. The creatinine clearance test is part of most batteries of quantitative urine tests. Creatinine clearance is measured together with other urinary components in order to interpret the overall excretion rate of the various urinary components.

Explanation of Test

The creatinine clearance test is a specific measurement of kidney function, primarily glomerular filtration. It measures the rate at which the kidneys clear creatinine from the blood. In a broad sense, clearance of a substance may be defined as the imaginary volume (milliliters) of plasma from which the substance would have to be completely extracted in order for the kidney to excrete that amount in 1 minute. In addition to estimating the GFR, this test is used to evaluate renal function in patients with wasting and to monitor the progression of renal disease.

Because the excretion of creatinine in a given person is relatively constant, the 24-hour urine creatinine level is used as a check on the completeness of a 24-hour urine collection.

Procedure

1. Properly label a 12-hour or 24-hour urine container.
2. Refrigerate or ice the specimen.
3. Follow general instructions for 24-hour urine collection (page 179).
4. Record exact starting and ending times on the specimen container and in the patient's health care record.
5. Send the entire specimen to the laboratory.
6. Also obtain a 5-ml venous blood sample for creatinine when the test begins.
7. Record the patient's height and weight on the container and in the patient's health care record. Creatinine clearance values are based on the body surface area, and these values are needed to calculate the surface area.

Clinical Implications

1. *Decreased* creatinine clearance is found in
   A. Impaired kidney function, intrinsic renal disease, glomerulonephritis, pyelonephritis, nephrotic syndrome, acute tubular dysfunction, amyloidosis, interstitial nephritis

B. Shock, dehydration
C. Hemorrhage
D. Chronic obstructive lung disease
E. Congestive heart failure
2. *Increased* creatinine clearance is found in
   A. State of high cardiac output
   B. Pregnancy
   C. Burns
   D. Carbon monoxide poisoning
3. *Increased* urine creatinine is found in
   A. Acromegaly
   B. Gigantism
   C. Diabetes mellitus
   D. Hypothyroidism
4. *Decreased* urine creatinine is found in
   A. Hyperthyroidism
   B. Anemia
   C. Muscular dystrophy
   D. Polymyositis, neurogenic atrophy
   E. Inflammatory muscle disease
   F. Advanced renal disease, renal stenosis
   G. Leukemia

Interfering Factors

1. Exercise may increase creatinine clearance.
2. Pregnancy substantially increases creatinine clearance.
3. Many drugs decrease creatinine clearance (see Appendix J).
4. The creatinine clearance overestimates the GFR when serum creatinine is elevated.
5. A diet high in meat may elevate the urine creatinine concentration.

> ▶ **Clinical Alert**
>
> Determination of urine creatinine is of little value for evaluating renal function unless it is done as part of a creatinine clearance test.

Patient Preparation

1. Instruct the patient about the purpose and procedure of the test and urine specimen collection. A written reminder may be helpful.
2. Allow food and encourage fluids for good hydration. Large urine volumes ensure optimal test results. Avoid tea and coffee (diuretics).
3. Avoid vigorous exercise during the test.
4. Drugs affecting the results should be stopped beforehand (especially cephalosporins). Check with physician.
5. Avoid eating large amounts of meat. Check with physician.
6. See Chapter 1 guidelines for safe, effective, informed *pretest* care.

Patient Aftercare

1. The patient may resume normal food, fluids, and activity.
2. Interpret test outcomes and monitor appropriately.
3. Follow Chapter 1 guidelines for safe, effective, informed *posttest* care.

URINE CYSTINE (RANDOM AND 24-HOUR) ●

Normal Values

Random specimen: Negative
24-h specimen, adult: <38 mg/24 h
24-h specimen, child: 5–31 mg/24 h

Background

Cystinuria is a condition characterized by increased amounts of the amino acid cystine in the urine. The presence of increased urinary cystine is caused not by a defect in the metabolism of cystine but rather by the inability of the renal tubules to reabsorb cystine filtered by the glomeruli. The tubules fail to reabsorb not only cystine but also lysine, ornithine, and arginine; this rules out the possibility of an error in metabolism, even though the condition is inherited.

Explanation of Test

These urine tests are useful for differential diagnosis of cystinuria, an inherited disease characterized by bladder calculi (cystine has low solubility). Patients with cystine stones face recurrent urolithiasis and repeated urinary infections.

Procedure

1. Obtain a random 20-ml urine specimen for a qualitative screening test.
2. When collecting a 24-hour urine specimen, the container needs a preservative (toluene). Follow general procedures for a 24-hour urine specimen (page 179).

Clinical Implications

1. Urine cystine is *increased* in cystinuria (up to 20 times normal).
2. Urine cystine is *decreased* in burn patients.

> **Clinical Alert**
>
> 1. Cystinosis, a different entity from cystinuria, is not detected by cystine studies. Most patients with infantile nephropathic cystinosis have neurologic defects that become apparent in infancy. Failure to thrive and renal dysfunction are evidence of this disease.
> 2. Patients with cystinosis have a defect in renal tubular reabsorption that develops into Fanconi's syndrome, which leads to a generalized amino aciduria. Cystine is elevated in the urine in the same proportion as all
>
> *(continued)*

(Clinical Alert continued)
> amino acids; the concentration is not high enough to form cystine stones. Plasma cystine is normal, but cystine is elevated in kidneys, eyes, spleen, and bone marrow; for purposes of diagnosis, it is usually measured in WBCs.

Patient Preparation
1. Explain test purpose and procedure for timed urine collection.
2. See Chapter 1 guidelines regarding safe, effective, informed *pretest* care.

Patient Aftercare
1. Interpret test outcomes and counsel appropriately.
2. Follow Chapter 1 guidelines for safe, effective, informed *posttest* care.

URINE HYDROXYPROLINE (TIMED URINE AND BLOOD) ●

Normal Values
Total hydroxyproline: 0–6 mg/24 h or 38–500 μmol/d
Free hydroxyproline: 0–2 mg/24 h or <30 μmol/d

Background
Hydroxyproline is an amino acid found only in collagen. It increases during periods of rapid growth, in bone diseases, and in some endocrine disorders. Urine hydroxyproline represents only 10% of total collagen breakdown and therefore correlates poorly with bone resorption.

Explanation of Test
Hydroxyproline is considered to be a marker for bone resorption, because 50% of human collagen resides in bone. This test indicates the presence of reabsorption of bone collagen in various disorders and evaluates the degree of destruction from primary or secondary bone tumors. It is used as an aid to diagnose hydroxyprolinemia, a rare genetic disorder characterized by mental retardation and thrombocytopenia.

Procedure
1. Obtain a 2-hour specimen after the patient has fasted overnight.
2. Notify the laboratory of the patient's age and sex.
3. If ordered, collect a 24-hour urine specimen. No preservative is required, but the specimen must be refrigerated or placed on ice.
4. Follow 24-hour urine collection procedures. The laboratory will record the total 24-hour volume.
5. The preferred method of testing in the first few months of life is blood sampling.

Clinical Implications
1. *Free hydroxyproline is increased in*

A. Hydroxyprolinemia, a hereditary autosomal recessive condition (rare)

B. Familial iminoglycinuria, also inherited

2. *Total hydroxyproline is increased* in

A. Hyperparathyroidism

B. Paget's disease

C. Marfan's syndrome

D. Acromegaly

E. Burns

Interfering Factors

Gelatin may affect test results (false-positive test).

Patient Preparation

1. Explain the test purpose and procedure for a timed urine collection. Fasting and special fluid requirements before testing are often required for a 2-hour timed procedure. Check with laboratory.

2. Avoid gelatin foods for several days before the test.

3. See Chapter 1 guidelines for safe, effective, informed *pretest* care.

Patient Aftercare

1. The patient may resume normal diet and activity.

2. Interpret test outcomes and counsel appropriately.

3. Follow Chapter 1 guidelines for safe, effective, informed *posttest* care.

URINE LYSOZYME (RANDOM, 24-HOUR URINE, AND BLOOD)

Normal Values

Blood plasma: 4–15.8 μg/ml or 0.28–1.10 μml/L

Urine, 24-h specimen: 0–1.4 μg/ml or 0–0.097 μmol/L

Background

Lysozyme (muramidase) in blood or urine is a bacteriolytic enzyme that comes from degradation of granulocytes and monocytes, but not lymphocytes. It is increased in leukemia owing to degradation of granulocytic or monocytic cells.

Explanation of Test

This blood and urine test differentiates acute myelogenous or monocytic leukemia from acute lymphatic leukemia. It is useful to monitor the response to treatment of acute myelogenous and active monocytic leukemia.

Procedure

1. Collect a 5-ml EDTA-anticoagulated blood sample or random urine specimen.

2. Follow general instructions for random urine specimen collection or 24-hour urine collections. *Transport the sample to the laboratory immediately after collection.*

Clinical Implications
1. *Lysozyme levels are increased* in
   A. Acute myelogenous leukemia (granulocytic)
   B. Acute monocytic leukemia
2. *Lysozyme levels may be increased* in
   A. Renal disorders and transplant rejection
   B. Tuberculosis
   C. Sarcoidosis (sarcoid lymph nodes)
   D. Crohn's disease
   E. Polycythemia vera
3. *Lysozyme levels are normal* in acute lymphatic leukemia.
4. *Lysozyme levels are decreased* in neutropenia with hypoplasia of bone marrow.

Patient Preparation
1. Explain the test purpose and procedure for urine or blood collection.
2. See Chapter 1 guidelines for safe, effective, informed *pretest* care.

Patient Aftercare
1. Interpret test outcomes and counsel appropriately.
2. Follow Chapter 1 guidelines for safe, effective, informed *posttest* care.

URINE AMINO ACIDS, TOTAL AND FRACTIONS
(RANDOM, 24-HOUR URINE, AND BLOOD)

Normal Values
Urine and blood amino acid values are age dependent.

Background
Many abnormalities in amino acid transport or metabolism can be detected by physiologic fluid analysis (urine, plasma, or cerebrospinal fluid). Free amino acids are found in urine and in acid filtrates of protein-containing fluids. Urine is used for initial screening of inborn metabolic errors. Both transport errors and metabolic errors can be detected by changes in observed amino acid patterns. In many cases, metabolic errors are detected when the amino acid or metabolite exceeds its renal threshold. Many intermediary metabolites have low renal thresholds.

Explanation of Test
This test is the initial screening test for inborn errors of metabolism and transport in cases of suspected genetic abnormalities in patients with mental retardation, reduced growth, or other unexplained symptoms. More than 50 aminoacidopathies are now recognized.

Procedure
1. A fasting blood specimen may need to be obtained.
2. Collect a random or 24-hour timed urine specimen. Keep the specimen refrigerated or on ice.

Clinical Implications

1. *Total serum amino acids are increased* in
   - **A.** Specific aminoacidopathies (see urine section)
   - **B.** Secondary causes
     - **(1)** Diabetes with ketosis
     - **(2)** Malabsorption
     - **(3)** Hereditary fructose intolerance
     - **(4)** Conditions with severe brain damage
     - **(5)** Reye's syndrome
     - **(6)** Acute and chronic renal failure
     - **(7)** Eclampsia
     - **(8)** Specific aminoacidopathies
2. *Total serum amino acids are decreased* in
   - **A.** Adrenocortical hyperfunction
   - **B.** Huntington's chorea
   - **C.** Phlebotomus fever
   - **D.** Nephritic syndrome
   - **E.** Rheumatoid arthritis
   - **F.** Hartnup's disease
   - **G.** Fever
   - **H.** Malnutrition
3. *Total urine amino acids are increased* in specific aminoacidurias:

Aminoacidurias

Aminoacidurias	Amino Acids Increased In Urine and Blood	Presence of Abnormal Enzymes
Phenylketonuria	Phenylketonuria	Phenylamine hydroxylase
Tyrosinosis	Tyrosine	p-Hydroxyphenyl-pyruvic acid oxidase
Histidinemia	Histidine	Histidase
Maple syrup urine disease	Valine, leucine, and isoleucine	Branched chain keto acid decarboxylase
Hypervalinemia	Valine	Probably valine transaminase
Hyperglycinemia	Glycine (lysine on high-protein diet)	Increased glycine and propionic acid
Hyperprolinemia		
Type I	Proline	Proline oxidase pyrroline-5-carboxylate dehydrogenase
Type II		
Hydroxyprolinemia	Hydroxyproline	Hydroxyproline oxidase

(continued)

Aminoacidurias *(Continued)*

Aminoacidurias	Amino Acids Increased In Urine and Blood	Presence of Abnormal Enzymes
Homocystinuria	Methionine, homocystine	Cystathionine synthetase
Hyperlysinemia	Lysine	Lysine-α-ketoglutarate reductase
Citrullinemia	Citrulline	Argininosuccinic acid synthetase
Alkaptonuria	Homogentisic acid (2:5 dihydroxyphenylacetic acid); no abnormal amino acid	Homogentisic acid oxidase
Oasthouse urine disease	Methionine, phenylalanine, valine, leucine, isoleucine, and tyrosine, and also α-hydroxybutyric acid in urine	Possibly methionine malabsorption syndrome

4. *Absence of amino acids* occurs in the following:

Disease	Amino Acids in Urine	Presence of Abnormal Enzyme
Argininosuccinic aciduria	Argininosuccinic acid (also citrulline)	Argininosuccinase
Cystathioninuria	Cystathionine	Cystathionines
Homocystineuria	Homocystine	Cystathionine synthetase
Hypophosphatasia	Phosphoethanolamine	Serum alkaline phosphate

5. *Renal transport aminoacidurias* include the following:

Disease	Amino Acids in Urine	Abnormality
Cystinuria (cystine stones)	Cystine; lysine; arginine, ornithine (basic amino acids)	Incomplete absorption of cystine, lysine, arginine, ornithine
Hartnup's disease	Monoaminomonocarboxylic (neutral) amino acids (proline, glycine, hydroxyproline, and methionine not increased)	Incomplete absorption of monoaminomono-carboxyamino acids
Glycinuria; renal type	Glycine—proline, hydroxyproline	Membrane transport defect
Familial iminoglycinuria		

Gardner LI. Endocrine and Genetic Diseases of Childhood and Adolescence, 2nd ed. Philadelphia: WB Saunders, 1975, p 1049.

6. *Secondary aminoacidurias* occur in the following:
   A. Viral hepatitis
   B. Multiple myeloma
   C. Hyperparathyroidism
   D. Rickets (vitamin D–resistant)
   E. Osteomalacia
   F. Hereditary fructose intolerance
   G. Galactosemia
   H. Uric disease
   I. Renal failure
   J. Wilson's disease
   K. Muscular dystrophy

Interfering Factors

1. Dilute urine (SG <1.010) affects test.
2. Hyperalimentation and intravenous therapy affect outcome.
3. Drugs such as amphetamines, norepinephrine, levodopa, and all antibiotics affect results.

Patient Preparation

1. Instruct the patient regarding the test purpose, collection procedure, and need for refrigeration. A written reminder may be helpful.
2. Allow foods and moderate amounts of fluids (do not overhydrate).
3. It may be necessary to consume proteins or carbohydrates for a challenge load to produce certain amino acid metabolites.
4. See Chapter 1 guidelines for safe, effective, informed *pretest* care.

Patient Aftercare

1. Interpret test outcomes and counsel appropriately. Genetic counseling may be necessary.
2. Follow Chapter 1 guidelines regarding safe, effective, informed *posttest* care.

BIBLIOGRAPHY

Ali A: Proteinuria: How much evaluation is appropriate? Postgrad Med 101: 173, 1997

Belsey R, Baer DM: Specimen collection for diagnosing UTI. Medical Laboratory Observer 28: 29, 1996

Cooper C: What color is that urine specimen. Am J Nurs 93(8): 37, 1990

Finnegan K: Correlating routine urinalysis with selected kidney disorders. Advances for Laboratory Professionals 2(12), June 1999

Goroll AH, May LA, Mully AG Jr: Primary Medicine, 3rd ed. Philadelphia, JB Lippincott, 1995

Klee GG: Maximizing Efficacy of Endocrine Tests: Importance of Decision-focused Testing Strategies and Appropriate Patient Preparation. Clinical Chemistry 45(8): 1323–1330. Special Issue 1999, Part 2 of 2, Proceedings of the Twenty-Second Annual Arnold O. Beckman Conference in Clinical chemistry Feb 21–22, 1999.

Kunin CM: Urinary tract infections: Detection, prevention, and management, 5th ed. Baltimore, Williams & Wilkins, 1996

Leavelle, DE: Interpretive Data for Diagnostic Laboratory Tests, Rochester, MN, Mayo Medical Laboratories, 1998

Lehmann CA (ed): Saunders Manual of Clinical Laboratory Science. Philadelphia, WB Saunders, 1988

Marchiondo K, Credit CE: A new look at urinary tract infections. Am J Nurs 98(3): 34–39, March 1998

McBride LJ: Textbook of Urinalysis and Body Fluids. Philadelphia, Lippincott, 1998

Newland JA: Cystitis in women, Am J Nurs 98(1): 16AAA, 1998

Speicher CE: The Right Test: A Physician's Guide to Laboratory Medicine, 3rd ed. Philadelphia, WB Saunders, 1998

Strasinger SK: Urinalysis and body fluids, 3rd ed. Philadelphia, FA Davis, 1994

Thompson WG: Things that go red in the urine; and others that don't. Lancet 347: 5, 1996

Young DS: Effects of Drugs on Clinical Laboratory Tests, 5th ed. Washington, DC, 1999

4

Stool Studies

●━━━━━━━━━━━━━━━━━━━━━━━━━━━━━━━━━━━━━

Formation and Composition of Feces

The elimination of digestive waste products from the body is essential to health. These excreted waste products are known as *stool* or *feces*. Stool examination is often done for evaluation of gastrointestinal (GI) disorders. These studies are helpful in detecting GI bleeding, GI obstruction, obstructive jaundice, parasitic disease, dysentery, ulcerative colitis, and increased fat excretion. (See Stool Analysis on p. 282.)

An adult excretes 100 to 200 g of fecal matter a day, of which as much as 75% may be water. The feces are what remains of the 8 to 10 L of digested fluid-like material that enters the intestinal tract each day, and oral food and fluids, saliva, gastric secretions, pancreatic juice, and bile add to the formation of feces.

Feces are composed of the following materials:

1. Waste residue of indigestible material (eg, cellulose) from food eaten during the previous 4 days.
2. Bile (pigments and salts): stool color is normally due to bile pigments that have been altered by bacterial action.
3. Intestinal secretions.
4. Water and electrolytes.
5. Epithelial cells that have been shed.
6. Large numbers of bacteria.
7. Inorganic material (10%–20%), chiefly calcium and phosphates.
8. Undigested or unabsorbed food (normally present in very small quantities).

The output of feces depends on a complex series of absorptive, secretory, and fermentative processes. Normal function of the colon involves three physiologic processes: (1) absorption of fluid and electrolytes; (2) contractions that churn and expose the contents to the GI tract mucosa and transport the contents to the rectum; and (3) defecation.

The small intestine is approximately 23 feet (7 m) long, and the large intestine is 4 to 5 feet (1.2–1.5 m) long. The small intestine degrades ingested fats, proteins, and carbohydrates to absorbable units and then absorbs them. Pancreatic, gastric, and biliary secretions exert their effects on the GI contents to prepare this material for active mucosal transport. Other active substances absorbed in the small intestine include fat-soluble vitamins, iron, and calcium. Vitamin B_{12}, after combining with intrinsic factors, is absorbed in the ileum. The small intestine also absorbs as much as 9.5 L of water and electrolytes for return to the bloodstream. Small intestine contents (ie, chyme) begin to enter the rectum as soon as 2 to 3 hours after a meal, but the process is not complete until 6 to 9 hours after eating.

The large intestine performs less complex functions than the small intestine. The proximal or right colon absorbs most of the water remaining after the GI contents have passed through the small intestine. Colonic absorption of water, sodium, and chloride is a passive process. Fecal water excretion is only about 100 ml/day. The colon mainly moves the luminal contents to and fro by seemingly random contractions of circular smooth muscle. Increased propulsive activity (ie, peristalsis) occurs after eating. Peristaltic waves are caused by the gastrocolic and duodenocolic reflexes, which are initiated after meals and stimulated by the emptying of the stomach into the duodenum. The muscles of the colon are innervated by the autonomic nervous system. Additionally, the parasympathetic nervous system stimulates movement, and the sympathetic system inhibits movement. Massive peristalsis usually occurs several times a day. Resultant distention of the rectum initiates the urge to defecate. In persons with normal motility and a mixed dietary intake, normal colon transit time takes 24 to 48 hours.

●STOOL ANALYSIS

Stool analysis determines the various properties of the stool for diagnostic purposes. Some of the more frequently ordered tests on feces include tests for leukocytes, blood, fat, ova and parasites, and pathogens. (Stool culture is explained in Chap. 7, Microbiologic Studies.) Stool is also examined by *chromatographic* analysis for the presence of gallstones. The recovery of a gallstone from feces provides the only proof that a common bile duct stone has been dislodged and excreted. Stool testing also screens for colon cancer and asymptomatic ulcerations or other masses of the GI tract and evaluates GI diseases in the presence of diarrhea and/or constipation. Stool testing is done in immunocompromised persons for parasitic diseases. Fat analysis is used as the gold standard to diagnose malabsorption syndrome.

Patients and health care personnel may dislike collecting and examining fecal material; however, this natural aversion must be overcome in light of the value of a stool examination for diagnosing disturbances and diseases of the GI tract, the liver, and the pancreas.

RANDOM COLLECTION AND TRANSPORT
OF STOOL SPECIMENS ●

1. Observe universal precautions (see Appendix A) when procuring and handling specimens to avoid pathogens (eg, hepatitis A, *Salmonella,* and *Shigella*).
2. Collect feces in a dry, clean, urine-free container that has a properly fitting cover.
3. The specimen should be uncontaminated with urine or other bodily secretions such as menstrual blood. Stool can be collected from the diaper of an infant or incontinent adult. Samples can be collected from temporary ostomy bags.
4. While wearing gloves, collect the entire stool specimen and transfer it to a container with a clean tongue blade or similar object. A sample 2.5 cm (1 inch) long or 64.7 mg (1 oz) of liquid stool may be sufficient for some tests.

5. For best results, cover specimens and deliver to the laboratory immediately after collection. Depending on the examination to be performed, the specimen should be either refrigerated or kept warm. If you are unsure of how to handle the specimen, contact the laboratory for detailed instructions concerning the disposition of the fecal specimen before collection is begun.

6. Post signs in bathrooms that say "DO NOT DISCARD STOOL" or "SAVE STOOL" to serve as reminders that fecal specimen collection is in progress.

COLLECTION AND TRANSPORT OF SPECIMENS FOR OVA AND PARASITES

1. Wear gloves. Observe standard precautions (see Appendix A). Collect feces in a dry, clean, urine-free container. If unsure of how to collect specimen, contact the laboratory before collection is begun.

2. Warm stools are best for detecting ova and parasites. Do *not* refrigerate specimens for ova and parasites.

3. Special vials that contain 10% formalin and polyvinyl alcohol (PVA) fixative may be used for collecting stool samples to test for ova and parasites. In this case, specimen storage temperature is not critical.

4. Due to the cyclic life cycle of parasites, three separate random stool specimens for analysis are recommended.

5. Place the specimen in a biohazard bag.

COLLECTION AND TRANSPORT OF SPECIMENS FOR ENTERIC PATHOGENS

1. While wearing gloves, collect feces in a dry, clean, urine-free container. If unsure of how to collect the specimen, contact the laboratory before collection is begun. Observe standard precautions.

2. Some coliform bacilli produce antibiotic substances that destroy enteric pathogens. Refrigerate the specimen immediately to prevent this from happening in the sample.

3. A diarrheal stool will usually give accurate results.

4. A freshly passed stool is the specimen of choice.

5. Collect stool specimens before antibiotic therapy is initiated and as early in the course of the disease as possible.

6. If mucus or blood is present, it definitely should be included with the specimen, because pathogens are more likely to be found in these substances. If only a small amount of stool is available, a walnut-sized specimen is usually adequate.

7. Accurately label all stool specimens with the patient's name, date, and tests ordered on the specimen. Keep the outside of the container free from contamination and immediately send the sealed container to the laboratory.

8. For best preservation and transport of pathogens, a Cary-Blair solution vial with indicator should be used.

Interfering Factors for All Types of Stool Collection

1. Stool specimens from patients receiving tetracyclines, antidiarrheal medications, barium, bismuth, oil, iron, or magnesium may not yield accurate results.
2. Bismuth found in paper towels and toilet tissue interferes with accurate results.
3. Do not collect or retrieve stool from the toilet bowl or use a specimen that has been contaminated with urine, water, or toilet bowl cleaner. A clean, dry bedpan may be the best receptacle for defecation.
4. Inaccurate test results may result if the sample is *not representative* of the entire stool evacuation.
5. Lifestyle, personal habits, travel, home and work environments, and bathroom accessibility are some of the factors that may interfere with proper sample procurement.

Patient Preparation

1. Explain the collection purpose, procedure, and interfering factors in language the patient understands. Because the specimen cannot be obtained on demand, it is important to provide detailed instructions before the test so that the specimen is collected when the opportunity presents itself. Provide written instructions if necessary.
2. Provide proper containers and other collection supplies. Instruct the patient to defecate in a large-mouthed plastic container, bag or clean bedpan. Provide for and respect the patient's privacy.
3. Instruct the patient *not to urinate* into the collecting container or bedpan.
4. No toilet paper should be placed in the container or bedpan because it interferes with testing.
5. If the patient has diarrhea, a large plastic bag attached by adhesive tape to the toilet seat may be helpful in the collection process. After defecation, the bag can be placed into a gallon container.
6. Specimens for most tests can be produced by a warm saline enema or Fleet Phospho-Soda enema.
7. Tests for both ova and parasites and cultures for enteric pathogens may be ordered together. In this case, the specimen should be divided into 2 samples, with one portion refrigerated for culture testing and one portion kept at room temperature for ova and parasite testing. There are commercial collection kits that require the stool to be divided and placed into separate vials for better recovery of ova and parasites and enteric pathogens. (See Chap. 7, Microbiologic Studies.)
8. Follow guidelines in Chapter 1 for safe, effective, informed *pretest* care.

Patient Aftercare

1. Provide patient privacy and the opportunity to cleanse perineal area and hands. Assist as necessary.
2. Follow guidelines in Chapter 1 for safe, effective, informed *posttest* care.

> **Clinical Alert**
>
> 1. Any stool collected may harbor highly infective pathogens. Use extreme caution and proper handling techniques at all times.
> 2. Instruct patients in proper hand-washing techniques after each use of the bathroom.

STOOL CONSISTENCY, SHAPE, FORM, AMOUNT, AND ODOR

Normal Values
100–200 g/d

Characteristic odor present; plastic, soft, formed; soft and bulky on a high-fiber diet; small and dry on a high-protein diet; seeds and visible undigested fiber and indigestible fiber present (Table 4-1).

Background
Inspection of the feces is an important diagnostic tool. The quantity, form, consistency, and color of the stool should be noted. When diarrhea is present, the stool is watery. Large amounts of mushy, frothy, foul-smelling stool is characteristic of steatorrhea. Constipation is associated with firm, spherical masses of stool. Feces have a characteristic odor that varies with diet and the pH of the stool.

Explanation of Test
Normally, evacuated feces reflect the shape and caliber of the colonic lumen as well as the colonic motility. The normal consistency is somewhat plastic and neither fluid, mushy, nor hard. Consistency can also be described as formed, soft, mushy, frothy, or watery. The odor of normal stool is caused by indole and skatole, formed by bacterial fermentation and putrefaction.

Procedure
Collect a random stool specimen in a plastic container (see p. 282).

Clinical Implications
1. Fecal consistency alterations
   a. Diarrhea due to:
      (1) Infection—*Salmonella, Shigella, Yersinia,* human immunodeficiency virus (HIV) enteropathy, *Campylobacter*
      (2) Inflammatory disorder—Crohn's disease, ulcerative colitis
      (3) Steatorrhea—sprue, celiac disease
      (4) Carbohydrate malabsorption—lactose or sucrose deficiency
      (5) Endocrine abnormalities—diabetes mellitus, hyperthyroid or hypothyroid, adrenal insufficiency
      (6) Hormone-producing tumors—Zollinger-Ellison syndrome, gastrinoma, medullary thyroid carcinoma, villous adenoma

TABLE 4-1
Normal Values in Stool Analysis

Macroscopic Examination	Normal Value
Amount	100–200 g/d
Color	Brown
Odor	Varies with pH of stool and depends on bacterial fermentation and putrefaction
Consistency	Plastic; not unusual to see fiber, vegetable skins and seeds; soft and bulky in high-vegetable diet; small and dry in high-meat diet
Size and shape	Formed
Gross blood	None
Mucus	None
Pus	None
Parasites	None

Microscopic Examination	Normal Values
Fat	Colorless, neutral fat (18%) and fatty acid crystals and soaps
Undigested food, meat fibers, starch, trypsin	None to small amount
Eggs and segments of parasites	None
Bacteria and viruses	None
Yeasts	None
Leukocytes	None

Chemical Examination	Normal Values
Water	Up to 75%
pH	Neutral to weakly alkaline (pH 6.5–7.5)
Occult blood	Negative
Urobilinogen	50–300 mg/24 h
Porphyrins	Corporphyrins: 400–1200 μg/24 h
	Uroporphyrins: 10–40 μg/24 h
Nitrogen	<2.5 g/24 h
APT test for swallowed blood	Negative in adults; positive in newborns
Trypsin	Positive in small amounts in adults; present in greater amounts in normal children
Osmolality, used with stool Na^+K to calculate osmotic gap	200–250 mOsm

(continued)

TABLE 4-1 *(Continued)*	
Chemical Examination	*Normal Values*
Sodium	5.8–9.8 mEq/24 h
Chloride	2.5–3.9 mEq/24 h
Potassium	15.7–20.7 mEq/24 h
Lipids (fatty acids)	0–6 g/24 h
Reducing substances	<0.25 g/dl

Reference values for electrolytes differ greatly from laboratory to laboratory.

    (7) Colon carcinoma
    (8) Infiltration of lesions due to lymphoma, scleroderma of bowel
    (9) Drugs, antibiotics, cardiac medications, chemotherapy
    (10) Osmotically active dietary items—sorbitol, psyllium fiber, caffeine, ethanol
    (11) GI surgery—gastrectomy, stomach stapling, intestinal resection
    (12) Factitious—self-induced laxative abuse associated with psychiatric disorders

  b. "Pasty" stool associated with high-fat content can be caused by:
    (1) Common bile duct obstruction
    (2) Celiac disease (sprue and steatorrhea); stool resembles aluminum paint
    (3) Cystic fibrosis—greasy "butter stool" appearance due to pancreatic involvement

  c. Bulky or frothy stool is usually due to steatorrhea and celiac disease.

2. Alterations in stool size or shape indicate altered motility or colon wall abnormalities.

  a. A narrow, ribbon-like stool suggests the possibility of spastic bowel, rectal narrowing or stricture, decreased elasticity, or a partial obstruction.

  b. Excessively hard stools are usually due to increased fluid absorption because of prolonged contact of luminal contents with colon mucosa during delayed transit time through the colon.

  c. A large-circumference stool indicates dilatation of the viscus.

  d. Small, round, hard stools (ie, scybala) accompany habitual, moderate constipation.

  e. Severe fecal retention can produce huge, firm, impacted stool masses with a small amount of liquid stool as overflow. These must be removed manually, occasionally under light anesthesia.

3. Fecal odor should be assessed whenever a stool specimen is collected.

  a. A foul odor is caused by degradation of undigested protein and is produced by excessive carbohydrate ingestion.

b. A sickly sweet odor is produced by volatile fatty acids and undigested lactose.

4. Mucus in stool occurs in constipation, malignancy, and colitis (see p. 295).

Patient Preparation

1. Barium procedures and laxative preparations should be avoided for 1 week before stool specimen collection.

2. Advise the patient of the purpose of test and instruct him or her in collection techniques and refrigeration of specimen.

3. Follow guidelines in Chapter 1 for safe, effective, informed *pretest* care.

Assessment of Diarrhea and Constipation

1. When performing a workup for the differential diagnosis of diarrhea or constipation, a patient history is most important. The following factors should be charted:

    a. An estimate of volume and frequency of fecal output

    b. Stool consistency and presence of blood, pus, mucus, oiliness, or bad odor in specimen; evaluate through direct observation

    c. Decrease or increase in frequency of defecation

    d. Sensations of rectal fullness with incomplete stool evacuation

    e. Painful defecation

2. Assess dietary habits and food allergies.

3. Assess emotional state of patient—psychological stress may be major cause of altered bowel habits.

4. Be alert for signs of laxative abuse.

Patient Aftercare

1. Evaluate outcome and record findings. If abnormalities are detected, counsel the patient appropriately. If the patient has watery diarrhea, note history of contact with affected family members, travel to a developing country, involvement in vacation/resort backpacking, community and municipal water supply, and contact with farm animals. Explain that additional testing may be necessary.

2. Follow guidelines in Chapter 1 for safe, effective, informed *posttest* care.

STOOL COLOR ●

Normal Values
Brown

Background
The brown color of normal feces is probably due to stercobilin (urobilin), a bile pigment derivative, which results from the action of reducing bacteria in bilirubin and other undetermined factors.

Explanation of Test

The first indication of GI disturbances is often a change in the normal brown color of the feces. A change in color can provide information about pathologic conditions, organic dysfunction, or intake of drugs. Color abnormalities may aid the clinician in selecting appropriate diagnostic chemical and microbiologic stool tests.

Procedure

Collect a random stool specimen (see p. 282). Observe standard precautions.

Clinical Implications

The color of feces changes in some disease states.

1. Yellow, yellow-green, or green: severe diarrhea
2. Black, with a "tarry" consistency: usually the result of bleeding in the upper GI tract (>100 ml blood)
3. Maroon, red, or pink: possibly the result of bleeding from the lower GI tract from tumors, hemorrhoids, fissures, or an inflammatory process
4. Clay-colored (tan-gray-white): biliary obstruction
5. Pale, with a greasy consistency: pancreatic deficiency causing malabsorption of fat

Clinical Alert

Grossly visible blood always indicates an abnormal state.

1. Blood streaked on the outer surface of stool usually indicates hemorrhoids or anal abnormalities.
2. Blood present in stool can also be caused by abnormalities higher in the colon. If transit time is sufficiently rapid, blood from the stomach or duodenum can appear as bright red, dark red, or maroon in stool.

Interfering Factors

1. Stool darkens on standing.
2. The color of stool is influenced by diet (certain foods), food dyes, and drugs (see Appendix J).
   a. Yellow-rhubarb or yellow to yellow-green color occurs in the stool of breast-fed infants who lack normal intestinal flora.
   b. Pale yellow, white, or gray stools are due to barium intake.
   c. Green color occurs in diets high in chlorophyll-rich green vegetables such as spinach or in some drugs (see Appendix J).
   d. Black color may be due to foods such as cherries, an unusually high proportion of dietary meat, artificially colored foods such as black jelly beans, or drugs and supplements such as charcoal, bismuth, or iron.
   e. Light-colored stool with little odor may be due to diets high in milk and low in meat.

f. Clay-like color may be due to a diet with excessive fat intake or barium intake.

g. Red color may be due to a diet high in beets or tomatoes, red food coloring, or peridium compound.

h. Certain color changes may result from specific drugs (see Appendix J).

Clinical Alert

A complete dietary and drug history will help to differentiate significant abnormalities from interfering factors.

Patient Preparation

1. Advise patient of purpose of test. Ask patient to notify clinician about stool color changes. Follow guidelines in Chapter 1 for safe, effective, informed *pretest* care.
2. Record dietary and drug history.
3. Laxatives and barium procedures should be avoided for 1 week prior to collection.

Patient Aftercare

1. Interpret and document abnormal appearance and colors of stool; counsel patient appropriately regarding the meaning of color changes.
2. Follow guidelines in Chapter 1 for safe, effective, informed *posttest* care.

BLOOD IN STOOL; OCCULT BLOOD

Normal Values
Negative for blood

Background
The most frequently performed fecal analysis is chemical screening for the detection of occult (ie, hidden) blood. Bleeding in the upper GI tract may produce a black, tarry stool. Bleeding in the lower GI tract may result in an overtly bloody stool. However, no visible signs of bleeding may be present with smaller amounts of blood found in early stages of GI diseases; thus, the chemical detection of occult blood is necessary to identify and treat disease early in its course.

Explanation of Test
An average, healthy person passes up to 2.0 ml of blood/150 g of stool into the GI tract daily. Passage of >2.0 ml of blood in the stool in 24 hours is pathologically significant. Detection of occult blood in the stool is very useful in detecting early disease of the GI tract. This test demonstrates the presence of blood produced by upper GI bleeding, as in the presence of gastric ulcer; it also screens for colonic carcinomas while they are still in the localized stages.

With proper medical follow-up, an 84% survival rate has been demonstrated for treated colonic carcinoma.

Procedure

1. Obtain a random stool specimen. Observe standard precautions. Tests for detecting fecal blood use the pseudoperoxidase activity of hemoglobin reacting with hydrogen peroxide to oxidize a colorless compound to a colored one (usually blue). Hemoccult II (Smith-Kline) is the most widely used commercial test with the lowest percentage of false-positive results (1%–12%). This test system uses guaiac-impregnated filter paper as the chromogen that produces the blue color in a positive reaction.
2. Using a wood applicator stick, a thin smear of stool is applied inside the indicated circle and allowed to dry. If stool is bloody, the collector may be at risk for hepatitis B, hepatitis C, or HIV infection.
3. Protect the Hemoccult slide from light, heat, and humidity.
4. The delay between smearing the stool and testing should not exceed 14 days. Do not refrigerate sample before testing.

Clinical Implications

1. Stool that appears dark red to tarry black indicates a loss of 50.0 to 75.0 ml of blood from the upper GI tract. Smaller quantities of blood in the GI tract can produce similar-appearing stools or appear as bright red blood.
2. A stool sample should be considered grossly bloody *only* after chemical testing for presence of blood. This will eliminate the possibility that abnormal coloring caused by diet or drugs may be mistaken for bleeding in the GI tract (see p. 289).
3. Positive testing for occult blood may be caused by the following conditions:
   a. Carcinoma of colon
   b. Ulcerative colitis
   c. Adenoma
   d. Diaphragmatic hernia
   e. Gastric carcinoma
   f. Rectal carcinoma
   g. Peptic ulcer

Clinical Alert

1. To be accurate, the test employed must be repeated three to six times on different stool samples; some bowel lesions may bleed intermittently.
2. The patient's diet should be free of meat and vegetable sources of peroxidase activity (eg, turnips, horseradish, red or rare meat, cauliflower, broccoli, cantaloupe, parsnips). Only after following this regimen can a positive series of tests be considered an indication for further patient evaluation and testing.

Interfering Factors

1. Drugs such as salicylates (aspirin), steroids, indomethacin, nonsteroidal antiinflammatory drugs (NSAIDs), anticoagulants, colchicine, and anti-metabolites are associated with increased GI blood loss in average, healthy persons and with more pronounced bleeding when disease is present. GI bleeding can also follow parenteral administration of the above-mentioned drugs and should be avoided 7 days before testing.
2. Drugs that may cause false-positive results for occult blood testing include the following:
   a. Boric acid
   b. Bromides
   c. Colchicine
   d. Iodine, povidone-iodine (Betadine)
   e. See Appendix J for other drugs.
3. Foods that may cause false-positive results for occult blood testing include the following:
   a. Meat, including processed meats and liver, which in the diet contains hemoglobin, myoglobin, and certain enzymes that can give false-positive tests for up to 4 days after consumption.
   b. Vegetables and fruits with peroxidase activity (eg, turnips, horseradish, mushrooms, broccoli, apples, radishes, bananas, cantaloupe).
4. Substances that cause false-negatives results for occult blood testing include the following:
   a. Ascorbic acid (vitamin C) in excess of 250 mg/day
   b. Vitamin C–enriched foods and juices
   c. Iron supplements that contain vitamin C in excess of 250 mg
   d. See Appendix J for other drugs.
5. Other factors affecting test results include the following:
   a. Bleeding hemorrhoids may produce erroneous results; take samples from center of stool to avoid this error
   b. Collection of specimen during menstrual period
   c. Hematuria (ie, blood in urine)
   d. Some long-distance runners (23%) have positive outcomes for occult blood
   e. Toilet bowl cleansers may interfere with the chemical reaction of the test; remove bowl cleaners and flush twice before proceeding with test

Patient Preparation

1. Explain the purpose, procedure, and interfering factors of the test, as well as the need to follow appropriate stool collection protocols.
2. It is recommended that the patient consume a high-residue diet starting 72 hours before and continuing throughout the collection period. Roughage in diet can increase test accuracy by helping to uncover silent lesions that bleed intermittently. The diet may include:
   a. Meats: only small amounts of chicken, turkey, and tuna
   b. Vegetables: generous amounts of both raw and cooked vegetables, in-

cluding lettuce, corn, spinach, carrots, and celery. Avoid vegetables with high peroxidase activity (see 3b above).

c. Fruits: plenty of fruits, especially prunes
d. Cereals: bran and bran-containing cereals
e. Moderate amounts of peanuts and popcorn daily. If any of the above foods are known to cause discomfort, the patient should consult the physician.

3. No barium enemas should be administered 72 hours prior to or during testing.
4. Patient instructions:

a. Do not collect samples during or until 3 days after your menstrual period, or while you have bleeding hemorrhoids or blood in your urine.
b. Do not consume the following medications, vitamins, and foods: for 7 days prior to and during the test period, avoid aspirin or other NSAIDs; for 72 hours prior to and during the test period, avoid vitamin C in excess of 250 mg/day (from all sources, dietary and supplementary), red meat (eg, beef, lamb) including processed meats and liver, raw fruits and vegetables (especially melons, radishes, turnips, and horseradish).
c. Remove toilet bowl cleaners from toilet tank and flush twice before proceeding.
d. Collect samples from three consecutive bowel movements or three bowel movements closely spaced in time.
e. Protect slides from heat, light, and volatile chemicals (eg, iodine, bleach). Keep cover flap of slides closed when not in use.

Patient Aftercare

1. Patient may resume normal diet after testing is complete.
2. Interpret occult blood test results and record findings. Counsel the patient regarding abnormal findings and monitor as necessary. Advise that further testing and follow-up may be required.
3. Follow guidelines in Chapter 1 for safe, effective, informed posttest care.

> **Clinical Alert**
>
> Blood in the stool is abnormal and should be reported and recorded.

APT TEST FOR SWALLOWED BLOOD

Normal Values

Test result will indicate whether blood present in newborn feces or vomitus is of maternal or fetal origin.

Background

Dr. L. Apt developed the test for identifying the swallowed blood syndrome. The swallowed blood syndrome refers to bloody stools usually passed on the second or third day of life. The blood may be swallowed during delivery or may be from a fissure of the mother's nipple in breast-fed infants. This condition must be differentiated from GI hemorrhage of the newborn. The test is based on the fact that the infant's blood contains largely fetal hemoglobin, which is alkali resistant. This blood can be differentiated from the mother's blood using laboratory methods.

Explanation of Test

The APT test is used to differentiate swallowed blood syndrome from infant GI hemorrhage. The test can be done on feces or vomitus. In the laboratory, the blood is dissolved and treated with NaOH for alkali denaturation. Fetal hemoglobin is alkali resistant, and the solution of blood remains pink. Swallowed blood of maternal origin contains adult hemoglobin, which is converted to brownish hematin when the alkali is added.

Procedure

1. Collect a random stool specimen from a newborn infant; observe universal precautions.
2. The following are acceptable specimens:
   a. Blood-stained diaper
   b. Grossly bloody stool
   c. Bloody vomitus or gastric aspiration
3. Place specimen or specimens in a biohazard bag and deliver to the laboratory as soon as possible. Refrigerate the specimen or specimens if there is any delay.

Clinical Implications

1. Fetal hemoglobin, which is pink in color, is present in gastric hemorrhage of the newborn.
2. Adult hemoglobin, which is brownish in color, is present in swallowed blood syndrome in the infant.

Interfering Factors

1. The test is invalid with black, tarry stools because the blood has already been converted to hematin.
2. The test is invalid if there is insufficient blood present; grossly visible blood must be present in the specimen.
3. Vomitus with pH <3.9 produces an invalid test result.
4. The presence of maternal thalassemia major produces a false-positive test result because of increased maternal hemoglobin F.

Patient Preparation

1. Advise parent or parents of the purpose of the test.
2. Follow guidelines in Chapter 1 for safe, effective, informed *pretest* care.

Patient Aftercare

1. Review test results and counsel the parent or parents regarding test outcome.

2. Follow guidelines in Chapter 1 for safe, effective, informed *posttest* care.

MUCUS IN STOOL ●

Normal Values
Negative for mucus

Background
The mucosa of the colon secretes mucus in response to parasympathetic stimulation.

Explanation of Test
Recognizable mucus in a stool specimen is abnormal and should be reported and recorded.

Procedure
Collect a random stool specimen (see p. 282). Observe and report findings of mucus.

Clinical Implications
1. Translucent gelatinous mucus clinging to the surface of formed stool occurs in the following conditions:
   a. Spastic constipation
   b. Mucous colitis
   c. Emotionally disturbed patients
   d. Excessive straining at stool
3. Bloody mucus clinging to the feces suggests the following conditions:
   a. Neoplasm
   b. Inflammation of the rectal canal
4. In villous adenoma of the colon, copious quantities of mucus may be passed (up to 3–4 L in 24 hours).
5. Mucus and diarrhea with white and red blood cells is associated with the following conditions:
   a. Ulcerative colitis (*Shigella*)
   b. Bacillary dysentery (*Salmonella*)
   c. Ulcerating cancer of colon
   d. Acute diverticulitis
   e. Intestinal tuberculosis
   f. Regional enteritis
   g. Amebiasis

Patient Preparation
1. Advise patient of purpose of observing for stool mucus.
2. Follow guidelines in Chapter 1 for safe, effective, informed *pretest* care.
3. Laxatives and barium procedures should be avoided for 1 week prior to test.

Patient Aftercare

1. Report and record presence, type, and amount of mucus.
2. Counsel patient appropriately. Monitor bowel habits. Explain that further testing and follow-up monitoring may be necessary.
3. Follow guidelines in Chapter 1 for safe, effective, informed *posttest* care.

STOOL pH

Normal Values

Neutral to slightly acid or alkaline: pH 6.5–7.5.
Newborns: pH 5.0–7.5

Background

Stool pH is diet dependent and is based on bacterial fermentation in the small intestine. Carbohydrate fermentation changes the pH to acid; protein breakdown changes the pH to alkaline.

Explanation of Test

Stool pH testing is done to evaluate carbohydrate and fat malabsorption and assess disaccharidase deficiency. Breast-fed infants have slightly acid stools; bottle-fed infants have slightly alkaline stools.

Procedure

Collect a fresh, random stool specimen in a plastic container with a tight-fitting lid (see p. 282). Refrigerate specimen.

Clinical Implications

1. Increased pH (alkaline)
   a. Secretory diarrhea without food intake
   b. Colitis
   c. Villous adenoma
   d. Antibiotic use (impaired colonic fermentation)
2. Decreased pH (acid)
   a. Carbohydrate malabsorption
   b. Fat malabsorption
   c. Disaccharidase deficiency

Interfering Factors

1. Barium procedures and laxatives affect test outcomes. They should be avoided for 1 week prior to stool sample collection.
2. Specimens contaminated with urine will invalidate the test.

Patient Preparation

1. Explain the purpose and procedure of the test following general guidelines in Chapter 1 for safe, effective, informed *pretest* care.

2. Advise patient that laxatives and barium procedures should be avoided for 1 week prior to stool sampling.

Patient Aftercare
1. Interpret pH outcome and record findings. If abnormal pH is found, assess dietary patterns and antibiotic use.
2. Monitor as appropriate for malabsorption syndrome.
3. A stool reducing substance test should be ordered if disaccharidase deficiency is suspected (see Stool Reducing Substances Test below).
4. Follow guidelines in Chapter 1 for safe, effective, informed *posttest* care.

STOOL REDUCING SUBSTANCES TEST

Normal Values
Normal: <0.25% or <0.25 g/dl reducing substances in stool
Questionable: 0.25%–0.5% or 0.25–0.50 g/dl reducing substances in stool
Abnormal: >0.5% or >0.5 g/dl reducing substances in stool

Background
Normally, sugars are rapidly absorbed in the upper small intestine. However, if this is not the case, they remain in the intestine and cause osmotic diarrhea due to osmotic pressure of the unabsorbed sugar in the intestine drawing fluid and electrolytes into the gut. The unabsorbed sugars are measured as reducing substances. Reducing substances that can be detected in the stool include glucose, fructose, lactose, galactose, and pentose. Carbohydrate malabsorption is a major cause of watery diarrhea and electrolyte imbalance seen in patients with the short bowel syndrome. Idiopathic lactase deficiency is common, occurring in 70% to 75% of Southern European Greeks and Italians, 70% of Black adults, >90% of Asian adults, and 5% to 20% of Caucasian American adults.

Explanation of Test
The finding of elevated levels of reducing substances in the stool is abnormal and suggests carbohydrate malabsorption. A presumptive diagnosis of disaccharide intolerance can be made with an elevated reducing substance level along with an acid (ie, low) pH.

Procedure
Collect a fresh random stool specimen and immediately deliver it to the laboratory (see p. 282).

Clinical Implications
Elevated reducing substances in stool are found in the following conditions:

1. Disaccharidase deficiency
2. Short bowel syndrome

3. Idiopathic lactase deficiency
4. Carbohydrate malabsorption abnormalities

Interfering Factors

1. Bacterial fermentation of sugars may give falsely low results if the stool is not tested immediately.
2. Newborns may normally have elevated results.

Patient Preparation

1. Explain the purpose of the test and interfering factors. Follow guidelines in Chapter 1 regarding safe, effective, informed *pretest* care.

Patient Aftercare

1. Interpret test outcomes. Follow guidelines in Chapter 1 for safe, effective, informed *posttest* care.
2. If outcome is positive, further testing may be necessary.

LEUKOCYTES IN STOOL ●

Normal Values
Negative for leukocytes

Background
Microscopic examination of the feces for the presence of white blood cells (leukocytes) is performed as a preliminary procedure in determining the cause of diarrhea.

Explanation of Test
The presence or absence of fecal leukocytes can provide diagnostic information prior to the isolation of a bacterial pathogen. Neutrophils (>3 neutrophils/high-power field) are seen in the feces in conditions that affect the intestinal wall (eg, ulcerative colitis, invasive bacterial pathogen infection). Bacteria that cause diarrhea by toxin production, viruses, and parasites do not cause neutrophils in the stool.

Procedure
Collect a random stool specimen (see p. 282). Mucus or a liquid stool specimen can be used.

Clinical Implications
1. Large amounts of leukocytes (primarily neutrophils) accompany the following conditions:
  a. Chronic ulcerative colitis
  b. Chronic bacillary dysentery
  c. Localized abscesses
  d. Fistulas of the sigmoid rectum or anus

2. Primarily neutrophilic leukocytes appear in the following conditions:
   a. Shigellosis
   b. Salmonellosis
   c. *Yersinia* infection
   d. Invasive *Escherichia coli* diarrhea
   e. Ulcerative colitis
3. Primarily mononuclear leukocytes appear in typhoid.
4. Absence of leukocytes is associated with the following conditions:
   a. Cholera
   b. Nonspecific diarrhea (eg, drug or food induced)
   c. Viral diarrhea
   d. Amebic colitis
   e. Noninvasive *E. coli* diarrhea
   f. Toxigenic bacteria (eg, *Staphylococcus, Clostridium*)
   g. Parasites (eg, *Giardia, Entamoeba*)

Patient Preparation
1. Explain the purpose of the test and the collection procedure. Follow guidelines in Chapter 1 for safe, effective, informed *pretest* care.
2. Barium procedures and laxatives should be avoided for 1 week before test.
3. Withhold antibiotic therapy until after collection.

Patient Aftercare
1. Interpret abnormal test results. Monitor for diarrhea. Counsel patient concerning the need for follow-up tests and treatment.
2. Follow guidelines in Chapter 1 for safe, effective, informed *posttest* care.

COLLECTION AND TRANSPORT OF 24-, 48-, AND 72-HOUR STOOL SPECIMENS ●

This method is used to test for fat, porphyrins, urobilinogen, nitrogen, and electrolytes.

Special Instructions for Submitting Individual Specimens
1. Collect all stool specimens for 1 to 3 days. The entire stool should be collected.
2. Label specimens with day of test (eg, *Day 1, Day 2, Day 3*), time of day collected, patient's name, and tests ordered.
3. Submit individual specimens to the laboratory as soon as they are collected.

Special Instructions for Submitting Total Specimens
1. Obtain a 1-gallon container from the laboratory (a 1-gallon paint tin or covered plastic pail is preferred).
2. Save all stool and place in the container. Keep refrigerated or in a container with canned ice and replace ice as needed.

3. At the end of the collection period, transfer the properly labeled container to the laboratory.
4. Record dates, duration of collection time period, tests to be performed, patient's name, and other vital information on the collection receptacle.

FAT IN STOOL; FECAL FAT STAIN

Normal Values

Qualitative
Neutral fat: <50 fat globules/high-power field
Fatty acids: <100 fat globules/high-power field

Quantitative
0.0–6.0 g/24 h

Background
Fecal fat is the gold standard test for diagnosing steatorrhea (malabsorption). The three major causes of steatorrhea, which is a pathologic increase in fecal fat, are impairment of intestinal absorption, deficiency of pancreatic digestive enzymes, and deficiency of bile.

Explanation of Test
Specimens from patients suspected of having steatorrhea can be screened microscopically for the presence of excess fecal fat. This procedure can also be used to monitor patients undergoing treatment for malabsorption disorders. In general, there is good correlation between the qualitative and quantitative fecal fat procedures. Lipids included in the microscopic examination of feces are neutral fats (triglycerides), fatty acid salts (soaps), fatty acids, and cholesterol. The presence of these lipids can be observed microscopically by staining with the dyes Sudan III, Sudan IV, or oil red O. The staining procedure consists of two parts: the neutral fat stain and the split fat stain.

Procedure
1. Collect a 48-hour to 72-hour specimen. A random specimen can be used for the qualitative test. Each individual stool specimen is collected and identified with the name of the patient, time and date of collection, and test to be performed. Also indicate the length (actual time frame) of the collection period. The specimen should be sent immediately to the laboratory.
2. Follow the procedure for the collection of 24-, 48-, or 72-hour specimens.

Clinical Implications
1. Increases in fecal fat and fatty acids are associated with malabsorption syndrome caused by the following conditions:
   a. Nontropical sprue
   b. Crohn's disease
   c. Whipple's disease
   d. Cystic fibrosis

2. Increases in fecal fat and fatty acids are also found in the following conditions:
    a. Enteritis and pancreatic diseases in which there is a lack of lipase (eg, chronic pancreatitis)
    b. Surgical removal of a section of the intestine
3. Fecal fat test does not provide a diagnostic explanation for the presence of steatorrhea.
    a. D-Xylose absorption test may be ordered for the differential diagnosis of malabsorption.

Interfering Factors

1. Increased neutral fat may occur under the following nondisease conditions:
    a. Use of rectal suppositories and/or oily creams applied to the perineum
    b. Ingestion of castor oil, mineral oil, or oily salad dressings
    c. Ingestion of dietetic low-calorie mayonnaise
    d. Ingestion of a high-fiber diet (>100 g/24 h)
    e. Use of psyllium-based stool softeners (eg, Metamucil)
2. Use of barium and bismuth interfere with test results.
3. Urine contaminates the specimen.
4. A random stool specimen is not an acceptable sample for the quantitative fat test.

Patient Preparation

1. Explain the purpose of the test, interfering factors, and the procedure for the collection of specimens. Follow guidelines in Chapter 1 concerning diverse patient needs and safe, effective, informed *pretest* care.
2. For a 72-hour stool collection, a diet containing 60 to 100 g of fat, 100 g of protein, and 180 g of carbohydrate is eaten for 6 days before and during the test.
3. Follow the procedure for the collection of 72-hour stool specimens (see p. 299).

Patient Aftercare

1. Resume normal diet.
2. Record appearance, color, and odor of all stools in persons suspected of having steatorrhea. The typical stool in patients with this condition is foamy, greasy, soft, pasty, and foul smelling.
3. Counsel patient concerning test outcome and possible need for further testing.
4. Follow guidelines in Chapter 1 for safe, effective, informed *posttest* care.

MEAT FIBERS IN STOOL; STOOL MUSCLE FIBER

Normal Values
Negative (no undigested meat fibers present in the normal stool)

Explanation of Test
The presence of undigested meat fibers (ie, muscle fibers) in stool implies impaired intraluminal digestion. There is positive correlation between the presence of meat/muscle fibers and the presence of fat excreted in the stool.

Procedure
1. The patient must eat 4 to 6 ounces of red meat for 24 to 72 hours before testing.
2. Collect a random specimen (see p. 282). Specimens obtained with a warm saline enema or Fleet Phospho-Soda are acceptable.
3. Record method and type of stool procurement.

Clinical Implications
Increased amounts of meat fibers are found in the following conditions:

1. Malabsorption syndromes caused by biliary obstruction
2. Pancreatic exocrine dysfunction (cystic fibrosis)
3. Gastrocolic fistula

Interfering Factors
1. Specimens should not be obtained with mineral oil, bismuth, or magnesium compounds.
2. Barium procedures and laxatives should be avoided for 1 week before collection.

Patient Preparation
1. Explain the purpose of the test and interfering factors.
2. Patient must eat a high-meat diet for 72 hours prior to test.
3. Follow guidelines in Chapter 1 for safe, effective, informed *pretest* care.

Patient Aftercare
1. Resume normal diet.
2. Interpret test outcomes.
3. Follow guidelines in Chapter 1 for safe, effective, informed *posttest* care.

UROBILINOGEN IN STOOL

Normal Values
50–300 mg/24 h or 100–400 Ehrlich units/100 g
Newborns–6 months: negative

Background
Increased destruction of red blood cells, as in hemolytic anemia, increases the amount of urobilinogen excreted. Liver disease, in general, reduces the flow of bilirubin to the intestine and thereby decreases the fecal excretion of uro-

bilinogen. In addition, complete obstruction of the bile duct reduces uro-bilinogen to very low levels.

Explanation of Test

This test investigates hemolytic diseases to determine if there is excess production of urobilinogen. Determination of stool urobilinogen is an estimate of the total excretion of bile pigments, which are the breakdown products of hemoglobin.

Procedure

Collect a random stool specimen (see p. 282). Protect the specimen from light, and immediately send it to the laboratory.

Clinical Implications

1. *Increased values* are associated with hemolytic anemias.
2. *Decreased values* are associated with the following conditions:
    a. Complete biliary obstruction
    b. Severe liver disease (eg, infectious hepatitis)
    c. Oral antibiotic therapy that alters intestinal bacterial flora
    d. Aplastic anemia, which results in decreased hemoglobin turnover

Interfering Factors

1. See Appendix J for drugs that affect test outcomes.

Patient Preparation

1. Explain purpose of test.
2. Patient should not be receiving oral antibiotic therapy for 1 week before test.
3. Laxatives and barium procedures should be avoided 1 week before test.
4. Follow guidelines in Chapter 1 for safe, effective, informed *pretest* care.

Patient Aftercare

1. Interpret test outcomes. Counsel patient appropriately regarding further testing. Monitor patient for liver disease, biliary obstruction, and diarrhea.
2. Follow guidelines in Chapter 1 for safe, effective, informed *posttest* care.

TRYPSIN IN STOOL: FECAL CHYMOTRYPSIN ●

Normal Values

Positive for small amounts in 95% of normal persons
Greater amounts in the stools of normal children

Background

Trypsin is a proteolytic enzyme formed in the small intestine. In older children and adults, trypsin is destroyed by bacteria in the GI tract.

Explanation of Test

This test is used as an indicator for pancreatic function and for evaluating the ability of trypsin to split carbohydrates, protein, and fats by this pancreatic enzyme. This test is more useful in evaluating malabsorption in children younger than age 4 years.

Procedure

1. Collect random specimens and send to the laboratory (see p. 282). Three separate, fresh stools are usually collected.
2. Specimen must be taken to the laboratory and tested within 2 hours.
3. In older children, a cathartic is given prior to obtaining a specimen (saline or Fleet only).

Clinical Implications

Decreased amounts of trypsin occur in the following conditions:

1. Pancreatic deficiency syndromes
2. Malabsorption
3. Cystic fibrosis (sweat chloride test is diagnostic)

Interfering Factors

1. No trypsin activity is detectable in constipated stools owing to prolonged exposure to intestinal bacteria, which inactivates trypsin.
2. Barium and laxatives used less than 1 week before test affect results.
3. In adults, the test is unreliable due to trypsin inactivation by intestinal flora.
4. Bacterial proteases may produce positive reactions when no trypsin is present.

Patient Preparation

1. Explain purpose of test and interfering factors.
2. Barium procedures and laxatives should be avoided for 1 week prior to stool collection.
3. Follow guidelines in Chapter 1 for safe, effective, informed *pretest* care.

Patient Aftercare

1. Interpret abnormal test results and counsel patient concerning possible need for follow-up testing.
2. Follow guidelines in Chapter 1 for safe, effective, informed *posttest* care.

> ▶ **Clinical Alert**
>
> 1. Diagnosis of pancreatic insufficiency should not be made until three separate specimens exhibit no trypsin activity.
> 2. Bacterial protease may produce positive reactions when no trypsin is present; therefore, both positive and negative reactions should be carefully interpreted.

STOOL ELECTROLYTES: SODIUM, CHLORIDE, POTASSIUM, AND OSMOLALITY ●

Normal Values

Sodium: 5.8–9.8 mEq/24 h; osmolality = 200–250 mOsm/kg or 250 mg/dl
Chloride: 2.5–3.9 mEq/24 h; osmotic gap = osmolality is 2 times sodium plus potassium
Potassium: 15.7–20.7 mEq/24 h (soldium plus potassium)

> **NOTE:** *Reference values vary from laboratory to laboratory. Check with your laboratory for normal values.*

Background

Normal colon function involves absorption of fluid and electrolytes.

Explanation of Test

Stool electrolyte tests are used to assess electrolyte imbalance in persons with diarrhea. Stool electrolytes must be evaluated along with the serum and urine electrolytes, as well as clinical findings in the patient. Stool osmolality is used in conjunction with blood serum osmolality to calculate the osmotic gap and to diagnose intestinal disaccharide deficiency.

Procedure

Collect a random or 24-hour stool specimen (see pp. 282 and 299). Keep the specimen covered and refrigerated.

Clinical Implications

1. Electrolyte abnormalities occur in the following conditions:
   a. Idiopathic proctocolitis: *Increased* sodium (Na) and Chloride (Cl), *normal* potassium (K).
   b. Ileostomy: *Increased* sodium (Na) and Chloride (Cl), *low* potassium (K).
   c. Cholera: *Increased* sodium (Na) and Chloride (Cl).
2. Chloride is greatly increased in stool in the following conditions:
   a. Congenital chloride diarrhea
   b. Acquired chloride diarrhea
   c. Secondary chloride diarrhea
   d. Idiopathic proctocolitis
   e. Cholera
3. Stool osmolality of 500 mg/dl per day is suspicious for factitious disorders (eg, laxative abuse, ingestion of rat poison). Higher levels indicate high amounts of stool reducing substances. The osmotic gap is increased in osmotic diarrhea caused by the following conditions:
   a. Saline laxatives
   b. Sodium or magnesium citrate
   c. Carbohydrates (lactulose or sorbitol candy)

Interfering Factors

1. Formed stools invalidate the results. Stools *must* be liquid for electrolyte tests.
2. The stool cannot be contaminated with urine.

3. Surreptitious addition of water to the stool specimen considerably lowers the osmolality. Stool osmolality must be <240 mOsm/kg to calculate the osmotic gap.

4. See Appendix J for drugs that cause increased values.

Patient Preparation

1. Explain purpose of test, procedure for stool collection, and interfering factors.

2. Barium procedures and laxatives should be avoided for 1 week before collection of specimen.

3. Follow guidelines in Chapter 1 for safe, effective, informed, *pretest* care.

Patient Aftercare

1. Interpret abnormal test outcomes. Monitor diarrhea episodes and record findings. Assess patient for electrolyte imbalances.

2. Follow guidelines in Chapter 1 for safe, effective, informed *posttest* care.

BIBLIOGRAPHY ●

Bakerman S: ABCs of Interpretive Laboratory Data, 3rd ed. Greenville, NC, Interpretive Laboratory Data, Inc., 1993

Bennett JC, Plum F (eds): Cecil Textbook of Medicine, 20th ed. Philadelphia, WB Saunders, 1996

Henry JB (ed): Clinical Diagnosis and Management by Laboratory Methods, 19th ed. Philadelphia, WB Saunders, 1996

Lehman CA (ed): Saunders Manual of Clinical Laboratory Science, Philadelphia, WB Saunders, 1998

Levin B, Hess K, Johnson C: Screening for colorectal cancer. A comparison of 3 fecal occult blood tests. Arch Intern Med 157:970, 1997

Novak RW: Identifying leukocytes in fecal specimens. Lab Med 27: 433, 1996

Speicher CE: The Right Test, A Physician's Guide to Laboratory Medicine, 3rd ed. Philadelphia, WB Saunders, 1998

Strasinger S: Urinalysis and Body Fluids, 3rd ed. Philadelphia, FA Davis, 1994

Wallach J: Interpretation of Laboratory Tests, Synopsis of Laboratory Medicine, 6th ed. Boston, Little, Brown & Co., 1996

Young DS: Effects of Drugs in Clinical Laboratory Tests, 5th ed. Washington, DC, AACC Press, 1999

5

Cerebrospinal Fluid Studies

●───────────────────────────

Description, Formation, and Composition of CSF

Cerebrospinal fluid (CSF) is a clear, colorless fluid formed within the cavities (ie, ventricles) of the brain. The choroid plexus produces about 70% of the CSF by ultrafiltration and secretion. The ependymal lining of the ventricles and cerebral subarachnoid space produce the remainder of the CSF total volume. Approximately 500 ml of CSF fluid is formed per day, although only 120 to 150 ml is present in the system at any one time. Reabsorption of CSF occurs at the arachnoid villi.

CSF circulates slowly from the ventricular system into the space surrounding the brain and spinal cord and serves as an hydraulic shock absorber, diffusing external forces to the skull that might otherwise cause severe injury. The CSF also helps to regulate intracranial pressure, supply nutrients to the nervous tissues, and remove waste products. The chemical composition of CSF does not resemble an ultrafiltrate of plasma. Certain chemicals in the CSF are regulated by specific transport systems (eg, K^+, Ca^{2+}, Mg^{2+}), whereas other substances (eg, glucose, urea, creatinine) diffuse freely. Proteins enter the CSF by passive diffusion at a rate dependent on the plasma-to-CSF concentration gradient. The term *blood-brain barrier* is used to represent the control and filtration of blood plasma components to the CSF and then to the brain.

Most CSF constituents are present in the same or lower concentrations as in the blood plasma, except for chloride concentrations, which are usually higher. Disease, however, can cause elements ordinarily restrained by the blood-brain barrier to enter the spinal fluid. Erythrocytes and leukocytes can enter the CSF from the rupture of blood vessels or from meningeal reaction to irritation. Bilirubin can be found in the spinal fluid after intracranial hemorrhage. In such cases, the arachnoid granulations and the nerve root sheaths will reabsorb the bloody fluid. Normal CSF pressure will consequently be maintained by the absorption of CSF in amounts equal to its production. Blockage causes an increase in the amount of CSF, resulting in hydrocephalus in infants or increased intracranial pressure in adults. Of the many factors that regulate the level of CSF pressure, venous pressure is the most important, because the reabsorbed fluid ultimately drains into the venous system.

Despite the continuous production (~0.3 ml/min) and reabsorption of CSF and the exchange of substances between the CSF and the blood plasma, considerable pooling occurs in the lumbar sac. The lumbar sac, located at L4 to L5, is the usual site used for puncture to obtain CSF specimens, because damage to the nervous system is less likely to occur in this area. In infants, the spinal cord is situated more caudally than in adults (L3-L4 until 9 months of age, when the cord ascends to L1-L2); therefore, a low lumbar puncture should be made in these patients.

NORMAL CSF VALUES

Volume	Adult: 90–150 ml; child: 60–100 ml
Appearance	Crystal clear, colorless
Pressure	Adult: 90–180 mm H_2O; child: 10–100 mm H_2O
Total cell count	Essentially free cells

(continued)

NORMAL CSF VALUES *(Continued)*

	Adults	*Newborn (0–14 d)*
WBCs	0–5 cells	0–30 cells
Differential		
Lymphocytes	40%–80%	5%–35%
Monocytes	15%–45%	50%–90%
Polys	0%–6%	0%–8%
RBCs (has limited diagnostic value)		
Specific gravity	1.006–1.008	
Osmolality	280–300 mOsm/kg	

CLINICAL TESTS

Glucose	45–80 mg/dl
Protein	
Lumbar	Adults: 15–45 mg/dl
	Neonates: 15–100 mg/dl
	Elderly (>60 y): 15–60 mg/dl
Cisternal	15–25 mg/dl
Ventricular	5–15 mg/dl
Lactic acid (lactate)	10–24 mg/dl
Glutamine	5–15 mg/dl
Albumin	10–35 mg/dl
Urea nitrogen	6–16 mg/dl
Creatinine	0.5–1.2 mg/dl
Cholesterol	0.2–0.6 mg/dl
Uric acid	0.5–4.5 mg/dl
Bilirubin	0 (none)
Phosphorous	1.2–2.0 mg/dl
Ammonia	10–35 µg/dl
Lactate dehydrogenase (LDH)	Adult: 0–40 U/L
	Newborn: 0–70 U/L

ELECTROLYES AND pH

pH	7.30–7.40
Lumbar	7.28–7.32
Cisternal	7.32–7.34
Chloride	115–130 mEq/L (mmol)
Sodium	135–160 mEq/L (mmol)
Potassium	2.6–3.0 mEq/L (mmol)
CO_2 content	20–25 mEq/L (mmol)
P_{CO_2}	44–50 mm Hg
P_{O_2}	40–44 mm Hg
Calcium	2.0–2.8 mEq/L (mmol)
Magnesium	2.4–3.0 mEq/L (mmol)
Osmolality	280–300 mOsm/kg

SEROLOGY AND MICROBIOLOGY

VDRL	Negative
Bacteria	None present
Viruses	None present

Explanation of Test

Cerebrospinal fluid is obtained by lumbar puncture. A lumbar puncture is done for the following reasons:

1. To examine the spinal fluid for diagnosis of four major disease categories:
   a. Meningitis
   b. Subarachnoid hemorrhage
   c. CNS malignancy
   d. Demyelinating diseases
2. To determine level of CSF pressure, to document impaired CSF flow, or to lower pressure by removing a volume of fluid. (Fluid removal should be done with caution.)
3. To introduce anesthetics, drugs, or contrast media used for radiographic studies into the spinal cord.

Certain observations are made each time lumbar puncture is performed:

1. CSF pressure is measured.
2. General appearance, consistency, and tendency of the CSF to clot are noted.
3. CSF cell count is performed to distinguish types of cells present; this must be done within 2 hours of obtaining the CSF sample.
4. CSF protein and glucose concentrations are determined.
5. Other clinical serologic and bacteriologic tests are done when the patient's condition warrants (eg, culture for aerobes and anaerobes or tuberculosis).
6. Tumor markers may be present in CSF; these test are useful as supplements to CSF cytology analysis (Table 5-1).

> **Clinical Alert**
>
> 1. Blood levels for specific substances should always be measured simultaneously with CSF determinations for meaningful interpretation of results.
> 2. Prior to lumbar puncture, check eyegrounds for evidence of papilledema, because its presence may signal potential problems or complications of lumbar puncture.
> 3. A mass lesion should be precluded by CT scan before lumbar puncture, because this can lead to brain stem herniation.
> 4. However, if increased pressure is found while performing the lumbar puncture, it should not be necessary to stop the procedure unless neurologic signs are present.

LUMBAR PUNCTURE (SPINAL TAP) ●

Procedure

1. The patient is usually placed in a side-lying position with the head flexed onto the chest and knees drawn up to, but not compressing, the abdomen

TABLE 5-1
Tumor Markers in CSF

Determination	Used in Diagnosis of	Normal Values*
α-fetoprotein (AFP)	CNS dysgerminomas and meningeal carcinomas	<1.5 mg/ml
β-Glucuronidase	Possible meningeal carcinomatosis	<49 mU/L (indeterminate, 49–70 mU/L; suspicious, >70 mU/L) <0.6 mg/ml
Carcinoembryonic antigen (CEA)	Meningeal carcinomatosis: intradural or extradural, or brain parenchymal metastasis from adenocarcinoma; although the assay appears to be specific for adenocarcinoma and squamous cell carcinoma, increased CEA values in CSF are not seen in all such tumors of the brain	
Human chorionic gonadotropin (HCG)	Adjunct in determining CNS dysgerminomas and meningeal carcinomatosis	<0.21 U/L
Lysozyme (muramidase)	CNS tumors, especially myoclonal and monocytic leukemia	4–13 µg/ml

*Normal values vary greatly; check with your reference laboratory.
NOTE: The value of tumor markers in CSF for routine clinical diagnosis has not been established.

to "bow" the back. This position helps to increase the space between the lower lumbar vertebrae so that the spinal needle can be inserted more easily between the spinal processes. However, a sitting position with the head flexed to the chest can be used. The patient is helped to relax and instructed to breathe slowly and deeply with his or her mouth open.

2. The puncture site is selected, usually between L4 and L5 or lower. There is a small bony landmark at the L5-S interspace known as the "surgeon's delight" that helps to locate the puncture site. The site is thoroughly cleansed with an antiseptic solution, and the surrounding area is draped with sterile towels in such a way that the drapes do not obscure important landmarks (Fig. 5-1).

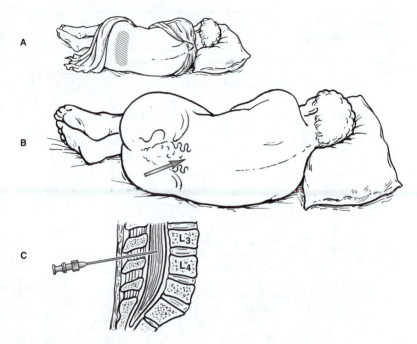

FIGURE 5-1
Spinal tap technique. The patient lies on his side with knees flexed and back arched to separate the lumbar vertebrae. The patient is surgically draped and an area overlying the lumbar spine is disinfected (A). The space between lumbar vertebrae L_3 and L_4 is palpated with the sterilely gloved forefinger (B) and the spinal needle is carefully directed between the spinous processes, through the infraspinous ligaments into the spinal canal (C).

3. A local anesthetic is injected slowly into the dermis around the intended puncture site.

4. A spinal needle with stylet is inserted into the midline between the spines of the lumbar space and slowly advanced until it enters the subarachnoid space. The patient may feel the entry as a "pop" of the needle through the dura mater. Once this happens, the patient can be helped to straighten his or her legs slowly to relieve abdominal compression.

5. With the needle remaining in the subarachnoid space, the stylet is removed, and a pressure manometer is attached to the needle to record the opening CSF pressure.

NOTE: *If the opening pressure is >200 mm H_2O in a relaxed patient, no more than 2 ml of CSF should be withdrawn.*

NOTE: *If the initial pressure is normal, the Queckenstedt's test may be done. (This test is not done if a central nervous system [CNS] tumor is suspected.)*

In this test, pressure is placed on both jugular veins to occlude them temporarily and to produce an acute rise in CSF pressure. Normally, pressure rapidly returns to average levels after jugular vein occlusion is removed. Total or partial spinal fluid blockage is diagnosed if the lumbar pressure fails to rise when both jugular veins are compressed or if the pressure requires >20 seconds to fall after compression is released.

6. A specimen consisting of up to 20 ml CSF is removed. Up to four samples of 2 to 3 ml each are taken, placed in separate sterile vials, and labeled sequentially. No. 1 is used for chemistry and serology; No. 2 is used for microbiology studies; No. 3 is used for hematology cell counts; and No. 4 is used for special studies such as cryptococcal antigens, syphilis testing (Venereal Disease Research Laboratory [VDRL]), protein electrophoresis, and other immunologic studies. A closing pressure reading may be taken before the needle is withdrawn. In cases of increased intracranial pressure (ICP), no more than 2 ml is withdrawn because of the risk that the brain stem may shift.

7. A small sterile dressing is applied to the puncture site.

8. Tubes should be correctly labeled with the proper sequential number (1, 2, 3, or 4), the patient's name, and the date of collection. Specimens of CSF must be immediately delivered to laboratory, where they should be given to laboratory personnel with specific instructions regarding the testing. CSF samples should never be placed in the refrigerator, because refrigeration alters the results of bacteriologic and fungal studies. Analysis should be started immediately. If viral studies are to be done, a portion of the specimen should be frozen.

9. Record procedure start and completion times, patient's status, CSF appearance, and CSF pressure readings.

Patient Preparation

1. Explain the purpose, benefits, and risks of lumbar puncture and explain tests to be performed on the CSF specimen; present a step-by-step description of the actual procedure. Emphasize the need for patient cooperation. Assess for contraindications or impediments such as arthritis.

2. Help the patient to relax by having him or her breath slowly and deeply. The patient must refrain from breath holding, straining, moving, and talking during the procedure.

3. Follow guidelines in Chapter 1 regarding safe, effective, informed *pretest* care.

Patient Aftercare

1. The patient should lie prone (flat or horizontal, or on the abdomen) for approximately 4 to 8 hours. Turning from side to side is permitted as long as the body is kept in a horizontal position.

2. Women may have difficulty voiding in this position. The use of a fracture bedpan may help.

3. Fluids are encouraged to help prevent or relieve headache, which is a possible result of lumbar puncture.

4. Interpret test outcomes. Assess and monitor for abnormal outcomes and complications such as paralysis (or progression of paralysis, as with spinal tumor), hematoma, meningitis, asphyxiation of infants owing to tracheal obstruction from pushing the head forward, and infection. Institute infection control precautions if test outcomes reveal an infectious process.

5. Observe for neurologic changes such as altered level of consciousness, change in pupils, change in temperature, increased blood pressure, irritability, and numbness and tingling sensations, especially in the lower extremities.

6. If headache should occur, administer analgesics as ordered and encourage a longer period of prone bed rest. If headache persists, a "blood patch" may need to be done, in which a small amount of the patient's own blood is introduced into the spinal canal at the same level that the canal was previously entered. For reasons not totally understood, this blood patch very effectively stops spinal headaches within a very short period.

7. Check the puncture site for leakage.

8. Document the procedure completion and any problems encountered or complaints voiced by the patient.

9. Follow guidelines in Chapter 1 regarding safe, effective, informed *posttest* care.

> **Clinical Alert**

1. Extreme caution should be used when performing lumbar puncture if ICP is elevated, especially in the presence of papilledema or split cranial sutures. However, with some cases of increased ICP, such as with a coma, intracranial bleeding, or suspected meningitis, the need to establish a diagnosis is absolutely essential and outweighs the risks of the procedure.

2. Contraindications to lumbar puncture include the following conditions:
   a. Suspected epidural infection
   b. Infection or severe dermatologic disease in the lumbar area, which may be introduced into the spinal canal
   c. Severe psychiatric or neurotic problems
   d. Chronic back pain
   e. Anatomic malformations, scarring in puncture site areas, or previous spinal surgery at the site

3. If there is CSF leakage at the puncture site, notify the physician immediately and document findings.

4. Follow standard precautions (see Appendix A) when handling CSF specimens.

CSF PRESSURE ●

Normal Values

Adult: 90–180 mm H_2O in the lateral recumbent position. (This value is height-dependent and will change with a horizontal or sitting posture.)

Child (≤8 years of age): 10–100 mm H_2O.

Background

The CSF pressure is directly related to pressure in the jugular and vertebral veins that connect with the intracranial dural sinuses and the spinal dura. In conditions such as congestive heart failure or obstruction of the superior vena cava, CSF pressure is increased, whereas in circulatory collapse, CSF pressure is decreased.

Explanation of Test

Pressure measurement is done to detect impairment of CSF flow or to lower the CSF pressure by removing a small volume of CSF fluid. Provided initial pressure is not elevated and there is no marked fall in pressure as fluid is removed, 10 to 20 ml of CSF may be removed without danger to the patient. Elevation of the opening CSF pressure may be the only abnormality found in patients with cryptococcal meningitis and pseudotumor cerebri. Repeated lumbar punctures are performed for ICP elevation in cryptococcal meningitis to decrease the CSF pressure.

Procedure

1. The CSF pressure should be measured before any fluid is withdrawn.
2. Up to four samples of 2 to 3 ml each are taken, placed in separate sterile vials, and labeled sequentially. No. 1 is used for chemistry and serology; No. 2 is used for microbiology studies; No. 3 is used for hematology cell counts; and No. 4 is used for special studies.

Clinical Implications

1. *Increases* in CSF pressure can be a significant finding in the following conditions:
   a. Intracranial tumors; abscess; lesions
   b. Meningitis (bacterial, fungal, viral, or syphilitic)
   c. Hypoosmolality as a result of hemodialysis
   d. Congestive heart failure
   e. Superior vena cava syndrome
   f. Subarachnoid hemorrhage
   g. Cerebral edema
   h. Thrombosis of venous sinuses
   i. Conditions inhibiting CSF absorption
2. *Decreases* in pressure can be a significant finding in the following conditions:
   a. Circulatory collapse
   b. Severe dehydration
   c. Hyperosmolality
   d. Leakage of spinal fluid
   e. Spinal-subarachnoid block
3. *Significant variations* between opening and closing CSF pressures can be found in the following conditions:
   a. Tumors or spinal blockage above the puncture site when there is a large pressure drop (no further fluid should be withdrawn)

b. Hydrocephalus when there is a small pressure drop that is indicative of a large CSF pool

Interfering Factors

1. Slight elevations of CSF pressure may occur in an anxious patient who holds his or her breath or tenses his or her muscles.
2. If the patient's knees are flexed too firmly against the abdomen, venous compression will cause an elevation in CSF pressure. This can occur in patients of normal weight and in those who are obese.

Patient Preparation

1. See page 313 for care prior to lumbar puncture.
2. Follow guidelines in Chapter 1 regarding safe, effective, informed *pretest* care.

Patient Aftercare

1. Interpret abnormal pressure levels and monitor and intervene appropriately to prevent complications.
2. See page 313 for care after lumbar puncture.
3. Follow guidelines in Chapter 1 regarding safe, effective, informed *posttest* care.

CSF COLOR AND APPEARANCE ●

Normal Values
Clear and colorless

Background
Normal CSF is crystal clear, with the appearance and viscosity of water. Abnormal CSF may appear hazy, cloudy, smokey, or bloody. Clotting of CSF is abnormal and indicates increased protein or fibrinogen levels.

Explanation of Test
The initial appearance of CSF can provide various types of diagnostic information. Inflammatory diseases, hemorrhage, tumors, and trauma produce elevated cell counts and corresponding changes in appearance.

Procedure
The CSF should be compared with a test tube of distilled water held against a white background. If there is no turbidity, newsprint can be read through normal CSF in the tube.

Clinical Implications

1. Abnormal appearance (Table 5-2)—causes and indications:
   a. Blood. The blood is evenly mixed in all three tubes in subarachnoid and cerebral hemorrhage. Table 5-3 describes differentiation of bloody

TABLE 5-2
Color Changes in CSF Suggestive of Disease States

Appearance	Condition
Opalescent, slightly yellow, with delicate clot	Tuberculous meningitis
Opalescent to purulent, slightly yellow, with coarse clot	Acute pyogenic meningitis
Slightly yellow; may be clear or opalescent, with delicate clot	Acute anterior poliomyelitis
Bloody, purulent, may be turbid	Primary amebic meningoencephalitis
Generally clear, but may be xanthochromic	Tumor of brain or cord
Xanthochromic	Toxoplasmosis
Viscous	Metastatic colon cancer, severe meningeal infection, cryptococcus, injury

spinal tap from cerebral hemorrhage. Clear CSF fluid does not rule out intracranial hemorrhage.
  b. Turbidity is graded from 1+ (slightly cloudy) to 4+ (very cloudy) and may be caused by the following conditions:
   (1) Leukocytes (pleocytosis)
   (2) Erythrocytes
   (3) Microorganisms such as fungi and amebae
   (4) Protein
   (5) Epidural fat aspirated (pale pink to dark yellow)
   (6) Contrast media
  c. Xanthochromia (pale pink to dark yellow) can be caused by the following conditions:
   (1) Oxhemoglobin from lysed red blood cells (RBCs) present in CSF before lumbar puncture
   (2) Methemoglobin
   (3) Bilirubin (>6 mg/dl)
   (4) Increased protein (>150 mg/dl)
   (5) Melanin (meningeae melanocarcinoma)
   (6) Carotene (systemic carotenemia)
   (7) Prior bleeding within 2–36 h (eg, traumatic puncture >72 h before)
  d. Yellow color (bilirubin >10 mg/dl) due to a prior hemorrhage (10 h–4 wk before)

Interfering Factors
1. CSF can look xanthochromic from contamination with methylate used to disinfect the skin.
2. If the blood in the specimen is due to a traumatic spinal tap, the CSF in the

TABLE 5-3
Differentiation of Bloody CSF Caused by Subarachnoid Hemorrhage Versus Traumatic Lumbar Puncture

CSF Findings	Subarachnoid Hemorrhage	Traumatic Lumbar Puncture*
CSF Pressure	Often increased	Normal
Blood in tubes for collecting CSF	Mixture with blood is uniform in all tubes	Earlier tubes more bloody than later tubes
CSF clotting	Does not clot	Often clots
Xanthochromia	Present if >8–12 h since cerebral hemorrhage	Absent unless patient is jaundiced
Immediate repeat of lumbar puncture at higher level	CSF same as initial puncture	CSF clear (if atraumatic)

*CSF with RBCs >6000 per mm³ appears grossly bloody

Clinical Alert for Table 5-3

1. Spinal fluid should be cultured for bacteria, fungi, and tuberculosis. In children, *Haemophilus influenzae* type B is the most common cause of bacterial meningitis; in adults, the most common bacterial pathogens for meningitis are meningococci and pneumococci.
2. Spinal fluid with any degree of cloudiness should be treated with extreme care, because this could be an indication of contagious disease.

third tube should be clearer than that in tube 1 or 2; a traumatic tap makes interpretation of results difficult.
3. Radioactive media produces an oily appearance.

Patient Preparation
1. Observations of color and appearance of CSF are always noted.
2. See page 313 for care prior to lumbar puncture.

Patient Aftercare
1. Recognize abnormal color and presence of turbidity and monitor patient appropriately.
2. See page 313 for care after lumbar puncture.

CSF MICROSCOPIC EXAMINATION OF CELLS;
TOTAL CELL COUNT; DIFFERENTIAL CELL COUNT   ●

Normal Values

Normal CSF is essentially free of cells.

Adults: 0–5 WBC/μg/L or 0–5 × 10^6 WBC/L
Newborn: 0–30 × 10^6 WBC/L

Differential:	*Adults*	*Newborn (0–14 days of age)*
Lymphocytes:	40%–80%	5%–35%
Monocytes:	15%–45%	50%–90%
Polys:	0%–6%	0%–8%

Major Cells Seen in Microscopic Examination of CSF

Cell Types	*Occurrence*	*Findings*
Blast forms	Acute leukemia	Lymphoblasts or myeloblasts
Ependymal and choroidal cells	Trauma (diagnostic procedures)	Clusters with distinct nuclei and distinct cell walls
Lymphocytes	Normal Viral, tubercular, and fungal meningitis Multiple sclerosis	All stages of development possible
Macrophages	Viral and tubercular meningitis RBCs in spinal fluid Contrast media	May contain phagocytized RBCs (appearing as empty vacuoles or ghost cells) and hemosiderin granules
Malignant cells	Metastatic carcinomas	Clusters with fusing of cell borders and nuclei
Monocytes	Chronic bacterial meningitis Viral, tubercular, and fungal meningitis Multiple sclerosis	Mixed with lymphocytes and neutrophils
Neutrophils	Bacterial meningitis Early cases of viral, tubercular, and fungal meningitis	Granules may be less prominent than in blood
Pia arachnoid mesothelial (PAM) cells	Normal, mixed reactions including lymphocytes, neutrophils, monocytes, and plasma cells	Resemble young monocytes with a round, not indented, nucleus
Plasma cells	Multiple sclerosis Lymphocyte reactions	Transitional and classic forms seen

Background

Normal CSF contains a small number of lymphocytes and monocytes in a ratio of approximately 70:30 in adults. A higher proportion of monocytes is present in young children. An increase in the number of white blood cells (WBCs) in CSF is termed *pleocytosis*. Disease processes may lead to abrupt increases or decreases in numbers of cells.

Explanation of Test

CSF is examined for the presence of RBCs and WBCs. The cells are counted and identified by cell type; the percentage of cell type is compared with the total number of white or red blood cells present. In general, inflammatory disease, hemorrhage, neoplasms, and trauma cause an elevated WBC count.

Procedure

Tube No. 3 is used for counting the cells present in the CSF sample. The cells are counted by a manual counting chamber or by electronic means. A CSF smear is made and various types of cells present are counted to determine differentiation of cells.

Clinical Implications

1. White cell counts $>500 \times 10^6$ usually arise from a purulent infection and are preponderantly granulocytes (ie, neutrophils). Neutrophilic reaction classically suggests meningitis caused by a pyogenic organism, in which case the white cell count can exceed 1000×10^6 and even reach $20,000 \times 10^6$.

   a. Increases in neutrophils are associated with the following conditions:
      (1) Bacterial meningitis
      (2) Early viral meningitis
      (3) Early tubercular meningitis
      (4) Fungal mycositic meningitis
      (5) Amebic encephalomyelitis
      (6) Early stages of cerebral abscess
   b. Noninfectious causes of neutrophilia include the following:
      (1) Reaction to central nervous system hemorrhage
      (2) Injection of foreign materials into the subarachnoid space (eg, x-ray contrast medium, anticancer drugs)
      (3) CSF infarct
      (4) Metastatic tumor in contact with CSF
      (5) Reaction to repeated lumbar puncture

Clinical Alert

Neutrophilic reaction classically suggests meningitis caused by a pyogenic organism.

2. White counts of 300 to 500 $\times$ 10^6 with preponderantly lymphocytes are indicative of the following conditions:
   a. Viral meningitis
   b. Syphilis of CNS (ie, meningoencephalitis)
   c. Tuberculous meningitis
   d. Parasitic infestation of the CNS
   e. Bacterial meningitis due to unusual organisms (eg, *Listeria*)
   f. Multiple sclerosis (reactive lymphs present)
   g. Encephalopathy caused by drug abuse
   h. Fifteen percent of Guillain-Barré syndrome
   i. Acute disseminated encephalomyelitis
   j. Sarcoidosis of meninges
   k. Human T-lymphotropic virus type III (HTLV III)
   l. Aseptic meningitis due to peptic focus adjacent to meninges
   m. Fungal meningitis
3. White cell counts with $\geq$40% monocytes occur in the following conditions:
   a. Chronic bacterial meningitis
   b. Toxoplasmosis and amebic meningitis
   c. Multiple sclerosis
4. Malignant cells (lymphocytes or histiocytes) may be present with primary and metastatic brain tumors, especially when there is meningeal extension.
5. Increased numbers of plasma cells occur in the following conditions:
   a. Acute viral infections
   b. Multiple sclerosis
   c. Sarcoidosis
   d. Syphilitic meningoencephalitis
   e. Subacute sclerosing panencephalitis
   f. Tuberculous meningitis
   g. Parasitic infestations of CSF
   h. Guillain-Barré syndrome
   i. Lymphocytic reactions
   Plasma cells are responsible for an increase in immunoglobulin G (IgG) and altered patterns in immunoelectrophoresis.
6. Macrophages are present in tuberculous or viral meningitis and in reactions to erythrocytes, foreign substances, or lipids in the CSF.
7. Glial, ependymal, and plexus cells may be present after surgical procedures or trauma to the CNS.
8. Leukemic cells appear in CSF when metastatic carcinoma is present.
9. Eosinophils are present in the following conditions:
   a. Parasitic infections
   b. Fungal infections
   c. Acute polyneuritis
   d. Idiopathic hypereosinophilic syndrome
   e. Reaction to foreign materials in CSF (eg, drugs, shunts)

Abnormal CSF Findings in Types of Meningitis

	Bacterial	*Viral*	*Tubercular*	*Fungal*
Total WBCs	Increased	Increased	Increased	Increased
Differential	Neutrophils present	Lymphocytes present	Lymphocytes and monocytes present	Lymphocytes and monocytes present
Protein	Marked increase	Moderate increase	Moderate to marked increase; clots occur with protein >150 mg/dl	Moderate to marked increase
Glucose	Markedly decreased	Normal	Decreased	Normal to decreased
Lactate	Increased	Normal	Increased	Increased
LDH fractions	LD isoenzymes 4 and 5 increased	LD isoenzymes 2 and 3 increased	—	—
Limulus amebocyte lysote indicator of crypto-coccus endotoxin produced by gram-negative bacteria	Positive	—	Pellicle formation when protein >150 mg/dl	Positive India ink with neoformans
Gram stain bacterial antigen and CIE serology	Positive for *Haemo-philus influenzae* menin–gococci	—	—	Latex serologic test positive

Patient Preparation

1. See page 313 for care prior to lumbar puncture.
2. Follow guidelines in Chapter 1 regarding safe, effective, informed *pretest* care.

Patient Aftercare
1. Interpret abnormal cell counts. Monitor, intervene, and counsel as appropriate for infection and malignancy.
2. See page 313 for care after lumbar puncture.
3. Follow guidelines in Chapter 1 regarding safe, effective, informed *posttest* care.

CSF GLUCOSE ●

Normal Values
Adult: 50–80 mg/dl
Child: 60–80 mg/dl
CSF/plasma glucose ratio = 0.4:0.8
CSF glucose level = 60% of blood glucose levels

Background
The CSF glucose level varies with the blood glucose levels. It is usually about 60% of the blood glucose level. A blood glucose specimen should be obtained at least 60 minutes before lumbar puncture for comparisons. Any changes in blood sugar are reflected in the CSF 1 to 3 hours later because of the lag in CSF glucose equilibrium time.

Explanation of Test
This measurement is helpful in determining impaired transport of glucose from plasma to CSF and increased use of glucose by the CNS, leukocytes, and microorganisms. The finding of a markedly decreased CSF glucose level accompanied by an increased white cell count with a large percentage of neutrophils is indicative of bacterial meningitis.

Procedure
One milliliter (1 ml) of CSF is placed in a sterile tube. The glucose test should be done on tube No. 1 when three tubes of CSF are taken. Accurate evaluation of CSF glucose requires a plasma glucose measurement. A blood glucose level ideally should be drawn 2 hours before the lumbar puncture.

Clinical Implications
1. Decreased CSF glucose levels are associated with the following conditions:
   a. Acute bacterial meningitis
   b. Tuberculosis, fungal and amebic meningitis
   c. Symptomatic hypoglycemia
   d. Increased use via anaerobic glucoses by brain tissue and impaired transport into the CSF
2. CSF glucose levels are uncommonly decreased in the following conditions:
   a. Malignant tumor with meningeal involvement
   b. Acute syphilitic meningitis

   c. Viral meningoencephalitis

   d. Sarcoidosis, trichinosis, and amebae

   e. Subarachnoid hemorrhage meningitis

   f. Rheumatoid meningitis

   g. Neoplasia

3. Increased CSF glucose levels are associated with diabetes, reflecting increased blood glucose levels within 2 hours of the lumbar tap.

Interfering Factors

1. Falsely decreased levels may be due to cellular and bacterial metabolism if the test is not performed immediately after specimen collection.

2. A traumatic tap may produce misleading results due to glucose present in blood.

3. See Appendix J for drugs that affect test outcomes.

> **Clinical Alert**
>
> **1.** All types of organisms consume glucose; therefore, decreased glucose levels reflect abnormal activity.
>
> **2.** The panic value for CSF glucose level is <20 mg/dl; below this level damage to the CNS will occur.

Patient Preparation

1. See page 313 for care prior to lumbar puncture.

2. Explain the need for a blood specimen test for glucose to compare with CSF glucose.

3. Follow guidelines in Chapter 1 regarding safe, effective, informed *pretest* care.

Patient Aftercare

1. Interpret abnormal CSF glucose levels and correlate with the presence of meningitis, cancer, hemorrhage, and diabetes. Monitor and intervene appropriately to prevent complications.

2. See page 313 for care after lumbar puncture.

CSF GLUTAMINE ●

Normal Values

5–15 mg/dl, or 0.4–1.1 μmol/ml

Background

Glutamine is synthesized in brain tissue from ammonia and alphaketoglutarate. Production of glutamine provides a mechanism for removing the ammonia, a toxic metabolic waste product, from the CNS.

Explanation of Test

The determination of CSF glutamine level provides an indirect test for the presence of excess ammonia in the CSF. As the concentration of ammonia in the CSF increases, the supply of alphaketoglutarate becomes depleted; consequently, glutamine can no longer be produced to remove the toxic ammonia, and coma ensues. A CSF glutamine test is therefore frequently requested for patients with coma of unknown origin.

Procedure

One milliliter (1 ml) of CSF is needed for the glutamine test. Tube No. 1 is used for this chemistry test. If cells are present, the samples must be centrifuged to remove the cells.

Clinical Implications

Increased CSF glutamine levels are associated with the following conditions:

1. Hepatic encephalopathy (glutamine values >35 mg/dl are diagnostic)
2. Reye's syndrome
3. Encephalopathy secondary to hypercapnia or sepsis
4. CSF pleocytosis

Patient Preparation

1. See page 313 for care prior to lumbar puncture.
2. Follow guidelines in Chapter 1 regarding safe, effective, informed *pretest* care.

Patient Aftercare

1. Interpret abnormal glutamine levels and correlate with clinical symptoms. Monitor and intervene appropriately to prevent complications.
2. See page 313 for care after lumbar puncture.
3. Follow guidelines in Chapter 1 regarding safe, effective, informed *posttest* care.

CSF LACTIC ACID

Normal Values

Adult: 10–25 mg/dl or 1.0–2.8 mmol/L
Newborn: 10–60 mg/dl or 1.1–6.7 mmol/L

Background

The source of CSF lactic acid is CNS anaerobic metabolism. Lactic acid in CSF varies independently with the level of lactic acid in the blood. Destruction of tissue within the CNS because of oxygen deprivation causes the production of increased CSF lactic acid levels. Thus, elevated CSF lactic acid levels can result from any condition that decreases the flow of oxygen to brain tissues.

Explanation of Test

The CSF lactic acid test is used to differentiate between bacterial and nonbacterial meningitis. Elevated CSF lactate levels are not limited to meningitis and can result from any condition that decreases the flow of oxygen to the brain. CSF lactate levels are frequently used to monitor severe head injuries.

Procedure

One-half milliliter (0.5 ml) of CSF is collected in a sterile test tube; tube No. 1 should be used. Refrigerate the sample.

Clinical Implications

Increased CSF glutamine levels are associated with the following conditions:

1. Bacterial meningitis (>3.3 mmol)
2. Brain abscess or tumor
3. Cerebral ischemia
4. Cerebral trauma
5. Seizures
6. Stroke (cerebral infarct)
7. Pleocytosis

Patient Preparation

1. See page 313 for care prior to lumbar puncture.
2. Follow guidelines in Chapter 1 regarding safe, effective, informed *pretest* care.

Patient Aftercare

1. Interpret test outcomes; monitor and intervene appropriately to detect CNS disease and prevent complications. Results must be interpreted in light of clinical symptoms.
2. See page 313 for care after lumbar puncture.
3. Follow guidelines in Chapter 1 regarding safe, effective, informed *posttest* care.

> ### Clinical Alert
>
> Increases in CSF lactic acid levels must be interpreted in light of the clinical findings and in conjunction with glucose levels, protein levels, and cell counts in the CSF. Equivocal results in some instances of aseptic meningitis may lead to erroneous diagnosis of a bacterial etiology.

CSF LACTATE DEHYDROGENASE (LD/LDH); CSF LACTATE DEHYDROGENASE (LDH) ISOENZYMES ●

Normal Values

Adults: 0–40 U/L
Newborns: 0–70 U/L

Background

Although many different enzymes have been measured in CSF, only lactate dehydrogenase (LDH) appears useful clinically. Sources of LDH in normal CSF include diffusion across the blood-CSF barrier, diffusion across the brain-CSF barrier, and LDH activity in cellular elements of the CSF such as leukocytes, bacteria, and tumor cells. Because brain tissue is rich in LDH, damaged central nervous system tissue can cause increased levels of LDH in the CSF.

Explanation of Test

High levels of LDH occur in about 90% of cases of bacterial meningitis and in only 10% of cases of viral meningitis. When high levels of LDH do occur in viral meningitis, the condition is usually associated with encephalitis and a poor prognosis. Tests of LDH isoenzymes have been used to improve the specificity of LDH measurements and are useful for making the differential diagnosis of viral versus bacterial meningitis. (See Chapter 6 for a complete description of isoenzymes.) Elevated LDH levels following resuscitation predict a poor outcome in patients with hypoxic brain injury.

Procedure

One milliliter (1 ml) of CSF is necessary for the LDH test, and the sample should be taken to the laboratory as quickly as possible. Tube No. 1 is used for LDH examination.

Clinical Implications

1. Increased CSF/LDH levels are associated with the following conditions:
   a. Bacterial meningitis (90% of cases)
   b. Viral meningitis (10% of cases)
   c. Massive cerebrovascular accident
   d. Leukemia or lymphoma with meningeal infiltration
   e. Metastatic carcinoma of the CNS
2. The presence of CSF/LDH isoenzymes 2 and 3 reflects a CNS lymphocytic reaction, suggesting viral meningitis.
3. The CSF/LDH isoenzyme pattern reflects a granulocytic (neutrophilic) reaction with LDH isoenzymes 4 and 5, suggesting bacterial meningitis.
4. High levels of CSF/LDH isoenzymes 1 and 2 suggest extensive CNS damage and a poor prognosis (ie, they are indicative of destruction of brain tissue).

Interfering Factors

For the LDH test to be valid, CSF must not be contaminated with blood. A traumatic lumbar tap will make results difficult to interpret.

Patient Preparation

1. See page 313 for care before lumbar puncture.
2. Follow guidelines in Chapter 1 regarding safe, effective, informed *pretest* care.

Patient Aftercare

1. Interpret abnormal LDH test patterns, and monitor and intervene appropriately to detect and prevent complications.
2. See page 313 for care after lumbar puncture.
3. Follow guidelines in Chapter 1 regarding safe, effective, informed *posttest* care.

CSF TOTAL PROTEIN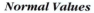

Normal Values

Results vary by method used; check with your laboratory for reference values.

Adults: 15–45 mg/dl (lumbar)
Adults: 15–25 mg/dl (cisternal)
Adults: 5–15 mg/dl (ventricular)
Neonates: 15–100 mg/dl (lumbar)
Elderly (>60 years of age): 15–60 mg/dl (lumbar)

Background

The CSF normally contains very little protein, because the protein in blood plasma does not cross the blood-brain barrier easily. Protein concentration normally increases caudally from the ventricles to the cisterns and finally to the lumbar sac.

Explanation of Test

The CSF protein is a nonspecific but reliable indication of CNS pathology such as meningitis, brain abscess, multiple sclerosis, and other degenerative processes causing neoplastic disease. Elevated CSF protein levels may be caused by increased permeability of the blood-brain barrier, decreased resorption of the arachnoid villi, mechanical obstruction of the CSF flow, or an increase of intrathecal immunologic synthesis.

Procedure

One milliliter (1 ml) of CSF is needed for protein analysis. Tube No. 1 should be used. Serum protein levels should be measured concurrently to interpret CSF protein values.

Clinical Implications

1. Increased CSF protein occurs in the following situations:
   a. Traumatic tap with normal CSF pressure: CSF initially streaked with blood, clearing in subsequent tubes
   b. Increased permeability of blood-CSF barrier: CSF protein 100–500 mg/dl.
   (1) Infectious conditions
   (a) Bacterial meningitis: Gram stain usually positive; culture may be negative if antibiotics have been administered
   (b) Tuberculosis: CSF protein 50–300 mg/dl; mixed cellular reaction typical

(c) Fungal meningitis: CSF protein 50–300 mg/dl; special stains helpful

(d) Viral meningitis: CSF protein usually <100 mg/dl

(2) Noninfectious conditions

(a) Subarachnoid hemorrhage: xanthochromia 2–4 h after onset

(b) Intracerebral hemorrhage: CSF protein 20–200 mg/dl; marked fall in pressure after removing small amounts of CSF; xanthochromia

(c) Cerebral thrombosis: slightly increased CSF protein in 40% of cases (usually <100 mg/dl)

(d) Endocrine disorders, diabetic neuropathy, myxedema, hyperadrenalism, hypoparathyroidism: CSF protein 50–150 mg/dl in ~50% of cases

(e) Metabolic disorders, uremia, hypercalcemia, hypercapnia, dehydration: CSF protein slightly elevated (usually <100 mg/dl)

(f) Drug toxicity, ethanol, phenytoin, phenothiazines: CSF protein slightly elevated in ~40% of cases (usually <200 mg/dl)

c. Obstruction to circulation of CSF occurs in the following circumstances:

(1) Mechanical obstruction (eg, tumor, abscess), herniated disc: rapid fall in pressure (yellow CSF, contains excess protein)

(2) Loculated effusion of CSF: repeated taps may show a progressive increase in CSF protein; diagnosis by myelography

d. Increased CSF/IgG synthesis occurs in the following conditions:

(1) Multiple sclerosis: CSF protein level slightly increased

(2) Subacute sclerosing panencephalitis: increased CSF protein

(3) Neurosyphilis: CSF protein normal or slightly increased (usually <100 mg/dl)

e. Increased CSF/IgG synthesis **and** increased permeability of blood-CSF barrier occurs in the following conditions:

(1) Guillain-Barré syndrome (infectious polyneuritis): CSF protein usually 100–400 mg/dl

(2) Collagen diseases (eg, periarteritis, lupus): CSF protein usually <400 mg/dl

(3) Chronic inflammatory demyelinating polyradiculopathy

f. Decreased CSF protein occurs in the following conditions:

(1) Leakage of CSF due to trauma

(2) Removal of a large volume of CSF

(3) Intracranial hypertension

(4) Hyperthyroidism

Clinical Alert

More than 1000 mg/dl of protein in CSF suggests subarachnoid block. In a complete spinal block, the lower the tumor location, the higher the CSF protein value.

Interfering Factors
1. Hemolyzed or xanthochromic drugs may falsely depress results.
2. Traumatic tap will invalidate the protein results.
3. See Appendix J for drugs that affect test outcomes.

Patient Preparation
1. See page 313 for care prior to lumbar puncture.
2. Follow guidelines in Chapter 1 regarding safe, effective, informed *pretest* care.

Patient Aftercare
1. Interpret abnormal CSF protein levels; monitor for both infectious and non-infectious conditions and intervene appropriately to prevent and detect complications.
2. See page 313 for care after lumbar puncture.
3. Follow guidelines in Chapter 1 regarding safe, effective, informed *posttest* care.

CSF ALBUMIN AND IMMUNOGLOBULIN G (IgG)

Normal Values
Albumin: 10–35 mg/dl
IgG: 0.5–6.0 mg/dl
CSF/serum albumin index: <9.0
IgG index: 0.28–0.66
CSF/IgG/albumin ratio: 0.09–0.25

Background
The albumin and IgG that are present in normal CSF are derived from the serum. Increased levels of either or both are indicative of damage to the blood-CNS barrier.

Explanation of Test
The combined measurement of albumin and IgG is used to evaluate the integrity and permeability of the blood-CSF barrier and to measure the synthesis of IgG within the CNS. The IgG index is the most sensitive method to determine local CNS synthesis of IgG and to detect increased permeability of the blood-CNS barrier.

$$\text{IgG Index} = \frac{\text{CSF IgG} \times \text{serum albumin}}{\text{CSF albumin} \times \text{serum IgG}}$$

The IgG index method is superior to the IgG/albumin ratio or measurement of IgG only. Normal persons usually have an index <0.60. With multiple sclerosis, the index is >0.77.

Procedure
One-half milliliter (0.5 ml) of CSF in a sterile tube is needed for this test. The sample must be frozen if the determination is not done immediately.

Clinical Implications
1. Increased CSF albumin occurs in the following conditions:
   a. Lesions of the choroid plexus
   b. Blockage of CSF flow
   c. Bacterial meningitis
   d. Guillain-Barré syndrome
   e. Many infectious diseases such as typhoid fever, tularemia, diphtheria, and septicemia
   f. Malignant neoplasms
   g. Polycythemia
   h. Hypothyroidism
   i. Diabetes mellitus
   j. Glomerulonephritis and other nephrotic syndromes
   k. Systemic lupus erythematosus
   l. Mercury poisoning and other toxic metals
   m. Electric shock
   n. Malaria, Rocky Mountain spotted fever
2. Increased CSF IgG/albumin index (increased IgG, normal albumin) occurs in the following conditions:
   a. Multiple sclerosis
   b. Subacute sclerosing leukoencephalitis
   c. Neurosyphilis
   d. Chronic phases of CNS infections (subacute sclerosing panencephalitis [SSPE])

Interfering Factors
A traumatic tap will invalidate the results.

Patient Preparation
1. See page 313 for care prior to lumbar puncture.
2. Follow guidelines in Chapter 1 regarding safe, effective, informed *pretest* care.

Patient Aftercare
1. Interpret test outcomes; monitor and intervene appropriately to prevent and detect complications.
2. See page 313 for care after lumbar puncture.
3. Follow guidelines in Chapter 1 regarding safe, effective, informed *posttest* care.

CSF PROTEIN ELECTROPHORESIS; OLIGOCLONAL BANDS; MULTIPLE SCLEROSIS PANEL ●

Normal Values
Oligoclonal banding: none present
IgG synthesis rate: 0.0–8.0 mg/d
IgG/albumin ratio: 0.09–0.25
Prealbumin: 2%–7%
Albumin: 56%–76%

Alpha$_1$: 2%–7%
Alpha$_2$: 4%–12%
Beta: 8%–18%
Gamma: 3%–12%

Background

Agarose gel electrophoresis of concentrated CSF is used to detect oligoclonal bands, defined as two or more discrete bands in the gamma region, and that are absent or of lesser intensity than in the concurrently tested patient's serum.

Explanation of Test

Fractionation (ie, electrophoresis) of CSF is used to evaluate bacterial and viral infections and tumors of the CNS. However, the most important application of CSF protein electrophoresis is the detection and diagnosis of multiple sclerosis (MS). Abnormalities of CSF in multiple sclerosis include an increase in total protein, primarily from IgG, which is the main component of the gamma globulin fraction. Abnormal immunoglobulins migrate as discrete, sharp bands called oligoclonal bands. This is the pattern observed in multiple sclerosis: a pattern of discrete bands within the gamma globulin portion of the electrophoretic pattern. However, oligoclonal bands are found in the CSF of patients with other types of nervous system disorders of the immune system, including human immunodeficiency virus (HIV).

Electrophoresis is also the method of choice to determine whether a fluid is actually CSF. Identification can be made based on the appearance of an extra band of transferrin (referred to as "TAV") which occurs in CSF and not in serum.

Procedure

1. Three milliliters (3 ml) of CSF is necessary for this test. Tube No. 1 is used. The sample must be frozen if test is not performed immediately.
2. CSF is concentrated approximately 80-fold by selective permeability. A sample of the concentrate is applied to a thin-layer agarose gel. The agarose gel is then subjected to electrophoresis. Serum electrophoresis must be done concurrently for interpretation of the bands.

Clinical Implications

1. Increases in CSF IgG or IgG/albumin index occur in the following conditions:
   a. Multiple sclerosis
   b. Subacute sclerosis leukoencephalitis
   c. Tumors of the brain and meninges
   d. Chronic CNS infections
   e. Some patients with meningitis, Guillain-Barré syndrome, lupus erythematosus involving the CNS, and other neurologic conditions
2. Increases in the CSF albumin index occur in the following conditions:
   a. Obstruction of CSF circulation
   b. Damage to the CNS blood-brain barrier
   c. Diabetes mellitus
   d. Systemic lupus erythematosus of the CNS
   e. Guillain-Barré syndrome
   f. Polyneuropathy
   g. Cervical spondylosis

3. Increased CSF gamma globulin and the presence of oligoclonal bands occur in the following conditions:
   a. Multiple sclerosis
   b. Neurosyphilis
   c. Subacute sclerosing panencephalitis
   d. Cerebral infarction
   e. Viral encephalitis
   f. Progressive rubella panencephalitis
   g. Cryptococcal meningitis
   h. Idiopathic polyneuritis
   i. Burkitt's lymphoma
   j. Bacterial meningitis
   k. Guillain-Barré syndrome
4. Increased CSF synthesis of IgG occurs in the following conditions:
   a. Multiple sclerosis (90% of definite cases)
   b. Inflammatory neurologic diseases

Clinical Alert

1. A serum electrophoresis must be done at the same time as the CSF electrophoresis. An abnormal result is the finding of two or more bands in the CSF that are *not* present in the serum specimen.
2. Oligoclonal bands are not specific for multiple sclerosis; however, the sensitivity is 83% to 94%.

Interfering Factors
1. A traumatic tap invalidates the results.
2. Recent myelography affects results.

Patient Preparation
1. See page 313 for care prior to lumbar puncture.
2. Follow guidelines in Chapter 1 regarding safe, effective, informed *pretest* care.

Patient Aftercare
1. Interpret test outcome; monitor for multiple sclerosis and other CNS disorders and intervene appropriately to prevent and detect complications.
2. See page 313 for care after lumbar puncture.
3. Follow guidelines in Chapter 1 regarding safe, effective, informed *posttest* care.

CSF SYPHILIS SEROLOGY

Normal Values
Negative (ie, nonreactive) for syphilis. Neurosyphilis is characterized by an increase in protein, an increase in the number of lymphocytes, and a positive

test for syphilis (see Chapter 8). Use CSF VDRL test to rule in, not rule out, neurosyphilis. Do not use VDRL to evaluate the results of syphilis therapy.

BIBLIOGRAPHY

Bakerman S: ABC's of Interpretive Laboratory Data, 3rd ed. Greenville, NC, Interpretive Laboratory Data, Inc., 1994

Bishop ML, Duben-Engelkirk JL, Fody EP: Clinical Chemistry—Principles, Procedures, Correlations, 3rd ed. Philadelphia, Lippincott-Raven, 1996

Henry JB (ed): Clinical Diagnosis and Management by Laboratory Methods, 19th ed. Philadelphia, WB Saunders, 1996

Leavelle DE (ed): Interpretive Handbook: Interpretive Data for Diagnostic Laboratory Tests. Rochester, MN, Mayo Medical Laboratories, 1999

Lehman CA (ed): Saunders Manual of Clinical Laboratory Science. Philadelphia, WB Saunders, 1998

Knight JA: Advances in the analysis of cerebral spinal fluid. Am Clin Lab Sci 27: 93, 1997

McBride LJ: Textbook of Urinalysis and Body Fluids. Philadelphia, Lippincott-Raven, 1998

Ryngsrud MK: Urinalysis and Body Fluids: a Color Text and Atlas. St. Louis, Mosby, 1998

Smith S, Forman D: Laboratory analysis of cerebrospinal fluid. Clin Lab Sci 7(4): 32–38, 1994

Strasinger S. Urinalysis and Body Fluids, 3rd ed. Philadelphia, FA Davis, 1994

Tietz NB (ed): Clinical Guide to Laboratory Tests, 3rd ed. Philadelphia, WB Saunders, 1995

Wallach J. Interpretation of Diagnostic Tests, 6th ed. Boston, Little, Brown & Co., 1996

Weiner WJ, Shulman LM (eds): Emergent and Urgent Neurology, 2nd ed. Philadelphia, Lippincott-Raven, 1998

Young DS: Effects of Drugs on Clinical Laboratory Tests, 5th ed. Washington, DC, AACC Press, 1999

6

Chemistry Studies

OVERVIEW OF CHEMISTRY STUDIES ●

Blood chemistry testing identifies many chemical blood constituents. It is often necessary to measure several blood chemicals to establish a pattern of abnormalities. A wide range of tests can be grouped under the headings of enzymes, electrolytes, blood sugar, lipids, hormones, vitamins, minerals, and drug investigation. Other tests have no common denominator. Selected tests serve as screening devices to identify target organ damage. When collecting specimens for chemistry studies, refer to standard precautions in Appendix A, latex precautions in Appendix B, Guidelines for specimen transport and storage in Appendix E, and **always** refer to Appendix J for drugs that affect test outcomes.

General Biochemical Profiles
Profiles are a group of select tests that screen for certain conditions. Some of the more common profiles or panels are listed in the following table.

Group Headings	Tests Suggested
Cardiac enzymes	CPK, AST, LDH, SGOT
Kidney functions/disease	BUN, phosphorus, LDH, creatinine, creatinine clearance, uric acid, total protein, A/G ratio, albumin, globulins, calcium, glucose, cholesterol
Lipids	Cholesterol, triglycerides, lipoprotein electrophoresis (LDL, VLDL, HDL)
Liver function/disease	Total bilirubin, alkaline phosphatase, cholesterol, GGT, total protein, A/G ratio, albumin, globulins, AST, LDH, viral hepatitis panel, PT
Thyroid function	T_2 uptake, Free T_4, Total T_4, T_7 FTI, TSH
Basic metabolic screen	Chloride, sodium, potassium, carbon dioxide, glucose, BUN, creatinine

A/G ratio, albumin/globulin ratio; AST, aspartate aminotransferase; BUN, blood urea nitrogen; CPK, creatine phosphokinase; FTI, free thyroxine index; HDL, high-density lipoproteins; LDH, lactate dehydrogenase; LDL, low-density lipoproteins; PT, prothrombin time; SGOT, serum glutamic-oxaloacetic transaminase; TSH, thyroid-stimulating hormone.

USE OF THE AUTOANALYZER

Sophisticated automated instrumentation makes it possible to conduct a wide variety of chemical tests on a single sample of blood and to report results in a timely manner. Results may be reported as normal, low, high, panic, toxic, or D (ie, fails Delta check). Computerized interfaces allow direct transmission of results between laboratory and clinical settings. "Hard copy" printouts can then become a permanent part of the health care record. Not only does this method of record keeping provide a baseline for future comparisons, but it can also allow unsuspected diseases to be uncovered and can lead to early diagnosis when symptoms are vague or absent.

NOTE: *Normal or reference values for any chemistry determination vary with the method or assay employed. For example, differences in substrates or temperature at which the assay is run will alter the "normal" range. Thus, "normal ranges" vary from laboratory to laboratory.*

The more commonly ordered chemistries include the following:

Albumin, Globulin
Alkaline phosphatase
Aspartate transaminase (AST)
Blood urea nitrogen (BUN) (Ca^{2+})
Calcium
Cholesterol
Creatinine

Glucose
Inorganic phosphorus
Total bilirubin
Total protein (TP) (see Chap. 8)
Triglycerides
Uric acid
Sodium, potassium, and chloride (electrolytes)

Patterns of abnormal values provide data for arriving at a definitive diagnosis.

USE OF MULTIPLE LABORATORIES ●

Certain tests may be sent out to reference or commercial laboratories. A certain percentage of these tests will fall into the category of being too sophisticated or of too low volume to obtain reliable results. This is one of the reasons why test results may not immediately be available for interpretation.

●ELECTROLYTE TESTS

CALCIUM (Ca^{2+}) ●

Normal Values

Total Calcium			Ionized Calcium		
Age	*mg/dl*	*mmol/L*	*Age*	*mg/dl*	*mmol/L*
0–10 d	7.6–10.4	1.90–2.60	Newborn	4.40–5.48	1.10–1.37
10 d–3 y	8.7–9.8	2.24–2.75	1–18 y	4.80–5.52	1.20–1.38
3–9 y	8.8–10.1	2.20–2.70	Adult	4.65–5.28	1.16–1.32
4–11 y	8.9–10.1				
11–13 y	8.8–10.6				
13–15 y	9.2–10.7	2.10–2.55			
15–18 y	8.4–10.7				
Adult	8.4–10.2				

Background

The bulk of body calcium (98%–99%) is stored in the skeleton and teeth, which act as huge reservoirs for maintaining blood levels of calcium. About 50% of blood calcium is ionized; the rest is protein-bound. Only ionized calcium can be used by the body in such vital processes as muscular contraction, cardiac function, transmission of nerve impulses, and blood clotting.

The amount of protein in the blood also affects calcium levels, because 50% of blood calcium is protein-bound. Thus, a decrease in serum albumin will result in a decrease in total serum calcium. The decrease, however, does not alter the concentration of the ionized form of calcium. Measurements of ionized calcium are done during open-heart surgeries, liver transplants, and other operations in which large volumes of blood anticoagulated with citrate are given. These tests are also used to monitor renal disease, renal transplantation, hemodialysis, hyperparathyroidism, hypoparathyroidism, pancreatitis, and malignancy. Parathyroid hormone (PTH), calcitonin, vitamin D, estrogens, androgens, carbohydrates, and lactose all are factors that influence calcium levels.

Explanation of Test

This test measures the concentration of total and ionized calcium in the blood to reflect parathyroid function, calcium metabolism, and malignancy activity.

> ### Clinical Alert
>
> Hyperparathyroidism and cancer are the most common causes of hypercalcemia. Hypoalbuminemia is the most common cause of decreased total calcium.

Procedure

A 5-ml venous blood sample provides sufficient serum for this test. Observe universal precautions. Citrated ethylenediaminetetra-acetic acid (EDTA) and oxalated blood gives falsely low values and should not be used. Heparinized samples are preferred for ionized calcium studies, and specimens should be placed on ice, be kept tightly capped, and be delivered immediately to the laboratory.

Clinical Implications

1. *Normal levels of total blood calcium* combined with other findings indicate the following conditions:
   a. Normal calcium levels with overall normal results in other tests indicate no problems with calcium metabolism.
   b. Normal calcium and abnormal phosphorus values indicate impaired calcium absorption due to alteration of PTH activity or secretion (eg, in rickets, the calcium level may be normal or slightly lowered and the phosphorus level depressed).
   c. Normal calcium and elevated blood urea nitrogen (BUN) levels indicate the following:
      (1) Possible secondary hyperparathyroidism: initially, lowered serum calcium results from uremia and acidosis. The reduced calcium level stimulates the parathyroid to release PTH, which acts on bone to release more calcium.
      (2) Possible primary hyperparathyroidism: excessive amounts of PTH cause elevation in calcium levels, but secondary kidney disease causes retention of phosphate and concomitant lower calcium levels.
   d. Normal calcium and decreased serum albumin indicates hypercalcemia. Normally, a decrease in calcium is associated with a decrease in albumin.
2. *Hypercalcemia (increased total calcium levels)* is caused by or associated with the following conditions:
   a. Hyperparathyroidism due to parathyroid adenoma, hyperplasia of parathyroid glands, or associated hypophosphatemia
   b. Cancer (PTH-producing tumors)
      (1) Metastatic bone cancers; cancers of lung, breast, thyroid, kidney, liver, and pancreas
      (2) Hodgkin's lymphoma, leukemia, and non-Hodgkin's lymphoma

(3) Multiple myeloma with extensive bone destruction, Burkitt's lymphoma

(4) Primary squamous cell carcinoma of lung, neck, and head

c. Granulomatous disease (eg, tuberculosis, sarcoidosis)

d. Thyroid toxicosis

e. Paget's disease of bone (also accompanied by high levels of alkaline phosphatase)

f. Idiopathic hypercalcemia of infancy

g. Bone fractures combined with bed rest, prolonged immobilization

h. Excessive intake of vitamin D, milk, antacids

i. Renal transplant

j. Milk-alkali syndrome (Burnett's syndrome)

3. *Hypocalcemia (decreased total calcium levels)* are commonly caused by or associated with the following conditions:

a. Pseudohypocalcemia, which reflects reduced albumin levels. The reduced protein is responsible for the low calcium level because 50% of the calcium total is protein-bound.

NOTE: *Excessive intravenous (IV) fluids decrease albumin levels and thus decrease calcium levels. Total serum protein and albumin should be measured at the same time as calcium for proper interpretation of calcium levels. Ionized calcium is not affected by albumin levels.*

b. Hypoparathyroidism due to surgical removal of parathyroid glands, irradiation, hypomagnesemia, gastrointestinal (GI) disorders, or renal wasting. The primary form is very rare.

c. Hyperphosphatemia due to renal failure, laxative intake, or cytotoxic drugs

d. Malabsorption due to sprue, celiac disease, or pancreatic dysfunction (fatty acids combine with calcium and are precipitated and excreted in the feces)

e. Acute pancreatitis

f. Alkalosis (calcium ions become bound to protein)

g. Osteomalacia (advanced)

h. Renal failure

i. Vitamin D deficiency, rickets

j. Malnutrition (inadequate nutrition)

k. Alcoholism, hepatic cirrhosis

Clinical Alert

Panic Values for Total Calcium

<6 mg/dl (1.5 mmol/L) may produce tetany and convulsions

>13 mg/dl (3.25 mmol/L) may cause cardiotoxicity, arrhythmias, and coma

Rapid treatment of hypercalcemia with calcitonin solution is indicated.

4. *Increased ionized calcium levels* occur in the following conditions:
   a. Hyperparathyroidism
   b. Ectopic PTH-producing tumors
   c. Increased vitamin D intake
   d. Malignancies
5. *Decreased ionized calcium levels* occur in the following conditions:
   a. Hyperventilation to control increased intracranial pressure (total Ca^{2+} may be normal)
   b. Administration of bicarbonate to control metabolic acidosis
   c. Acute pancreatitis (eg, diabetic acidosis, sepsis)
   d. Hypoparathyroidism
   e. Vitamin D deficiency
   f. Magnesium deficiency
   g. Multiple organ failure
   h. Toxic shock syndrome

Clinical Alert

Panic Values for Ionized Calcium
<2.0 mg/dl (0.78 mmol/L) may produce tetany or life-threatening complications
2.0–3.0 mg/dl (<1.00 mmol/L) in cases of multiple blood transfusions (this is an indication to administer calcium)
>7.0 mg/dl (>1.58 mmol/L) may cause coma

Interfering Factors

1. Thiazide diuretics may impair urinary calcium excretion and result in hypercalcemia (most common drug-induced factor).
2. For patients with renal insufficiency undergoing dialysis, a calcium-ion exchange resin is sometimes used for hyperkalemia. This resin may increase calcium levels.
3. Increased magnesium and phosphate uptake and excessive use of laxatives may lower blood calcium level because of increased intestinal calcium loss.
4. When decreased calcium levels are due to magnesium deficiency (as in poor bowel absorption), the administration of magnesium will correct the calcium deficiency.
5. If a patient is known to have or suspected of having a pH abnormality, a concurrent pH test with ionized calcium level should be requested.
6. Many drugs may cause increased or decreased levels of calcium. Calcium supplements taken shortly before specimen collection will cause falsely high values.
7. Elevated serum protein increases calcium; decreased protein decreases calcium.

Patient Preparation

1. Explain purpose and procedure. Encourage relaxation.
2. Tourniquet application should be as brief as possible when drawing ionized calcium to prevent venous stasis and hemolysis.
3. Calcium supplements should not be taken within 8 to 12 hours before the blood sample is drawn.
4. Follow guidelines in Chapter 1 for safe, effective, informed *pretest* care.

Patient Aftercare

1. Resume normal activities.
2. Interpret test results and monitor appropriately for calcium abnormalities.
3. Follow guidelines in Chapter 1 for safe, effective, informed *posttest* care.

CHLORIDE (Cl^-)   ●

Normal Values

Adult: 98–106 mmol/L or mEq/L
Newborn: 98–113 mmol/L or mEq/L

Background

Chloride, a blood electrolyte, is an anion that exists predominantly in the extracellular spaces as part of sodium chloride or hydrochloric acid. Chloride maintains cellular integrity through its influence on osmotic pressure and acid-base and water balance. It has the reciprocal power of increasing or decreasing in concentration in response to concentrations of other anions. In metabolic acidosis, there is a reciprocal rise in chloride concentration when the bicarbonate concentration drops. Similarly, when aldosterone directly causes an increase in the reabsorption of sodium (the positive ion), the indirect effect is an increase in the absorption of chloride (the negative ion).

Chlorides are excreted with cations (positive ions) during massive diuresis from any cause and are lost from the GI tract when vomiting, diarrhea, or intestinal fistulas occur.

Explanation of Test

Alteration of sodium chloride level is seldom a primary problem. Measurement of chlorides is usually done for inferential value and is helpful in diagnosing disorders of acid-base and water balance. Because of the relatively high chloride concentrations in gastric juices, prolonged vomiting may lead to considerable chloride loss and lowered serum chloride levels.

In an emergency, chloride is the least important electrolyte to measure. However, it is especially important in the correction of hypokalemic alkalosis. If potassium is supplied without chloride, hypokalemic alkalosis may persist.

Procedure

Obtain a 5-ml venous blood sample in a heparinized Vacutainer tube. Serum can also be used.

Clinical Implications

> **NOTE:** *Whenever serum chloride levels are much lower than 100 mEq/L, urinary excretion of chlorides is also low.*

1. *Decreased blood chloride levels* occur in the following conditions:
   a. Severe vomiting
   b. Gastric suction
   c. Chronic respiratory acidosis
   d. Burns
   e. Metabolic alkalosis
   f. Congestive failure
   g. Addison's disease
   h. Salt-losing diseases (syndrome of inappropriate antidiuretic hormone [SIADH])
   i. Overhydration or water intoxication
   j. Acute intermittent porphyria
2. *Increased blood chloride levels* occur in the following conditions:
   a. Dehydration
   b. Cushing's syndrome
   c. Hyperventilation, which causes respiratory alkalosis
   d. Metabolic acidosis with prolonged diarrhea
   e. Hyperparathyroidism (primary)
   f. Select kidney disorders (eg, renal tubular acidosis)
   g. Diabetes insipidus
   h. Salicylate intoxication
   i. Head injury with hypothalamic damage

Interfering Factors

1. The plasma chloride concentration in infants is usually higher than that in children and adults.
2. Certain drugs may alter chloride levels.
3. Increases are associated with excessive IV saline infusions.

Clinical Alert

Panic Values for Serum Chloride
<70 or >120 mEq/L or mmol/L

Patient Preparation

1. Explain test purpose and blood collection procedure.
2. If possible, the patient should fast at least 8 to 12 hours before the test.
3. Follow guidelines in Chapter 1 for safe, effective, informed *pretest* care.

Patient Aftercare

1. Resume normal activities and diet.
2. Interpret test results and monitor appropriately.

3. If an electrolyte disorder is suspected, daily weight and accurate fluid intake and output should be recorded.
4. Follow guidelines in Chapter 1 for safe, effective, informed *posttest* care.

PHOSPHATE (P); INORGANIC PHOSPHORUS (PO$_4$) ●

Normal Values
Adult: 2.5–4.5 mg/dl or 0.87–1.45 mmol/L
Child: 4.5–5.5 mg/dl or 1.45–1.78 mmol/L
Newborn: 4.5–9.0 mg/dl or 1.45–2.91 mmol/L

Background
Of the human body's total phosphorus content, 85% is combined with calcium in the bone, and the remainder resides within the cells. Most of the phosphorus in the blood exists as phosphates or esters. Phosphate is required for generation of bony tissue and functions in the metabolism of glucose and lipids, in the maintenance of acid-base balance, and in the storage and transfer of energy from one site in the body to another. Phosphorus enters the red blood cells with glucose and therefore is lowered in the plasma after carbohydrate ingestion or infusion.

Explanation of Test
Phosphate levels are always evaluated in relation to calcium levels because there is an inverse relation between the two elements. When calcium levels are decreased, phosphorus levels are increased, and when phosphorus levels are decreased, calcium levels are increased. An excess of one electrolyte in serum causes the kidneys to excrete the other electrolyte. Many of the causes of elevated calcium levels are also causes of decreased phosphorus levels. As with calcium, the controlling factor is PTH.

Procedure
Obtain a fasting, 5-ml, venous blood sample. Serum is preferred, but heparinized blood is acceptable. Serum should be removed from clot as soon as possible after collection.

Clinical Implications
1. *Hyperphosphatemia* (increased blood phosphorus levels) is most commonly found in association with kidney dysfunction and uremia. This is because phosphate is so minutely regulated by the kidneys. These conditions include the following:
   a. Renal insufficiency and severe nephritis (accompanied by elevated BUN and creatinine) and renal failure
   b. Hypoparathyroidism (accompanied by elevated phosphorus, decreased calcium, and normal renal function) and pseudohypoparathyroidism
   c. Hypocalcemia

d. Milk-alkali syndrome
e. Excessive intake of vitamin D
f. Fractures in the healing stage
g. Bone tumors and metastases
h. Addison's disease
i. Acromegaly
j. Liver disease and cirrhosis
k. Cardiac resuscitation

2. *Hypophosphatemia* (decreased phosphorus level) occurs in the following conditions:
   a. Hyperparathyroidism
   b. Rickets (childhood) or osteomalacia (adult) and vitamin D deficiency
   c. Diabetic coma (increased carbohydrate metabolism)
   d. Hyperinsulinism
   e. Continuous administration of IV glucose in a nondiabetic patient (phosphorus follows glucose into the cells)
   f. Liver disease and acute alcoholism
   h. Vomiting and severe diarrhea
   i. Severe malnutrition and malabsorption
   j. Gram-negative septicemia
   k. Hypercalcimia of any cause
   l. Prolonged hypothermia

Interfering Factors

1. Phosphorus levels are normally high in children.
2. Phosphorus levels can be falsely increased by hemolysis of blood; therefore, separate serum from cells as soon as possible.
3. Drugs can be the cause of decreases in phosphorus.
4. The use of laxatives or enemas containing large amounts of sodium phosphate will cause increased phosphorus levels. With oral laxatives, the blood phosphorus level may increase as much as 5 mg/dl 2 to 3 hours after intake. This increased level is only temporary (5–6 hours), but this factor should be considered when abnormal levels are seen that cannot otherwise be explained.
5. Seasonal variations exist in phosphorus levels (maximum levels in May and June, lowest levels in winter).

Patient Preparation

1. Explain test purpose and blood sampling procedures. The patient should fast before the test.
2. Note on test requisition if any catastrophic stressful events have taken place which may cause high phosphorus levels.
3. Note time of day test is drawn; levels are highest in the morning and lowest in the evening.
4. Follow guidelines in Chapter 1 regarding safe, effective, informed *pretest* care.

Patient Aftercare

1. Resume normal activities.

2. Interpret test outcomes and monitor as appropriate for calcium imbalances. When phosphorus rises rapidly, calcium drops; watch for arrhythmias and muscle twitching. The signs and symptoms of phosphate depletion may include manifestations in the neuromuscular, neuropsychiatric, GI, skeletal, and cardiopulmonary systems. Manifestations usually are accompanied by serum levels <1 mg/dl.

3. Follow guidelines in Chapter 1 for safe, effective, informed *posttest* care.

Clinical Alert

Panic Value For Phosphate
<1.0 mg/dl

MAGNESIUM (Mg^{2+})

Normal Values
Adult: 1.6–2.6 mg/dl or 0.66–1.07 mmol/L
Child: 1.7–2.1 mg/dl or 0.70–0.86 mmol/L
Newborn: 1.5–2.2 mg/dl or 0.62–0.91 mmol/L

Background
Magnesium in the body is concentrated in the bone, cartilage, and within the cell itself and is required for the use of adenosine triphosphate (ADP) as a source of energy. It is therefore necessary for the action of numerous enzyme systems such as carbohydrate metabolism, protein synthesis, nucleic acid synthesis, and contraction of muscular tissue. Along with sodium, potassium, and calcium ions, magnesium also regulates neuromuscular irritability and the clotting mechanism.

Magnesium and calcium are intimately linked in their body functions, and deficiency of either one has a significant effect on the metabolism of the other because of magnesium's importance in the absorption of calcium from the intestines and in calcium metabolism. Magnesium deficiency will result in the drift of calcium out of the bones, possibly resulting in abnormal calcification in the aorta and the kidney. This condition responds to administration of magnesium salts. Normally, 95% of the magnesium that is filtered through the glomerulus is reabsorbed in the tubule. When there is decreased kidney function, greater amounts of magnesium are retained, resulting in increased blood serum levels.

Explanation of Test
Magnesium measurement is used to evaluate renal function and electrolyte status and to evaluate magnesium metabolism.

Procedure

Obtain a fasting, 5-ml, venous blood sample. Avoid hemolysis, and separate serum from cells as soon as possible. Heparinized blood may be used.

Clinical Implications

1. *Reduced blood magnesium levels* occur in the following conditions:
   a. Hypercalcemia of any cause
   b. Diabetic acidosis
   c. Hemodialysis
   d. Chronic renal disease (glomerulonephritis)
   e. Chronic pancreatitis
   f. Hyperaldosteronism
   g. Pregnancy (second and third trimester)
   h. Hypoparathyroidism
   i. Excessive loss of body fluids (eg, sweating, lactation, diuretic abuse, chronic diarrhea)
   j. Malabsorption syndromes
   k. Chronic alcoholism (hepatic cirrhosis)
   l. Long-term hyperalimentation
   m. Inappropriate secretion of antidiuretic hormone (ADH)

   NOTE: *In magnesium deficiency states, urinary magnesium decreases before the serum magnesium. Serum magnesium levels may remain normal even when total body stores are depleted up to 20%.*

2. *Increased blood magnesium levels* occur in the following conditions:
   a. Renal failure or reduced renal function (acute and chronic)
   b. Dehydration
   c. Hypothyroidism
   d. Addison's disease
   e. Adrenalectomy (adrenocortical insufficiency)
   f. Diabetic acidosis (severe)
   g. Use of antacids containing magnesium (eg, Milk of Magnesia), administration of magnesium salts

Interfering Factors

1. Prolonged salicylate therapy, lithium, and magnesium products (eg, antacids, laxatives) will cause falsely increased magnesium levels, particularly if there is renal damage.
2. Calcium gluconate, as well as a number of other drugs, can interfere with testing methods and cause falsely decreased results.
3. Hemolysis will invalidate results, because about three fourths of the magnesium in the blood is found intracellularly in the red blood cells.

Patient Preparation

1. Explain test purpose and blood-drawing procedure.
2. Patient should be fasting if possible, and be in a prone position when blood is drawn. An upright position increases the magnesium level by 4%.

3. Follow guidelines in Chapter 1 regarding safe, effective, informed *pretest* care.

Patient Aftercare

1. Interpret test results and monitor as appropriate. Treatment of diabetic coma often results in low plasma magnesium levels. This change occurs because magnesium moves with potassium into the cells after insulin administration.

2. Measure serum magnesium in persons receiving aminoglycosides and cyclosporine. There is a known association between these therapies and hypermagnesemia. Treatment of hypermagnesemia involves withholding source of magnesium excess, promoting excretion, giving calcium salts, and performing hemodialysis.

3. Magnesium deficiency may cause apparently unexplained hypocalcemia and hypokalemia. In these instances, patients may have neurologic and/or GI symptoms. Observe for the following signs and symptoms:
   a. Muscle tremors, twitching, tetany
   b. Hypocalcemia
   c. Hyperactive deep tendon reflexes
   d. Electrocardiogram (ECG): prolonged P-R and Q-T intervals; broad, flat T waves; premature ventricular tachycardia and fibrillation
   e. Anorexia, nausea, vomiting
   f. Insomnia, delirium convulsions

4. Observe for signs of too much magnesium (which acts as a sedative):
   a. Lethargy, flushing, nausea, vomiting, slurred speech
   b. Weak or absent deep tendon reflexes
   c. ECG: prolonged PR and Q-T intervals; widened QRs; bradycardia
   d. Hypotension, drowsiness, respiratory depression

5. Follow guidelines in Chapter 1 for safe, effective, informed *posttest* care.

Clinical Alert

Panic Values for Magnesium
Hypomagnesemia: <1.0 mg/dl (tetany occurs)
Hypermagnesemia: >5.0 mg/dl
   5.0–10.0 mg/dl: central nervous system (CNS) depression, nausea, vomiting, fatigue
   10–15 mg/dl: coma, ECG changes, respiratory paralysis
   30 mg/dl: complete heart block
   34–40 mg/dl: cardiac arrest

POTASSIUM (K⁺)

Normal Values
Adult: 3.5–5.3 mmol/L or mEq/L
Child (1–18 y): 3.4–4.7 mmol/L or mEq/L

Infant (7 d–1 y): 4.1–5.3 mmol/L or mEq/L
Neonate (0–7 d): 3.7–5.9 mmol/L or mEq/L

Background

Potassium is the principal electrolyte (cation) of intracellular fluid and the primary buffer within the cell itself. Ninety percent of potassium is concentrated within the cell; only small amounts are contained in bone and blood. Damaged cells release potassium into the blood.

The body is adapted for efficient potassium excretion. Normally, 80% to 90% of the cells' potassium is excreted in the urine by the glomeruli of the kidneys; the remainder is excreted in sweat and in the stool. Even when no potassium is taken into the body (as in a fasting state), 40 to 50 mEq are still excreted daily in the urine. The kidneys do not conserve potassium, and when an adequate amount of potassium is not ingested, a severe deficiency will occur. Potassium balance is maintained in adults on an average dietary intake of 80 to 200 mEq/day. Normal intake, minimal needs, and maximum tolerance for potassium are almost the same as those for sodium.

Potassium plays an important role in nerve conduction, muscle function, acid-base balance, and osmotic pressure. Along with calcium and magnesium, potassium controls the rate and force of contraction of the heart and, thus, the cardiac output. Evidence of a potassium deficit can be noted on an ECG by the presence of a U wave.

Potassium and sodium ions are particularly important in the renal regulation of acid-base balance because hydrogen ions are substituted for sodium and potassium ions in the renal tubule. Potassium is more important than sodium because potassium bicarbonate is the primary intracellular inorganic buffer. In potassium deficiency, there is a relative deficiency of intracellular potassium bicarbonate, and the pH is relatively acid. The respiratory center responds to the intracellular acidosis by lowering P_{CO_2} through the mechanism of hyperventilation. The potassium concentration is greatly affected by the adrenal hormones. Potassium deficiency will cause a significant reduction in protein synthesis.

Explanation of Test

This test evaluates changes in body potassium levels and diagnoses acid-base and water imbalances. The level of potassium is not an absolute value; it varies with circulatory volume and other factors. Because a totally unsuspected potassium imbalance can suddenly prove lethal, its development must be anticipated. Thus, it is important to check the potassium level in severe cases of Addison's disease, uremic coma, intestinal obstruction, acute renal failure, GI loss in the administration of diuretics, steroid therapy, and cardiac patients on digitalis. Potassium levels should be monitored during treatment of acidosis, including ketoacidosis of diabetes mellitus.

Procedure

1. Collect a 5-ml venous blood sample using serum or heparinized Vacutainer tube. Observe universal precautions. Avoid hemolysis in obtaining the sample.
2. The sample must be delivered to the laboratory and centrifuged immediately to separate cells from serum. Potassium leaks out of the cell and levels in the sample will be falsely elevated later than 4 hours postcollection.

Clinical Implications

1. *Decreased blood potassium (hypokalemia)* levels are associated with shifting of K^+ into cells, K^+ loss from GI and biliary tracts, renal K^+ excretion, and reduced K^+ intake, as can occur in the following conditions:
   a. Diarrhea, vomiting sweating
   b. Starvation, malabsorption
   c. Bartter's syndrome
   d. Draining wounds
   e. Cystic fibrosis
   f. Severe burns
   g. Primary aldosteronism
   h. Alcoholism
   i. Osmotic hyperglycemia
   j. Respiratory alkalosis
   k. Renal tubular acidosis
   l. Diuretic, antibiotic, and mineralocorticoid administration
   m. Barium chloride poisoning
   n. Treatment of megaloblastic anemia with vitamin B_{12} or folic acid
2. Potassium levels of 3.5 mEq/L are more commonly associated with deficiency rather than normality. A falling trend (0.1–0.2 mEq/day) is indicative of a developing potassium deficiency.
   a. The most frequent cause of potassium deficiency is GI loss.
   b. The most frequent cause of potassium depletion is IV fluid administration without adequate potassium supplements
3. *Increased potassium levels (hyperkalemia)* occur when K^+ shifts from cells to intracellular fluid, with inadequate renal excretion, and with excessive K^+ intake, as can occur in the following conditions:
   a. Renal failure, dehydration, obstruction and trauma
   b. Cell damage, as in burns, accidents, surgery, chemotherapy, disseminated intravascular coagulation (damaged cells release potassium into the blood)
   c. Metabolic acidosis (drives potassium out of the cells), diabetic ketoacidosis
   d. Addison's disease
   e. Pseudohypoaldosteronism
   f. Uncontrolled diabetes, decreased insulin
   g. Primary acquired hyperkalemia, such as systemic lupus erythematosus, sickle cell disease, interstitial nephritis, and tubular disorders

Interfering Factors

1. Hemolyzed blood may not be used; K^+ values are elevated to as much as 50% over normal with moderate hemolysis. Opening and closing the fist 10 times with a tourniquet in place results in an increase in potassium level by 10% to 20%. For this reason, it is recommended that the blood sample be obtained without a tourniquet, or that the tourniquet be released after the needle has entered the vein.

2. Drug usage

   a. IV administration of potassium penicillin may cause hyperkalemia; penicillin sodium may cause increased excretion of potassium.

   b. Glucose administered during tolerance testing or the ingestion and administration of large amounts of glucose in patients with heart disease may cause a decrease of as much as 0.4 mEq/L in potassium blood levels.

   c. A number of drugs raise potassium levels, especially potassium-sparing diuretics and nonsteroidal antiinflammatory drugs, especially in the presence of renal disease.

   d. Excessive intake of licorice decreases potassium levels.

3. Leukocytosis, as occurs in leukemia, raises potassium levels.

4. Patients who have thrombocytosis due to polycythemia vera or a myeloproliferative disease may have spuriously high potassium levels. This falsely elevated level is caused by a high number of platelets, which release potassium during coagulation. Therefore, heparinized samples, rather than clotted serum samples, should be used in these patients.

Patient Preparation

1. Explain test purpose and blood-drawing procedure. Do not have patient open and close fist while drawing blood.

2. Follow guidelines in Chapter 1 for safe, effective, informed *pretest* care.

Clinical Alert

1. Panic values for potassium:

   <2.5 mEq/L causes ventricular fibrillation.

   >7.0 mEq/L causes muscle irritability including myocardial irritability.

2. The most common cause of hypokalemia in patients receiving IV fluids is water and sodium chloride administration without adequate replacement for K⁺ lost in urine and drainage fluids. A patient receiving IV fluids needs K⁺ every day. The minimum daily dose should be 40 mEq, but the optimum daily dose ranges between 60 and 120 mEq. Potassium needs are greater in persons with tissue injury, wound infection, and gastric intestinal or biliary drainage. If adequate amounts of potassium (40 mEq/day) are not given in IV solution, hypokalemia will eventually develop. Patients receiving <10 mEq KCl in 100 ml of IV solution should be monitored by ECG for potential arrhythmia if the IV rate is ≥100/h. Concentrated doses of IV potassium should always be administered via volume-controlled IV infusion devices. A burning sensation felt at the site of needle insertion may indicate that the concentration is toxic, and the IV rate can be reduced. Some physicians order a small dose of lidocaine to be

(continued)

(Clinical Alert continued)
added to IV potassium to eliminate the burning sensation some patients experience. Always be sure to check for lidocaine allergies prior to administration of this local anesthetic.
3. Closely monitor for hypokalemia in patients taking digitalis and diuretics, because cardiac arrhythmias can occur. Hypokalemia enhances the effect of digitalis preparations, creating the possibility of digitalis intoxication from even an average maintenance dose. Digitalis, diuretics, and hypokalemia are a potentially lethal combination.

Patient Aftercare

1. Interpret test results, monitor changes in body potassium, and intervene as appropriate.
2. Recognizing signs and symptoms of hypokalemia and hyperkalemia is very important. Many of these originate in the nervous and muscular systems and are usually nonspecific and similar.
3. The potassium blood level rises 0.6 mEq/L for every 0.1 decrease in blood pH.
4. Follow guidelines in Chapter 1 for safe, effective, informed *posttest* care.

HYPERKALEMIA (EXCESS K^+)

1. Record fluid intake and output. Check blood volume and venous pressure, which will give clues to dehydration or circulatory overload. Identify ECG changes. In *hyperkalemia*, these include the following:
   a. Elevated T wave heart block
   b. Flattened P wave
   c. Cardiac arrest may occur without warning other than ECG changes.
2. Observe for slow pulse, oliguria, neuromuscular alterations such as muscle irritability and impaired muscle function, flaccid paralysis, tremors, and twitching preceding actual paralysis.
3. Hyperkalemia can be treated with sodium bicarbonate, glucose, and insulin.

HYPOKALEMIA (DEFICIENCY OF K^+)

1. Record fluid intake and output. Check blood volume and venous pressure, which will give clues to circulatory overload or dehydration. Identify ECG changes. In *hypokalemia,* these include the following:
   a. Depressed T waves
   b. Peaking of P waves
2. Observe for dehydration caused by severe vomiting, hyperventilation, sweating, diuresis, or nasogastric tube with gastric suction. Accurately record state of hydration or dehydration.
3. Observe for neuromuscular changes such as fatigue, muscle weakness, muscle pain, flabby muscles, paresthesia, hypotension, rapid pulse, respiratory

muscle weakness leading to paralysis, cyanosis, respiratory arrest, anorexia, nausea, vomiting, paralytic ileus, apathy, drowsiness, tetany, and coma.

4. Hypokalemia may be treated with a K^+ rice diet, K^+-sparing diuretics. Kayexalate, a sodium-potassium exchange resin, can be administered orally, nasogastrically, or rectally. Use salt substitutes containing potassium chloride and administer IV oral potassium chloride supplements.

Clinical Alert

1. Be on the alert for the following arrhythmias, which may occur with hyperkalemia:
   a. Sinus bradycardia
   b. Sinus arrest
   c. First-degree atrioventricular block
   d. Nodal rhythm
   e. Idioventricular rhythm
   f. Ventricular tachycardia
   g. Ventricular fibrillation
   h. Ventricular arrest
2. Be on the alert for the following arrhythmias, which may occur with hypokalemia:
   a. Ventricular premature beats
   b. Atrial tachycardia
   c. Nodal tachycardia
   d. Ventricular tachycardia
   e. Ventricular fibrillation

SODIUM (Na^+)

Normal Values

Adult: 135–145 mmol/L or mEq/L
Child (1–16 y): 135–145 mmol/L or mEq/L
Full-term infant: 133–142 mmol/L or mEq/L
Premature infant: 132–140 mmol/L or mEq/L

Background

Sodium is the most abundant cation (90% of the electrolyte fluid) and the chief base of the blood. Its primary functions in the body are to chemically maintain osmotic pressure and acid-base balance and to transmit nerve impulses. The body has a strong tendency to maintain a total base content, and only slight changes are found even under pathologic conditions. Mechanisms for maintaining a constant sodium level in the plasma and extracellular fluid include renal blood flow, carbonic anhydrase enzyme activity, aldosterone, action of other steroids whose plasma level is controlled by the anterior pituitary gland, renin enzyme secretion, ADH, and vasopressin secretion.

Explanation of Test

Determinations of plasma sodium levels detect changes in water balance rather than sodium balance. Sodium levels are used to determine electrolytes, acid-base balance, water balance, water intoxication, and dehydration.

Procedure

Obtain a 5-ml venous blood sample. Heparinized blood can be used. Avoid hemolysis. Observe standard precautions.

Clinical Implications

1. *Hyponatremia* (decreased sodium levels) reflect a relative excess of body water rather than low total body sodium. *Reduced* sodium levels (hyponatremia) are associated with the following conditions:
    a. Severe burns
    b. Congestive heart failure (predictor of cardiac mortality)
    c. Excessive fluid loss (eg, severe diarrhea, vomiting, sweating)
    d. Excessive IV induction of nonelectrolyte fluids (eg, glucose)
    e. Addison's disease (impairs sodium reabsorption)
    f. Severe nephritis (nephrotic syndrome)
    g. Pyloric obstruction
    h. Malabsorption syndrome
    i. Diabetic acidosis
    j. Drugs such as diuretics
    k. Edema (dilutional hyponatremia)
    l. Large amounts of water by mouth (water intoxication)
    m. Stomach suction accompanied by water or ice chips by mouth
    n. Hypothyroidism
    o. Excessive ADH production
2. *Hypernatremia* (increased sodium levels) are uncommon, but when they do occur, they are associated with the following conditions:
    a. Dehydration and insufficient water intake
    b. Conn's syndrome
    c. Primary aldosteronism
    d. Coma
    e. Cushing's disease
    f. Diabetes insipidus
    g. Tracheobronchitis

Clinical Alert

Panic Values for Sodium

<120 mEq/L (weakness, dehydration)
90–105 mEq/L (severe neurologic symptoms, vascular cause)
>155 mEq/L (cardiovascular and renal symptoms)
>160 mEq/L (heart failure)

Interfering Factors

1. Many drugs affect levels of blood sodium.
   a. Anabolic steroids, corticosteroids, calcium, fluorides, and iron can cause increases in sodium level.
   b. Heparin, laxatives, sulfates, and diuretics can cause decreases in sodium level.
2. High triglycerides or low protein cause artificially low sodium values.

Patient Preparation

1. Explain test purpose and procedure.
2. Follow guidelines in Chapter 1 for safe, effective, informed *pretest* care.

Patient Aftercare

1. Interpret test outcomes and monitor for fluid and sodium imbalances.
2. IV therapy considerations are as follows:
   a. Sodium balance is maintained in adults with an average dietary intake of 90 to 250 mEq/day. The maximum daily tolerance to an acute load is 400 mEq/day. If a patient is given 3 L of isotonic saline in 24 hours, he will receive 465 mEq of sodium. This amount exceeds the average, healthy adult's tolerance level. It will take a *healthy* person 24 to 48 hours to excrete the excess sodium.
   b. After surgery, trauma, or shock, there is a decrease in extracellular fluid volume. Replacement of extracellular fluid is essential if water and electrolyte balance is to be maintained. The ideal replacement IV solution should have a sodium concentration of 140 mEq/L.
3. Monitor for signs of edema or hypertension, and record and report these if present.
4. Follow guidelines in Chapter 1 regarding safe, effective, informed *posttest* care.

OSMOLALITY AND WATER-LOAD TEST (WATER-LOADING ANTIDIURETIC HORMONE SUPPRESSION TEST) ⬤

Normal Values

Serum Osmolality
Adult: 275–295 mOsm/kg H_2O or mmol/kg H_2O
Newborn: as low as 266 mOsm/kg H_2O or mmol/kg H_2O

Urine Osmolality
Adult
24-h: 300–900 mOsm/kg H_2O or mmol/kg H_2O
Random: 50–1200 mOsm/kg H_2O or mmol/kg H_2O
After 12-h fluid restriction: >850 mOsm/kg H_2O or mmol/kg H_2O
Ratio of urine/serum osmolality: 0.2–4.7 (average, 1.0–3.0)
Ratio after fluid restriction: 3:1 or a range of 0.2 to 4.7:1

Osmolal Gap
Serum: 5–10 mOsm/kg H_2O or mmol/kg H_2O
Urine: 80–100 mOsm/kg H_2O or mmol/kg H_2O

Background

Osmolality, which is the measure of the number of dissolved solute particles in solution, increases with dehydration and decreases with overhydration. In general, the same conditions that reduce or increase serum sodium affect osmolality.

Explanation of Test

This test is used as an evaluation of water and electrolyte balance. It is helpful in assessing hydration status, seizures, liver disease, ADH function, and coma, and it is used in toxicology workups for ethanol, ethylene glycol, isopropanol, and methanol ingestions.

> **Clinical Alert**
>
> 1. Simultaneous determination of urine and serum osmolalities facilitates interpretation of results. High urinary/serum (U/S) ratio is seen in concentrated urine. Normal ranges for the U/S ratio are ~0.2 to 4.7 and may be >3 with overnight dehydration. With poor concentrating ability, the ratio is low but is still >1. In SIADH, sodium and urine osmolalities are high for the serum osmolality.
> 2. Determination of the urine osmolar gap is used to characterize metabolic acidosis and is described as the sum of urinary concentrations of sodium, potassium, bicarbonate, chloride, glucose and urea compared with measured urine osmolality.

Procedure for Determining Osmolality

1. Obtain a 5-ml venous blood sample. Serum or heparinized plasma is acceptable. Observe universal precautions.
2. A 24-hour urine specimen may be collected concurrently and kept on ice.
3. Osmolality is determined in the laboratory using the freezing point depression methodology for both serum and urine.

Procedure for Determining Water-Loading Antidiuretic Hormone Suppression

1. The ideal position during the testing period is the recumbent position, because the response to water loading is reduced in persons in the upright position.
2. One hour before testing, the patient is given 300 ml of water to replace fluid lost during the overnight fast. This water is not counted as part of the test load.
3. The patient drinks a test load of water (20 ml/kg body weight) within 30 minutes.
4. After the test load of water is consumed, all urine is collected for the next 4 to 5 hours, and each voiding is checked for volume osmolality and spe-

cific gravity. Hourly blood samples are obtained for osmolality, and the entire volume of urine obtained is checked for osmolality.

5. Normal values for water-loading antidiuretic hormone suppression test are excretion of >90% of water-load within 4 hours. Urine osmolality falls to <100 mOsm/kg. Specific gravity falls to 1.003.

6. Plasma ADH should also be determined at hourly intervals.

Clinical Implications

1. In *decreased renal function,* <80% of fluid is excreted, and urine specific gravity may not fall below 1.010. This phenomenon occurs in the following conditions:
   a. Adrenocortical insufficiency
   b. Malabsorption syndrome
   c. Edema
   d. Ascites
   e. Obesity
   f. Hypothyroidism
   g. Dehydration
   h. Congestive heart failure
   i. Cirrhosis

2. Disorders with *increased ADH secretion (SIADH)* give an inadequate response; <90% of water is excreted, and urine osmolality remains >100 mOsm/kg H_2O. Plasma ADH measured at 90 minutes confirms diagnosis of SIADH.

Patient Preparation for Water-Loading Test

1. Explain the test purpose and procedure. The test takes 5 to 6 hours to complete.

2. No food, alcohol, medications, or smoking are allowed for 8 to 10 hours before testing. No muscular exercise is allowed during the test.

3. The patient may experience nausea, abdominal fullness, fatigue, and desire to defecate.

4. Discard first morning urine specimen.

5. Follow guidelines in Chapter 1 for safe, effective, informed *pretest* care.

Patient Aftercare for Water-Loading Test

1. Observe for adverse reactions to water-loading test such as extreme abdominal discomfort, shortness of breath, or chest pain.

2. If water clearance is impaired, the water load will not induce diuresis, and maximum urinary dilution will not occur.

3. Accurate results may not be obtained if nausea, vomiting, or diarrhea occur or if a disturbance in bladder emptying is present. Note on chart if any of these effects occur.

5. Follow guidelines in Chapter 1 regarding safe, effective, informed *posttest* care.

> ▶ **Clinical Alert**
>
> In patients with impaired ability to tolerate the water-loading test, seizures or fatal hyponatremia may occur.

Clinical Implications

1. *Increased values (hyperosmolality)* are associated with the following conditions:
   a. Dehydration
   b. Diabetes insipidus (central or nephrogenic)
   c. Hypercalcemia
   d. Diabetes mellitus, hyperglycemia, diabetic ketoacidosis
   e. Hypernatremia
   f. Cerebral lesions
   g. Alcohol ingestion (ethanol, methanol, ethylene glycol)
   h. Mannitol therapy
   i. Azotemia
   j. Inadequate water intake
   k. Chronic renal disease
2. *Decreased values (hypoosmolality)* are associated with the following conditions:
   a. Loss of sodium with diuretics and low-salt diet (hyponatremia)
   b. Renal losses
   c. Adrenocortical insufficiency
   d. Inappropriate secretion of ADH, as may occur in trauma and lung cancer
   e. Excessive water replacement (overhydration, water intoxication)
   f. Panhypopituitarism

Clinical Implications of Osmolol Gap

1. Abnormal levels (>10 mOsm/kg H_2O) can occur in the following conditions:
   a. Methanol
   b. Ethanol
   c. Isopropol alcohol
   d. Mannitol
   e. Severely ill patients, especially those in shock, lactic acidosis, and renal failure
2. Ethanol glycol, acetone, and paraldehyde have relatively small osmolol gaps, even at lethal levels.

Interfering Factors

1. Decreases in osmolol gap are associated with altitude, diurnal variation with water retention at night, and some drugs.
2. Some drugs also cause increases in osmolol gap.
3. Hypertriglyceridemia and hyperproteinemia cause an elevated osmolol gap.

Patient Preparation

1. Explain test purpose and procedure.
2. No alcohol may be ingested during the 24 hours before the test.
3. Follow guidelines in Chapter 1 for safe, effective, informed *pretest* care.

Patient Aftercare

1. Interpret test results and monitor appropriately. A patient receiving IV fluids should have a normal osmolality. If the osmolality increases, the fluids contain relatively more electrolytes than water. If it falls, relatively more water than electrolytes is present.
2. If the ratio of serum sodium to serum osmolality falls below 0.43, the outlook is guarded. This ratio may be distorted in cases of drug intoxication.
3. Follow guidelines in Chapter 1 for safe, effective, informed *posttest* care.

> ### Clinical Alert
>
> 1. Panic serum osmolality values are results <240 or >321. A value of 385 relates to stupor in hyperglycemia. Values of 400 or 420 are associated with grand mal seizures. Values >420 are fatal.
> 2. A water-loading ADH suppression test may be ordered to investigate impaired renal excretion of water.

SWEAT TEST

Normal Values

Sweat Sodium
Normal: 10–40 mmol/L or mEq/L
Cystic fibrosis: 70–190 mmol/L or mEq/L

Sweat Chloride
Normal: 5–35 mmol/L or mEq/L
Cystic fibrosis: 60–200 mmol/L or mEq/L

Potassium Sweat
Normal male: 4.4–9.7 mEq/L or mmol/L
Normal female: 7.6–15.6 mEq/L or mmol/L
Cystic fibrosis: 14–30 mEq/L or mmol/L

Explanation of Test

This test is done to diagnose cystic fibrosis. Abnormally high concentrations of sodium and chloride appear in the secretions of eccrine sweat glands in persons with cystic fibrosis. This condition is present at birth and persists throughout life. This study uses sweat-inducing techniques (eg, pilocarpine iontophoresis) followed by chemical analysis to determine sodium, chloride, and potassium content of collected sweat.

Procedure

1. The forearm is the preferred site for stimulation of sweating, but in thin or small babies, the thigh, back, or leg may be used. It may be necessary to stimulate sweating in two places to obtain sufficient sweat for testing, especially in young infants. At least 100 µl of sweat is necessary. In cold weather, or if the testing room is cold, a warm covering should be placed over the arm or other site of sweat collection.
2. Sweat production is stimulated by skin application of gauze pads or filter paper saturated with a measured amount of pilocarpine and attachment of electrodes through which a current of 4 to 5 mAmp is delivered at intervals for a total of 5 minutes.
3. The electrodes and pad are removed, and the area is thoroughly washed with distilled water and carefully dried.
4. Successful iontophoresis is indicated by a red area about 2.5 cm in diameter that appears where the electrode was placed.
5. The skin is scrubbed thoroughly with distilled water and dried carefully. The area for sweat collection must be completely dry, free from contamination by powder or antiseptic, and free of any area that might ooze.
6. Collection of sweat occurs by applying preweighed filter or sweat collection cups that are taped securely over the red spot. The inside surfaces of the collecting device should never be touched.
7. The paper is left on for at least 1 hour before removal and is then placed in a preweighed flask to avoid evaporation. The flask is again weighed. The desired volume of sweat is 200 mg; the minimum volume necessary is 100 mg.
8. If a cup is used, it is left in place for 1 hour and then carefully removed by scraping it across the iontophoresed area. This "puddles" the sweat in the cup to reduce evaporation and to redissolve any salts left by the evaporation. Suction capillary tubes are used to remove sweat from the collection cups.

Clinical Implications

1. Children with cystic fibrosis have sodium and chloride values of >60 mEq/L.
2. Borderline or gray-zone cases are those with values between 40 and 60 mEq/L for both sodium and chloride. These persons require retesting. Potassium values do not assist in differentiating borderline cases.
3. In adolescence and adulthood, chloride levels of >80 mEq/L usually indicate cystic fibrosis.
4. Elevated sweat electrolytes also can be associated with the following conditions:
   a. Addison's disease
   b. Congenital adrenal hyperplasia
   c. Vasopressin-resistant diabetes insipidus

d. Glucose-6-phosphatase deficiency (G6PD)
e. Hypothyroidism
f. Familial hypoparathyroidism
g. Alcoholic pancreatitis

Interfering Factors

1. The sweat test is not valuable after puberty because levels may vary over a very wide range among individuals.
2. Dehydration and edema, particularly of areas where sweat is collected, may interfere with test results.
3. A gap of >30 mEq/L between sodium and chloride values indicates calculation or analysis error or contamination of the sample.
4. Sweat testing is not considered accurate until the third or fourth week of life because infants <3 weeks of age may not sweat enough to provide a sufficient sample.
5. Test may be falsely normal in patients with salt depletion, as in periods of hot weather.

Clinical Alert

1. The test should always be repeated if the result, the clinical features, or other diagnostic tests do not fit together.
2. The test can be used to exclude the diagnosis of cystic fibrosis in siblings of diagnosed patients.
3. There have been reports of cystic fibrosis patients with normal sweat electrolyte levels.
4. Sweat potassium testing is not diagnostically valuable.

Patient Preparation

1. Explain test purpose and procedure. The sweat test is indicated for the following persons:
   a. Infants who pass initial meconium late; who have intestinal obstruction in newborn, failure to thrive, steatorrhea, chronic diarrhea, rapid respiration and retraction with chronic cough, asthma, hypoproteinemia (especially on soybean formula), atelectasis or hyperaeration on x-ray, hyperprothrombinemia, or rectal prolapse; who taste salty; or who are offspring of a parent with cystic fibrosis (ie, the obligate heterozygote).
   b. Persons suspected of having cystic fibrosis or celiac disease, all siblings of patients with cystic fibrosis, or persons with disaccharide intolerance, recurrent pneumonia, chronic atelectasis, chronic pulmonary disease, bronchiolectasis chronic cough, nasal polyposis, cirrhosis of liver and hypertension.
   c. Any parents who request a sweat test on their child.
2. Inform the patient that a slight stinging sensation is usually experienced, especially in fair-skinned persons.

3. Follow guidelines in Chapter 1 regarding safe, effective, informed *pretest* care.

Patient Aftercare
1. After the cup is removed, carefully wash and dry the skin to prevent irritation caused by collection cups.
2. Resume normal activities.
3. Interpret test results and counsel and monitor patient as appropriate. Provide genetic counseling. Cystic fibrosis is transmitted as an autosomal recessive trait. The Caucasian carrier rate is 1 in 20, and the African American carrier rate is 1 in 60 to 1 in 100.
4. Follow guidelines in Chapter 1 for safe, effective, informed *posttest* care.

●BLOOD GLUCOSE AND RELATED TESTS

C-PEPTIDE ●

Normal Values
Fasting: 0.78–1.89 ng/ml or 0.26–0.63 mmol/L
60-Min postglucagon: 2.73–5.64 ng/ml

Background
C-peptide is formed during the conversion of pro-insulin to insulin. C-peptide serum levels correlate with insulin levels in blood, except in islet cell tumors and possibly in obese patients.

Explanation of Test
The main use of C-peptide is to evaluate hypoglycemia. C-peptide levels provide reliable indicators for pancreatic, β, and secretory functions and insulin secretions. In a patient with insulin-dependent diabetes mellitus (IDDM), C-peptide measurements can mark endogenous β-cell activity. C-peptide levels can also be used to confirm suspected surreptitious insulin injections (ie, factitious hypoglycemia). Findings in these patients reveal that insulin levels are usually high, insulin antibodies may be high, but C-peptide levels are low or undetectable. This test also monitors the patient's recovery after excision of an insulinoma. Rising C-peptide levels suggest insulinoma tumor recurrence or metastases.

Procedure
1. A 1-ml venous blood sample is drawn from a fasting patient using red-topped chilled tube. Serum is needed for test.
2. The blood is separated in a 4-degree centigrade and frozen if it will not be tested until later.
3. A sample for glucose testing is usually drawn at the same time.

Clinical Implications

1. *Increased C-peptide* values occur in the following conditions:
   a. Endogenous hyperinsulinism (insulinemia)
   b. Oral hypoglycemic drug ingestion
   c. Pancreas or β-cell transplant
   d. Renal failure
   e. Type II diabetes mellitus (non–insulin-dependent)
2. *Decreased C-peptide* valves occur in the following conditions:
   a. Factitious hypoglycemia (surreptitious insulin administration)
   b. Radical pancreatectomy
   c. Insulin-dependent diabetes (type I)
3. C-peptide stimulation test can determine the following:
   a. Distinguishes between insulin-dependent (type I) and non–insulin-dependent diabetes (type II).
   b. Patients with diabetes whose C-peptide stimulation values are >1.8 ng/ml can be managed without insulin treatment.

> ▶ **Clinical Alert**
>
> To differentiate insulinoma from factitious hypoglycemia, an insulin/C-peptide ratio can be performed.
> <1.0 Ratio: increased, endogenous insulin secretion
> >1.0 Ratio: exogenous insulin

Patient Preparation

1. Explain the test purpose and blood-drawing procedure.
2. The patient must fast, except for water, for 8 to 12 hours before blood is drawn.
3. Radioisotope testing, if necessary, should take place *after* blood is drawn for C-peptide levels.
4. If the C-peptide stimulation test is done, IV glucagon must be given after a baseline value blood sample is drawn.
5. Follow guidelines in Chapter 1 for safe, effective, informed *pretest* care.

Patient Aftercare

1. Resume normal activities.
2. Interpret test results and monitor as appropriate.
3. Follow guidelines in Chapter 1 for safe, effective, informed *posttest* care.

GLUCAGON ●

Normal Values

Adult: 20–100 pg/ml or ng/L
Child: 0–148 pg/ml
Newborn: 0–1750 pg/ml

NOTE: *During a glucose tolerance test (GTT) in healthy persons, glucagon levels will decline significantly compared with baseline fasting levels as normal hyperglycemia takes place during the first hour of testing.*

Background

Glucagon is a peptide hormone that originates in the α-cells of the pancreatic islets of Langerhans. This hormone promotes glucose production in the liver. Normally, insulin opposes this action. Glucagon provides a sensitive, coordinated control mechanism for glucose production and storage. For example, low blood glucose levels cause glucagon to stimulate glucose release into the bloodstream, whereas elevated blood glucose levels reduce the amount of circulating glucagon to ~50% of that found in the fasting state. The kidneys also affect glucagon metabolism. Elevated fasting glucagon levels in the presence of renal failure return to normal levels following successful renal transplantation. Abnormally high glucagon levels drop toward normal once insulin therapy effectively controls diabetes. However, when compared with a healthy person, glucagon secretion in the person with diabetes does not decrease after eating carbohydrates. Moreover, in healthy persons, arginine infusion causes increased glucagon secretion.

Explanation of Test

This test measures glucagon production and metabolism. A glucagon deficiency reflects pancreatic tissue loss. Failure of glucagon levels to rise during arginine infusion confirms glucagon deficiency. Hyperglucagonemia (ie, elevated glucagon levels) occurs in diabetes, acute pancreatitis, and situations in which catecholamine secretion is stimulated (eg, pheochromocytoma, infection).

Procedure

A 5-ml blood sample is drawn from a fasting person into an EDTA Vacutainer tube containing Trasylol proteinase inhibitor. Special handling is required, because glucagon is very prone to enzymatic degradation. Tubes used to draw blood must be chilled before the sample is collected and placed on ice afterward, and plasma must be frozen as soon as possible after centrifuging. Observe standard precautions.

Clinical Implications

1. *Increased glucagon levels* are associated with the following conditions:
   a. Acute pancreatitis (eg, pancreatic α-cell tumor)
   b. Diabetes mellitus: persons with severe diabetic ketoacidosis are reported to have fasting glucagon levels five times normal despite marked hyperglycemia.
   c. Glucagonoma (familial) may be manifested by three different syndromes:
      (1) The first syndrome exhibits a characteristic skin rash, necrolytic migratory erythema, diabetes mellitus or impaired glucose tolerance, weight loss, anemia, and venous thrombosis. This form usually shows elevated glucagon levels >1000 pg/ml.

(2) The second syndrome occurs with severe diabetes.

(3) The third form is associated with multiple endocrine neoplasia syndrome and can show relatively lower glucagon levels as compared with the others.

d. Chronic renal failure

e. Hyperlipidemia

f. Stress (trauma, burns, surgery)

g. Uremia

h. Hepatic cirrhosis

i. Hyperosmolality

2. *Reduced levels of glucagon* are associated with the following conditions:

a. Loss of pancreatic tissue

(1) Pancreatic neoplasms

(2) Pancreatectomy

b. Chronic pancreatitis

c. Cystic fibrosis

Patient Preparation

1. Explain purpose of test and blood-drawing procedure. A minimum 8-hour fast is necessary before the test.

2. Promote relaxation in a low-stress environment; stress alters normal glucagon levels.

3. No radioisotopes should be administered within 1 week before the test.

4. Follow guidelines in Chapter 1 for safe, effective, informed *pretest* care.

Patient Aftercare

1. Resume normal activities.

2. Interpret test outcome and monitor for the three different syndromes of glucagonoma.

3. Follow guidelines in Chapter 1 for safe, effective, informed *posttest* care.

INSULIN

Normal Values

Immunoreactive
Adult: 0–35 µU/ml or 0–243 pmol/L
Child: 0–10 µU/ml or 0–69 pmol/L

Free
Adult: 0–17 µU/ml or 0–118 pmol/L
Child (prepubertal): 0–13 µU/ml or 0–90 pmol/L

Background

Insulin, a hormone produced by the pancreatic β-cells of the islets of Langerhans, regulates carbohydrate metabolism together with contributions from the liver, adipose tissue, and other target cells. Insulin is responsible for maintaining blood glucose levels at a constant level within a defined range. The rate of insulin secretion is primarily regulated by the level of blood glucose perfusing the pancreas; however, it can also be affected by hormones, the autonomic nervous system, and nutritional status.

Explanation of Test
Insulin levels are valuable for establishing the process of an insulinoma (ie, tumor of the islets of Langerhans). This test is valuable for investigating the causes of fasting hypoglycemic states and neoplasm differentiation. The insulin study can be done in conjunction with a GTT or fasting blood glucose test.

Procedure
1. Obtain a 4-ml blood sample from a fasting person; serum is preferred. Observe standard precautions.
2. If done in conjunction with a GTT, the specimens should be drawn before administering oral glucose and again at 30, 60, and 120 minutes after glucose ingestion (the same times as the GTT).

Clinical Implications
1. *Increased insulin values* are associated with the following conditions:
   a. Insulinoma (pancreatic islet tumor). Diagnosis is based on the following findings:
      (1) Hyperinsulinemia with hypoglycemia (glucose <30 mg/dl)
      (2) Persistent hypoglycemia together with hyperinsulinemia (>20 μU/ml) after tolbutamide injection (rapid rise and rapid fall)
      (3) Failed C-peptide suppression with a plasma glucose level ≤30 mg/dl and an insulin/glucose ratio >0.3.
   b. Non–insulin-dependent (type II) diabetes mellitus (NIDDM), untreated
   c. Acromegaly
   d. Cushing's syndrome
   e. Endogenous administration of insulin
   f. Obesity (most common cause)
2. *Decreased insulin values* are found in the following conditions:
   a. Insulin-dependent (type I) diabetes mellitus (IDDM), severe
   b. Hypopituitarism

Interfering Factors
1. Surreptitious insulin or oral hypoglycemic agent ingestion or injection causes elevated insulin levels.
2. Oral contraceptives and other drugs cause falsely elevated values.
3. Recently administered radioisotopes affect test results.

Patient Preparation
1. Explain test purpose and procedure.
2. The patient should fast from all food and fluid except water unless otherwise directed.

3. Because insulin release from an insulinoma may be erratic and unpredictable, it may be necessary for the patient to fast for as long as 72 hours before the test.
4. Follow guidelines in Chapter 1 for safe, effective, informed *pretest* care.

Patient Aftercare

1. Resume normal activity and diet.
2. Interpret test results and counsel appropriately. Obese patients may have insulin resistance and unusually high fasting and postprandial insulin levels.
3. Follow guidelines in Chapter 1 regarding safe, effective, informed *posttest* care.

Clinical Alert

A potentially fatal situation may exist if the insulinoma secretes unpredictably high levels of insulin. In this case, the blood glucose may drop to such dangerously low levels as to render the person comatose and unable to self-administer oral glucose forms. Patients and their families must learn how to deal with such an emergency and to be vigilant until the problem is treated.

FASTING BLOOD GLUCOSE (FBG); FASTING BLOOD SUGAR (FBS)

Normal Values
Adult: 65–110 mg/dl or 3.5–6.1 nmol/L
Child (6–18 y): 70–106 mg/dl or 3.9–6.0 nmol/L
Young child (7 d–6 y): 74–127 mg/dl or 4.2–7.0 nmol/L
Neonate (0–7 d): 30–100 mg/dl or 1.7–5.6 nmol/L

Background
Glucose is formed from carbohydrate digestion and conversion of glycogen to glucose by the liver. The two hormones that directly regulate blood glucose are glucagon and insulin. Glucagon accelerates glycogen breakdown in the liver and causes the blood glucose level to rise. Insulin increases cell membrane permeability to glucose, transports glucose into cells (for metabolism), stimulates glycogen formation, and reduces blood glucose levels. Driving insulin into the cells requires insulin and insulin receptors. For example, after a meal, the pancreas releases insulin for glucose metabolism, provided there are enough insulin receptors. Insulin binds to these receptors on the surface of target cells such as are found in fat and muscle. This opens the channels so that glucose can pass into cells, where it can be converted to energy. As cellular glucose metabolism occurs, blood glucose levels fall. Adrenocorticotropic hormone (ACTH), adrenocorticosteroids, epinephrine, and thyroxine also play key roles in glucose metabolism.

Explanation of Test

Fasting blood glucose is a vital component of diabetes management. Abnormal glucose metabolism may be caused by inability of pancreatic islet β-cells to produce insulin, reduced numbers of insulin receptors, faulty intestinal glucose absorption, inability of the liver to metabolize glycogen, or altered levels of hormones that play a role in glucose metabolism (eg, ACTH).

In most cases, significantly elevated fasting blood sugar levels (ie, >140 mg/dl; hyperglycemia) are, in themselves, usually diagnostic for diabetes. However, mild, borderline cases may present with normal fasting glucose values. If diabetes is suspected, a GTT can confirm the diagnosis. Occasionally, other diseases may produce elevated blood sugar levels; therefore, a comprehensive history, physical examination, and workup should be done before a definitive diagnosis of diabetes is established.

> ### ▶ Clinical Alert
>
> New NIH guidelines endorse diabetic testing of all adults ≥ 45 years every 3 years.

Procedure

1. A 5-ml venous blood sample is drawn from a fasting person. In known cases of diabetes, blood drawing should precede insulin or oral hypoglycemic administration. Observe standard precautions. Serum is acceptable if separated from red cells. A gray-topped tube, which contains sodium chloride, is acceptable for 24 hours without separation.
2. Self-monitoring of blood glucose by the person with diabetes can be done by fingerstick blood drop sampling several times per day if necessary. Several devices are commercially available for this procedure; they are relatively easy to use and have been established as a major component in satisfactory diabetes control.
3. Noninvasive methods using skin pads to check blood sugar level are being developed for self monitoring that eliminate the dreaded finger prick test, for example a Gluco-watch (developed by Cygnes of Redwood City, CA), worn on the wrist and powered by a AAA battery.

Patient Checklist

Testing Your Blood Sugar
This list is a general outline. Each brand of meter has its own instructions. Read the instructions on each new meter carefully to get accurate results.

Make sure your hands are clean and dry.
Prick your finger with the lancet.
Squeeze out a drop of blood.
Drop the blood onto the test strip or sensor.
Wait for the test strip or sensor to develop.

Compare the test strip to the chart or insert it in the meter.

Safely dispose of your lancet in an approved sharps container.

Record blood glucose results with date and time.

If you have IDDM, you should also monitor your urine for ketones to alert you to possibly dangerous complications such as diabetic ketoacidosis.

Test more often on days when you are ill, when your blood glucose is too high, when your meal or exercise plan changes, when you travel, or if you feel that your blood glucose is low.

Clinical Implications

1. *Elevated blood sugar (hyperglycemia)* occurs in the following conditions:

    a. Diabetes mellitus: a fasting glucose of >140 mg/dl on more than one occasion is usually diagnostic for diabetes mellitus. An oral GTT is not usually necessary in this instance.

    b. Other conditions that produce elevated blood glucose levels include the following:

        (1) Cushing's disease (increased glucocorticoids cause elevated blood sugar levels)

        (2) Acute emotional or physical stress situations (eg, myocardial infarction [MI], cerebrovascular accident, convulsions)

        (3) Pheochromocytoma

        (4) Pituitary adenoma (increased secretion of growth hormone causes elevated blood glucose levels)

        (5) Hemochromatosis

        (6) Pancreatitis (acute and chronic)

        (7) Glucagonoma

        (8) Advanced liver disease

        (9) Chronic renal disease

        (10) Vitamin B deficiency

        (11) Pregnancy (may signal potential for onset of diabetes later in life)

2. *Decreased blood glucose (hypoglycemia)* occurs in the following conditions:

    a. Pancreatic islet cell carcinoma (insulinomas)

    b. Extrapancreatic stomach tumors (carcinoma)

    c. Addison's disease (adrenal insufficiency)

    d. Hypopituitarism, hypothyroid

    e. Starvation, malabsorption

    f. Liver damage (alcoholism, chloroform poisoning, arsenic poisoning)

    g. Premature infant; infant delivered of a diabetic mother

    h. Enzyme-deficiency diseases (eg, galactosemia, inherited maple syrup disease, von Gierke's syndrome)

    i. Insulin overdose (accidental or deliberate)

    j. Reactive hypoglycemia, including alimentary hyperinsulinism, prediabetes, endocrine deficiency

    k. Postprandial hypoglycemia may occur after GI surgery and is described with hereditary fructose intolerance, galactosemia, and leucine sensitivity

Interfering Factors

A. *Elevated glucose*

1. Steroids, diuretics, other drugs (see Appendix J)
2. Pregnancy (a slight blood glucose elevation normally occurs)
3. Surgical procedures and anesthesia
4. Obesity or sedentary lifestyle
5. Parenteral glucose administration (eg, from total parenteral nutrition)
6. IV glucose (recent or current)
7. Heavy smoking

B. *Decreased glucose*

1. Hematocrit >55%
2. Intense exercise
3. Toxic doses of aspirin and acetaminophen
4. Other drugs, including ethanol, quinine, and haloperidol

Patient Preparation

1. Explain test purpose and blood-drawing procedure.
2. The test requires at least an overnight fast; water is permitted. Instruct the patient to defer insulin or oral hypoglycemics until after blood is drawn, unless specifically instructed to do otherwise.
3. The last time the patient ate must be noted in the record and on the laboratory requisition.
4. Follow guidelines in Chapter 1 for safe, effective, informed *pretest* care.

Patient Aftercare

1. The patient may eat and drink after blood is drawn.
2. Interpret test results and monitor appropriately for hyperglycemia and hypoglycemia. Counsel regarding necessary lifestyle changes (eg, diet, exercise, glucose monitoring, medication).

Patient Checklist

Take special care of your feet.

Use a lubricant or unscented hand cream on dry, scaly skin.

Look for calluses on your soles. Rub them gently with a pumice stone.

Make sure new shoes fit properly; wear freshly washed socks or stockings.

Never go barefoot.

Avoid using hot water bottles, tubs of hot water, or heating pads on your feet.

Trim your toenails straight across.

Make sure your doctor inspects your feet as part of every visit.

Use a team approach to help you make decisions about your care. The team may include your doctor, a diabetes educator, a dietitian, your dentist, and your family.

Use other health professionals to help with your care. These may include an eye doctor (ophthalmologist or optometrist), an exercise physiologist, a podiatrist (a foot specialist), and a psychologist.

Follow the most healthful lifestyle you can.

3. Persons with glucose levels ≥200 mg/dl should be placed on a strict intake and output program.

Clinical Alert

1. If a person with known or suspected diabetes experiences headaches, irritability, dizziness, weakness, fainting, or impaired cognition, a blood glucose test or fingerstick test must be done before giving insulin. Similar symptoms may be present for both hypoglycemia and hyperglycemia. If a blood glucose level cannot be obtained and one is uncertain regarding the situation, glucose may be given in the form of orange juice, sugar-containing soda, or candy (eg, "Life-Savers"). Make certain the person is sufficiently conscious to manage eating or swallowing. In the acute care setting, IV glucose may be given in the event of severe hypoglycemia. A glucose "gel" is also commercially available and may be rubbed on the inside of the mouth by another person if the person with diabetes is unable to swallow or to respond properly. Instruct persons prone to hypoglycemia to carry sugar-type items on their person and to wear a necklace or bracelet that identifies the person as diabetic.

2. Frequent blood glucose monitoring, including self-monitoring, allows better control and management of diabetes than urine glucose monitoring.

3. When blood glucose values are >300 mg/dl, urine output increases, as does the risk of dehydration.

4. Panic values/critical values for fasting blood glucose:
   <40 mg/dl may cause brain damage
   >470 mg/dl may cause coma

5. Diabetes is a "disease of the moment": persons living with diabetes are continually affected by fluctuations in blood glucose levels and must learn to manage and adapt their lifestyle within this framework. For some, adaptation is relatively straightforward; for others, especially those identified as being "brittle," lifestyle changes and management are more complicated, and these patients require constant vigilance, attention, encouragement, and support.

4. Follow guidelines in Chapter 1 for safe, effective, informed *posttest* care.

NOTE: *Each person with diabetes may experience certain symptoms in their own unique way and in a unique pattern.*

2-HOUR POSTPRANDIAL BLOOD SUGAR/GLUCOSE (2-h PPBS)

Normal Values
65–139 mg/dl or 3.5–7.7 mmol/L

Explanation of Test
A postprandial test is performed 2 hours after a meal. Glucose concentration in a 2-hour blood specimen after a meal is rarely elevated in nondiabetic persons but is significantly increased in diabetic patients.

Procedure

Two hours after the patient eats, a 5-ml venous blood sample is obtained. Observe universal precautions. Serum is acceptable, as is use of a gray-topped tube.

Clinical Implications

1. *Elevated levels:*
   a. 140–200 mg/dl indicates impaired glucose tolerance
   b. >200 mg/dl (>11.1 mmol/L) is diagnostic for diabetes mellitus
   c. >150 mg/dl (>8.3 mmol/L) in a pregnant woman indicates gestational diabetes (follow-up with a 3-hour glucose tolerance test to confirm diagnosis)
2. Normal persons return to baseline glucose levels 2 to 3 hours after eating; patients taking insulin have lower values.

Interfering Factors

1. Vomiting, gum chewing, and snacking during the 2-hour test interval invalidates the test result.

Patient Preparation

1. Fasting blood glucose determination and glucose 2-hour postprandial are recommended to establish the diagnosis of diabetes mellitus. Glycosylated hemoglobin is recommended for monitoring diabetes control.
2. Explain purpose and procedure of test. The patient must fast overnight before blood is drawn. Only water may be ingested.
3. Ideally, the patient should be on a high-carbohydrate diet 2 to 3 days before testing.
4. After fasting, a high-carbohydrate meal is eaten.
5. The test is timed from the beginning of the meal. Document time in the patient's record.
6. The patient should rest during the 2-hour interval. Smoking is not permitted during this time.
7. Follow guidelines in Chapter 1 regarding safe, effective, informed *pretest* care.

Patient Aftercare

1. After blood is drawn, the patient may resume eating and activity.
2. Interpret test results and counsel appropriately.
3. Follow guidelines in Chapter 1 for safe, effective, informed *posttest* care.

Clinical Alert

1. Blood glucose values of 140 to 200 mg/dl indicate decreased glucose tolerance; a follow-up GTT should be done.
2. Test results are reliable only to the extent that the patient is properly prepared.
3. The test is contraindicated in the presence of obvious diabetes mellitus.

O'SULLIVAN TEST (1-h GESTATIONAL DIABETES SCREEN)

Normal Values
130–140 mg/dl (1 h after 50 g glucose)

Background
Glucose intolerance during pregnancy is associated with an increase in perinatal morbidity and mortality, especially in women who are aged >25 years, overweight, or hypertensive. Additionally, more than one half of all pregnant patients with an abnormal GTT do not have any of the same risk factors. It is therefore recommended that all pregnant women be screened for gestational diabetes.

Explanation of Test
The O'Sullivan test is done to detect gestational diabetes. During pregnancy, abnormal carbohydrate metabolism is evaluated by screening all pregnant women at ~24 to 28 weeks of gestation. An oral glucose load of 50 g is administered, and blood is examined for glucose levels 1 hour after administration. Women with a family history of diabetes or previous gestational diabetes should undergo the O'Sullivan test at 15 to 19 weeks of gestation and again at 24 to 28 weeks of gestation.

Clinical Implications
Abnormal O'Sullivan test result is >140 mg/dl glucose.

1. A 3-hour gestational GTT must then be done.
2. A positive result in a pregnant woman means she is at much greater risk (7 times) of having gestational diabetes.

Procedure
A 50-ml venous blood sample (EDTA plasma) is drawn after glucose load. Observe standard precautions.

Patient Preparation
1. Explain test purpose (to evaluate abnormal carbohydrate metabolism) and procedure. No fasting is required.
2. Instruct the woman about obtaining a urine sample for glucose testing to check prior to drinking the glucose load. Positive urine glucose should be checked with the physician prior to glucose load. Those with glycosuria >250 mg/dl must have a blood glucose test prior to O'Sullivan testing.
3. Give the patient 50 g of glucose beverage (150 ml of 100-g glucose [Trutol or Orange DEX]).
4. Explain to the patient that no eating, drinking, or gum chewing is allowed during the test. The patient should not leave the office. She may void if necessary.
5. After 1 hour, the patient is to have 1 EDTA tube (5-ml venous blood) drawn using standard venipuncture technique.

Patient Aftercare
1. Normal activities, eating, and drinking may be resumed.
2. Interpret test results and explain to patient that a normal outcome is <140 mg/dl.
3. A follow-up 3-hour gestational GTT is indicated for all abnormal screenings.

GLUCOSE TOLERANCE TEST (GTT); ORAL GLUCOSE TOLERANCE TEST (OGTT) ●

Normal Values

Fasting
Adult: 70–110 mg/dl or 3.9–6.1 mmol/L
Child: <130 mg/dl or <72 mmol/L

30-Minute
Adult: 110–170 mg/dl or 6.1–9.4 mmol/L

60-Minute (1-Hour)
Adult: 120–170 mg/dl or 6.7–9.4 mmol/L
Child: <140 mg/dl or <7.8 mmol/L

120-Minute (2-Hour)
Adult: 70–120 mg/dl or 3.9–6.7 mmol/L
Child: <140 mg/dl or <7.8 mmol/L

3-Hour
Adult: 70–120 mg/dl or 3.9–6.7 mmol/L

All four blood values must be within normal limits to be considered normal.

Background
In a healthy individual, the insulin response to a large oral glucose dose is almost immediate. It peaks in 30 to 60 minutes and returns to normal levels within 3 hours when sufficient insulin is present to metabolize the glucose ingested at the beginning of the test.

Explanation of Test
If fasting and postprandial glucose test results are borderline, the GTT can support or rule out a diagnosis of diabetes mellitus; it can also be a part of a workup for unexplained hypertriglyceridemia, neuropathy, impotence, renal diseases, or retinopathy. This test may be ordered when there is sugar in the urine or when the fasting blood sugar level or 2-hour postprandial blood sugar level is significantly elevated. The GTT should ***not*** be used as a screening test for nonpregnant adults or children (Table 6-1).

TABLE 6-1
International Classifications for Diabetes Mellitus and Other Glucose Intolerance Categories

Five Major Clinical Classes					Two Statistical Classes	
Type 1	Type 2	Type 3	Type 4	Type 5	No. 1	No. 2
Insulin-dependent diabetes mellitus (IDDM)	Non-insulin-dependent diabetes mellitus (NIDDM) A. Nonobese B. Obese	Diabetes mellitus with other conditions or syndromes	Impaired glucose tolerance (IGT) A. Nonobese B. Obese C. Associated with other diseases or conditions	Gestational diabetes (GDM)	Previous abnormality of glucose tolerance (Prev AGT)	Potential abnormality of glucose tolerance (Pot AGT)
Diagnostic Criteria						
Types 1 and 2		Type 3	Type 4	Type 5	Nos. 1 and 2	
Adults Classic symptoms and unequivocal elevation of plasma glucose *or* Fasting plasma glucose >140 mg/dl more than once *or* Oral glucose tolerance test (challenge dose, 75 g) >200 mg/dl at 1 and 2 h, confirmed by repetition		Same as for IDDM including associated conditions or syndromes	**Adults** Fasting plasma glucose <140 mg/dl; oral glucose tolerance test >200 mg/dl at 1 h; 140–199 mg/dl at 2 h	Two of the following minimum levels: fasting plasma glucose >105 mg/dl; oral glucose tolerance test (challenge dose 100 g) >190 mg/	**Adults** Fasting plasma glucose <115 mg/dl; oral glucose tolerance test <200 mg/dl at 1 h; <140 mg/dl at 2 h **Children** Fasting plasma glucose <130 mg/dl; oral glucose tolerance <140 mg/dl at 2 h	

(continued)

TABLE 6-1 *(Continued)*

<table>
<tr><td colspan="5" align="center">*Diagnostic Criteria*</td></tr>
<tr><td>*Types 1 and 2*</td><td>*Type 3*</td><td>*Type 4*</td><td>*Type 5*</td><td>*Nos. 1 and 2*</td></tr>
<tr>
<td>**Children**
Classic symptoms and random plasma glucose >200 mg/dl
or
Fasting plasma glucose >140 mg/dl more than once
and
Oral glucose tolerance test (challenge dose, 1.75 g/kg ideal body weight, up to a maximum of 75 g) >200 mg/dl at 1 and 2 h, confirmed by repetition</td>
<td></td>
<td>**Children**
Fasting plasma glucose <140 mg/dl; oral glucose tolerance test >140 mg/dl at 2 h</td>
<td>dl at 1 h; >165 mg/dl at 2 h, >145 mg/dl at 3 h</td>
<td></td>
</tr>
</table>

From the National Diabetes Data Group, National Institutes of Health, Bethesda, MD.

Indications for Test

The GTT should be done on certain patients, particularly those with the following indications (few indications still meet wide acceptance):

1. Family history of diabetes
2. Obesity
3. Unexplained episodes of hypoglycemia
4. History of recurrent infections (boils and abscesses)
5. In women, history of delivery of large infants, stillbirths, neonatal death, premature labor, and spontaneous abortions.
6. Transitory glycosuria or hyperglycemia during pregnancy, surgery, trauma, stress, MI, and ACTH administration.

Procedure

This is a timed test. A 2-hour test is done for detecting diabetes in individuals other than pregnant women; the 3-hour test is done for pregnant women; and the 5-hour test evaluates possible hypoglycemia.

1. A diet of ≥150 g of carbohydrates should be eaten for 3 days before the test.
2. The following drugs may influence test results and should be discontinued 3 days before the test:
   a. Hormones, oral contraceptives
   b. Salicylates
   c. Diuretic agents
   d. Hypoglycemic agents
3. Insulin and oral hypoglycemics should be withheld until the test is completed.
4. Record the patient's weight.
   a. Pediatric doses of glucose are based on body weight, calculated as 1.75/kg of body weight to 75 g/kg weight.
   b. Pregnant women: 100 g glucose.
   c. Nonpregnant adult: 75 g glucose.
   d. Possible gestational diabetes: 100g glucose.
5. A 5-ml sample of venous blood is drawn. Serum or gray-topped tubes are used. The patient should fast 12 to 16 hours before testing. After the blood is drawn, the patient drinks all of a specially formulated glucose solution within a 5-minute time frame.
6. Blood samples are obtained at 30 minutes, 1 hour, 2 hours, and 3 hours after glucose ingestion.
7. Specimens taken 4 and 5 hours after ingestion are significant for detecting hypoglycemia and may be ordered.
8. Tolerance tests can also be performed for pentose, lactose, galactose, and D-xylose.
9. The GTT is **not** indicated in these situations:
   a. Persistent fasting hyperglycemia >140 mg/dl
   b. Persistent fasting normal glucose
   c. Patients with overt diabetes mellitus

10. Test has limited value in diagnosis of diabetes mellitus in children and is rarely indicated for that purpose.

Clinical Implications

1. The presence of abnormal GTT values (decreased tolerance to glucose) is based on the International Classification for Diabetes Mellitus and the following glucose intolerance categories:

   a. At least 2 GTT values must be abnormal for a diagnosis of diabetes mellitus to be validated.

   b. In cases of overt diabetes, no insulin is secreted; abnormally high glucose levels persist throughout the test.

   c. Glucose values that fall above normal values but below the diagnostic criteria for diabetes or impaired glucose tolerance (IGT) should be considered nondiagnostic.

2. Interpretation of glucose tolerance levels:

Fasting Adult	140 mg/dl
Adult diabetes mellitus 1-h glucose	>200 mg/dl
and 2-h glucose	>200 mg/dl
Fasting Adult	140 mg/dl
Adult impaired glucose tolerance 1-h glucose	>200 mg/dl
and 2-h glucose	>140–200 mg/dl
Juvenile diabetes mellitus (fasting glucose)	>140 mg/dl
and 1-h glucose	>200 mg/dl
and 2-h glucose	>200 mg/dl
Impaired glucose tolerance in children (fasting glucose) mg/dl	
and 2-h glucose	>140 mg/dl

3. A diagnosis of gestational diabetes is based on the following blood glucose results (≥2 tests must be met and exceeded): fasting, >105 mg/dl; 1-hour, >190 mg/dl; 2-hour, >165 mg/dl; and 3-hour, >145 mg/dl.

   a. All **pregnant** women should be tested for gestational diabetes with a 50-g dose of glucose at 24 to 28 weeks of gestation.

   b. If abnormal results occur during pregnancy, repeat GTT at the first postpartum visit.

   c. During labor, maintain maternal glucose levels at 80 to 100 mg/dl; beware of markedly increased insulin sensitivity in the immediate postpartum period.

4. Decreased glucose tolerance occurs with high glucose values in the following conditions:

   a. Diabetes mellitus
   b. Postgastrectomy
   c. Hyperthyroidism
   d. Excess glucose ingestion
   e. Hyperlipidemia types III, IV, and V
   f. Hemochromatosis
   g. Cushing's disease (steroid effect)

h. CNS lesions

i. Pheochromocytoma

5. Decreased glucose tolerance with hypoglycemia can be found in persons with von Gierke's disease, severe liver damage, or increased epinephrine levels.

6. Increased glucose tolerance with flat curve (ie, glucose does not increase, but may decrease to hypoglycemic levels) occurs in the following conditions:

   a. Pancreatic islet cell hyperplasia or tumor

   b. Poor intestinal absorption caused by diseases such as sprue, celiac disease, or Whipple's disease

   c. Hypoparathyroidism

   d. Addison's disease

   e. Liver disease

   f. Hypopituitarism, hypothyroidism

Interfering Factors

1. Smoking increases glucose levels.

2. Altered diets (eg, weight reduction) before testing can diminish carbohydrate tolerance and suggest "false diabetes."

3. Glucose levels normally tend to increase with aging.

4. Prolonged oral contraceptive use causes significantly higher glucose levels in the second hour or in later blood specimens.

5. Infectious diseases, illnesses, and operative procedures affect glucose tolerance. Two weeks of recovery should be allowed before performing the test.

6. Certain drugs impair glucose tolerance levels (This list is not all inclusive. See Appendix J for other drugs.):

   a. Insulin

   b. Oral hypoglycemics

   c. Large doses of salicylates

   d. Thiazide diuretics

   e. Oral contraceptives

   f. Corticosteroids

   g. Estrogens

   h. Heparin

   i. Nicotinic acid

   j. Phenothiazines

   k. Lithium

   l. Metyrapone (Metopirone)

   If possible, these drugs should be discontinued for at least 3 days before testing. Check with clinician for specific orders.

7. Prolonged bed rest influences glucose tolerance results. If possible, the patient should be ambulatory. A glucose tolerance on a hospitalized patient has limited value.

Patient Preparation

1. Explain test purpose and procedure. A written reminder may be helpful.

   a. A diet high in carbohydrates (150 g) should be eaten for 3 days preceding the test. Instruct the patient to abstain from alcohol.

b. The patient should fast for at least 12 but not more than 16 hours before the test. Only water may be ingested during fasting time and test time. Use of tobacco products is not permitted during testing.

c. Patients should rest or walk quietly during the test period. They may feel weak, faint, or nauseated during the test. Vigorous exercise alters glucose values and should be avoided during testing.

2. Collect blood specimens at the prescribed times and record exact times collected. Urine glucose testing is no longer recommended.

3. Follow guidelines in Chapter 1 for safe, effective, informed *pretest* care.

Patient Aftercare

1. The patient may resume normal diet and activities at the end of the test. Encourage eating complex carbohydrates and protein if permitted.

2. Administer prescribed insulin or oral hypoglycemics when the test is done. Arrange for the patient to eat within a short time (30 minutes) after these medications are taken.

3. Interpret test results and counsel appropriately. Patients newly diagnosed with diabetes will need diet, medication, and lifestyle modification instructions.

4. Follow guidelines in Chapter 1 for safe, effective, informed *posttest* care.

Clinical Alert

1. Glucose tolerance testing is contraindicated in patients with a recent history of surgery, MI, or labor and delivery; these conditions can produce invalid values.

2. If fasting glucose is >140 mg/dl on two separate occasions, or if the 2-hour postprandial blood glucose is >200 mg/dl on two separate occasions, GTT is not necessary for a diagnosis of diabetes mellitus to be established.

3. The GTT is of limited diagnostic value for children.

4. The GTT should be postponed if the patient becomes ill, even with common illnesses such as the flu or a severe cold.

5. Record and report any reactions during the test. Weakness, faintness, and sweating may occur between the second and third hours of the test. If this occurs, a blood sample for a glucose level should be drawn immediately and the GTT aborted.

6. Should the patient vomit the glucose solution, the test is declared invalid; it can be repeated in 3 days (~72 hours).

GLYCOSYLATED HEMOGLOBIN (Hb A$_{1c}$); GLYCOHEMOGLOBIN (G-Hb); DIABETIC CONTROL INDEX

Normal Values

Results are expressed as percentage of total hemoglobin.

G-Hb: 4.8%–7.8%

Hb A$_{1c}$: 4.4%–64.0%

Background

Glycohemoglobin is a normal, minor type of hemoglobin. Glycosylated hemoglobin is formed at a rate proportional to the average glucose concentration by a slow, nonenzymatic process within the red blood cells (RBCs) during their 120-day circulating life span. Glycohemoglobin is blood glucose bound to hemoglobin. In the presence of hyperglycemia, an increase in glycohemoglobin causes an increase in Hb A_{1c}. If the glucose concentration increases because of insulin deficiency, then glycosylation is irreversible.

Explanation of Test

Glycosylated hemoglobin values reflect average blood sugar levels for the 2- to 3-month period before the test. This test provides information for evaluating diabetic treatment modalities, is useful in determining treatment for juvenile-onset diabetes with acute ketoacidosis, and tracks control of blood glucose in milder cases of diabetes. It can be a valuable adjunct in determining which therapeutic choices and directions (eg, oral antihypoglycemic agents, insulin, B-cell transplants) will be most effective. A blood sample can be drawn at any time. The measurement is of particular value for specific groups of patients: diabetic children, diabetics in whom the renal threshold for glucose is abnormal, unstable insulin-dependent diabetics in whom blood sugar levels vary markedly from day to day, type II diabetics who become pregnant, and persons who, before their scheduled appointments, change their usual habits, dietary or otherwise, so that their metabolic control appears better than it actually is.

Procedure

Obtain a 3-ml venous blood sample with EDTA anticoagulant additive. Serum may not be used. Observe standard precautions.

Clinical Implications

1. Values are frequently increased in persons with poorly controlled or newly diagnosed diabetes.
2. With optimal control, the Hb A_{1c} moves toward normal levels.
3. A diabetic patient who recently comes under good control may still show higher concentrations of glycosylated hemoglobin. This level declines gradually over several months as nearly normal glycosylated hemoglobin replaces older RBCs with higher concentrations.
4. Increases in glycosylated hemoglobin occur in the following conditions:
   a. Iron-deficiency anemia
   b. Splenectomy
   c. Alcohol toxicity
   d. Lead toxicity
5. Decreases in glycosylated hemoglobin occur in the following conditions:
   a. Hemolytic anemia
   b. Chronic blood loss
   c. Pregnancy
   d. Chronic renal failure

Interfering Factors

1. Presence of Hb F, S, and H causes falsely elevated values.
2. Presence of Hb S, C, E, D, G and Lepore causes falsely decreased values.

Patient Preparation

1. Explain test purpose and blood-drawing procedure. Observe universal precautions. Fasting is not required.
2. Note that this test is *not* meant for short-term diabetes mellitus management; instead, it assesses the efficacy of long-term management modalities over several weeks or months.
3. Follow guidelines in Chapter 1 for safe, effective, informed *pretest* care.

Patient Aftercare

1. Interpret test outcome and counsel patient appropriately for management of diabetes. If test results are not consistent with clinical findings, check the patient for Hb F, which elevates the A_{1c} results.
2. Follow guidelines in Chapter 1 regarding safe, effective, informed *posttest* care.

> **Clinical Alert**
>
> A number of different tests can determine glycosylated hemoglobin levels. The most specific of these measures is Hb A_{1c}. There are different expected values for each test. Keep in mind that Hb A_1 is always 2% to 4% higher than Hb A_{1c}. When interpreting results, be certain of the specific test used.

LACTOSE TOLERANCE; BREATH HYDROGEN TEST ●

Normal Values

Change in glucose from normal value of >30 mg
    Inconclusive: 20–30 mg/dl
    Abnormal: <20 mg/dl
Hydrogen (breath): <25 ppm increase from baseline

Background

Lactose intolerance often begins in infancy, with symptoms of diarrhea, vomiting, failure to thrive, and malabsorption. The patient becomes asymptomatic when lactose is removed from the diet. This syndrome is caused by a deficiency of sugar-splitting enzymes (lactase) in the intestinal tract.

Explanation of Test

This test is actually a GTT done to diagnose intestinal disaccharidase (lactase) deficiency. Breath samples reveal increased hydrogen levels, which are caused by lactose buildup in the intestinal tract.

Procedure
1. Follow instructions given for the GTT.
2. A blood specimen is drawn from a fasting patient. The patient then drinks 50 g of lactose mixed with 200 ml of water.
3. Blood lactose samples are drawn at 0, 30-, 60-, and 90-minute intervals.
4. Hydrogen breath samples are taken at the same time intervals as the blood specimens. Contact your laboratory for collection procedures.

Clinical Implications
1. Lactose intolerance occurs as follows:
   a. A "flat" lactose tolerance finding (ie, no rise in glucose) points to a deficiency of sugar-splitting enzymes, as in irritable bowel syndrome. This type of deficiency is more prevalent in American Indians, African Americans, Asians, and Jews.
   b. A monosaccharide tolerance test such as the glucose/galactose tolerance test should be done as a follow-up.
      (1) The patient ingests 25 g of both glucose and galactose.
      (2) A normal increase in glucose indicates a lactose deficiency.
   c. The hydrogen breath test is abnormal in the lactose deficiency test because:
      (1) Malabsorption causes hydrogen (H_2) production through the process of fermentation in the colon.
      (2) The H_2 formed is directly proportional to the amount of test dose lactose **not** absorbed.
   d. In diabetes, blood glucose values may show increases of >20 mg/dl despite impaired lactose absorption.

Patient Preparation
1. Explain test purpose and procedure. The patient must fast for 12 hours prior to the test.
2. No dark bread, peas, beans, sugars, or high-fiber foods should be eaten within 24 hours of the test.
3. Smoking is not permitted during the test and for 8 hours prior to testing.
4. No antibiotics should be taken for 2 weeks prior to the test unless specifically ordered.
5. Follow guidelines in Chapter 1 for safe, effective, informed *pretest* care.

Patient Aftercare
1. Resume normal diet and activity.
2. Interpret test results and counsel appropriately. Patients with irritable bowel syndrome with gas, bloating, abdominal pain, constipation, and diarrhea have lactose deficiency. Restricting milk intake relieves symptoms.
3. Follow guidelines in Chapter 1 regarding safe, effective, informed *posttest* care.

● END PRODUCTS OF METABOLISM AND OTHER TESTS

AMMONIA (NH$_3$)   ●

Normal Values
Adult: 9–33 μmol/L
Child: 21–50 μmol/L
Infant (<2 wk): 56–92 μmol/L
Neonate: 64–107 μmol/L

Values test somewhat higher in capillary blood samples. Values can vary greatly with testing method used.

Background
Ammonia, an end product of protein metabolism, is formed by bacteria acting on intestinal proteins together with glutamine hydrolysis in the kidneys. The liver normally removes most of this ammonia via the portal vein circulation and converts the ammonia to urea. Because any appreciable level of ammonia in the blood affects the body's acid-base balance and brain function, its removal from the body is essential. The liver accomplishes this by synthesizing urea so that it can be excreted by the kidneys.

Explanation of Test
Blood ammonia levels are used to diagnose Reye's syndrome, to evaluate metabolism, and to determine the progress of severe liver disease and its response to treatment. Blood ammonia measurements are useful in monitoring patients on hyperalimentation therapy.

Procedure
1. Obtain a 3-ml venous plasma sample from a fasting patient. Heparinize the sample. Observe standard precautions.
2. Place the sample in an iced container, and perform the test within 20 minutes.
3. Note all antibiotics the patient is receiving; these drugs lower ammonia levels.

Clinical Implications
1. *Increased ammonia levels* occur in the following conditions:
   a. Reye's syndrome
   b. Liver disease, cirrhosis
   c. Hepatic coma (does not reflect degree of coma)
   d. GI hemorrhage
   e. Renal disease
   f. Shock

g. Transient hyperammonemia of newborn

h. Certain inborn errors of metabolism (eg, argininosuccinicaciduria)

i. GI tract infection with distention and stasis

2. *Decreased ammonia levels* occur in hyperornithinemia.

Interfering Factors

1. Ammonia levels vary with protein intake and many drugs.

2. Exercise may cause an increase in ammonia levels.

3. Ammonia levels may be increased by use of a tight tourniquet or by tightly clenching the fist while samples are drawn.

Patient Preparation

1. Explain test purpose and procedure. Instruct the patient to fast (if possible) for 8 hours before the blood test. Water is permitted.

2. Follow guidelines in Chapter 1 regarding safe, effective, informed *pretest* care.

Patient Aftercare

1. Interpret test outcomes, monitor appropriately, and begin treatment.

2. In patients with impaired liver function demonstrated by elevated ammonia levels, the blood ammonia level can be lowered by reduced protein intake and by use of antibiotics to reduce intestinal bacteria counts.

3. Follow guidelines in Chapter 1 for safe, effective, informed *posttest* care.

> ### Clinical Alert
>
> Ammonia should be measured in all cases of unexplained lethargy and vomiting, in encephalitis, or in any neonate with unexplained neurologic deterioration.

BILIRUBIN

Normal Values

Adult

Total: 0.2–1.3 mg/dl or 3.4–17.1 μmol/L

Conjugated (direct): 0.0–0.2 mg/dl or 0.0–3.4 μmol/L

Background

Bilirubin results from the breakdown of hemoglobin in the red blood cells and is a byproduct of hemolysis (ie, red blood cell destruction). It is produced by the reticuloendothelial system. Removed from the body by the liver, which excretes it into the bile, it gives the bile its major pigmentation. Usually, a small amount of bilirubin is found in the serum. A rise in serum bilirubin levels occurs when there is an excessive destruction of red blood cells or when the liver is unable to excrete the normal amounts of bilirubin produced.

There are two forms of bilirubin in the body: indirect or unconjugated bilirubin, which is protein bound, and direct or conjugated bilirubin, which circulates freely in the blood until it reaches the liver, where it is conjugated with glucuronide transferase and then excreted into the bile. An increase in protein-bound bilirubin (unconjugated bilirubin) is more frequently associated with increased destruction of red blood cells (hemolysis); an increase in free-flowing bilirubin is more likely seen in dysfunction or blockage of the liver. A routine examination measures only the total bilirubin. A normal level of total bilirubin rules out any significant impairment of the excretory function of the liver or excessive hemolysis of red cells. Only when total bilirubin levels are elevated will there be a call for differentiation of the bilirubin levels by conjugated and unconjugated types.

Explanation of Test
The measurement of bilirubin allows evaluation of liver function and hemolytic anemias. This test is not suitable for infants younger than 15 days (see Neonatal Bilirubin).

Procedure
1. Obtain a 5-ml non-hemolyzed sample from a fasting patient. Observe standard precautions. Serum is used.
2. Protect the sample from ultraviolet light (sunlight).
3. Avoid air bubbles and unnecessary shaking of the sample during blood collection.
4. If the specimen cannot be examined immediately, store it away from light and in a refrigerator.

Clinical Implications
1. *Total bilirubin elevations accompanied by jaundice* may be due to hepatic, obstructive, or hemolytic causes.
   a. *Hepatocellular jaundice* results from injury or disease of the parenchymal cells of the liver and can be caused by the following conditions:
      (1) Viral hepatitis
      (2) Cirrhosis
      (3) Infectious mononucleosis
      (4) Reactions of certain drugs such as chlorpromazine
   b. *Obstructive jaundice* is usually the result of obstruction of the common bile or hepatic ducts due to stones or neoplasms. The obstruction produces high conjugated bilirubin levels due to bile regurgitation.
   c. *Hemolytic jaundice* is due to overproduction of bilirubin resulting from hemolytic processes that produce high levels of unconjugated bilirubin. Hemolytic jaundice can be found in the following conditions:
      (1) After blood transfusions, especially those involving many units
      (2) Pernicious anemia
      (3) Sickle cell anemia
      (4) Transfusion reactions (ABO or Rh incompatibility)

    (5) Crigler-Najjar syndrome (a severe disease that results from a ge-
netic deficiency of a hepatic enzyme needed for the conjugation
of bilirubin)

    (6) Erythroblastosis fetalis (see Neonatal Bilirubin)

2. *Elevated indirect* **unconjugated** *bilirubin levels* occur in the following
conditions:

    a. Hemolytic anemias due to a large hematoma

    b. Trauma in the presence of a large hematoma

    c. Hemorrhagic pulmonary infarcts

    d. Crigler-Najjar syndrome (rare)

    e. Gilbert's disease (conjugated hyperbilirubinemia; rare)

3. *Elevated direct* **conjugated** *bilirubin levels* occur in the following conditions:

    a. Cancer of the head of the pancreas

    b. Choledocholithiasis

    c. Dubin-Johnson syndrome

Interfering Factors

1. A 1-hour exposure of the specimen to sunlight or high-intensity artificial
light at room temperature will decrease the bilirubin content.

2. No contrast media should be administered 24 hours before measurement;
a high-fat meal may also cause decreased bilirubin levels by interfering with
the chemical reactions.

3. Air bubbles and shaking of the specimen may cause decreased bilirubin
levels.

4. Certain foods (eg, carrots, yams) and drugs (see Appendix J) increase the
yellow hue in the serum and can falsely increase bilirubin levels when tests
are done using certain methods (eg, spectrophotometer).

5. Prolonged fasting raises the bilirubin level, as does anorexia.

Clinical Alert

Panic Value for Bilirubin in Adults
>12 mg/dl

Patient Preparation

1. Explain test purpose and procedure and relation of results to jaundice.

    Jaundice/Icterus: Excessive amounts of bilirubin eventually seep into the
tissues, which assume a yellow hue as a result. This yellow color is a clinical
sign of jaundice. In newborns, signs of jaundice may indicate hemolytic anemia or congenital icterus. Total bilirubin must be >2.5 mg/dl to detect jaundice in adults.

2. The patient should be fasting, if possible.

3. Follow guidelines in Chapter 1 for safe, effective, informed *pretest* care.

Patient Aftercare

1. Interpret test outcome and monitor appropriately.
2. Resume normal activities.
3. Follow guidelines in Chapter 1 for safe, effective, informed *posttest* care.

NEONATAL BILIRUBIN, TOTAL AND FRACTIONATED
("BABY BILI")

Normal Values

Newborn (0–7 d)
  Total: 1.0–10.0 mg/dl
  Conjugated (direct): 0.0–0.8 mg/dl
  Unconjugated (indirect): 0.0–10.0 mg/dl
  Cord blood total: <2.0 mg/dl

Background

In newborns, signs of jaundice may indicate hemolytic anemia or congenital icterus. If bilirubin levels reach a critical point in the infant, damage to the CNS may occur in a condition known as *kernicterus*. Therefore, in these infants, the level of bilirubin is the deciding factor in whether or not to perform an exchange transfusion. Total bilirubin must be >5.0 mg/dl to detect jaundice in newborns.

Jaundice may also be seen in babies who are breast-feeding due to low milk intake and subsequent lack of vitamin K–dependent clotting factors. This condition usually resolves within 1 week.

Explanation of Test

Neonatal bilirubin is used to monitor erythroblastosis fetalis (hemolytic disease of the newborn), which usually causes jaundice in the first 2 days of life. All other causes of neonatal jaundice, including physiologic jaundice, hematoma/ hemorrhage, liver disease, and biliary disease should also be monitored. Normal, full-term neonates experience a normal, neonatal, physiologic, transient hyperbilirubinemia by the third day of life which rapidly falls by the fifth to tenth day of life.

Procedure

1. Draw blood from heel of newborn using a capillary pipette and amber Microtainer tube; 0.5 ml of serum is needed. Cord blood may also be used.
2. Protect sample from light.

Clinical Implications

1. *Elevated total bilirubin* (neonatal) is associated with the following conditions:
   a. Erythroblastosis fetalis occurs as a result of blood incompatibility between mother and fetus.
     (1) Rh (D) antibodies and other Rh factors
     (2) ABO antibodies
     (3) Other blood groups, including KIDD, KELL, and DUFFY (see Chapter 8).

b. Galactosemia

c. Sepsis

d. Infectious diseases (eg, syphilis, toxoplasmosis, cytomegalovirus)

e. Red blood cell enzyme abnormalities

    (1) G6PD

    (2) Pyruvate kinase (PK) deficiency

    (3) Spherocytosis

f. Subdural hematoma, hemangiomas

2. *Elevated unconjugated (indirect) neonatal bilirubin* is associated with the following conditions:

a. Erythroblastosis fetalis

b. Hypothyroidism

c. Crigler-Najjar syndrome

d. Obstructive jaundice

e. Infants of diabetic mothers

3. *Elevated conjugated (direct) neonatal bilirubin* is associated with the following conditions:

a. Biliary obstruction

b. Neonatal hepatitis

c. Sepsis

Clinical Alert

Panic Value for Neonatal Bilirubin
>15 mg/dl (mental retardation can occur)

Patient Preparation

1. Explain test purpose and procedure and its relation to jaundice to the mother.

Patient Aftercare

1. Interpret test outcome and monitor appropriately.

2. For slight elevations (ie, <10.0 mg/dl), phototherapy may be initiated.

3. Monitor neonatal bilirubin levels to determine indication for exchange transfusion. Test should be done every 12 hours in jaundiced newborns.

Indications for Exchange Transfusion

Birth Weight (g)	Serum Bilirubin (mg/dl)
<1000	10.0
1001–1250	13.0
1251–1500	15.0
1501–2000	17.0
2001–2500	18.0
>2500	20.0

Transfuse at one step earlier in the presence of the following conditions:

Serum protein <5 g/dl
Metabolic acidosis (pH <7.25)
Respiratory distress (with O_2 <50 mm Hg)
Certain clinical findings (eg, hypothermia, CNS, or other clinical deterioration; sepsis; hemolysis)

Other criteria for exchange transfusion are suddenness and rate of bilirubin increase and when such an increase occurs; for example, an increase of 3 mg/dl in 12 hours, especially after bilirubin has already leveled off, must be followed by frequent serial determinations, especially if it occurs on the first or seventh day of life rather than on the third day. Beware of a rate of bilirubin increase of >1 mg/dl during the first day of life. Serum bilirubin of 10 mg/dl after 24 hours or 15 mg/dl after 48 hours despite phototherapy usually indicates that serum bilirubin will reach 20 mg/dl.

BLOOD UREA NITROGEN (BUN, UREA NITROGEN)

Normal Values
Adult: 7–18 mg/dl or 2.5–6.4 mmol/L
Elderly (>60 y): 8–20 mg/dl or 2.9–7.5 mmol/L
Child: 5–18 mg/dl or 1.8–6.4 mmol/L

Background
Urea forms in the liver and, along with CO_2, constitutes the final product of protein metabolism. The amount of excreted urea varies directly with dietary protein intake, increased excretion in fever, diabetes, and increased adrenal gland activity.

Explanation of Test
The test for BUN, which measures the nitrogen portion of urea, is used as an index of glomerular function in the production and excretion of urea. Rapid protein catabolism and impairment of kidney function will result in an elevated BUN level. The rate at which the BUN level rises is influenced by the degree of tissue necrosis, protein catabolism, and the rate at which the kidneys excrete the urea nitrogen. A markedly increased BUN is conclusive evidence of severe impaired glomerular function. In chronic renal disease, the BUN level correlates better with symptoms of uremia than does the serum creatinine.

Procedure
Obtain a 5-ml venous blood sample. Serum is preferred. Observe universal precautions.

Clinical Implications
1. *Increased BUN levels (azotemia)* occur in the following conditions:
   a. Impaired renal function caused by the following conditions:
      (1) Congestive heart failure
      (2) Salt and water depletion

(3) Shock

(4) Stress

(5) Acute MI

b. Chronic renal disease such as glomerulonephritis and pyelonephritis.

c. Urinary tract obstruction

d. Hemorrhage into GI tract

e. Diabetes mellitus with ketoacidosis

f. Excessive protein intake or protein catabolism as occurs in burns or cancer.

2. *Decreased BUN levels* are associated with the following conditions:

a. Liver failure (severe liver disease) such as that resulting from hepatitis, drugs, or poisoning

b. Acromegaly

c. Malnutrition, low-protein diets

d. Anabolic steroid use

e. Impaired absorption (celiac disease)

f. Nephrotic syndrome (occasional)

g. SIADH

Interfering Factors

1. A combination of a low-protein and high-carbohydrate diet can cause a decreased BUN level.

2. The BUN is normally lower in children and women because they have less muscle mass than adult men.

3. Decreased BUN values normally occur in late pregnancy because of increased plasma volume (physiologic hydremia).

4. Older persons may have an increased BUN when their kidneys are not able to concentrate urine adequately.

5. IV feedings only may result in overhydration and increased BUN levels.

6. Many drugs may cause increased or decreased BUN levels.

Clinical Alert

1. If a patient is confused, disoriented, or has convulsions, the BUN level should be checked. If the level is high, it may help to explain these signs and symptoms.

2. Panic value for BUN is >100 mg/dl.

Patient Preparation

1. Explain test purpose and blood-drawing procedure. Assess dietary history.

2. Follow guidelines in Chapter 1 for safe, effective, informed *pretest* care.

Patient Aftercare

1. Interpret test outcome and monitor as appropriate for impaired kidney function.

2. In patients with an elevated BUN level, fluid and electrolyte regulation may be impaired.
3. Follow guidelines in Chapter 1 for safe, effective, informed *posttest* care.

CHOLINESTERASE, SERUM (PSEUDOCHOLINESTERASE); CHOLINESTERASE, RED BLOOD CELL ●

Normal Values
Serum cholinesterase: 4.9–11.9 U/ml or kU/L
Dibucaine inhibition: 79%–84%
RBC cholinesterase: 6700–10,000 U/L

Values vary with substrate and method. These are two different tests.

Background
The cholinesterase of serum is referred to as pseudocholinesterase to distinguish it from the true cholinesterase of the red blood cell (RBC). Both of these enzymes act on acetylcholine and other cholinesters. Alkylphosphates are potent inhibitors of both serum and RBC cholinesterase.

Patients who are homozygous for the atypical gene that controls serum cholinesterase activity have low levels of cholinesterase that are not inhibited by dibucaine. Persons with normal serum cholinesterase activity show 70% to 90% inhibition by dibucaine.

Explanation of Test
These are two separate tests. The primary use of serum cholinesterase measurement (pseudocholinesterase) is to monitor the effect of muscle relaxants (eg, succinylcholine), which are used in surgery. Patients for whom suxamethonium anesthesia is planned should be tested using the dibucaine inhibition test for the presence of atypical cholinesterase variants which are incapable of hydrolyzing this widely used muscle relaxant.

The RBC cholinesterase test is used when poisoning by pesticides such as Parathion or Malathion is suspected. Severe insecticide poisoning causes headaches, visual distortions, nausea, vomiting, pulmonary edema, confusion, convulsions, respiratory paralysis, and coma.

Procedures
1. Serum cholinesterase: obtain a 5-ml blood sample; 3 ml of serum is needed. The test must be performed within 48 hours of collection. Observe standard precautions.
2. RBC cholinesterase: a blood sample is drawn using sodium heparin as an anticoagulant; serum cannot be used. Observe standard precautions.

Clinical Implications
1. *Decreased or no serum cholinesterase* occurs in the following conditions:
   a. Congenital inherited recessive disease. These patients are not able to hydrolyze drugs such as muscle relaxants used in surgery. These patients

may have a prolonged period of apnea and possibly die if they are given succinylcholine.

b. Poisoning from organic phosphate insecticides

c. Liver diseases, hepatitis, cirrhosis with jaundice

d. Conditions that may have decreased blood albumin, such as malnutrition, anemia, infections, skin diseases, and acute MI

e. Congestive heart failure

2. *Decreased RBC cholinesterase levels* occur in the following conditions:

a. Congenital inherited recessive disease

b. Organic phosphate poisoning

c. Evaluation of paroxysmal nocturnal hemoglobinemia

d. Anemia

e. Tuberculosis

f. Hypoproteinemia

g. Uremia

h. Shock

3. *Increased serum cholinesterase* is found in in the following conditions:

a. Type IV hyperlipidemia

b. Nephrosis

c. Obesity

d. Diabetes

4. *Increased RBC cholinesterase* is associated with reticulocytosis.

Patient Preparation

1. Explain test purpose and procedure.

2. Draw blood for serum cholinesterase 2 days before surgery.

3. Blood should not be drawn in the recovery room; prior administration of surgical drugs and anesthesia invalidates the test results.

4. Follow guidelines in Chapter 1 for safe, effective, informed *pretest* care.

Patient Aftercare

1. Interpret test outcome and counsel appropriately.

2. Patients exhibiting <70% inhibition should be considered as an atypical cholinesterase variant, and the administration of succinylcholine or similar type drugs may pose a risk.

3. Follow guidelines in Chapter 1 for safe, effective, informed *posttest* care.

Clinical Alert

1. In industrial exposure, workers should not return to work until cholinesterase values rise to at least 75% of normal. Red blood cell cholinesterase regenerates at the rate of 1% per day. Plasma cholinesterase regenerates at the rate of 25% in 7 to 10 days and returns to baseline in 4 to 6 weeks.

2. Cholinesterase activity is completely and irreversibly inhibited by organophosphate pesticides.

CREATININE ●

Normal Values
Adult: 0.6–1.5 mg/dl or 62–125 μmol/L
Child (3–18 y): 0.5–1.0 mg/dl or 44–88 μmol/L
Young child (0–3 y): 0.3–0.7 mg/dl or 27–62 μmol/L
BUN/creatinine ratio: 10:1 to 20:1

Background
Creatinine is a byproduct in the breakdown of muscle creatine phosphate resulting from energy metabolism. It is produced at a constant rate depending on the muscle mass of the person and is removed from the body by the kidneys. Production of creatinine is constant as long as muscle mass remains constant. A disorder of kidney function reduces excretion of creatinine, resulting in increased blood creatinine levels.

Explanation of Test
This test diagnoses impaired renal function. It is a more specific and sensitive indicator of kidney disease than BUN, although in chronic renal disease, both BUN and creatinine are ordered to evaluate renal problems, because the BUN/creatinine ratio provides more information.

Procedure
Obtain a 5-ml venous blood sample. Serum is preferred, but heparinized blood can be used. Observe standard precautions.

Clinical Implications
1. *Increased blood creatinine levels* occur in the following conditions:
   a. Impaired renal function
   b. Chronic nephritis
   c. Obstruction of urinary tract
   d. Muscle disease
      (1) Gigantism
      (2) Acromegaly
      (3) Myasthenia gravis
      (4) Muscular dystrophy
      (5) Poliomyelitis
   e. Congestive heart failure
   f. Shock
   g. Dehydration
   h. Rhabdomyolysis
2. *Decreased creatinine levels* occur in the following conditions:
   a. Small stature
   b. Decreased muscle mass
   c. Advanced and severe liver disease
   d. Inadequate dietary protein

   e. Pregnancy (0.4–0.6 mg/dl is normal; >0.8 mg/dl is abnormal and should be noted)

3. *Increased ratio* (>20:1) with normal creatinine occurs in the following conditions:

   a. Increased BUN (prerenal azotemia), heart failure, salt depletion, dehydration

   b. Catabolic states with tissue breakdown

   c. GI hemorrhage

   d. Impaired renal function plus excess protein intake, production, or tissue breakdown

4. *Increased ratio* (>20:1) with elevated creatinine occurs in the following conditions:

   a. Obstruction of urinary tract

   b. Prerenal azotemia with renal disease

5. *Decreased ratio* (<10:1) with decreased BUN occurs in the following conditions:

   a. Acute tubular necrosis

   b. Decreased urea synthesis as in severe liver disease or starvation

   c. Repeated dialysis

   d. SIADH

   e. Pregnancy

6. *Decreased ratio* (<10:1) with increased creatinine occurs in the following conditions:

   a. Phenacemide therapy (accelerates conversion of creatine to creatinine)

   b. Rhabdomyolysis (releases muscle creatinine)

   c. Muscular patients who develop renal failure

Interfering Factors

1. High levels of ascorbic acid and cephalosporin antibiotics can cause a falsely increased creatinine level; these agents also interfere with BUN/creatinine ratio.

2. Drugs that influence kidney function plus other medications can cause a change in the blood creatinine level (see Appendix J).

3. A diet high in meat can cause increased creatinine levels.

4. Creatinine is falsely decreased by bilirubin, glucose, histidine, and quinidine compounds.

5. Ketoacidosis may increase serum creatinine substantially.

▶ Clinical Alert

1. Panic value is 10 mg/dl in nondialysis patients.

2. Creatinine level should always be checked before administering nephrotoxic chemotherapeutics such as methotrexate, cisplatin, cyclophosphamide, mithramycin, and semustine.

Patient Preparation

1. Explain test purpose and procedure.
2. Assess diet for meat intake.
3. Follow guidelines in Chapter 1 for safe, effective, informed *pretest* care.

Patient Aftercare

1. Interpret test results and monitor as appropriate for impaired renal function.
2. Follow guidelines in Chapter 1 for safe, effective, informed *posttest* care.

URIC ACID ●

Normal Values

Men: 3.5–7.2 mg/dl or 0.21–0.42 mmol/L
Women: 2.6–6.0 mg/dl or 0.154–0.35 mmol/L
Children: 2.0–5.5 mg/dl or 0.12–0.32 mmol/L

Background

Uric acid is formed from the breakdown of nucleonic acids and is an end product of purine metabolism. A lack of the enzyme uricase allows this poorly soluble substance to accumulate in body fluids. Two thirds of the uric acid produced daily is excreted by the kidneys, whereas the remaining one third exits by the stool. The basis for this test is that an overproduction of uric acids occurs when there is excessive cell breakdown and catabolism of nucleonic acids (as in gout), excessive production and destruction of cells (as in leukemia), or an inability to excrete the substance produced (as in renal failure).

Explanation of Test

Measurement of uric acid is used most commonly in the evaluation of renal failure, gout, and leukemia. In hospitalized patients, renal failure is the most common cause of elevated uric acid levels, and gout is the least common cause.

Procedure

Obtain a 5-ml venous blood sample. Serum is preferred; heparinized blood is acceptable. Observe standard precautions.

Clinical Implications

1. *Elevated uric acid levels (hyperuricemia)* occur in the following conditions:
    a. Gout (the amount of increase is not directly related to the severity of the disease)
    b. Renal diseases and renal failure, prerenal azotemia
    c. Alcoholism
    d. Down syndrome

    e. Lead poisoning
    f. Leukemia, multiple myeloma
    g. Lymphoma
    h. Starvation, weight-loss diets
    i. Metabolic acidosis
    j. Toxemia of pregnancy (serial determination to follow therapy)
    k. Liver disease
    l. Hyperlipidemia, obesity
    m. Hypoparathyroidism, hypothyroidism
    n. Hemolytic anemia, sickle cell anemia
    o. Following excessive cell destruction, as in chemotherapy and radiation treatment
    p. Psoriasis
2. *Decreased levels of uric acid* occur in the following conditions:
    a. Fanconi's syndrome
    b. Wilson's disease
    c. SIADH
    d. Some malignancies (eg, Hodgkin's disease, multiple myeloma)
    e. Xanthinuria (deficiency of xanthine oxidase)

Interfering Factors

1. Stress and strenuous exercise will falsely elevate uric acid.
2. Many drugs cause increase or decrease of uric acid (see Appendix J).
3. Purine-rich diet (eg, liver, kidney, sweetbreads) increases uric acid levels.
4. High levels of aspirin decrease uric acid levels.

Patient Preparation

1. Advise patient of test purpose and blood-drawing procedure.
2. Promote relaxation; avoid strenuous exercise.
3. Follow guidelines in Chapter 1 for safe, effective, informed *pretest* care.

Patient Aftercare

1. Resume normal activities.
2. Interpret test results and monitor appropriately for renal failure, gout, or leukemia. Uric acid level should fall in patients who are treated with uricosuric drugs such as allopurinol, probenecid, and sulfinpyrazone.
3. Follow guidelines in Chapter 1 for safe, effective, informed *posttest* care.

Clinical Alert

1. Monitor uric acid levels during treatment of leukemia.
2. Acute, dangerous levels may occur following administration of cytotoxic drugs.

LEAD (Pb)

Normal Values
0–10 µg/dl

Background
Lead is absorbed into the body through both the respiratory and GI tracts. It also moves transplacentally to the fetus. Absorption through these different routes varies and is affected by age, nutritional status, particle size, and chemical form of the lead. Absorption is inversely proportional to particle size; this factor that makes lead-bearing dust important. Adults absorb 6% to 10% of dietary lead and retain very little of it; however, children from birth to 2 years of age have been shown to absorb 40% to 50% and to retain 20% to 25% of dietary lead. Spontaneous excretion of lead in urine by infants and young toddlers is normally about 1 µg/kg/24 hours, which may increase somewhat in cases of acute poisoning. Dietary intake of lead is <1 µg/kg, which provides a margin of safety in the sense that a child goes into positive lead balance when intake exceeds 5 µg/kg of body weight. Early symptoms of lead poisoning include anorexia, apathy or irritability, fatigue, and anemia. Toxic effects include GI distress, joint pain, colic, headache, stupor, convulsions, and coma. Another test that may be used to evaluate lead intoxication is free erythrocyte protoporphyrin. However, a blood lead assay is the definitive test.

Explanation of Test
The blood lead assay is used to screen adults and children for lead poisoning (plumbism). In adults, high levels are caused mainly by industrial exposure from lead-based paints, gasoline, and ceramics. High-risk children usually are aged 3 to 12 years and live in or visit old, dilapidated housing with lead-based paint.

Procedure
Obtain a sample by fingerstick using lead-free heparinized capillary tubes or venous blood drawn in a 3-ml trace element–free tube. Do not separate plasma from cells. Refrigerate the sample. Observe standard precautions.

Clinical Implications
1. Blood lead levels in adults:
   a. <10 µg/dl is normal without occupational exposure.
   b. <20 µg/dl is acceptable with occupational exposure.
   c. 25 µg/dl: report to state occupational agency.
   d. >60 µg/dl: remove from occupational exposure and begin chelation therapy.

U.S. Centers for Disease Control and Prevention		
Class	*Blood Lead**	*Action*
I	<10 μg/dl	Not lead poisoned
IIA	10–14 μg/dl	Rescreen frequently and consider prevention activities
IIB	15–19 μg/dl	Institute nutritional and educational interventions
III	20–44 μg/dl	Evaluate environment and consider chelation therapy
IV	45–69 μg/dl	Institute environmental intervention and chelation therapy
V	>69 μg/dl	Medical emergency

*Owing to possible contamination during collection, elevated levels should be confirmed with a second specimen before therapy is instituted.

Interfering Factors
1. Failing to use lead-free Vacutainer tubes invalidates results.

Clinical Alert

1. Critical values:
   a. <15 years of age, >20 μg/dl; ≥15 years of age, >30 μg/dl
   b. Blood lead concentrations ≥70 μg/dl whole blood (class V) should be hospitalized immediately and treated as medical emergencies.
   c. A single lead determination cannot distinguish between chronic and acute exposure.

Patient Preparation
1. Explain test purpose and procedure.
2. Explain the importance of follow-up if lead levels are elevated.

Patient Aftercare
1. Resume normal activities.
2. Interpret test results and counsel appropriately for elevated lead levels.
   a. Parental compliance is necessary. Parent education about lead poisoning can be given face-to-face, by pamphlet distribution, or in both ways.
   b. The most important component of medical management is to facilitate reduction in the child's exposure to the environmental lead. In providing intervention for the child with an elevated blood lead level, the initial step is to obtain a detailed environmental history. The causes of childhood lead poisoning are multiple and must take into account potential environmental hazards as well as characteristics of the individual child. Once a child is found to have lead intoxication, all potential sources must be identified.

c. The recommended diet for a child with lead toxicity is simply a good diet with adequate protein and mineral intake and limitation of excess fat. It is no longer necessary to exclude canned foods and beverages when the cans are manufactured in the United States, because the manufacture of cans with lead-soldered seams ended in the U.S. in 1991.

d. Iron deficiency can enhance absorption and toxicity of lead and often coexists with overexposure to lead. All children with a blood lead concentration ≥20 μg/dl whole blood should have appropriate testing for iron deficiency.

e. In class IV lead intoxication, chelation is necessary. Chelation therapy must be done in conjunction with eliminating the source of the lead poisoning. Chelation therapy, when promptly administered, can be life-saving and can reduce the period of morbidity associated with lead toxicity.

● HORMONE TESTS

ANDROSTANEDIONE ●

Normal Values
Child: 0.08–0.5 ng/ml
Woman: 0.47–2.68 ng/ml
Man: 0.57–2.65 ng/ml
Postmenopausal woman: <1.0 ng/ml

Background
Androstanedione is one of the major androgens produced by the ovaries in females, and to a lesser extent in the adrenals in both genders. This hormone is converted to estrogens by hepatic enzymes.

Explanation of Test
This hormone measurement is helpful in the evaluation of conditions characterized by hirsutism and virilization.

Procedure
1. Obtain a 5-ml venous blood sample in the morning and place on ice. Observe standard precautions.
2. In women, collect this specimen 1 week before or after the menstrual period. Record date of last menstrual period on the laboratory form.

Clinical Implications
1. *Increased androstanedione values* are associated with the following conditions:
   a. Stein-Leventhal syndrome
   b. Cushing's syndrome

   c. Certain ovarian tumors

   d. Ectopic ACTH-producing tumor

   e. Late-onset congenital adrenal hyperplasia

   f. Ovarian stromal hyperplasia

2. *Decreased androstanedione values* are found in the following conditions:

   a. Sickle-cell anemia

   b. Adrenal and ovarian failure

Patient Preparation

1. Explain purpose of test and blood-drawing procedure.

2. Patient should be fasting and blood should be drawn at peak production (7:00 AM).

3. Collect specimen 1 week before menstrual period in women.

4. Follow guidelines in Chapter 1 for safe, effective, informed *pretest* care.

Patient Aftercare

1. Resume normal activities.

2. Interpret test results and counsel appropriately for ovarian and adrenal dysfunction.

3. Follow guidelines in Chapter 1 for safe, effective, informed *posttest* care.

ALDOSTERONE   ●

Normal Values

Adult: 7–30 ng/dl or 0.19–0.83 nmol/L
Adolescent: 4–48 ng/dl or 0.11–1.33 nmol/L
Child: 5–80 mg/dl or 0.14–2.22 nmol/L
Low-sodium diet: values 3–5 times higher

Background

Aldosterone is a mineralocorticoid hormone produced in the adrenal zona glomerulosa under complex control by the renin-angiotensin system. Its action is on the renal distal tubule, where it increases resorption of sodium and water at the expense of increased potassium excretion.

Explanation of Test

This test is useful in detecting primary or secondary aldosteronism. Patients with primary aldosteronism characteristically have hypertension, muscular pains and cramps, weakness, tetany, paralysis, and polyuria. It is also used to evaluate causes of hypertension.

Procedure

1. Plasma is taken with the patient in an upright position for 2 hours and with unrestricted salt intake.

2. Obtain a 5-ml venous blood specimen in a heparinized or EDTA Vacutainer tube. The cells must be separated from plasma immediately. Obtain the specimen in the morning after the patient has been upright for at least 2 hours. Blood should be drawn with patient sitting. Observe standard precautions.

3. Specify and record the time of the venipuncture. Circadian rhythm exists in normal subjects, with levels of aldosterone peaking in the morning.
4. A 24-hour urine specimen with boric acid preservative may also be ordered. Refrigerate immediately following collection.

Clinical Implications

1. *Elevated levels of aldosterone (primary aldosteronism)* occur in the following conditions:
   a. Aldosterone-producing adenoma (Conn's disease)
   b. Adrenocortical hyperplasia (pseudoprimary aldosteronism)
   c. Indeterminate hyperaldosteronism
   d. Glucocorticoid remediable hyperaldosteronism
2. *Secondary aldosteronism,* in which aldosterone output is elevated due to external stimuli or because of greater activity in the renin-angiotensin system, occurs in the following conditions:
   a. Salt depletion
   b. Potassium loading
   c. Laxative abuse
   d. Cardiac failure
   e. Cirrhosis of liver with ascites
   f. Nephrotic syndrome
   g. Bartter's syndrome
   h. Diuretic abuse
   i. Hypovolemia and hemorrhage
   j. After 10 days of starvation
   k. Toxemia of pregnancy
3. *Decreased aldosterone levels* are found in the following conditions:
   a. Aldosterone deficiency
   b. Addison's disease
   c. Syndrome of renin deficiency (very rare)
   d. Low aldosterone levels associated with hypertension are found in Turner's syndrome, diabetes mellitus, and alcohol intoxication

Interfering Factors

1. Values are increased by upright posture.
2. Recently administered radioactive medications affect test outcomes.
3. Heparin therapy causes levels to fall. See Appendix J for drugs that increase and decrease levels.
4. Thermal stress, late pregnancy, and starvation cause levels to rise.
5. Aldosterone levels decrease with age.

Clinical Alert

1. The simultaneous measurement of aldosterone and renin is helpful in differentiating primary from secondary hyperaldosteronism. Renin

(continued)

(Clinical Alert continued)
  levels are high in secondary aldosteronism and low in primary aldosteronism.
2. Potassium deficiencies should be corrected before testing for aldosterone.

Patient Preparation
1. Explain test purpose and procedures. If 24-hour urine specimen is required, follow protocols in Chapter 3.
2. Diuretic agents, progestational agents, estrogens, and licorice should be discontinued for 2 weeks before the test.
3. The patient's diet for 2 weeks before the test should be normal (other than the previously listed restrictions) and should include 3 g/day (135 mEq/L/day) of sodium. Check with your laboratory for special protocols.
4. Follow guidelines in Chapter 1 for safe, effective, informed *pretest* care.

Patient Aftercare
1. Resume normal activities and diet.
2. Interpret test results and monitor appropriately for aldosteronism and aldosterone deficiency.
3. Follow guidelines in Chapter 1 for safe, effective, informed *posttest* care.

ANTIDIURETIC HORMONE (ADH); ARGININE VASOPRESSIN HORMONE ●

Normal Values
0.0–4.7 pg/ml or 1.5 mg/L

Background
ADH is excreted by the posterior pituitary gland. When ADH activity is present, small volumes of concentrated urine are excreted. When ADH is absent, large amounts of diluted urine are produced.

Explanation of Test
Measurement of the level of ADH is useful in the differential diagnosis of polyuric and hyponatremic states. ADH testing aids in diagnosis of urine concentration disorders, especially diabetes insipidus, SIADH, psychogenic water intoxication, and syndromes of ectopic ADH production.

Procedure
1. Venous blood samples are drawn into prechilled tubes and put on ice. Observe standard precautions. Plasma with EDTA anticoagulant is needed.
2. Patient should be in a sitting position and calm during blood collection.

Clinical Implications

1. *Increased secretion of ADH* is associated with the following conditions:
   a. SIADH (with respect to plasma osmolality)
   b. Ectopic ADH production (systemic neoplasm)
   c. Nephrogenic diabetes insipidus
   d. Acute intermittent porphyria
   e. Guillain-Barré syndrome
   f. Brain tumor, diseases, injury, neurosurgery
   g. Pulmonary diseases
2. *Decreased secretion of ADH* occurs in the following conditions:
   a. Central diabetes insipidus (hypothalamic or neurogenic)
   b. Psychogenic polydipsia (water intoxication)
   c. Nephrotic syndrome

Interfering Factors

1. Recently administered radioisotopes cause spurious results.
2. Many drugs affect results, (eg, thiazide, diuretics, oral hypoglycemia, and narcotics.) See Appendix J.

Patient Preparation

1. Explain test purpose and procedure.
2. Encourage relaxation before and during blood-drawing procedure.
3. Follow guidelines in Chapter 1 for safe, effective, informed *pretest* care.

Patient Aftercare

1. Resume normal activities.
2. Interpret test results and counsel appropriately for urine concentration disorders and polyuria.
3. Follow guidelines in Chapter 1 for safe, effective, informed *posttest* care.

> ### Clinical Alert
>
> To distinguish SIADH from other conditions that cause dilutional hyponatremia, other tests must be done such as plasma osmolality, plasma sodium, and water-loading test.

ATRIAL NATRIURETIC FACTOR (ANF) ●

Normal Values
20–77 pg/ml

Background
ANF is a hormone secreted by the heart during acute and chronic cardiac volume and pressure overload. The discovery of ANF indicates that the heart is

an endocrine gland and confirms speculation that there is a mechanism in or near the heart that regulates body fluid hemostasis.

Explanation of Test
This test is useful in diagnosing congestive heart failure. It is not useful for diagnosing other heart conditions.

Procedure
1. Obtain a plasma sample by venipuncture from a fasting patient. Use a lavender-topped KEDTA tube. If a nonfasting sample is obtained, notify laboratory.
2. Prechill the tube at 4° centigrade before drawing sample. After drawing sample, chill tube in wet ice for 10 minutes.

Clinical Implications
Increased ANF levels occur in congestive heart failure.

Interfering Factors
See Appendix J for drugs that affect test outcomes.

Patient Preparation
1. Explain test purpose and need to fast. Assess for signs and symptoms indicating need for testing (eg, chronic fatigue, cough, heart palpitations, high blood pressure).
2. Withhold cardiovascular medications per physician's order (eg, β and calcium antagonists, cardiac glycosides, diuretics, vasodilators) prior to drawing specimen.
3. Follow guidelines in Chapter 1 for safe, effective, informed *pretest* care.

Patient Aftercare
1. Medications and usual diet may be restarted per physician's order.
2. Evaluate patient outcomes and monitor appropriately for congestive heart failure.
3. In collaboration with physician, explain need for possible follow-up tests and medication therapy.
4. Follow guidelines in Chapter 1 for safe, effective, informed *posttest* care.

CORTISOL (HYDROCORTISONE) ●

Normal Values

Cortisol
8:00 AM: 5–23 µg/dl or 138–635 mmol/L
4:00 PM: 3–16 µg/dl or 83–441 mmol/L
Newborn: 2–11 µg/dl or 55–304 mmol/L

After first week of life cortisol levels attain adult values.

Suppression
8:00 AM: 5–23 µg/dl or 138–635 mmol/L
4:00 PM: 3–16 µg/dl or 83–441 mmol/L
8:00 AM following administration of dexamethasone: <5 µg/dl (AM value).

Stimulation

Baseline: at least 5 µg/dl

After Cortrosyn administration: rise of at least 10 µg/dl

Background

Cortisol (hydrocortisone/compound F) is a glucocorticosteroid of the adrenal cortex and affects metabolism of proteins, carbohydrates, and lipids. Cortisol stimulates glucogenesis by the liver, inhibits the effect of insulin, and decreases the rate of glucose use by the cells. In health, the secretion rate of cortisol is higher in the early morning (6:00–8:00 AM) and lower in the evening (4:00–6:00 PM). This variation is lost in patients with Cushing's syndrome and in persons under stress.

Explanation of Test

The cortisol test evaluates adrenal hormone function. Cortisol is elevated in adrenal hyperfunction and decreased in adrenal hypofunction. Suppression and stimulation tests may also be done. Cortisol (dexamethasone) suppression test screens for Cushing's syndrome and identifies depressed persons who are likely to respond to antidepressants or electroshock therapy. It is based on the fact that ACTH production is suppressed in healthy persons after a low dose of dexamethasone, whereas it is not in persons with Cushing's syndrome or in some depressed persons.

Procedure

Obtain 5-ml venous blood samples at 8:00 AM and at 4:00 PM. Serum is preferred. Heparin anticoagulant may be used. Observe standard precautions.

Clinical Implications

1. *Decreased cortisol levels* are found in the following conditions:
   a. Adrenal hyperplasia
   b. Addison's disease
   c. Anterior pituitary hyposecretion (pituitary destruction)
   d. Hypothyroidism (hypopituitarism)
   e. Hepatitis and cirrhosis
2. *Increased cortisol levels* are found in the following conditions:
   a. Hyperthyroidism
   b. Stress (trauma, surgery)
   c. Carcinoma (extreme elevation in the morning and no variation later in the day)
   d. Cushing's syndrome (high on rising but no variation later in the day)
   e. Overproduction of ACTH due to tumors (oat cell cancers)
   f. Adrenal adenoma
   g. Obesity

Interfering Factors

1. Pregnancy will cause an increased value.
2. There is no normal diurnal variation in patients under stress.

3. Drugs such as spironolactone and oral contraceptives will give falsely elevated values (see Appendix J).
4. Decreased levels occur in persons taking dexamethasone, prednisone, or prednisolone (steroids) (see Appendix J).

Patient Preparation
1. Explain test purpose and blood-drawing procedure. Blood must be drawn at 8:00 AM and 4:00 PM.
2. Encourage relaxation.
3. No radioisotopes should be administered within 1 day before the test.
4. Follow guidelines in Chapter 1 for safe, effective, informed *pretest* care.

Patient Aftercare
1. Resume normal activities.
2. Interpret test results and counsel appropriately for adrenal dysfunction.
3. Follow guidelines in Chapter 1 for safe, effective, informed *posttest* care.

CORTISOL SUPPRESSION
(DEXAMETHASONE SUPPRESSION; DST) ●

Normal Values
<5 µg/dl

Explanation of Test
See foregoing cortisol test for purpose and indications. Test helps to differentiate causes of elevated cortisol.

Procedure
1. Obtain venous blood samples the day following administration of dexamethasone. Serum or heparinized plasma are acceptable. Observe standard precautions.
2. Late evening or bedtime, dexamethasone tablets are administered by mouth. Usually, 1 mg is given.

Clinical Implications
No diurnal variation or suppression occurs in persons with Cushing's syndrome (>10 µg/dl) or endogenous depression (50% of cases).

Interfering Factors
1. False suppression can occur in the following conditions:
    a. Pregnancy
    b. High doses of estrogens
    c. Anorexia nervosa
    d. Uncontrolled diabetes
    e. Trauma, high stress, fever, dehydration
    f. Phenytoin (Dilantin) (see Appendix J for other drugs)

Patient Preparation

1. Explain test purpose and procedure. Fasting is required for the 8:00 AM test.
2. Discontinue all medications for 24 to 48 hours before the study. Especially important are spironolactone, estrogens, birth control pills, cortisol, tetracycline, stilbestrol, and phenytoin. Check with the physician.
3. Weigh the patient and record weight.
4. Have baseline blood cortisol drawn at 8:00 AM and 4:00 PM. Give 1 mg dexamethasone at 11:00 PM the same day. Draw blood at 8:00 AM the next day.
5. No radioisotopes should be administered within 1 week before test.
6. Follow guidelines in Chapter 1 regarding safe, effective, informed *pretest* care.

Patient Aftercare

1. Resume normal activities.
2. Interpret test results and counsel appropriately for Cushing's syndrome or endogenous depression.
3. Follow guidelines in Chapter 1 for safe, effective, informed *posttest* care.

CORTISONE STIMULATION (COSYNTROPIN; CORTROSYN STIMULATION); ADRENOCORTICOTROPIN HORMONE (ACTH) STIMULATION ●

Normal Values

Cortisol: >10 μg/dl rise after Cortrosyn administration

Explanation of Test

This detects adrenal insufficiency after Cortrosyn administration. Cortrosyn is a synthetic subunit of ACTH that exhibits the full corticosteroid-stimulating effect of ACTH in healthy persons. Failure to respond is an indication of adrenal insufficiency. See foregoing cortisol tests for values.

Procedure

1. Obtain a 4-ml fasting venous blood sample at 8:00 AM. Observe standard precautions.
2. Administer Cortrosyn intramuscularly (IM) or intravenously as prescribed.
3. Obtain additional 4-ml blood specimens 30 and 60 minutes after administration of Cortrosyn. Serum or heparinized blood is acceptable.

Clinical Implications

Absent or blunted response to cortisol stimulation occurs in the following conditions:

1. Addison's disease (adrenal insufficiency)
2. Hypopituitarism (secondary adrenal insufficiency)

Interfering Factors

1. Prolonged steroid administration
2. Estrogens (see Appendix J)

Patient Preparation

1. Explain test purpose and procedure. Fasting during test is required. Blood specimens are obtained before or after IM injection of Cortrosyn.
2. Follow guidelines in Chapter 1 for safe, effective, informed *pretest* care.

Patient Aftercare

1. Resume normal activities.
2. Interpret test results and monitor appropriately for adrenal insufficiency.
3. Follow guidelines in Chapter 1 for safe, effective, informed *posttest* care.

> **Clinical Alert**
>
> In adrenal hyperplasia, there is increase cortisol of 3 to 5 times the normal; in adrenal carcinoma, there is no increase.

GASTRIN

Normal Values

Man: <100 pg/ml or ng/L   Child: 10–125 pg/ml or ng/L
Woman: <75 pg/ml or ng/L

Background

Gastrin, a hormone secreted by the antral G cells in stomach mucosa, stimulates gastric acid production and affects antral motility and secretion of pepsin and intrinsic factor. Gastrin values follow a circadian rhythm and fluctuate physiologically in relation to meals.

Explanation of Test

Measurement of serum gastrin is generally used to diagnose stomach disorders such as gastrinoma and Zollinger-Ellison syndrome in the presence of hyperacidity. (Gastric hyperacidity must be documented.)

Procedure

Obtain a 5-ml venous blood sample from a fasting patient. Serum is preferred. Observe standard precautions.

Clinical Implications

1. *Increased gastrin levels* are found in the following conditions:
   a. Stomach carcinoma (reduction of gastric acid secretion)
   b. Gastric and duodenal ulcers
   c. Zollinger-Ellison syndrome (>500 pg/ml)
   d. Pernicious anemia (low secretion of hydrochloric acid results in elevated gastrin levels)

    e. End-stage renal disease (gastrin metabolized by the kidneys)
    f. Antral G-cell hyperplasia
    g. Vagotomy without gastric resection
    h. Hyperparathyroidism
    i. Pyloric obstruction
2. *Decreased gastrin levels* occur in the following conditions:
    a. Antrectomy with vagotomy
    b. Hypothyroidism

Interfering Factors
Values will be falsely increased in nonfasting patients, the elderly, and diabetics taking insulin, as well as in persons after gastroscopy and those taking H_2 secretion blockers (cimetidine), steroids, and calcium.

Patient Preparation
1. Explain test purpose and procedure.
2. Fasting is required for 12 hours preceding the test. Water is permitted.
3. Follow guidelines in Chapter 1 for safe, effective, informed *pretest* care.

Patient Aftercare
1. Resume normal activities.
2. Interpret test results and monitor appropriately. Follow-up testing using gastric stimulation or gastrin suppression may be indicated.
3. Follow guidelines in Chapter 1 for safe, effective, informed *posttest* care.

GROWTH HORMONE (hGH); SOMATOTROPIN

Normal Values
Adult: <5 ng/ml or <5 μg/L
Child: 0–10 ng/ml or 0–10 μg/L
Newborn: 5–40 ng/ml or μg/L

Stimulation Test (using arginine, glucagon or insulin)
>5 ng/ml (rise from baseline)
>10 ng/ml peak response from baseline

Suppression Test (using 100 g glucose)
0–2 ng/ml

> **NOTE:** *Because of marked fluctuations in hGH, a random specimen has limited value. Stimulation or inhibitor tests provide more information.*

Background
Human growth hormone (somatotropin, hGH) is essential to the growth process and has an important role in the metabolism of adults. It is secreted by the pituitary gland in response to exercise, deep sleep, hypoglycemia,

glucagon, insulin, and vasopressin. It also stimulates the production of ribonucleic acid (RNA), mobilizes fatty acids from fat deposits, and is intimately connected with insulinism. If the pituitary gland secretes too little or too much hGH in the growth phase of life, dwarfism or giantism will result, respectively. An excess of growth hormone during adulthood leads to acromegaly.

Explanation of Test
The test confirms hypopituitarism or hyperpituitarism so that therapy can be initiated as soon as possible. Challenge or stimulation tests are generally used to detect hGH deficiency and are more informative. Much controversy surrounds the use of growth hormone stimulation tests, and the diagnosis should be considered in the context of the clinical picture.

Procedure
1. Obtain a 5-ml venous blood sample from a fasting patient. Observe standard precautions. Serum or plasma may be used.
2. Check with your laboratory for specific challenge protocols for stimulation tests such as insulin-induced hypoglycemia, arginine transfusion, glucagon infusion, L-dopa, and propranolol with exercise.

Clinical Implications
1. *Increased hGH levels* are associated with the following conditions:
   a. Pituitary giantism
   b. Acromegaly
   c. Laron dwarfism (hGH resistant)
   d. Uncontrolled diabetes mellitus
2. *Decreased hGH levels* are associated with the following conditions:
   a. Pituitary dwarfism
   b. Hypopituitarism
   c. Adrenocortical hyperfunction
3. Following stimulation testing, no response (or an inadequate response) is seen in hGH and ACTH deficiencies (hypopituitarism).
   a. Blood glucose must fall to <40 mg/dl.
   b. Adrenergic signs must be observed.
4. Following suppression tests, there is no or incomplete suppression in persons with giantism or acromegaly.
   a. Paradoxical rises in hGH may occur in patients with acromegaly.
   b. Partial suppression is sometimes seen in anorexia nervosa.
   c. In children, a rebound-stimulation effect may be seen 2 to 5 hours following administration of glucose (suppression test).

Interfering Factors
1. *Increased levels* are associated with the use of oral contraceptives, estrogens, arginine, glucagon, levodopa, low glucose, and insulin.
2. Levels will rise to 15 times normal by the second day of starvation; levels also rise after deep sleep.

3. *Decreased levels* are associated with obesity and the use of corticosteroids.
4. Many drugs interfere with test results (see Appendix J).
5. Recently administered radioisotopes interfere with test results.

Patient Preparation

1. Explain test purpose and blood-drawing procedure.
2. Fasting from food for 8 to 10 hours is required; water is permitted. For accurate levels, the patient should be free of stress and at complete rest in a quiet environment for at least 30 minutes before specimen collection.
3. The patient's physiologic state (eg, feeding, fasting, sleep, and/or activity) at testing should be noted in the health care record.
4. Stimulation tests: 1 tube collected before stimulation and at timed intervals (eg, 10, 20, 30, 45, and 60 minutes) after stimulation. Suppression tests: 1 tube collected before suppression and at 30, 60, 90, and 120 minutes after suppression.
5. For initial testing of hGH deficiency, a vigorous exercise test is considered to be a simple, risk-free screening test, especially for children.
6. Follow guidelines in Chapter 1 for safe, effective, informed *pretest* care.

Patient Aftercare

1. Resume normal activities.
2. Interpret test results and monitor appropriately. A glucose challenge test may be indicated for follow-up.
3. Follow guidelines in Chapter 1 for safe, effective, informed *posttest* care.

PARATHYROID HORMONE ASSAY; PARATHYRIN; PARATHORMONE (PTH–C-TERMINAL)

Normal Values

N-terminal: 8–24 pg/ml or ng/L
Intact molecule: 10–65 pg/ml or ng/L
Calcium: 8.5–10.9 mg/dl (calcium must be tested to properly interpret results)
C-terminal (biomolecule): 50–330 pg/ml

Background

Parathormone (PTH), a polypeptide hormone produced in the parathyroid gland, is one of the major factors in the regulation of calcium concentration in extracellular fluid. Three molecular forms of PTH exist: intact (also called native or glandular hormone); multiple N-terminal fragments; and C-terminal fragments.

Explanation of Test

This test studies altered calcium metabolism, establishes a diagnosis of hyperparathyroidism, and distinguishes nonparathyroid from parathyroid causes of hypercalcemia. A decrease in the level of ionized calcium is the primary stimulus for PTH secretions, whereas a rise in calcium inhibits secretions. This normal relation is lost in hyperthyroidism, and PTH will be inappropriately high in relation to calcium. Acute changes in secretory activity are better reflected by the PTH, N-terminal assay. PTH and N-terminal levels are usually decreased when hypercalcemia is due to neoplastic secretions (prostaglandins). PTH and N-terminal levels may be a more reliable indication of secondary hyperparathyroidism in patients with renal failure. Creatinine level is determined concurrently with all PTH assays to determine kidney function and for meaningful interpretation of results.

Procedure

1. Obtain a 10-ml venous blood sample from a patient who has fasted for 10 hours. Collect the sample in chilled vials and keep on ice. Observe standard precautions. Serum or EDTA plasma is used.
2. Immediately take specimen to the laboratory and centrifuge in at 4-degrees centigrade after blood has clotted.

Clinical Implications

1. *Increased PTH values* occur in primary hyperparathyroidism and in pseudo-hyperparathyroidism when there is a primary defect in renal tubular responsiveness to PTH (secondary hyperparathyroidism).
2. *Decreased PTH values* occur in the following conditions:
   a. Hypoparathyroidism (Graves' disease)
   b. Nonparathyroid hypercalcemia
   c. Secondary hypoparathyroidism (surgical)
   d. Magnesium deficiency
   e. Sarcoidosis
   f. Hyperthyroidism
   g. DiGeorge syndrome
3. *Increased PTH–N-terminal values* occur in the following conditions:
   a. Primary hyperparathyroidism
   b. Secondary hyperparathyroidism (more reliable than PTH–C-terminal)
4. *Decreased PTH–N-terminal values* occur in the following conditions:
   a. Hypoparathyroidism
   b. Nonparathyroid hypercalcemia
   c. Aluminum-associated osteomalacia
   d. Severely impaired bone mineralization
5. *Increased PTH–C-terminal values* occur in the following conditions:
   a. Primary hyperparathyroidism (very specific for)
   b. Some neoplasms with elevated calcium
   c. Renal failure (even if parathyroid disease is absent)
6. *Decreased PTH–C-terminal values* occur in the following conditions:
   a. Hypoparathyroidism
   b. Nonparathyroid hypercalcemia

Interfering Factors

1. Elevated blood lipids and hemolysis interfere with test methods.
2. Milk-alkali syndrome may falsely lower PTH levels (Burnett's syndrome).

3. Recently administered radioisotopes (see Appendix J).
4. Vitamin D deficiency will increase PTH levels.
5. Many drugs alter results; phosphates raise PTH levels up to 125%, and vitamin A and D overdose decrease PTH levels (see Appendix J).

Patient Preparation

1. Explain test purpose and procedure.
2. Fasting for at least 10 hours is required. Draw blood by 8:00 AM because of circadian rhythm changes. Concurrently also draw blood for testing of calcium level.
3. Follow guidelines in Chapter 1 for safe, effective, informed *pretest* care.

Patient Aftercare

1. Resume normal activities.
2. Interpret test results and monitor appropriately for calcium imbalance and hypoparathyroidism or hyperparathyroidism.
3. Follow guidelines in Chapter 1 for safe, effective, informed *posttest* care.

SOMATOMEDIN-C; INSULIN-LIKE GROWTH HORMONE

Normal Values

Age	Male (U/ml)	Female (U/ml)
0–2 y	0.8–1.10	0.11–2.20
3–5 y	0.12–1.60	0.18–2.40
6–10 y	0.22–2.80	0.41–4.50
11–12 y	0.28–3.70	0.99–6.80
13–14 y	0.90–5.60	1.20–5.90
15–17 y	0.91–3.10	0.71–4.10
>18 y	0.34–1.90	0.45–2.20

Background

Somatomedin-C, a polypeptide hormone produced by the liver and other tissues, mediates growth hormone activity and glucose metabolism. It is carried in the blood and is bound to a protein carrier that prolongs its half-life.

Explanation of Test

This test is used to monitor the growth of children as well as to diagnose acromegaly and hypopituitarism. Normal somatomedin-C results rule out a deficiency of growth hormone. Testing of somatomedin-C is preferable to growth hormone tests because its levels are more constant.

Procedure

1. It is preferred that the patient be fasting. Obtain a 5-ml plasma venous blood sample using EDTA anticoagulant. Observe standard precautions. Serum may also be used.

2. Blood-drawing tubes must be chilled before and placed on ice immediately after obtaining specimen. Spin the sample in a refrigerated centrifuge.

Clinical Implications

1. *Increased somatomedin-C levels* are associated with the following conditions:
   a. Acromegaly (some cases)
   b. Hypoglycemia associated with non–islet cell tumors
   c. Hepatoma
   d. Wilms' tumor
2. *Decreased somatomedin-C levels* are associated with the following conditions:

   a. Dwarfism
   b. Hypopituitarism
   c. Hypothyroidism
   d. Kwashiorkor
   e. Laron dwarfism
   f. Cirrhosis of liver and other hepatocellular diseases
   g. Malnutrition and anorexia
   h. Diabetes mellitus
   i. Emotional deprivation syndrome

Interfering Factors

1. Somatomedin-C levels are *increased* 2 to 3 times in pregnancy.
2. Somatomedin-C levels are *decreased* in the following conditions:
   a. Acute illness   b. Normal aging

Patient Preparation

1. Explain test purpose and procedure. Fasting is not required.
2. No radioisotopes should be administered within 1 week of testing.
3. Follow guidelines in Chapter 1 for safe, effective, informed *pretest* care.

Patient Aftercare

1. Resume normal activities.
2. Interpret test results and monitor appropriately for abnormal growth and development.
3. Follow guidelines in Chapter 1 for safe, effective, informed *posttest* care.

●FERTILITY TESTS

Fertility denotes the ability of a man and a woman to reproduce; conversely, infertility denotes the lack of fertility—an involuntary reduction in the ability to produce children. When a couple has been engaging in regular, unprotected sexual intercourse for at least 1 year without conceiving, the couple is considered infertile. In about one third of cases, a male factor is the predominant cause; in another one third, the female factor predominates; and in another one third, no cause is found in either partners.

The workup for infertility starts with a complete history and physical for both the woman and the man, including their sexual history. A rational approach is to put each partner through a series of tests which generally uncovers a vast majority of the contributing factors of infertility. These tests usually take 2 to 3 months to complete.

Standard pre- and posttest care for couples undergoing fertility testing includes the following: Provide information and suppport. Be sensitive to couple's need for privacy and confidentiality. Maintain a communication network about new procedures, tests, and treatments. Help couples deal with feelings of sadness and loss. Assist couples to deal with the effects of stress and the financial burden during the diagnostic process. Assist couples in arranging work and testing schedules with the least amount of disruption for the couple. Arrange for counseling with experts who understand the different ways infertility affects someone's life.

Tests include evaluation of amenorrhea, anovulation, sperm count (angiosperm, oligospermia), hormone testing, hysterosalpingogram, laparoscopy, and hysteroscopy, semen analysis, postcoital test, endometrial biopsy, and chromosome karyotype to exclude Kallmann's syndrome. Hormone testing rules pregnancy in or out (eg, chorionic gonadotropin, prolactin, luteinizing hormone (LH), follicle-stimulating hormone (FSH), thyroid-stimulating hormone (TSH), postcoital test, and antisperm antibodies). Also see estrogen testing in Chapter 3.

> **NOTE:** *A postcoital examination is done to assess cervical mucus and competent sperm motility. A specimen is obtained from the endocervical canal within 2 to 12 hours of coitus and is examined for viscosity (stretching to 6 cm is normal) and for firming effect of estrogen. The presence of ≥ 5 motile sperm confirms male competence.*

CHORIONIC GONADOTROPIN; HUMAN CHORIONIC GONADOTROPIN (hCG) β-SUBUNIT; PREGNANCY TEST ●

Normal Values

Qualitative (for Routine Pregnancy Tests)
Urine- or serum-negative (not pregnant)

Quantitative (for Nonroutine Detection of hCG)
Men: <5.0 IU/L or mIU/L
Nonpregnant women: <5.0 IU/L or mIU/ml
Pregnant women:
    1 wk of gestation: 5–50 mIU/ml or IU/L
    2 wk of gestation: 50–500 mIU/ml or IU/L
    3 wk of gestation: 100–10,000 mIU/ml or IU/L
    4 wk of gestation: 1080–30,000 mIU/ml or IU/L
    6–8 wk of gestation: 3500–115,000 mIU/ml or IU/L
    12 wk of gestation: 12,000–270,000 mIU/ml or IU/L
    13–16 wk of gestation: up to 200,000 mIU/ml or IU/L
    17–40 wk of gestation: gradual fall to 4000 mIU/ml or IU/L

Background
The glycoprotein hormones hCG, luteinizing hormone (LH), follicle-stimulating hormone (FSH), and thyroid-stimulating hormone (TSH) are composed of

two different subunits. The α-subunit is similar in all of the glycoprotein hormones, and the β-subunit is unique to each hormone. Highly specific assays allow hCG to be measured in the presence of other glycoprotein hormones. The increased sensitivity of the β-hCG test detects pregnancy as early as 6 to 10 days after implantation of the oocyte. A variety of poorly differentiated or undifferentiated neoplasms may produce ectopic chorionic gonadotropin. Assay for total hCG, both α- and β-subunits, or β-hCG may detect ectopic tumors (eg, choriocarcinoma, hydatidiform mole, germinal testicular tumors). In these neoplasms, hCG is usually the product of syncytiotrophoblastic cells.

Explanation of Test

This qualitative test detects normal pregnancy. It is quicker but less sensitive (sensitivity, 20–50 mIU/ml) than the quantitative test. This test can be expected to become positive within 3 days of implantation (ie, just after the first missed menstrual period). Cross-reactivity with LH is low, and false-positive results are rare. Occasionally, a patient with very high LH levels will give a borderline reaction. The qualitative test is usually done using urine.

The quantitative β-hCG test is used for nonroutine detection of hCG. It is sensitive to 1 to 3 mIU/L. This test provides the most sensitive **and** specific test for the detection of early pregnancy, estimation of gestational age, and diagnosis of ectopic pregnancy or threatened spontaneous abortion. This test is also useful in the workup and management of testicular tumors. High levels may be found in choriocarcinoma, embryonal cell carcinoma, and ectopic pregnancy. hCG levels are extremely useful in following germ cell neoplasms that produce hCG, especially trophoblastic neoplasms. There is little cross-reactivity with LH.

Procedure

Obtain a 5-ml venous blood sample. Serum is used for the test. Observe standard precautions. Urine may be used for the qualitative test. First morning specimen is recommended.

Clinical Implications

1. *Increased hCG values* occur in the following conditions:
   a. Pregnancy
   b. Successful therapeutic insemination and in vitro fertilization
   c. Hydatidiform mole
   d. Choriocarcinoma
   e. Seminoma
   f. Ovarian and testicular teratomas
   g. Ectopic pregnancy
   h. Certain neoplasms of the lung, stomach, and pancreas
2. *Decreased hCG values* occur in threatened spontaneous abortion and ectopic pregnancy.

Interfering Factors

1. Lipemia, hemolysis, and radioisotopes administered within 1 week of testing may affect results.

2. Test results can be positive up to 1 week after a complete abortion.
3. False-negative and false-positive results can be caused by many drugs (see Appendix J).

> **Clinical Alert**
>
> Because there is great variability in hCG concentration among pregnant women, a single test determination cannot be used to accurately date the gestational age. Serial determinations may be helpful when abnormal pregnancy is suspected.

Patient Preparation
1. Explain test purpose and procedure.
2. Determine and record date of last menstrual period in women.
3. Follow guidelines in Chapter 1 for safe, effective, informed *pretest* care.

Patient Aftercare
1. Resume normal activities.
2. Interpret test results and counsel appropriately for pregnancy or gestational problems.
3. Follow guidelines in Chapter 1 for safe, effective, informed *posttest* care.

FOLLICLE-STIMULATING HORMONE (FSH); LUTEINIZING HORMONE (LH)

Normal Values

Luteinizing Hormone (LH)		Follicle Stimulating Hormone (FSH)	
	mIU/ml		*mIU/ml*
FEMALE		*FEMALE*	
Excluding midcycle peak	3.6–29.4	Excluding midcyle peak	2.8–17.2
Midcycle peak	58–204	Midcycle peak	15–35
Postmenopausal	35–129	Postmenopausal	24–170
NORMAL MALE	3.9–22.6	*NORMAL MALE*	1.6–18.6
Testicular failure	13–173	Testicular failure	7–180
Ovarian failure	30–154	Ovarian failure	31–205

Contact your laboratory for reference values in infants and children. Normal values may vary with method of testing.

Background
FSH and LH are glycoprotein pituitary hormones produced and stored in the anterior pituitary. They are under complex regulation by hypothalamic go-

nadotropin-releasing hormone and by gonadal sex hormones (estrogen and progesterone in females and testosterone in males). FSH acts on granulosa cells of the ovary and the Sertoli cells of the testis, and LH acts on Leydig (interstitial) cells of the gonads. Normally, FSH increases occur at earlier stages of puberty, 2 to 4 years before LH reaches comparable levels. In males, FSH and LH are necessary for spermatozoa development and maturation. In females, follicular formation in the early stages of the menstrual cycle is stimulated by FSH; then the midcycle surge of LH causes ovulation of the FSH-ripened ovarian follicles to occur.

Explanation of Test

This test measures the gonadotropic hormones FSH and LH and may help determine whether a gonadal deficiency is of primary origin or is due to insufficient stimulation by the pituitary hormones.

Evaluation of FSH supports other studies related to determining causes of hypothyroidism in women and endocrine dysfunction in men. In primary ovarian failure or testicular failure, FSH levels are increased. Measuring the levels of FSH and LH are of value in studying children with endocrine problems related to precocious puberty.

In the case of anovulatory fertility problems, the presence or absence of the midcycle peak can be established through a series of daily blood specimens.

Procedure

1. Obtain a 5-ml venous blood sample. Serum is needed for the test.
2. In women, date of last menstrual period is recorded.
3. It is important to measure both FSH and LH.

Clinical Alert

Sometimes multiple blood specimens are necessary because of episodic releases of FSH from the pituitary gland. An isolated sample may not indicate the actual activity; therefore, pooled blood specimens or multiple single blood specimens may be required.

Clinical Implications

1. *Decreased FSH levels* occur in the following conditions:
   a. Feminizing and masculinizing ovarian tumors when FSH production is inhibited because of increased estrogen secretion.
   b. Failure of hypothalamus to function properly (Kallman's syndrome)
   c. Pituitary LH or FSH deficiency
   d. Neoplasm of testes or adrenal glands that influences secretion of estrogens or androgens
   e. Polycystic ovarian disease
   f. Hemochromatosis
2. *Decreased FSH and LH* occur in pituitary or hypothalamic failure.

3. *Increased FSH levels* occur in the following conditions:
   a. Turner's syndrome (ovarian dysgenesis); ~50% of patients with primary amenorrhea have Turner's syndrome.
   b. Hypopituitarism
   c. Sheehan's syndrome
   d. Precocious puberty, either idiopathic or secondary to a CNS lesion
   e. Klinefelter's syndrome
   f. Castration
   g. Alcoholism
   h. Menopause and menstrual disorders
4. *Both FSH and LH are increased* in the following conditions:
   a. Hypogonadism
   b. Complete testicular feminization syndrome
   c. Gonadal failure
   d. Congenital absence of testicle or testicles (anorchia)
   e. Menopause
5. Elevated basal LH with an LH/FSH ratio >2 and some increase of ovarian androgen in an essentially nonovulatory adult woman is presumptive evidence of Stein-Leventhal syndrome.

Interfering Factors
1. Recently administered radioisotopes
2. Hemolysis of blood sample
3. Estrogens or oral contraceptives, testosterone
4. Several drugs affect test outcomes—see Appendix J.
5. Pregnancy

Patient Preparation
1. Instruct the patient regarding test purpose and procedure.
2. For women, record date of last menstrual period.
3. Follow guidelines in Chapter 1 for safe, effective, informed *pretest* care.

Patient Aftercare
1. Interpret test outcomes and counsel appropriately.
2. Follow guidelines in Chapter 1 for safe, effective, informed *posttest* care.

PROLACTIN (hPRL)   ●

Normal Values
Nonpregnant women: 0–17 ng/ml or µg/L
Pregnant women: 34–386 ng/ml or µg/L by third trimester
Adult men: 0–15 ng/ml or µg/L
Children: 3.2–20 ng/ml or µg/L

Background
Prolactin is a pituitary hormone essential for initiating and maintaining lactation. The gender difference in prolactin does not occur until puberty, when in-

creased estrogen production results in higher prolactin levels in females. Circadian changes in prolactin concentration in adults are marked by episodic fluctuation and a sleep-induced peak in the early morning hours.

Explanation of Test

This test may be helpful in the diagnosis, management, and follow-up of a prolactin-secreting tumor accompanied by secondary amenorrhea or galactorrhea, hyperprolactinemia, and infertility. It is also useful in the management of hypothalamic disease and in monitoring the effectiveness of surgery, chemotherapy, and radiation treatment of prolactin-secreting tumors.

Procedure

The patient should fast for 12 hours before testing. Obtain a 5-ml venous blood sample. Serum is used. Procure specimens in the morning, 3 to 4 hours after awakening. Observe standard precautions.

Clinical Implications

1. *Increased prolactin values* are associated with the following conditions:
   a. Galactorrhea or amenorrhea
   b. Diseases of the hypothalamus and pituitary (acromegaly)
   c. Prolactin-secreting pituitary tumors
   d. Sexual precocity in children
   e. Ectopic production of prolactin from tumors, carcinoma, and leukemia
   f. Hypothyroidism (primary)
   g. Renal failure, liver failure
   h. Anorexia nervosa
   i. Insulin-induced hypoglycemia
2. *Decreased prolactin values* are found in the following conditions:
   a. Sheehan's syndrome (pituitary apoplexy)
   b. Idiopathic hypogonadotropic hypogonadism

Interfering Factors

1. Increased values are associated with newborns, pregnancy, postpartum period, stress, exercise, sleep, nipple stimulation, and lactation.
2. Drugs (eg, estrogens, methyldopa, phenothiazines, opiates) may increase values. See Appendix J for other drugs.
3. Dopaminergic drugs inhibit prolactin secretion. Administration of L-dopa can normalize prolactin levels in galactorrhea, hyperprolactinemia, and pituitary tumor. See Appendix J for other drugs.

▶ Clinical Alert

Levels >200 ng/ml in a nonlactating female indicates a prolactin-secreting tumor; however, a normal prolactin level does not rule out pituitary tumor.

Patient Preparation

1. Explain test purpose. Fasting is required. Obtain blood specimen between 8:00 AM and 10:00 AM (3–4 hours after patient has awakened).
2. Avoid stress, excitement, or stimulation; venipuncture itself can sometimes elevate prolactin levels.
3. If possible, discontinue all prescribed medications for 2 weeks before test.
4. Follow guidelines in Chapter 1 for safe, effective, informed *pretest* care.

Patient Aftercare

1. Resume normal activities.
2. Interpret test outcome and counsel regarding repeat testing to monitor treatment. Magnetic resonance imaging may be indicated.
3. Follow guidelines in Chapter 1 for safe, effective, informed *posttest* care.

PROGESTERONE

Normal Values

Man: 0–0.4 ng/ml

Woman

Follicular: 0.1–1.5 ng/ml
Luteal: 2.5–28.1 ng/ml
1st trimester: 9–47 ng/ml
2nd trimester: 16.8–146 ng/ml
3rd trimester: 55–255 ng/ml

Midluteal: 5.7–28.1 ng/ml
Oral contraceptives:
 0.1–0.3 ng/ml
Elderly (>60 y): 0–0.2 ng/ml
Prepubertal: 0.1–0.3 ng/ml

Background

Progesterone, a female sex hormone, is primarily involved in the preparation of the uterus for pregnancy and its maintenance during pregnancy. The placenta begins producing progesterone at 12 weeks of gestation. Progesterone level peaks in the midluteal phase of the menstrual cycle. In nonpregnant women, progesterone is produced by the corpus luteum. Progesterone is the single best test to determine whether ovulation has occurred.

Explanation of Test

This test is part of a fertility study to confirm ovulation, evaluate corpus luteum function, and assess risk for early spontaneous abortion. Testing of several samples during the cycle is necessary. Ovarian production of progesterone is low during the follicular (first) phase of the menstrual cycle. After ovulation, progesterone levels rise for 4 to 5 days and then fall. During pregnancy, there is a gradual increase from the week 9 to week 32 of gestation, often to 100 times the level in the nonpregnant woman. Levels of progesterone in twin pregnancy are higher than in a single pregnancy.

Procedure

1. Obtain a venous blood sample. Observe standard precautions. The test request should include gender, day of last menstrual period, and length of gestation in women.
2. Urine tests can also be done.

Clinical Implications

1. *Increased progesterone levels* are associated with the following conditions:
   a. Congenital adrenal hyperplasia
   b. Lipid ovarian tumor
   c. Molar pregnancy
   d. Chorionepithelioma of ovary
2. *Decreased progesterone levels* are associated with the following conditions:
   a. Threatened spontaneous abortion
   b. Galactorrhea-amenorrhea syndrome

Interfering Factors

See Appendix J for drugs that affect test outcomes.

Patient Preparation

1. Explain test purpose and procedure. Note date of last menstrual period/ length of gestation.
2. No radioisotopes should be administered within 1 week before the test.
3. Follow guidelines in Chapter 1 for safe, effective, informed *pretest* care.

Patient Aftercare

1. Resume normal activities.
2. Interpret test results, and counsel and monitor appropriately regarding fertility and pregnancy.
3. Follow guidelines in Chapter 1 for safe, effective, informed *posttest* care.

TESTOSTERONE, TOTAL AND FREE ●

Normal Values

Total Testosterone
Man: 270–1070 ng/dl
Woman: 6–86 ng/dl
   Pregnant woman: 3–4 times normal
   Postmenopausal woman: one half of normal
Child: 2–20 ng/dl

Free Testosterone

Age	Men	Women
20–29 y	19–41 pg/ml	0.9–3.2 pg/ml
30–39 y	18–39 pg/ml	0.8–3.0 pg/ml
40–49 y	16–33 pg/ml	0.6–2.5 pg/ml
50–59 y	13–31 pg/ml	0.3–2.7 pg/ml
>60 y	9–26 pg/ml	0.2–2.2 pg/ml

Background

Testosterone is responsible for the development of male secondary sexual characteristics. It is secreted by the adrenal glands and testes in men and by the adrenal glands and ovaries in women. Excessive production induces premature puberty in men and masculinity in women. Testosterone exists in serum as both unbound (free) fractions and bound fractions to albumin: sex hormone–binding globulin (SHBG), and testosterone-binding globulin. Unbound (free) testosterone is the active portion. Testosterone levels undergo large and rapid fluctuations; levels peak in early morning for males. Females show a cyclic elevation 1 to 2 days midcycle.

Explanation of Test

Testosterone measurements in men assess hypogonadism, pituitary gonadotropin function, impotency, and cryptorchidism; these measurements are also useful in the detection of ovarian tumors and virilizing conditions in women. In prepubertal boys, it can assess special precocity. This test may be part of fertility workup.

Procedure

1. Obtain a 5-ml venous blood sample; serum is preferred. Observe standard precautions.
2. Indicate age and gender on laboratory requisition.

Clinical Implications

1. Men: *decreased total testosterone levels* occur in the following conditions:
   a. Hypogonadism (pituitary failure)
   b. Klinefelter's syndrome
   c. Hypopituitarism (primary and secondary)
   d. Orchidectomy
   e. Hepatic cirrhosis
   f. Down syndrome
   g. Delayed puberty
2. Men: *decreased free testosterone levels occur* in hypogonadism and elderly men.
3. Men: *increased total testosterone levels* occur in the following conditions:
   a. Hyperthyroidism
   b. Syndromes of androgen resistance
   c. Adrenal tumors
   d. Precocious puberty and adrenal hyperplasia in boys
4. Women: *increased total testosterone levels* are associated with the following conditions:
   a. Adrenal neoplasms
   b. Ovarian tumors, benign or malignant (virilizing)
   c. Trophoblastic disease during pregnancy
   d. Idiopathic hirsutism
   e. Hilar cell tumor

5. Women: *increased free testosterone levels* are associated with the following conditions:
   a. Female hirsutism
   b. Polycystic ovaries
   c. Virilization

> **Clinical Alert**
>
> 1. Testosterone levels are normal in cryptorchidism, azoospermia, and oligospermia.
> 2. In general, there appears to be little advantage in doing urine testosterone measurements compared with (or in addition to) serum measurements; the serum test is recommended.

Interfering Factors
1. Alcoholism in males decreases testosterone levels.
2. Estrogen therapy increases testosterone levels (see Appendix J).
3. Many drugs, including androgens and steroids, decrease testosterone levels (see Appendix J).

Patient Preparation
1. Explain test purpose and procedure. Draw blood at 7:00 AM for highest levels.
2. Multiple pooled samples drawn at different times throughout the day may be necessary for more reliable results.
3. No radioisotopes should be administered within 1 week before the test.
4. Multiple samples drawn at different times throughout the day and pooled will give a more reliable result.
5. Follow guidelines in Chapter 1 regarding safe, effective, informed *pretest* care.

Patient Aftercare
1. Resume normal activities.
2. Interpret test results and counsel appropriately regarding hormone dysfunction.
3. Follow guidelines in Chapter 1 for safe, effective, informed *posttest* care.

●ENZYME TESTS

ACID PHOSPHATASE; PROSTATIC ACID PHOSPHATASE (PAP) ●

Normal Values
0–3.1 ng/ml

Background
Acid phosphatases are enzymes that are widely distributed in tissues, including the bone, liver, spleen, kidney, red blood cells, and platelets. However,

their greatest diagnostic importance involves the prostate gland, where acid phosphatase activity is 100 times higher than in other tissues. Immunochemical methods are highly specific for determining the prostatic fraction; however, since PAP is not elevated in early prostatic disease, this test is not recommended for screening.

Explanation of Test

This test monitors the effectiveness of treatment for cancer of the prostate. Elevated levels of acid phosphatase are seen when prostate cancer has metastasized beyond the capsule to the other parts of the body, especially the bone. Once the carcinoma has spread, the prostate starts to release acid phosphatase, resulting in an increased blood level. The prostatic fraction procedure specifically measures the concentration of prostatic acid phosphatase secreted by cells of the prostate gland. Acid phosphatase is also present in high concentration in seminal fluid. Tests for presence of this enzyme on vaginal swabs may be used to investigate rape.

Procedure

Obtain a 5-ml venous blood sample. Serum is used. Seminal fluid may also be tested. Observe standard precautions.

Clinical Implications

1. A significantly elevated acid phosphatase value is almost always indicative of metastatic cancer of the prostate. If the tumor is successfully treated, this enzyme level will drop within 3 to 4 days after surgery or 3 to 4 weeks after estrogen administration.
2. Moderately elevated values also occur in the absence of prostate carcinoma in the following conditions:
   a. Niemann-Pick disease
   b. Gaucher's disease
   c. Prostatitis (benign prostatic hypertrophy)
   d. Urinary retention
   e. Any cancer that has metastasized to the bone

Interfering Factors

1. Various drugs may cause increased and decreased PAP levels.
2. Palpation of the prostate gland and prostate biopsy prior to testing causes increases in PAP levels.

Patient Preparation

1. Explain test purpose and procedure.
2. No palpation of or procedures on the prostate gland and no rectal examinations should be performed 2 to 3 days before test.
3. Follow guidelines in Chapter 1 for safe, effective, informed *pretest* care.

Patient Aftercare

1. Resume normal activities.
2. Interpret test results and counsel appropriately regarding repeat testing. When elevated values are present, retesting and biopsy are considered.
3. Follow guidelines in Chapter 1 for safe, effective, informed *posttest* care.

PROSTATE-SPECIFIC ANTIGEN (PSA) ●

Normal Values

Men: 0–4.0 ng/ml or μg/L

Background

Prostate-specific antigen (PSA) is functionally and immunologically distinct from prostatic acid phosphatase. PSA is localized in both normal prostatic epithelial cells and prostatic carcinoma cells. PSA has proven to be the most prognostically reliable marker for monitoring recurrence of prostatic carcinoma; however, this test does not have the sensitivity or specificity to be considered an ideal tumor marker.

The most useful approach to date may be age-specific PSA reference ranges, which is based on the concept that blood PSA concentration is dependent on patient age. The increase in PSA with advancing age is attributed to four major factors: prostate enlargement, increasing inflammation, presence of microscopic but clinically insignificant cancer, and leakage of PSA into the serum.

Suggested Age-Specific PSA Reference Ranges	
Age (y)	*PSA Range (ng/ml)*
40–49	0.0–2.5
50–59	0.0–3.5
60–69	0.0–4.5
70–79	0.0–6.5

From Oesterling JE, Jacobsen SJ, Chute CG, et al: Serum prostate-specific antigen in a community-based population of healthy men: establishment of age-specific reference ranges. JAMA 270(7): 860–864, 1993

Explanation of Test

Testing for both PSA and PAP increases detection of early prostate cancer. PSA testing determines the effectiveness of therapy for prostate cancer and is used as an early indicator of prostate cancer recurrence. The greatest value of PSA is as a marker in the follow-up of patients at high risk for disease progression.

Procedure

Obtain a 5-ml venous blood sample. Serum is needed. Observe standard precautions. Record patient's age.

Clinical Implications

1. *PSA increases* occur in prostate cancer (80% of patients).
2. Patients with benign prostatic hypertrophy often demonstrate values between 4.0 and 8.0 μg/L. Results between 4.0 and 8.0 μg/L may represent benign prostatic hypertrophy or possible cancer of the prostate. Results >8.0 μg/L are highly suggestive of prostatic cancer.
3. Increases to >4.0 ng/ml have been reported in about 8% of patients with no prostatic malignancies and no benign diseases.
4. If a prostate tumor is completely and successfully removed, *no* antigen will be detected.

Interfering Factors

Transient increases in PSA occur following prostate palpation or rectal examination.

Patient Preparation

1. Explain test purpose and procedure.
2. Do not schedule any prostatic examinations, including rectal examination, prostate biopsy, or surgical transurethral resection of prostate (TURP), for 3 days before the blood test is performed.
3. Follow guidelines in Chapter 1 for safe, effective, informed *pretest* care.

Patient Aftercare

1. Resume normal activities.
2. Interpret test results, and monitor and counsel as appropriate for response to treatment and progression or remission of prostate cancer.
3. Follow guidelines in Chapter 1 for safe, effective, informed *posttest* care.

> ### Clinical Alert
>
> 1. PSA is not a definitive diagnostic marker to screen for carcinoma of the prostate because it is also found in men with benign prostatic hypertrophy.
> 2. Digital rectal examination (DRE) is recommended by the American Cancer Society as the primary test for detection of prostatic tumor. Recent studies indicate that serum PSA may offer additional information. PSA should be used in conjunction with DRE.

ALANINE AMINOTRANSFERASE (AMINOTRANSFERASE, ALT); SERUM GLUTAMIC-PYRUVIC TRANSAMINASE (SGPT)

Normal Values

Adult: 10–60 U/L
Child: 5–30 U/L
Newborn: 1–25 U/L

ALT values are slightly higher in males and black persons. Normal values vary with testing method. Check with your laboratory for reference values.

Background
ALT is an enzyme. High concentrations occur in the liver, and relatively low concentrations are found in the heart, muscle, and kidney.

Explanation of Test
This test is primarily used to diagnose liver disease and to monitor the course of treatment for hepatitis, active postnecrotic cirrhosis, and the effects of later drug therapy. ALT also differentiates between hemolytic jaundice and jaundice due to liver disease.

Procedure
1. Obtain a 5-ml venous blood sample. Serum is needed for the test. Observe standard precautions.
2. Avoid hemolysis during collection of the specimen.

Clinical Implications
1. *Increased ALT levels* are found in the following conditions:
   a. Hepatocellular disease (moderate to high increase)
   b. Active cirrhosis (mild increase)
   c. Metastatic liver tumor (mild increase)
   d. Obstructive jaundice or biliary obstruction (mild to moderate increase)
   e. Viral, infectious or toxic hepatitis (30–50 times normal)
   f. Infectious mononucleosis
   g. Pancreatitis (mild increase)
   h. Myocardial infarction
   i. Polymyositis
   j. Severe burns
   k. Trauma to striated muscle
   l. Severe shock
2. Aspartate transaminase (AST)/ALT comparison: Although the AST level is always increased in acute MI, the ALT level does not always increase proportionately. The ALT is usually increased more than the AST in acute extrahepatic biliary obstruction. ALT is less sensitive than AST to alcoholic liver disease.
3. *Decreased ALT* levels occur in the following conditions:
   a. Genitourinary tract infection
   b. Malnutrition

Interfering Factors
1. Many drugs may cause falsely increased and decreased ALT levels (see Appendix J).
2. Salicylates may cause decreased or increased ALT levels.

> **Clinical Alert**
>
> There is a correlation between the presence of elevated serum ALT and abnormal antibodies to the hepatitis B virus core antigen. Persons with elevated ALT levels should not donate blood.

Patient Preparation

1. Explain test purpose and blood-drawing procedure.
2. Follow guidelines in Chapter 1 for safe, effective, informed *pretest* care.

Patient Aftercare

1. Resume normal activities.
2. Interpret test results and monitor as appropriate for liver disease.
3. Follow guidelines in Chapter 1 for safe, effective, informed *posttest* care.

ALKALINE PHOSPHATASE (ALP), TOTAL; 5'-NUCLEOTIDASE ●

Normal Values

Age	Males	Females
4 y	324–803 U/L	368–809 U/L
5 y	389–904 U/L	352–772 U/L
6 y	390–906 U/L	367–805 U/L
7 y	374–881 U/L	398–875 U/L
8 y	367–871 U/L	433–956 U/L
9 y	381–893 U/L	461–1,018 U/L
10 y	415–945 U/L	468–1,034 U/L
11 y	402–1,103 U/L	388–1,144 U/L
12 y	403–1,222 U/L	290–1,055 U/L
13 y	395–1,276 U/L	260–976 U/L
14 y	361–1,241 U/L	333–787 U/L
15 y	299–1,110 U/L	163–595 U/L
16 y	221–906 U/L	133–573 U/L
17 y	151–677 U/L	
17–23 y		114–312 U/L
18 y	113–485 U/L	
≥19 y	98–251 U/L	
24–45 y		81–213 U/L
46–50 y		84–218 U/L
51–55 y		90–234 U/L
56–60 y		99–257 U/L
61–65 y		108–282 U/L
≥66 y		119–309 U/L

NOTE: *Values may vary with method of testing. Check with your laboratory for reference values.*

Background

Alkaline phosphatase is an enzyme originating mainly in the bone, liver and placenta, with some activity in the kidney and intestines. It is called *alkaline* because it functions best at a pH of 9. ALP levels are age and gender dependent.

Explanation of Test

Alkaline phosphatase is used as an index of liver and bone disease when correlated with other clinical findings. In bone disease, the enzyme level rises in proportion to new bone cell production resulting from osteoblastic activity and the deposit of calcium in the bones. In liver disease, the blood level rises when excretion of this enzyme is impaired as a result of obstruction in the biliary tract.

Procedure

1. Obtain a 5-ml fasting venous blood sample. Serum is used for this test. Anticoagulants may not be used. Observe standard precautions.
2. Refrigerate sample as soon as possible.
3. Note age and gender on test requisition.

Clinical Implications

1. *Elevated levels of ALP in liver disease* (correlated with abnormal liver function tests) occur in the following conditions:
   a. Obstructive jaundice (gallstones obstructing major biliary ducts; accompanying elevated bilirubin)
   b. Space-occupying lesions of the liver such as cancer (hepatic carcinoma) and malignancy with liver metastasis
   c. Hepatocellular cirrhosis
   d. Biliary cirrhosis
   e. Intrahepatic and extrahepatic cholestasis
   f. Hepatitis, infectious mononucleosis
   g. Diabetes mellitus (causes increased synthesis)
2. *Bone disease and elevated ALP levels* occur in the following conditions:
   a. Paget's disease (osteitis deformans; levels 10 to 25 times normal)
   b. Metastatic bone tumor
   c. Osteogenic sarcoma
   d. Osteomalacia (elevated levels help differentiate between osteomalacia and osteoporosis, in which there is no elevation), rickets
   e. Healing factors (osteogenesis imperfecta)
3. Other diseases involving *elevated ALP levels* include the following:
   a. Hyperparathyroidism (accompanied by hypercalcemia)
   b. Pulmonary and myocardial infarctions
   c. Hodgkin's disease
   d. Cancer of lung or pancreas
   e. Ulcerative colitis
   f. Sarcoidosis
   g. Perforation of bowel (acute infarction)
   h. Amyloidosis
   i. Chronic renal failure

    j. Primary hypophosphatemia

    k. Hyperphosphatasia

4. *Decreased levels of ALP* occur in the following conditions:

    a. Hypophosphatasia (congenital)

    b. Malnutrition, scurvy

    c. Hypothyroidism, cretinism

    d. Pernicious anemia and severe anemias

    e. Magnesium deficiency

    f. Milk alkali (Burnett's syndrome)

    g. Celiac sprue

    h. Magnesium and zinc deficiency

Interfering Factors

1. A variety of drugs produce mild to moderate increases or decreases in ALP levels. See Appendix J for drugs that affect outcomes.

2. Young children, those experiencing rapid growth, pregnant women, and postmenopausal women have physiologically high levels of ALP; this level is slightly increased in older persons.

3. After IV administration of albumin, there is sometimes a marked increase in ALP for several days.

4. ALP levels increase at room temperature.

5. ALP levels decrease if blood is anticoagulated.

Patient Preparation

1. Explain test purpose and blood-drawing procedure. Fasting is required.

2. Follow guidelines in Chapter 1 for safe, effective, informed *pretest* care.

Patient Aftercare

1. Resume normal activities.

2. Interpret test results and monitor appropriately for liver or bone disease and evidence of tumor. Testing for 5′-nucleotidase provides supportive evidence in the diagnosis of liver disease. When ALP and 5′-nucleotidase test results are evaluated, they provide definitive diagnosis of Paget's disease and rickets, in which high levels of ALP accompany normal (0–5 U/L) or marginally increased 5′-nucleotidase activity. 5′-Nucleotidase is increased in liver disease (eg, hepatic carcinoma, biliary cirrhosis, extrahepatic obstruction, metastatic neoplasia of liver). 5′-Nucleotidase level usually does not increase in skeletal disease.

3. Follow guidelines in Chapter 1 for safe, effective, informed *posttest* care.

ALKALINE PHOSPHATASE ISOENZYMES (ISO)

Normal Values

AP-1, α_2: values (liver) reported as weak, moderate, or strong or 24–158 μ/L

AP-2, β_1: values (bone) reported as weak, moderate, or strong or 24–146 μ/L

AP-3, β_2: values (intestines) reported as weak, moderate, or strong or 0–22 μ/L

AP-4: values (placental) reported as present weak, moderate, or strong. Placental is found only in pregnant women.

Background

The isoenzymes of ALP are produced in various tissues. AP-1, α_2 is produced in the liver and by proliferating blood vessels. AP-2, β_1 is produced by bone and placental tissue. The intestinal isoenzyme AP-3, β_2 is present in small quantities in group O and B individuals who are Lewis-positive secretors. Placental ALP is present in the last trimester of pregnancy.

Explanation of Test

Any patient with an elevation of serum total alkaline phosphatase is a candidate for ALP isoenzyme study. The ALP ISO is mainly used to distinguish between bone and liver elevations of alkaline phosphatase.

Procedure

Obtain a 5-ml fasting venous blood sample in a plain red-topped tube or ISST tube. Serum is needed. Observe standard precautions. Centrifuge blood promptly 30 minutes after draw.

Clinical Implications

1. Liver (AP-1, α_2) isoenzymes are elevated in hepatic and biliary diseases such as the following conditions:
   a. Cirrhosis (hepatic)
   b. Hepatic carcinoma
   c. Biliary obstruction, primary biliary cirrhosis
2. Bone (AP-2, β_1) isoenzymes are elevated in the following conditions:
   a. Paget's disease
   b. Hyperparathyroidism
   c. Bone cancer, rickets
   d. Osteomalacia
   e. Celiac disease
   f. Certain renal disorders
3. Intestinal (AP-3, β_2) isoenzymes are elevated in the following conditions:
   a. Intestinal infarction
   b. Ulcerative lesions of stomach, small intestine, and colon
   c. May be increased in cirrhosis of liver
   d. Patients undergoing hemodialysis
4. Placental AP-4 isoenzymes are increased in the following conditions:
   a. Pregnant women (late in third trimester to onset of labor)
   b. Complications of pregnancy such as hypertension and preeclampsia
   c. Placental-like isoenzymes occur in some cancers:
      (1) Regan isoenzyme
      (2) Nagao isoenzyme

Clinical Alert

1. This test should not be done if the total alkaline phosphatase level is normal.

(continued)

(Clinical Alert continued)

2. For evaluation of the biliary tract, alternatives tests such as GGT, leucine aminopeptidase (LAP), and 5′-nucleotidase studies are recommended over ALP ISO test.
3. Alkaline phosphatase isoenzymes have little value in children and adolescents because bone and liver fractions are normally elevated.
4. A hemolyzed specimen is not acceptable.

Interfering Factors

Same as for alkaline phosphatase.

Patient Preparation and Patient Aftercare

See total alkaline phosphatase patient preparation and aftercare on p. 432. The same guidelines apply to alkaline phosphatase isoenzyme testing.

ALDOLASE (ALD)

Normal Values

Adult: 1.5–8.1 U/L
Child (1 month–6 y): 3.0–16 U/L
Neonate (0–1 month): 6.0–32.0 U/L

Background

Aldolase is an enzyme present primarily in heart and skeletal muscle. Small amounts are also present in liver, kidneys, and brain in isoenzymatic forms.

Explanation of Test

This test is helpful in complex diagnostic situations to evaluate muscle wasting process and skeletal muscle degeneration. In the progressive dystrophies, aldolase levels may be 10 to 15 times normal when muscle mass is relatively intact, as in early stages of the disease. When advanced muscle wasting is present, ALD values decline. In the inflammatory myopathies (eg, dermatomyositis), serum aldolase (as well as creatinine kinase [CK]) levels may be applied to monitoring response to steroid therapy.

Procedure

Obtain a 5-ml venous blood sample. Fasting is required. Serum or plasma may be used. Observe standard precautions.

Clinical Implications

1. Highest aldolase levels are found in Duchenne's muscular dystrophy.
2. Lesser ALD elevations are found in the following conditions:
   a. Dermatomyositis
   b. Polymyositis
   c. Limb-girdle muscular dystrophy
   d. Acute hepatitis and other liver diseases
   e. Eosinophilia-myalgia syndrome
   f. Gangrene

g. Some carcinomas with liver metastases

h. Delirium tremens, burns

i. CNS tumors

j. Acute psychosis or schizophrenia

k. Granulocytic and megaloblastic anemias

l. Myocardial infarction

3. Normal aldolase values are found in neurogenic atrophies, multiple sclerosis, and myasthenia gravis.

4. Decreased levels of ALD are found in hereditary fructose intolerance.

Patient Preparation

1. Explain test purpose and procedure. Fasting from midnight until the specimen is obtained is required. Water is permitted.

2. Follow guidelines in Chapter 1 for safe, effective, informed *pretest* care.

Patient Aftercare

1. Resume normal activities.

2. Interpret test results and counsel appropriately. Aldolase is not specific for muscle disease. The CK assay has been the preferred test for muscle disease. CK isoenzymes have a specific band for skeletal muscle.

3. Follow guidelines in Chapter 1 for safe, effective, informed *posttest* care.

ANGIOTENSIN-CONVERTING ENZYME (ACE)

Normal Values

5–21 nmol/ml/min

Background

Angiotensin I is produced by the action of renin on angiotensinogen. Angiotensin I–converting enzyme (ACE) catalyzes the conversion of angiotensin I to the vasoactive peptide angiotensin II. Angiotensin I is concentrated in the proximal tubules.

Explanation of Test

This test is used primarily to evaluate the severity and activity of sarcoidosis. Serial determinations may be helpful in following the clinical course of the disease.

Procedure

Obtain a 5-ml venous blood sample. Serum is used. Observe standard precautions. Specimen must be frozen if test is not performed immediately.

Clinical Implications

1. *Increased ACE levels* are associated with the following conditions:

   a. Sarcoidosis (ACE levels reflect the severity of the disease, with 68% positivity in stage 1 disease, 86% in stage 2, and 92% in stage 3)

    b. Gaucher's disease
    c. Leprosy
    d. Acute and chronic bronchitis
    e. Connective tissue diseases
    f. Amyloidosis
    g. Pulmonary fibrosis
    h. Fungal diseases and histoplasmosis
2. *Decreased ACE levels* occur in the following conditions:
    a. Following prednisone treatment for sarcoidosis
    b. Advanced lung neoplasms

Interfering Factors

This test should not be done on persons <20 years of age because they normally have a very high level of ACE. About 5% of the normal adult population have elevated ACE levels.

Patient Preparation

1. Explain test purpose and blood-drawing procedure.
2. Follow guidelines in Chapter 1 for safe, effective, informed *pretest* care.

Patient Aftercare

1. Interpret test results and monitor as appropriate for sarcoidosis and amyloid disease.
2. Follow guidelines in Chapter 1 for safe, effective, informed *posttest* care.

AMYLASE AND LIPASE   ●

Normal Values

Amylase	Lipase
Newborn: 6–65 U/L	Adult: 10–140 U/L
Adult: 25–125 U/L	Elderly (>60 y): 18–180 U/L
Elderly: 21–160 U/L	

    Normal values vary widely according to method of testing. Check with your laboratory for reference ranges.

Background

Amylase, an enzyme that changes starch to sugar, is produced in the salivary glands, pancreas, liver, and fallopian tubes. If there is an inflammation of the pancreas or salivary glands, much amylase enters the blood. Amylase levels in the urine reflect blood changes by a time lag of 6 to 10 hours (see Amylase Excretion/Clearance, Chap. 3). Lipase changes fats to fatty acids and glycerol. The pancreas is the major source of this enzyme. Lipase appears in the blood following pancreatic damage.

Explanation of Test
Amylase and lipase tests are used to diagnose and monitor treatment of acute pancreatitis and to differentiate pancreatitis from other acute abdominal disorders (80% of patients with acute pancreatitis will have elevated amylase and lipase levels; lipase stays elevated longer).

Procedure
Obtain a 5-ml venous blood sample. Serum is used. EDTA anticoagulant interferes with lipase testing. Observe standard precautions.

Clinical Implications
1. *Greatly increased amylase levels* occur in acute pancreatitis early in the course of the disease. The increase begins in 3 to 6 hours after the onset of pain.
2. *Increased amylase levels* also occur in the following conditions:
   a. Chronic pancreatitis, pancreatic trauma
   b. Partial gastrectomy
   c. Obstruction of pancreatic duct
   d. Perforated peptic ulcer
   e. Alcohol poisoning
   f. Cerebral trauma
   g. Obstruction or inflammation of salivary duct or gland and mumps
   h. Acute cholecystitis (common duct stone)
   i. Intestinal obstruction with strangulation
   j. Ruptured tubal pregnancy and ectopic pregnancy
   k. Ruptured aortic aneurysm
   l. Macroamylasia
3. *Decreased amylase levels* occur in the following conditions:
   a. Pancreatic insufficiency
   b. Hepatitis, severe liver disease
   c. Advanced cystic fibrosis
   d. Pancreatectomy
4. *Elevated lipase levels* occur in pancreatic disorders (eg, pancreatitis, pancreatic carcinoma). Elevations of lipase may not occur until 24 to 36 hours after onset of illness and may remain elevated for up to 14 days. Lipase elevation occurs later and persists longer than blood amylase changes.
5. *Increased lipase values* also are associated with the following conditions:
   a. Cholecystitis
   b. Organ transplant
   c. Strangulated or infarcted bowel
   d. Peritonitis
6. Serum lipase levels are normal in patients with elevated amylase who have peptic ulcer, salivary adenitis, inflammatory bowel disease, intestinal obstruction, and macroamylasemia. Coexistence of increased serum amylase and normal lipase levels may be a helpful clue to the presence of macroamylasemia.

> ◗ **Clinical Alert**
>
> *Panic Level for Lipase*
> >600 IU/L

Interfering Factors
1. Amylase
   a. Anticoagulated blood gives lower results.
   b. Lipemic serum interferes with test.
   c. Increased levels are found in alcoholics and pregnant women and in diabetic ketoacidosis.
   d. Many drugs can interfere with this test (see Appendix J).
2. Lipase
   a. EDTA anticoagulant interferes with test.
   b. Lipase is increased in ~50% of patients with chronic renal failure.
   c. Lipase increases in patients undergoing hemodialysis.
   d. Many drugs can affect outcomes. See Appendix J.

Patient Presentation
1. Explain test purpose and procedure. Amylase and lipase testing are done together in the presence of abdominal pain, epigastric tenderness, nausea, and vomiting. These findings characterize acute pancreatitis as well as other acute surgical emergencies.
2. If amylase/creatinine clearance testing is also being done, a single, random urine sample is collected at the same time blood is drawn.
3. Follow guidelines in Chapter 1 regarding safe, effective, informed *pretest* care.

Patient Aftercare
1. Resume normal activities.
2. Interpret test results and monitor as appropriate for pancreatitis or other acute abdominal conditions.
3. Follow guidelines in Chapter 1 for safe, effective, informed *posttest* care.

ASPARTATE TRANSAMINASE (AMINOTRANSFERASE, AST); SERUM GLUTAMIC-OXALOACETIC TRANSAMINASE (SGOT)

Normal Values

0–5 d: 35–140 U/L	6–12 y: 10–50 U/L
6 d–3 y: 20–60 U/L	12–18 y: 10–40 U/L
3–6 y: 15–50 U/L	Adult (>18 y): 5–40 U/L

Background
Aspartate transaminase (AST) is an enzyme present in tissues of high metabolic activity and decreasing concentration AST in the heart, liver, skeletal mus-

cle, kidney, brain, pancreas, spleen, and lungs. The enzyme is released into the circulation following the injury or death of cells. Any disease that causes change in these highly metabolic tissues will result in a rise in AST levels. The amount of AST in the blood is directly related to the number of damaged cells and the amount of time that passes between injury to the tissue and the test. Following severe cell damage, the blood AST level will rise in 12 hours and remain elevated for ~5 days.

Explanation of Test
This test is used to evaluate liver and heart diseases.

Procedure
Obtain a 5-ml venous sample. Serum is used. Observe standard precautions. Hemolysis should be avoided.

Clinical Implications
1. *Increased AST levels* occur in MI.
   a. In MI, the AST level may be increased to 4 to 10 times the normal values.
   b. The AST level reaches a peak in 24 hours and returns to normal by day 3 or 4 post-MI. Secondary rises in AST levels suggest extension or recurrence of MI.
   c. The AST curve in MI parallels that of creatinine phosphokinase (CPK) (see p. 441).
2. *Increased AST levels* occur in liver diseases (10–100 times normal).
   a. Acute hepatitis and chronic hepatitis
   b. Active cirrhosis (drug induced)
   c. Infectious mononucleosis
   d. Hepatic necrosis and metastasis
   e. Primary or metastatic carcinoma
   f. Alcoholic hepatitis
   g. Reye's syndrome
3. Other diseases associated with *elevated AST levels* include the following:
   a. Acute pancreatitis (may be normal)
   b. Trauma and irradiation of skeletal muscle
   c. Dermatomyositis
   d. Polymyositis
   e. Trichinosis
   f. Cardiac catheterization
   g. Recent brain trauma with brain necrosis, cerebral infarction
   h. Crushing and traumatic injuries
   i. Progressive muscular dystrophy (Duchenne's)
   j. Pulmonary emboli
   k. Gangrene

l. Malignant hyperthermia, heat angiography
m. Mushroom poisoning
n. Congestive heart failure
o. Hemolytic anemia, exhaustion, heat stroke
4. *Decreased AST levels* occur in the following conditions:
   a. Azotemia
   B. Chronic renal dialysis

Interfering Factors
1. Slight decreases occur during pregnancy, when there is abnormal metabolism of pyridoxine.
2. Many drugs can cause elevated or decreased levels (see Appendix J). Alcohol ingestion affects results.
3. Exercise and IM injections do not affect results.
4. False decreases occur in diabetic ketoacidosis, severe liver disease, and uremia.

Patient Preparation
1. Explain test purpose and blood-drawing procedure. For diagnosis of MI, AST testing should be done on 3 consecutive days because the peak is reached in 24 hours and levels return to normal in 3 to 4 days.
2. Follow guidelines in Chapter 1 for safe, effective, informed *pretest* care.

Patient Aftercare
1. Interpret test results and monitor appropriately for heart and liver diseases.
2. Unexplained AST elevations should be further investigated with ALT and GGT tests.
3. Follow guidelines in Chapter 1 for safe, effective, informed *posttest* care.

CARDIAC TROPONIN T (cTnT); TROPONIN I (cTnI)   ●

Normal Values
Negative

Values may vary depending on the testing method used. Check with your laboratory for reference values.

Background
Cardiac troponin is unique to the heart muscle and is highly concentrated in cardiomyocytes. This protein is released with very small areas of myocardial damage as early as 1 to 3 hours postinjury, and levels return to normal within 14 to 15 days.

Explanation of Test

This test is used in the early diagnosis of small myocardial infarcts that are undetectable by conventional diagnostic methods. Cardiac troponin levels are also used later in the course of MI because they remain elevated for 14 to 15 days postinjury. This test is used to monitor healing and reperfusion.

Procedure

1. Obtain a 5-ml venous blood sample in a red-topped tube within hours after onset of chest pain. Observe standard precautions.

Clinical Implications

1. Positive or elevated cardiac troponin levels indicate small infarcts; increases remain for 14 to 15 days.

Interfering Factors

1. Cardiac troponin levels may possibly be increased in chronic muscle or renal disease and trauma.
2. Levels are not affected by orthopedic or lung surgery.

Patient Preparation

1. Explain that the test is a sensitive marker for minor myocardial injury in unstable angina.
2. Follow guidelines in Chapter 1 for safe, effective, informed *pretest* care.

Patient Aftercare

1. Interpret test results, and counsel and monitor appropriately. Additional testing may be necessary (eg, cardiac myogen light classes, glycogen phosphorylcholine BB [GPBB]).
2. Follow guidelines in Chapter 1 for safe, effective, informed *posttest* care.

CREATINE PHOSPHOKINASE (CPK); CREATINE KINASE (CK); CPK AND CK ISOENZYMES

Normal Values

Men: 38–174 U/l	MM CK_3: 96%–100%
Women: 26–140 U/l	MB CK_2: 0%–4%
Isoenzymes:	BB CK_1: 0%

NOTE: *Normal values may vary with method of testing and reaction temperature. Check with your laboratory.*

NOTE: *Healthy African-American persons have higher CK levels than do Caucasian or Hispanic persons.*

Background

Creatine kinase (CPK/CK) is an enzyme found in higher concentrations in the heart and skeletal muscles and in much smaller concentrations in brain tissue. Because CK exists in relatively few organs, this test is used as a specific index of injury to myocardium and muscle. CPK can be divided into three isoenzymes: MM or CK_3, BB or CK_1, and MB or CK_2. CK-MM is the isoenzyme that constitutes almost all the circulatory enzymes in healthy persons. Skeletal muscle contains primarily MM; cardiac muscle contains primarily MM and MB; and brain tissue, GI system, and genitourinary tract contain primarily BB. Normal CK levels are virtually 100% MM isoenzyme. A slight increase in total CPK is reflected from elevated BB from CNS injury. CPK isoenzyme studies help distinguish whether the CPK originated from the heart (MB) or the skeletal muscle (MM).

Explanation of Test

The CK (CPK) test is used in the diagnosis of MI and as a reliable measure of skeletal and inflammatory muscle diseases. CK levels can prove helpful in recognizing muscular dystrophy before clinical signs appear. CK levels may rise significantly with CNS disorders such as Reye's syndrome. The determination of CK isoenzymes may be helpful in making a differential diagnosis. Elevation of MB, the cardiac isoenzyme, provides a more definitive indication of myocardial cell damage than total CK alone. MM isoenzyme is an indicator of skeletal muscle damage. Newer tests, such as CK isoforms, allow for earlier detection of MI than is possible with CK-MB.

Procedure

Obtain a 5-ml venous blood sample. Serum must be used. Observe standard precautions. If a patient has been receiving multiple injections IM, note this fact on the laboratory requisition. Avoid hemolysis.

Clinical Implications of Total CK Levels

1. *Increased CK/CPK levels* occur in the following conditions:
   a. Acute myocardial infarction
      (1) With MI, the rise starts soon after an attack (~4–6 hours) and reaches a peak of at least several times normal within 24 hours. CK returns to normal in 48 to 72 hours.
      (2) CK and CK-MB (CK_2 MB) peaks about 1 day following onset, as does AST.
      (3) Lactate dehydrogenase (LD) usually peaks at 2 days following onset, when the LD_1-LD_2 inversion (flip) is found.
      (4) CK-MB, LD_1, LD_1:LD_2 ratio, total CK, and total LD classically increase with acute MI. CK-MB and LD_1 increase both in percentage and absolutely (each isoenzyme percentage times the respective total enzyme), peak, and then decrease.

(5) AST testing with LD and LD isoenzymes is advocated when the patient reaches medical attention 48 to 72 hours after onset of a possible acute MI.

b. Severe myocarditis
c. After open heart surgery
d. Cardioversion (cardiac defibrillation)

2. Other diseases and procedures that cause increased CK/CPK levels include the following:

a. Acute cerebrovascular disease
b. Progressive muscular dystrophy (levels may reach 20–200 times normal), Duchenne's muscular dystrophy, female carriers of muscular dystrophy
c. Dermatomyositis and polymyositis
d. Delirium tremens and chronic alcoholism
e. Electric shock, electromyography
f. Malignant hyperthermia
g. Reye's syndrome
h. Convulsions, ischemia, or subarachnoid hemorrhage
i. Last weeks of pregnancy and during childbirth
j. Hypothyroidism
k. Acute psychosis
l. CNS trauma, extensive brain infarction
m. Neoplasms of prostate, bladder, or GI tract

3. Normal values are found in myasthenia gravis and multiple sclerosis.
4. Decreased values have no diagnostic meaning and may be caused by low muscle mass and bed rest (overnight values can drop 20%).

Clinical Implications of CK Isoenzymes

1. *Elevated MB (CK_2) isoenzyme levels* occur in the following conditions:

a. Myocardial infarct (rises 4–6 hours after MI; not demonstrable after 24–36 hours; ie, peak with rapid fall)
b. Myocardial ischemia, angina pectoris
c. Duchenne's muscular dystrophy
d. Subarachnoid hemorrhage
e. Reye's syndrome
f. Muscle trauma, surgery (postoperative)
g. Circulatory failure and shock
h. Infections of heart and skeletal muscle
i. Chronic renal failure
j. Hypothymia, malignant hyperthermia

2. BB (CK_1) elevations occur in the following conditions:

a. Reye's syndrome
b. Some breast, bladder, lung, uterus, testes, and prostate cancers
c. Severe shock syndrome
d. Brain injury, neurosurgery

    e. Hypothermia
    f. Following coronary bypass surgery
    g. Newborns
3. MM (CK_1) is elevated in most conditions in which total CK is elevated.

Clinical Alert

1. After an MI, MB appears in the serum in 6 to 12 hours and remains for about 18 to 32 hours. The finding of MB in a patient with chest pain is diagnostic of MI. In addition, if there is a negative CK-MB for $\geq$48 hours following a clearly defined episode, it is clear that the patient has not had an MI.

2. CK-MB, LD_1, LD_1:LD_2 ratio, total CK, and total LD classically increase with acute MI. CK-MB and LD_1 increase both in percentage and absolutely (each isoenzyme percent times the respective total enzyme), peak, then decrease.

Interfering Factors

1. Strenuous exercise, weight-lifting, and surgical procedures that damage skeletal muscle may cause increased levels of CK.
2. Alcohol and other drugs of abuse increase CK levels.
3. Athletes have a higher CK value because of greater muscle mass.
4. Multiple IM injections may cause increased or decreased CK levels (see Appendix J).
5. Many drugs may cause increased CK levels.
6. Childbirth may cause increased CK levels.
7. Hemolysis of blood sample causes increased CK levels.

Patient Preparation

1. Explain test purpose and need for at least three consecutive blood draws following episode.
2. Note on requisition when suspected cardiac episode occurred.
3. No exercise is allowed before test.
4. Follow guidelines in Chapter 1 for safe, effective, informed *pretest* care.

Patient Aftercare

1. Resume normal activities.
2. Interpret test results and monitor as appropriate for MI, muscular dystrophy, and other causes of abnormal test outcomes.
3. Follow guidelines in Chapter 1 for safe, effective, informed *posttest* care.

GALACTOSE-1-PHOSPHATE URIDYLTRANSFERASE (GPT); GALACTOKINASE

Normal Values
Galactose-1-phosphate uridyltransferase: 18.5–28.5 U/g of hemoglobin
Galactokinase: 18–39 µmol/h/g of hemoglobin

Background
The enzyme galactose-1-phosphate uridyltransferase is needed in the use of galactose-1-phosphate so that it does not accumulate in the body. A very rare genetic disorder resulting from an inborn (inherited or acquired during intrauterine development) error of galactose metabolism may occur.

Explanation of Test
This measurement is used to identify galactose defects, which can result in widespread tissue damage and abnormalities such as cataracts, liver disease, and renal disease. It also causes failure to thrive and mental retardation.

Procedure
Obtain a 5-ml venous blood sample. Anticoagulate with heparin or EDTA. Observe standard precautions.

Clinical Implications
Decreased values are associated with galactosemia, a rare genetic disorder transmitted in an autosomal recessive fashion. The resulting accumulation of galactitol and/or galactose-1-phosphate can result in juvenile cataracts, liver failure, failure to thrive, and mental retardation in persons with galactose-1-phosphate uridyltransferase deficiency.

Patient Preparation
1. Explain test purpose and procedure. Genetic counseling may be necessary.
2. Follow guidelines in Chapter 1 for safe, effective, informed *pretest* care.

Patient Aftercare
1. Interpret test results and counsel appropriately.
2. Parents of infants and children with positive test results should be instructed that the disease can be effectively treated by removing galactose-containing foods, especially milk, from the diet. With dietary galactose restriction, liver and lens changes are reversible.
3. Follow guidelines in Chapter 1 for safe, effective, informed *posttest* care.

HEXOSAMINIDASE, TOTAL AND ISOENZYME A

Normal Values

Hexosaminidase A	*Total Hexosaminidase*
Noncarrier: 7.2–9.88 U/L	Noncarrier: 9.83–15.95 U/L
Heterozygous: 3.30–5.39 U/L	Heterozygous: 3.30–5.39 U/L
Tay-Sachs: 0 U/L	Homozygous Tay-Sachs: 17.1 U/L

Normal values vary with method of testing used. Check with your laboratory for reference values.

Background

Three isoenzymes of hexosaminidase have been identified in serum: A (acid form), B (base form), and S. Hexosaminidase A is a lysosomal isoenzyme, deficiency of which characterizes patients with Tay-Sachs disease. Homozygotes have no hexosaminidase A and a large increase in hexosaminidase B and S. Heterozygotes have a moderate decrease in hexosaminidase A and a slight increase of hexosaminidase B and S.

Explanation of Test

Hexosaminidase A is used as a diagnostic test for Tay-Sachs disease and can be of help in identifying carriers among persons with no family history of Tay-Sachs. This condition is due to an autosomal recessive trait found predominantly, but not exclusively, in Ashkenazi Jews and is characterized by the appearance during infancy of psychomotor deterioration, blindness, cherry red spot on the macula, and an exaggerated extension response to sound. In the brains of affected children, the level of ganglioside is increased 100 times owing to the deficiency of this enzyme.

Procedure

Obtain a 5-ml venous blood sample. The test uses serum. If the test is not performed immediately, serum must be frozen.

Clinical Implications

1. *Decreased hexosaminidase A.* An almost total deficiency of the A component is diagnostic of Tay-Sachs disease or GM_2 gangliosidosis. The total hexosaminidase is of no value in Tay-Sachs.
2. *Decreased hexosaminidase A and B.* In a variant of Tay-Sachs disease known as Sandhoff's disease, both A and B isoenzymes are defective, causing an absence of this enzyme. The total hexosaminidase level is also decreased in Sandhoff's disease.
3. *Increased total hexosaminidase* occurs in the following conditions:
   a. Hepatic disease (biliary obstruction)
   b. Gastric cancer
   c. Myeloma
   d. Myocardial infarction
   e. Vascular complications of diabetes mellitus

Interfering Factors

1. Total values are increased in pregnancy (5 times normal).
2. Oral contraceptives falsely increase values.

> **Clinical Alert**
>
> *Critical Values for Hexosaminidase A*
> <50% of total activity indicates Tay-Sachs disease

Patient Preparation
1. Explain test purpose and procedure.
2. Pregnancy and/or oral contraceptives are contraindications for testing.
3. Follow guidelines in Chapter 1 for safe, effective, informed *pretest* care.

Patient Aftercare
1. Interpret test results and be prepared to perform genetic counseling of patient and family.
2. Follow guidelines in Chapter 1 for safe, effective, informed *posttest* care.

LACTIC ACID DEHYDROGENASE (LD, LDH)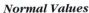

Normal Values
0–5 y: 425–975 U/L   14–16 y: 370–645 U/L
5–12 y: 370–840 U/L   Adult (>16 y): 313–618 U/L
12–14 y: 370–785 U/L

Normal values vary with method of testing used. Check with your laboratory for reference values.

Background
Lactic acid dehydrogenase is an intracellular enzyme that is widely distributed in the tissues of the body, particularly in the kidney, heart, skeletal muscle, brain, liver, and lungs. Increases in the reported value usually indicate cellular death and leakage of the enzyme from the cell.

Explanation of Test
Although elevated levels of LDH are nonspecific, this test is useful in confirming myocardial or pulmonary infarction when viewed in relation to other test findings. For example, LD remains elevated longer than CK in MI. LDH level is also helpful in the differential diagnosis of muscular dystrophy and pernicious anemia. More specific findings may be found by breaking down the LDH into its five isoenzymes. (When LD values are reported or quoted, *total* LDH is meant.)

Procedure
1. Obtain a 5-ml venous blood sample. Serum is used. Observe standard precautions.
2. Avoid hemolysis in obtaining blood sample.

Clinical Implications

A. *Increased LDH (LD)* occurs in the following conditions:

1. High levels occur within 36 to 55 hours after MI and continue longer than elevations of SGOT or CPK (3–10 days). Differential diagnosis of acute MI may be accomplished with LDH isoenzymes.

2. In pulmonary infarction, increased LDH occurs within 24 hours of pain onset. The pattern of normal SGOT and elevated LDH that levels off 1 to 2 days after an episode of chest pain is indicative of pulmonary infarction.

3. *Elevated levels of LDH* are also observed in various other conditions:
   a. Congestive heart failure
   b. Liver diseases (eg, cirrhosis, alcoholism, acute viral hepatitis)
   c. Malignant neoplasms, cancer, leukemias, lymphoma
   d. Hypothyroidism
   e. Lung diseases (pulmonary infarction)
   f. Skeletal muscle diseases (muscular dystrophy), muscular damage
   g. Megaloblastic and pernicious anemias, hemolytic anemia, sickle cell disease
   h. Delirium tremens
   i. Shock, hypoxia
   j. Hyperthermia
   k. Renal infarct

4. Angina and pericarditis do *not* produce LDH elevations.

B. *Decreased LDH levels* are associated with a good response to cancer therapy.

Interfering Factors

1. Strenuous exercise and the muscular exertion involved in childbirth cause increased LDH levels.

2. Skin diseases can cause falsely increased LDH levels.

3. Hemolysis of red blood cells due to freezing, heating, or shaking the blood sample will cause falsely increased LDH levels.

4. Various drugs may cause increased or decreased LDH levels (see Appendix J).

> ### Clinical Alert
>
> LDH is found in nearly every tissue of the body; therefore, elevated levels are of limited diagnostic value by themselves. Differential diagnoses may be accomplished with LD isoenzyme determination.

Patient Preparation

1. Explain test purpose and blood-drawing procedure.

2. Follow guidelines in Chapter 1 for safe, effective, informed *pretest* care.

Patient Aftercare

1. Resume normal activities.

2. Interpret test results and monitor for myocardial and pulmonary infarction

and other diseases related to abnormal results. LD isoenzymes may be ordered.

3. Follow guidelines in Chapter 1 for safe, effective, informed *posttest* care.

LACTIC ACID DEHYDROGENASE (LDH, LD) ISOENZYMES (ELECTROPHORESIS) ●

Normal Values

LDH_1: 17%–27% of total
LDH_2: 29%–39% of total
LDH_3: 19%–27% of total

LDH_4: 8%–16% of total
LDH_5: 6%–16% of total

Background

Electrophoresis, or separation, of LDH identifies the five isoenzymes or fractions of LDH, each with its own physical characteristics and electrophoretic properties. Fractionating the LDH activity sharpens its diagnostic value, because LDH is found in many organs. LD isoenzymes are released into the bloodstream when tissue necrosis occurs. The isoenzymes are elevated in terms of patterns established, not on the basis of the value of a single isoenzyme. The origins of the LDH isoenzymes are as follows: LD_1 and LD_2 are present in cardiac tissue and erythrocytes; LD_3 originates mainly from lung, spleen, pancreas, and placenta; and LD_4 and LD_5 originate from skeletal muscle and liver.

Explanation of Test

The five isoenzyme fractions of LDH show different patterns in various disorders. Abnormalities in the pattern suggest which tissues have been damaged. This test is useful in the differential diagnosis of acute MI, megaloblastic anemia (eg, folate deficiency, pernicious anemia), hemolytic anemia, and very occasionally, renal infarct. These entities are characterized by LD_1 increases, often with LD_1:LD_2 inversion (flip).

Procedure

Obtain a 5-ml venous blood sample. Serum is needed. Avoid hemolysis. Observe standard precautions.

Clinical Implications

1. Abnormal LD_1 and LD_2 patterns reflect damaged tissues (see display regarding Abnormal LD Isoenzyme Patterns).
   a. The appearance of an LD flip (ie, when LD_1 level is higher than LD_2 level) is extremely helpful in the diagnosis of MI. The presence of an LD flip 1 day following incident or with the detection of CK-MB is essentially diagnostic of MI if baseline cardiac enzymes/isoenzymes are normal and if rises and falls are as anticipated for the diagnosis of acute MI.

   b. Persistent LD_1:LD_2 flip following acute myocardial infarct may represent reinfarction. When acute MI is complicated by shock, a normal pattern may be found. LD_1:LD_2 inversion commonly appears subsequent to the isomorphic pattern in instances of acute MI.

   c. The LDH pattern in hemolytic megaloblastic and sickle cell anemia is essentially the same as in MI and other anemias. This is because red blood cells have an isoenzyme pattern similar to that of heart muscle. The time elapsed to peak values may help to differentiate these conditions.

2. LD_3 increases occur in advanced cancer and malignant lymphoma; this level should decrease following effective therapy. LD_3 is occasionally elevated in pulmonary infarction or pneumonia.

3. LD_5 is *increased* in the following conditions:

   a. Liver disease, hepatitis

   b. Congestive heart failure

   c. Striated muscle trauma, burns

4. LD_5 increase is more significant when LD_5/LD_4 ratio is increased.

5. In most cancers, one to three of the bands (LD_2, LD_3 and LD_4) are frequently increased. A notable exception is in seminomas and dysgerminomas, in which LD_1 is increased. Frequently, an increase in LD_3 may be the first indication of the presence of cancer.

6. All LD isoenzymes are increased in systemic diseases (eg, carcinomatous collagen vascular, disseminated intravascular coagulation, sepsis).

Abnormal LD Isoenzyme Patterns

Disease	LD_1	LD_2	LD_3	LD_4	LD_5
Myocardial infarction	X	X			
Pulmonary infarction*				X	X
Congestive heart failure				X	X
Viral hepatitis				X	X
Toxic hepatitis				X	X
Leukemia, granulocytic		X	X		
Pancreatitis		X	X		
Carcinomatosis (extensive)		X	X		
Megaloblastic anemia	X	X			
Hemolytic anemia	X	X			
Muscular dystrophy**	X	X			

Clinical Alert

1. LD isoenzyme testing should be reserved for diagnosis of complex cases. In 5% to 20% of patients with acute MI, the expected reversal of LD_1/LD_2 does not occur; in these patients, there is often simply an increase in LD_1.

2. LDH isoenzymes should be interpreted in light of the clinical findings.

7. Increased total LD with normal distribution of isoenzymes may be seen in coronary artery disease (CAD) with chronic heart failure and various combinations of acute and chronic diseases.

Patient Preparation

1. Explain test purpose and procedure. Repeat testing on 3 consecutive days is likely.
2. Follow guidelines in Chapter 1 for safe, effective, informed *pretest* care.

Patient Aftercare

1. Resume normal activities.
2. Interpret test results and monitor appropriately for abnormal LD patterns.
3. Follow guidelines in Chapter 1 for safe, effective, informed *posttest* care.

RENIN (ANGIOTENSIN); PLASMA RENIN ANGIOTENSIN (PRA)

Normal Values

Adult normal-sodium diet
    Supine: 0.15–2.33 ng/ml/h
    Standing: 1.31–3.95 ng/ml/h
Adult low-sodium diet
    Supine: renin levels increase 2 times normal.
    Standing: renin levels increase 6 times normal.

Background

Renin is an enzyme that converts angiotensinogen to angiotensin I. Derived from the liver, angiotensinogen is an α_2-globulin in the serum. Angiotensin I is then converted in the lung to angiotensin II. Angiotensin II is a potent vasopressor agent responsible for hypertension of renal origin, as well as a powerful releaser of aldosterone from the adrenal cortex. Both angiotensin II and aldosterone increase blood pressure. Renin levels increase when there is decreased renal perfusion pressure. The renin-aldosterone axis regulates sodium and potassium balance and blood volume and pressure. Renal reabsorption of sodium affects plasma volume. Low plasma volume, low blood pressure, low sodium, and increased potassium induce renin release, causing increased aldosterone through stimulation of angiotensin. Potassium loss, acute blood pressure increases, and increased blood volumes suppress renin release.

Explanation of Test

This test is most useful in the differential diagnosis of hypertension, whether essential, renal, or renovascular. In primary hyperaldosteronism, the findings will demonstrate that aldosterone secretion is exaggerated and secretion of renin is suppressed.

Procedure

1. Obtain a 5-ml venous blood sample. Fasting is required. Collect specimen with scrupulous attention to detail. Use EDTA as the anticoagulant to aid in preservation of any angiotensin formed before examination. Observe standard precautions.

2. Draw blood in chilled tubes and place samples on ice. Transport samples to laboratory immediately.
3. Record posture and dietary status of patient at time of blood drawing.
4. A 24-hour urine sodium should be done concurrently to aid in diagnosis.

Clinical Implications

1. *Increased renin levels* occur in the following conditions:
   a. Secondary aldosteronism with malignant hypertension
   b. Renovascular hypertension
   c. Reduced plasma volume due to low-sodium diet, diuretics, Addison's disease, or hemorrhage
   d. Chronic renal failure
   e. Salt-losing status owing to GI disease
   f. Renin-producing tumors of kidney
   g. Few patients (15%) with essential hypertension
   h. Bartter's syndrome (high renin hypertension)
   i. Pheochromocytoma
2. *Decreased renin levels* are found in the following conditions:
   a. Primary aldosteronism (98% of cases)
   b. Unilateral renal artery stenosis
   c. Administration of salt-retaining steroids
   d. Congenital adrenal hyperplasia with 17-hydroxylase deficiency

Interfering Factors

1. Levels vary in healthy persons and increase under influences that tend to shrink the intravascular fluid volume.
2. Random specimens may be difficult to interpret unless dietary and salt intake of patient is regulated.
3. Values are higher when the patient is in an upright position, when the test is performed early in the day, when the patient is on a low-salt diet, during pregnancy, and with drugs such as diuretics and antihypertensives and foods such as licorice. See Appendix J for other drugs that affect outcomes.
4. Recently administered radioisotopes interfere with test results.
5. Indomethacin and salicylates decrease renin levels.

Patient Preparation

1. Explain test purpose and procedure.
2. A regular diet that contains 180 mEq of sodium and 100 mEq of potassium must be maintained for 3 days before the specimen is obtained. A 24-hour urine sodium and potassium should also be done to evaluate salt balance.
3. Instruct the patient that it is necessary to be in a supine position for at least 2 hours before obtaining the specimen. The specimen is drawn with patient in the supine position.
4. Antihypertensive drugs, cyclic progestogens, estrogens, diuretics, and licorice should be terminated at least 2 weeks and preferably 4 weeks before a renin-aldosterone workup.
5. If a standing specimen is ordered, the patient must be standing for 2 hours

prior to testing and blood should be drawn with the patient in the sitting position.

6. No caffeine may be ingested the morning before or during the test.

7. Follow guidelines in Chapter 1 for safe, effective, informed *pretest* care.

Patient Aftercare

1. Interpret test results and counsel appropriately regarding hypertension.

2. Resume normal activities.

3. Follow guidelines in Chapter 1 for safe, effective, informed *posttest* care.

RENIN STIMULATION/CHALLENGE TEST ●

Challenge Test

A challenge test distinguishes primary from secondary hyperaldosteronism on the basis of renin levels. The test is performed with the patient in both the recumbent and upright positions and after the patient has been maintained on a low-salt diet. In normal persons and in those with essential hypertension, renin concentration is increased by the reduction in volume due to sodium restriction and the upright position. In primary aldosteronism, volume depletion does not occur, and renin concentration remains low.

General Procedure for Renin Stimulation Test

1. The patient should be admitted to the hospital for this test. On admission, obtain and record the patient's weight.

2. A reduced-sodium diet supplemented with potassium is given for 3 days, along with diuretics (eg, furosemide, chlorothiazide), as ordered.

3. Weigh patient again on the third day, record data, and ensure that the patient remains upright for 4 hours and participates in normal activities.

4. A venous heparinized blood sample for renin is obtained at 11:00 AM, when renin is usually at its maximum level. Place specimen on ice, and send it immediately to the laboratory.

Interpretation of Renin Stimulation Test

In healthy persons and most hypertensive patients, the stimulation of a low-salt diet, a diuretic, and upright posture will raise renin activity to very high levels and result in weight loss. However, in primary aldosteronism, the plasma level is expanded and remains so. In these patients, there is little if any weight loss, and the renin level is very low or undetectable. A response within the normal range can occur in the presence of aldosterone.

Patient Preparation

1. Explain test purpose and procedure. The purpose of the preparation is to deplete the patient of sodium.

2. Check with individual laboratory for specific practices.

3. Follow guidelines in Chapter 1 for safe, effective, informed *pretest* care.

Patient Aftercare

1. Resume normal activities.

2. Interpret test results and counsel appropriately regarding hypertension.

3. Follow guidelines in Chapter 1 for safe, effective, informed *posttest* care.

γ-GLUTAMYLTRANSFERASE
(γ-GLUTAMYL TRANSPEPTIDASE, GGT, γGT)   ●

Normal Values
Men: 5–85 U/L   Women: 5–55 U/L

Background
The enzyme γ-glutamyl transpeptidase is present mainly in the liver, kidney, and pancreas. Despite the fact that the kidney has the highest level of this enzyme, the liver is considered the source of normal serum activity. γGT has no origin in bone or placenta.

Explanation of Test
This test is used to determine liver cell dysfunction and to detect alcohol-induced liver disease. Because the GGT is very sensitive to the amount of alcohol consumed by chronic drinkers, it can be used to monitor the cessation or reduction of alcohol consumption in chronic alcoholics and early risk drinkers. GT activity is elevated in all forms of liver disease. This test is much more sensitive than either the alkaline phosphatase test or the transaminase test (ie, SGOT, SGPT) in detecting obstructive jaundice, cholangitis, and cholecystitis. It is also indicated in the differential diagnosis of liver disease in children and pregnant women who have elevated levels of LDH and alkaline phosphatase. γGT is also useful as a marker for prostatic cancer and hepatic metastasis from breast and colon.

Procedure
Obtain a 5-ml venous blood sample. Serum is used. Observe standard precautions.

Clinical Implications
A. *Increased γGT levels* are associated with the following conditions:
1. Liver diseases
   a. Hepatitis (acute and chronic)
   b. Cirrhosis (obstructive and familial)
   c. Liver metastasis and carcinoma
   d. Cholestasis (especially during or following pregnancy)
   e. Chronic alcoholic liver disease, alcoholism
   f. Infectious mononucleosis
2. γGT levels are also increased in the following conditions:
   a. Pancreatitis
   b. Carcinoma of prostate
   c. Carcinoma of breast and lung
3. In MI, γGT is usually normal. However, if there is an increase, it occurs ~4 days after MI and probably implies liver damage secondary to cardiac insufficiency.
4. Hyperthyroidism.

B. *Decreased γGT levels* are found in hypothyroidism.

C. γGT values are normal in bone disorders, bone growth, pregnancy, skeletal muscle disease, strenuous exercise, and renal failure.

Interfering Factors

1. Various drugs, (eg, phenothiazines and barbituates affect test outcomes. See Appendix J)
2. Alcohol (ethanol)

Patient Preparation

1. Explain test purpose and blood-drawing procedure. No alcohol is allowed before the test.
2. Follow guidelines in Chapter 1 for safe, effective, informed *pretest* care.

Patient Aftercare

1. Resume normal activities.
2. Interpret test results and monitor as appropriate for liver, pancreatic, or thyroid disease and/or cancer recurrence.
3. Follow guidelines in Chapter 1 for safe, effective, informed *posttest* care.

HOMOCYSTEINE   ●

Normal Values
4–17 μmol/L for fasting specimens

Background
Homocysteine is an amino acid resulting from the synthesis of cysteine from methionine and enzyme reaction of cobalamin and folate. Large quantities of homocysteine are excreted and assimilated in the blood plasma of patients with homocysteinemia associated with:

1. Increased risk of vascular disease
2. Increased risk of venous thromboses
3. Elevated homocysteine with a direct toxic effect on endothelium

Folic acid deficiency is characterized by elevated plasma homocysteine; folic acid supplementation reduces plasma homocysteine. Elevated plasma homocysteine levels due to aberrant B_{12} respond favorably to vitamin B_{12} supplementation.

Explanation of Test
This test measures the blood plasma level of homocysteine. It is useful for diagnosing individuals with potential increased risk factors for CAD and thromboses, for providing a functional assay for folic acid deficiency, and for diagnosing homocysteinemia. Homocysteine is retained by persons with reduced renal function.

Procedure

Obtain a venous blood sample. Fasting is necessary. Observe standard precautions.

Clinical Implications

Increased or elevated homocysteine levels occur in the following conditions:
1. Folic acid deficiency
2. Abnormal vitamin B_{12} metabolism and deficiency
3. Homocystinuria

> **Clinical Alert**
>
> Homocysteine values and their relation to CAD are still being investigated. The methionine load test is also currently investigative and has not yet been approved as a routine test.

Interfering Factors

1. Penicillamine reduces plasma levels of homocysteine.
2. Nitrous oxide, methotrexate deficiency, and azauridine increase plasma levels of homocysteine.

Patient Preparation

1. Explain test purpose and blood-drawing procedure.
2. The test requires fasting.
3. Evaluate renal function in patients with homocystinuria.
4. Follow guidelines in Chapter 1 for safe, effective, informed *pretest* care.

Patient Aftercare

1. The patient may eat and drink after blood is drawn.
2. Interpret test results and counsel appropriately.
3. Evaluate for other cardiovascular risk factors, compare test results, and monitor appropriately. Promote lifestyle changes accordingly.
4. Monitor for folic acid or vitamin B_{12} deficiency and provide supplements as needed.
5. Follow guidelines in Chapter 1 for safe, effective, informed *posttest* care.

α_1-ANTITRYPSIN (AAT) ●

Normal Values by Rate Nephelometry

110–200 mg/dl

If result is <125 mg/dl, phenotype will be determined to confirm homozygous and heterozygous deficiencies.

Background

α_1-Antitrypsin is a protein produced by the liver which inhibits the protease released into body fluids by dying cells. This protein deficiency is associated with pulmonary emphysema and liver disease. Human serum contains at least three inhibitors of protease. Two of the best known are α_1-antitrypsin and α_2-macroglobulin. Total antitrypsin levels in blood are composed of about 90% AAT and 10% α_2-macroglobulins.

Explanation of Test

This is a nonspecific method to diagnose inflammation, severe infection, and necrosis. AAT measurement is important for diagnosing respiratory disease and cirrhosis of the liver because of its direct relation to pulmonary and other metabolic disorders. Pulmonary problems such as emphysema occur when antitrypsin-deficient persons are unable to ward off the action of endoproteases. Those who are deficient in AAT develop emphysema at a much earlier age than do other emphysema patients.

Procedure

Obtain a 7-ml serum sample. Use a red-topped tube. Observe standard precautions.

Clinical Implications

1. Interpretation of AAT levels is based on the following:
   a. High levels are generally found in normal persons.
   b. Intermediate levels are found in persons with a predisposition to pulmonary emphysema.
   c. Low levels are found in patients with obstructive pulmonary disease and in children with cirrhosis of the liver.
2. *Increased AAT levels* occur in the following conditions:
   a. Acute and chronic inflammatory disorders
   b. After injections of typhoid vaccine
   c. Cancer
   d. Thyroid infections
   e. Oral contraceptive use
   f. Stress syndrome
   g. Hematologic abnormalities
3. *Decreased AAT levels* are associated with these progressive diseases:
   a. Adult, early onset, chronic pulmonary emphysema
   b. Liver cirrhosis in children
   c. Pulmonary disease
   d. Severe hepatic damage
   e. Nephrotic syndrome
   f. Malnutrition

Interfering Factors

α_1-Antitrypsin is an acute-phase reactant, and any inflammatory process will elevate serum levels.

Patient Preparation

1. Explain test purpose and procedure. Fasting is required if the patient's history shows elevated cholesterol and/or triglyceride levels.
2. Follow guidelines in Chapter 1 for safe, effective, informed *pretest* care.

Patient Aftercare

1. Interpret test results and counsel appropriately. Advise patients with decreased levels to avoid smoking and, if possible, occupational hazards such as dust, fumes, and other respiratory pollutants.
2. Because AAT deficiencies are inherited, genetic counseling may be indicated. Follow-up AAT phenotype testing can be performed on family members to determine the homozygous or heterozygous nature of the deficiency.
3. Follow guidelines in Chapter 1 for safe, effective, informed *posttest* care.

●DRUG MONITORING

THERAPEUTIC DRUG MONITORING   ●

Normal Values

See Table 6-2 for maintenance levels.

Explanation of Test

Therapeutic drug monitoring is a reliable and practical approach to managing drug therapy in individual patients. Determination of drug levels is especially important when the potential for drug toxicity is significant or when an inadequate or undesirable response follows the use of a standard dose. Therapeutic drug monitoring provides an easier and more rapid estimation of dosage requirements than does observation of the drug effects themselves. For some drugs, monitoring is routinely useful (eg, digoxin); for others, it can be helpful in certain situations (eg, antibiotics). The plasma level of drugs needed to control the patient's symptoms is called the therapeutic concentration, which at a steady state, the rate of drug administration is equal to the rate of drug elimination, and the concentration of the drug remains constant. Monitoring at intervals minimizes the possibility of the development of dose-related side effects. If single-drug therapy is not effective, therapeutic monitoring allows the physician to select supplementary medication and monitor its effect on the primary drug.

Indications for Testing

1. Verify correct drug dosage and level. The drug source, dose, or regimen is changed.
2. Noncompliance (nonadherence) is suspected, and patient motivation to maintain medication is poor.

TABLE 6-2
Blood Plasma Concentration of Commonly Monitored Drugs

Therapeutic Drug	*Therapeutic/ Maintenance Dose*	*Toxic (Panic or Critical) Value*
Acetaminophen (Tylenol)	10–30 ug/ml or 66–199 umol/l	>200 ug/ml or >1324 umol/l
Alcohol (ethanol)	Driving while intoxicated 100 mg/dl or 21.7 mmol/l	>200 mg/dl or 43.4 mmol/l
Amikacin (Amikin)	Therapeutic peak Life threatening infections (43–51 umol/l) Serious infections 20–25 ug/ml (34–43 umol/l)	Trough Life threatening—4–8 ug/ml (7–14 umol/l)
	Urinary tract infections 15–20 ug/ml (26–34 umol/l)	Serious infections 4–8 ug/ml (7–14 umol/l)
Amiodarone (Cordarone)	0.5–2.5 ug/ml (1–4 umol/l)	≥3.5 ug/ml (≥6 umol/l)
Druk	Therapeutic/Maintenance Dose	Toxic (panic or critical value)
Amitriptyline (Elavil)	100–250 ng/ml or SI: 390–900 nmol/l	500 ng/ml or SI: 1805 nmol/l
Caffeine	5–15 ug/ml SI: 26–77 umol/l	≥30 ug/ml or SI: 155 umol/l
Carbamazepine (Tegretol)	6–12 ug/ml or SI: 25–51 umol/l	>15 ug/ml or >64 umol/l
Chloramphenicol (Chloromycetin)	Therapeutic peak 15–20 ug/ml or SI: 46–62 umol/l	>40 ug/ml or SI: >124 umol/l
Chlordiazepoxide (Librium)	0.1 ug–3 ug/ml SI: 0–10 umol/l	>23 ug/ml SI: >77 umol/l
Clonazepam (Clonopin)	20–80 ng/ml SI: 63 nmol–254 nmol/l	>80 ng/ml SI: >254 nmol/l
Clorazepate	0.12–1.00 ug/ml or 0.36–3.0 umol/l	Not defined
Cyclosporine	100–400 ng/ml or 83–333 nmol/l	≥400 ng/ml or >333 nmol/l
Desipramine (Norpramin)	75–300 ng/ml or 281–1125 nmol/l	>400 ng/ml or >1500 nmol/l
Diazepam (Valium)	0.2–1.5 ug/ml (SI: .7–5.3 umol/l)	Check with laboratory
Digitoxin (cyrstodigin) Digitaline (Canadian brand name)	20–35 ng/ml or 26–46 nmol/l	>45ng/ml or >59 nmol/l
Digoxin (Lanoxin)	0.5–2.2 ng/ml SI: .64–2.8 nmol/l	≥3.0 ng/ml SI: 3.84 nmol/l

(continued)

TABLE 6-2 *(Continued)*

Therapeutic Drug	Therapeutic/ Maintenance Dose	Toxic (Panic or Critical) Value
Disopyramide (Norpace)	Atrial arrhythmias 2.8–3.2 ug/ml Ventricular arrhythmias 3.3–7.5 ug/ml	>7 ug/ml
Doxepin (Sinequan)	30–150 ng/ml SI: 107–537 nmol/l	>500 ng/ml SI: 1790 nmol/l
Ethchlorvynol (Placidyl)	2–8 ug/ml or 14–55 umol/l	>20 ug/ml or >138 umol/l
Ethosuximide (Zarontin)	40–100 ug/ml SI: 280–710 umol/l	>150 ug/ml SI: 1062 umol/l
Fenoprotein (Nalfon)	20 65 ug/ml SI: 83–268 umol/l	Check with laboratory
Flecainide (Tambocor)	0.2–1 ug/ml SI: Check with laboratory	>1.0 ug/ml SI: Check with laboratory
Fluoxetine (Prozac)	100–800 ng/ml SI: 289–2314 nmol/l	Fluoxetine + Norfluoxetine >2000 ng/ml
Gentamicin (Garamycin)	Serious infections 6–8 ug/ml (12–17 umol/l) Life-threatening—8–10 ug/ml (17–21 umol/l) Urinary tract infections— 4–6 ug/ml (8–12 umol/l)	Trough Serious infections—0.5–1 ug/ml (1–2.0 umol/l) Life-threatening Infections—1–2 ug/ml (2–4 umol/l)
Haloperidol (Haldol)	5–15 ng/ml (Psychiatric disorders—less for Tourette's and mania. SI: 10–30 nmol/l	>42 ng/ml SI: 84 nmol/l
Ibuprofen (eg. Advil, Motrin)	10–50 ug/ml or 49–243 umol/l	100–700 ug/ml or 485–3394 umol/l
Imipramine (Tofranil) (Desipramine is an active metabolite of imipramine.)	Therapeutic maintenance value: imipramine and desipramine: 150–250 ng/ml (SI: 530–890 nmol/l) Desipramine: 150–300 ng/ml (SI: 560–1125 nmol/l) Utility of serum level monitoring of imipramine is controversial.	>500 ng/ml (SI: 446–893 nmol/l)
Isoniazid	1–7 ug/ml or 7–51 umol/l	20–710 ug/ml or 146–5176 umol/l
Kanamycin (Kantrex)	Peak: 25–35 ug/ml SI: 51.5–72.1 umol/l Trough: 4–8 ug/ml SI: 8–16 umol/l	Toxic peak: >35 ug/ml >72.1 umol/l Toxic trough: >10 ug/ml >21 umol/l
Lidocaine (Lignocaine, Xylocaine)	1.5–6.0 ug/ml or 6.4–25.6 umol/l	>8 ug/ml or >35.0 umol/l
Lithium (Eskalith)	0.6–1.2 mEq/l or 0.6–1.2 nmol/l	>2.0 mEq/l or 2 nmol/l
Meperidine (Demerol)	70–500 ng/ml SI: 283–2020 nmol/l	>1000 ng/ml SI: >4043 nmol/l

TABLE 6-2 *(Continued)*

Therapeutic Drug	Therapeutic/ Maintenance Dose	Toxic (Panic or Critical) Value
Meprobamate	6–12 ug/ml or 28–55 umol/l	≥60 ug/ml or >275 umol/l
Methotrexate	Variable	48 h after high dose: >0.5 umol/l
Mexiletin (Mexitil)	0.5–2 ug/ml	>2 ug/ml
Procainamide	4–10 ug/ml; SI: 17–42 umol/l	Procainamide >10–12 ug/ml; SI: 42–51 umol/l
Combined (n-acetyl-procainamide) NAPA	15–25 ug/ml 10–30 ug/ml	
Nortriptyline (Pamelor, Aventyl)	50–150 ng/ml SI: 190–570 nmol/l	>500 ng/ml SI: 1900 nmol/l
Oxazepam (Serax)	0.2–1.4 ug/ml or 0.70–4.9 umol/l	Check with laboratory
Pentobarbital (Nembutal)	Hypnotic: 1–5 ug/ml (SI: 4–22 umol/l) Coma: 10–50 ug/ml (SI: 44–221 umol/l)	>10 ug/ml SI: >44
Phenobarbital (Luminal)	20–40 ug/ml SI: 86–172 umol/l	>40 ug/ml Slowness ataxia, nystagmus—35–80 ug/ml; SI:150–344 umol/l Coma with reflexes: 65–117 ug/ml; SI: 279–502 umol/l Coma without reflexes: >100 ug/ml; SI: >430 umol/l
Phenytoin (Dilantin)	10–20 ug/ml SI: 40–79 umol/l	Varies time: 20–40 ug/ml SI: 79–158 umol/l
Primidone (Mysoline)	5–12 ug/ml or SI: 23–55 umol/l	>15 ug/ml or >69 umol/l
Procainamide (Pronestyl)	4–10 ug/ml or 17–52 umol/l	10–12 ug/ml or 42–51 umol/l
Propanolol (Inderal)	50–100 ng/ml or 193–386 nmol/l	Check with laboratory
Propoxyphene (Darvon) and propoxyphene hapsylate (Darvocet-N)	0.1–0.4 ug/ml or 0.3–1.2 umol/l	>0.5 ug/ml or >1.5 umol/l
Protriptyline (Vivactil)	70–250 ng/ml or 266–950 nmol/l	>500 ng/ml or >1900 nmol/l
Quinidine	2–5.0 ug/ml SI: 6–15 umol/l	≥7.0 ug/ml SI: 22 umol/l

TABLE 6-2 *(Continued)*

Therapeutic Drug	Therapeutic/ Maintenance Dose	Toxic (Panic or Critical) Value
Salicylates (acetylsalicylic acid, aspirin)	150–300 ug/ml or 1086–2172 umol/l	>300 ug/ml or >2172 umol/l (severely acid, toxic) >50 mg/dl at 24 h postingestion
Theophylline [Aminophylline	Bronchodilator: 8–20 ug/dl or 44–111 umol/l	>20 ug/ml or >111 umol/l
(Theophylline ethylenediamine)—79% theophylline] Aminophylline is a xanthine derivative—Theophylline ethylenediamine which is 79% theophylline). Nitroprusside is converted to cyanide ions in the blood stream—decomposes to prussic acid which in the presence of sulfur donor is converted to ethiocyanate half lite. Parent drug (nitroprusside) <10 minutes.		
Thiocyanide	2.7–7 days 1–4 ug/ml or 17–69 umol/l	≥60 ug/ml or >69 umol/l
Nitroprusside (Nitropress)	Monitor thiocyanate levels if requiring prolonged infusion >4 days or ≥4 ug/kg/minute	
Thiocyanate	6–29 ug/ml	35–100 ug/ml
Thioridazine (Mellaril)	1.0–1.5 ug/ml or 2.7–4.1 umol/l	>10 ug/ml or >27.0 umol/l
Tobramycin (Nebain)	Therapeutic peak: Serious infections: 6–8 ug/ml (SI: 12–17 mg/l)	>12 ug/ml
	Life-threatening infections: 8–10 ug/ml (SI: 17–21 mg/l) UTI: 4–6 ug/ml (SI: 7–12 mg/l)	
	Therapeutic trough: Serious infections: 0/5–1 ug/ml Life-threatening: 1–2 ug/ml	>4 ug/ml
Tocainide (Tonocard)	5–12 ug/ml	≥15 ug/ml
Trazodone (Desyrel)	0.5–2.5 ug/ml	Potentially toxic >2.5 ug/ml Toxic >4 ug/ml
Tolbutamide (Orinase)	Fasting blood glucose: <120 mg/dl Adults: 80–140 mg/dl Geriatrics: 100–150 mg/dl Glycosylated hemoglobin: <7%	
Valproic acid (Depakene)	50–100 ug/ml or 347–693 umol/l	100 ug/ml or 693 umol/l
Vancomycin	Peak: 20–40 ug/ml Trough: 5–10 ug/ml	Peak: 40 ug/ml Trough: 15 ug/ml
Verapamil (Isoptin)	50–200 ng/ml (SI: 100–410 nmol/l)	≥400 ng/ml (peak)
Urine:		
Methanol	No evidence	20 mg/dl
Ethanol	No evidence	>300 mg/dl
Isopropanol	No evidence	50 mg/dl

TABLE 6-2 *(Continued)*

Therapeutic Drug	Therapeutic/ Maintenance Dose	Toxic (Panic or Critical) Value
Warfarin (Coumadin)	Therapeutic: 2–5 ug/ml (SI: 6.5–16.2 umol/l)	Check with laboratory.

Prothrombin time should be 1.5 to 2 × the control or INR should be increased 2 to 3 × based upon indication. Normal prothrombin time 10–13 seconds.

Volatile drug screen

Blood:

Methanol	No evidence	20 mg/dl
Ethanol	No evidence	>300 mg/dl
		>400 mg/dl severe toxicity
Isopropanol	No evidence	>1000 mg/l coma

Therapeutic value refers to expected drug concentration associated with desirable clinical effects in the majority of the patient population treated.

Critical (toxic) value refers to the drug concentration associated with undesirable effects or, in certain cases, death.

Peak drug level refers to maximum drug concentration achieved following administration of a single dose. For a specific drug, both the concentration achieved and time interval between dosing and peak drug level required may vary considerably from patient to patient.

Trough drug level refers to minimum drug concentration preceding administration of a single dose.

Toxic (panic or critical) values denote a serious condition associated with undesirable effects or in certain cases, death, and require quick action when test results are outside of prescribed limits.

3. Physiologic status is altered by factors such as weight, menstrual cycle, body water, stress, age, and thyroid function.

4. Co-administered (multiple) drugs may cause either synergistic or antagonistic drug reactions.

5. Pathology may influence drug absorption and elimination.
   a. Cardiovascular dysfunction
   b. Liver clearance
   c. Renal clearance (urinary output and pH)
   d. Poor GI absorption
   e. Altered plasma protein binding or change in blood proteins that carry drug

6. Some drugs have a very small safety range (ie, therapeutic window or concentration). Factors that affect concentration include absorption, metabolism, excretion, tissue storage, and site of action.

Procedure

1. Obtain a venous sample of blood. Serum or plasma can be used depending on the drug being tested and laboratory protocols.

2. Serum-separation tubes may not be used for drug monitoring because small amounts of the drug adhere to the separator gel barrier.

3. The time the specimen is drawn is extremely important in respect to determining peak and trough values.

Patient Preparation

1. Explain test purpose and procedure. Recommended regimen for drawing specimens for therapeutic drug testing follows.

Trough	*Immediately After*
Draw immediately prior to the next dose.	

Peak	
Draw 30 minutes after IM injection (normal renal function); draw 30 minutes after 30-minute IV infusion (normal renal function).	Draw immediately after 60-minute IV infusion (normal renal function).

12 Hours After	
Twelve hours after initiating therapy for arrhythmia prophylaxis; then every 24 hours thereafter. Additionally, every 12 hours when evidence of cardiac or hepatic insufficiency exists, whenever toxicity is suspected, and whenever ventricular arrhythmias occur despite lidocaine administration.	Immediately after IV loading dose: 2 hours after start of IV maintenance infusion; 6 to 12 hours after start of IV maintenance therapy; three steady-state samples over one oral dosing interval at time of administration; two more at equally spaced intervals.

Prior to IV Infusion	
	Prior to IV infusion (if patient received theophylline therapy): 30 minutes after completion of IV loading dose; 12 to 24 hours after start of IV infusion. Repeat as needed to ensure concentration is maintained within the therapeutic range. Peak depends upon oral preparation. Solution or solid with rapid dissolution characteristics: Peak—1 hour past dose after at least one day of therapy; 2 hours after oral dose; slow-release formulations: 4 hours after oral dose; Theo-Dur: 4 hours after at least one day of therapy.

Trough	
Immediately prior to the next oral dose.	

2. Follow guidelines in Chapter 1 for safe, effective, informed *pretest* care.

Patient Aftercare

1. Interpret test results, and counsel and monitor appropriately. Assess changes in patient's condition. Knowledge of drug interactions aid in the interpretation of test results. The importance of sampling time in obtaining values from therapeutic drug monitoring data cannot be understated. Whatever sampling procedure is used (eg, peak or maximum concentration, trough or minimum drug concentration), it is important that the same time interval between sampling and dose administration be used consistently when comparing results from serial samples on the same patient.

2. Elimination half-life refers to the length of time required to eliminate drug from the body after the initial distribution phase is complete. The elimination of half-life is the time taken for the plasma concentration as well as the amount of the drug in the body to fall by one-half. It takes 4 to 3 half-lifes to reach a steady state or in other words, for the drug concentration to remain constant. Under certain conditions, elimination half-life dates are useful in estimating how long to wait following initiation of therapy before sampling.

> **Clinical Alert**
>
> Factors influencing drug and chemical concentrations in living patients are frequently altered significantly after death.

BLOOD ALCOHOL CONTENT
(BAC; ETHANOL [ETHYL ALCOHOL, ETOH])

Normal Values
Negative: no alcohol detected

Background
Ethanol is absorbed rapidly from the GI tract, with peak blood levels usually occurring within 40 to 70 minutes of ingestion on an empty stomach. Food in the stomach depresses alcohol absorption. Ethanol is metabolized by the liver to acetaldehyde. Once peak blood ethanol levels are reached, disappearance is linear; a 70-kg man metabolizes 7 to 10 g alcohol/hour (15 + 5 mg/dl/hour). Symptoms of intoxication in the presence of low alcohol levels could indicate a serious acute medical problem requiring immediate attention.

Explanation of Test
Quantitation of alcohol level may be performed for medical or legal purposes, to diagnose alcohol intoxication, and to determine appropriate therapy. Alcohol level must be tested as a possible cause of unknown coma because alcohol intoxication mimics diabetic coma, cerebral trauma, and drug overdose. This test is also used to screen for alcoholism and to monitor ethanol treatment for methanol intoxication.

Procedure

1. Obtain a 5-ml venous blood sample from the arm in living persons. From dead persons, take samples from the aorta. Observe standard precautions.
   a. Use a nonalcohol solution (eg, Betadine) for cleansing the venipuncture site.
   b. Sodium fluoride or oxalate anticoagulant is recommended. Serum can also be used.
   c. Keep blood sample tightly stoppered.
2. A 20-ml sample of urine or gastric contents can also be used.
3. A breath analyzer measures ethanol content at the end of expiration following a deep inspiration.

Clinical Implications

1. At levels of 50 to 100 mg/dl, certain signs and symptoms are reported (eg, flushing, slowing of reflexes, impaired visual acuity).
2. At levels >100 mg/dl, CNS depression is reported. In many states, this is the cutoff level for driving under the influence of alcohol.
3. Blood levels of 300 mg/dl are associated with coma.
4. Death has been reported at levels >400 mg/dl.
5. Properly collected urine samples will have an alcohol content similar to that of blood. Saliva samples will have an alcohol content 1.2 times that of blood.

Interfering Factors

1. Increased blood ketones, as in diabetic ketoacidosis, can falsely elevate blood or breath test results.
2. Ingestion of other alcohols such as isopropanol or methanol may affect results.

Clinical Alert

1. Panic value is >300 mg/dl. Report and initiate overdose treatment at once.
2. Symptoms of intoxication in the presence of low blood alcohol could indicate a serious medical problem requiring immediate medical attention.

Patient Preparation

1. Explain test purpose and procedure. Proper collection, handling, and storage of the blood alcohol specimen is essential when the question of sobriety is raised.
2. Advise patient of legal rights in cases involving question of sobriety.
3. A witnessed, signed consent form may have to be obtained.
4. Follow guidelines in Chapter 1 for safe, effective, informed *pretest* care.

Patient Aftercare

1. Interpret test results and monitor as appropriate.
2. If alcohol levels are high, initiate treatment at once.

3. Follow guidelines in Chapter 1 for safe, effective, informed *posttest* care.

●LIPOPROTEIN TESTS

Lipoprotein measurements are diagnostic indicators for hyperlipidemia and hypolipidemia. Hyperlipidemia is classified as types I, IIa, IIb, III, IV, and V. Lipids are fatty substances made up of cholesterol, cholesterol esters (liquid compounds), triglycerides, nonesterized fatty acids, and phospholipids. Lipoproteins are unique plasma proteins that transport otherwise insoluble lipids. They are categorized as chylomicrons, β-lipoproteins (low-density lipoproteins [LDL]), pre–β-lipoproteins (very-low-density lipoproteins [VLDL]), and α-lipoproteins (high-density lipoproteins [HDL]). Apolipoprotein A is mainly composed of HDL, chylomicrons, and VLDL. Apolipoprotein B is the main component of LDL. Lipids provide energy for metabolism, serve as precursors of steroid hormones (adrenals, ovaries, testes) and bile acids, and play an important role in cell membrane development. A lipid profile usually includes cholesterol, triglycerides, LDL, and HDL levels.

CHOLESTEROL

Normal Values
Normal values vary with age, diet, and geographical/cultural region.

Adult
    Desirable level: 140–199 mg/dl or <5.18 mmol/L
    Borderline high: 200–239 mg/dl or 5.18–6.19 mmol/L
    High: ≥240 mg/dl or >6.20 mmol/L
Child and adolescent (12–18 y):
    Desirable level: <170 mg/dl or <4.39 mmol/L
    Borderline high: 170–199 mg/dl or 4.40–5.16 mmol/L
    High: >200 mg/dl or >5.18 mmol/L

Background
Cholesterol is a steroid alcohol (sterol) found in animal fats and oils. It is widely distributed throughout the body, especially in the blood, brain, liver, kidneys, and nerve fiber myelin sheaths, and it is an essential component of cell membrane development and production of bile acids, adrenal steroids, and sex hormones.

Explanation of Test
Cholesterol testing evaluates the risk of arthrosclerosis, myocardial occlusion, and coronary arterial occlusion. Cholesterol relates to coronary heart disease (CHD) and is an important screening test for risk factors. It is part of the lipid

profiles. Elevated cholesterol levels are a major component in the hereditary hyperlipoproteinemias. Cholesterol studies are also frequently a part of thyroid and liver function studies.

Procedure
Obtain a 5-ml venous blood sample. Fasting is required. Serum is needed. Observe standard precautions.

Clinical Implications
1. Total blood cholesterol levels are the basis for classifying CHD risk.
   a. Levels >240 mg/dl are considered high and should include follow-up lipoprotein analysis. Borderline high levels (200–239 mg/dl) in the presence of CHD or two other CHD risk factors should also include lipoprotein analysis/profiles.
   b. CHD risk factors include male gender, family history of premature CHD (MI or sudden death before age 55 years in a parent or sibling), smoking (>10 cigarettes/day), hypertension, low HDL-cholesterol levels (<35 mg/dl confirmed by repeat measurement), diabetes mellitus, history of definite cerebrovascular or occlusive peripheral vascular disease, and severe obesity (>30% overweight).
   c. In public screening programs, all patients with cholesterol levels >200 mg/dl should be referred to their physicians for further evaluation.
2. *Elevated cholesterol levels (hypercholesterolemia)* occur in the following conditions:
   a. Type II familial hypercholesterolemia
   b. Hyperlipoproteinemia types I, IV, and V
   c. Hepatocellular disease, biliary cirrhosis
   d. Cholestasis
   e. Nephrotic syndrome glomerulonephritis
   f. Chronic renal failure
   g. Pancreatic and prostatic malignant neoplasms
   h. Hypothyroidism
   i. Poorly controlled diabetes mellitus
   j. Alcoholism
   k. Glycogen storage disease (von Gierke's disease)
   l. Werner's syndrome
   m. Diet high in cholesterol and fats
   n. Obesity
3. *Decreased cholesterol levels (hypocholesterolemia)* occur in the following conditions:
   a. α-Hypoprotein deficiency (Tangier disease)
   b. Severe hepatocellular disease
   c. Myeloproliferative diseases
   d. Hyperthyroidism
   e. Malabsorption syndrome, malnutrition

f. Megaloblastic or sideroblastic anemia (chronic anemias)
g. Severe burns, inflammation
h. Conditions of acute illness, infection
i. Chorionic obstructive lung disease

Interfering Factors

1. Estrogens decrease plasma cholesterol levels; pregnancy increases these levels.
2. Certain drugs increase or decrease cholesterol levels.
3. Seasonal variations in cholesterol levels have been observed; levels are higher in fall and winter and lower in spring and summer.
4. Positional variations occur; levels are lower when sitting versus standing and lower when recumbent versus sitting.

Patient Preparation

1. Explain test purpose and procedure. An overnight fast before testing is recommended, although nonfasting specimens may be taken. Pretest, a normal diet should be consumed for 7 days. The patient should abstain from alcohol for 48 hours before testing. Prolonged fasting with ketosis increases values.
2. Document drugs the patient is taking.
3. Encourage the patient to relax.
4. Follow guidelines in Chapter 1 for safe, effective, informed *pretest* care.

Patient Aftercare

1. Interpret test results and counsel appropriately. Cholesterol levels are influenced by heredity, diet, body weight, and physical activity. Some lifestyle changes may be necessary to reduce elevated levels.
2. Cholesterol levels >200 mg/dl should be retested and the results averaged. If the two results differ by >10%, a third test should be done.
3. Once hyperlipidemia has been established, the diet should be lower in animal fats and should replace saturated fats with polyunsaturated fats. Fruits, vegetables (especially greens), and whole-grain products should be increased. Patients with diabetes, as well as others, should seek counsel from a dietitian regarding diet management if necessary. Therapy for hyperlipidemia should always begin with diet modification.
4. The American Heart Association and National Cholesterol Education Programs have excellent resources for providing diet and lifestyle management information.
5. At least 6 months of dietary therapy should be tried before initiating cholesterol-reducing drug therapy.
6. A comprehensive lipoprotein analysis should be done if cholesterol levels are not lowered within 6 months after start of therapy.

> **Clinical Alert**
>
> Cholesterol measurement should not be done immediately after MI. A 3-month wait is suggested.

HIGH-DENSITY LIPOPROTEIN CHOLESTEROL (HDL-C) ●

Normal Values

Men: 37–70 mg/dl
Women: 40–85 mg/dl
<25 mg/dl of HDL: CHD risk at dangerous level
26–35 mg/dl of HDL: high CHD risk
36–44 mg/dl of HDL: moderate CHD risk
45–59 mg/dl of HDL: average CHD risk
60–74 mg/dl of HDL: below average CHD risk
>75 mg/dl of HDL: no risk (associated with longevity)

Background

HDL-C is a class of lipoproteins produced by the liver and intestines. HDL is comprised of phospholipids and 1 or 2 apolipoproteins. It plays a role in the metabolism of the other lipoproteins and in cholesterol transport from peripheral tissues to the liver. LDL and HDL may combine to maintain cellular cholesterol balance through the mechanism of LDL moving cholesterol into the arteries and HDL removing it from the arteries. Decreased HDL levels are atherogenic, whereas elevated HDL levels protect against arthrosclerosis by removing cholesterol from vessel walls and transporting it to the liver where it is removed from the body.

Explanation of Test

HDL-C is used to assess CAD risk and monitor persons with known low HDL levels. HDL-C levels are inversely proportional to CHD risk and is a primary independent risk factor. The measurement of HDL-C is a good reflection of the status of CAD at all times, not for just the day the sample was drawn, because it has a diurnal variation of ~8%.

Procedure

Obtain a 5-ml venous blood sample. Fasting is necessary. The HDL is precipitated out from the total cholesterol for analysis. A cholesterol/HDL-C ratio can be calculated from these values.

Clinical Implications

1. *Increased HDL-C values* occur in the following conditions:
   a. Familial hyper–α-lipoproteinemia (HDL excess)
   b. Chronic liver disease (cirrhosis, alcoholism, hepatitis)
   c. Long-term aerobic or vigorous exercise

2. *Decreased HDL-C values* are associated with increased risk for CHD and premature CHD and occur in the following conditions:

a. Premature CHD

b. Familial hypo–α-lipoproteinemia (Tangier disease)

c. Apo C-III deficiency

d. Hypertriglyceridemia (familial)

e. Poorly controlled diabetes mellitus

f. Hepatocellular diseases

g. Nephrotic syndrome, uremia

h. Chronic renal failure, uremia

i. In the United States, 3% of men have low HDL levels for unknown reasons, even though cholesterol and triglyceride values are normal and they are at risk for CAD.

j. Niemann-Peck disease

k. Certain rare genetic HDL deficiencies

Interfering Factors

1. Increased HDL level is associated with estrogen therapy, moderate intake of alcohol and other drugs (especially androgenic and related steroids), and insulin therapy.

2. Decreased HDL levels are associated with the following:

a. Certain drugs such as steroids, antihypertensive agents, diuretics, β-blockers, and triglycerides

b. Stress and recent illness

c. Starvation and anorexia

d. Obesity, lack of exercise

e. Smoking

Patient Preparation

1. Explain test purpose. A 12-hour fast is recommended, but nonfasting specimens may be taken. Alcohol should not be consumed for at least 24 hours before the test.

2. If possible, all medication should be withheld for at least 24 hours before testing. Check with physician.

3. Encourage relaxation.

4. Follow guidelines in Chapter 1 for safe, effective, informed *pretest* care.

Patient Aftercare

1. Interpret test results and counsel appropriately (see cholesterol patient aftercare).

2. Low HDL levels can be raised by diet management, exercise, weight loss, and smoking cessation. Many resources are available through the American Heart Association and other organizations.

3. Drug therapy may be necessary if other methods fail to raise HDL levels.

4. Follow guidelines in Chapter 1 for safe, effective, informed *posttest* care.

> **Clinical Alert**
>
> Cholesterol and HDL-C levels should not be done immediately after MI. A 3-month wait is suggested.

> **Clinical Alert**
>
> The cholesterol/HDL ratio provides more information than does either value alone. The higher the cholesterol/HDL ratio, the greater the risk for developing atherosclerosis. This ratio should be reported with total cholesterol values, along with the %HDL-C.

VERY-LOW-DENSITY LIPOPROTEINS (VLDL); LOW-DENSITY LIPOPROTEINS (LDL)

Desirable Values

Adult
Desirable LDL-cholesterol: <130 mg/dl or <3.4 mmol/L
Borderline high-risk cholesterol: 140–159 mg/dl or 3.4–4.1 mmol/L
High-risk LDL-cholesterol: >160 mg/dl or >4.1 mmol/L

Child and Adolescent:
Desirable: <110 mg/dl or <2.8 mmol/L
Borderline high-risk: 110–129 mg/dl or 2.8–3.4 mmol/L
High-Risk: >130 mg/dl or >3.4 mmol/L

Background
Most serum cholesterol is present in the LDL. LDLs are the cholesterol-rich remnants of the VLDL lipid transport vehicle. Because LDL has a longer half-life (3–4 days) than its precursor VLDL, LDL is more prevalent in the blood. It is mainly catabolized in the liver and possibly in nonhepatic cells as well. The VLDLs are major carriers of triglycerides. Degradation of VLDL is a major source of LDL. Circulating fatty acids form triglycerides in the liver, and these are packaged with apoprotein and cholesterol to be exported into the blood as VLDLs. Therefore, LDH is the test of choice because of its longer half-life and the fact that VLDLs are extremely hard to measure.

Explanation of Test
This test is specifically done to determine CHD risk. LDLs are closely associated with increased incidence of atherosclerosis and CHD.

Procedure

1. VLDL calculated (estimation): triglycerides/5.
2. LDL cholesterol levels are calculated by using the Friedwald formula:

$$LDL\ cholesterol = total\ cholesterol - HDL\ cholesterol - \left(\frac{triglycerides}{5}\right)$$

3. The formula is valid only if the cholesterol and triglyceride values are from a fasting specimen and the triglyceride value is >400 mg/dl.
4. Lipoprotein analysis measures fasting levels of total cholesterol, total triglycerides, and HDL-cholesterol. LDL-cholesterol is calculated from these values.
5. There is a nondirect test for LDH that may be ordered if triglycerides are >400 mg/dl.

Clinical Implications

1. *Increased LDL levels* are caused by the following conditions:
   a. Familial type II hyperlipidemia, familial hypercholesterolemia
   b. Secondary causes include the following:
   (1) Diet high in cholesterol and saturated fat
   (2) Hyperlipidemia secondary to hypothyroidism
   (3) Nephrotic syndrome
   (4) Multiple myeloma and other dysglobulinemias
   (5) Hepatic obstruction or disease
   (6) Anorexia nervosa
   (7) Diabetes mellitus
   (8) Chronic renal failure
   (9) Porphyria
   (10) Premature CHD
2. *Decreased LDL levels* occur in the following conditions:
   a. Hypolipoproteinemia
   b. Tangier's disease
   c. Type I hyperlipidemia
   d. Apo C-II deficiency
   e. Hyperthyroidism
   f. Chronic anemias
   g. Severe hepatocellular disease
   h. Reye's syndrome
   i. Acute stress (burns, illness)
   j. Inflammatory joint disease
   k. Chronic pulmonary disease

Interfering Factors

1. Increased LDLs are associated with pregnancy and certain drugs such as steroids, progestins, and androgens.
2. Not fasting may cause false elevation.
3. Decreased LDLs are found in women taking oral estrogen therapy.

Patient Preparation

Same as for HDL patient preparation.

Patient Aftercare

1. Interpret test results and counsel appropriately.
2. If patient has high LDH levels, repeat the test in 2 to 8 weeks and average the values to establish an accurate baseline from which to devise a treatment plan.
3. The National Cholesterol Education Program offers excellent resource materials for patient education.

	Initiation Level	*Minimal Goal*
DIETARY TREATMENT		
Without CHD or 2 other risk factors	>160 mg/dl	<160 mg/dl
With CHD or 2 other risk factors	>130 mg/dl	<130 mg/dl
DRUG TREATMENT		
Without CHD or 2 other risk factors	>190 mg/dl	160 mg/dl
With CHD or 2 other risk factors	>160 mg/dl	<130 mg/dl

NOTE: *Patients need a lower initiation level and goal if they are at high risk because of existing CHD or any two of the following risk factors: male gender, family history of premature CHD, smoking, hypertension, low HDL-cholesterol, diabetes mellitus, cerebrovascular or peripheral vascular disease, or severe obesity.*

4. A comprehensive history and physical, together with analysis of test results, determines whether high LDL-cholesterol is secondary to another disease or drug or is the result of a familial lipid disorder. The patient's total coronary risk profile, clinical status, age, and gender are considered when prescribing a cholesterol-lowering treatment program.

Clinical Alert

Another method for assessing CAD/CHD risk is by calculating the LDH/HDL ratio (LDL-C − HDL-C).

LDL-C/HDL-C RATIO

Risk Level	*Men*	*Women*
Low	1.00	1.47
Average	3.55	3.22
Moderate	6.25	5.03
High	7.99	6.14

APOLIPOPROTEIN A AND B (APO A, APO B) ●

Normal Values

	Men	*Women*
Apo A$_1$	94–178 mg/dl	101–199 mg/dl
Apo B	63–133 mg/dl	60–126 mg/dl
Apo A$_1$/Apo B ratio	0.80–1.33	0.94–2.63

Background

Hypolipoproteins/apolipoproteins are surface proteins of lipoprotein particles and are important in the study of atherosclerosis. Apolipoprotein A is the main component of HDLs, and a small amount is from chylomicrons and VLDLs. Apolipoprotein B is the main component of LDL and is important in regulating cholesterol synthesis and metabolism.

Explanation of Test

This test is used to diagnose CAD. Apo A$_1$ deficiencies are often associated with premature cardiovascular disease. Apo B plays an important role in LDL catabolism. The ratio of Apo A to Apo B correlates more closely with increased risk of CAD than do cholesterol levels or LDL/HDL ratio.

Procedure

Obtain a 5-ml venous blood sample. Serum is needed. Do not freeze the specimen.

Clinical Implications

1. *Increased Apo A$_1$* is associated with familial (inherited) hyper–α-lipoproteinemia.
2. *Decreased Apo A$_1$* is associated with the following conditions:
   a. B-lipoproteinemia
   b. Apo C-II deficiency
   c. Apo A$_1$ Melano disease
   d. Apo A$_1$–C-III deficiency
   e. Hypertriglyceridemia
   f. Poorly controlled diabetes
   g. Premature CHD
   h. Hepatocellular disease
   i. Nephrotic syndrome and renal failure
3. *Increased Apo B* is associated with the following conditions:
   a. Hyperlipoproteinemia types IIa, IIb, and V
   b. Premature CHD

    c. Diabetes mellitus
    d. Hypothyroidism
    e. Nephrotic syndrome, renal failure
    f. Hepatic disease and obstruction
    g. Dysglobulinemia
    h. Porphyria
    i. Cushing's syndrome
    j. Werner's syndrome

3. *Decreased Apo B* occurs with the following conditions:

a. Tangier disease	**f.** Malnutrition/malabsorption
b. Hypo-B-lipoproteinemia	**g.** Chronic anemias
c. Type I hyperlipidemia	**h.** Reye's syndrome
d. Apo C-II deficiency	**i.** Acute stress (burns, illness)
e. Hypothyroidism	**j.** Inflammatory joint disease

Interfering Factors

1. *Decreased Apo A-I* is associated with a diet high in polyunsaturated fats, smoking, and some drugs. See Appendix J.
2. *Decreased Apo B* is associated with a diet high in polyunsaturated fats and low-cholesterol diets, and many drugs.
3. *Increased apolipoprotein levels* can be caused by various drugs.

> **Clinical Alert**
>
> An adverse Apo A-I/Apo B ratio in early life is a potential marker for CHD risk.

Patient Preparation

1. Explain test purpose and procedure. A 12-hour fast is required, but water may be taken. Smoking is prohibited.
2. Encourage relaxation.
3. Follow guidelines in Chapter 1 for safe, effective, informed *pretest* care.

Patient Aftercare

1. Resume normal activities.
2. Interpret test results and counsel appropriately regarding CAD risk and potential lifestyle changes.
3. Follow guidelines in Chapter 1 for safe, effective, informed *posttest* care.

TRIGLYCERIDES ●

Normal Values

Age	Male	Female
0–9 y	30–100 mg/dl	35–110 mg/dl
9–14 y	32–125 mg/dl	37–131 mg/dl
14–20 y	37–148 mg/dl	39–124 mg/dl
>20 y	40–160 mg/dl	35–135 mg/dl

Values are related to age and diet.

Background

Triglycerides account for >90% of dietary intake and comprise 95% of fat stored in tissues. Because they are insoluble in water, they are the main plasma glycerol ester. Normally stored in adipose tissue as glycerol, fatty acids, and monoglycerides, the liver reconverts these to triglycerides. Of the total, 80% of triglycerides are in VLDL, and 15% are in LDL.

Explanation of Test

This test evaluates suspected atherosclerosis and measures the body's ability to metabolize fat. Elevated triglycerides, together with elevated cholesterol, are atherosclerotic disease risk factors. Because cholesterol and triglycerides can vary independent of each other, measurement of both values is more meaningful. Diurnal variation causes triglycerides to be lowest in the morning and highest around noon.

Procedure

Obtain a 5-ml venous blood sample. Fasting for 12 to 14 hours is required. Observe standard precautions. Serum or plasma may be used. Do not use glycerinated tubes.

Clinical Implications

1. *Increased triglycerides* occur with the following conditions:
   a. Hyperlipoproteinemia type I, IIb, III, IV, and B
   b. Liver disease, alcoholism
   c. Nephrotic syndrome, renal disease
   d. Hypothyroidism
   e. Poorly controlled diabetes mellitus
   f. Pancreatitis
   g. Glycogen storage disease (von Gierke's disease)
   h. Myocardial infarction (elevated levels may persist for several months)
   i. Gout
   j. Werner's syndrome
   k. Down syndrome

2. *Decreased triglyceride* levels occur with the following conditions:
   a. Congenital α-β-lipoproteinemia
   b. Malnutrition
   c. Hyperthyroidism
   d. Recent weight loss
   e. Chronic obstructive lung disease

NOTE: *Certain levels of triglycerides are associated with certain disorders:*

1. <250 mg/dl: Not associated with a disease state
2. 250–500 mg/dl: Associated with peripheral vascular disease and may be a marker for genetic forms of hyperlipoproteinemias that need specific therapy
3. >500 mg/dl: Associated with high risk of pancreatitis
4. >1000 mg/dl: Associated with type I or type V hyperlipidemia and substantial risk of pancreatitis
5. >5000 mg/dl: Associated with eruptive xanthoma, corneal arcus, lipemia retinalis, and enlarged liver and spleen

Interfering Factors
1. A transient increase occurs following a heavy meal or alcohol ingestion; a transient decrease occurs after strenuous exercise.
2. Increased values are associated with pregnancy and oral contraceptive use.
3. Values may be increased in acute illness, colds, or flu.
4. Many drugs cause increases and decreases. See Appendix J.

Patient Preparation
1. Explain test purpose and procedure. Fasting for at least 12 hours overnight is required, but water may be ingested.
2. The patient should be on a normal diet for 1 week pretest. No alcohol is permitted for at least 24 to 48 hours before testing.
3. Follow guidelines in Chapter 1 for safe, effective, informed *pretest* care.

Patient Aftercare
1. Interpret test results and counsel appropriately. Weight reduction, a low-fat diet, and an exercise program can reduce high triglyceride levels.
2. Advise that triglycerides are not a strong predictor of CHD and, as such, are not an independent risk factor if <250 mg/dl. However, increased levels may increase cardiovascular disease risk.
3. Follow guidelines in Chapter 1 for safe, effective, informed *posttest* care.

> ### Clinical Alert
>
> **1.** Panic values of >500 mg/dl indicate hypertriglyceridemia in the presence of diagnosed pancreatitis.
> **2.** Values of >1000 mg/dl present a substantial risk of pancreatitis.
>
> *(continued)*

(Clinical Alert continued)

3. Chylomicronemia, although associated with pancreatitis, is not accompanied by increased atherogenesis. Chylomicrons are not seen in normal fasting serum but instead are found as exogenous triglycerides in healthy persons after a fatty meal has been eaten.

LIPOPROTEIN ELECTROPHORESIS ●

Normal Values

For 12- to 14-hour fasting specimen:
   Chylomicrons: 0%–2%
   β or LDL: 33%–52% (mass fraction of total lipoprotein)
   Pre-β or VLDL: 7%–28% (mass fraction of total lipoprotein)
   α or HDL: 10%–30% (mass fraction of total lipoprotein)
   Plasma appearance: clear

Background

Lipoproteins are comprised of hydrophobic lipids bound to protein, which produces a liquid-soluble complex. Chylomicrons primarily transport dietary triglycerides from the intestines. They are proteins derived from dietary sources, and if significantly increased, they can extend into the pre-β area. In hyperchylomicronemia, chylomicrons represent dietary fat in transport. The standing plasma contains a cream layer over a clear layer in type I hyperlipidemia (where chylomicrons are elevated), but not in type IV (where both chylomicrons and triglycerides are elevated). VLDLs transport cholesterol and triglycerides that have been synthesized in the liver. LDLs are the major cholesterol-transporting lipoproteins. Atherosclerotic plaque cholesterol is derived from LDLs, and LDL elevations are associated with an increased CAD risk. Conversely, HDLs provide protection against atherosclerosis by reversing cholesterol transport mechanisms. Levels of plasma HDL cholesterol are inversely proportional to the risk of heart disease.

Explanation of Test

Lipoprotein electrophoresis evaluates hyperlipidemia and determines abnormal serum lipoprotein distribution and concentration.

Procedure

Obtain a 5-ml sample of venous blood. Fasting is required. Serum is used. Do not freeze. Observe standard precautions.

Clinical Implications

1. Patients may be phenotyped using Frederickson's Classification System. Triglyceride, cholesterol and lipoprotein levels are considered in this system.
2. Lipoproteins are decreased in the following conditions:

   a. β-Lipoproteinemia
   b. Tangier disease
   c. Hypo–β-lipoproteinemia
3. Lipoproteins are increased in the following conditions:
   a. Hyper–β-lipoproteinemia
   c. Hyper–α-lipoproteinemia

Interfering Factors

1. Lipid phenotypes are affected by stress or dietary changes
2. Phenotyping is invalid in the presence of secondary disorders such as diabetes mellitus, renal failure, or nephritis
3. Certain drugs may alter electrophoretic mobilizing of lipoproteins
4. Heparinized blood is not acceptable; test results are not reliable during heparin therapy.

Patient Preparation

1. Explain test purpose and blood-drawing procedure. A 12-hour fast is required before blood is drawn.
2. The patient should be on a normal diet for 2 weeks before test.
3. Follow guidelines in Chapter 1 for safe, effective, informed *pretest* care.

Patient Aftercare

1. Interpret test results and counsel appropriately regarding dietary and drug therapy. The National Cholesterol Education Program and other organizations have many resources available. (National Cholesterol Education Program, National Institutes of Health, 9000 Rockville Pike, Bethesda, MD 20184).
2. Follow guidelines in Chapter 1 for safe, effective, informed *posttest* care.

FREE FATTY ACIDS; FATTY ACID PROFILE ●

Normal Values

Adult: 8–25 mg/dl or
Child: <31 mg/dl or obese adult: <31 mg/dl

Fatty Acid Profile
Linolate: >25% of total fatty acids
Arachnidate: 0%–6%
Oleic: 26%–35%
Palmitate: 23%–25%
Linoleic: 8%–16%
Steric: 10%–14%

Phytanic Acid
Normal: >0.3%
Borderline: 0.3%–0.5%
Refsum's disease: >0.5%

Background

Free fatty acids are formed by lipoprotein and triglyceride breakdown. The amount of free fatty acids and triglycerides present in blood comes from dietary sources, from fat deposits, or is synthesized by the body. Carbohydrates can be converted to fatty acids and then stored in fat cells as triglycerides.

Explanation of Test

Fatty acid and carbohydrate metabolism is altered in the fat breakdown process (eg, when fasting). Unusually high levels are associated with untreated diabetes. Disorders identified with excess fatty acids are also usually associated with high VLDL levels.

Specific fatty acid measurement can be useful for monitoring nutritional status in the presence of malabsorption, starvation, and long-term parenteral nutrition. It is also valuable for the differential diagnosis of polyneuropathy when Refsum's disease is suspected. In this disease, the enzyme that degrades phytanic acid is lacking.

Procedure

Obtain a 5-ml blood sample. Fasting is required. The blood serum should be separated from blood cells within 45 minutes of collection and should be placed on ice. Observe standard precautions. Serum or EDTA plasma may be used.

Clinical Implications

1. *Increased free fatty acid values* are associated with the following conditions:
   a. Poorly controlled diabetes mellitus
   b. Pheochromocytoma
   c. Hyperthyroidism
   d. Huntington's chorea
   e. von Gierke's disease
   f. Alcoholism
   g. Acute myocardial infarction
   h. Reye's syndrome
2. *Increased phytanic acid* occurs in the following conditions:
   a. Refsum's disease (>50%; repeat the test to confirm)
   b. β-lipoproteinemia
3. *Decreased fatty acids* are found in:
   a. Cystic fibrosis
   b. Malabsorption (acrodermatitis enteropathica)
   c. Zinc deficiency (linoleate and arachnidate low)

Interfering Factors

1. Values are elevated by exercise, anxiety, hypothermia, certain drugs, and long-term fasting. See Appendix J.
2. Values are decreased by long-term IV or parenteral nutrition therapy and certain drugs. See Appendix J.
3. Prolonged fasting or starvation (as much as 3 times normal) affects levels.

Patient Preparation

1. Explain test purpose and blood-drawing procedure. Fasting is required, but water may be taken.
2. Patients receiving heparin therapy should not be tested.

3. Discontinue strenuous exercise before the test. Encourage relaxation.
4. Follow guidelines in Chapter 1 for safe, effective, informed *pretest* care.

Patient Aftercare
1. Resume normal activities.
2. Interpret test results and monitor appropriately.
3. Follow guidelines in Chapter 1 for safe, effective, informed *posttest* care.

● THYROID FUNCTION TESTS

Laboratory determinations of thyroid function are useful in distinguishing patients with euthyroidism (normal thyroid gland function) from those with hyperthyroidism (increased function) or hypothyroidism (decreased function).

PATIENT CARE FOR THYROID TESTING ●

Patient Preparation
1. Explain test purpose and blood specimen collection procedure. To understand the thyroid function tests, it is necessary to understand the following basic concepts. The thyroid gland takes iodine from the circulating blood, combines it with the amino acid tyrosine, and converts it to the thyroid hormones T_4 and T_3. Iodine comprises about two thirds of the weight of the thyroid hormones. The thyroid gland stores T_3 and T_4 until they are released into the bloodstream under the influence of TSH from the pituitary gland. Only a small amount of the hormones is not bound to protein. However, it is the free portion of the thyroid hormones that is the true determinant of the thyroid status of the patient.
2. Assess for signs and symptoms of thyroid disease and note thyroid and iodine medications. Fasting is required for some tests.
3. A typical thyroid panel includes the following tests:
   a. T_3 uptake (TU)
   b. Free T_4
   c. Total T_4
   d. T_3 total
   e. Free thyroxine index (FTI, T_7)
   f. TSH
4. The most useful laboratory tests to confirm or exclude hyperthyroidism are total thyroxine (T_4), free thyroxine index (FTI), total triiodothyronine (T_3), and the ultrasensitive TSH. The most useful tests to detect hypothyroidism are total T_4, free thyroxine index (FTI) and thyroid-stimulating hormone (TSH, thyrotropin). A thyrotropin-releasing hormone (TRH)

stimulation test can be valuable in establishing the thyroid status in some patients with equivocal signs of thyroid dysfunction and borderline laboratory values. It should be kept in mind that values obtained for the assessment of thyroid function can be influenced by factors other than disease, such as age, current illness, binding capacity of serum proteins, and some drugs.

5. Follow guidelines in Chapter 1 for safe, effective, informed *pretest* care.

Patient Aftercare

1. Interpret test results, counsel and monitor appropriately for abnormal thyroid function and disease. Follow-up testing may be required.

2. Thyroid antibody testing can also be done for diagnosis of autoimmune thyroid testing.

3. Follow guidelines in Chapter 1 for safe, effective, informed *posttest* care.

CALCITONIN

Normal Values

Men: <19 pg/ml or ng/L
Women: <14 pg/ml or ng/L

Calcium Infusion (2.4 mg of calcium/kg)
Men: <190 pg/ml or ng/L
Women: <130 pg/ml or ng/L

Pentagastrin Injection (0.5 µg/kg)
Men: <110 pg/ml or ng/L
Women: <35 pg/ml or ng/L

Background

Calcitonin, a hormone secreted by the C cells (parafollicular) of the thyroid gland, inhibits bone resorption by regulating the number and activity of osteoblasts. Calcitonin is secreted in direct response to high blood calcium levels and helps to prevent abrupt changes in calcium levels and the excessive loss of calcium.

Explanation of Test

Measurement of calcitonin is used preoperatively to diagnose familiar medullary thyroid carcinoma and postoperatively to detect recurrence or metastasis of thyroid carcinoma. This test is done to measure increases in immunoreactive calcitonin after stimulation with calcium and/or pentagastrin. Early detection of elevated calcitonin leads to diagnosis of tumor or abnormally secreting C cells before cancer spreads.

Procedure

Obtain a 5-ml venous blood specimen. Fasting is necessary. The blood should be heparinized and chilled immediately. If testing is not performed immediately, blood should be frozen.

Clinical Implications

1. *Increased levels of calcitonin* are associated with the following conditions:
   a. Medullary thyroid cancers
   b. C-cell hyperplasia
   c. Chronic renal failure
   d. Pernicious anemia
   e. Zollinger-Ellison syndrome
   f. Cancer of lung (oat cell lung marker)
   g. Carcinoid syndrome
   h. Alcoholic cirrhosis
   i. Patients with pancreatitis and thyroiditis
   j. Hypercalcemia of any etiology
   k. Carcinoma of breast, islet cell or ovary in some patients (ectopic calcitonin)
2. In a small portion of patients who do have medullary cancer, the fasting level of calcitonin is normal. In these instances, a provocative test using calcium or pentagastrin should be done.
   a. Very high levels >1000 mg/L are evidence of medullary thyroid carcinoma.
   b. These stimulation tests are not needed if the basal calcitonin test is diagnostically high.
   c. In patients with elevated calcitonin levels who do not have medullary thyroid carcinoma, the response is not as vigorous.

Interfering Factors

1. Levels are normally increased in pregnancy at term and in newborns.
2. Gross lipemia and hemolysis interfere with test.

Clinical Alert

1. Screening of families with the calcitonin test of patients with proven medullary cancer of the thyroid is recommended because the tumor has both sporadic and familial incidence.
2. If the calcitonin test is normal in family members, it is advisable to repeat the calcium provocative test periodically (over a period of months or years).
3. Some patients do not respond to the stimulation test who have medullary thyroid carcinoma.

Patient Preparation

1. Explain test purpose and procedure.
2. Fasting from food overnight is required. Water is permitted.
3. If the provocative tests using calcium and pentagastrin are to be done, the patient is to be fasting, also.
   a. *Pentagastrin* is injected 0.5 μg/kg IV push. Blood samples are drawn

before the injection to determine baseline value of calcitonin. A blood sample is drawn 1.5, 2, and 5 minutes after the injection.

b. *Calcium* is injected 2.0 mg/kg after baseline sample is drawn. A blood sample is drawn 5 and 10 minutes after injection.

4. Follow guidelines in Chapter 1 for safe, effective, informed *pretest* care.

NOTE: *A combined calcium and pentagastrin test may be more effective and reliable than either test by itself.*

Patient Aftercare

1. Interpret test outcome and monitor appropriately.

2. The patient may experience transient nausea or fatigue after injection and may experience chest pain for a short time.

3. Resume normal activities when symptoms abate.

4. Follow guidelines in Chapter 1 for safe, effective, informed *posttest* care.

FREE THYROXINE T$_4$ (FT$_4$)

Normal Values

0.7–2.0 ng/dl or 10–26 pmol/L

For patients taking Synthroid, up to 5.0 ng/dl

Background

Free thyroxine (FT$_4$) comprises a small fraction of total thyroxine. The free FT$_4$ is unbound to protein and available to the tissues, and it is the metabolically active form of this hormone. This fraction constitutes ~5% of the circulatory thyroxine T$_4$.

Explanation of Test

FT$_4$ has diagnostic value in situations in which total hormone levels do not correlate with the thyrometabolic state, and there is suspected abnormality in thyroxine-binding globulin (TBG) levels. It provides a more accurate picture of the thyroid status in persons with abnormal thyroxine binding globulin levels in pregnancy and in those who are receiving estrogens, hydrogens, phenytoin, or salicylates.

Procedure

Obtain a 5-ml venous blood sample. Accurate results can be obtained with as little as 0.5 ml of blood in pediatric cases. Serum is needed for this test. Observe standard precautions.

Clinical Implications

1. *Increased FT$_4$ levels* are associated with the following conditions:

a. Graves' disease (hyperthyroidism)

b. Hypothyroidism treated with thyroxine

c. Euthyroid sick syndrome

2. *Decreased FT$_4$ levels* are associated with the following conditions:
   a. Primary hypothyroidism
   b. Secondary hypothyroidism (pituitary)
   c. Tertiary hypothyroidism (hypothalamic)
   d. Hypothyroidism treated with triiodothyronine

Interfering Factors
1. Values are increased in infants at birth. This value rises even higher after 2 to 3 days of life.
2. Many drugs affect test outcomes. See Appendix J.
3. Heparin causes falsely elevated FT$_4$ values.
4. Levels can fluctuate in patients with severe or chronic illness.
5. Levels fluctuate in pregnancy

Patient Preparation and Aftercare
See patient care for thyroid testing. The same protocols prevail in FT$_4$ testing.

FREE TRIIODOTHYRONINE (FT$_3$) ●

Normal Values
Adult: 260–480 pg/dl or 4.0–7.4 pmol/L

Explanation of Test
This is one of the determinations used to evaluate thyroid function and measure that fraction of the circulatory T$_3$ that exists in the free state in the blood, unbound to protein. FT$_3$ is done to rule out T$_3$ toxicosis, to evaluate thyroid replacement therapy, and to clarify protein-binding abnormalities.

Procedure
Obtain a 5-ml venous blood sample. Observe standard precautions.

Clinical Implications
1. *Increased FT$_3$ values* are associated with the following conditions:
   a. Hyperthyroidism
   b. T$_3$ toxicosis
   c. Peripheral resistance syndrome
2. *Decreased FT$_3$ values* are associated with the following conditions:
   a. Hypothyroidism (primary and secondary)
   b. Third trimester of pregnancy

   NOTE: *In nonthyroidal illness, a low FT$_3$ level is a nonspecific finding.*

Interfering Factors
1. Recently administered radioisotopes and some drugs in Appendix J
2. High altitude

Patient Preparation and Aftercare
See patient care for thyroid testing. The same protocols prevail for FT$_3$.

FREE THYROXINE INDEX (FTI, T₇) ●

Normal Values
Adult: 1.5–4.5 index (these are arbitrary units)

Check with your laboratory for their normal values.

Explanation of Test
The free thyroxine index (FTI) is a mathematical calculation used to correct the estimated total thyroxine (T_4) for the amount of thyroxine-binding globulin (TBG) present. To perform this calculation, two results are needed: the T_4 value and the T_3 uptake ratio. The product of these two values is the free thyroxine index (FTI). The FTI is useful in the diagnosis of hyperthyroidism and hypothyroidism, especially in patients with known or suspected abnormalities in thyroxine-binding protein levels. In such cases, blood levels and clinical signs may seem contradictory unless both T_4 and TBG are considered as interrelated parameters of thyroid status. Measurement of FT_4 also gives a more accurate picture of the thyroid status when the TBG is abnormal in pregnant women or persons being treated with estrogen, androgens, phenytoin, or salicylates.

Procedure
A calculation is made based on results of T_3 uptake and T_4 total.

$$FTI = T_4 \text{ total} \times T_3 \text{ uptake (\%)}/100.$$

The FTI permits meaningful interpretation by balancing out most nonthyroidal factors. In recent years, this parameter has lost popularity and is of dubious value.

Clinical Implications
Application of the equation of the FTI includes the following:

Status	*TBG*	*T₃ Uptake*	×	*T₄*	=	*FTI*
Euthyroid	Normal	35%		9.0		3.1
Euthyroid	Low	52%		4.0		2.1
Euthyroid	High	13%		16.0		2.8
Hypothyroid	High	24%		4.0		0.9
Hyperthyroid	Low	46%		13.0		6.0

This is a mathematical calculation that does not involve the patient.

Interfering Factors
1. Levels fluctuate in pregnancy
2. See Appendix J for drugs that affect test outcomes.

NEONATAL THYROTROPIN-RELEASING HORMONE (TRH) ●

Normal Values
Newborn screen: <20 μU/ml

TRH surges at birth, peaking at 30 minutes of life at a level of 25 to 160 μU/ml. It declines and reaches adult levels by the first week of life.

Background
Neonatal primary hypothyroidism is characterized not only by low T_4 levels in blood serum but also by elevated thyrotropin-releasing hormone (TRH) levels (so as to differentiate from TSH test).

Explanation of Test
This measurement is used as a confirmatory test for infants with positive T_4 screens or low blood serum T_4 levels. Although TRH measurement has been suggested as the primary screening test for neonatal hypothyroidism, infants with secondary (hypothalamic or hypopituitary) hypothyroidism, who constitute about 10% of all neonatal hypothyroid cases, would be missed in such a screening system.

Procedure
1. Cleanse the infant's heel with an antiseptic and puncture with a sterile disposable lancet. Collect this blood specimen 3 to 7 days after birth.
2. If bleeding is slow, it helps to hold the leg dependent for a short time before blotting the blood on the filter paper.
3. The circles on the filter paper must be completely filled. This can best be done by placing one side of the filter paper against the infant's heel and watching for the blood to appear on the front side of the paper and completely fill the circle.
4. Air dry the filter paper for 1 hour, fill in all information, and send to the laboratory immediately. Do not expose samples to extreme heat or light.

Clinical Implications
An elevated TRH test is associated with neonatal hypothyroidism.

Patient Preparation
1. Inform the parent or parents about test purpose and method of specimen collection.
2. See patient care for thyroid testing.

Patient Aftercare
1. Be prepared to counsel parent or parents regarding steps to take if the TRH test is abnormal.

NEONATAL THYROXINE (T$_4$); NEONATAL SCREEN FOR HYPOTHYROIDISM

Normal Values

Neonate (1–5 d): >7.5 µg/dl
Neonate (6–8 d): >6.5 µg/dl

Background

Normal brain growth and development cannot take place without adequate thyroid hormone. Congenital hypothyroidism (cretinism) is characterized by low levels of T$_4$ and elevated levels of TSH.

Explanation of Test

This is a screening test of thyroxine (T$_4$) activity to detect neonatal hypothyroidism. Specimens should be obtained after the first 24 hours of protein feeding or within the first week of life. Thyroxine is obtained from whole blood blotted on filter paper using a radioimmunoassay technique.

Procedure

1. Cleanse the infant's heel with an antiseptic and puncture the skin with a sterile disposable lancet.
2. If bleeding is slow, it helps to hold the leg dependent for a short time before blotting the blood on the filter paper.
3. The circles on the filter paper must be completely filled. This can best be done by placing one side of the filter paper against the infant's heel and watching for the blood to appear on the front side of the paper and completely fill the circle. Do not damage filter paper.
4. Air dry for 1 hour, fill in all requested information, and send to laboratory immediately. Protect specimen from extreme heat and light.

Clinical Implications

1. Low values are associated with hypothyroidism.
2. A number of nonthyroid conditions can result in depressed T$_4$ levels (eg, low birth weight, prematurity, twinning, fetal distress, deficient TBG levels).

Patient Preparation and Aftercare

Refer to neonatal TRH testing for care. The same protocols prevail for neonatal T$_4$.

Clinical Alert

1. Do not interpret this test in terms of the adult serum T$_4$ values. This is an entirely different procedure using a different type of specimen.

(continued)

(Clinical Alert continued)
2. Notify attending physician and the infant's parent or parents of positive results within 24 hours.
3. If T_4 results are abnormal, a TRH (TSH) test should be done.
4. Normal T_4, and in some cases, normal TSH, screening results do not ensure against failure of normal development due to presence of hypothyroidism. Of all cases of infantile hypothyroidism, 6% to 12% have normal screening hormone levels.

THYROGLOBULIN (Tg) ●

Normal Values
Adult: 3–42 ng/ml or µg/L
Newborn (48 h): 36–48 ng/ml

NOTE: *8% of normal adults have serum values of Tg < 10 ng/ml.*

Background
Thyroglobulin is composed of glycoprotein and the iodinated secretions of epithelial cells of the thyroid. These iodinated secretions contain both the precursors of T_4 and T_3 and the hormones themselves.

Explanation of Test
This test is helpful in the differential diagnosis of hyperthyroidism and in monitoring the course of differentiated or metastatic thyroid cancer. It is not useful in the diagnosis of thyroid cancer. Levels decrease following successful initial treatment, and in recurrence of metastasis, the level will again rise. Lack of sensitivity and specificity limits the value of this test.

Procedure
Obtain a 5-ml venous blood sample. Serum is needed. Observe standard precautions.

Clinical Implications
1. *Increased thyroglobulin levels* are associated with the following conditions:
   a. Untreated and metastatic differentiated thyroid cancers (not medullary carcinoma)
   b. Hyperthyroidism (not good correlation with elevated T_4)
   c. Subacute thyroiditis
   d. Benign adenoma (some cases)
   e. Occurrence of metastases after initial treatment
2. *Decreased thyroglobulin levels* are associated with the following conditions:
   a. Thyrotoxicosis factitia
   b. Infants with goitrous hypothyroidism.

Interfering Factors
1. Newborns have high Tg levels which drop to adult levels by 2 years of age.
2. Autoantibodies to Tg cause decreased values. Thyroglobulin antibody test may have to be done to confirm decreased levels.

Patient Preparation
1. See patient care for thyroid testing on page 482.
2. Patient should be off of thyroid medication for 6 weeks prior to specimen collection.
3. Determination of Tg levels may be substituted for I^{131} scans in patients at low risk for thyroid cancer.

Patient Aftercare
1. Resume thyroid medication and normal activities.
2. Monitor as appropriate for metastatic thyroid cancer.
3. Refer to patient aftercare instructions for thyroid testing on p. 483. The same protocols prevail for Tg testing.

THYROID-STIMULATING HORMONE (THYROTROPIN; TSH)

Normal Values
Adult: 0.2–5.4 mU/L
Neonate: 3–20 μIU/L by day 3 of life

Background
The thyroid is unique among the endocrine glands because it has a large store of hormone and a slow rate of normal turnover. Stimulation of the thyroid gland by the TSH, which is produced by the anterior pituitary gland, causes the release and distribution of stored thyroid hormones. TSH stimulates secretion of T_4 and T_3. TSH secretion is physiologically regulated by T_3 and T_4 (feedback inhibition) and is stimulated by thyrotropin-releasing hormone (TRH) from the hypothalamus. TSH is the single most sensitive test for primary hypothyroidism. If there is clear evidence of hypothyroidism and the TSH is not elevated, then an implication of possible hypopituitarism exists.

Explanation of Test
This measurement is used in the diagnosis of primary hypothyroidism when there is thyroid gland failure due to intrinsic disease, and it is used to differentiate primary from secondary hypothyroidism by determining the actual circulatory level of TSH. TSH levels are high in primary hypothyroidism. Low TSH levels occur in hyperthyroidism. This is the single most sensitive test for primary hypothyroidism.

TSH measurements with sufficient sensitivity to distinguish low levels from normal levels have become the preferred test for hyperthyroidism. The high-sensitivity TSH test is useful for diagnosing sick euthyroid patients and in differentiating mild hyperthyroidism from Graves' disease. With the new, sensitive assays, a TRH stimulation test is no longer necessary.

Procedure

Obtain a 5-ml venous blood sample. Place specimen in a biohazard bag.

Clinical Implications

1. *Increased TSH levels* are seen in the following conditions:
   a. Adults and neonates with primary hypothyroidism
   b. Thyrotropin-producing tumor (eg, ectopic TSH secretion from lung, breast tumors)
   c. Hashimoto's thyroiditis
   d. Thyrotoxicosis due to pituitary tumor
   e. TSH antibodies
   f. Hypothyroid patients receiving insufficient thyroid replacement hormone
2. *Decreased TSH levels* are associated with the following conditions:
   a. Primary hyperthyroidism
   b. Secondary and tertiary hypothyroidism
   c. Treated Graves' disease
   d. Euthyroid sick disease
   e. Overreplacement of thyroid hormone in treatment of hypothyroidism

Interfering Factors

1. Values are normally high in neonatal cord blood. There is hypersecretion of TSH in newborns up to 2 to 3 times normal. The TSH level approaches normal by the first week of life.
2. Values are suppressed during treatment with thyroxine and corticosteroids. See Appendix J for other drugs.
3. Values are abnormally increased with lithium, potassium iodide, amphetamine abuse and iodine-containing drugs.
4. Radioisotopes administered within 1 week before test invalidate the result.
5. Values may be decreased in the first trimester of pregnancy.

Patient Preparation

1. Explain test purpose and procedure.
2. Follow guidelines in Chapter 1 for safe, effective, informed *pretest* care.

Patient Aftercare

1. Resume normal activities.
2. Interpret test results and counsel as appropriate for hypothyroidism or hyperthyroidism.
3. Follow guidelines in Chapter 1 for safe, effective, informed *posttest* care.

THYROXINE-BINDING GLOBULIN (TBG) ●

Normal Values

Men: 15–30 μg/dl

Women	2nd trimester: 41.4–63.9 μg/dl
Nonpregnant: 11.5–32.2 μg/dl	3rd trimester: 31.0–73.6 μg/dl
1st trimester: 19.8–64.7 μg/dl	Oral contraceptives: 23.1–47.9 μg/dl

Background

Almost all of the thyroid hormones in the blood are protein bound: albumin, thyroid-binding prealbumin, and most important, thyroxine-binding globulin (TBG). Variations in TBG levels have a major effect on bound and free (metabolically active) forms of T_4 and T_3.

Explanation of Test

This measurement is useful to distinguish between hyperthyroidism causing high T_4 and euthyroid patients with increased binding by TBG who have increased T_4 and normal levels of free hormones, to identify hereditary deficiency or increase of TBG, to workup thyroid disease in hypothyroid populations, and when the mean TBG concentration is significantly higher than the mean level in normal thyroid populations. In hyperthyroid populations, the mean TBG level concentration is lower than the mean level in normal thyroid populations.

Procedure

Obtain a 2-ml venous blood specimen. Place specimen in a biohazard bag.

Clinical Implications

1. The *TBG test is increased* in the following conditions:
   a. Genetically determined high TBG
   b. Hypothyroidism (some cases)
   c. Infectious hepatitis and other liver diseases
   d. Acute intermittent porphyria
   e. Estrogen-producing tumors
2. The *TBG test is decreased* in the following conditions:
   a. Genetic deficiency of TBG
   b. Nephrotic syndrome
   c. Major illness, surgical stress
   d. Acromegaly
   e. Severe acidosis
   f. Testosterone producing tumors
   g. Hepatic disease
   h. Marked hypoproteinemia, malnutrition

Interfering Factors

1. Many drugs increase (eg, estrogens, oral contraceptives) or decrease (eg, phenytoin and steroids) values. See Appendix J.
2. Neonates have higher values.
3. Recently administered radioisotopes affect results.

Patient Preparation and Aftercare
1. See patient care for thyroid testing (pp. 482 and 483).

THYROXINE; TOTAL T$_4$ ●

Normal Values
Adult: 5.4–11.5 µg/dl or 57–148 nmol/L
Child: 6.4–13.3 µg/dl or 83–172 nmol/L

If testing is done by radioimmunoassay, it is reported as T$_4$ RIA.

Background
Thyroxine is the thyroid hormone with four atoms of iodine; hence, it is called T$_4$. The combination of the serum T$_4$ and T$_3$ uptake as an assessment of TBG helps to determine whether an abnormal T$_4$ value is due to alterations in serum TBG or to changes of thyroid hormone levels. Deviations of both tests in the same direction usually indicate that an abnormal T$_4$ level is due to abnormalities in thyroid hormone. Deviations of the two tests in opposite directions provide evidence that an abnormal T$_4$ may relate to alterations in TBG.

Explanation of Test
Thyroxine, one of the thyroid function panel tests, is a direct measurement of the concentration of T$_4$ in the blood serum. Total T$_4$ level is a good index of thyroid function when the TBG is normal. The increase in TBG levels normally seen in pregnancy and with estrogen therapy increases total T$_4$ levels. The decrease of TBG levels in persons receiving anabolic steroids, in chronic liver disease, and in nephroses decreases the total T$_4$ value. This test is commonly done to rule out hyperthyroidism and hypothyroidism. The T$_4$ test also can be used as a guide in establishing maintenance doses of thyroid in the treatment of hypothyroidism. In addition, it also can be used in hyperthyroidism to follow the results acheived with antithyroid drug administration.

Procedure
Obtain a 5-ml venous blood sample. If the patient is already receiving thyroid treatment, it must be discontinued 1 month before the test. Observe standard precautions.

Interfering Factors
1. Total thyroxine levels increase during the second or third month of pregnancy as a result of increased estrogen production.
2. Total thyroxine levels increase with the use of drugs such as estrogens, heroin, and methadone. See Appendix J.
3. Contrast agents used for x-rays and other diagnostic procedures affect results.
4. Values are decreased with salicylates and anticonvulsants.

Clinical Implications

1. *Increased T₄ values* are found in the following conditions:
   a. Hyperthyroidism
   b. Clinical status that increases TBG
   c. Thyrotoxicosis factitia
   d. Acute thyroiditis
   e. Hepatitis, liver disease
   f. Neonates
   g. D-Thyroxine therapy
2. *Decreased T₄ values* are found in the following conditions:
   a. Hypothyroidism
   b. Disorders of decreased TBG
   c. Hypoproteinemia
   d. Treatment with triiodothyronine

Patient Preparation

1. Explain test purpose and procedure. T_4 is usually the first test used in the diagnosis of hypothyroidism or hyperthyroidism.
2. Avoid strenuous exercise.
3. No radiopaque contrast should be administered for 1 week prior to testing.
4. If patient is on thyroid therapy, discontinue treatment for 1 month before testing to determine baseline values.
5. Follow guidelines in Chapter 1 for safe, effective, informed *pretest* care.

Patient Aftercare

1. Resume normal activities.
2. See patient care for thyroid testing on page 483.

CLINICAL ALERT
T_4 values are higher in neonates due to elevated TBG. Values rise abruptly in the first few hours after birth and decline gradually until the age of 5 years.

TRIIODOTHYRONINE (T₃), TOTAL ●

Normal Values
Age >24 y: 80–200 ng/dl
Age 15–23 y: 100–220 ng/dl
Age 1–14 y: 125–250 ng/dl

If radioimmunoassay is used, the result is reported as T_3 RIA.

Background
T_3 has three atoms of iodine, compared with four atoms in T_4. T_3 is more active metabolically than T_4, but its effect is shorter. There is much less T_3 than T_4 in the serum, and it is bound less firmly to TBG.

Explanation of Test

This measurement is a quantitative determination of the total T_3 concentration in the blood and is the test of choice in the diagnosis of T_3 thyrotoxicosis. *It is not the same as the T_3 uptake test that measures the unsaturated TBC in serum*. It can also be very useful in the diagnosis of hyperthyroidism. T_3 thyrotoxicosis refers to a variant of hyperthyroidism in which a thyrotoxic patient has elevated T_3 values and normal T_4 values. This test is of limited value in diagnosing hypothyroidism.

Procedure

Obtain a 5-ml venous blood sample. Observe standard precautions.

Clinical Implications

1. *Increased T_3 values* are associated with the following conditions:
   a. Hyperthyroidism
   b. T_3 thyrotoxicosis
   c. Daily dosage of $\geq$25 μg of T_3
   d. Acute thyroiditis
   e. TBG elevation from any cause
   f. Daily dosage of $\geq$300 μg of T_4
2. *Decreased T_3 valves* are associated with the following conditions:
   a. Hypothyroidism; however, some clinically hypothyroid patients will have normal levels
   b. Starvation and state of nutrition, acute illness
   c. TBG decrease from any cause

Interfering Factors

1. Values are increased in pregnancy and with the use of drugs such as estrogens, methadone, and heroin. See Appendix J.
2. Values are decreased with the use of drugs such as anabolic steroids, androgens, large doses of salicylates, and phenytoin.
3. Fasting causes T_3 level to decrease.

> **Clinical Alert**
>
> Panic values of <50 ng/dl or >300 ng/dl.

Patient Preparation and Aftercare

Care is the same as for T_4 testing (see pp. 482 and 483).

TRIIODOTHYRONINE UPTAKE (T_3UP) (T_3U) ●

Normal Values

0.8–1.30 (ratio between patient specimen and the standard control)
25%–35% uptake (these are arbitrary units)

Explanation of Test

This test is an indirect measurement of unsaturated thyroxine-binding globulin (TBG) in blood. This determination, expressed in arbitrary terms, is inversely proportional to the TBG. For this reason, low T_3U levels are indicative of situations that result in elevated levels of TBG uptake. For example, in hypothyroidism, when insufficient T_4 is available to produce saturation of TBG, UTBG is elevated, and T_3U values are low. Similarly, in pregnant patients or those receiving estrogen, TBG levels are increased proportionately more than are T_4 levels, resulting in high levels of UTBG, which are reflected in low T_3U results. This test should not be ordered alone; it is useful only when T_4 is done. It is also used to calculate the T_7 or free thyroxine index (FTI).

Clinical Implications

1. See Explanation of Test.

Interfering Factors

1. *Decreased T_3U levels* occur in normal pregnancy, and with drugs such as estrogens, antiovulatory drugs, methadone, and heparin.
2. *Increased T_3U levels* occur with drugs such as dicumarol, heparin, androgens, anabolic steroids, phenytoin, and large doses of salicylates.

Patient Preparation and Aftercare

See patient care for thyroid testing (pp. 482 and 483). Pretest and posttest care is the same as for T_4 testing (see p. 495).

Clinical Alert

1. This test has nothing to do with the actual T_3 blood level despite its name, which is sometimes confusingly abbreviated to the T_3 test. It is emphasized that the T_3U and the true T_3 are entirely different tests. The T_3U gives only an indirect measurement of overall binding.
2. This test should be used only in conjunction with the T_4 test to calculate the free thyroxine index (FTI).
3. Some methods of determining T_3U have a direct relation with T_4. Check the reference values of your laboratory.

BIBLIOGRAPHY ●

Amann ST, DiMagno E, Rubin W: Pancreatitis: diagnostics and therapeutic interventions. Patient Care 31: 200, 1997

American Diabetes Association: Clinical practice recommendations 1998. Diabetes Care 21(Suppl 1):, 1998

Apple FS: Clinical and analytical standardization issues confronting cardiac troponin I. Clinical chemistry 45(1): 18, 1999

Carter HB, Epstein JI, Chan DW, Fozard JL, Pearson JD: Recommended prostate-specific antigen testing intervals for the detection of curable prostate cancer. JAMA 277: 1456–1460, 1997

Dougas M, Strelnick A: Testing intervals for PSA test. J Fam Pract 45(2): 98–106, 1997

Fox GN, Sabovic Z: Chromium picolinate supplementation for diabetes mellitus. J Fam Pract 46(1): 83–86, 1998

Frizzell J: The PSA test. AJN 98(4): 14–15, 1998

Henry J: Clinical Diagnosis and Management by Laboratory Methods, 19th ed. Philadelphia, WB Saunders, 1996

Hlatky MA, Owens DK: Cost effectiveness of tests to assess the risk of sudden death after acute myocardial infarction. J Am Coll Cardiol 31(7): 1490–1492, 1998

Kaplan MM: Clinical perspectives in the diagnosis of thyroid disease. Clinical Chemistry 45(8): 1377–1383. Special Issue Part 2 of 2, Proceedings of the Twenty-Second Annual Arnold O. Beckman Conference in Clinical Chemistry, February 21–22, 1999.

Lebovitz HE: Type 2 Diabetes: An Overview. Clinical Chemistry 45(8): 1339–1346. Special Issue 1999 Part 2 of 2, Proceedings of the Twenty-Second Annual Arnold O. Beckman Conference in Clinical Chemistry, February 21–22, 1999.

Lee NA, Reasner CA: Beneficial effect of chromium supplementation on serum triglyceride levels in NIDDM. Diabetes Care 17(12): 1449–1452, 1994

Lehmann CH (ed): Saunders Manual of Clinical Laboratory Science. Philadelphia. WB Saunders, 1998

Lernmark A: Type I Diabetes. Clinical Chemistry 45(8): 1331–1338. Special Issue 1999 Part 2 of 2 Proceedings of the Twenty-Second Annual Arnold O. Beckman Conference in Clinical Chemistry, February 21–22, 1999.

MacKenzie HA: Recent advances in photoacoustic, non-invasive disease testing: Oak Ridge Conferences, April 23 & 24, 1999. Sponsor: American Association for Clinical Chemistry

Neiblum DR, Boynton RF: Evaluation and treatment of chronic hepatitis C infection. Primary Care 23(3): 535–547, 1996

Prescott M, Lenokes JG, Anderson AC (eds): Lead poisoning in childhood. Baltimore. Paul A Brookes Co., 1996

Report of the Expert Committee on the Diagnosis and Classification of Diabetes Mellitus. Diabetes Care 20: 1183–1197, 1997

Sunheimer R: Advances in cholesterol testing. Advance for Laboratory Administrators 8(6), June 1999

Tietz NW: Clinical Guide to Laboratory Tests, 3rd ed. Philadelphia, WB Saunders, 1996

Trundle D: Troublesome questions about thyroid tests. Medical Laboratory Observer 28(10), October 1996

U.S. Department of Health and Human Services: Detection, Evaluation and Treatment of High Cholesterol in Adults. NIH Pub. #93–3036. Washington, DC, U.S. Government Printing Office, September, 1993

Wallace J: Interpretation of Diagnostic Tests: A Synopsis of Laboratory Medicine, 6th ed. Boston, Little, Brown & Co., 1996

Watts NB: Clinical Utility of Biochemical Markers of Bone Remodeling. Clinical Chemistry 45(8): 1359–1368. Special Issue 1999 Part 2 of 2, Proceedings of the Twenty-Second Annual Arnold O. Beckman Conference in Clinical Chemistry, Februrary 21–22, 1999

Winter W, Schatz D, Kenndy L, Venecor F: The new ADA Diabetes Guidelines: Implications for the Clinical Laboratory. Internet course at www.aacc.org. 1998/1999

Young DS: Effects of Drugs on Clinical Laboratory Tests, 5th ed. Washington, DC, AACC Press, 1999

7

Microbiologic Studies

Diagnostic Testing and Microbes

In diagnostic testing, microorganisms are referred to as *pathogens*. The word *pathogenic* is usually defined as "causing infectious disease"; however, organisms that are pathogenic under one set of conditions may, under other conditions, reside within or on the surface of the body without causing disease. When these organisms are present but do not cause harm to the host, they are considered *commensals*. Once they begin to multiply and to cause tissue damage, they are considered pathogens, with the potential for causing or increasing a pathogenic process (Table 7-1). Many newly discovered organisms are clinically relevant. Some of these organisms, formerly considered to be insignificant contaminants or commensals, have taken on roles as causative agents for opportunistic diseases in patients with human immunodeficiency virus (HIV) infection or other immunodeficiency syndromes or diseases associated with a compromised health state. Consequently, virtually any organism recovered in pure culture from a body site must be considered a *potential pathogen*.

Basic Concepts of Infectious Disease

Infectious diseases cause pathologic conditions. Infectious processes demonstrate observable physiologic and other human responses to the invasion and multiplication of the offending microorganisms. Once an infectious disease is suspected, appropriate cultures should be done or nonculture techniques—such as serologic testing for antigens and antibodies, monoclonal antibodies, and DNA probes—should be used. Proper specimen collection and appropriate blood and skin tests are necessary to detect and diagnose the presence of the microorganism.

Opportunity for infection depends on host resistance, organism volumes, the ability of the organism to find a portal of entry, and its ability to overcome host defenses, invade tissues, and produce toxins. Organisms may become seated in susceptible persons through inhalation, ingestion, direct contact, inoculation, breaks in natural skin or mucous membrane barriers, changes in organism volumes, alterations in normal flora balances, or changes in other host defense mechanisms.

Host Factors

The development of an infectious disease is influenced by the patient's general health, normal defense mechanisms, previous contact with the offending organism, past clinical history, and type and location of infected tissue. Mechanisms of host resistance are detailed in the following lists:

Primary Host Defenses
1. Anatomic barriers
    A. Intact skin surfaces
    B. Nose hairs
    C. Respiratory tract cilia
    D. Coughing and flow of respiratory tract fluids and mucus
    E. Swallowing and gastrointestinal tract peristalsis
2. Physiologic barriers
    A. High or low pH and oxygen tension (prevents proliferation of organisms)

TABLE 7-1
Pathogens Detectable in Body Tissues and Fluids by Diagnostic Methods

NASOPHARYNX AND OROPHARYNX	SPUTUM	FECES
β-Hemolytic streptococci	*Blastomyces dermatitidis*	*Candida albicans*
Bordetella pertussis	*Bordetella pertussis*	*Campylobacter jejuni*
Mycoplasma spp.	*Candida albicans*	*Clostridium botulinum*
Branhamella catarrhalis	*Coccidiodes immitis*	*Entamoeba histolytica*
Herpes simplex virus	Influenza viruses	*Escheria coli* (toxogenic strains)
Pseudomonas spp.	*Streptococcus pneumoniae*	*Mycobacterium tuberculosis*
Candida albicans	*Pseudomonas* spp.	*Pseudomonas* (large counts)
Corynebacterium diphtheriae	*Haemophilus influenzae*	*Salmonella* spp.
Hemophilus influenzae (large counts)	Hemolytic streptococci	*Shigella* spp.
Meningococci	*Histoplasma capsulatum*	Staphylococci
Pneumococci (large counts)	*Klebsiella* spp.	*Vibrio cholerae*
Staphylococcus aureus	*Mycobacterium tuberculosis*	*Vibrio comma*
Enterobacteriaceae	*Yersinia pestis*	*Vibrio para-haemolyticus*
Capnocytophaga spp.	*Francisella tularensis*	*Yersinia enterocolitica*
Cryptococcus neoformans	*Staphylococcus aureus*	*Clostridium difficile*
	Mycoplasma spp.	Rotavirus
	Eikenella corrodens	Hepatitis A, B, and C
	Legionella spp.	*Giardia lamblia*
		Cryptosporidium spp.

URINE

β-Hemolytic streptococci, groups B and D

Coliform bacilli (counts of ≥100,000), including *Escherichia coli, Klebsiella, Enterobacter,* and *Serratia*

Enterococci *(Streptococcus faecalis)*

Gonococci *(Neisseria gonorrhoeae)*

Mycobacterium tuberculosis

Pseudomonas aeruginosa

Staphylococcus aureus

Staphylococcus saprophyticus

Salmonella and *Shigella* spp.

Trichomonas vaginalis

Candida albicans and other yeasts

Staphylococcus epidermidis

(continued)

TABLE 7-1 *(Continued)*

SKIN	*EAR*
Bacteroides spp.	*Aspergillus fumigatus*
Clostridium spp.	*Candida albicans* and other fungi
Coliform bacilli	Coliform bacilli
Fungi	Hemolytic streptococci
Proteus spp.	*Proteus* spp.
Pseudomonas spp.	Pneumococci *(Streptococcus pneumoniae)*
Staphylococcus aureus	*Pseudomonas aeruginosa*
Streptococcus pyogenes	*Staphylococcus aureus*
Varicella zoster virus	*Haemophilus influenzae*
Herpes simplex virus	*Moraxella catarrhalis*
	Mycoplasma pneumoniae
	Peptostreptococcus spp.
	Bacteroides fragilis
	Fusobacterium nucleatum
	Influenza virus
	Respiratory syncytial virus (RSV)

CEREBROSPINAL FLUID	*VAGINAL DISCHARGE*	*URETHRAL DISCHARGE*
Bacteroides spp.	β-Hemolytic streptococci	*Chlamydia trachomatis*
Brucella abortus	*Candida albicans*	Coliform bacilli
Coccidiodes immitis	Coliform bacilli	Cytomegalovirus
Histoplasma capsulatum	Enterococci	*Hemophilus ducreyi*
Blastomyces dermatitidis	*Gardnerella vaginalis*	Herpes simplex virus
Candida spp.	*Listeria monocytogenes*	*Neisseria gonorrhoeae*
Nocardia spp.	*Mycoplasma* spp.	*Treponema pallidum*
Actinomyces spp.	Human papilloma virus	*Trichomonas vaginalis*
Salmonella spp.	*Neisseria gonorrhaeae*	*Mycoplasma* spp.
Cryptococcus neoformans	*Treponema pallidum*	Cytomegalovirus
Hemophilus influenzae	*Hemophilus ducreyi*	Human papilloma virus
Leptospira spp.	*Chlamydia trachomatis*	
Mycobacterium tuberculosis	Herpes simplex virus	
	Trichomonas vaginalis	

TABLE 7–1 *(Continued)*	
CEREBROSPINAL FLUID	***VAGINAL DISCHARGE***
Neisseria meningitidis	*Ureaplasma urealyticum*
Pneumococci	*Mobiluncus* spp. and
(Streptococcus	other anaerobes
pneumoniae)	Cytomegalovirus
Pseudomonas spp.	
Staphylococci	
Streptococci	

B. Chemical inhibitors to bacterial growth (eg, proteases)
C. Bile acids
D. Active lysozymes in saliva and tears
E. Fatty acids on skin surfaces

Secondary Host Defenses (Physiologic Barriers)
1. Responses of complement, lysozymes, opsonins, and secretions
2. Phagocytosis
3. Immunoglobulin A (IgA), IgG, and IgM antibody formation
4. Cell-mediated immune responses

Factors Decreasing Host Resistance
1. Age: The very young and the very old are more susceptible.
2. Presence of chronic disease (eg, cancer, cardiovascular disease, diabetes)
3. Use or history of certain therapeutic modalities such as radiation, chemotherapy, corticosteroids, antibiotics, or immunosuppressants
4. Toxins, including alcohol, street drugs, legitimate therapeutic drugs, venom or toxic secretions from a reptile or insect, or other nonhuman bites or punctures
5. Others, including excessive physical or emotional stress states, nutritional state, and presence of foreign material at the site

COLLECTION AND TRANSPORT OF SPECIMENS

General Principles
The health care professional is responsible for collecting specimens for diagnostic examinations. Because procedures vary, check institutional protocols for specimen retrieval, transport, preservation, and reporting of test results.

Specimens for bacterial culture should be representative of the disease process. Also, sufficient material must be collected to ensure an accurate examination. As an example, serous drainage from a diabetic foot ulcer with possible osteomyelitis may yield inaccurate results. In this case, a bone biopsy or purulent drainage of infected tissue would be a better specimen. Likewise, if there is a lesion of the skin and subcutaneous tissue, material from the margin of the lesion rather than the central part of the lesion would be more desirable. If a purulent sputum sample cannot be obtained to aid in the diagnosis of pneumonia, blood cultures, pleural fluid examination, and bronchoalveolar lavage specimens are also acceptable.

It is imperative that material be collected where the suspected organism is most likely to be found, with as little outside contamination as possible. For this reason, certain precautions must be followed routinely:

1. Observe standard precautions. Clean the skin starting centrally and going out in larger circles. Repeat several times, using a clean swab or wipe each time. If 70% alcohol is used, it should be applied for 2 minutes. Tincture of iodine requires only 1 minute of cleansing.
2. Bypass areas of normal flora; culture only for a specific pathogen.
3. Fluids, tissues, skin scrapings, and urine should be collected in sterile containers with tight-fitting lids. Polyester-tipped swabs in a collection system containing an ampule of Stuart's transport medium ensure adequacy of the specimen for 72 hours at room temperature.
4. Place the specimen in a biohazard bag.

> ### Clinical Alert
>
> 1. Without routine precautions for collecting and handling specimens, the patient's condition may be incorrectly diagnosed, laboratory time may be wasted, effective treatment may be delayed, or pathogenic organisms may be transmitted to health care workers and other patients.
> 2. It is important to report all identified diseases, conditions, and outbreaks according to state and federal guidelines (Chart 7-1).

Sources of Specimens

Microbiologic specimens may be collected from many sources, such as blood, pus or wound exudates or drainage, urine, sputum, feces, genital discharges or secretions, cerebrospinal fluid (CSF), and eye or ear drainage. During specimen collection, these general procedures should be followed:

1. Label specimens properly with the following information (institutional requirements may vary):
   A. Patient's name, age, sex, address, hospital identification number, and physician's full name
   B. Specimen source (eg, throat, conjunctiva)
   C. Time of collection—time completed
   D. Specific studies ordered
   E. Clinical diagnosis; suspected microorganisms
   F. Patient's history
   G. Patient's immune state

CHART 7-1 ▌
Reportable Diseases, Conditions and Outbreaks—
State of Wisconsin*

CATEGORY I

The following diseases are of urgent public health importance. Report **IMMEDIATELY** by telephone to your patient's local health officer on identification of a case or suspected case. Complete and mail an Acute and Communicable Diseases Case Report within 24 hours.

Anthrax
Botulism
Botulism, infant
Chlorea
Diphtheria
Food- or water-borne
  outbreaks

Hepatitis, viral type A
Measles
Pertussis
Plague
Poliomyelitis
Rabies (human)
Rubella

Rubella (congenital
  syndrome)
Tuberculosis
Yellow fever

CATEGORY II

The following diseases must be reported to the local health officer on an Acute and Communicable Diseases Case Report or by telephone within 72 hours after the identification of a case or suspected case.

Acquired
  immunodeficiency
  syndrome (AIDS)
Amebiasis
Blastomycosis
Brucellosis
Campylobacter enteritis
Encephalitis, viral
  (specify etiology)
Giardiasis
Hepatitis, viral types
  B, C (type A is in
  Category I)
Histoplasmosis
Kawasaki syndrome
Legionnaire's disease
Leprosy
Leptospirosis
Lyme disease
Malaria
Meningitis, aseptic
  (specify ethiology)
Meningitis, bacterial
  (specify etiology)

Meningococcal disease
Mumps**
Nontuberculosis
  mycobacterial disease
  (specify etiology)
Psittacosis
Q fever
Reye's syndrome
Rheumatic fever
  (newly diagnosed)
Rocky Mountain
  spotted fever
Salmonellosis
Sexually transmitted
  Chancroid
  Chlamydia trachomatis
  Genital herpes
    infection (primary first
    clinical episode only)
  Gonorrhea
  Granuloma inguinale
  Lymphogranuloma
    venereum
  Nongonococcal cervicitis
  Nongonococcal urethritis
  Sexually transmitted
    pelvic inflammatory disease
  Syphilis
  Shigellosis

Tetanus**
Toxic shock
  syndrome
Toxic substance–
  related diseases:
    Infant methe-
      moglobinemia
    Lead intoxication
      (specify Pb
      levels), metal
      poisonings,
      and organic
      chemical
      poisonings
    Pesticide poisoning
Toxoplasmosis
Tularemia
Typhoid fever
Typhus fever
Yersiniosis

(continued)

CHART 7-1 *(continued)*

Also: Suspected outbreaks of other acute or occupationally-related diseases should be reported.

CATEGORY III
Human immunodeficiency virus (HIV) infection: report within 72 hours to the State Epidemiologist.

CATEGORY IV
Report number of chickenpox cases each week, Saturday through Friday.

*Wisconsin Statute Chapter 143 and Administrative Rule Chapter HSS 145 require reporting of communicable diseases.

  H. Previous and current infections
  I. Previous or current antibiotic therapy
  J. Isolation status—state type of isolation (eg, respiratory, wound)
  K. Other requested information pertinent to testing
2. Avoid contaminating the specimen; maintain aseptic or sterile technique as required:
  A. Special supplies may be required:
    (1) For anaerobes, sterile syringe aspiration of pus or other body fluid
    (2) Carbon dioxide–containing transport medium for selected tissue specimens
  B. Sterile specimen containers
  C. Precautions to take during specimen collection include
    (1) Care to maintain clean outside container surfaces
    (2) Use of appropriately fitting covers or plugs for specimen tubes and bottles
    (3) Replacement of sterile plugs and caps that have become contaminated
    (4) Observation of standard precautions
3. Preservation of specimens: Prompt delivery to the laboratory is desirable, although many specimens may be refrigerated (not frozen) for a few hours without any adverse effects. Note the following exceptions:
  A. Urine culture samples must be *refrigerated*.
  B. CSF specimens should be transported to the laboratory as soon as possible. If this is problematic, the culture should be *incubated* (meningococci do not withstand refrigeration).
4. Transportation of specimens: Specimen material should be transported quickly to the laboratory to prevent desiccation of the specimen and death of the microorganisms.

A. For anaerobic microbe cultures, no more than 10 minutes should elapse between time of collection and culture. Anaerobic specimens should be placed into a butyl rubber-stoppered, gased-out glass tube.

B. Urine specimens should be *refrigerated* until tested.

C. Feces suspected of harboring *Salmonella* or *Shigella* organisms should be placed in a special transport medium, such as buffered glycerol–saline, if culturing of the specimen will be delayed.

5. Specimen quantity: With few exceptions, the quantity of the specimen should be as large as possible. When only a small quantity is available, swabs should be moistened with sterile saline just before collection, especially for nasopharyngeal cultures.

6. Specimen collection

A. Whenever possible, specimens should be collected before antibiotic regimens are instituted; for example, complete all blood culture sampling before starting antibiotic therapy.

B. Collection must be geared to the rise in symptoms such as fever. (The practitioner should be familiar with the clinical course of the suspected disease.)

Transport of Specimens by Mail

Several kits containing transport media are available for use when there is a significant delay between collection and culturing. Culturette swabs (Becton-Dickinson Microbiology Systems) are available for bacterial, viral, and anaerobic collection of specimens. Some laboratories provide Cary-Blair and polyvinyl alcohol (PVA) fixative transport vials for stool collection for culture and ova and parasite examination. Depending on the request, some specimens may have to be shipped in a Styrofoam box with refrigerant packs. This is especially true for specimens to be tested for viral examination. It is prudent to consult the reference laboratory to which specimens will be sent for information on proper collection and shipment.

According to the Code of Federal Regulations, a viable organism or its toxin or a diagnostic specimen (volume <50 ml) must be placed in a secure, closed, watertight container that is then enclosed in a second secure, watertight container. Biohazard labels should be placed on the outside of the container.

Specimens that are to be transported within an institution should be placed in a sealed biohazard bag. Ideally, the requisition should accompany the specimen but not be sealed inside the bag.

DIAGNOSIS OF BACTERIAL DISEASE ●

Bacteriologic studies try to trace the specific organism causing an infection (Table 7-2). This organism may be specific to one disease, such as *Mycobacterium tuberculosis* for tuberculosis (TB), or it may cause a variety of infections, such as those associated with *Staphylococcus* species. Antibiotic sensitivity studies then determine the responses of the specific organism to various classes and types of antibiotics. An antibiotic that inhibits bacterial growth is the logical choice for treating the infection.

TABLE 7-2
Bacterial Diseases and Their Laboratory Diagnosis

Disease	Causative Organism	Source of Specimen	Diagnostic Tests
Anthrax	*Bacillus anthracis*	Blood, sputum, sore	Blood, sputum, skin smear and culture; specific serologic test; biopsy, ELISA technique
Brucellosis (undulant fever)	*Brucella melitensis, Brucella abortus, Brucella suis*	Blood, bone marrow, CSF, tissue, lymph node, urine	Culture, specific serologic test, ELISA technique
Bubonic plague	*Yersinia pestis*	Buboes (enlarged and inflamed lymph nodes), blood, sputum	Skin, blood, and sputum smear; culture; agglutination test
Chancre	*Haemophilus ducreyi*	Genital lesion	Lesion smear and culture; biopsy; serologic test
Cholera	*Vibrio cholerae*	Feces	Stool smear and culture; skin biopsy
Psittacosis	*Chlamydia psittaci*	Blood, sputum, lung	Culture, smears, serologic tests (immunofluorescent and enzyme immunoassay)
Diphtheria	*Corynebacterium diphtheriae*	Nasopharynx	Nasopharyngeal smear and culture
Erysipeloid	*Erysipelothrix rhusiopathiae*	Lesion, blood	Culture
Gonorrhea	*Neisseria gonorrhoeae*	Vagina, urethra, CSF, blood, joint fluid, throat	Smear, culture, and fluorescent antibody test
Granuloma inguinale (donovanosis)	*Calymmatobacterium granulomatis*	Groin lesion	Smears and culture from lesion
Gastritis, gastric ulcer	*Helicobacter pylori*	Gastric tissue biopsy	Culture
Relapsing fever	*Borrelia recurrentis*	Peripheral blood	Direct examination
Lyme disease	*Borrelia burgdorferi*	Blood, CSF, skin lesion	Serologic test

508

Disease	Organism	Specimen	Test
Legionnaires' disease	*Legionella pneumophila*	Sputum	Culture, direct fluorescent antibody, serology
Leprosy (Hansen's disease)	*Mycobacterium leprae*	Skin scrapings	Skin smear, biopsy, serologic test
Lymphogranuloma venereum	*Chlamydia trachomatis*	Genital swab, conjunctiva swab	Culture and smear, immunofluorescent test
Listeriosis	*Listeria monocytogenes*	Stool, blood, CSF, amniotic fluid, placenta, vagina	Smears and culture, serologic test
Pneumonia	*Haemophilus influenzae, Klebsiella pneumoniae, Staphylococcus aureus, Streptococcus pneumoniae*	Bronchoscopy secretions, sputum, blood, lung aspirate or biopsy, pleural fluid	Smear and culture
Strep throat, scarlet fever, impetigo	*Streptococcus pyogenes*	Throat, lesion	Culture, serology
Tetanus	*Clostridium tetani*	Wound	Wound smear and culture
Toxic shock syndrome	*Staphylococcus aureus*	Tissue	Culture; latex agglutination
Tuberculosis	*Mycobacterium tuberculosis*	Sputum, gastric washings, urine, CSF	Smear and culture of sputum, gastric washings, urine, and CSF; skin test
Tularemia	*Francisella tularensis*	Skin, lymph node, ulcer tissue biopsy, sputum, bone marrow	Serologic test; ELISA technique
Typhoid	*Salmonella typhi*	Blood (after first week of infection); feces (after second week of infection)	Culture and serologic test
Whooping cough	*Bordetella pertussis*	Nasopharyngeal swab	Culture, fluorescent antibody test, serology, enzyme immunoassay
Nocardiosis	*Nocardia asteroides*	Sputum, lesion	Culture
Mycoplasma	*Mycoplasma pneumoniae*	Blood, sputum, nasopharyngeal and throat swabs	Serology, culture

Some questions that need to be asked when searching for bacteria as the cause of a disease process include the following: (1) Are bacteria responsible for this disease? (2) Is antimicrobial therapy indicated? Most bacteria-related diseases have a febrile course. From a practical standpoint during evaluation of the febrile patient, the sooner a diagnosis can be reached and the sooner a decision can be made concerning antimicrobial therapy, the less protracted the period of recovery.

Anaerobic bacterial infections are commonly associated with localized necrotic abscesses: they may yield several different strains of bacteria. Because of this, the term *polymicrobic disease* is sometimes used to refer to anaerobic bacterial diseases. This view is in sharp contrast to the "one organism—one disease" concept that characterizes other infections, such as typhoid fever, cholera, or diphtheria. Isolation and identification of the different strains of anaerobic bacteria through sensitivity studies is desirable so that appropriate therapy may be given.

STUDIES OF THE SENSITIVITY (SUSCEPTIBILITY) OF BACTERIA TO ANTIMICROBIAL AGENTS ●

A sensitivity (susceptibility) test detects the type and amount of antibiotic or chemotherapeutic agent required to inhibit bacteria growth. Often, culture and sensitivity tests are ordered together. Sensitivity studies also may be indicated when an established regimen or treatment is to be altered.

The most common and useful test for evaluating antibiotic sensitivity is the disk method. A basic set of antibiotic-impregnated disks on agar is inoculated with a culture derived from the specific bacteria being tested. After a suitable period of incubation, the degree of bacterial growth within the different antibiotic zones on the disks is determined by microscopic observation and measurement. Growth zone diameters, measured in millimeters, are compared against set standards to determine whether the organism is truly sensitive to the antibiotic or falls into the intermediate category. The drug zone showing the least amount of bacterial growth is considered to be the drug of choice for treatment.

Clinical Implications

1. The terms *sensitive* and *susceptible* imply that an infection caused by the bacterial strain tested will respond favorably in the presence of the indicated antimicrobial agent.
2. The terms *intermediate, partially resistant,* and *moderately susceptible* mean that the bacterial strain tested is not completely inhibited by therapeutic concentrations of a test drug.
3. *Indeterminant* means that the bacterial organism may be either susceptible or resistant to the antibiotic test sample. Usually these organisms are susceptible to high blood levels of selected antibiotics.
4. The term *resistant* implies that the organism is not inhibited by the antibiotic.

5. Clinicians tend to rely more on published reports of an antibiotic's effectiveness than on the sensitivity report. Sensitivity is an *in vitro* test (in a test tube), whereas the antibiotic will be working *in vivo* (in the body).

6. Some antimicrobial agents act in a *bactericidal* manner, meaning that they kill the organism. Others act in a *bacteriostatic* manner, meaning that they inhibit growth of the organism but do not necessarily kill it. Emergence of strains of penicillin-resistant *Neisseria gonorrhoeae,* methicillin (or oxacillin)–resistant *Staphylococcus aureus,* amikacin-resistant *Pseudomonas* spp. or other gram negative rods, and vancomycin-resistant *Enterococcus* spp. present challenges to the clinician in regard to treatment. Many hospitals screen for methicillin-resistant *S. aureus* (MRSA) and vancomycin-resistant *Enterococcus* (VRE) species so as to isolate patients infected with these organisms.

Bactericidal Agents	*Bacteriostatic Agents*
Aminoglycoside	Chloramphenicol
Cephalosporins	Erythromycin
Metronidazole	Sulfonamides
Penicillins	Tetracycline
Quinolones	
Rifampin	
Vancomycin	

DIAGNOSIS OF MYCOBACTERIAL INFECTIONS ●

The genus *Mycobacterium* contains several species of bacteria that are pathogenic to humans (Table 7-3). For example, *M. tuberculosis* is spread from person to person through inhalation of airborne respiratory secretions containing mycobacteria expelled during coughing, sneezing, or talking. In patients with the acquired immunodeficiency syndrome (AIDS), *Mycobacterium avium-intracellulare* (MAI complex) is acquired via the gastrointestinal tract, often through ingestion of contaminated water or food.

The disease progression of mycobacteriosis, particularly in patients with AIDS, is rapid (a few weeks). This short time span has led to new methods for rapid recovery and identification of mycobacteria so that antibiotic therapy can be instituted promptly. These newer techniques involve the use of certain radiometric instruments that shorten the growth period for mycobacteria to 1 to 2 weeks. Isotopic nucleic acid probes are available for culture identification of *M. tuberculosis,* MAI complex, *Mycobacterium kansasii,* and *Mycobacterium gordonae.* Polymerase chain reaction (PCR) techniques, which use DNA technology to directly detect mycobacteria in clinical specimens, is also available to clinical laboratories.

A disturbing problem that has arisen since the resurgence of TB among persons with AIDS is the appearance of multiple drug–resistant *M. tuberculosis* strains. The Bactec System is a rapid radiometric detection method that enables

TABLE 7-3
Mycobacterial Infections and Their Laboratory Diagnosis

Causative Organism	Source of Specimen	Diagnostic Test
Mycobacterium tuberculosis	Sputum, urine, CSF, tissue, bone marrow	Culture and smear; skin test; DNA probe
Mycobacterium avium-intracellulare	Sputum, stool, CSF, tissue, blood, semen, lymph nodes	Culture and smear; DNA probe
Mycobacterium kansasii	Skin, joint, lymph nodes, sputum, tissue	Culture and smear
Mycobacterium leprae	CSF, skin, bone marrow, lymph nodes	Histopathologic examination of lesion
Mycobacterium marinum	Joint lesion	Culture and smear
Mycobacterium xenopi	Sputum	Culture and smear
Mycobacterium fortuitum	Surgical wound, bone, joint, tissue, sputum	Culture and smear
Mycobacterium chelonei	Surgical wound, sputum, tissue	Culture and smear

mycobacteria to grow in 1 to 2 weeks, compared with the 3 to 4 weeks required with conventional methods. A rapid test (NAP) is available to presumptively identify *M. tuberculosis* and also can perform a mycobacterial susceptibility test. This system, in conjunction with DNA probe technology for mycobacteria, can provide more rapid presumptive identification and susceptibility results.

Collection of Specimens

1. Sputum and bronchial aspirates and lavages produce the best samples for diagnosis of pulmonary infection. Purulent sputum (5 to 10 ml) from the first productive cough of the morning should be expectorated into a sterile container. If the specimen is not processed immediately, it should be refrigerated. Pooled specimens collected over several hours are not acceptable. For best results, 3 to 5 specimens should be collected over several days. A prerequisite of good specimen collection is the use of sterile, sturdy, leakproof containers placed into biohazard bags.

2. If the patient is unable to produce sputum, an early-morning gastric sample may be aspirated and cultured. This specimen must be hand-delivered to the laboratory to be processed or neutralized immediately.

3. Patients with suspected renal disease should provide early-morning urine specimens collected for 3 to 5 days in a row. Pooled 24-hour urine collections are not recommended. Unless processed immediately, the specimen should be refrigerated.

4. If TB meningitis is suspected, at least 10 ml of CSF should be obtained.
5. Sterile body fluids, tissue biopsies, and aspirated material from skin lesions are acceptable specimens for mycobacterial cultures. The least desirable specimen is one obtained on a swab. Tissue should be placed in a neutral transport medium to avoid desiccation.
6. Feces are commonly the first specimen to be positive for MAI complex. An acid-fast stain is usually performed on the direct smear. Culture is performed only if the smear tests positive.
7. MAI complex organisms are isolated from the blood of immunosuppressed patients. The Bactec System provides a special blood culture bottle for blood and bone marrow samples obtained for radiometric growth of mycobacteria. Septi-Chek (Becton-Dickinson) is a biphasic blood culture system for mycobacteria. Blood can also be drawn in Isolator tubes and held for prolonged periods without loss of MAI complex; this allows drawing of the specimen distant from the laboratory.

DIAGNOSIS OF RICKETTSIAL DISEASE ●

Rickettsiae are small, gram-negative coccobacilli that structurally resemble bacteria but are one tenth to one half as large. Polychromatic stains (Giemsa stain) are better than simple stains or the Gram stain for demonstrating rickettsiae in cells.

Rickettsiosis is the general name given to any disease caused by rickettsiae (Table 7-4). These organisms are considered to be *obligate intracellular parasites;* that is, they cannot exist anywhere except inside the bodies of living organisms. Diseases caused by rickettsiae are transmitted by *arthropod vectors,* such as lice, fleas, ticks, or mites (Table 7-5). Rickettsial diseases are divided into the following general groups:

1. Typhus-like fevers
2. Spotted fever
3. Scrub typhus
4. Q fever
5. Other rickettsial diseases

Q fever, caused by *Coxiella burnetii,* is characterized by an acute febrile illness, severe headache, rigors, and possibly pneumonia or hepatitis. It can cause encephalitis in children and has been isolated in breast milk and in the placenta of infected mothers, making it possible for a fetus to be infected in utero. Both complement fixation and fluorescent antibody tests can detect antibodies to the organism. *C. burnetii* displays an antigenic variation during an infection. Phase I antibodies are preponderant during the chronic phase, whereas Phase II antibodies predominate during the acute phase. A diagnosis is made when the phase I titer in a convalescent serum specimen is 4 times greater than that in an acute serum specimen.

Early diagnosis of rickettsial infection is usually based on observation of clinical symptoms such as fever, rash, and exposure to ticks. Biopsy specimens of skin tissue from a patient with suspected Rocky Mountain spotted fever can

TABLE 7-4
Rickettsial Diseases and Their Laboratory Diagnosis

Disease		Geographic Distribution	Natural Cycle		Transmission to Humans	Serologic Diagnosis
Group/Type	Agent		Antropod	Mammal		
Typhus epidemic*	*Rickettsia prowazekii*	Worldwide	Body louse	Human	Infected louse feces into broken skin	Positive group- and type-specific agglutination IgG antibody
Endemic (marine)	*Rickettsia typhi*	Worldwide	Flea	Rodents	As above	Specific immunofluorescent pattern
Spotted fever, Rocky Mountain spotted fever	*Rickettsia rickettsii*	Western hemisphere	Ticks	Wild rodents, dogs	Tick bite	Immunofluorescent latex agglutination
North Asian tick-borne rickettsiosis	*Rickettsia sibirica*	Siberia, Mongolia	Ticks	Wild rodents	Tick bite	Complement fixation
Boutonneuse fever	*Rickettsia conorii*	Africa, Europe, Mideast, India	Ticks	Wild rodents	Tick bite	Positive group- and type-specific
Ehrlichiosis	*Ehrlichia canis, Ehrlichia sennetsu*		Ticks	Human		Polymerase chain reaction (PCR) amplification
Queensland tick typhus	*Rickettsia australis*	Australia	Ticks	Marsupials, wild rodents	Tick bite	Complement fixation

Disease	Organism	Geographic distribution	Blood-sucking	Reservoir	Transmission	Microimmunofluorescence
Rickettsial pox	Rickettsia akari	North America, Europe		Mouse, other rodents	Mite bite	Microimmunofluorescence
Scrub typhus	Rickettsia tsutsugamushi	Asia, Australia, Pacific Islands	Tromiculid	Wild rodents	Mite bite	Specific complement fixation positive in about 50% of patients, and indirect immunofluorescence
Q fever	Coxiella burnetii	Worldwide	Ticks	Small mammals, cattle, sheep, and goats	Inhalation of dried, infected material, milk, products of conception	Positive for complement fixation phases I and II
Trench fever	Rochalimaea quintana	Europe, Africa, North America	Body louse	Human	Infected louse feces into broken skin	Specific complement fixation reaction
Oroya fever	Bartonella bacilliformis	Peru, Ecuador, Columbia, Brazil	Sand fly	Human	Bite of sand fly	Specific complement fixation reaction

*Recurrence years after original attack of epidemic typhus.

TABLE 7-5
Modes of Transmission of the Major Rickettsial Diseases

Disease in Humans	Etiologic Agent	Chain of Transmission
Epidemic typhus	*Rickettsia prowazekii*	Human→louse→human→louse
Endemic typhus	*Rickettsia typhi*	Rat→rat flea→rat→rat flea→rat→human
Rocky Mountain spotted fever (boutonneuse fever, other spotted fevers)	*Rickettsia rickettsii*	Tick→tick→tick→tick→dog→ human→tick→human
Scrub typhus (tsutsugamushi fever)	*Rickettsia tsutsugamushi*	Mite→field mouse→mite→ field mouse→human
Rickettsial pox	*Rickettsia akari*	Mite→house mouse→mite→ house mouse→human
Q fever	*Coxiella burnetii*	Tick→small mammal→tick→ cattle→(airborne)→human

be tested with an immunofluorescent stain and diagnosed 3 to 4 days after symptoms appear.

Signs and Symptoms
1. Fever
2. Skin rashes
3. Parasitism of blood vessels
4. Prostration
5. Stupor and coma
6. Headache
7. Ringing in the ears
8. Dizziness

NOTE: *Rickettsial diseases are often characterized by an incubation period of 10 to 14 days, followed by an abrupt onset of the signs and symptoms listed, in a patient with a history of arthropod bites. Cultures of rickettsia are performed only in reference laboratories. Rickettsial infections usually are diagnosed by serologic methods, using acute and convalescent serum specimens. A 4-fold rise in serum antibody titer is preferable, but a single titer greater than 1:64 is highly suggestive of infection (see Chapter 8).*

DIAGNOSIS OF PARASITIC DISEASE ●

Many parasitic infections are asymptomatic or produce only mild symptoms. Routine blood and stool examinations uncover many unsuspected infections (Table 7-6).

Approximately 70 species of animal parasites commonly infect the human

TABLE 7-6
Parasitic Diseases and Their Laboratory Diagnosis

Disease	Causative Organism	Source of Specimen	Diagnostic Tests
Amebiasis	*Entamoeba histolytica*	Stool, liver	Stool smear, rectal biopsy, and serologic test
Ascariasis	*Ascaris lumbricoides*	Stool, sputum	Stool and sputum smear; serologic test
Cestodiasis of intestine (tapeworm disease)	*Taenia saginata, Taenia solium, Diphyllobothrium, Hymenolepsis nana, Hymenolepsis diminuta*	Stool	Stool smear and Scotch tape test
Chagas disease	*Trypanosoma cruzi*	Blood, spinal fluid	Blood and spinal fluid smear; animal inoculation
Cryptosporidiosis	*Cryptosporidium parvum*	Stool, lung, gallbladder	Stool, lung and gallbladder smear
Cysticercosis	*Taenia solium* larvae	Muscle and brain	Muscle and brain cyst biopsy
Echinococcosis	*Echinococcus granulosus*	Sputum and urine, liver, spleen	Sputum and urine smear; serologic test; Casoni skin test; liver and bone biopsy
Enterobiasis (pinworm disease)	*Enterobius vernicularis*	Stool	Scotch tape smear
Filariasis	*Wucheria bancrofti, Brugia malayi, Loa loa*	Blood	Blood smear; lymph node biopsy; serologic test
Giardiasis	*Giardia lamblia*	Stool, duodenal aspirate or biopsy	Stool smear; Enterotest, immunologic test
Hookworm disease	*Ancylostoma duodenale, Necator americanus*	Stool	Stool smear

(continued)

TABLE 7-6 *(Continued)*

Disease	Causative Organism	Source of Specimen	Diagnostic Tests
Isospora	*Isospora belli*	Stool	Stool smear
Kala-azar	*Leishmania donovani*	Liver, bone marrow, blood	Liver, bone marrow and blood smear and culture; lymph node and spleen biopsy
Malaria	*Plasmodium falciparum* *Plasmodium malariae* *Plasmodium vivax* *Plasmodium ovale*	Blood, bone marrow	Blood and bone marrow smear and serologic test
Acanthamoebiasis	*Acanthamoeba culbertsoni*	CSF, corneal biopsy or scraping	Smear and tissue culture
Naegleriosis	*Naegleria fowleri*	CSF	Smear
Sarcocystis	*Sarcocystis hominis* or *Sarcocystis suishiominis*	Stool	Smear
Blastocystis	*Blastocystis homonis*	Stool	Smear
Pneumocystosis	*Pneumocystis carinii*	Lung biopsy, broncho-alveolar lavage	Smear; serologic test
Onchocerciasis	*Onchocerca volvulus*	Skin	Skin biopsy
Paragonimiasis	*Paragonimus westermani*	Sputum; stool	Sputum and stool smear; serologic test; skin test
Scabies	*Sarcoptes scabiei*	Skin	Skin smear, serologic test, skin test
Schistosomiasis of intestine and bladder	*Schistosoma mansoni, Schistosoma japonicum, Schistosoma haematobium*	Stool, urine	Urine and stool smear; serologic test; skin test, rectal, bladder and liver biopsy

TABLE 7-6 *(Continued)*

Disease	Causative Organism	Source of Specimen	Diagnostic Tests
Strongyloidiasis	*Strongyloides stercoralis*	Stool, duodenal aspirate	Stool and gastric smear; serologic test
Toxoplasmosis	*Toxoplasma gondii*	Blood, tissue, CSF	Serologic test; skin test; tissue smear
Trichinosis	*Trichinella spiralis*	Muscle	Serologic test; skin test; muscle biopsy
Trichomoniasis	*Trichomonas vaginalis*	Vagina; bladder, urethra	Vaginal and urethral smear and culture
Trichuriasis	*Trichuris trichiura*	Stool	Stool smear
Trypanosomiasis	*Trypanosoma rhodesiense, Trypanosoma gambiense*	Blood; spinal fluid, lymph node	Blood, spinal fluid and lymph node smear; serologic test
Visceral larva migrans	*Toxocara canis, Toxocara cati*	Liver	Serologic test; skin test; liver biopsy
Trematodes	*Fasciola hepatica Clonorchis sinensis Fasciolopsis buskii*	Stool	Stool smear

body. More than half of these can be detected by examination of stool specimens because the parasites inhabit the gastrointestinal tract and its environs. Of the parasites that can be diagnosed by stool examinations, approximately one third are single-celled protozoa and two thirds are multicellular worms. Only 6 or 7 types of intestinal protozoa are clinically important, but almost all of the worm classes are potentially pathogenic.

Diagnosis for parasites begins with ova and parasite examination. Other diagnostic options include sigmoidoscopy smears, biopsies, barium radiologic studies, and serologic tests. Collection of fecal specimens for parasites should be done before administration of barium sulfate, mineral oil, bismuth, antimalarial drugs, and some antibiotics (eg, tetracycline). For ova and parasite examination, ideally, 1 specimen should be collected every other day for a total of 3 specimens. At the most, these specimens should be gathered within 10 days.

For detection of *Giardia,* other diagnostic tests such as the Entero-Test capsule (string test) and duodenal aspiration or biopsy may be necessary. The Entero-Test consists of a gelatin capsule containing a coiled length of nylon yarn. The capsule is swallowed, the gelatin dissolves, and the weighted string is carried into the duodenum. After about 4 hours, the string is withdrawn, and the accompanying mucus is examined microscopically for *Giardia*. Duodenal fluid also can be submitted by the physician to be examined for *Giardia* and *Strongyloides stercoralis*. The specimen should contain no preservatives and should be examined for organisms within 1 hour after collection.

Cryptosporidium parvum has long been recognized as an animal parasite but is also capable of infecting humans, especially physically compromised patients. Organisms have been recovered from the gallbladder, the lungs, and the stool.

Another protozoan infecting humans is *Pneumocystis carinii*. This organism causes pneumonia in the physically compromised patient, especially in the presence of HIV infection. An open-lung biopsy or a specimen from bronchoalveolar lavage are the specimens of choice. For extraintestinal diagnosis of amebiasis, tests include hepatic scans, ultrasound studies, and needle aspiration.

Collection of Specimens

1. Generally, it is not possible to accurately identify a parasite from a single specimen.
2. Most parasites found in humans are identified in blood or feces but may also be evident in urine, sputum, tissue fluids, or biopsy tissues.
3. Fecal specimens should not be contaminated with water or urine. All specimens should be labeled with the patient's name, clinician's name, identification number (if applicable), and date and time collected. Various commercial collection systems are available to allow collection of specimens at home, in a nursing institution, or in a hospital setting. Clear instructions should be communicated and given in writing to the patient to ensure proper collection.
4. When sputum is collected for ova and parasites, it should be a "deep sputum" from the lower respiratory tract. It should be collected early in the morning, before the patient eats or brushes the teeth, and immediately delivered to the laboratory.

Clinical Alert

In the diagnosis of parasitic worms, the most important factor is the number of worms harbored.

Clinical Considerations

1. General considerations
   A. *Eosinophilia* is considered a definite indicator for parasitic infection. Protozoa also may produce associated eosinophilia.
   B. Protozoa and helminths, particularly larvae, may be found in organs, tissues, and blood.
2. Specimen-related considerations
   A. *Hepatic puncture* can reveal visceral leishmaniasis. Liver biopsy may yield toxocaral larvae and schistosomal worms and eggs. Hepatic ab-

scess material taken from the peripheral area may reveal more organisms than the necrotic center.

B. *Bone marrow* may be positive for trypanosomiasis and malaria when blood samples produce negative results. Bone marrow specimens are obtained through puncture of the sternum, iliac crest, vertebral processes, trochanter, or tibia.

C. Puncture or biopsy samples from a *lymph node* may be examined for the presence of trypanosomiasis, leishmaniasis, toxoplasmosis, and filariasis.

D. *Mucous membrane* lesion or *skin samples* may be obtained through scraping, needle aspiration, or biopsy.

E. *CSF* may contain trypanosomes and *Toxoplasma* organisms.

F. *Sputum* may reveal *Paragonimus westermani* (lung fluke) eggs. Occasionally, the larvae and hookworm of *S. stercoralis* or *Ascaris lumbricoides* may be expectorated during pulmonary migration. In pulmonary *echinococcosis* (hydatid disease), hydatid cyst contents may be found in sputum.

G. Specimens taken from *cutaneous ulcers* should be aspirated below the ulcer bed rather than at the surface. A few drops of saline may be introduced by needle and syringe to aspirate the intracellular leishmanial organisms.

H. *Corneal* scrapings or biopsy specimens can be examined histologically or cultured for the presence of *Acanthamoeba*. This organism is rare but can cause keratitis among contact lens wearers.

I. Films for *blood parasites* are usually prepared when the patient is admitted. Samples should be taken at 6- to 18-hour intervals for at least 3 successive days.

DIAGNOSIS OF FUNGAL DISEASE ●

Fungal diseases, also known as *mycoses,* are believed to be more common now than in the past because of increased use of antibacterial and immunosuppressive drugs (Table 7-7). Fungi prefer the debilitated host, the person with chronic disease or impaired immunity, or a patient who has been receiving prolonged antibiotic therapy.

Of >200,000 species of fungi, approximately 200 species are generally recognized as being pathogenic for humans. Fungi live in soil enriched by decaying nitrogenous matter and are capable of maintaining a separate existence through a parasitic cycle in humans or animals. The systemic mycoses are not communicable in the usual sense of human-to-human or animal-to-animal transfer. Humans become accidental hosts through inhalation of spores or by introduction of spores into tissues through trauma. Altered susceptibility may result in fungal lesions; this frequently occurs in patients who have a debilitating disease, diabetes, or impaired immunologic responses due to steroid or antimetabolite therapy. Prolonged administration of antibiotics can result in a fungal superinfection.

TABLE 7-7
Fungal Diseases and Their Laboratory Diagnosis

Disease	Causative Organism	Source of Specimen	Diagnostic Tests
Actinomycosis	*Actinomyces israelii*	Skin, subcutaneous tissue, sputum	Culture, smear
Aspergillosis	*Aspergillus fumigatus, Aspergillus flavus, Aspergillus terreus*	Sputum, tissue, ear, corneal scraping	Culture, smear, serologic test, chest x-ray, computed tomography
Blastomycosis	*Blastomyces dermatitidis*	Skin lesion, sputum, bone, joint	Smear and culture; serologic test, skin test
Candidiasis	*Candida albicans*	Mucous membrane, sputum, blood, tissue, urine, CSF	Culture and smear
Coccidiodomycosis	*Coccidioides immitis*	Sputum, bone, skin, joint, CSF	Smear, culture, serology skin biopsy
Cryptococcosis	*Cryptococcus neoformans*	CSF, sputum, urine	Serology, culture, smear
Histoplasmosis	*Histoplasma capsulatum*	Sputum, urine, blood, bone marrow	Smear, culture
Mucormycosis	Members of order Mucorales (*Absidia, Rhizopus, Mucor*)	Nose, pharynx, stool, CSF, sputum, ear	Culture
Nocardiosis	*Nocardia asteroides, Nocardia caviae*	Sputum, spinal fluid, tissue, abscess drainage	Sputum, spinal fluid culture, smear; biopsy
Paracoccidioidomycosis	*Paracoccidioides brasiliensis*	Lung tissue, sputum, bone, CSF	Culture, serology
Pseudollescheria	*Allescheria boydii*	Lesions of skin, bone, brain, joint	Culture
Sporotrichosis	*Sporotrix schenckii*	Skin lesion, CSF, bone marrow, ear	Skin culture, biopsy; serologic test

Tinea pedis (athlete's foot)	*Epidermophyton* spp. and *Candida albicans*, *Trichophyton mentagrophytes*, *Trichophyton rubrum*	Skin	Hair, skin, nail scrapings for culture
Tinia capitis (ringworm of scalp)	*Microsporum* (any spp.) and *Trichophyton* (all except *T. concentricum*)	Skin, hair	Hair/skin scrapings for culture
Tinea barbae (ringworm of beard, barber's itch)	*Trichophyton* and *Microsporum* spp.	Skin, hair	As above
Tinea cruris (jock itch)	*Epidermophyton* spp. and *Candida albicans*	Skin	As above
Tinea corporis (ringworm of the body)	*Trichophyton rubrum*, *Trichophyton tonsurans*	Skin	Skin scrapings for culture
Tinea unguum (nail)	*Trichophyton rubrum*, *Trichophyton tonsurans*, *Trichophyton verrucosum*, *Epidermophyton* spp.	Nail	Culture

523

Fungal diseases may be classified according to the type of tissues involved:

1. *Dermatophytoses* include superficial and cutaneous mycoses, such as athlete's foot, ringworm, and "jock itch." Species of *Microsporum, Epidermophyton,* and *Trichophyton* are the causative organisms.
2. *Subcutaneous mycoses* involve the subcutaneous tissues and muscles.
3. *Systemic mycoses* involve the deep tissues and organs and are the most serious of the 3 groups.

Amphotericin B, introduced into practice in 1958, was for many years the only drug available to treat invasive fungal infections. Now ketoconazole, fluconazole, intraconazole, and lipid formulations of amphotericin B provide alternative choices when treatment of fungal disease is warranted.

Collection of Hair and Skin Specimens

1. Clean the suspected area with 70% alcohol to remove bacteria.
2. Scrape the peripheral erythematous margin of putative "ringworm" lesions with a sterile scalpel or wooden spatula and place the scrapings in a covered sterile container.
3. Clip samples of infected scalp or beard hair and place in a covered sterile container.
4. Pluck hair stubs out with tweezers, because the fungus is usually found at the base of the hair shaft. Use of a Wood's light in a darkened room helps identify the infected hairs.
5. Samples from infected nails should be procured from beneath the nail plate to obtain softened material from the nail bed. If this is not possible, collect shavings from the deeper portions of the nail and place them in a covered sterile container.

Common Diagnostic Methods for Fungal Diseases

1. Direct microscopic examination of tissue samples placed on a slide is performed to determine whether a fungus is actually present.
2. A Wood's light is used to determine presence of a fungus. A Wood's light is a lamp that uses ultraviolet rays of 3660Å. In a darkened room, infected hairs fluoresce a bright yellow-green under the Wood's light.
3. The potassium hydroxide (KOH) test to determine the presence of mycelial fragments, arthrospores, spherules, or budding yeast cells involves mixing the specimen with KOH on a glass slide, covering the slide, and exposing it to gentle heat. The slide is then microscopically examined for fungal elements.
4. Cultures are done to identify the specific type of fungus. Fungi are slow-growing and are subject to overgrowth by contaminating and more rapidly growing organisms. Fungemia (fungus in the blood) is an opportunistic infection, and often a blood culture reveals the earliest suggestion of the causative organism. Use of the DuPont Isolator System, a lysis-centrifugation system, not only shortens the time necessary for detection but also improves the rate of detection.
5. A fluorescent brightener, calcofluor white, fluoresces when exposed to ultraviolet light. This reagent stains the fungi, causing them to exhibit a fluo-

rescence that can be detected microscopically. It can be used on tissue and has the same sensitivity as KOH. Moreover, it allows for easier and faster detection of fungal elements. Calcofluor white–stained specimens can also be examined under bright-field or phase-contrast microscopy.

6. For fungal serology tests, single titers greater than 1:32 usually indicate the presence of disease. A 4-fold or greater rise in titer of samples drawn 3 weeks apart is significant. However, serologic diagnosis of *Candida* and *Aspergillus* species can be disappointing. The latex serology test for *Cryptococcus* antigen detects 95% of cryptococcal meningitis cases. Complement fixation tests for *histoplasmosis* and *coccidioidomycosis* can aid diagnosis of these diseases. The immunodiffusion test is helpful for diagnosis of *blastomycosis*.

Types of Specimens

1. Skin
2. Nails
3. Hair
4. Ulcer scrapings
5. Pus
6. CSF
7. Urine
8. Blood
9. Bone marrow
10. Stool
11. Bronchial washings
12. Tissue biopsies
13. Prostatic secretions
14. Sputum

DIAGNOSIS OF SPIROCHETAL DISEASE ●

Spirochetes appear as spiral and curved bacteria. The 4 genera of spiral and curved bacteria—*Borrelia, Treponema, Leptospira,* and *Spirillum* (Table 7-8)—include several human pathogens. Most spirochetes multiply within a living host. Pathogenic *Treponema* are transmitted from person to person through direct contact. *Borrelia* pass through an arthropod vector. *Leptospira* are usually contracted accidentally by humans through water contaminated with animal urine or a bite by an infected animal.

Clinical Considerations

BORRELIA

1. *Borrelia* appear in the blood at the onset of various forms of relapsing fever. Louse-borne relapsing fever is caused by *Borrelia recurrentis,* tick-borne relapsing fever by several other *Borrelia* species, and Lyme disease by *Borrelia burgdorferi.*
2. *Treponema (Borrelia) vincentii* is the species responsible for ulcerative gingivitis (trench mouth).

TREPONEMA

1. *Treponema pallidum* is the species responsible for venereal syphilis in humans.
2. *Treponema pallidum* subsp. *pertenue* is the causative agent of yaws.
3. *Treponema carateum* causes pinta (carate).
4. *Treponema pallidum* subsp. *endemicum* is the cause of endemic nonvenereal syphilis (bejel).

TABLE 7-8
Spirochetal Diseases and Their Laboratory Diagnosis

Disease	Causative Organism	Source of Specimen	Diagnostic Tests
Pinta	*Treponema carateum*	Skin	Skin smear, serologic test
Rat-bite fever	*Spirillum minor, Streptobacillus moniliformis*	Blood, joint fluid, abscess	Culture serology
Relapsing fever	*Borrelia recurrentis*	Blood	Blood smear
Syphilis	*Treponema pallidum*	Skin lesion	Skin smear, treponema immobilization test (TPI), and fluorescent treponemal antibody absorption (FTA-A6) test
Weil's disease (leptospiral jaundice)	*Leptospira interrogans*	Urine, blood, CSF	Culture serology
Yaws	*Treponema pertenue*	Skin	Culture, serologic test
Lyme disease	*Borrelia burgdorferi*	Skin lesion, blood, CSF	Skin, smear, and serologic test
Nonvenereal syphilis	*Treponema endemicum*	Skin, blood	Serologic test, characteristic erythema, chronicum migrans lesion

LEPTOSPIRA

1. *Leptospira* is the genus of microorganism responsible for Weil's disease (infectious jaundice), swamp fever, swineherd's disease, and canicola fever.
2. The organism is widely distributed in the infected person and appears in the blood early in the disease process.
3. After 10 to 14 days the organisms appear in considerable numbers in the urine.
4. Patients with Weil's disease show striking antibody responses; serologic testing is useful for diagnosis of this disease.

SPIRILLUM

Streptobacillus moniliformis and *Spirillum minor* are the species responsible for rat-bite fever. Although this condition occurs worldwide and is common in Japan and Asia, it is uncommon in North and South America and most European countries. Cases in the United States have been tied to bites by laboratory rats.

DIAGNOSIS OF VIRAL AND MYCOPLASMAL DISEASE ●

Viral diseases are the most common of all human infections. Once thought to be confined to the childhood years, viral infections in adults have increasingly been recognized and implicated as the cause for many cases of morbidity and death. Viruses can be responsible for such infectious diseases as hepatitis, AIDS, and other sexually transmitted diseases (STDs); they are being considered as possible etiologic agents in cancer. They also affect immunosuppressed patients and the elderly (Chart 7-2).

Viruses are submicroscopic, filterable, infectious organisms that exist as intracellular parasites. They are divided into 2 groups according to the type of nucleic acid they contain: RNA or DNA. The *mycoplasmas* are scotobacteria without cell walls that are surrounded by a single triple-layered membrane; they are also known as *pleuropneumonia-like* organisms (PPLO).

Viruses and mycoplasmas are infectious agents small enough to pass through bacteria-retaining filters. Although small size is the only property they have in common, viruses and mycoplasmas cause illnesses that are often indistinguishable from each other in terms of clinical signs and symptoms; in addition, both frequently occur together as a double infection. Therefore, the serologic (antigen-antibody) procedures commonly used for diagnosing viral disease are also used for diagnosing mycoplasmal infections (Table 7-9).

Physiologically, mycoplasmal diseases are considered to be intermediate between those caused by bacteria and those caused by rickettsiae. One species, *Mycoplasma pneumoniae,* is recognized as the causative agent of primary atypical pneumonia and bronchitis. Other species are suspected as possible causal agents for urethritis, infertility, early-term spontaneous abortion, rheumatoid arthritis, myringitis, and erythema multiforme.

Approach to Diagnosis

1. Isolation of the virus in tissue culture remains the gold standard for detection of many common viruses. Diagnostic modalities include the following:
   A. Tissue culture
   B. Use of special culture media
   C. Typing, as for herpes simplex
   D. Use of identification reagents, immunofluorescence and immunoperoxidase, latex agglutination, or enzyme-linked immunosorbent assay (ELISA)
   E. Visualization through an electron microscope
   F. Direct nucleic acid probe and PCR-DNA technology
2. Serologic studies for antigen-antibody detection are valuable in regard to viral disease. Epstein-Barr virus (EBV) and human hepatitis viruses are routinely serodiagnosed. Classically, a 4-fold rise in antibody titer is used to identify a particular infectious agent, provided that the pathogenesis of the agent agrees with the symptoms of the infected patient. An acute-phase serum is collected within the first several days after symptom onset. A convalescent-phase serum is collected 2 to 4 weeks later. A 4-fold difference in antibody titer between the 2 sera is statistically significant.

CHART 7–2. ▶
Viral Infections in Infants, Children, and Adults

DISEASE OR SYNDROME	SUSPECTED VIRAL AGENTS
Infants and children	
Upper respiratory tract infection	Rhinovirus, coronavirus, parainfluenza, adenovirus, respiratory syncytial virus, influenza
Pharyngitis	Adenovirus, coxsackie A, herpes simplex, Epstein-Barr, rhinovirus, parainfluenza, influenza
Croup	Parainfluenza, respiratory syncytial
Bronchitis	Parainfluenza, respiratory syncytial
Bronchiolitis	Respiratory syncytial, parainfluenza
Pneumonia	Respiratory syncytial, adenovirus, influenza, parainfluenza
Gastroenteritis	Rotavirus, adenovirus 40–41, calicivirus, astrovirus
Adults	
Upper respiratory tract infection	Rhinovirus, coronavirus, adenovirus, influenza, parainfluenza
Pneumonia	Coxsackie B
Gastroenteritis	Norwalk-like virus
All persons	
Parotitis	Mumps, parainfluenza
Myocarditis/pericarditis	Coxsackie and echoviruses
Keratitis/conjunctivitis	Herpes simplex, varicella-zoster, adenovirus
Pleurodynia	Coxsackie B
Herpangina	Coxsackie A
Febrile illness with rash	Echo and coxsackie viruses
Infectious mononucleosis	Epstein-Barr, cytomegalovirus
Meningitis	Echo and coxsackie viruses, lymphocytic choriomeningitis, herpes simplex virus 2
Encephalitis	Herpes simplex, togaviruses, bunyaviruses, flaviviruses, rabies, enteroviruses, measles, HIV, JC virus

(continued)

CHART 7-2 *(continued)*

DISEASE OR SYNDROME	SUSPECTED VIRAL AGENTS
All persons	
Hepatitis	Hepatitis A; B; C; non-A, non-B; delta agent; E
Hemorrhagic cystitis	Adenovirus
Cutaneous infection with rash	Herpes simplex, varicella-zoster, enteroviruses, Epstein-Barr, measles, rubella, parvovirus, human herpes virus 6
Hemorrhagic fever	Ebola, Marburg, Lassa, hantavirus, and other viruses
Acute respiratory failure	Hantavirus

3. Available cell cultures vary greatly in their sensitivity to different viruses. One cell type or species may be more sensitive than another for detecting the virus in low titers. For example, human embryonic kidney or monkey kidney (1 MK) can be used for adenovirus, enterovirus, herpes simplex, measles, influenza, parainfluenza, and rubella; however, human embryonic kidney (HEK) cannot be used for cytomegalovirus (CMV) or myxovirus.

4. The critical first step in successful viral diagnosis is the timely and proper collection of specimens. The choice of which specimen to collect depends on typical signs and symptoms and the suspected virus. Improper specimen choice and collection is 1 of the biggest factors in diagnostic delays.

Specimen Collection

1. Collect specimens for viruses as early as possible during the course of the illness, preferably within the first 4 days after symptom onset. If specimen collection is delayed for 7 or more days after symptoms appear, diagnosis will be compromised. Virus titers are highest in the early part of the illness, when the host has not yet mounted a robust immune response. Little neutralizing antibody is present. Detection of a virus by culture, direct detection, or serology is greatly enhanced when the virus titers are high.

2. Sampling procedure
  A. For localized infection:
    (1) Direct sampling of affected site (eg, throat swab, skin scraping)
    (2) Indirect sampling. For example, if CSF is the target sample in a central nervous system infection, the indirect approach would involve obtaining throat or rectal swabs for culture.
  B. Sampling from more than one site—for example, in disseminated disease or with nonspecific clinical findings
  C. The type of applicator used to obtain specimens may affect accurate results. Do not use wooden applicators or cotton swabs, because they are

text continues on page 535

TABLE 7-9
Viral Infections and Their Laboratory Diagnosis

Infection Type and Virus Information	Throat	Stool/Rectal Swab	CSF	Urine	Vesicle fluid/swab	Conjunctival swab/scraping	Other	Blood Serology	Additional Information
RESPIRATORY									
Adenovirus	X							Yes	
Enterovirus	X							No*	
Herpes simplex virus	X							Yes	
Influenza virus	X							Yes	
Mumps virus	X			X				Yes	
Parainfluenza virus	X							Yes	
Respiratory syncytial virus	X						Nasopharyngeal aspirate	Yes	
Rhinovirus	X						Nasal		Nasal specimen preferred
RASH									
Maculopapular									
Adenovirus	X	X						Yes	
Enterovirus	X	X						No*	
Rubella virus	X			X			Viral culture rarely done	Yes	Special culture required
Measles (rubeola)	X						Viral culture rarely done	Yes	Special culture required

530

Infection Type and Virus Information	Throat	Stool/Rectal Swab	CSF	Urine	Vesicle fluid/swab	Conjunctival swab/scraping	Other	Blood Serology	Additional Information
Vesicular									
Coxsackievirus A or echovirus	X	X			X			No*	Many strains of type A coxsackievirus do not grow in tissue culture
Herpes simplex virus					X			Yes	
Varicella-zoster virus					X			Yes	
Vaccinia and other poxviruses					X			No	
Central nervous system (aseptic meningitis, encephalitis)									
Arbovirus							Blood	Yes	
Enterovirus	X	X	X	X				No	
Herpes simplex virus			X				Brain biopsy	Yes	Recovery of HSV type 1 from CSF is rare except in neonates
Mumps virus	X		X	X				Yes	
Rabies virus							Blood	Yes	Skin biopsy of neck for fluorescent assay

(continued)

TABLE 7-9
Viral Infections and Their Laboratory Diagnosis

Infection Type and Virus Information	Throat	Stool/ Rectal Swab	CSF	Urine	Vesicle fluid/ swab	Conjunctival swab/ scraping	Other	Blood Serology	Additonal Information
CONGENITAL AND PERINATAL									
CMV	X			X			Blood (leukocytes)	Yes	
Enterovirus	X	X	X				Blood	No*	
HSV	X	X	X				Blood	Yes	
GASTROINTESTINAL									
Adenovirus		X						Yes	Parvoviruses and rotaviruses cannot be cultivated in the usual cell cultures used for diagnostic virology but can be seen with EM or detected immunologically
Parvovirus (Norwalk-like agents)								Research laboratories only	
Rotavirus								Research laboratories only	

Infection Type and Virus Information	Throat	Stool/Rectal Swab	CSF	Urine	Vesicle fluid/swab	Conjunctival swab/scraping	Other	Blood Serology	Additional Information
EYE									
Adenovirus	X					X		Yes	Other viruses that can cause infections: CMV and VZV
Enterovirus	X					X		No*	
Herpes simplex virus	X					X		Yes	
HEART									
Coxsackie virus B	X	X					Pericardial fluid	No*	Mumps, measles (rubeola) are rare causes of heart disease
Cytomegalovirus	X			X			Pericardial fluid	Yes	
Influenza A, V	X			X				Yes	
Infectious mononucleosis	X							Yes	
Cytomegalovirus	X			X			Blood (leukocytes)	Yes	
Epstein-Barr virus								Yes	
Immunodeficient patient CMV	X			X			Blood (leukocytes)	Yes	Many other viruses, such as adenovirus, and enterovirus, can cause severe disease in immunologically compromised patients

TABLE 7-9
Viral Infections and Their Laboratory Diagnosis

Infection Type and Virus Information	Throat	Stool/ Rectal Swab	CSF	Urine	Vesicle fluid/ swab	Conjunctival swab/ scraping	Other	Blood Serology	Additional Information
HEPATITIS									
CMV	X			X			Liver	Yes	
EBV								Yes	
HEPATITIS A, B, AND C							Liver biopsy	Yes	See Chapter 8
GENITAL									
HSV					X		Endocervical swab	Yes	See Chapter 8
URINARY									
Adenovirus				X				Yes	
CMV				X				Yes	

*Enterovirus serology is not routinely available but can be performed with selected antigens under special circumstances.

toxic to viruses. A self-contained transport system is recommended to ensure that the specimen remains moist.

3. When transporting specimens:
   A. Keep in mind that viral specimens are unstable and rapidly lose infectivity outside of living cells. Prompt delivery to the laboratory is essential. Samples must be refrigerated or placed on ice or cold packs while in transit.
   B. Freezing and thawing of specimens diminishes the quantity of available viable virus.
4. Accurate patient information must accompany the specimen to the laboratory. In addition to the required patient identification information, the requisition should include
   A. Pertinent information that would influence processing of the specimen (eg, patient is immunocompromised due to renal transplantation)
   B. Exact nature of the specimen
   C. Patient demographics
   D. Contact person or clinic so as to expedite the notification of positive results
5. Specimens of small volume (eg, vesicular fluid, fine-needle aspiration, biopsies) should be transported in a liquid medium. Suggested viral transport media are Hanks' balanced salt solution, 0.2 mol/L sucrose-phosphate, and bacteriologic broth (tryptic soy or veal infusion).

Often a complete microbiologic workup of a specimen (tissue, bronchoscopy) is requested along with a viral workup. Because viral transport media contain antibiotics, sterile saline is recommended. Personnel in the laboratory can then divide the specimen for workup within the microbiology subsections.

Specimens of a liquid nature (urine, CSF, sputum, body fluids) are collected in a sterile container. For patients with suspected viremia, a viral culture of the buffy coat of peripheral blood is submitted. Blood specimens are collected in evacuated tubes containing heparin or ethylene diamine tetraacetic acid (EDTA).

Clinical Considerations

1. Herpes simplex is the virus most frequently isolated and diagnosed in the laboratory.
2. Acute viral titers are the most common serologic tests requested.
3. Viral culture results are normally available within 3 to 5 days, although rapid test results (24 hours) are accurate and available for certain viruses, such as CMV.
4. Significance of viral cultures
   A. Positive viral culture results from the following sources are *diagnostically accurate:*
      (1) Autopsy specimens
      (2) Blood (leukocyte buffy coat)
      (3) Biopsy

(4) CSF
(5) Other body fluids
(6) Cervix
(7) Eye
(8) Skin lesions
(9) Fine-needle aspirates
(10) Bronchial alveolar wash brushing

B. *Probably diagnostically accurate* (diagnostic if confirmed by serology):
(1) Throat
(2) Urine
(3) Sputum
(4) Genital (cervical, penile)
(5) Nasal aspirates or washes
(6) Vesicular
(7) Skin (mouth, lip)

C. *Possibly diagnostically accurate:* stool or rectal swab

D. Viruses do not compromise normal bacterial flora in the body. However, bacterial or fungal contamination of specimens can occur.

DIAGNOSIS OF SEXUALLY TRANSMITTED DISEASE ●

STDs present a serious and increasing public health problem. They are caused by a variety of etiologic agents (Table 7-10). Some conditions, such as chlamydial and nongonococcal urethritis, have reached epidemic proportions. Although nongonococcal urethritis is a nonreportable disease in the United States, it is estimated that >2 million new cases occur each year. Manifestations of these infections range from the carrier state (asymptomatic) to diseases with obvious symptoms such as cervicitis, conjunctivitis, endometritis, epididymitis, infertility, pharyngitis, proctitis, lymphogranuloma venereum, salpingitis, trachoma, urethritis and, in the neonate, conjunctivitis and pneumonia.

The causative agent of *lymphogranuloma venereum* is *Chlamydia trachomatis.* The primary lesion associated with lymphogranuloma venereum appears as a small, painless vesicle. Other signs and symptoms include manifestations of pelvic inflammatory disease, inguinal lymphadenopathy, fever, chills, and malaise. Occasionally, a genitoanorectal syndrome with signs of a bloody, mucopurulent rectal discharge occurs within this disease. Diagnosis usually is made by isolation of the causative organism; complement fixation and macroimmunofluorescence tests also can be helpful.

Suggested Specimens

1. Urine
2. Semen
3. Urethral, vaginal, cervical, or oral swabs
4. Prostatic secretion
5. Tissue biopsy
6. Blood
7. Stool

TABLE 7-10
Sexually Transmitted Diseases and Their Laboratory Diagnoses

Disease	Causative Agents*	Diagnosis
Chancroid	*Haemophilus ducreyi*	Culture of lesion or aspirate. Differential diagnosis should include syphilis, herpes and LAV monoclonal antibody test
Gonorrhea	*Neisseria gonorrhoeae*	Gram stain of male urethra, culture of male urethra or female cervix, rectum, or pharynx. When indicated, urogenital swab tested for direct antigen
Granuloma inguinale (Donovanosis)	*Calymmatobacterium granulomatis* (formerly *Donovania granulomatis*)	Wright's Giemsa stain of lesion, tissue biopsy
Hepatitis B	Hepatitis B virus (HBV)	Serologic testing HB, AG—most infectious state of disease. HB, AG: presence and persistence of infectivity and chronicity usually appear before symptoms.
Genital herpes	Herpes simplex virus (HSV) types 1 and 2	Culture from unroofed blister, scrapings examined by fluorescent microscopy or cytologic stains; viral culture
Lymphogranuloma venereum (LGV)	*Chlamydia trachomatis* serotypes L_1, L_2 and L_3	Culture of aspirate of bubo, serologic tests of blood (immunofluorescence and enzyme immunoassay)
Molluscum contagiosum	Molluscum contagiosum virus	Clinical appearance of lesions (pearly white, painless, umbilicated papules), microscopic examination of scrapings
Chlamydia	*Chlamydia trachomatis* serotypes D–K	Cell culture, urogenital swabs for direct antigen test, or fluorescent microscopy; DNA probe technology
Candidosis (monilia)	*Candida albicans*	Culture, KOH wet mount, gram stain

(continued)

TABLE 7-10 *(Continued)*

Sexually Transmitted Diseases and Their Laboratory Diagnoses

Disease	Causative Agents*	Diagnosis
Pelvic inflammatory disease (PID)	*Neisseria gonorrhoeae, Chlamydia trachomatis*	Clinical symptoms, cervical culture, laparoscopy or culdocentesis
Pediculosis pubis	*Phthirus pubis* (pubic or crab louse)	Adult lice or nits appear on body hairs
Scabies	*Sarcoptes scabiei*	Characteristic lesions, scrapings for microscopy
Syphilis	*Treponema pallidum*	Darkfield microscopy, serology
Trichomoniasis	*Trichomonas vaginalis*	Vaginal, urethral, prostatic secretion examined microscopically in a drop of saline for motile *Trichomonas*; culture; speculum examination reveals foamy, greenish discharge and presence of bright red dots in vaginal wall and cervix
Nonspecific urethritis (nongonococcal urethritis—NGU)	*Chlamydia trachomatis* (50% of cases), *Ureaplasma urealyticum,* a human T-strain mycoplasma (*Mycoplasma hominis*), *Trichomonas vaginalis, Candida albicans,* herpes simplex virus	Failure to demonstrate *N. gonorrhoeae* in cell culture of genital specimen, tissue, urine
Nonspecific vaginitis	*Gardnerella vaginalis, Mobiluncus cortisii, Mobiluncus mulieris*	Wet mount for "clue" cells or Pap smear; fishy smell is released when specimen fluid is mixed with 10% KOH. Culture or enzyme immunoassay to rule out gonorrhea
Condylomata acuminata (venereal warts)	Human papilloma DNA virus	Typical clinical lesion; cauliflower-like, soft, pink growth around vulva, anus, labia, vagina, glans penis, urethra and perineum; rule out syphilis
Acquired immunodeficiency syndrome (AIDS)	Human immunodeficiency virus (HIV)	Serology

TABLE 7-10
Sexually Transmitted Diseases and Their Laboratory Diagnoses

Disease	Causative Agents*	Diagnosis
Gastrointestinal (giardiasis, amebiasis, shigellosis campylobacteriosis, and anorectal infections)	Enteric infections: *Giardia lamblia, entamoeba histolytica* and *Cryptosporidum* spp	Stool—polyvinyl alcohol fixative or formalin ethyl acetate sedimentation (FES). Stool stain; ova and parasite examination
	Shigella spp.	Rectal stool swab culture
	Campylobacter fetus	Rectal stool swab culture
	Strongyloids spp. (worms)	Stool (FES); ova and parasite examination
	Anorectal: *Neisseria gonorrhoeae*	Anal swab specimen, culture
	Chlamydia trachomatis	Anal swab or rectal biopsy culture
	Treponema pallidum	Darkfield microscopy plus serology, lesion swab, culture
	Herpes simplex virus	Signs and symptoms, tissue culture
	Human papilloma virus	Signs and symptoms, tissue culture

*The pathogens causing sexually transmitted diseases span the full range of medical microbiology; their only common characteristic is that they may cause genital disease or be transmitted by genital contact.

Common Diagnostic Methods

1. Viral isolation in tissue cell cultures
2. Specific serologic antibody assays and syphilis detection tests
3. Cytologic techniques, such as Papanicolaou (Pap) and Tzanck smears to demonstrate giant cells associated with herpesvirus infection
4. Gram stain and bacterial culture; saline wet prep
5. ELISA and immunoperoxidase assay to detect causative agent
6. Fluorescein or enzyme-tagged monoclonal antibodies to detect and identify etiologic agents

Clinical Considerations

1. Patients presenting with 1 STD are frequently infected with other types of sexually transmitted pathogens.
2. Asymptomatic carriers are more common than generally realized.
3. Tracing and testing of sexual partners is a very important part of diagnosis and treatment.

4. The disease may recur if the patient becomes reinfected by the nontreated sexual partner.

5. Genital tract infections caused by sexually transmitted organisms in children are often the result of sexual abuse. Cultures should always be obtained, especially for *Chlamydia,* because antigen detection methods are less sensitive in children than in adults.

6. For suspected herpetic lesions, the virus is best recovered from the base of an active lesion. The older the lesion, the less likely it is to yield viable virus. Open the vesicle with a small-gauge needle or Dacron swab. Rub the base of the lesion vigorously to recover infected cells onto the swab, and place the swab in a viral transport medium. Alternatively, a swab collection system specifically for recovery of virus may be used. If large vesicles are present, aspirate material directly by needle and syringe. A separate swab can be collected for a Tzanck preparation (histology stain).

7. For darkfield examination (eg, syphilis) cleanse the area around the lesion with sterile saline. Abrade the surface with sterile dry gauze until blood is expressed. Continue to blot until blood ceases; squeeze the area until serous fluid is expressed. Touch the material to a clean glass slide, add a coverslip, and examine the specimen immediately for motile spirochetes.

8. Infections that can be acquired by infants as they pass through an infected birth canal include herpes, CMV, gonorrhea, group B streptococcus sepsis, and chlamydial conjunctivitis. Laboratory diagnosis of these infections is by direct detection or culture of the organisms or by specific serologic IgM tests. Specific IgM tests are available for the TORCH (toxoplasma, rubella, CMV, and herpes) organisms. CMV can also be detected by urine culture for the virus. Tissue culture or direct fluorescent antibody stain can diagnose neonatal herpes. Group B streptococcus antigen can be detected in serum, CSF, and urine from neonates.

9. Complications for untreated STDs include ectopic (tubal) pregnancy, infertility, chronic pelvic pain, and poor pregnancy outcomes.

● DIAGNOSTIC PROCEDURES

Five different categories of laboratory tests are used for the diagnosis of infectious diseases: smears and stains, cultures, tissue biopsy, serologic testing, and skin testing. Cultures and skin testing are described in detail in this chapter; serologic testing is described in Chapter 8. A brief description of each of these procedures follows.

The Smear and Stain

A smear specimen for microscopic study is prepared by rolling a small quantity of the specimen material across a glass slide. If the material is also to be stained, it is generally fixed to the slide by quick passage of the slide through the flame of a Bunsen burner. Smears also can be fixed in a methanol solution. For direct examination of unstained material, phase-contrast microscopy is used.

Smears are most often observed after they have been stained. Stains are salts composed of a positive and a negative ion, 1 of which is colored. Structures present in the specimen pick up the stain and make the organism visible under the light microscope. One staining procedure, called the *negative stain,* colors the background but leaves the organisms themselves uncolored. The gross structure of the organisms can then be studied.

TYPES OF STAINS

Bacterial stains are of 2 major types: simple and differential. A *simple stain* consists of a coloring agent such as gentian violet, crystal violet, carbol-fuchsin, methylene blue, or safranine O. A thin smear of sampled organisms is stained and then observed under an oil-immersion lens. A *differential stain* is one in which 2 chemically different stains are applied to the same smear. Organisms that are physiologically different pick up different stains.

The *Gram stain* is the most important of all bacteriologic differential stains. It divides bacteria into 2 physiologic groups: gram-positive and gram-negative organisms. The staining procedure consists of 4 major steps: (1) staining the smear with gentian or crystal violet; (2) washing off the violet stain and flooding the smear with an iodine solution; (3) washing off the iodine solution and flooding the smear with 95% alcohol; and (4) counterstaining the smear with safranine O, a red dye. The Gram stain permits morphologic study of the sampled bacteria and divides all bacteria according to their ability or inability to pick up 1 or both of the stains. Gram-positive and gram-negative bacteria exhibit different properties, which helps to identify and differentiate them.

Stains other than the Gram stain are used for examining bacteriologic smears. Some, such as the *acid-fast stain,* can identify organisms of the genus *Mycobacterium.* Other stains differentiate certain structures, such as capsules, endospores, or flagella.

Cultures

Preparation of a culture involves growing microorganisms or living tissue cells on a special medium that supports the growth of a given material. Cultures may be maintained in test tubes, Petri dishes, dilution bottles, or other suitable containers. The container holds a food (call the *culture medium*) that is either solid, semisolid, or liquid. Each organism has its own special requirements for growth (proper combination of nutritive ingredients, temperature, and presence or absence of oxygen). The culture is prepared in accordance with the food needs of the organism. Later, it is either refrigerated or incubated, according to the temperature requirements for supporting growth.

Tissue Biopsy

At times, microorganisms are isolated from small quantities of body tissue that have been surgically removed. Such tissue is removed with the use of full aseptic technique and transferred to a sterile container to be rapidly transported to the laboratory for analysis. Generally, the specimens are finely ground in a sterile homogenizer and then plated out.

Serologic Testing

Infectious diseases can be diagnosed by detection of an immunologic response specific to an infecting agent in a patient's serum. Normal humans produce both IgM (first-response antibodies) and IgG (antibodies that may persist long after an infection) to most pathogens. For most pathogens, a 4-fold increase in the patient's antibody titer is considered to be diagnostic of current infection. If the infecting agent is rare or previous exposure is unlikely (eg, rabies virus, botulin), the presence of specific antibody in a single serum specimen can be diagnostic. Methods for detecting the presence of antibodies include counterimmunoelectrophoresis, immunodiffusion assay, complement fixation, ELISA, indirect fluorescent antibody, radioimmunoassay, and Western blot immunoassay (see Chapter 8).

Skin Testing

Skin testing determines hypersensitivity to the toxic products formed in the body by pathogens. In general, three types of skin tests are performed: scratch tests, patch tests, and intradermal tests.

BLOOD CULTURES ●

Normal Values

Negative for pathogens

Explanation of Test

Blood for culture is probably the single most important specimen submitted to the microbiologic laboratory for examination. Blood cultures are collected whenever there is reason to suspect bacteremia or septicemia. Although mild transitory bacteremia is a frequent finding in many infectious diseases, a persistent, continuous, or recurrent bacteremia indicates a more serious condition that may require immediate treatment. The expeditious detection and identification of pathogens (bacteria, fungi, viruses, and parasites) in the blood may aid in making a clinical and etiologic diagnosis.

Indications for Blood Culture

1. Bacteremia
2. Septicemia
3. Unexplained postoperative shock
4. Postoperative shock after genitourinary tract manipulation or surgery
5. Unexplained fever of several days' duration
6. Chills and fever in patients with
   A. Infected burns
   B. Urinary tract infection
   C. Rapidly progressing tissue infection
   D. Postoperative wound sepsis
   E. Indwelling venous or arterial catheter
7. Debilitated patients receiving
   A. Antibiotics
   B. Corticosteroids

C. Immunosuppressives

D. Antimetabolites

E. Parenteral hyperalimentation

NOTE:

1. During an acute febrile illness, immediately draw 2 separate blood samples from opposite arms and promptly begin antibiotic therapy.

2. For fever of unknown origin, 2 blood cultures can initially be drawn 45 to 60 minutes apart. If necessary, 2 more sets of samples can be drawn 24 to 48 hours later.

3. In cases of acute endocarditis, 3 separate samples should be drawn during the first 1 to 2 hours of evaluation. Then therapy should begin. In cases of suspected endocarditis, obtain 3 samples, at least 30 minutes apart, on the first day. If results are negative, 2 more sets of samples may be obtained on subsequent days.

4. Parasites in the blood (Plasmodium, Trypanosoma, and Babesia) are usually detected by direct microscopic observation. Viruses that circulate in the blood include EBV, CMV, HIV, and other human retroviruses.

5. For infants and small children, only 1 to 5 ml of blood can safely be drawn for culture. Quantities < 1 ml may be insufficient to detect bacterial organisms.

Procedure for Obtaining Blood Culture

During venipuncture, because of the high potential for infecting the patient, aseptic technique must be used. Key points are listed as follows:

1. Observe standard precautions. The proposed puncture site should be scrubbed with an antiseptic agent such as povidone-iodine or 70% alcohol. Allow to dry for 1 to 2 minutes.

2. The rubber stoppers of culture bottles should be cleansed with iodine and allowed to air dry. They should then be cleansed with 70% alcohol.

3. Venipuncture should be performed with a sterile syringe and needle; avoid contamination of the cleansed puncture site.

4. Approximately 10 to 20 ml of blood should be withdrawn into a 20-ml syringe or directly into the culture tubes. Because of the danger of accidental needle sticks, the practice of changing needles to transfer the specimen into blood culture bottles has been replaced by direct injection with the original phlebotomy needle.

5. If 2 culture bottles are to be inoculated (1 anaerobic and 1 aerobic), the anaerobic bottle should be inoculated before the aerobic bottle.

6. Both bottles should be mixed gently to vent the aerobic bottle; use a cotton-plugged needle specially designed for that purpose.

7. Properly label the specimens and immediately transfer them to the laboratory.

8. After the venipuncture, the site should be cleansed with alcohol, because some patients are sensitive to iodine.

> ### Clinical Alert
>
> 1. Handle all blood specimens according to universal precautions.
> 2. After disinfection, *do not* palpate the venipuncture site unless sterile gloves are worn. Palpation is the greatest potential cause of blood culture contamination.
> 3. The attending physician should be notified immediately about positive culture results so that appropriate treatment may be started.
> 4. Specimens can be drawn from 2 or 3 different sites to exclude a skin-contaminating organism. Taking >3 blood culture samples in a 24-hour period does not produce significantly increased positive results.
> 5. It is recommended to draw blood below an intravenous line (if possible) to prevent dilution of the sample.

9. In special situations, (those patients who have already received antibacterial therapy) certain enzymes can be incorporated into the growth medium to eliminate the activity of the antibacterial agent on the blood sample.

Clinical Implications

1. *Negative* cultures

   If all cultures, subcultures, and Gram-stained smears are negative, the blood culture may be reported as "no growth, aerobic *or* anaerobic, after a 3-day incubation," followed by "Final report: No growth after 7 to 14 days of incubation."
2. *Positive* cultures: Pathogens most commonly found in blood cultures include
   A. *Bacteroides* spp.
   B. *Brucella* spp. (hold cultures for 4 weeks)
   C. Coliform bacilli
   D. *Pseudomonas aeruginosa*
   E. *Haemophilus influenzae*
   F. *Listeria monocytogenes*
   G. *Streptococcus pneumoniae*
   H. Enterococci
   I. *S. aureus, Staphylococcus epidermidis*
   J. *Streptococcus pyogenes*
   K. *Salmonella* spp.
   L. *Candida albicans*
   M. *Clostridium perfringens*

Interfering Factors

1. Blood cultures are subject to contamination, especially by skin bacteria. These skin organisms should be identified if possible.
2. Nonfilterable blood contains abnormal proteins.

Patient Preparation
Explain culture purpose and procedure. See Chapter 1 guidelines for safe, effective, informed *pretest* care.

Patient Aftercare
1. Interpret test results; monitor for bacteremia, septicemia, and other febrile illness; and counsel appropriately about treatment.
2. Follow Chapter 1 guidelines for safe, effective, informed *posttest* care.

URINE CULTURES ●

Normal Values
Negative

Explanation of Test
Urine cultures are most commonly used to diagnose bacterial urinary tract infection (kidneys, ureter, bladder, and urethra). Urine is an excellent culture and growth medium for most organisms that infect the urinary tract. The combination of pyuria (pus in the urine) and significant bacteriuria strongly suggests the presence of a urinary tract infection.

Collection of Specimens for Culture: General Principles
1. Early-morning specimens should be obtained whenever possible, because bacterial counts are highest at that time.
2. A clean-voided urine specimen of at least 3 to 5 ml should be collected into a sterile container. Catheterization and aspiration of a suprapubic or indwelling catheter are alternative methods for procuring urine specimens.
3. Urine specimens for culture must never be retrieved from a urine collection bag that is part of an indwelling catheter drainage system.

> ### Clinical Alert
> Catheterization heightens the risk of introducing a urinary tract infection. If possible, avoid collecting urine by this method. *Do not* catheterize when only a bacteriologic specimen is needed.

4. Ideally, urine should be taken to the laboratory and examined as soon as possible. When this is not possible, the urine can be refrigerated for up to 24 hours before being cultured.
5. Two successive clean-voided or midstream urine specimens should be collected to establish that true bacteriuria is present.

6. Whenever possible, specimens should be obtained before antibiotic or antimicrobial therapy begins.
7. Professional health personnel should instruct the patient concerning proper specimen collection technique. Failure to isolate a causative organism is frequently the result of faulty cleansing or collection techniques that can come from misinformation about the proper collection procedure.
8. Provide proper supplies and privacy for cleansing and urine collection. Instruct patients in proper cleansing techniques. The patient who is unable to comply with instructions should be assisted by health care personnel.
9. The urine specimen should be properly covered and labeled. Pertinent information includes
   A. Patient's identification information
   B. Physician's name
   C. Suspected clinical diagnosis
   D. Method of collection
   E. Precise time obtained
   F. Whether forced fluids or intravenous fluids have been administered
   G. Specific chemotherapeutic agents being administered

Procedure for Collection of Clean-Catch Urine Specimen or Midstream Specimen

> **Clinical Alert**
>
> 1. Urine is an excellent culture medium. At room temperature it promotes the growth of many organisms. Specimen collection should be as aseptic as possible. Samples should be transported to the laboratory and examined as soon as possible. The specimen must be refrigerated if there is a delay in examination.
> 2. In the case of suspected urinary TB, three consecutive early-morning specimens should be collected. Special care should be taken when cleaning the external genitalia to reduce the risk of contamination with commensal acid-fast *Mycoplasma Smegmatis*.

1. For women:
   A. Remove lower undergarments and clothing.
   B. Thoroughly wash and dry hands.
   C. Remove the cap from the sterile container and place it so that only the outer surface touches whatever it is placed on.
   D. Cleanse the area around the urinary meatus from front to back with an antiseptic sponge.
   E. With 1 hand, spread and keep the labia apart. Hold the sterile container in the other hand, using care not to contaminate the inside surface.
   F. Void the first 25 ml into the toilet, then catch the rest of the urine directly into the sterile container without stopping the urine stream until sufficient quantity is collected. Hold the collection cup in such a way

that it avoids contact with the legs, vulva, or clothing. Keep fingers away from the rim and inner surface of the container.

G. Recap the specimen container, taking care not to contaminate the inside surface of the cap.

H. Wash and dry hands thoroughly.

I. Health care personnel should observe universal precautions when handling specimens.

2. For men:

A. Thoroughly wash and dry hands; remove the cap from the sterile container and place it so that only the outer surface touches whatever it is placed on.

B. Completely retract the foreskin to expose the glans.

C. Cleanse the area around the meatus with antiseptic sponges.

D. Void the first 25 ml of urine directly into the toilet and then void a sufficient amount of urine into the sterile specimen container. Do not collect the last few drops of urine.

E. Recap the specimen container, taking care not to contaminate the inside surface of the cap; wash and dry hands thoroughly.

F. Health care personnel should observe universal precautions when handling specimens.

3. For infants and young children:

A. Urine may be collected in a suitable plastic collection apparatus. Because the collection bag touches skin surfaces and picks up commensal organisms, the specimen must be analyzed as soon as possible.

B. Before applying the collection bag, thoroughly cleanse and dry the urethral area.

C. Cover collection bag with a diaper or undergarment to prevent dislodging.

Clinical Implications

1. A bacterial count of ≥100,000 CFU (colony forming units)/ml indicates infection. A mixed bacterial count of <10,000 CFU/ml does not necessarily indicate infection but rather possible contamination. However, growth of a single potential pathogen >10,000 CFU/ml may be clinically significant. A pure culture of *S. aureus* or yeast is significant regardless of the colony count.

2. The following organisms, when present in the urine in sufficient titers, may be considered pathogenic:

A. *Escherichia coli*

B. Enterococci

C. *N. gonorrhoeae*

D. *Klebsiella-Enterobacter-Serratia* spp.

E. *M. tuberculosis*

F. *Proteus* spp.

G. *P. aeruginosa*

H. Staphylococci (coagulase-positive and coagulase-negative)

I. Streptococci (β-hemolytic, usually group B)

J. *Trichomonas vaginalis*

K. *C. albicans* and other yeasts

3. Urine samples obtained by straight catheterization, suprapubic aspiration, or cystoscopy or during surgery represent bladder urine. Growth of *any* isolate is considered clinically significant.

Interfering Factors
1. Patients who are receiving forced fluids may have urine that is sufficiently dilute to reduce the bacterial count to <100,000 CFU/ml.
2. Bacterial contamination comes from sources such as
  A. Perineal hair
  B. Bacteria beneath the prepuce in male patients
  C. Bacteria from vaginal secretions, from the vulva, or from the distal urethra in female patients
  D. Bacteria from the hands, skin, or clothing

Patient Preparation
1. Explain the purpose and procedure of the test.
2. The cleansing procedure must be done correctly to remove contaminating organisms from the vulva, urethral meatus, and perineal area so that any bacteria found in the urine can be assumed to have come only from the bladder and urethra.
3. See Chapter 1 guidelines for safe, effective, informed *pretest* care.

Patient Aftercare
1. Interpret test outcomes, monitor for urinary tract infection, and counsel appropriately about treatment and possible further testing.
2. Follow Chapter 1 guidelines for safe, effective, informed *posttest* care.

> **Clinical Alert**
>
> The urine culture sample should *not* be taken from a urinal or bedpan and should *not* be brought from home. The urine should be collected directly into the sterile container that will be used for culture.

EYE AND EAR CULTURES

Normal Values

Low counts of *Staphylococcus epidermidis, Lactobacillus* spp., and *Propionibacterium acnes* may be found in eye cultures.
The same is true for the flora of the external ear.

Explanation of Test
Bacterial conjunctivitis, caused by *S. pneumoniae, S. aureus,* and *S. epidermidis,* is the most common type of infectious conjunctivitis. Inflammation of the cornea usually follows some type of trauma to the ocular surface.

Acute otitis media occurs in the form of a pustule and is often caused by *S. aureus.* Swimmer's ear is related to maceration of the ear from swimming or hot, humid weather; it often is caused by *P. aeruginosa.* Otitis media often begins as a viral infection, with a bacterial infection occurring soon afterward. In children, the most common pathogens are *S. pneumoniae, H. influenzae,* and group A streptococci.

Procedure for Eye Cultures

1. Observe standard precautions. Purulent material from the lower conjunctival sac or inner canthus of the eye is collected on a sterile swab and placed in transport medium. The 2 eyes should be cultured separately.
2. In cases of keratitis, scrapings of the cornea with a heat-sterilized platinum spatula are made directly onto the medium (blood or chocolate agar, brain-heart infusion medium for fungi, or thioglycollate broth). For viral culture, the material is placed into viral transport broth.
3. Specimens should not be refrigerated or transported on ice. They should be delivered to the laboratory as soon as possible after collection.

Procedure for Ear Cultures

1. In cases of external otitis, the ear should be cleansed with a mild germicide to exclude contaminating skin flora.
2. Use a sterile swab or syringe and needle to collect middle ear fluid. Cultures from the mastoid usually are taken during surgery.
3. Specimens should not be refrigerated and should be delivered to the laboratory as soon as possible after collection.

Patient Preparation

1. Explain the purpose and procedure for the culture.
2. See Chapter 1 guidelines for safe, effective, informed *pretest* care.

Patient Aftercare

1. Interpret test outcomes, monitor site of infection, and counsel appropriately.
2. Follow Chapter 1 guidelines for safe, effective, informed *posttest* care.

● RESPIRATORY TRACT CULTURES

Normal Values

The following organisms may be present in the nasopharynx of apparently healthy persons:

1. *C. albicans*
2. Diphtheroid bacilli
3. *Haemophilus hemolyticus*
4. Staphylococci (coagulase-negative)
5. Streptococci (α-hemolytic)
6. Streptococci (nonhemolytic)
7. Micrococci
8. *Lactobacillus* spp.
9. *Veillonella* spp.

Explanation of Test
Four major types of culture may be used to diagnose infectious respiratory tract diseases: sputum, throat swabs, nasal swabs, and nasopharyngeal swabs. At times, the purposes for which certain tests are ordered overlap.

Clinical Alert

1. Twenty percent of normal adults carry *S. aureus;* 10% are carriers of group A hemolytic streptococci.
2. A rapid strep test gives results after 10 minutes instead of 24 to 48 hours. It has a false-negative rate of 5% to 10%, about the same as traditional methods. It permits rapid diagnosis and treatment.
3. Both throat and urine cultures are done to detect EBV and CMV.

SPUTUM CULTURES

Normal Values
Negative for infection

Explanation of Test
Sputum is *not* material from the postnasal region and *is not* spittle or saliva. A sputum specimen comes from deep within the bronchi. Effective coughing usually enables the patient to produce a satisfactory sputum specimen.

Indications for Collection
Sputum cultures are important for diagnosis of the following conditions:

1. Bacterial pneumonia
2. Pulmonary TB
3. Chronic bronchitis
4. Bronchiectasis
5. Suspected pulmonary mycotic infections
6. Mycoplasmal pneumonia
7. Suspected viral pneumonia

Procedure
Good sputum samples depend on thorough health care worker education and patient understanding during the collection process. Patients should be instructed to provide a deep coughed specimen into a sterile container. Expectorated material of 1 to 3 ml is sufficient for most examinations. Often an early-morning specimen is best. Specimens should not be refrigerated but should be delivered to the laboratory as soon as possible. Label speci-

mens properly and note the suspected disease on the accompanying requisition.

Patient Preparation

1. Instruct the patient that this test requires tracheobronchial sputum from deep in the lungs. Instruct the patient to take 2 or 3 deep breaths, then to take another deep breath and forcefully cough with exhalation.
2. If the cough is not productive, the patient may be assisted by respiratory therapy personnel to obtain an "aerosol-induced" specimen. Patients breathe aerosolized droplets of a sodium chloride–glycerin solution until a strong cough reflex is initiated. The specimen often appears watery but is in fact material directly from alveolar spaces. It should be noted on the requisition as being "aerosol-induced."
3. When pleural empyema is present, thoracentesis fluid and blood culture are excellent diagnostic specimens. Bronchial washings, bronchoalveolar lavage, and bronchial brush cultures are excellent for detecting most major pathogens of the respiratory tract.
4. See Chapter 1 guidelines for safe, effective, informed *pretest* care.

Patient Aftercare

1. Interpret test outcomes, counsel about treatment, and monitor for respiratory tract infections.
2. Follow Chapter 1 guidelines for safe, effective, informed *posttest* care.

THROAT CULTURES (SWAB OR WASHINGS)

Normal Values

Negative: no growth

Explanation of Test

1. Throat cultures are important for diagnosis of the following conditions:
   A. Streptococcal sore throat
   B. Diphtheria—obtain both throat and nasopharyngeal cultures
   C. Thrush (candidal infection)
   D. Viral infection
   E. Tonsillar infection
   F. Gonococcal pharyngitis
   G. *Bordetella pertussis*
2. Throat cultures can establish the focus of infection in
   A. Scarlet fever
   B. Rheumatic fever
   C. Acute hemorrhagic glomerulonephritis

3. Throat cultures can be used to detect the carrier state of persons harboring such organisms as
   A. β-Hemolytic streptococcus
   B. *Neisseria meningitidis*
   C. *Corynebacterium diphtheriae*
   D. *S. aureus*

Clinical Implications
Positive findings are associated with infection in the presence of

1. Group A β-hemolytic streptococci
2. *N. gonorrhoeae*
3. *C. diphtheriae*
4. *B. pertussis*
5. Adenovirus and herpesvirus
6. *Mycoplasma* and *Chlamydia*

Procedure
1. For adult patients:
   A. Place the patient's mouth in good visual light.
   B. Use a sterile throat culture kit with a polyester-tipped applicator or swab and a sterile container or tube of culture medium.
   C. Depress the patient's tongue with a tongue blade and visualize the throat as well as possible. Rotate the swab firmly and gently over the back of the throat, around both tonsils or fossae, and on areas of inflammation, exudation, or ulceration.
      (1) Avoid touching the tongue or lips with the swab.
      (2) Because most patients gag or cough, the collector should wear a face mask for protection.
   D. Place the swab into the designated receptacle so that it comes in contact with the culture medium. Immediately send the specimen to the laboratory.
   E. A throat culture can be refrigerated if examination is delayed.
2. For pediatric patients:
   A. Seat the patient in the adult's lap.
   B. Have the adult encircle the child's arms and chest to prevent the child from moving.
   C. The collector should place 1 hand on the child's forehead to stabilize the head and to prevent movement.
   D. Proceed with the technique used for collection of the throat and nose culture as described for adults.
3. For throat washings:
   A. The patient should gargle with 5 to 10 ml of sterile saline solution and should then expectorate it into a sterile cup.
   B. This method provides more specimen than a throat swab and is more definitive for viral isolation.

Patient Preparation

1. Explain purpose and procedure to patient or parents.
2. See Chapter 1 guidelines for safe, effective, informed *pretest* care.

Patient Aftercare

1. Interpret test outcomes, monitor for throat infection, and counsel appropriately.
2. Follow Chapter 1 guidelines for safe, effective, informed *posttest* care.

NASAL AND NASOPHARYNGEAL CULTURES (SWAB) ●

Indications for Collection

1. Patients with acute leukemia
2. Transplant recipients
3. Patients receiving intermittent dialysis
4. Tracing and tracking epidemics

Procedure

Swab both external nares and the deeper, more moist recesses of the nose. Both nose and throat specimens are preferred for diagnosis of paramyxoviruses. Refer to pediatric procedures on page 552. Nasopharyngeal swabs are better suited for recovery of respiratory syncytial virus, parainfluenza virus, *B. pertussis,* and viruses causing rhinitis. Specimens should be transported in a protein fluid and refrigerated if not cultured within a few hours.

● OTHER CULTURES AND SMEARS

WOUND AND ABSCESS CULTURES ●

Normal Values

Clinical specimens taken from wounds can harbor any of the following microorganisms. Pathogenicity depends on the quantity of organisms present. Quantitative or semiquantitative reporting of culture results may provide information on the relative importance of the various organisms present in the lesion and also the response of the infection to antibiotic therapy.

1. *Actinomyces* spp.
2. *Bacteroides* and *Fusobacterium* spp.
3. *C. perfringens* and other species
4. *E. coli*
5. Other gram-negative enteric bacilli
6. *Mycobacterium marinum*
7. *Nocardia* spp.
8. *Pseudomonas* spp.
9. *S. aureus*
10. Coryneform JK bacillus
11. *Enterococci*
12. Streptococci (β-hemolytic)
13. *Candida* spp.

Explanation of Test

Wound infections and abscesses occur as complications of surgery, trauma, or disease that interrupts a skin surface. Material from infected wounds reveals a variety of aerobic and anaerobic microorganisms. Because anaerobic microorganisms are the preponderant microflora in humans and are consistently present in the upper respiratory, gastrointestinal, and genitourinary tracts, they are also likely to invade other parts of the body to cause severe, and sometimes fatal, infections. Blood cultures should always be drawn from patients with bullous lesions, burn infections, or significant myonecrosis.

Clinical Implications

Clinically significant pathogens are likely to be present in the following specimens:

1. Pus from deep wounds or abscesses, especially if associated with a foul odor
2. Necrotic tissue or débrided material from suspected gas gangrene infection
3. Samples from infections bordering mucous membranes
4. Postoperative wound drainage
5. Lower-extremity ulcers from diabetic patients
6. Decubitus ulcers from elderly or bedridden patients

Procedure

PROCEDURE FOR WOUND CULTURE

1. Observe standard precautions.
2. Most wounds need some form of preparation to reduce the risk of introducing extraneous organisms into the collected specimen. In the presence of moderate to heavy pus or drainage, irrigate the wound with sterile saline until all visible debris has been washed away. When culturing chronically present wounds (pressure sores), débride the wound surface of any loose necrotic, sloughed material before culturing.
3. Next, apply sterile gauze pads to absorb excess saline and to expose the culture site. Always culture highly vascular areas of granulation tissue. Wearing sterile gloves, separate margins of deep wounds with thumb and forefinger to permit insertion of the swab deep into the wound cavity. Press and rotate the swab several times over the clean wound surfaces to extract tissue fluid containing the potential pathogen. Avoid touching the swab to intact skin at the wound edges.
4. Immediately place the swab into the appropriate transport container.

PROCEDURE FOR ANAEROBIC COLLECTION OF ASPIRATED MATERIAL

1. The culture site should first be decontaminated with surgical soap and 70% ethyl or isopropyl alcohol.
2. Aspirate at least 1 ml of fluid using a sterile 3-ml syringe and a needle of appropriate gauge. Immediately transfer the aspirate to an anaerobic transport medium.

3. Aspiration cultures are commonly done for closed wounds, such as soft tissue abscesses, cellulitis, or infected skin flaps. Tissue biopsies are more often performed during surgery, when infected tissue is more easily accessible.

INFORMATION FOR THE MICROBIOLOGY LABORATORY

Properly label the specimen with the following:

1. Patient identification information
2. Physician's name
3. Date and time the specimen was collected.
4. Anatomic site or specific source of the specimen
5. Type of specimen (eg, granulation tissue, abscess fluid, postsurgical wound)
6. Examination requested
7. Patient's diagnosis
8. Current antibiotic therapy

> ### Clinical Alert
>
> A microscopic examination of pus and wound exudates can be very helpful in diagnosing a pathogenic organism. Consider the following:
> **1.** Pus from streptococcal infections is thin and serous.
> **2.** Pus from staphylococcal infections is gelatinous.
> **3.** Pus from *P. aeruginosa* infections is blue-green.
> **4.** Actinomycosis infections show "sulfur" granules.
> **5.** Bronze discoloration of the skin and fluid-filled blisters are present in gas gangrene.

Patient Preparation

1. Explain purpose and wound culture procedure.
2. See Chapter 1 guidelines for safe, effective, informed *pretest* care.

Patient Aftercare

1. Interpret test outcomes, monitor site of infection, and counsel appropriately about treatment.
2. Follow Chapter 1 guidelines for safe, effective, informed *posttest* care.

SKIN CULTURES ●

Normal Values

The following organisms may be present on the skin of a healthy person. When present in low numbers, some of these organisms may be considered normal commensals; at other times, when they multiply to excess, these same organisms may become pathogens.

1. *Clostridium* spp.	**6.** *Proteus* spp.
2. Coliform bacilli	**7.** Staphylococci
3. Diphtheroids	**8.** Streptococci
4. Enterococci	**9.** Yeasts and fungi
5. Mycobacteria	

Explanation of Test

The most common bacteria implicated in skin infections are *S. aureus* and streptococci (group A). The common abnormal skin conditions include

1. Pyoderma
   A. Staphylococcal impetigo, characterized by bullous lesions with thin, amber, varnish-like crusts
   B. Streptococcal impetigo, characterized by thick crusts
2. Erysipelas
3. Folliculitis
4. Furuncles
5. Carbuncles
6. Secondary invasion of burns, scabies, and other skin lesions
7. Dermatophytes, especially athlete's foot, scalp and body ringworm, and "jock itch"

Procedure for Obtaining Scrapings from Vesicular Lesions or Skin

1. Observe standard precautions.
2. Clean the affected site with sterile saline, wipe gently with alcohol, and allow it to air dry.
3. Aspirate a fluid sample from fresh, intact vesicles with a 25-gauge needle attached to a tuberculin syringe, and transfer the specimen to the transport medium by ejecting it from the syringe.
4. If fluid cannot be aspirated, open the vesicles and use a cotton-, rayon-, or Dacron-tipped applicator to swab the base of the lesion to collect infected cells. Place the swab directly into transport medium.
5. To make smears for stains, use a scalpel blade to scrape the base of the lesion, taking care not to macerate the cells. Spread scraped material in a thin layer on a slide.
6. Place the specimen in biohazard bag. Immediately transport the specimen to the laboratory for bacterial, fungal, or viral cultures.

▶ **Clinical Alert**

The most useful and common specimens for analysis are skin scrapings, nail scrapings, and hairs (see Diagnosis of Fungal Disease).

Clinical Implications

1. When present on the skin in significant quantities, the following organisms may be considered pathogenic and indicative of an abnormal condition:

A. *Bacteroides* spp.
B. *Clostridium* spp.
C. Coliform bacilli
D. Fungi *(Sporotrichum, Actinomyces, Nocardia, C. albicans, Trichophyton, Microsporum, Epidermophyton)*
E. *S. aureus*
F. *Streptococcus pyogenes*
G. *P. aeruginosa*
H. Varicella-zoster virus
I. Herpes simplex virus

Patient Preparation
1. Explain purpose and wound culture procedure.
2. See Chapter 1 guidelines for safe, effective, informed *pretest* care.

Patient Aftercare
1. Interpret test outcomes, monitor site of infection, and counsel appropriately about treatment.
2. Follow Chapter 1 guidelines for safe, effective, informed *posttest* care.

STOOL AND ANAL CULTURES AND SMEARS

Normal Values
1. The following organisms may be present in the stool of apparently healthy people:
  A. *C. albicans*
  B. Clostridia
  C. Enterococci
  D. *E. coli*
  E. *Proteus* spp.
  F. *P. aeruginosa*
  G. Anaerobic streptococci
  H. Staphylococci
2. Several newly recognized gastrointestinal pathogens include
  A. *Helicobacter pylori*
  B. *Aeromonas* spp.
  C. *Blastocystitis hominis*
  D. *E. coli* O157:H7
  E. Adenovirus

Explanation of Test
Stool cultures are commonly done to identify parasites, enteric disease organisms, and viruses in the intestinal tract. Of all specimens collected, feces are likely to contain the greatest number and greatest variety of organisms. For a routine stool culture, the stool is examined to detect and to rule out *Salmonella, Shigella, Campylobacter, Yersinia, E. coli* O157:H7, and pure cultures of *Staphylococcus*.

A single negative stool culture should not be considered the endpoint in testing. At least 3 stool cultures are recommended if the patient's clinical picture suggests bacterial involvement, despite previous negative cultures. Moreover, once a positive diagnosis has been made, the patient's personal contacts should also be tested to prevent a potential spread of infection.

Procedure

PROCEDURE FOR STOOL SPECIMEN COLLECTION

1. Observe standard precautions.
2. Feces should be collected into a dry container or a clean, dry bedpan. Do not mix stool with urine.
3. A freshly passed stool is best. The entire stool volume should be collected.
4. Only a small amount of stool is needed. A stool the size of a walnut is usually adequate; however, the entire passed stool should be sent for examination.
5. Diarrheal stool usually gives acceptable results.
6. Stool must not be retrieved from the toilet for specimen use.
7. Do not place toilet tissue with the specimen. It may contain bismuth, which interferes with laboratory tests.
8. Transfer stool specimens from the bedpan to the container with tongue blades.
9. Properly label the sealed specimen container and immediately send it to the laboratory.
10. If a delay of >2 hours for stool culture is anticipated (from time of collection until receipt in the laboratory), the specimen should be placed in a transport medium, such as Cary-Blair medium. Specimens processed within 2 hours of collection do not require added preservatives.

PROCEDURE FOR OBTAINING A RECTAL SWAB

1. Observe standard precautions.
2. Gently insert the swab into the rectum (to a depth of at least 3 cm) and rotate it to retrieve a visible amount of fecal material (Fig. 7-1).
3. Place the swab into the receptacle containing transport medium, such as Cary-Blair medium.
4. Properly label the specimen and send it in a biohazard bag to the laboratory as soon as possible.

Clinical Alert

Fecal specimens are far superior to rectal swab specimens. Often rectal swabs reach only the anal canal and provide material of limited diagnostic significance.

PROCEDURE FOR PERFORMING CELLOPHANE TAPE TEST

1. Observe standard precautions.
2. The tape test is indicated in cases of suspected enterobiasis (pinworms).

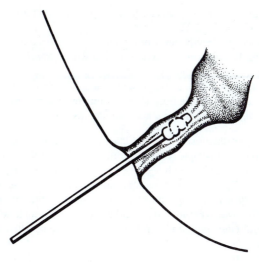

FIGURE 7-1
Method for obtaining the rectal culture

3. Apply a strip of clear cellophane tape (not micropore or adhesive type tape) to the perineal region. Remove and spread the tape on a slide for microscopic examination.

4. A paraffin-coated swab can be used in place of the cellophane tape test. If used, place the swab within a stoppered test tube.

5. It may be necessary to make 4 to 6 examinations on consecutive days before ruling out the presence of pinworms.

6. Test for pinworm eggs in the morning, before the patient has defecated or bathed. For small children, it is best to collect the specimen just before the child awakens.

7. In about one third of infected children, pinworm eggs can be obtained from beneath the fingernails. Follow instructions on the testing kit.

Clinical Implications

1. *C. albicans, S. aureus,* and *P. aeruginosa,* found in large numbers in the stool, are considered pathogenic in the setting of previous antibiotic therapy. Alterations of normal flora by antibiotics often change the "environment" so that normally harmless organisms become pathogens.

2. *Cryptosporidiosis* is a cause of severe, protracted diarrhea in immunosuppressed patients.

3. *H. pylori* has been associated with gastritis and peptic ulcer disease. *H. pylori* is found only on the mucus-secreting epithelial cells of the stomach. Detection of *H. pylori* in gastric biopsy specimens necessitates collection of the specimens in sterile containers. Smears and cultures should be examined for the presence of this organism. Initial culture incubation requires 7

days. Therefore, results of gastric biopsy specimen cultures may take 8 to 10 days to obtain.

4. *Clostridium difficile:* Whenever normal flora are reduced by antibiotic therapy or other host factors, the syndrome known as *pseudomembranous colitis* occurs. This condition is often caused by the anaerobic organism known as *C. difficile.* It may be present in small numbers in the normal person, or it may occur in the hospital environment. When normal flora are reduced, *C. difficile* can multiply and produce its toxins.

The definitive diagnosis of *C. difficile*–associated diarrhea is based on clinical criteria. Endoscopic visualization of a characteristic pseudomembrane or plaque, together with a history of antibiotic therapy, is diagnostic for *C. difficile.* Three laboratory tests are also available. These include stool culture for *C. difficile* (nonspecific; requires at least 48 hours); tissue culture for detection of cytotoxin (48 hours); and rapid tests that include enzyme immunoassay and latex agglutination, both of which are sensitive and specific for *C. difficile.*

Interfering Factors
Feces from patients receiving barium, bismuth, mineral oil, or antibiotics are not satisfactory specimens for identifying protozoa.

Patient Preparation for Stool Specimen Collection
1. Explain purpose and procedure. Instruct the patient to defecate into a clean, dry bedpan or large-mouthed container.
2. The patient should not defecate into the toilet bowl or urinate into the bedpan or collecting container, because urine has an adverse effect on protozoa.
3. Do not place toilet paper into the bedpan or collection container; it may contain bismuth, which can interfere with testing.
4. See Chapter 1 guidelines for safe, effective, informed *pretest* care.

Patient Aftercare
1. Interpret test outcomes, monitor for intestinal infection, and counsel appropriately about treatment and possible further testing.
2. Follow Chapter 1 guidelines for safe, effective, informed *posttest* care.

Clinical Alert

1. In the institutional setting, patients with diarrhea should remain in isolation until the cause for the diarrhea is determined.
2. When pathogens are found in the diarrheic stool, the patient usually remains isolated until the stool becomes formed and antibiotic therapy is completed.

CEREBROSPINAL FLUID (CSF) CULTURES AND SMEARS

Normal Values
Flora are not normally present in CSF. However, the specimen may be contaminated by normal skin flora during the process of CSF procurement.

Indications for Collection
1. Viral meningitis
2. Pyogenic meningitis
3. TB meningitis
4. Chronic meningitis

Explanation of Test
Bacteriologic examination of CSF is an essential step in the diagnosis of any case of suspected meningitis. Acute bacterial meningitis is an infection of the meninges (the membrane covering the brain and spinal cord). It is a rapidly progressive, fatal disease if left untreated or if treated inadequately. Death can occur within hours of symptom onset. Prompt identification of the causative agent is necessary for appropriate antibiotic therapy and aggressive treatment. Meningitis is caused by a variety of gram-positive and gram-negative microorganisms. Bacterial meningitis also can be secondary to infections in other areas of the body.

A smear and culture should be done on all CSF specimens obtained from persons with suspected meningitis, whether the CSF fluid appears clear (normal) or cloudy.

In bacterial meningitis (except TB meningitis), the CSF shows the following characteristics:

1. Purulence (usually)
2. Increased numbers of leukocytes
3. Preponderance of polymorphonuclear cells
4. Decreased CSF glucose concentration in relation to serum glucose
5. Elevated CSF protein concentration

In meningitis caused by the tubercle bacillus, viruses, fungi, or protozoa, the CSF shows the following characteristics:

1. Nonpurulent (usually)
2. Decreased mononuclear white cell count; increased lymphocytes
3. Normal or decreased CSF glucose concentration
4. Elevated CSF protein concentration

In those persons with suspected meningitis, the CSF fluid is generally submitted for chemical and cytologic examinations as well as culture.

Procedure
1. The specimen must be collected under sterile conditions, sealed immediately to prevent leakage or contamination, and sent to the laboratory

without delay. Three or 4 tubes of CSF should be collected. The final tube is used for cell count and differential; the others can be used for microbiologic and chemical studies.

> **Clinical Alert**
>
> In cases of suspected meningitis, a culture should be done and a diagnosis made as quickly as possible. This is important because some causative organisms cannot tolerate temperature changes.
>
> If a viral cause is suspected, a portion of the CSF fluid should be refrigerated (0°C to 4°C). Freezing is not recommended unless inoculation into tissue culture will take longer than 5 days.

2. Label the specimen properly. Alert laboratory staff so that the specimen can be examined immediately.

> **Clinical Alert**
>
> Newborns have the highest prevalence of meningitis of any age group. Organisms causing disease in the newborn (usually acquired during the birth process) include group B streptococcus, *E. coli,* and *L. monocytogenes*.

3. Notify the attending physician as soon as results are obtained so that appropriate treatment can be started in a timely fashion.

Clinical Implications

1. Pathogens found in CSF include
   - **A.** *Cryptococcus* and other fungi
   - **B.** *H. influenzae*
   - **C.** *Naegleria* or *Acanthamoeba* spp.
   - **D.** Viruses (usually enteroviruses)
   - **E.** *L. monocytogenes*
   - **F.** *M. tuberculosis*
   - **G.** *N. meningitidis*
   - **H.** Streptococcal pneumococci
   - **I.** Staphylococci
   - **J.** *Streptococcus* (group B)
   - **K.** *T. pallidum*
   - **L.** *Toxoplasma gondii*
2. Positive CSF cultures occur in
   - **A.** Meningitis
   - **B.** Trauma
   - **C.** Abscess of brain or ependyma of spine
   - **D.** Septic thrombophlebitis of venous sinuses

Maintenance of Culture

1. If the CSF specimen cannot be delivered to the laboratory immediately, the container should be stored at room temperature.
2. No more than 4 hours should elapse before laboratory analysis takes place

because of the low survival rates of the organisms causing meningitis (especially *H. influenzae* and the meningococcus).

Patient Preparation

1. Explain purpose and lumbar puncture procedure (see Chapter 4).
2. See Chapter 1 guidelines for safe, effective, informed *pretest* care.

Patient Aftercare

1. Interpret test outcomes, monitor for meningitis, and counsel appropriately (see Chapter 4).
2. Follow Chapter 1 guidelines for safe, effective, informed *posttest* care.

CERVICAL, URETHRAL, ANAL, AND OROPHARYNGEAL CULTURES AND SMEARS FOR GONORRHEA AND OTHER SEXUALLY TRANSMITTED DISEASES ●

Normal Values

Negative cultures for sexually transmitted diseases

Explanation of Test

These tests are done for patients with genital ulcers, vaginal lymphadenopathy, lesions affecting epithelial surfaces, signs and symptoms of bacterial STDs, pelvic inflammatory disease, urethritis, or abnormal discharge and itching.

Procedures for Obtaining Cultures

CERVICAL CULTURE (FEMALE PATIENTS)

The cervix is the best site from which to obtain a culture specimen (Fig. 7-2).

1. Observe standard precautions.
2. Moisten the vaginal speculum with warm water; *do not* use a lubricant. Remove cervical mucus, preferably with a cotton ball held in a ring forceps.
3. Insert a sterile, cotton-tipped swab into the endocervical canal; move the swab from side to side; allow 30 seconds for absorption of organisms by the swab.

Because *T. vaginalis* may be present in urethral or vaginal discharge, material for culture should be collected as described; however, an additional swab should be placed in a tube containing 0.5 ml of sterile saline and be delivered to the laboratory immediately.

Swabs for culture should be transported to the laboratory in Stuart's transport medium and should be held at room temperature until processed. If specimens are not processed within 12 hours, they should be refrigerated. Recovery of a pathologic organism may be more difficult because of delay in processing.

URETHRAL CULTURE (MALE PATIENTS)

1. Use a sterile swab to obtain the specimen from the anterior urethra by gently scraping the urethral mucosa (Fig. 7-3).

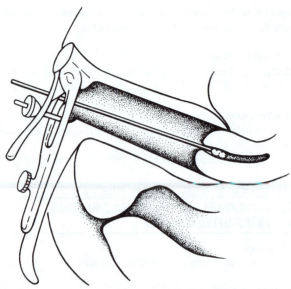

FIGURE 7-2
Method for obtaining the endocervical culture.

2. For *Chlamydia,* the swab should be rotated 360 degrees to dislodge some of the epithelial cells. *N. gonorrhoeae* organisms inhabit the exudate, whereas *C. trachomatis* organisms are intracellular (within the epithelial cells).

ANAL CANAL CULTURE
This site is most likely to be positive when a cervical culture is negative.

> ### Clinical Alert
>
> If the male urethral culture is negative but gonorrhea is still suspected, prostatic massage may produce an increased number of organisms in the urethral discharge. The first morning specimen before urination may be the best.

NOTE: *In a female patient, the anal canal specimen can be obtained after the cervical specimen without changing the patient's position and without using the anoscope. Observe universal precautions.*

1. Insert a sterile, cotton-tipped swab approximately 2.5 cm into the anal canal. (If the swab is inadvertently pushed into feces, use another swab to obtain the specimen.)
2. Move the swab from side to side in the anal canal to sample the crypts; allow several seconds for absorption of organisms by the swab.

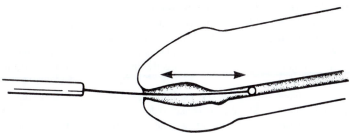

FIGURE 7–3
Method for obtaining the urethral culture.

OROPHARYNGEAL CULTURE
Culture specimens should also be obtained from the oropharynx for those persons who engage in oral sex.

Clinical Alert

The finding of repeated negative cultures for gonococci does not always exclude a diagnosis of gonorrhea.

Patient Preparation
1. Explain culture purpose and collection procedure.
2. Place the patient in the dorsal lithotomy position and appropriately drape for genital procedures. Provide as much privacy as possible.
3. Follow standard precautions.
4. See Chapter 1 guidelines for safe, effective, informed *pretest* care.

Patient Aftercare
1. Interpret test outcomes and counsel appropriately.
2. Explain need for possible follow-up testing and treatment.
3. See Chapter 1 guidelines for safe, effective, informed *posttest* care.

TISSUE, BONE, AND BODY FLUID CULTURES ●

Normal Values
Negative for pathogens

Explanation of Test
Types of fluid collected for bacterial, viral, or fungal culture include pleural, ascitic, synovial, and pericardial fluid. Tissues may have to be minced or ground to release trapped bacteria before culturing.

Procedure for Collection of Specimens

1. Body fluids should be transported to the laboratory in a sterile tube or sterile capped syringe. Ten to 20 ml of fluid is adequate for culture examination.
2. Bone is collected during surgery and sent to the laboratory in a sterile container. Fragments can be placed directly onto the agar surface or into enrichment broth.
3. Pieces of tissue usually are collected during surgery or during needle biopsy procedures. They should be collected in a sterile specimen cup. A small amount of sterile nonbacteriostatic saline may be added to keep specimen moist.

Patient Preparation

1. Explain the purpose and procedure for the culture.
2. See Chapter 1 guidelines for safe, effective, informed *pretest* care.

Patient Aftercare

1. Interpret test outcomes; monitor site of collection, and counsel appropriately.
2. Follow Chapter 1 guidelines for safe, effective, informed *posttest* care.

● SKIN TESTS

Normal Values

Positive reactions indicate lack of immunity to a specific disease (eg, TB-producing agent) or sensitivity to a specific allergen (eg, mold).

Explanation of Test

Skin testing is done for 3 major reasons: (1) to detect sensitivity to allergens such as dust and pollen, (2) to determine sensitivity to microorganisms believed to cause disease, and (3) to determine whether cell-mediated immune functions are normal. The test that detects sensitivity to allergens is mentioned only briefly in this chapter on page 567; most of this discussion focuses on skin tests used to determine sensitivity to pathogens.

INTRADERMAL TESTS

The substance being tested is injected into the layers of skin with a tuberculin syringe fitted with a short-bevel, 26- or 27-gauge needle. A positive reaction produces a red, inflamed area at the site of the injection within a given time period (eg, 72 hours for the Mantoux test for TB).

Skin tests that indicate hypersensitivity to a toxin from a disease-producing agent may also signal immunity to the disease. Positive reactions may also indicate an active or inactive phase of the disease under study. Skin tests can be categorized according to their nature and purpose as follows:

1. Tests to reveal a present or past exposure to the infectious agent; for example, tuberculin test (positive reaction = presence of active or inactive TB).
2. Tests to show sensitivity to materials toward which a person may react in

an exaggerated manner; for example, allergenic extracts such as house dust and pollen (positive reaction = sensitivity to allergen extracts).

3. Tests to detect impaired cellular immunity. Intradermal skin testing with several common antigenic microbial substances (eg, purified protein derivative [PPD] tuberculin, mumps virus, *C. albicans,* streptokinase-streptodornase) can determine whether immune function is normal. This would be important in treating leukemia and cancer with chemotherapy. (Negative reaction to any intradermal antigen = impaired immunity.)

Procedure for Skin Tests

1. Most diagnostic skin tests are prepackaged as sterile kits. Follow the manufacturer's instructions carefully.
2. Generally, 0.1 ml of the test material is injected intradermally on the volar aspect of the forearm.
3. A positive reaction is manifested by redness or swelling of >1 cm in diameter at the injection site. A central area of necrosis is a highly significant finding.

Clinical Alert

Material for diagnostic skin tests may be inadvertently injected into subcutaneous tissue rather than intradermal tissue. A subcutaneous injection yields a false-negative result.

TUBERCULIN SKIN TEST (TB TEST); TWO-STEP TB TEST ●

Normal Values
Reaction negative or not significant

Explanation of Test
The intradermal tuberculin skin test detects TB infection; it does not distinguish active TB from dormant TB. PPD tuberculin is a protein fraction of the tubercle bacilli; when it is introduced into the skin of a person with active or dormant TB infection, it causes a localized skin erythema and induration at the injection site because of accumulated small, sensitized lymphocytes.

The Mantoux test is the test of choice. The tuberculin is injected into the intradermal skin layer with a syringe and fine-gauge needle. The multiple puncture test (tine test) is used for screening purposes for asymptomatic persons, but the Mantoux test is far more accurate.

The 2-step TB skin test is done to reduce the likelihood that a "boosted" reaction will be interpreted as a recent infection. The 2-step skin test is not routine for contact case investigation.

Indications for Testing
1. Persons who exhibit signs (x-ray film abnormality) or symptoms (eg, cough, hemoptysis, weight loss) suggestive of TB.

2. Recent close contacts with persons known to have or suspected of having TB.
3. Persons who show abnormal chest radiographs compatible with past TB exposure.
5. Members of groups at high risk for *M. tuberculosis* infection, such as immigrants from Asia, Africa, and Latin America; poverty-prone and "skid row" populations; personnel and long-term residents of health care facilities and institutions (eg, nursing homes, mental institutions, prisons).
6. The 2-step test is indicated for noninfected new employees and new residents of institutions (eg, nursing homes, hospitals, homeless shelters, correctional institutions, alcohol and drug treatment centers), persons 55 years of age and older, and persons born in countries with high prevalence.

Procedure for Intradermal Skin Test (Mantoux)

1. Observe universal precautions. Draw up PPD tuberculin into a tuberculin syringe (follow manufacturer's directions carefully) with a 0.5-inch, 26- or 27-gauge needle. Use 0.1 ml (5 tuberculin units) for each test.
2. Cleanse the skin on the volar or dorsal aspect of the forearm with alcohol and allow to dry.
3. Stretch the skin taut.
4. Hold the tuberculin syringe close to the skin so that the hub of the needle touches the skin as the needle is introduced under the skin. A discrete, pale elevation of the skin (wheal) 6 to 10 mm in diameter should be produced when the prescribed amount of PPD tuberculin is injected into the intradermal skin layer.
5. For the *2-step test,* administer the Mantoux intradermal skin test, as described, for all persons for whom testing is indicated. Strictly enforce reading of results in 48 to 72 hours. If the result is positive, do not administer a second PPD dose but refer the patient for follow-up. If induration is present but does not classify as positive, retest immediately on the patient's other arm and read the results in 48 to 72 hours. If the result of the first Mantoux test is negative, retest in 1 to 2 weeks, using the same PPD dose and the same arm as for the first test. Read the results in 48 to 72 hours. If the reaction at second test is negative (no induration), perform no further testing now. Make plans to administer the 1-step Mantoux test yearly (or every 3 to 6 months if the patient is at high risk).
6. Document site of test for follow-up reading of results.

Clinical Implications

1. The test should be read at 48 to 72 hours after injection. The larger the area of the skin reaction, the more likely it is to represent TB infection. Positive tests show an indurated area of 5 to 15 mm. However, a significant reaction to the skin test does not necessarily signify the presence of TB.
2. A significant reaction does not distinguish between active and dormant TB infection; the stage of infection can be determined from the results of clinical bacteriologic sputum tests and chest roentgenograms.
3. A significant reaction in a clinically ill patient means that active TB should be considered as a cause for illness. With HIV infection, a reaction of 5 mm or more is considered positive.

4. A significant reaction in a healthy person usually signifies either healed TB or an infection caused by a different mycobacterium. Chest roentgenograms can confirm the absence of an active disease process.

Interfering Factors

False-negative results may occur even in the presence of active TB or whenever sensitized T lymphocytes are temporarily depleted in the body.

Reading the Test Results

1. The test should be read 48 to 72 hours after injection.
2. Examine the injection site in good light.
3. The patient should flex the forearm at the elbow.
4. Inspect the skin for induration (hardening or thickening).
5. Rub a finger lightly from the normal skin area to the indurated zone (if present).

Clinical Alert

1. Tuberculin test material should never be transferred from 1 container to another.
2. Intradermal skin tests should be given immediately after the tuberculin is drawn up.
3. The greatest value of tuberculin skin testing is in the negative results; a negative test result in the presence of signs and symptoms of lung disease is strong evidence against active TB in most cases.
4. A presumptive diagnosis of TB must be bacteriologically confirmed.
5. In the United States, the incidence of TB is higher among older persons, men, nonwhites, and the foreign-born.
6. Typical new case scenario: born in 1930s, infected in 1940s, developed TB in 1980s.
7. Sixteen percent of TB cases are extrapulmonary.
8. TB is acquired through close, frequent, and prolonged exposure to infected persons.
9. A person diagnosed with TB has on average 9 contacts, of whom 21% are infected.
10. Persons who have received bacille Calmette-Guérin (BCG) vaccine prophylactically or for bladder cancer treatment test positive for TB. Reactions of 5 to 10 mm may be caused by BCG vaccination. However, unless the vaccination was very recent, tuberculin reactions greater than 10 mm should not be attributed to BCG.
11. Periodic chest x-ray films are valuable adjuncts for monitoring patients who test positive, because there is no sure way of predicting who will develop active TB.

(continued)

(Clinical Alert continued)

12. BCG is a freeze-dried preparation of a live, attenuated bovine strain of mycobacteria. It is used for TB immunization in children (eg, infant with a negative TB test who lives in a household with untreated or ineffectively treated cases of TB).

13. Clinicians in contact with suspected or confirmed TB must wear a properly fitted, high-efficiency, dust- and mist-proof mask.

6. Circle the zone of induration with a pencil and measure the diameter in millimeters perpendicularly to the long axis of the forearm. Disregard erythema; it is clinically insignificant.

7. Large reactions may still be evident 7 days after the test.

Interpreting the Test Results

1. The test interpretation is based on the presence or absence of induration.

2. Negative or insignificant reaction: zone of induration smaller than 5 mm in diameter. Positive or significant reaction: zone of induration ≥10 mm in diameter.

3. For persons in good health with no risk factors, an induration of 15 to 20 mm usually is considered positive. However, because those who are at increased risk for TB (in poor health) have decreased hypersensitivity, a 5-mm induration may be considered positive. Retest within 3 weeks.

Classification of the Tuberculin Skin Test Reaction

An induration of **5 or more millimeters** is considered positive for	An induration of **10 or more millimeters** is considered positive for	An induration of **15 or more millimeters** is considered for persons who do not have any risk factors for TB
—HIV-infected persons	—foreign-born persons	
—close contacts of a person with infectious TB	—HIV-negative persons who inject drugs	
—persons who have abnormal chest radiographs	—medically underserved, low-income populations	
—persons who inject drugs and whose HIV status is unknown	—residents of long-term care facilities	
	—persons with certain medical conditions*	
	—children <4 years old without any other risk factors	
	—staff of long-term care facilities and health care facilities	

*eg, diabetes mellitus, prolonged corticosteroid therapy, immunosuppressive therapy, gastrectomy, some hematologic and reticuloendothelial diseases, end-stage renal disease, silicosis, and body weight that is 10% or more below ideal.

From Centers for Disease Control and Prevention (CDC), Tuberculosis Information, Diagnosis of TB Infection and TB Disease, August 25, 1997, Document 250102.

Potential Causes of False-Negative Results

Reactions can be categorized according to the following factors:

FACTORS RELATED TO PERSON BEING TESTED

Presence of infections
Viral (measles, mumps, chickenpox)
Live virus vaccinations (measles, mumps, polio)
Nutritional factors (severe protein depletion)
Diseases affecting lymphoid organs (Hodgkin's disease, lymphoma, chronic lymphocytic leukemia, sar coidosis)
Drugs (corticosteroids, other im munosuppressive agents)
Age (newborns, elderly patients with "waned" sensitivity)
Recent or overwhelming *M. tubercu losis* infection

FACTORS RELATED TO TUBERCULIN INJECTED

Improper storage (exposure to light, heat)
Improper dilution
Chemical denaturation
Contamination
Adsorption (partially controlled by adding Tween-80)
Outdated material

FACTORS RELATED TO METHOD OF ADMINISTRATION

Injection of too little or too much antigen
Delayed administration after drawing up dose
Injection too deep or too shallow

FACTORS RELATED TO TEST INTERPRETATION AND RECORDING OF RESULTS

Test not read within prescribed time frame
Inexperienced reader
Conscious or unconscious bias
Recording error
Measurement error

Patient Preparation

1. Explain TB skin test purpose and procedure and the necessity of returning for "reading" of the skin reaction.
2. See Chapter 1 guidelines for safe, effective, informed *pretest* care.

Patient Aftercare

1. Interpret test outcomes at the prescribed time; monitor and counsel appropriately about need for chest radiograph and sputum cultures for those with positive TB skin tests. Discuss initial and continued therapy and institute infection and case control as required. The possibility of TB disease must be ruled out before preventive therapy can start.
2. Follow Chapter 1 guidelines for safe, effective, informed *posttest* care.

MUMPS TEST

Normal Values

As described in Clinical Implications

Background

Mumps, the common disease that produces swelling and tenderness of the parotid glands, is caused by a myxovirus.

Explanation of Test

An antigen made from infected monkeys or chickens is injected intradermally. A positive mumps skin test may indicate either a previous infection or an existing infection; therefore, it is not very effective as a diagnostic tool. The test is used primarily as part of a battery of skin tests to determine immunocompetence.

Procedure

1. Observe standard precautions. Before injecting antigen, assess for allergy to eggs. Persons who are allergic to eggs are at risk for an anaphylactic reaction to mumps antigen.
2. Inject mumps antigen intradermally.

Clinical Implications

1. A positive reaction indicates resistance to the mumps virus.
2. A negative reaction indicates susceptibility to mumps virus.

Interpretation of the Test Results

1. Read the test 48 hours after the time of injection.
2. Positive reaction: erythema and a lesion >10 mm in diameter.
3. Negative reaction: no erythema and a lesion <10 mm in diameter.

Patient Preparation

1. Explain skin test purpose and procedure.
2. See Chapter 1 guidelines for safe, effective, informed *pretest* care.

Patient Aftercare

1. Interpret test outcomes regarding immunocompetence.
2. Follow Chapter 1 guidelines for safe, effective, informed *posttest* care.

CANDIDA AND TETANUS TOXOID TESTS   ●

Candida and tetanus toxoid are additional skin tests that can be done to detect delayed-type hypersensitivity. The *Candida* antigen is a mixture of trichophytin and *Oidium.* Both antigens are administered in a manner similar to the tuberculin skin test.

To interpret these skin tests for anergy, the following Centers for Disease Control and Prevention guidelines are recommended. For high-risk patients (HIV infection, intravenous drug abuse, immunocompromise), an induration area of ≥5 mm is considered positive. For patients at moderate risk (institutionalized patients, health care workers), an indurated area of ≥10 mm is significant. In patients with no significant risk factors, an indurated area of 15 mm or larger is considered positive.

These additional skin tests are helpful in evaluating a negative PPD test in an immunosuppressed person. No reaction to mumps, tetanus, or *Candida* testing may indicate a false-negative PPD test. However, an induration of >2 mm with the mumps, *Candida,* or tetanus antigen confirms the negative PPD result.

BIBLIOGRAPHY ●

Beaumont E: Technology score card: Focus on infection control. Am J Nurs 97(12): 51–54, 1997

Borton D: Isolation precautions. Nursing '97 January: 49–52, 1997

Brewer TF, et al: An effectiveness and cost analysis of presumptive treatment of *Mycobacterium tuberculosis.* Am J Infect Control 26(3): 232–238, 1998

Culter AF: Testing for *Helicobacter pylori* in clinical practice. Am J Med 20: 35–39, 1996

Friedman RB, Yancy DS: Effects of Disease on Clinical Laboratory Tests, 3rd ed. Washington, DC, American Association for Clinical Chemistry Press, 1997

Heymann SJ, Brewer TF, Ettling M: Effectiveness and cost of rapid and conventional laboratory methods for *Mycobacterium tuberculosis* screening. Public Health Rep 112: 513–523, 1997

Koneman EW, et al: Color Atlas and Textbook of Diagnostic Microbiology, 5th ed. Philadelphia, Lippincott-Raven, 1997

National Academy of Science: The Hidden Epidemic: Confronting Sexually Transmitted Diseases. Washington, DC, National Academy Press, 1997

Newland JA: Gonorrhea in women. Am J Nurs 97(8): 16AA, 1997

Sharts-Hopko NC: STDs in woman: What you need to know. Am J Nurs 97(4): 46–54, 1997

Skelskey C, Lesham A: Tuberculosis surveillance in long-term care. Am J Nurs 97(10): 16BBBB–16DDDD, 1997

Speicher CE: The Right Test: A Physician's Guide To Laboratory Medicine, 3rd ed. Philadelphia, WB Saunders, 1998

Sugar AM, Lyman CA: A Practical Guide to Medically Important Fungi and the Diseases They Cause. Philadelphia, Lippincott-Raven, 1997

US Department of Health and Human Services: Care Curriculum in Tuberculosis. Atlanta, Centers for Disease Control and Prevention, 1994

US Preventive Services Task Force: Guide to Clinical Preventive Services, 2nd ed. Baltimore, Williams & Wilkins, 1996

Wisconsin Medicine Pubic Health Update: Tuberculosis (TB). Bureau of Health Care Financing with the Bureau of Public Health, Wisconsin Department of Health and Family Services, Madison, WI, October 15, 1996

Woods ML II, McGee ZA: Sexually transmitted diseases: Highlights of the revised CDC management guidelines. Consultant 35: 1298, 1995

8

Immunodiagnostic Studies

OVERVIEW OF IMMUNODIAGNOSTIC STUDIES   ●

Immunodiagnostic or serodiagnostic testing studies antigen-antibody reactions for diagnosis of infectious disease, autoimmune disorders, immune allergies, and neoplastic disease. These modalities also test for blood groups and types, tissue and graft transplant matching, and cellular immunology. Blood serum is tested for antibodies against particular antigens, hence the term blood serology testing.

Antigens are substances that stimulate and subsequently react with the products of immune response. They may be enzymes, toxins, microorganisms (eg, bacterial, viral, parasitic, fungal), tumors, or autoimmune factors. *Antibodies* are proteins produced by the body's immune system in response to an antigen or antigens. The antigen-antibody response is the body's natural defense against invading organisms. Red blood cell groups contain almost 400 antigens. Immune reactions to these antigens result in a wide variety of clinical disorders which can be tested (eg, Coombs test).

Pathologically, *autoimmune disorders* are produced by autoantibodies—that is, antibodies against *self*. Examples include rheumatoid disease and lupus erythematosus.

Immunodeficiency diseases exhibit a lack of one or more basic components of the immune system, which includes B lymphocytes, T lymphocytes, phagocytic cells, and the complement system. These diseases are classified as primary (eg, congenital, Di George syndrome) and secondary (eg, acquired immunodeficiency syndrome [AIDS]).

Hypersensitivity reactions are documented using immediate hypersensitivity tests and are defined as abnormally increased immune responses to some allergens (eg, allergic reaction to bee stings or pollens). Delayed hypersensitivity skin tests are commonly used to evaluate cell-medicated immunity. Histocompatibility antigens (transplantation antigens) and tests for human leukocyte antigen (HLA) are important diagnostic tools to detect and prevent immune rejection in transplantation.

Types of Tests

Many methods of varying sophistication are used for immunodiagnostic studies (see the table below).

Some Tests That Determine Antigen-Antibody Reactions			
Name of Test	**Observable Reaction**	**Visible Change**	**Tests For**
1) Agglutination, hemagglutination (HA), immune hemagglutination assay (IHA)	Particulate antigen reacts with corresponding antibody; antigen may be in form of RBCs (hemagglutination, latex, or charcoal coated with antigen)	Clumping	Rubella; thyroid cold agglutin antibodies
2) Precipitation (eg, immunodiffusion [ID], counter immunoelectrophoresis [CIE])	Soluble antigen reacts with corresponding antibody by immunodiffusion (ID) or count	Precipitates	Fungal antibodies food poisoning;
3) Complement fixation (CF)	Competition between two antigen-antibody systems (test and indicator systems)	Complement activation, hemolysis	Viral antibodies
4) Immunofluorescence (eg, indirect fluorescent antibody [IFA])	Fluorescent-tagged antibody reacts with antigen-antibody complex in the presence of ultraviolet light	Visible microscopic fluorescence	Antinuclear antibodies (ANAs); antimitochondrial antibodies (AMAs)

(continued)

Some Tests That Determine Antigen-Antibody Reactions *(Continued)*

Name of Test	Observable Reaction	Visible Change	Tests For
5) Enzyme immunoassay (EIA)	Enzymes are used to label induced antigen-antibody reactions	Chromogenic fluorescent or luminescent change in substrate	Extractable nuclear antigens (ENAs); antiribonucleo-proteins (RNPs)
6) Enzyme-linked immunosorbent assay (ELISA)	Indirect EIA for quantification of an antigen or antibody enzyme and substrate	Color change indicates enzyme substrate reaction	Amyloid β-protein in Alzheimer's disease
7) Immunoblot (eg, Western blot [WB])	Electrophoresis separation of antigen subspecies	Detection of antibodies of specific mobility	Confirms HIV-1
8) Polymerase chain reaction (PCR)	Amplifies low levels of specific DNA sequences; each cycle doubles the amount of specific DNA sequence	Exponential accumulation of DNA fragment being amplified; defects in DNA appear as mutations	Slightest trace of infection can be detected; more accurate than traditional tests for chlamydia; genetic disorders
9) Rate nephelometry	Measures either antigen or antibody in solution through the scattering of a light beam; antibody reagent used to detect antigen IgA, IgG, IgM; concurrent controls are run to establish amount of background scatter in reagents and test samples	Light scatter propor-tionately increases as numbered size of immune complexes increase	Quantitative immunoglob-ulins IgA, IgG, IgM recorded in mg/dl or IU/ml.
10) Flow cytometry	Blood cells types are identified with monoclonal antibodies (mABs) specific for cell	Light scatter identifies cell size and granularity of	Lymphocyte immuno-phenocytology differentiates B cells from

(continued)

Name of Test	Observable Reaction	Visible Change	Tests For
	markers by means of a flow cytometer with an argon laser beam; as the cells pass the beam, they scatter the light; light energy is converted into electrical energy cells and stained with green (fluorescence) or orange (phycoerythrin).	lymphocytes, monocytes, and granulocytes; color fluoro-chromes tagged to monoclonal antibodies bend to specific surface antigens for simultaneous detection of lymphocyte subsets	T cells and T-helper cells from T-suppressor cells
11) Restriction fragment length polymorphism (RFLP)	DNA-based typing technique		Epidemiology of nosocomial and community-acquired infections
12) cDNA probes	Uses cDNA probes directed against ribosomal RNA	Amplifies nucleic acid to identify presence of bacterial or viral load	Infectious diseases such as TB, HCV, and HIV.

Some Tests That Determine Antigen-Antibody Reactions *(Continued)*

HCV, human cytomegalovirus; HIV, human immunodeficiency virus; TB, tuberculosis.

Collection of Serum for Immunologic Tests

Specific antibodies can be detected in serum and other body fluids (eg, synovial fluid, cerebrospinal fluid).

1. *Procure samples.* For diagnosis of infectious disease, one blood sample using red-topped tubes should be obtained at illness onset (acute phase), and the other sample should be drawn 3 to 4 weeks later (convalescent phase). In general, serologic test usefulness depends on a titer increase in the time interval between the acute and the convalescent phase. For some serologic tests, one serum sample may be adequate if the antibody presence indicates an abnormal condition or the antibody titer is unusually high. See Appendix A for standard precautions and Appendix B for latex precautions.
2. *Perform the serologic test before doing skin testing.* Skin testing often induces antibody production and could interfere with serologic test results.
3. *Label the sample properly and submit requested information.* Place specimen

in biohazard bag. Send samples to the laboratory promptly. Hemolyzed samples cannot yield accurate results. Hemoglobin in the serum sample can interfere with complement-fixing antibody values.

Interpreting Results of Immunologic Tests

The following factors affect test results:

1. History of previous infection by the same organism
2. Previous vaccination (determine time frame)
3. Anamnestic reactions caused by heterologous antigens: an *anamnestic reaction* is the appearance of antibodies in the blood after administration of an antigen to which the patient has previously developed a primary immune response
4. Cross-reactivity: antibodies produced by one species of an organism can react with an entirely different species (eg, *Tularemia* antibodies may agglutinate *Brucella* and vice versa, rickettsial infections may produce antibodies reactive with *Proteus* OX19)
5. Presence of other serious illness states (eg, lack of immunologic response in agammaglobulinemia, cancer treatment with immunosuppressant drugs)
6. Seroconversion

Serologic Versus Microbiologic Methods

Serologic testing for microbial immunology evaluates antigens of bacteria, viruses, fungi, and parasites. The best means of establishing infectious disease etiology is by isolation and confirmation of the involved pathogen. Serologic methods can assist or confirm microbiologic analysis when the patient is tested late in the disease course, antimicrobial therapy has suppressed organism growth, or culture methods cannot verify a causative agent.

Serologic Tests of Bacterial, Viral, Fungal, and Parasitic Diseases

● BACTERIAL TESTS

SYPHILIS DETECTION TESTS   ●

Normal Values

Nonreactive: negative for syphilis

Background

Syphilis is a venereal disease caused by *Treponema pallidum,* a spirochete with closely wound coils approximately 8 to 15 μm long. Untreated, the disease progresses through three stages that can extend over many years.

Explanation of Tests

Antibodies to syphilis begin to appear in the blood 4 to 6 weeks after infection (Table 8-1). Nontreponemal tests determine the presence of reagin, which is a nontreponemal autoantibody directed against cardiolipin antigens. These tests include rapid plasma reagin (RPR) and Venereal Disease Research Laboratory (VDRL). The U.S. Centers for Disease Control and Prevention (CDC) recommend these tests for syphilis screening; however, they may show negative results in some cases of late syphilis. Biologic false-positive results can also occur (Table 8-2).

Conversely, treponemal (ie, specific) tests detect antibodies to *T. pallidum*. These tests include the particle agglutination *Treponema pallidum* test (TP-PA) and the fluorescent treponemal antibody test (FTA-ABS). These tests confirm syphilis when a positive nontreponemal test result is obtained. Because these tests are more complex, they are not used for screening.

Procedure

1. Collect a 5-ml blood serum sample in a red-topped tube. Observe standard precautions. Fasting is usually not required.

Clinical Implications

1. Diagnosis of syphilis requires correlation of patient history, physical findings, and results of syphilis antibody tests. *T. pallidum* is diagnosed when *both* the screening and the confirmatory tests are reactive.

TABLE 8-1
Sensitivity of Commonly Used Serological Tests for Syphilis

Test	Stage		
	Primary (%)	Secondary (%)	Late (%)
NONTREPONEMAL (REAGIN) TESTS			
Venereal Disease Research Laboratory test (VDRL)	70	99	1*
Rapid plasma reagin card test (RPR); automated reagin test (AERT)	80	99	0
SPECIFIC TREPONEMAL TESTS			
Fluorescent treponemal antibody absorption test (FTA-ABS)	85	100	98
Treponema pallidium particle agglutination (TP-PA) (This new procedure has sensitivity similar to MHA-TP.)	65	100	95

*Treated late syphilis
Modified from Tramont EC: *Treponema pallidum*. In Mandell GL, Douglas RE, Bennett JE (eds): *Principles and Practice of Infectious Diseases*. New York, John Wiley & Sons, 1985, p. 1329.
Also product insert Serodia TP-PA, Fujirebio, Inc., Tokyo, Japan, 1997.

TABLE 8-2
Nonsyphilitic Conditions Giving Biologic False-Positive
Results (BFPs) Using VDRL and RPR Tests

Disease	Approximate Percentage BFPs
Malaria	100
Leprosy	60
Relapsing fever	30
Active immunization in children	20
Infectious mononucleosis	20
Lupus erythematosus	20
Lymphogranuloma venereum	20
Pneumonia, atypical	20
Rat-bite fever	20
Typhus fever	20
Vaccinia	20
Infectious hepatitis	10
Leptospirosis (Weil's disease)	10
Periarteritis nodosa	10
Trypanosomiasis	10
Chancroid	5
Chickenpox	5
Measles	5
Rheumatoid arthritis	5–7
Rheumatic fever	5–6
Scarlet fever	5
Subacute bacterial endocarditis	5
Pneumonia, pneumococcal	3–5
Tuberculosis, advanced pulmonary	3–5
Blood loss, repeated	? (low)
Common cold	? (low)
Pregnancy	? (low)

2. Treatment of syphilis may alter both the clinical course and the serologic pattern of the disease. Treatment related to tests that measure *reagin* (RPR and VDRL) includes the following measures:

   a. If the patient is treated at the seronegative primary stage (eg, after the appearance of the syphilitic chancre but before appearance of reaction or reagin), the VDRL remains nonreactive.

   b. If the patient is treated in the seropositive primary stage (eg, after the appearance of a reaction), the VDRL usually becomes nonreactive within 6 months of treatment.

   c. If the patient is treated during the secondary stage, the VDRL usually becomes nonreactive within 12 to 18 months.

   d. If the patient is treated ≥10 years after disease onset, the VDRL usually remains unchanged.

3. A negative serologic test may indicate one of the following circumstances:
   a. The patient does not have syphilis.
   b. The infection is too recent for antibodies to be produced. Repeat tests should be performed at 1-week, 1-month, and 3-month intervals to establish presence or absence of disease.
   c. The syphilis is in a latent or inactive phase.
   d. The patient has a faulty immunodefense mechanism.
   e. Laboratory techniques were faulty.

False-Positive and False-Negative Reactions

A positive reaction is not conclusive for syphilis. Several conditions produce biologic false-positive results for syphilis. Biologic false-positive reactions are by no means "false." They may reveal the presence of other serious diseases. It is theorized that reagin (reaction) is an antibody against tissue lipids. Lipids are presumed to be liberated from body tissue in the normal course of activity. These liberated lipids may then induce antibody formation. Nontreponemal biologic false-positive reactions can occur in the presence of drug abuse, lupus erythematosus, mononucleosis, malaria, leprosy, viral pneumonia, recently immunized persons, or on rare occasions, during pregnancy. False-negative reactions may occur early in the disease course or during inactive or later stages of disease.

Interfering Factors

1. Excess chyle in the blood interferes with test results.

> ### Clinical Alert
> Avoid drawing the blood sample immediately after a meal.

2. Alcohol decreases reaction intensity in tests that detect reagin; therefore, alcohol ingestion should be avoided for at least 24 hours before blood is drawn.

Patient Preparation

1. Explain test purpose and procedure. Assess for interfering factors. Instruct the patient to abstain from alcohol for at least 24 hours before the blood sample is drawn.
2. Follow guidelines in Chapter 1 regarding safe, effective, informed *pretest* care.

Patient Aftercare

1. Interpret test results and counsel appropriately. Explain biologic false-positive or false-negative reactions. Advise that repeat testing may be necessary.
2. Follow guidelines in Chapter 1 regarding safe, effective, informed *posttest* care.

Clinical Alert

1. Sexual partners of patients with syphilis should be evaluated for the disease.
2. After treatment, patients with early stage syphilis should be tested at 3-month intervals for 1 year to monitor for declining reactivity.

LYME DISEASE TEST

Normal Values

Indirect fluorescent antibody (IFA) titer: <1:256
Enzyme-linked immunosorbent assay (ELISA): nonreactive or negative for Lyme disease

Background

Lyme disease is transmitted by the bite of tiny deer ticks which reside on deer and other wild animals. Lyme disease is present worldwide, but certain geographic areas show higher incidences. Transmission to humans is highest during the spring, summer, and early fall months. The tick bite usually produces a characteristic rash, termed erythema chronicum migrans. If untreated, sequelae lead to serious joint, cardiac, and central nervous system (CNS) symptoms.

Explanation of Test

This test diagnoses Lyme disease, a multisystem disorder caused by the spirochete *Borrelia burgdorferi*. Tests for antibodies include IFA, ELISA, Western blot (WB; confirmatory), and polymerase chain reaction (PCR). Antibody formation takes place in the following manner: IgM is detected 3 to 4 weeks after Lyme disease onset, peaks at 6 to 8 weeks after onset, and then gradually disappears. IgG is detected 2 to 3 months after infection and may remain elevated for years.

Procedure

1. Collect a 5-ml blood serum sample in a red-topped tube. Observe standard precautions. Cerebrospinal fluid may also be used for the test. Place specimen in a biohazard bag.

Interfering Factors

1. False-positive results may occur with high levels of rheumatoid factors or in the presence of other spirochete infections such as syphilis (cross-reactivity).
2. Asymptomatic individuals who spend time in endemic areas may have already produced antibodies to *B. burgdorferi*.

Clinical Implications

1. Serologic tests lack the degree of sensitivity, specificity, and standardization necessary for diagnosis in the absence of clinical history. The antigen detection assay for bacterial proteins is of limited value in early stages of disease.
2. In patients presenting with a clinical picture of Lyme disease, negative serologic tests are inconclusive during the first month of infection.
3. Repeat paired testing should be performed if borderline values are reported.
4. The CDC states that the best clinical marker for Lyme disease is the initial skin lesion erythema migrans (EM), which occurs in 60% to 80% of patients.
5. CDC laboratory criteria for the diagnosis of Lyme disease include the following factors:
   a. Isolation of *B. burgdorferi* from a clinical specimen
   b. IgM and IgG antibodies in blood or CSF
   c. Paired acute and convalescent blood samples showing significant antibody response to *B. burgdorferi*

Patient Preparation

1. Assess patient's clinical history, exposure risk, and knowledge regarding the test. Explain test purpose and procedure as well as possible follow-up testing.
2. Follow guidelines in Chapter 1 regarding safe, effective, informed *pretest* care.

Patient Aftercare

1. Interpret test outcomes for a positive test. Refer to page •• for interpretation of immunologic test results. Advise that follow-up testing may be required to monitor response to antibiotic therapy.
2. Patients with a negative test result and clinical findings suggestive of Lyme disease should also receive antibiotic treatment. Repeat testing may be necessary because patients in early stages may test negative.
3. Follow guidelines in Chapter 1 regarding safe, effective, informed *posttest* care.

LEGIONNAIRE'S DISEASE ANTIBODY TEST

Normal Values

Negative for Legionnaire's disease by IFA or ELISA

Background

Legionnaire's disease is a respiratory condition caused by *Legionella pneumophila*. It is best diagnosed by organism culture; however, the organism is difficult to grow.

Explanation of Test

Detection of *L. pneumophila* in respiratory specimens by means of direct fluorescent antibody (DFA) technique is useful for rapid diagnosis but lacks sensitivity when only small numbers of organisms are available. Serologic tests should be used only if specimens for culture are not available or if culture and DFA produce negative results.

Procedure

1. Collect a 5-ml blood serum sample in a red-topped tube. Observe standard precautions.
2. Follow-up testing is usually requested 3 to 6 weeks after initial symptom appearance.
3. A urine specimen may be required if antigen testing is indicated.

Clinical Implications

1. A dramatic rise of titer to levels >1:128 in the interval between acute- and convalescent-phase specimens occurs with recent infections.
2. Serologic tests are not the method of choice because they indicate retrospective values weeks after the acute phase.
3. Serologic testing is valuable because it provides a confirmatory diagnosis of *L. pneumophila* infection when other tests have failed. IFA is the serologic test of choice because it can detect all classes of antibodies.
4. Demonstration of *L. pneumophila* antigen in urine by ELISA is indicative of infection.

Patient Preparation

1. Assess clinical history and knowledge about the test. Explain purpose and procedure of blood test.
2. Follow guidelines in Chapter 1 regarding safe, effective, informed *pretest* care.

Patient Aftercare

1. Interpret test outcomes and significance. Advise that negative results do not rule out *L. pneumophila*. Follow-up testing is usually needed.
2. Follow guidelines in Chapter 1 regarding safe, effective, informed *posttest* care.

CHLAMYDIA ANTIBODY IgG TEST

Normal Values

Negative for chlamydia antibody by complement-fixation (CF), IFA, and PCR tests

Background

Chlamydia is caused by a genus of bacteria (*Chlamydia* spp.) that require living cells for growth and are classified as obligate cell parasites. Recognized species include *Chlamydia psittaci* and *Chlamydia trachomatis*. *C. psittaci* causes psittacosis in birds and humans. *C. trachomatis* is grouped into three serotypes. One group causes lymphogranuloma venereum (LGV), a venereal disease. Another group causes trachoma, an eye disease. The third group causes genital tract infections different from LGV. Culture of the organism is definitive for chlamydiae.

Explanation of Test

Because *Chlamydia* organisms are difficult to culture and grow, antibody testing aids in diagnosis of chlamydial infection.

Procedure

1. Collect a 5-ml blood serum sample in a red-topped tube. Observe standard precautions.

Clinical Implications

1. Presence of antibody titer indicates past chlamydial infection. A fourfold or greater rise in antibody titer between acute and convalescent specimens indicates recent infection. Serologic tests cannot differentiate among the species of *Chlamydia*.
2. Infection with psittacosis is revealed in an elevated antibody titer. History will reveal contact with infected birds (pets or poultry).
3. LGV in males is characterized by swollen and tender inguinal lymph nodes. In females, swelling occurs in the intraabdominal, perirectal, and pelvic lymph nodes. *Chlamydia* causes urethritis in males. It can infect the female urethra and endocervix and it is also a cause of pelvic inflammatory disease in females. Eye disease caused by *Chlamydia* is endemic in parts of Africa, the Middle East, and Southeast Asia, although its presence is established worldwide. Culture and stained smear identification of the organism is diagnostic.

Interfering Factors

Depending on geographic location, nonspecific titers can be found in the general healthy population.

Patient Preparation

1. Assess patient knowledge regarding the test and explain purpose and procedure. Elicit history regarding possible exposure to organism.
2. Follow guidelines in Chapter 1 regarding safe, effective, informed *pretest* care.

Patient Aftercare

1. Interpret test outcomes and significance of test results. Refer to page 579 for interpretation of immunodiagnostic test results.
2. Follow guidelines in Chapter 1 regarding safe, effective, informed *posttest* care.

STREPTOCOCCAL ANTIBODY TESTS: ANTISTREPTOLYSIN O TITER (ASO), STREPTOZYME, ANTI-DNASE B (ADB, STREPTODORNASE) ●

Normal Values

ASO titer: <166 Todd units (or <200 IU)
Anti-DNase B (ADB)
Birth–4 years: <170 U
5–19 years <480 U

≥20 years: < 340 U
Streptozyme: negative for streptococcal antibodies

Background

Group A β-hemolytic streptococci are associated with streptococcal infections or illness.

Explanation of Test

These tests detect antibodies to enzymes produced by organisms. Group A β-hemolytic streptococci produce several enzymes including streptolysin O, hyaluronidase, and DNase B. Serologic tests that detect these enzyme antibodies include antistreptolysin O titer (ASO), which detects streptolysin O; streptozyme, which detects antibodies to multiple enzymes; and anti-DNase B (ADB), which detects DNase B. Serologic detection of streptococcal antibodies helps to establish prior infection but are of no value for diagnosing acute streptococcal infections. Acute infections should be diagnosed by direct streptococcal cultures or the presence of streptococcal antigens.

The ASO test aids in the diagnosis of several conditions associated with streptococcal infections such as rheumatic fever, glomerulonephritis, endocarditis, and scarlet fever. Serial rising titers over several weeks are more significant than a single result. Anti DNase B antibodies may appear earlier than ASO in streptococcal pharyngitis and this test is more sensitive for streptococcal pyoderma.

Procedure

1. Collect a 5-ml blood serum sample in a red-topped tube. Observe standard precautions. Place specimen in a biohazard bag.
2. Repeat testing 10 days after the first test is recommended.

Clinical Implications

1. In general, a titer of >166 Todd units is considered a definite elevation.
2. The ASO or the ADB test alone are positive in 80% to 85% of group A streptococcal infections (eg, streptococcal pharyngitis, rheumatic fever, pyoderma, glomerulonephritis).
3. When ASO and ADB tests are run concurrently, 95% of streptococcal infections can be detected.
4. A repeatedly low titer is good evidence for the absence of active rheumatic fever. Conversely, a high titer does not necessarily mean rheumatic fever or glomerulonephritis is present; however, it does indicate the presence of a streptococcal infection.
5. ASO production is especially high in rheumatic fever and glomerulonephritis. These conditions show marked ASO titer increases during the symptomless period preceding an attack. Also, ADB titers are particularly high in pyoderma.

Interfering Factors

1. An increased titer can occur in healthy carriers.
2. Antibiotic therapy suppresses streptococcal antibody response.

3. Increased β-lipoprotein levels inhibit streptolysin O and produce falsely high ASO titers.

> **Clinical Alert**
>
> The ASO test is impractical in patients who have recently received antibiotics or who are scheduled for antibiotic therapy because the treatment suppresses the antibody response.

Patient Preparation
1. Assess patient's clinical history and test knowledge. Explain test purpose and procedure.
2. Follow guidelines in Chapter 1 regarding safe, effective, informed *pretest* care.

Patient Aftercare
1. Interpret test outcomes. Refer to page 579 for interpretation of immunologic test results. Explain test results. Inform patient that repeat testing is frequently required.
2. Advise patient that prior antibiotic therapy may suppress antibody formation. If antibiotics have been prescribed, explain the importance of taking the entire amount.
3. Follow guidelines in Chapter 1 regarding safe, effective, informed *posttest* care.

HELICOBACTER PYLORI IgG ANTIBODY TEST

Normal Values
Negative for *Helicobacter pylori* by ELISA indicates no detectable IgG antibody
A positive result indicates the presence of detectable IgG antibody

Background
H. pylori is a bacterium associated with gastritis, duodenal and gastric ulcers, and possibly gastric carcinoma. The clinician orders this test when screening a patient for possible *H. pylori* infection. The organism is present in 95% to 98% of patients with duodenal ulcers and 60% to 90% of patients with gastric ulcers. A person with gastrointestinal symptoms with evidence of *H. pylori* colonization (eg, presence of specific antibodies, positive breath test, positive culture, positive biopsy) is considered to be infected with *H. pylori*. A person without gastrointestinal symptoms having evidence of the presence of *H. pylori* is said to be colonized rather than infected.

Explanation of Test
Traditionally, the presence of *H. pylori* has been detected through biopsy specimens obtained by endoscopy. As with any invasive procedure, there is risk and discomfort to the patient.

Noninvasive methods of detection include the following:

1. A urea breath test, which uses radiopharmaceuticals (still under investigation)
2. Serology
3. Stool: *H.pylori* stool antigen test (HpSa)

The presence of *H. pylori*–specific IgG antibodies in human serum has been shown to be an accurate indicator of *H. pylori* colonization.

ELISA testing relies on the presence of *H. pylori* IgG–specific antibody to bind to antigen on the solid phase, forming an antigen-antibody complex which undergoes further reactions to produce a color indicative of the presence of antibody and is quantified using a spectrophotometer or ELISA microweld plate reader.

Procedure

1. Collect a 7-ml blood serum sample in a red-topped tube. Observe standard precautions.
2. A random stool specimen may be ordered to test for the presence of *H. pylori* antigen.

Clinical Implications

1. This assay is intended for use as an aid in the diagnosis of *H. pylori* infection in persons with gastrointestinal symptoms. Studies have shown that a large proportion of healthy people have antibodies against *H. pylori*, and additionally, false-negatives may occur. The clinical diagnosis should not be based on serology alone, but on a combination of serology, symptoms, and gastric biopsy-based tests as warranted.
2. The stool antigen test is used to monitor response during therapy and to test for cure after treatment.

Patient Preparation

1. Explain test purpose and procedure.
2. Follow guidelines in Chapter 1 regarding safe, effective, informed *pretest* care.

Patient Aftercare

1. Interpret test outcomes in light of patient's history, including other clinical and laboratory findings.
2. Follow guidelines in Chapter 1 regarding safe, effective, informed *posttest* care.

●VIRAL TESTS

INFECTIOUS MONONUCLEOSIS TESTS: ROUTINE, HETEROPHILE ANTIBODY TITER TEST, EPSTEIN-BARR VIRUS (EBV) ANTIBODY TESTS ●

Normal Values

Negative for infectious mononucleosis (IM) and Epstein-Barr virus (EBV) antibodies

Background

Epstein-Barr virus (EBV) is a herpesvirus found throughout the world. The most common symptomatic manifestation of EBV infection is a disease known as infectious mononucleosis (IM). This disease induces formation of increased numbers of abnormal lymphocytes in the lymph nodes and stimulates increased heterophile antibody formation. IM occurs most often in young adults who have not been previously infected, through contact with infectious oropharyngeal secretions. Symptoms include fever, pharyngitis, and lymphadenopathy. EBV is also thought to play a role in the etiology of Burkitt's lymphoma, nasopharyngeal carcinoma, and chronic fatigue syndrome.

Explanation of Test

The most common test for Epstein-Barr virus (EBV) is the rapid slide test (Monodist) for heterophile antibody agglutination. The heterophile antibody agglutination test is not specific for EBV and therefore is not useful for evaluating chronic disease. If the heterophile test is negative in the presence of acute IM symptoms, specific EBV antibodies should be determined. These include antibodies to viral capsid antigen (anti-VCA) and antibodies to EBV nuclear antigen (EBNA) using IFA and ELISA tests.

Diagnosis of IM is based on the following criteria: clinical features compatible with IM, hematologic picture of relative and absolute lymphocytosis, and presence of heterophile antibodies.

Procedure

1. Collect a 5-ml blood serum sample in a red-topped tube. Observe standard precautions. Place specimen in a biohazard bag.

Clinical Implications

1. The presence of heterophile antibodies (Monospot), along with clinical signs and other hematologic findings, is diagnostic for IM.
2. Heterophile antibodies remain elevated for 8 to 12 weeks after symptoms appear.
3. Approximately 90% of adults have antibodies to the virus.

Patient Preparation

1. Assess patient's clinical history, symptoms, and test knowledge. Explain test purpose and procedure. If preliminary tests are negative, follow-up tests may be necessary.
2. Follow guidelines in Chapter 1 regarding safe, effective, informed *pretest* care.

Patient Aftercare

1. Interpret test outcomes. Refer to page 579 for interpretation of immunologic test results. Explain treatment. After primary exposure, a person is considered immune. Recurrence of IM is rare.
2. Resolution of IM usually follows a predictable course: pharyngitis disappears

within 14 days after onset, fever subsides within 21 days, and fatigue, lymphadenopathy, and liver and spleen enlargement regress by 21 to 28 days.
3. Follow guidelines in Chapter 1 regarding safe, effective, informed *posttest* care.

RUBELLA ANTIBODY TESTS

Normal Values
Hemagglutination inhibition (HAI) titer <1:10: susceptible to rubellavirus
HAI titer >1:10: immune to rubellavirus
ELISA-negative: not immune
ELISA-positive: immune
Latex agglutination–negative: not immune
Latex agglutination–positive: immune

Background
Rubellavirus causes German measles, a contagious disease characterized by fever and rash. Rubella acquired by a pregnant woman during the first trimester of pregnancy is associated with congenital fetal abnormalities, miscarriage, and stillbirth.

Explanation
These tests determine susceptibility and immunity to rubellavirus. Women of childbearing age and others such as health care workers should be tested to identify rubella immune or carrier status. Testing for the IgM antibody is also indicated with any low-birth-weight newborn who also has symptoms of congenital rubella. Rubella infection induces IgM and IgG antibody formation. Presence of an IgM antibody titer in an infant is diagnostic for congenital rubella infection (rubella antibodies do not cross the placenta). Tests for rubellavirus include hemagglutination inhibition (HAI), ELISA, and latex agglutination.

Procedure
1. Collect a 5-ml blood serum sample in a red-topped tube. Observe standard precautions. Place specimen in a biohazard bag.
2. Follow-up testing may be required.

Clinical Implications
1. A fourfold rise in titer values for IgG between the acute and convalescent samples together with clinical symptoms is diagnostic of recent rubella infection. IgM is detectable soon after clinical symptoms occur and reaches peak levels at 10 days.
2. After infection, titer remains high for many years. Repeat infections are rare.
3. Rubella vaccine immunization produces formation of rubella antibodies.
4. Negative titers indicate no previous rubella infection and, therefore, no

immunity to disease. Positive titers indicate past rubella infection and immunity to the disease.

5. Passively acquired rubella antibody levels in the infant decrease markedly within 2 to 3 months postinfection.

Patient Preparation

1. Assess patient's test knowledge. Explain test purpose and procedure. Advise pregnant women that rubella acquired in the first trimester of pregnancy is associated with an increased incidence of miscarriage, stillbirth, and congenital abnormalities.

2. Follow guidelines in Chapter 1 regarding safe, effective, informed *pretest* care.

Patient Aftercare

1. Interpret test outcome and counsel appropriately. Advise women of childbearing age who test negative to be immunized before becoming pregnant. Immunization is contraindicated during pregnancy. Advise patients who test positive that they are naturally immune to further rubella infection.

2. Follow guidelines in Chapter 1 regarding safe, effective, informed *posttest* care.

HEPATITIS TESTS ●

Normal Values

Negative for hepatitis A, B, C, D, or E by radioimmunoassay (RIA), ELISA, or microparticle enzyme immunoassay (MEIA)

Test Findings in Various Disease Stages					
Disease Stages	*HVA*	*HVB*	*HVC*	*HVD*	*HVE*
Acute	IgM anti-HAV	IgM anti-HBc, HBsAg	anti-HCV	HDAg	IgM anti-HVE
Chronic	None	HBsAg	anti-HCV	Total anti-HVD	None
Infectivity	None	HBeAg, HBsAg, HBV-DNA	anti-HCV	Total anti-HVD	None
Recovery	None	anti-HBe, anti-HBs	None	None	None
Carrier state	None	HBsAg	None	HDAg, anti-HD	None
Screening immunity	Total anti-HAV	anti-HBs, total anti-HBc	None	None	Uncertain

Background

Hepatitis can be caused by viruses and several other agents including drugs and toxins. Approximately 95% of hepatitis cases are due to five major virus types: hepatitis A, B, C, D, and E (Table 8-3). Diagnosing the specific virus is difficult because the symptoms presented by each viral type are similar. Additionally, some individuals may be asymptomatic or have very mild symptoms that are ascribed to the "flu." Serologic tests for hepatitis virus markers have made it easier to define the specific type.

Hepatitis A virus (HAV), which is acquired through enteric transmission, infects the gastrointestinal tract and is eliminated through the feces. Serologically, presence of the IgM antibody to hepatitis A virus (IgM anti-HAV) and the total antibody to hepatitis A virus (total anti-HAV) identifies the disease.

Hepatitis B virus (HBV) demonstrates a central core containing the core antigen and a surrounding envelope containing the surface antigen. Detection of core antigen (HBcAg), envelope antigen (HBeAg), and surface antigen (HBsAg) or their corresponding antibodies comprises hepatitis B serologic assessment. Viral transmission occurs through exposure to contaminated blood or blood products through an open wound (eg, needlesticks, lacerations).

Hepatitis C virus (HCV), formerly known as non-A, non-B hepatitis, is also transmitted parenterally. Hepatitis C infection is characterized by presence of antibodies to hepatitis C (anti-HCV) and levels of alanine aminotransferase (ALT) which fluctuate between normal and markedly elevated. Levels of anti-HCV remain positive for many years; therefore, a reactive test indicates infection with HCV but not infectivity or immunity. PCR, which detects HCV RNA, should be used to confirm infection when acute hepatitis C is suspected.

Hepatitis D virus (HDV) is encapsulated by the hepatitis B surface antigen (HBsAg). Without the HBsAg coating, HDV cannot survive. Because HDV can cause infection only in the presence of active HBV infection, it is usually found where a high incidence of HBV occurs. Transmission is parenteral. Serologic HDV determination is made by detection of the hepatitis D antigen (HDAg) early in the course of the infection and by detection of anti-HDV antibody (anti-HDV) in the later stages of the disease.

Hepatitis E virus (HEV) is transmitted enterically and is associated with poor hygienic practices and unsafe water supplies, especially in developing countries. It is quite rare in the United States. Specific serologic tests include detection of IgM and IgG antibodies to hepatitis E (anti-HEV).

Glossary of Terms

ALT (alanine aminotransferase): an enzyme normally produced by the liver; blood levels may increase in cases of liver damage.

Anti-HBc: antibody to hepatitis B core antigen.

Anti-HBe: antibody to hepatitis B envelope antigen.

Anti-HBs: antibody to hepatitis B surface antigen.

Antibody: a Y-shaped protein molecule (immunoglobulin) in serum or body fluid that either neutralizes an antigen or tags it for attack by other cells or

TABLE 8-3
Summary of Clinical and Epidemiologic Features of Viral Hepatitis Agents

Features	Hepatitis A	Hepatitis B	Hepatitis C	Hepatitis D	Hepatitis E
Incubation period	2–6 wk	8–24 wk	2–52 wk	3–13 wk	3–6 wk
Onset	Abrupt	Insidious	Insidious	Abrupt	Abrupt
Symptoms					
Jaundice	Children: 10% Adults: 70%–80%	25%	25%	Varies	Unknown
Asymptomatic patients	Most children	Most children Adults: 50%	About 75%	Rare	Rare
Routes of transmission					
Fecal/oral	Yes	No	No	No	Yes
Parenteral	Rare	Yes	Yes	Yes	No
Sexual	No	Yes	Possible	Yes	No
Perinatal	No	Yes	Possible	Possible	No
Water/food	Yes	No	No	No	Yes
Chronic state	No	Adults: 6%–10% Children: 25%–50% Infants: 70%–90%	50%	10%–15%	No
Case fatality rate	0.6%	1.4%	1%–2%	30%	1%–2% Pregnant women: 20%

chemicals; acts by uniting with and firmly binding to an antigen. The prefix *anti-* followed by initials of a virus refers to specific antibody against the virus.

Chronic hepatitis: a condition in which symptoms and/or signs of hepatitis persist for >6 months.

Cirrhosis: irreversible scarring of the liver that may occur after acute or chronic hepatitis.

Delta agent: a unique RNA virus that causes acute or chronic hepatitis; requires hepatitis B virus for replication and infects only patients who are HBsAg-positive; comprised of a delta antigen core and a hepatitis B surface antigen (HBsAg) coat; also known as hepatitis D virus.

Endemic: present in a community at all times but occurring in a small number of cases.

Enteric route: the spread of organisms via the oral-intestinal-fecal cycle.

Flavivirus: a family of small RNA viruses; HCV is similar to members of the Flavivirus family.

Fulminant hepatitis: the most severe form of hepatitis; may lead to acute liver failure and death.

HBcAg: hepatitis B core antigen.

HBsAg: hepatitis B surface antigen.

Hepatotropic: having an affinity for or exerting a specific effect on the liver.

IgG: a form of immunoglobulin that occurs late in an infectious process.

IgM: a form of immunoglobulin that occurs early in an infectious process.

IgM anti-HAV: M class immunoglobulin antibody to hepatitis A virus.

IgM anti-HBc: M class immunoglobulin antibody to hepatitis B core antigen.

Immune globulin: a sterile solution of water-soluble proteins that contains those antibodies normally present in adult human blood; used as a passive immunizing agent against various viruses such as HAV.

Negative-sense RNA virus: a virus in which the viral proteins are encoded by messenger RNA molecules that are complementary to the viral genome.

Non-A, non-B hepatitis: viral hepatitis caused by viruses other than A, B, or D (eg, C, E).

Parenteral: entering the body subcutaneously, intramuscularly, or intravenously, or other means whereby the organisms reach the bloodstream directly.

Positive-sense RNA virus: a virus in which the parenteral (or genomic) RNA serves as the messenger RNA for protein synthesis.

Recombinant antigen: an antigen that results from the recombination of genetic components which then are artificially introduced into a cell, leading to synthesis of a new protein.

Viral load: the amount or concentration of virus in the circulation.

New viruses—GBV-A, GBV-B and GBV-C: may be causative agents in non–A through E hepatitis.

Explanation of Test

These measurements are used for differential diagnosis of viral hepatitis. Serodiagnosis of viral hepatitis is complex because of the number of serum markers necessary to determine the stage of illness. Testing methods include RIA, ELISA, and MEIA.

Procedure

1. Collect a 5-ml blood serum sample in a red-topped tube. Observe standard precautions. Place specimen in a biohazard bag.

Clinical Implications

1. Individuals with hepatitis may have generalized symptoms resembling the "flu" and may dismiss their illness as such.
2. A specific type of hepatitis cannot be differentiated by clinical observations alone. Testing is the only sure method to define the category.
3. Rapid diagnosis of acute hepatitis is essential for the patient so that treatment can be instituted and for those who have close patient contact so that protective measures can be taken to prevent disease spread.
4. Persons at higher risk for acquiring hepatitis A include patients and staff in health care and custodial institutions, people in day care centers, intravenous drug abusers, and those who travel to undeveloped countries or regions where food and water supplies may be contaminated.
5. Persons at higher risk for hepatitis B include those with a history of drug abuse, those who have sexual contact with infected persons, and those who have household contact with infected persons and especially those with skin and mucosal surface lesions (eg, impetigo, saliva from chronic HBV persons on toothbrush racks and coffee cups in their homes); additionally, infants born to infected mothers (during delivery), hemodialysis patients, and health care employees are at higher risk of infection. Of all persons with HBV infection, 38% to 40% contract HBV during early childhood.
6. Health care workers should be periodically tested for hepatitis exposure and should always observe standard precautions when caring for patients.
7. Persons at risk for hepatitis C include those who have received blood transfusions, engage in intravenous drug abuse, undergo hemodialysis, have had organ transplantation, or have sexual contact with an infected person; hepatitis C can also be transmitted during delivery from mother to neonate. Most people are asymptomatic at time of diagnosis for hepatitis C.

The following hepatitis markers appear after infection.

Serological Marker	Time Marker Appears After Infection	Clinical Implications
HEPATITIS A VIRUS		
HAV-Ab/IgM	4–6 wk	Positive for acute stage of hepatitis A; develops early in disease course

(continued)

(Continued)

Serological Marker	Time Marker Appears After Infection	Clinical Implications
HAV-Ab/IgG	8–12 wk	Indicates previous exposure and immunity to hepatitis A
HEPATITIS B VIRUS		
HBsAg-hepatitis B virus	12 wk	Positive in acute stage of hepatitis B; earliest indicator of acute antigen infection; also indicates chronic infection
HBeAg	4–12 wk	Positive in acute active stage with viral replication (infectivity factor); highly infectious
HBcAB, hepatitis B core antibody	6–14 wk	This marker may remain in serum for a longer time; together with HBsAB represents convalescent stage; indicates past infection
ABcAbIgM	6–14 wk	Indicates acute infection
HBeAb antibody	8–16 wk	Indicates acute infection resolution
HBsAb antibody	4–10 mo	Indicates previous exposure, clinical recovery, immunity to hepatitis B; not necessarily to other types of hepatitis; marker for permanent immunity to hepatitis B

Patient Preparation

1. Assess patient's social and clinical history and knowledge of test. Explain test purpose and procedure.
2. Follow guidelines in Chapter 1 regarding safe, effective, informed *pretest* care.

Patient Aftercare

1. Explain significance of test results and counsel appropriately regarding presence of infection, recovery, and immunity. Counsel health care workers and family regarding protective and preventive measures necessary to avoid transmission. Instruct patient to alert health care workers and others regarding their hepatitis history in situations in which exposure to body fluids and wastes may occur.
2. Pregnant women may need special counseling.
3. Follow guidelines in Chapter 1 regarding safe, effective, informed *posttest* care.

Clinical Alert

1. Observe enteric and standard precautions for 7 days after onset of symptoms and/or jaundice in hepatitis A. Hepatitis A is most contagious before symptoms and/or jaundice appear.
2. Use standard blood and body fluid precautions with hepatitis B and hepatitis B antigen carriers. Precautions apply until the patient is HBsAg-negative and anti-HBs appear. Avoid "sharps" (eg, needles, scalpel blades) injuries. Should accidental injury occur, encourage some bleeding and wash area well with a germicidal soap. Report injury to proper department and follow-up with necessary interventions. Put on gown when blood splattering is anticipated. A private hospital room and bathroom may be indicated.
3. If patient has had a blood transfusion, he or she should not donate blood for 6 months. Transfusion-acquired hepatitis may not show up for 6 months posttransfusion. Persons who test positive for HBsAg should *never* donate blood or plasma.
4. Persons who have sexual contact with hepatitis B–infected individuals run a greater risk of acquiring the infection. HBsAg appears in most body fluids including saliva, semen, and cervical secretions.
5. Standard precautions must be observed in all cases of suspected hepatitis until the diagnosis and hepatitis type are confirmed.
6. Immunization of persons exposed to the infection should be done as soon as possible. In the case of contact with hepatitis B, both hepatitis B immunoglobulin (HBIG) and HBV vaccine should be administered within 24 hours of skin break contact and within 14 days of last sexual contact. For hepatitis A, IG should be given within 2 weeks of exposure. In day care centers, IG should be given to all contacts (children and personnel).

INDICATIONS FOR HEPATITIS B VACCINE

Family members of adoptees from foreign countries who are HBsAg-positive.

Health care workers (dentist, DO, MD, RN, and trainees in health care fields).

Hemodialysis patients or patients with early renal failure.

Household or sexual contacts of persons chronically infected with hepatitis B.

Immigrants from Africa or Southeast Asia. Recommended for children <11 years old and all susceptible household contacts of persons chronically infected with hepatitis B.

Injection drug users.

Inmates of long-term correctional facilities.

Clients and staff of institutions for the developmentally disabled.

International travelers to countries of high or intermediate HBV endemicity.

Laboratory workers.

Public safety workers (eg, police, fire fighters)

Recipients of clotting factors. Use a fine needle (≤23 gauge) and firm pressure at injection site for ≥2 minutes.

Persons with sexually transmitted diseases or multiple sexual partners in previous 6 months, commercial sex workers (prostitutes), homosexual and bisexual men.

Postvaccination blood testing is recommended for sexual contacts of HBsAg-positive persons; health care workers at high risk, recipients of clotting factors, those who are HBsAg-positive.

Persons in nonresidential day care programs should be vaccinated if an HBsAg-positive classmate behaves aggressively or has special medical problems that increase the risk of exposure to blood. Staff in nonresidential day care programs should be vaccinated if a client is HBsAg-positive.

a. Observe enteric and standard precautions for 7 days after onset of symptoms and/or jaundice with hepatitis B. Hepatitis A is most contagious before symptoms and/or jaundice appear.

b. Use standard blood and body fluid precautions for type B hepatitis and hepatitis B antigen carriers. Precautions apply until the patient is HBsAG-negative and the anti-HBs appear. Avoid "sharps" (eg, needles, scalpel blades) injuries. Should accidental injury occur, encourage some bleeding and wash area well with a germicidal soap. Report injury to proper department and follow-up with necessary interventions. Put on gown when blood splattering is anticipated. A private hospital room and bathroom may be indicated.

2. Persons with a history of receiving blood transfusion should not donate blood for 6 months. Transfusion-acquired hepatitis may not show up for 6 months posttransfusion. Persons who test positive for HBsAg should *never* donate blood or plasma.

3. Persons who have sexual contact with hepatitis B–infected individuals run a greater risk of acquiring that same infection. HBsAg appears in most body fluids such as saliva, semen, and cervical secretions.

4. Observe standard precautions in all cases of suspected hepatitis until the diagnosis and hepatitis type are confirmed.

Differential Diagnosis of Viral Hepatitis				
Virus	*Transmission*	*Incubation Period*	*Test for Active Infection*	*Social and Clinical History*
Hepatitis A	Fecal-oral by person-to-person contact or ingestion of contaminated food	Average, 30 d (range, 15–50 d)	IgM antibody to hepatitis A capsid proteins	Household or sexual contact with an infected person, day care centers, and *(continued)*

Differential Diagnosis of Viral Hepatitis *(Continued)*

Virus	Transmission	Incubation Period	Test for Active Infection	Social and Clinical History
				common source outbreaks from contaminated food
Hepatitis B	Sexual, blood and other body fluids	Average, 120 d (range, 45–160 d)	HBsAg; the best test for acute or recent infection is IgM antibody to HBcAg	Sexual promiscuity, male-to-male-to-female sexual practices, injection drug use, birth to an infected mother
Hepatitis C	Blood	Commonly 6–9 wk (range, 2 wk–6 mo)	ELISA is the initial test to show if ever infected; it should be confirmed by another test such as PCR	Injection drug use, occupational exposure to blood hemo-dialysis transfusion, possibly sexual transmission
Hepatitis D	Sexual, blood and other body fluids	2–8 wk (from animal studies)	Total antibody to delta hepatitis shows if ever infected; IgM test is in research laboratories; ELISA.	Requires active infection with HBV. Injection drug users and persons receiving clotting factor concentrates are at highest risk of infection

Differential Diagnosis of Viral Hepatitis *(Continued)*

Virus	*Transmission*	*Incubation Period*	*Test for Active Infection*	*Social and Clinical History*
Hepatitis E	Fecal-oral	Average, 26–42 d (range, 15–64 d)	Research laboratories	No known cases originated in the United States; international travelers are the only high-risk group to date

Tests for the following viruses are incuded because the clinical signs and symptoms mimic hepatitis

Virus	*Transmission*	*Incubation Period*	*Test for Active Infection*	*Social and Clinical History*
Epstein-Barr virus (EBV)	Oropharyngeal (saliva)	4–6 wk	IgM antibody to EBV viral capsid	Seroconversion by age 5 y in 50% of persons in the United States; children with an acutely infected sibling are at greater risk
Cytomegalovirus (CMV, human herpes virus 5)	Intimate contact with infected fluids; sexual, perinatal, blood transfusion, and infected breast milk	About 3–8 wk for transfusion-acquired CMV	Culture, monoclonal antibody to early antigen	Household sexual contact with an infected person, male-to-male sexual practices, day care centers, perinatal transmission

ELISA, enzyme-linked immunosorbent assay; PCR, polymerase chain reaction.

VIRAL ANTIBODY TESTS ●

Normal Values
Negative titer for viral disease: <1:8 by CF

Background
Viruses produce antibodies that can be detected by blood serum tests. Although the primary diagnosis for most viral infections is cell culture in many instances, blood serum study is the only practical approach. Antibodies to many viral antigens remain for months or years after an acute infection. A significant rise in antibody titer is considered diagnostic of recent viral infection.

Explanation of Test
These antibody studies establish the presence of various viral diseases. Viral diseases are classified according to site as respiratory, gastrointestinal, CNS, and exanthem (skin eruption). Acute and convalescent specimens are required.

Procedure
1. Collect a 5-ml blood serum sample in a red-topped tube. Observe standard precautions. Place specimen in a biohazard bag.
2. A follow-up convalescent-stage serum test is required. Spinal fluid can be tested for CNS viral determinants.

Clinical Implications
1. A fourfold increase in antibody titer values from acute-stage to convalescent-stage serum specimens indicates presence of viral infection.

Patient Preparation
1. Assess patient's clinical history and knowledge regarding test. Explain test purpose and procedure.
2. Follow guidelines in Chapter 1 regarding safe, effective, informed *pretest* care.

Patient Aftercare
1. Interpret test outcome. Refer to page 579 for interpretation of immunologic test results. Explain significance of results to patient and necessity for repeat testing.
2. Follow guidelines in Chapter 1 regarding safe, effective, informed *posttest* care.

RABIES ANTIBODY TESTS ●

Normal Values
IFA <1:16 or DFA examination of the animal brain for presence of the virus

Explanation of Test
Serologic testing is diagnostic for the presence of rabies in animals. It also indicates the degree of antibody responses to rabies immunization (eg, for people who routinely work with animals).

Procedure for Humans

1. Collect a 5-ml blood serum sample in a red-topped tube. Observe standard precautions. Place specimen in a biohazard bag.

Procedure for Animals

1. If the suspect animal exhibits abnormal behavior, standard procedure is to sacrifice it and examine its brain for Negri body inclusions in the neurons.
2. Rabies testing is usually performed in a public health laboratory.

Clinical Implications

1. An elevated titer in humans indicates an adequate response after immunization. A rabies titer of 1:16 or greater is considered protective.

> **Clinical Alert**
>
> 1. Prevention: pre-exposure vaccine (human diploid cell rabies vaccine [HDCV]) should be given to persons at high-risk such as veterinarians, wildlife personnel, zoo workers, quarantine kennels workers, and those employed in laboratories that use animals.
> 2. Postbite: administer rabies immunoglobulin (RIG) as soon as possible after the bite, regardless of time interval, to neutralize the virus in the wound. HDCV in five 1-ml intramuscular doses should be given in the deltoid muscle. The first HDCV dose is given concurrently with the RIG, and subsequent doses are given 3, 7, 14, and 28 days after the first dose.
> 3. The animal brain should be tested as soon as possible. Holding the animal for observation is not recommended.

Patient Preparation

1. Explain test purpose and procedure.
2. Follow guidelines in Chapter 1 regarding safe, effective, informed *pretest* care.

Patient Aftercare

1. Interpret test results after immunization.
2. Follow guidelines in Chapter 1 regarding safe, effective, informed *posttest* care.

ANTIBODY TO HUMAN IMMUNODEFICIENCY VIRUS (HIV-1/2); ACQUIRED IMMUNODEFICIENCY SYNDROME (AIDS) TEST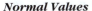

Normal Values

Negative; nonreactive for HIV types 1 and 2 by ELISA, WB, and IFA

Explanation of Test

These tests detect human immunodeficiency viruses types 1 and 2 (HIV-1/2) which cause acquired immunodeficiency syndrome (AIDS). Infection with

HIV-1 is most prevalent in the United States and Western Europe. Most cases associated with HIV-2 are reported in West Africa. Tests to detect the presence of HIV-1 antibody screen blood and blood products that will be used for transfusion. They are also used to test people at risk for developing AIDS such as intravenous drug users, sexual partners of HIV-infected persons, and infants born to HIV-infected women. The diagnosis of AIDS must be clinically established. Tests used to determine the presence of antibodies to HIV-1 include ELISA, WB, and IFA.

A single reactive ELISA test by itself cannot be used to diagnose AIDS. The test should always be repeated in duplicate using the same blood sample. If repeatedly reactive, follow-up tests using WB or IFA should be done. A positive WB or IFA is considered confirmatory for HIV. The combination HIV-1/2 test has replaced the HIV-1 test for screening blood and blood products for transfusion. It is also used for testing potential organ transplant donors.

Procedure
1. Collect a 5-ml blood serum sample in a red-topped tube. Observe standard precautions. Place specimen in biohazard bag.
2. Saliva specimens may be collected; usually indicated in clinic settings or outreach environments.

Clinical Implications
1. A positive ELISA that fails to be confirmed by WB or IFA should not be considered negative, especially in the presence of symptoms or signs of AIDS. Repeat testing in 3 to 6 months is suggested.
2. A positive result may occur in noninfected persons because of unknown factors.
3. Negative tests tend to rule out AIDS in high-risk patients who do not have the characteristic opportunistic infections or tumors.
4. An HIV infection is described as a continuum of stages that range from the acute, transient, mononucleosis-like syndrome associated with seroconversion to asymptomatic HIV infection to symptomatic HIV infection and, finally, to AIDS. AIDS is end-stage HIV infection.
5. Treatments are more effective and less toxic when begun early in the course of HIV infection.
6. HIV PCR method to determine viral load may be performed during HIV treatment to monitor patient prognosis and treatment.
7. Diagnosis of HIV in neonates is difficult because maternally acquired antibodies may be present until the child is 18 months of age. Additionally, PCR to detect antigen is usually not successful until the child is 6 months of age.

Interfering Factors
1. Nonreactive HIV test results occur during the acute stage of disease when the virus is present but antibodies are not sufficiently developed to be detected. It may take up to 6 months for the test result to become positive. During this stage, the test for the HIV antigen may confirm an HIV infection.
2. Test kits for HIV are extremely sensitive. As a result, nonspecific reactions

> **Clinical Alert**
>
> 1. Issues of confidentiality surround HIV testing. Access to test results should be given judiciously on a need-to-know basis unless the patient specifically expresses otherwise. Interventions to block general computer access to this information are necessary; each health care facility must determine how best to accomplish this.
> 2. Conversely, health care workers directly involved with the care of an HIV/AIDS patient have a right to know the diagnosis so that they may protect themselves from exposure.
> 3. All results, both positive and negative, must be somehow entered in the patient's health care records while maintaining confidentiality. People are more likely to test voluntarily when they trust that inappropriate disclosure of HIV testing information will not occur. Long-term implications include potential loss of jobs, housing, insurance coverage, and personal relationships.
> 4. The clinician must sign a legal form stating that the patient has been informed regarding test risks.
> 5. A person who exhibits HIV antibodies is presumed to be HIV-infected; appropriate counseling, medical evaluation, and health care interventions should be discussed and instituted.
> 6. Positive test results must be reported to the state public health authorities according to prescribed state regulations and protocols.
> 7. Anonymous testing and reporting is available, such as commercial home tests.

may occur if the tested person has been previously exposed to HIV human cells or the growth media.

Patient Preparation

1. An informed, witnessed consent form must be properly signed by any person being tested for HIV/AIDS. This consent form must accompany the patient and the specimen (see Appendix H for sample form).
2. It is essential that counseling precede and follow the HIV antibody test. This test should not be performed without the subject's informed consent, and persons who need to legitimately access results must be mentioned. Discussion of the clinical and behavioral implications derived from the test results should address the accuracy of the test and should encourage behavioral modifications (eg, sexual contact, shared needles, blood transfusions).
3. Infection control measures mandate use of standard precautions (see Appendix A).
4. Follow guidelines in Chapter 1 regarding safe, effective, informed *pretest* care.

Patient Aftercare

1. Interpret test outcomes. Explain significance of test results. Advise patient that screening tests must be confirmed before the results are reported as HIV reactive. Provide options for immediate counseling if necessary.

2. Follow guidelines in Chapter 1 regarding safe, effective, informed *posttest* care.

HIV Oral Testing

Noninvasive oral HIV testing uses methods to identify high levels of IgG in the gingival crevice of the mouth. This crevice secretes a fluid or transudate that contains a relatively high concentration of IgG in HIV-positive persons.

Procedure for Oral Testing

1. Use a special testing kit such as the commercial Orasure Testing System. The kit's components consist of a specially treated cotton pad on a nylon stick and a vial containing preservative solution. Salt solution in the pad facilitates absorption of the required fluid.

2. Use precise technique. Place pad between the lower cheek and gum, rub back and forth until moistened, and leave in place for 2 minutes. Remove specially treated pad and place it in the vial of special antimicrobial preservative solution. Place specimen container in a biohazard bag and transport to laboratory.

3. The Omni Sal device used in Europe employs a different collection method in which a cotton pad is placed under the tongue. An indicator in the collecting device changes color when an adequate amount of oral fluid has been collected.

4. Recent food intake, smoking, oral hygiene, or treatment with anticholinergic drugs do not affect test results.

Additional Applications for Oral Specimen Testing

Test for HIV-1 and HIV-2

Viral hepatitis A, B, and C

H. pylori

Measles

Mumps

Rubella

Syphilis

CMV

Autoimmune diseases

Cancer (CEA, PSA, CA125)

Diabetes types I and II

Therapeutic drug and hormone monitoring and detection of other drugs

HERPES SIMPLEX VIRUS (HSV) ANTIBODIES (HSV-1 AND HSV-2 TESTS)

Normal Values

Some level of antibodies can be found in the normal population

Negative for HSV-1 and HSV-2 IFA, EIA, and IHA tests

Background

Two types of herpes simplex virus exist. Herpes simplex virus type 1 (HSV-1) causes orofacial herpes; type 2 (HSV-2) causes genital and neonatal herpes. Serologic differentiation is difficult; therefore, type-specific antibody tests are required.

Explanation of Test

These tests identify the herpes simplex infections. Human herpes simplex virus (HSV) infections are found worldwide. The clinical course is variable, and symptoms may be mild enough to go unrecognized. Major signs and symptoms include oral and skin eruptions, genital tract infections and lesions, and neonatal herpes. Herpes simplex is also common in individuals with immune system deficiencies (eg, cancers, HIV/AIDS, chemotherapy treatment). HSV antibody testing is also widely used for bone marrow recipients and donors.

Procedure

1. Collect a 5-ml blood serum sample in a red-topped tube. Observe standard precautions. Place specimen in biohazard bag.
2. Follow-up testing is usually required.

Clinical Implications

1. Most persons in the general population have been infected with HSV by 20 years of age. After the primary infection, antibody levels fall and stabilize until a subsequent infection occurs.
2. Diagnosis of current infection is related to determining a significant increase in antibody titers between acute-stage and convalescent-stage blood samples.
3. Serologic tests cannot indicate the presence of active genital tract infections. Instead, direct examination with procurement of lesion cultures should be done.
4. Newborn infections are acquired during delivery through the birth canal and may present as localized skin lesions or more generalized organ system involvement.

Patient Preparation

1. Assess patient's knowledge regarding the test. Explain test purpose and procedure.
2. Follow guidelines in Chapter 1 regarding safe, effective, informed *pretest* care.

Patient Aftercare

1. Interpret test outcomes. Refer to page 579 for interpretation of immunologic test results. Advise pregnant women that the newborn may be infected during birth when active genital-area infection is present. Explain need for repeat testing.
2. Follow guidelines in Chapter 1 regarding safe, effective, informed *posttest* care.

CYTOMEGALOVIRUS (CMV) ANTIBODY TEST ●

Normal Values

Negative for CMV antibodies by immunofluorescent assay (IFA), ELISA, and related agglutination

Background

Cytomegalovirus (CMV) is a ubiquitous human viral pathogen that belongs to the herpesvirus family. Infection with CMV is usually asymptomatic and can persist in the host as a chronic or latent infection. Cytomegalovirus has been linked with sexually transmitted infections. Blood banks routinely screen for CMV antibodies and report these as CMV-negative or CMV-positive.

Explanation of Test

This test determines the presence of CMV antibodies and is routinely done in congenitally infected newborns, immunocompromised patients, and sexually active persons who present with mononucleosis-like symptoms. Antibody titers must be evaluated in the context of the patient's current clinical symptoms and viral culture results. Tests to detect CMV antigen are available and aid in early detection. Viral culture confirms CMV infection.

Procedure

1. Collect a 5-ml blood serum sample in a red-topped tube. Observe standard precautions. Place specimen in biohazard bag.
2. It is recommended that posttransplant titers be monitored at weekly intervals, particularly following bone marrow transplant.

Clinical Implications

1. Infants who acquire CMV during primary infection of the mother are prone to develop severe cytomegalic inclusion disease (CID). CID may be fatal or may cause neurologic sequelae such as mental retardation, deafness, microcephaly, or motor dysfunction.
2. Transfusion of CMV-infected blood products or transplantation of CMV-infected donor organs may produce interstitial pneumonitis in an immunocompromised recipient.
3. Seroconversion or a significant rise in titer may indicate presence of a recent infection; however, it cannot differentiate between a primary or a recurrent antibody response.

Patient Preparation

1. Explain test purpose and procedure.
2. Follow guidelines in Chapter 1 regarding safe, effective, informed *pretest* care.

Patient Aftercare

1. Interpret test results. Refer to page 579 for interpretation of immunologic test results. Counsel appropriately.
2. Follow guidelines in Chapter 1 regarding safe, effective, informed *posttest* care.

HUMAN T-CELL LYMPHOTROPIC VIRUS TYPE I (HTLV-I) ANTIBODY TEST ●

Normal Values
Negative for human T-cell lymphotropic virus type I (HTLV-I) antibodies

Explanation of Test
This test detects antibodies to HTLV-I, a retrovirus associated with adult T-cell leukemia (ATL) and demyelinating neurologic disorders. The presence of HTLV-I antibodies in an asymptomatic person excludes that person from donating blood; However, this finding does not mean that a leukemia or a neurologic disorder exists or will develop.

Procedure
1. Collect a 5-ml blood serum sample in a red-topped tube. Observe standard precautions. Place specimen in a biohazard bag.

Clinical Implications
1. Positive results (antibodies to HTLV-I) occur in the presence of HTLV-I infection. Infection transmitted to recipients of HTLV-I–infected blood is well documented.
2. The presence of antibodies to HTLV-I bears no relation to the presence of antibodies to HIV-1; its presence does not put a person at risk of HIV/AIDS, but they often occur concurrently because of similar risk factors.
3. HTLV-I is endemic to the Caribbean, Southeastern Japan, and some areas of Africa.
4. In the United States, HTLV-I has been detected in persons with adult T-cell leukemia (ATL), intravenous drug users, and healthy persons, as well as in donated blood products. Transmission can also take place through ingestion of breast milk, sexual contact, and sharing of contaminated intravenous drug paraphernalia.

Patient Preparation
1. Assess patient's knowledge about test. Explain test purpose and procedure.
2. Follow guidelines in Chapter 1 regarding safe, effective, informed *pretest* care.

Patient Aftercare
1. Interpret test results. Refer to page 579 for interpretation of immunologic test results. Counsel patient appropriately.
2. Follow guidelines in Chapter 1 regarding safe, effective, informed *posttest* care.

PARVOVIRUS B-19 ANTIBODY TEST ●

Normal Values
Negative for parvovirus B-19–specific IgM and IgG antibodies by ELISA and IFA

Explanation of Test

These tests detect parvovirus B-19, the only parvovirus known to cause human disease. The B-19 virus destroys red blood cell precursor cells and interferes with normal red blood cell production. In young children, it is associated with erythema infectiosum, a mild, self-limiting disease characterized by a low-grade fever and rash. Recently, it has been associated with aplastic crisis in patients with chronic hemolytic anemia and in immunodeficient patients who have bone marrow failure.

Procedure

1. Collect a 5-ml blood serum sample in a red-topped tube. Observe standard precautions. Place sample in a biohazard bag.

Clinical Implications

Positive parvovirus B-19 infection has been implicated in aplastic anemia associated with organ transplants. It is recommended, therefore, that this test be included in the serologic assessment of prospective organ donors.

Patient Preparation

1. Assess patient's knowledge regarding test. Explain purpose and blood test procedure. Advise any prospective organ donor that this test is part of a panel of tests performed prior to organ donation to protect the organ recipient from potential infection.
2. Follow guidelines in Chapter 1 regarding safe, effective, informed *pretest* care.

Patient Aftercare

1. Interpret test outcome. Refer to page 579 for interpretation of immunologic test results. Explain significance of test results.
2. Follow guidelines in Chapter 1 regarding safe, effective, informed *posttest* care.

Clinical Alert

Repeatedly positive tests must be confirmed by WB.

● FUNGAL TESTS

FUNGAL ANTIBODY TESTS: HISTOPLASMOSIS, BLASTOMYCOSIS, COCCIDIOIDOMYCOSIS ●

Normal Values

Negative for fungal antibodies
CF titer: <1:8
Immunodiffusion: negative

Background

Certain fungal species are associated with human respiratory diseases acquired by inhaling spores from sources such as dust, soil, and bird droppings. Serologic tests may be used for diagnosis. Fungal diseases are categorized as either superficial or deep. For the most part, superficial mycoses are limited to the skin, mucous membranes, nails, and hair. Deep mycoses involve the deeper tissues and internal organs. Histoplasmosis, coccidioidomycosis, and blastomycosis are caused by deep mycoses.

Explanation of Test

These tests detect serum precipitin antibodies and CF antibodies present in the fungal diseases of coccidioidomycosis, blastomycosis, and histoplasmosis. Coccidioidomycosis, also known as desert fever, San Joaquin fever, and valley fever, is contracted through inhalation of *Coccidioides immitis* spores found in dust or soil. Blastomycosis is caused by infection with organisms of the genus *Blastomyces.* Histoplasmosis is a granulomatous infection caused by *Histoplasma capsulatum.*

Procedure

1. Collect a 5-ml blood serum sample in a red-topped tube. Observe standard precautions. Place in a biohazard bag.

Clinical Implications

1. Antibodies to *Coccidioides, Blastomyces,* and *Histoplasma* appear early in the course of the disease (weeks 1–4) and then disappear.

Interfering Factors

1. Antibodies to fungi may be found in blood samples from apparently healthy people.
2. When testing for blastomycosis, cross-reactions with histoplasmosis may occur.

Patient Preparation

1. Explain test purpose and procedure.
2. Follow guidelines in Chapter 1 regarding safe, effective, informed *pretest* care.
3. Specimens for culture of the organism may also be required.

Patient Aftercare

1. Interpret test results. Refer to page 579 for interpretation of immunologic test results. Counsel appropriately.
2. Follow guidelines in Chapter 1 regarding safe, effective, informed *posttest* care.

CANDIDA ANTIBODY TEST

Normal Values

Negative for *Candida* antibodies; precipitins are occasionally found in the normal population

Background

Candidiasis is usually caused by *Candida albicans* and affects the mucous membranes, skin, and nails. Compromised individuals with depressed T-cell function are most likely to have invasive disease.

Explanation of Test

Identifying the *Candida* antibody can be helpful when the diagnosis of systemic candidiasis cannot be shown by culture or tissue sample. Clinical symptomatology must be present for the test to be meaningful. Tests used include counterimmunoelectrophoresis (CIE), which is particularly valuable on CSF and urine specimens, and latex agglutination.

Procedure

1. Collect a 5-ml blood serum sample in a red-topped tube. Observe standard precautions. Place in biohazard bag.

Clinical Implications

1. A titer greater than 1:8 by latex agglutination indicates systemic infection.
2. A fourfold rise in titers of paired blood samples 10 to 14 days apart indicates acute infection.
3. Patients on long-term intravenous therapy treated with broad-spectrum antibiotics and diabetics commonly have disseminated infections caused by *Candida albicans*. The disease also occurs in bottle-fed newborns and in the urinary bladder of catheterized patients.
4. Vulvovaginal candidiasis, common in late pregnancy, can transmit candidiasis to the infant via the birth canal.

Interfering Factors

1. Approximately 25% of the normal population tests positive for the presence of *Candida*.
2. Cross-reaction can occur with latex agglutination testing in persons who have cryptococcosis or tuberculosis.
3. Positive results can occur in the presence of mucocutaneous candidiasis or severe vaginitis.

Patient Preparation

1. Explain test purpose and procedure.
2. Follow guidelines in Chapter 1 regarding safe, effective, informed *pretest* care.
3. Specimens for culture of the organism may also be required.

Patient Aftercare

1. Interpret test results. Refer to page 579 for interpretation of immunologic test results. Counsel patient appropriately. Repeat testing is usually indicated.
2. Follow guidelines in Chapter 1 regarding safe, effective, informed *posttest* care.

ASPERGILLUS ANTIBODY TEST

Normal Values
Negative for *Aspergillus* antibody by immunodiffusion

Background
The aspergilli, especially *Aspergillus fumigatus, A. flavus,* and *A. niger,* are associated with pulmonary infections and invasive fatal disease sequelae in immunosuppressed patients. Manifestations of *Aspergillus* infections include allergic bronchopulmonary disease, lung mycetoma, endophthalmitis, and disseminated brain, kidney, heart, and bone disease.

Explanation of Test
This test detects antibodies present in aspergillosis.

Procedure
1. Collect a 5-ml blood serum sample in a red-topped tube. Cerebrospinal fluid can also be tested. Observe standard precautions. Place specimen in a biohazard bag.

Clinical Implications
1. Positive test results are associated with pulmonary infections in compromised patients and *Aspergillus* infections of prosthetic heart valves.
2. If blood serum exhibits one to four bands, aspergillosis is strongly suspected. Weak bands suggest an early disease process or hypersensitivity pneumonitis.

Patient Preparation
1. Explain test purpose and procedure.
2. Follow guidelines in Chapter 1 regarding safe, effective, informed *pretest* care.
3. Specimens for culture of the organism may also be required.

Patient Aftercare
1. Interpret test outcome. Refer to page 579 for interpretation of immunologic test results. Counsel appropriately.
2. Follow guidelines in Chapter 1 regarding safe, effective, informed *posttest* care.

CRYPTOCOCCUS ANTIBODY TEST

Normal Values
Negative for *Cryptococcus* antibody

Background
Cryptococcus neoformans, a yeast-like fungus, causes a lung infection thought to be acquired by inhalation. The organism has been isolated from several natural environments, especially where weathered pigeon droppings accumulate.

Symptoms include fever, headache, dizziness, ataxia, somnolence, and occasionally cough.

Explanation of Test
This test detects antibodies present in *Cryptococcus* infections. It appears that ~ 50% of patients who present with antibodies have a predisposing condition such as lymphoma or sarcoidosis or are being treated with steroid therapy. Infection with *C. neoformans* has long been associated with Hodgkin's disease and other malignant lymphomas. In fact, *C. neoformans,* in conjunction with malignancy, occurs to such a degree that some researchers have raised the question regarding the possible etiologic relation between the two diseases. Tests ordered for this disease include latex agglutination testing for antigens or antibodies.

Procedure
1. Collect a 5-ml blood serum sample in a red-topped tube. A 2-ml spinal fluid sample may also be used. Observe standard precautions. Place specimen in a biohazard bag.

Clinical Implications
1. Positive *C. neoformans* tests are associated with infections of the lower respiratory tract via inhalation of aerosols containing *C. neoformans* cells disseminated by the fecal droppings of pigeons.

Patient Preparation
1. Explain test purpose and procedure. Obtain clinical history and assess for exposure.
2. Follow guidelines in Chapter 1 regarding safe, effective, informed *pretest* care.
3. Specimens for culture of the organism may also be required.

Patient Aftercare
1. Interpret test results. Refer to page 579 for interpretation of immunologic test results. Counsel patient appropriately.
2. Follow guidelines in Chapter 1 regarding safe, effective, informed *posttest* care.

● PARASITIC TESTS

TOXOPLASMOSIS (TPM) ANTIBODY TESTS ●

Normal Values
Titer <1:16: no previous infection (*except* for ocular infection) by IFA
Titer 1:16–1:256: prevalent in general population

Background

Toxoplasmosis is caused by the sporozoan parasite *Toxoplasma gondii* and is a severe, generalized, granulomatous CNS disease. It may be either congenital or acquired and is found in humans, domestic animals (eg, cats), and wild animals. Humans may acquire the infection through ingestion of inadequately cooked meat or other contaminated material. Congenital toxoplasmosis may cause fetal death. Symptoms of subacute infection may appear shortly after birth or much later. Complications of congenital toxoplasmosis include hydrocephaly, microcephaly, convulsions, and chronic retinitis. It is believed that one fourth to one half of the adult population is asymptomatically infected with toxoplasmosis. The CDC recommends serologic testing during pregnancy.

Explanation of Test

The IFA test helps to differentiate toxoplasmosis from infectious mononucleosis. Toxoplasmosis antibodies appear within 1 to 2 weeks of infection and peak at 6 to 8 months. IFA is also a valuable screening test for latent toxoplasmosis.

Procedure

1. Collect a 5-ml blood serum sample in a red-topped tube. Observe standard precautions. Place specimen in a biohazard bag.

Clinical Implications

The IFA test is considered positive under any of the following conditions:

1. Titer of 1:256 or higher indicates recent exposure or current infection; rising titer is of greatest significance.
2. Any titer value is significant in a newborn infant.
3. Titer of 1:1024 or greater is significant for active disease.
4. Titer of 1:16 or less occurs with ocular toxoplasmosis.

Patient Preparation

1. Explain test purpose and procedure.
2. Follow guidelines in Chapter 1 regarding safe, effective, informed *pretest* care.

Patient Aftercare

1. Interpret test results. Refer to page 579 for interpretation of immunologic test results. Counsel appropriately.
2. Follow guidelines in Chapter 1 regarding safe, effective, informed *posttest* care.

AMEBIASIS (*ENTAMOEBA HISTOLYTICA*) ANTIBODY TEST ●

Normal Values

Negative for *Entamoeba* antibodies by indirect hemagglutination, latent agglutination, and counterimmunoelectrophoresis (CIE)

Explanation of Test

Entamoeba histolytica, the causative agent of amebiasis, is a pathogenic intestinal parasite. The *E. histolytica* test determines the presence or absence of specific serum antibodies to this parasite. Stool examination is considered the definitive diagnostic tool; however, the absence of detectable stool organisms does not necessarily rule out the disease. Antibiotic therapy, oil enemas, and barium may interfere with the ability to isolate this organism in the stool.

Procedure

1. Collect a 5-ml blood serum sample in a red-topped tube. Observe standard precautions. Place specimen in a biohazard bag.

Clinical Implications

1. Positive test of ≥1:128 indicates active or recent infection.

   NOTE: *A positive test may only reflect past but not current infections.*

2. Amebic liver abscess and amebic dysentery indicate the presence of amebiasis.
3. Titers range from 1:256 to 1:2048 in the presence of current active amebiasis.
4. Titers ≤1:32 generally exclude amebiasis.

Patient Preparation

1. Explain test purpose and procedure.
2. Follow guidelines in Chapter 1 regarding safe, effective, informed *pretest* care.

Patient Aftercare

1. Interpret test results. Refer to page 579 for interpretation of immunologic test results. Counsel patient appropriately.
2. Follow guidelines in Chapter 1 regarding safe, effective, informed *posttest* care.

● MIXED TESTS

TORCH TEST ●

Normal Values

Negative for *Toxoplasma,* rubella, cytomegalovirus, and herpes simplex antibodies

Background

TORCH is an acronym that stands for *Toxoplasma,* rubella, cytomegalovirus, and herpes simplex virus. These pathogens are frequently implicated in congenital or neonatal infections that are not clinically apparent but which may result in serious CNS impairment.

Explanation of Test

Both mothers and newborn infants are tested for exposure to these agents. The test differentiates acute, congenital, and intrapartum infections caused by *Toxoplasma gondii,* rubella virus, cytomegalovirus, and herpesvirus. The presence of IgM-associated antibodies in newborns reflects actual fetal antibody production. High levels of IgM at birth indicate fetal in utero response to an antigen. In this instance, an intrauterine infection should be considered. TORCH is more useful in excluding rather than establishing etiology.

Procedure

1. Collect a 5-ml blood serum sample in a red-topped tube. Observe standard precautions. Place specimen in a biohazard bag.

Clinical Implications

1. Persistent rubella antibodies in an infant >6 months of age highly suggests congenital infection. Congenital rubella is characterized by neurosensory deafness, heart anomalies, cataracts, growth retardation, and encephalitic symptoms.
2. A diagnosis of toxoplasmosis is established through sequential testing rather than by a single positive result. Sequential examination reveals rising antibody titers, changing titers, and the conversion of serologic tests from negative to positive. A titer of 1:256 suggests recent infection. About one third of infants who acquire infection in utero show signs of cerebral calcifications and chorioretinitis at birth; the rest are born without symptoms.
3. A marked and persistent rise in CF antibody titer over time is consistent with a diagnosis of rubella in infants <6 months of age.
4. Presence of herpes antibodies in CSF, together with signs of herpetic encephalitis and persistent HSV-1 or HSV-2 antibody levels in a newborn showing no obvious external lesions is consistent with a diagnosis of herpes simplex.

Patient Preparation

1. Explain test purpose and procedure.
2. Follow guidelines in Chapter 1 regarding safe, effective, informed *pretest* care.

Patient Aftercare

1. Interpret test results. Refer to page 579 for interpretation of immunologic test results. Monitor and counsel appropriately for intrauterine and congenital infections.
2. Follow guidelines in Chapter 1 regarding safe, effective, informed *posttest* care.

COLD AGGLUTININ TESTS
(ACUTE AND CONVALESCENT STUDIES)

●

Normal Values
≤1:16 by red cell agglutination at 4°C

Background
Cold agglutinins are usually IgM autoantibodies that cause agglutination of the patient's own red blood cells at temperatures in the range of 0 to 10°C. These antibodies are called cold agglutinins because they have maximum activity at temperatures <37°C, and they are found in small amounts in the blood of normal persons.

Explanation of Test
This test most commonly diagnoses primary atypical viral pneumonia caused by *Mycoplasma pneumoniae;* it is used to diagnose certain hemolytic anemias (eg, cold agglutination disease) as well. The diagnosis depends on demonstrating a fourfold or higher increase in antibody titers between an early acute-phase blood serum sample and a blood serum sample taken in the convalescence phase, 7 to 10 days after the first sample. Positive reaction frequency and titer elevation both appear to be directly related to infection severity.

Procedure
1. Collect a 10-ml blood serum sample in a red-topped tube. Observe standard precautions. Place specimen in a biohazard bag.
2. The sample should be prewarmed to 37°C for at least 15 minutes before the serum is separated from the cells. This allows the cold agglutinating antibodies to be collected from the red cell membranes so they can be detected in the agglutination procedure using O-negative indicator cells (pooled group O donors).

Clinical Implications
1. In viral pneumonia, the titer rises 8 to 10 days after onset, peaks in 12 to 25 days, and decreases 30 days after onset. Up to 90% of people with severe illness exhibit positive titers.
2. Chronic increased titer levels are associated with the following conditions:
   a. Cold antibody hemolytic anemia
   b. Chronic cold agglutinin disease
   c. Paroxysmal cold hemoglobinuria
   d. Severe Raynaud's phenomenon (may lead to gangrene)
   e. B-cell chronic lymphocytic leukemia
3. More important than any single high value is the rise in titer during the course of illness. The titer usually decreases by 4 to 6 weeks after the onset of illness.
4. Transient increases in titers are associated with primary atypical viral pneumonia, infectious mononucleosis, congenital syphilis, hepatic cirrhosis, and trypanosomiasis.

Interfering Factors

1. A high cold agglutinin titer interferes with blood typing and crossmatching.
2. High titers are sometimes spontaneous in older persons and may persist for years.
3. Antibiotic therapy may interfere with cold agglutinin development.

Patient Preparation

1. Explain test purpose and procedure.
2. Follow guidelines in Chapter 1 regarding safe, effective, informed *pretest* care.

Patient Aftercare

1. Interpret test results. Refer to page 579 for interpretation of immunologic test results. Counsel appropriately. Cold agglutinin titers rise during the second and third week of illness before rapidly returning to baseline levels. The test should be repeated at appropriate intervals.
2. Follow guidelines in Chapter 1 regarding safe, effective, informed *posttest* care.

C-REACTIVE PROTEIN (CRP) TEST ●

Normal Values

<0.8 mg/dl by rate nephelometry

Background

During any inflammatory process, a specific abnormal protein named C-reactive protein (CRP) appears in the blood. This protein is virtually absent from the blood serum of healthy persons. CRP rapidly appears in blood and body fluids in response to injurious stimuli.

CRP is thought to be mainly synthesized in the liver. Large amounts appear in peritoneal, pleural, pericardial, and synovial body fluids. CRP is the classical and most dramatic acute-phase reactant, with levels that increase up to 1000-fold and then decline rapidly when the inflammatory process regresses.

Explanation of Test

The CRP test is nonspecific for evaluating inflammatory disease course and severity in conditions in which there is tissue necrosis, such as in myocardial infarction, malignancy, or rheumatoid arthritis. Blood serum CRP can be detected within 18 to 24 hours after the onset of tissue damage. CRP is useful for following the progress of rheumatic fever therapy and for interpreting the sedimentation rate. It also has a place in monitoring the wound healing process, especially with internal incisions, burns, and organ transplantation.

Procedure

1. Collect a 5-ml blood serum sample in a red-topped tube. Observe standard precautions. Place specimen in a biohazard bag.

Clinical Implications

1. CRP is positive in the following conditions:
   a. Rheumatic fever
   b. Rheumatoid arthritis
   c. Myocardial infarction
   d. Malignancy (active, widespread)
   e. Bacterial and viral infections (acute)
   f. Postoperatively (with no complications; declines after fourth postoperative day)
2. The presence of CRP has added significance over and above elevated erythrocyte sedimentation rates (ESR), which may be influenced by altered physiologic states.
3. CRP tends to increase before rises in antibody titers and ESR levels occur. CRP levels also tend to decrease sooner than ESR levels.

Patient Preparation

1. Explain test purpose and procedure. Instruct the patient to fast for 8 to 12 hours before test if required. Water may be taken.
2. Follow guidelines in Chapter 1 regarding safe, effective, informed *pretest* care.

Patient Aftercare

1. Interpret test results, counsel, and monitor appropriately. Repeat testing is often necessary. A positive test indicates active inflammation but not its cause. It is an excellent tool for monitoring disease activity.
2. In rheumatoid arthritis, the test becomes negative with successful treatment and indicates that the inflammatory reaction has subsided, even though the sedimentation rate may be abnormal.
3. Follow guidelines in Chapter 1 regarding safe, effective, informed *posttest* care.

Immunologic Tests for Immune Dysfunction and Related Disorders of the Immune System

PROTEIN ELECTROPHORESIS, SERUM AND URINE ●

Normal Values: Serum Protein Electrophoresis (SPE)

Total protein	Albumin
Adult: 6.0–8.0 g/dl	Adult: 3.8–5.0 g/dl
<5 days: 5.4–7.0 g/dl	Newborn: 2.6–3.6 g/dl
1–3 years: 5.9–7.0 g/dl	1–3 years: 3.4–4.2 g/dl
4–6 years: 5.9–7.8 g/dl	4–6 years: 3.5–5.2 g/dl
7–9 years: 6.2–8.1 g/dl	7–9 years: 3.7–5.6 g/dl
10–19 years: 6.3–8.6 g/dl	10–19 years: 3.7–5.6 g/dl

α_1-Globulin: 0.1–0.3 g/dl
α_2-Globulin: 0.6–1.0 g/dl
β-Globulin: 0.7–1.4 g/dl
Gamma globulin: 0.7–1.6 g/dl

Reference Values: Urine Protein Electrophoresis (UPE)

A descriptive report is prepared by the pathologist.

Background

Serum proteins represent a diverse microenvironment. They are a source of nutrition and a buffer system. Immunoglobulins and related proteins function as immunologic agents. Carrier proteins (eg, haptoglobin, prealbumin, transferrin) transport certain ions and molecules to their destinations. Antiproteases (eg, α_1-antitrypsin, α_2-macroglobulin) regulate the activity of various proteolytic enzymes, and other classes of proteins regulate oncotic pressure, genetic component pressures (eg, chromosomal), and metabolic substances (eg, hormones). Blood serum and urine are commonly screened for the monoclonal immunoglobulin component by means of serum protein electrophoresis (SPEP). Immunoglobulins are the major component of the serum gamma globulin fraction. In health, the immunoglobulins are polyclonal instead of monoclonal. When a monoclonal band is observed, it frequently signals a neoplastic process such as multiple myeloma or Waldenstrom's macroglobulinemia. SPEP enhances follow-up procedures such as specific protein quantification of immunoglobulins (IgA, IgG, IgM) and immunofixation. It provides one of the best tools for general screening of the human health state.

Explanation of Test

These tests can diagnose some inflammatory and neoplastic states, nephrotic syndromes, liver disease, and immune dysfunctions and can evaluate nutritional states and osmotic pressures in edematous and malnourished patients. SPEP produces electrophoretic separation of the five major protein fractions (albumin, α_1-globulin, α_2-globulin, β-globulin, and gamma globulin) in serum and urine specimens so that a more definitive diagnosis can be made. Major components present in each protein fraction or zone exhibit characteristic, unique electrophoretic patterns and are defined as the albumin zone (albumin); the α_1 zone (α_1-lipoproteins, high-density lipoprotein, α_1-antitrypsin); the α_2 zone (α_2-macroglobulin, haptoglobin, β-lipoprotein); the β zone (transferrin, C3 [complement]); and the gamma zone (fibrinogen, IgA, IgM, IgG).

Procedure

1. Collect a 7-ml blood serum sample in a red-topped tube. Observe standard precautions.
2. First voided morning urine specimen or 24-hour timed urine specimen is preferred. A 100-ml sample from a 24-hour urine collection is submitted for a urine protein electrophoresis.
3. If blood or urine sample demonstrates the presence of a paraprotein, a follow-up or confirmatory immunofixation electrophoresis (IFE; see p. 627)

can be performed on the same specimen submitted for the protein electrophoresis.

4. To quantify the amount of protein in each fraction, separate proteins are scanned and separated according to net molecular charge by means of a densitometer and are expressed in grams per deciliter (g/dl).

Clinical Implications

1. The following are the most frequent protein abnormalities in protein quantification and SPEP:
   a. Total serum protein (the sum of circulating serum proteins) *increases* (hyperproteinemia) in dehydration and hemoconcentration states due to fluid loss (eg, vomiting, diarrhea, poor kidney function); increases are also found in the following conditions:
   (1) Liver disease
   (2) Multiple myeloma and other gammopathies
   (3) Waldenstrom's macroglobulinemia
   (4) Tropical disease
   (5) Sarcoidosis and other granulomatous diseases
   (6) Collagen disorders such as systemic lupus erythematosus (SLE) and rheumatoid arthritis (RA)
   (7) Chronic inflammatory states
   (8) Chronic infections
   b. Total serum protein *decreases* (hypoproteinemia) in the following conditions:
   (1) Insufficient nutritional intake (starvation or malabsorption)
   (2) Severe liver disease or alcoholism
   (3) Renal disease, nephrotic syndrome
   (4) Diarrhea (Crohn's disease, ulcerative colitis)
   (5) Severe skin diseases or burns
   (6) Severe hemorrhage (when plasma volume is replaced more rapidly than protein)
   (7) Heart failure
   (8) Hypothyroidism
   (9) Prolonged immobilization (trauma, orthopedic surgery)
   c. Serum albumin *increases* with intravenous infusions and dehydration (elevated hemoglobin and hematocrit indicate higher albumin levels).
   d. Serum albumin *decreases* in the following conditions:
   (1) Decreased synthesis states such as liver diseases, alcoholism, malabsorption syndromes, Crohn's disease, other protein-losing enteropathies, starvation states, and congenital analbuminemia
   (2) *Increased* albumin loss (eg, nephrotic syndrome, third-degree burns)
   (3) Poor nutrition states and inadequate iron intake
   (4) Low albumin-to-globulin (A/G) ratio (eg, collagen disease, chronic inflammation, liver diseases, macroglobulinemia, severe infections, cachexia, burns, ulcerative colitis)

e. α_1-Globulin *increases* with infections (acute and chronic) and febrile reactions.

f. α_1-Globulin *decreases* with nephrosis and alpha/antitrypsin difference.

g. α_2-Globulin *increases* in the following conditions:
   (1) Biliary cirrhosis
   (2) Obstructive jaundice
   (3) Nephrosis
   (4) Multiple myeloma (rare)
   (5) Ulcerative colitis

h. α_2-Globulin *decreases* in acute hemolytic anemia.

i. β-Globulin *increases* in biliary cirrhosis, obstructive jaundice, and multiple myeloma (occasional).

j. β-Globulin *decreases* in nephrosis.

k. Gamma globulin increases in the following conditions:
   (1) Chronic infections
   (2) Hepatic diseases
   (3) Autoimmune diseases
   (4) Collagen diseases
   (5) Multiple myeloma
   (6) Waldenstrom's macroglobulinemia
   (7) Leukemia and other cancers

l. Gamma globulin *decreases* in the following conditions:
   (1) Agammaglobulinemia
   (2) Hypogammaglobulinemia
   (3) Nephrotic syndrome

Interfering Factors

1. Decreased albumin can be seen with rapid intravenous fluid infusions and hydration and during all trimesters of pregnancy.

2. Excessive hemolysis decreases albumin 0.5 g/ml when patients are in the supine position. Conversely, hemolysis and dehydration elevate the total serum protein.

3. Prolonged bed rest and the last trimester of pregnancy produces lower total protein levels.

Patient Preparation

1. Explain test purpose and specimen collection procedure.

2. If a 24-hour urine specimen is to be collected, the patient will require specific instructions, an appropriate container, and a receptacle for catching the voided urine (see Chap. 3, Urine Studies).

3. Follow guidelines in Chapter 1 regarding safe, effective, informed *pretest* care.

Patient Aftercare

1. Interpret test outcome and monitor appropriately. Very low levels of protein and albumin are associated with edema and hypocalcemia. Assess the patient for signs and symptoms related to these conditions and report and document same. Rarely is any one type of electrophoretic analysis used to diagnose a gammopathy. Follow-up testing may include IFE, quantitative immunoglobulins, and bone marrow studies.

2. Follow guidelines in Chapter 1 regarding safe, effective, informed *posttest* care.

Clinical Alert

1. Normally, very little protein is excreted in the urine; however, relatively large amounts may be excreted in certain disease states. In the presence of lipoid nephrosis, selective proteinuria produces excess albumin excretion. With nonselective proteinuria (eg, glomerulonephritis), all types of serum proteins usually appear in the urine. Urine protein electrophoresis can identify Bence-Jones proteins, which migrate in the β-globulin and gamma globulin regions. See Chapter 3 for a complete explanation of urine protein and albumin.

QUANTITATIVE IMMUNOGLOBULINS: IgA, IgG, IgM ●

Normal Values

Adults
IgG: 700–1500 mg/dl
IgA: 60–400 mg/dl
IgM: 60–300 mg/dl
These values are derived from rate nephelometry.

Children

IgA (boys and girls)
  0–4 months: 5–64 mg/dl
  5–8 months: 10–87 mg/dl
  9–14 months: 17–94 mg/dl
  15–23 months: 22–178 mg/dl
  2–3 years: 24–192 mg/dl
  4–6 years: 26–232 mg/dl
  7–9 years: 33–258 mg/dl
  10–12 years: 45–285 mg/dl
  13–15 years: 47–317 mg/dl
  16–17 years: 55–377 mg/dl
IgM (boys)
  0–4 months: 14–142 mg/dl
  5–8 months: 24–167 mg/dl
  9–23 months: 35–200 mg/dl
  2–3 years: 41–200 mg/dl
  4–17 years: 47–200 mg/dl

IgM (girls)
  0–4 months: 14–142 mg/dl
  5–8 months: 24–167 mg/dl
  9–23 months: 35–242 mg/dl
  2–3 years: 41–242 mg/dl
  4–17 years: 56–242 mg/dl
IgG (boys and girls)
  0–4 months: 141–930 mg/dl
  5–8 months: 250–1190 mg/dl
  9–11 months: 320–1250 mg/dl
  1–3 years: 400–1250 mg/dl
  4–6 years: 560–1307 mg/dl
  7–9 years: 598–1379 mg/dl
  10–12 years: 638–1453 mg/dl
  13–15 years: 680–1531 mg/dl
  16–17 years: 724–1611 mg/dl

Background

Five classes of immunoglobulins (antibodies)—IgA, IgG (with 4 subclasses, IgG_1, IgG_2, IgG_3, and IgG_4) IgM, IgD, and IgE—have been isolated. Immunoglobulins function to neutralize toxic substances, support phagocytosis, and destroy microorganism functions. For example, IgA takes two forms: serum and secretory. Serum IgA is present in blood serum; secretory IgA is found in saliva, tears, colostrum, and bronchial, gastrointestinal, and genitourinary secretions, where it can protect against microorganism invasion.

IgG, the only immunoglobulin that can cross the placenta, is responsible for protection of the newborn during the first months of life. IgM possesses antibody activity against gram-negative organisms and rheumatoid factors and forms natural antibodies such as the ABO blood group. IgM does not cross the placenta and is therefore usually absent in the newborn. It is observed ~ 5 days after birth.

Explanation of Test

Quantitative immunoglobulin measurements can monitor the course of a disease and its treatment. If there is a monoclonal protein or M component present on SPEP, a quantitative measurement of IgA, IgG, and IgM can identify the specific immunoglobulin. IgD and IgE are present in trace amounts.

Procedure

1. Collect a 7-ml blood serum sample in a red-topped tube. Observe standard precautions.

Clinical Implications

1. IgA accounts for 10%–15% of total immunoglobulin. *Increases* occur in the following conditions:
   a. Chronic, nonalcoholic liver diseases, especially primary biliary cirrhosis (PBC)
   b. Obstructive jaundice
   c. Exercise
   d. Alcoholism
   e. Subacute and chronic infections
2. IgA *decreases* occur in the following conditions:
   a. Ataxia-telangiectasia
   b. Chronic sinopulmonary disease
   c. Congenital deficit
   d. Late pregnancy
   e. Prolonged exposure to benzene immunosuppressive therapy
   f. Abstinence from alcohol after a period of 1 year
   g. Drugs and dextrin
   h. Protein-losing gastroenteropathies

> **Clinical Alert**
>
> Persons with IgA deficiency are predisposed to autoimmune disorders and can develop antibody to IgA, with possible anaphylaxis occurring if transfused with blood containing IgA.

3. IgG constitutes 75%–80% of total immunoglobulins. *Increases* occur in the following conditions:
   a. Chronic granulomatous infections
   b. Hyperimmunization
   c. Liver disease
   d. Malnutrition (severe)
   e. Dysproteinemia
   f. Disease associated with hypersensitivity granulomas, dermatologic disorders, and IgG myeloma
   g. Rheumatoid arthritis

4. IgG *decreases* occur in the following conditions:
   a. Agammaglobulinemia
   b. Lymphoid aplasia
   c. Selective IgG, IgA deficiency
   d. IgA myeloma
   e. Bence-Jones proteinemia
   f. Chronic lymphoblastic leukemia

5. IgM constitutes 5% to 10% of total antibody. *Increases* in adults occur in the following conditions:
   a. Waldenstrom's macroglobulinemia
   b. Trypanosomiasis
   c. Malaria
   d. Infectious mononucleosis
   e. Lupus erythematosus
   f. Rheumatoid arthritis
   g. Dysgammaglobulinemia (certain cases)

> **Clinical Alert**
>
> In the newborn, a level of IgM >20 mg/dl indicates in utero stimulation of the immune system (eg, rubella virus, cytomegalovirus, syphilis, toxoplasmosis).

6. IgM *decreases* occur in the following conditions:
   a. Agammaglobulinemia
   b. Lymphoproliferative disorders (certain cases)
   c. Lymphoid aplasia

   d. IgG and IgA myeloma
   e. Dysgammaglobulinemia
   f. Chronic lymphoblastic leukemia

Patient Preparation

1. Explain test purpose and specimen collection procedure.
2. Follow guidelines in Chapter 1 regarding safe, effective, informed *pretest* care.

Patient Aftercare

1. See posttest care for protein electrophoresis. The same guidelines prevail on p. 620.
2. Interpret test outcome. Follow-up immunoglobulin testing may be necessary, along with serum viscosity, to monitor a patient with monoclonal gammopathy.
3. Follow guidelines in Chapter 1 regarding safe, effective, informed *posttest* care.

IMMUNOFIXATION ELECTROPHORESIS (IFE), SERUM AND URINE ●

Normal Values

No abnormality present

Background

Monoclonal immunoglobulins consist of heavy and light chains. IFE identifies the presence or absence of a monoclonal protein and determines its heavy-chain and light-chain types.

Explanation of Test

This test measures immune status and competence by identifying monoclonal and particle protein band immunoglobulins involved in the immune response. IFE is a follow-up test performed when a monoclonal spike is observed on SPEP or when a monoclonal gammopathy is suspected on the basis of the patient's immunoglobulin concentrations.

Procedure

1. Collect a 7-ml blood serum sample in a red-topped tube and/or a 24-hour urine specimen. Observe standard precautions. Submit 25 ml from a 24-hour urine collection if a urine IFE is to be run simultaneously.
2. If the IFE is a follow-up to a paraprotein being demonstrated by protein electrophoresis (see p. 620), the same specimen (blood, urine, or both) used for the electrophoresis can be used for this procedure as well.
3. In IFE, high-resolution electrophoresis produces stained bands. By comparing the location of the stained immunofixed band with a band in the same location in the SPEP reference pattern, a particular protein band can be identified.

Clinical Implications

1. *Monoclonal* protein in the serum or urine suggests a neoplastic process; a *polyclonal* increase in immunoglobulins is seen in chronic liver disease, connective tissue disease, and infection.
2. In multiple myeloma, 99% of patients have a monoclonal protein in the serum or urine. Waldenstrom's macroglobulinemia is characterized by the presence of a serum monoclonal IgM protein in all cases.
3. A monoclonal light chain (K or Bence-Jones protein) is found in the urine of ~ 75% of patients with multiple myeloma. Approximately 75% of patients with Waldenstrom's macroglobulinemia have a monoclonal light chain in the urine. Heavy-chain fragments as well as free light chains may be seen in the urine of patients with multiple myeloma or amyloidosis.

Patient Preparation

1. Explain test purpose and specimen collection procedure.
2. If a blood sample is needed, the same specimen submitted for the serum protein electrophoresis can be used. If the test is to be performed separately, then another 7ml blood sample collected in a red-topped tube is required. Note patient's age; this procedure is seldom indicated in patients <30 years of age because monoclonal proteins are rarely identified in this age group.
3. A 24-hour urine specimen is preferred. Provide instructions and a 24-hour collection container (see Chap. 3, Urine Studies, for protocols).
4. Follow guidelines in Chapter 1 regarding safe, effective, informed *pretest* care.

Patient Aftercare

1. Interpret test outcomes and monitor appropriately for neoplasms, infection, and liver and connective tissue disease.
2. Follow guidelines in Chapter 1 regarding safe, effective, informed *posttest* care.

CRYOGLOBULIN TEST ●

Normal Values

Negative for cryoglobulin
If positive after 3 to 5 days at 4°C, IFE of the cryoprecipitate is performed to identify the protein complex

Background

Cryoimmunoglobulins are protein complexes that undergo reversible precipitation at low temperatures and redissolve on warming in the body or under laboratory conditions.

Explanation of Test

This test provides additional diagnostic information about certain disorders such as malignant B-cell diseases, collagen disorders, acute and chronic infections, and primary cryoglobulinemia in persons with cold hypersensitivity. Detection of cryoglobulins is highly specific for immune complexes.

Procedure

1. Collect a 15-ml blood serum sample in a red-topped tube. Observe standard precautions. Keep the specimen at 37°C until the cells are separated.

Clinical Implications

1. Disorders associated with cryoglobulinemia include the following:
   a. Malignant B-cell diseases (eg, multiple myeloma, Waldenstrom's macroglobulinemia, chronic lymphocytic leukemia)
   b. Collagen diseases (eg, rheumatoid arthritis, Sjögren's syndrome, SLE)
   c. Acute and chronic infections:
      (1) Syphilis
      (2) Subacute bacterial endocarditis
      (3) Infectious mononucleosis
      (4) Cytomegalovirus disease
   d. Sarcoidosis
   e. Acute poststreptococcal glomerulonephritis
   f. Cirrhosis
   g. Hemolytic anemia

Patient Preparation

1. Explain test purpose and procedure.
2. Follow guidelines in Chapter 1 regarding safe, effective, informed *pretest* care.

Patient Aftercare

1. Interpret test results. Counsel and monitor appropriately for infections, collagen disorders, and malignant blood cell disease. Follow-up testing is usually needed.
2. Follow guidelines in Chapter 1 regarding safe, effective, informed *posttest* care.

COLLAGEN, RHEUMATIC, AND CONNECTIVE TISSUE DISEASE TESTS

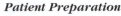

Patient Preparation

Explain test purpose and procedure. A number of laboratory tests are ordered to diagnose complex problems and to assess and monitor the course of collagen, rheumatic, and connective tissue disorders. These diseases include SLE, rheumatoid arthritis, Sjögren's syndrome, progressive systemic sclerosis (PSS), and mixed connective tissue disease. The following is a list of several of these tests:

a. Antinuclear antibody	**h.** Anti–Scl-70 antibody
b. Anticentrome antibody	**i.** CH50 (total hemolytic complement)
c. Anti-dsDNA antibody	**j.** C3 complement component
d. Anti-RNP antibody	**k.** C4 complement component
e. Anti-Sm antibody	**l.** C1 esterase inhibitor
f. Anti-SSA antibody	**m.** Rheumatoid factor
g. Anti-SSB antibody	

Patient Aftercare

1. Interpret test results. Monitor and counsel patient about follow-up tests and treatment. These are chronic diseases that must be dealt with on a continuing basis and may require significant lifestyle changes. Repeat testing evaluates the effectiveness of therapy. Minor symptoms, in the absence of major organ involvement, are frequently treated with non-steroidal antiinflammatory drugs (NSAIDs) such as salicylates. Cutaneous manifestations respond to topical corticosteroid treatments. Short-acting corticosteroids (eg, prednisone) are necessary if acute serologic changes and severe clinical manifestations appear. Short courses of moderate-dose corticosteroids suppress the symptoms of the acute disease, shorten time periods of exacerbation, normalize serologic parameters, and prevent or delay disease progression to its more serious stages. Evidence of rapid reduction of anti-dsDNA antibody levels following initiation of therapy suggests that nonimmune mechanisms operate to clear immune system aberrations. This is especially important for SLE, in which the accumulation of these immune complexes can lead to eventual renal failure.

2. Long-term, moderate- to high-dose corticosteroids are central regimens prescribed for diffuse proliferative glomerulonephritis as well as rheumatoid arthritis.

3. Corticosteroid dosage may be reduced and renal disease may be favorably managed by adding immunosuppressive drugs (eg, cyclophosphamide aza-thioprine) to the therapy regimen. Infection secondary to immunosuppressive treatment is a leading cause of death for patients with SLE. Patient education plays a major role in prevention of infection. Emphasize that the outlook is favorable for improvements in the diagnosis, treatment, and understanding of these diseases.

4. Follow guidelines in Chapter 1 regarding safe, effective, informed *posttest* care.

ANTINUCLEAR ANTIBODY (ANA) TEST ●

Normal Values
Negative for ANA by indirect immunofluorescence (IFA)
If positive, pattern is reported and serum is titered

Background
The diagnosis of SLE is difficult because clinical signs and symptoms are extremely varied and may mimic several connective tissue diseases such as rheumatoid arthritis or other systemic autoimmune disorders. SLE is characterized by a profuse production of different autoantibodies, some of which are pathogenic. SLE is a multisystem disease which can affect every organ system in the body (especially the kidney). It varies in its clinical manifestations in different persons or at different times. The IFA test for antinuclear antibodies

(ANAs) is one of the most useful tests currently available for SLE. ANAs are gamma globulins that react with cell nuclei of all organs, human or animal. ANAs usually belong to more than one immunoglobulin class. An effective fluorescent ANA test detects ~ 95% of SLE cases.

Explanation of Test

This test is used in the differential diagnosis of rheumatic diseases and to detect antinucleoprotein factors and patterns associated with certain autoimmune diseases. One particular antibody pattern is associated with SLE; another antibody pattern correlates with scleroderma, another with Sjögren's syndrome or with Raynaud's disease, and so forth. Although the ANA titer may not correlate with the clinical disease picture in all cases, most SLE patients produce high ANA titers with homogeneous and peripheral (rim) staining patterns. Speckled and nucleolar patterns may be associated with SLE at lower frequencies.

Procedure

1. Collect a 7-ml blood serum sample in a red-topped tube. Observe standard precautions.

Clinical Implications

1. ANA test is positive at a titer of 1:40 or 1:80 depending on the laboratory. Indirect immunofluorescence is the most common test for ANA.
2. A positive result does not necessarily confirm a disease; lower titers of ANAs are present in some apparently normal persons.
3. Percentages of positive test results according to disease process are: SLE and lupoid hepatitis, >95%; scleroderma, 60% to 70%; rheumatoid arthritis, 25% to 30%; Sjögren's disease, 50% to 60%; dermatomyositis, 10% to 50%; and polyarteritis, 10%.
4. A negative total ANA test is strong evidence against the presence of SLE.
5. Sera from some healthy elderly persons contain low titers of ANA (usually <1:160) in the absence of disease.

Interfering Factors

Certain drugs may cause positive ANA tests (eg, procainamide, hydralazine).

Patient Preparation

See special section for collagen and rheumatic disease testing on p. 629.

Patient Aftercare

1. See special section for collagen and rheumatic disease testing (p. 630).
2. Other confirmatory SLE tests include anti-dsDNA, CH50, and kidney or skin biopsy.
3. Follow-up tests for positive ANA results include anti-dsDNA; antibodies to extractable nuclear antigens (anti-RNP, anti-Sm); anti-SSA, also known as anti-Ro; anti-SSB, also known as anti-La; antiscleroderma (Scl-70); and anticentromere, also known as CREST antibody.

ANTICENTROMERE ANTIBODY TEST ●

Normal Values
Negative for anticentromere antibody by indirect immunofluorescence
If positive, serum is titered

Explanation of Test
A variant of scleroderma, the CREST syndrome, is characterized by calcinosis, Raynaud's phenomenon, esophageal dysfunction, sclerodactyly, and telangiectasia. Characteristically, anticentromere antibodies appear in ~ 90% of patients. This antibody is detected by using Hep-2 cells in various stages of cell division. The centromere region of the cell chromosomes will stain if an anticentromere antibody is present.

Procedure
1. Collect a 7-ml blood serum sample in a red-topped tube. Observe standard precautions.

Clinical Implications
Positive results are associated with the CREST syndrome in scleroderma.

Patient Preparation and Aftercare
See special section on collagen and rheumatic disease tests (pp. 629 and 630).

ANTI-dsDNA ANTIBODY TEST, IgG ●

Normal Values
Negative: <25 IU by ELISA
Borderline: 25–30 IU
Positive: 31–200 IU
Strongly positive: >200 IU

Background
Although not completely understood, the primary mechanism of tissue injury in SLE and related autoimmune disease is the formation of antigen-antibody immune complexes. Not all ANAs are pathogenic. For the few that are harmful, pathogenicity depends on the specific immunoglobulin class, ability to activate complement, size of the immune complex, and site of tissue deposition. For example, studies of immune complex–mediated tissue injury in the kidney have shown a clear relation between deposition of immune complexes and glomerular disease.

Explanation of Test
The anti-dsDNA test is done specifically to identify or differentiate native (ie, double-stranded) DNA antibodies, found in 40% to 60% of patients with SLE

during the active phase of their disease, from other nonnative DNA antibodies found in other rheumatic diseases. The presence of antibodies to dsDNA generally correlates with lupus nephritis. An anti-dsDNA test supports a diagnosis, allows monitoring of disease activity and response to therapy, and establishes a prognosis for SLE.

Procedure
1. Collect a 7-ml blood serum sample in a red-topped tube. Observe standard precautions.

Clinical Implications
1. Anti-dsDNA concentrations may decrease with successful therapy and may increase with an acute recurrence of SLE.
2. DNA–anti-dsDNA immune complexes play a role in SLE pathogenesis through the deposit of these complexes in the kidney and other tissues.

Interfering Factors
The Farr assay, an RIA method, detects both single-stranded (ss) as well as double-stranded (ds) DNA antibodies. Antibodies to ssDNA are nonspecific but are associated with various other rheumatic diseases.

Patient Preparation and Aftercare
See special section for collagen and rheumatic disease tests (pp. 629 and 630).

ANTIBODIES TO EXTRACTABLE NUCLEAR ANTIGENS (ENAs): ANTIRIBONUCLEOPROTEIN (RNP); ANTI-SMITH (Sm); ANTI–SJÖGREN'S SYNDROME (SSA, SSB) ●

Normal Values
Expected Valves by ELISA:
Negative: <20 Units
Borderline: 20–25 Units
Positive: ≥26 Units

Background
The extractable nuclear antigens (ENAs), another group of nuclear antigens (nonhistone proteins) to which autoantibodies may develop, are so named because of their presence in saline solution extracts of certain nonhuman cells. The most common ENAs are ribonucleoprotein (RNP) and Smith (Sm). Antibodies to RNP are present in patients with a combination of overlapping rheumatologic symptoms known as mixed connective tissue disease (MCTD).

Explanation of Test
These tests are indicated for differential diagnosis of SLE, scleroderma, rheumatoid arthritis, and Sjögren's syndrome. They are done to correctly identify a

specific autoantibody directed against nuclear antigens composed of nonhistone proteins. All four of these antibodies produce a finely speckled pattern of nuclear fluorescence in the ANA test. Anti-RNP detection is helpful in the differential diagnosis of systemic rheumatic disease and is a useful follow-up for collagen vascular autoimmune disorders. The test for anti-Sm is highly diagnostic of SLE and is also used as a follow-up test for collagen vascular disorders. SSA and SSB antibody detection is particularly useful when an "ANA-negative" case of SLE is expected.

Procedure

1. Collect a 7-ml blood serum sample in a red-topped tube. Observe standard precautions.

Clinical Implications

1. A high level of RNP antibodies is an outstanding feature of MCTD.
2. Antibodies to the Sm antigen occur in SLE and are a specific marker for the disease.
3. The SSA/Ro and SSB/La antigens have a physical affinity for each other; patients frequently have antibodies to both. SSA antibodies may be found in Sjögren's syndrome alone or in Sjögren's syndrome associated with SLE. Persons with both Sjögren's and rheumatoid arthritis have neither SSA or SSB antibodies. They tend to develop antibodies against the Epstein-Barr virus associated with rheumatoid arthritis nuclear antigen (RANA).

Patient Preparation and Aftercare

See special section on collagen, rheumatic, and connective tissue diseases tests (pp. 629 and 630).

ANTISCLERODERMA (Scl-70) ANTIBODY TEST ●

Normal Values

Expected values by ELISA:
Negative: < 20 Units
Borderline: 20–25 Units
Positive: ≥26 Units

Background

Scl-70 is a nuclear antigen which may cause autoantibodies to develop against it. It is a nonhistone protein. Anti–Scl-70 antibodies are commonly found in scleroderma patients with extensive cutaneous disease and interstitial pulmonary fibrosis.

Explanation of Test

This is a follow-up test for diagnosing vascular collagen diseases, especially for cases of suspected scleroderma. Scl-70 antibodies are seen in up to 60% of patients with diffuse scleroderma. These antibodies produce a fine speckled pattern, with or without nucleolar staining, in the fluorescent ANA test.

Procedure

1. Collect a 7-ml blood serum sample in a red-topped tube. Observe standard precautions.

Clinical Implications

1. The Scl-70 antibody is present in scleroderma but is rarely present in other rheumatic diseases (eg, SLE, rheumatoid arthritis, Sjögren's syndrome). Testing is not useful in patients without demonstrable antinuclear antibodies.

Patient Preparation and Aftercare

See special section on collagen and rheumatic disease tests (pp. 629 and 630).

TOTAL HEMOLYTIC COMPLEMENT (CH50) ●

Normal Values

25–110 U/ml by hemolytic tube titration

Background

Complement (C) is a complex sequential cascade system in which inactive proteins become active and interact very much like the clotting system. The complement system is very important as part of the body's defense mechanism against infection. Activation of complement results in cell lysis, release of histamine from mast cells and platelets, increased vascular permeability, contraction of smooth muscle, and chemotaxis of leukocytes. These inactive proteins constitute about 10% of the globulins in normal blood serum. The complement system is also interrelated with the coagulation, fibrinolytic, and kinin systems. The action of complement, however, is not always beneficial. The potent reactions mediated by this complex system are not always contained. In the presence of gram-negative bacteremia, the complement can escape its built-in control mechanisms, causing severe damage to the body. It is not clear how this happens, but it is known that complement abnormalities develop before shock occurs.

Explanation of Test

This test screens for certain autoimmune diseases, estimates the extent of immune complex formation, and detects all inherited and most acquired immune deficiencies. Serial measurements monitor disease course and treatment in SLE, rheumatoid arthritis, and glomerulonephritis. It is a useful adjunct for rheumatoid factor and SLE testing when immune complexes appear to be the primary mediators of tissue injury.

Procedure

1. Collect a 7-ml blood serum sample in a red-topped tube. Observe standard precautions. A joint fluid specimen of at least 1 ml can also be used and should be collected in a tube that does not contain additives.

> **Clinical Alert**
>
> Complement deteriorates at room temperature in serum or fluid; samples should be brought to the laboratory as soon as possible. Separate serum from clot and freeze at ~ 70°C until test is performed. Both blood and fluid must be processed and frozen within 2 hours after specimen collection. Failure to process the specimen in this manner may lead to falsely decreased functional activity levels.

Clinical Implications

1. *Increased total complement values* are associated with most inflammatory responses; these acquired elevations are usually transient, and concentrations return to normal when the situation is resolved.
2. *Decreased total complement values* are associated with hereditary defects of specific complement components. In C2 deficiency, autoimmune disorders occur as SLE, and C1q deficiency may cause agammaglobulinemia. Lack of one of the complement system inhibitors such as cholinesterase inhibitor occurs in hereditary angioedema.
   a. Complement consumption by activation of the alternative pathway, an amplification of the classical pathway not requiring an "immunologic" stimulus, can be seen in the following conditions:
      (1) Gram-negative septicemia
      (2) Subacute bacterial endocarditis
      (3) Acute poststreptococcal glomerulonephritis
      (4) Membranoproliferative glomerulonephritis
   b. Complement consumption due to activation of the classical pathway by immune complex formation occurs in the following conditions:
      (1) SLE
      (2) Serum sickness
      (3) Acute vasculitis
      (4) Severe rheumatoid arthritis
      (5) Hepatitis
      (6) Cryoglobulinemia

Patient Preparation and Patient Aftercare

See special section on collagen and rheumatic disease diagnosis on pp. 629 and 630.

C3 COMPLEMENT COMPONENT

Normal Values

70–150 mg/dl by rate nephelometry

Background

C3 comprises 70% of the total protein in the complement system and is essential to the activation of both classical and alternative pathways. Along with the other components of the complement system, C3 may be used up in re-actions that occur in some antigen-antibody reactions. C3 is synthesized in liver, macrophages, fibroblasts, lymphoid cells, and skin.

Explanation of Test

This test is done when it is suspected that individual complement component concentrations are abnormally reduced. This test, along with C1q and C4, are the most frequently ordered complement measurements. There is a correlation between most forms of nephritis, the degree of nephritis severity, and C3 levels.

Procedure

1. Collect a 7-ml blood serum sample in a red-topped tube. Observe standard precautions. This amount is sufficient for both C3 and C4 testing.

Clinical Implications

1. *Decreased C3 levels* are associated with most active diseases with immune complex formation.
   a. Severe recurrent bacterial infections due to C3 homozygous deficiency
   b. Absence of C3b inactivator factor
   c. Acute poststreptococcal glomerulonephritis
   d. Immune complex disease
   e. Active SLE
   f. Membranoproliferative glomerulonephritis
   g. Autoimmune hemolytic anemia
   h. Nephritis
   i. Rheumatoid arthritis
   j. Disseminated intravascular coagulation disorder
   k. Liver disease
2. *Increased levels* are found in numerous inflammatory states.

Patient Preparation and Patient Aftercare

See special section on collagen and rheumatic disease diagnosis on pp. 629 and 630.

> ### Clinical Alert
>
> Patients with low C3 levels are in danger of shock leading to death.

C4 COMPLEMENT COMPONENT

Normal Values

10–30 mg/dl by rate nephelometry

Background

C4 is another of the components of the complement system and is synthesized in bone and lung tissue. C4 may be bypassed in the alternative complement pathway when immune complexes are not involved, or it may be used up in the very complicated series of reactions that follow many antigen-antibody reactions.

Explanation of Test
This is a follow-up test done when total complement levels are abnormally decreased.

Procedure
Collect a 7-ml blood serum sample in a red-topped tube. Observe standard precautions. This amount is sufficient for both C3 and C4 testing.

Clinical Implications
1. *Decreased C4 levels* are associated with the following conditions:
   a. Acute SLE
   b. Early glomerulonephritis
   c. Immune complex disease
   d. Cryoglobulinemia
   e. Inborn C4 deficiency
   f. Hereditary angioneurotic edema
2. *Increased C4 levels* are associated with malignancies.

Patient Preparation and Patient Aftercare
See special section on collagen and rheumatic disease diagnosis on pp. 629 and 630.

C′1 ESTERASE INHIBITOR (C′1 INH) ●

Normal Values
Values are determined by radical immunodiffusion (RID); results are reported as functional or nonfunctional. A nonfunctional result is consistent with hereditary angioedema.

Background
C′1 esterase inhibitor is a glycoprotein. It acts as a regulatory brake on the complement activation process. Decreased production of this glycoprotein results in hereditary angioedema (HAE).

Explanation of Test
This determination is an important tool for diagnosing HAE, a disorder caused by a low concentration of C esterase inhibitor or by an abnormal structure of the protein. Affected persons are apparently heterozygous for the condition. It is also used in the differential diagnosis of the more prevalent but less serious allergic and nonfamilial angioedema.

Procedure
1. Collect a 7-ml blood serum sample in a red-topped tube. Observe standard precautions.

2. Spin down, separate from clot, and freeze 1.0 ml of serum at $-70°C$ until testing is performed.

Clinical Implications

1. Decreased values are associated with HAE, a genetic disease characterized by acute edema of subcutaneous tissue, gastrointestinal tract, or upper respiratory tract. During acute attacks of the disease, C4 and C2 components can be markedly reduced.

Patient Preparation and Patient Aftercare

1. See special section on collagen and rheumatic disease diagnosis on pp. 629 and 630.

Clinical Alert

Prednisolone and transfusions of fresh frozen plasma have been successfully used to treat HAE.

RHEUMATOID FACTOR (RHEUMATOID ARTHRITIS [RA] FACTOR)

Normal Values

Nonreactive: 0–39 IU/ml based on rate nephelometry
Weakly reactive: 40–79 IU/ml
Reactive: >80 IU/ml

Background

The blood of many persons with rheumatoid arthritis contains a macroglobulin-type antibody called rheumatoid factor (RF). Evidence indicates that rheumatoid factors are anti–gamma globulin antibodies; however, until a specific antigen that produces RF is discovered, the exact nature of RF can only be speculated. Even more uncertain is the role that RF plays in rheumatoid arthritis. Although RF may cause or perpetuate the destructive changes associated with rheumatoid arthritis, it may also be incidental to these changes or may even serve some beneficial purpose. RF is sometimes found in blood serum from patients with other diseases, even though RF incidence and values are higher in patients with rheumatoid arthritis.

Explanation of Test

This test is useful in the diagnosis of rheumatoid arthritis. It measures rheumatoid factors (antibodies directed against the Fc fragment of IgG). These are usually IgM antibodies, but they may also be IgG or IgA. Four of the following clinical criteria must be present to diagnose rheumatoid arthritis.

Revised American College of Rheumatology Criteria for Rheumatoid Arthritis
1. Morning stiffness for at least 6 weeks

2. Pain on motion or tenderness in at least one joint for at least 6 weeks
3. Swelling in at least one joint for at least 6 weeks
4. Swelling in at least one other joint for at least 6 weeks
5. Symmetrical joint swelling with simultaneous involvement of the same joint on both sides of the body
6. Subcutaneous nodules
7. X-ray changes, including bony decalcification

Procedure
1. Collect a 7-ml blood serum sample in a red-topped tube. Observe standard precautions.

Clinical Implications
1. When a patient who tests positive improves, subsequent tests also remain positive unless titers were initially low.
2. A positive RA factor test result often supports a tentative diagnosis of early-onset rheumatoid arthritis (eg, versus rheumatic fever).
3. Rheumatoid factors frequently occur in a variety of other diseases such as SLE; endocarditis; tuberculosis; syphilis; sarcoidosis; cancer; viral infections; diseases affecting the liver, lung, or kidney; and Sjögren's syndrome and in patients who have received skin and renal allografts.
4. Absence of RA factor does not exclude the diagnosis or existence of rheumatoid arthritis.

Interfering Factors
The result is normally higher in older patients and in those who have received multiple vaccinations and transfusions.

Patient Preparation and Aftercare
See special section on collagen and rheumatic disease tests (pp. 629 and 630).

THYROID ANTIBODY GROUP, ANTITHYROGLOBULIN AND ANTIMICROSOMAL ●

Normal Values
Antimicrosomal: <1:100 by gelatin particle agglutination
Antithyroglobulin: <1:100 by gelatin particle agglutination

Background
Antibodies to thyroid gland components occur in various thyroid disorders (70%–90% with chronic thyroiditis; lesser percentages in other thyroid diseases). A number of autoantibodies are involved, including one reaction against thyroglobulin and another against the microsomal component of thyroid epithelial cells. In certain destructive thyroid diseases, intact thyroglobulin may be released

from the thyroid gland, stimulating antibody formation. These antibodies may be responsible for further destruction of this gland. Antibody production may exist only in lymphocytes within the thyroid, and serum may be negative.

Explanation of Test

These studies detect elevated thyroid antibodies in certain thyroid diseases such as Hashimoto's disease and primary myxedema. When tests for both thyroglobulin antibodies and thyroid microsomal antibodies are done in combination, the specificity for detection of thyroid autoimmune antibodies is greatly increased and is more sensitive than a single test when used for detection. Patients with low thyroid antibody titers should be tested periodically, because the presence of the antibody may be an early sign of autoimmune disease. Both tests should be performed together before thyroid surgery.

Procedure

Collect a 7-ml blood serum sample in a red-topped tube. Observe standard precautions.

Clinical Implications

1. High titers of both antibodies (>1:400) are found in Hashimoto's disease, but elevations can also be seen in other autoimmune diseases. Patients with Hashimoto's thyroiditis have a higher frequency of other autoimmune disorders (eg, Sjögren's syndrome, SLE).
2. Increased thyroid antibodies also occur in the following conditions:
   a. Graves' disease
   b. Thyroid carcinoma
   c. Idiopathic myxedema
   d. Pernicious anemia
   e. SLE, RA, Sjögren's syndrome
   f. Subacute thyroiditis
   g. Nontoxic nodular goiter
3. The presence of microsomal antibodies indicates an increased risk for later development of hypothyroidism.
4. The absence of both thyroglobular and microsomal antibodies rules out autoimmune thyroid disease.
5. The microsomal antibody test is more sensitive than the thyroglobulin test for Hashimoto's or Graves' disease.

Interfering Factors

1. About 10% of the normal population may have low titers of thyroid antibodies with no symptoms of disease. Incidence of low titer is higher in women and increases with age.
2. Excessive specimen hemolysis and lipemic or chylous specimens alter results.
3. Antibody production may be confined to lymphocytes within the thyroid, resulting in negative serum test results.

Patient Preparation

1. Explain test purpose. Thyroid antibody group testing is done to confirm diagnosis and monitor the course of disease activity.
2. Follow guidelines in Chapter 1 regarding safe, effective, informed *pretest* care.

Patient Aftercare

1. Interpret test outcomes and determine the need for possible follow-up testing. Diagnosis of autoimmune thyroiditis is made on the basis of clinical observations, thyroid function tests (see Chap. 6), and the presence of circulating autoantibodies (eg, antithyroglobulin, antimicrosomal).
2. Follow guidelines in Chapter 1 regarding safe, effective, informed *posttest* care.

ANTI–SMOOTH MUSCLE ANTIBODY (ASMA) TEST

Normal Values

Negative by indirect immunofluorescence
If positive, serum is titered

Background

ASMA is associated with liver and bile duct autoimmune diseases. The immune response itself is believed to be responsible for the disease process.

Explanation of Test

This measurement differentiates chronic active hepatitis and primary biliary cirrhosis from other liver diseases in which ASMAs are seldom present (eg, SLE).

Procedure

1. Collect a 7-ml blood serum sample in a red-topped tube. Observe standard precautions. This amount is sufficient for both ASMA and antimitochondrial antibody (AMA) testing.

Clinical Implications

1. ASMAs are found in chronic active hepatitis, a progressive disease of unknown etiology found predominantly in young women. It has factors characteristic of both acute and chronic hepatitis (80% of patients). If this disease is associated with a positive ANA test, the disease is often called lupoid hepatitis.
2. ASMAs are seldom present in the following conditions:
   a. Extrahepatic biliary obstruction
   b. Drug-induced liver disease
   c. Acute alcoholic hepatitis
   d. Hepatoma

TABLE 8-4
Prevalence of Autoantibodies in Liver Disease

Disease	Anti–Smooth Muscle (%)	Antimitochondrial (%)	ANA (%)
Chronic active hepatitis	70–90	30–60	60
Chronic persistent hepatitis	45	15–20	15–30
Acute viral hepatitis	10–30	5–20	20
Acute alcoholic hepatitis	0	0	0
Biliary cirrhosis	30	60–70	5
Cryptogenic cirrhosis	15	30	0
Alcoholic (Laennec's) cirrhosis	0	0	0
Extrahepatic biliary obstruction	5–10	5–10	5

Patient Preparation

1. Explain test purpose and procedure.
2. Follow guidelines in Chapter 1 regarding safe, effective, informed *pretest* care.

Patient Aftercare

1. Interpret test outcomes and monitor appropriately. Detection of ASMA by immunofluorescence assists in determining the presence of chronic active hepatitis and need for therapy when used in conjunction with other laboratory tests such as those used to evaluate liver enzymes, ANAs, and IgG levels. All of these are elevated in the majority of patients with chronic active hepatitis.
2. Follow guidelines in Chapter 1 regarding safe, effective, informed *posttest* care.

ANTIMITOCHONDRIAL ANTIBODY (AMA) TEST

Normal Values

Negative by indirect immunofluorescence
If positive, serum is titered

Background

AMA is non–organ- and non–species-specific and is directed against a lipoprotein in the inner mitochondrial membrane. The AMAs are predominantly of the IgG class; however, they have not been proven directly to cause liver cell or bile duct destruction.

Explanation of Test

This measurement aids in the diagnosis of primary biliary cirrhosis (PBC). PBC is a progressive disease most commonly seen in women in the second half of their reproductive years.

Procedure

1. Collect a 7-ml blood serum sample in a red-topped tube. Observe standard precautions. This amount is sufficient for both AMA and ASMA testing.

Clinical Implications

1. Elevated concentrations of AMAs are present in >80% of patients with primary biliary cirrhosis.
2. High titers are also associated with long-standing hepatic obstruction, chronic hepatitis, and cryptogenic cirrhosis.
3. Elevated levels are occasionally present in the following conditions:
   a. SLE
   b. Rheumatoid arthritis
   c. Thyroid disease
   d. Pernicious anemia
   e. Idiopathic Addison's disease

Patient Preparation

1. Explain test purpose and procedure.
2. Follow guidelines in Chapter 1 regarding safe, effective, informed *pretest* care.

Patient Aftercare

1. Interpret test outcomes and monitor appropriately. Immunofluorescence testing, along with quantitation of IgM and liver enzymes, both of which tend to be elevated in PBC, are reliable follow-up protocols.
2. Follow guidelines in Chapter 1 regarding safe, effective, informed *posttest* care.

ANTIPARIETAL CELL ANTIBODY (APCA) TEST

Normal Values

Negative for APCA by indirect immunofluorescence
If positive, serum is titered

Background

The disruption of normal intrinsic factor production or function due to autoimmune processes can lead to pernicious anemia. Antibodies to two antigens of the gastric parietal cell—antiparietal cell antibodies (APCAs) and intrinsic factor antibodies—are found in pernicious anemia.

Explanation of Test

This measurement is helpful in diagnosing chronic gastric disease and differentiating autoimmune pernicious anemia from other megaloblastic anemias. Persons with other anemias do not have detectable APCAs.

Procedure

1. Collect a 7-ml blood serum sample in a red-topped tube. Observe standard precautions.

Clinical Implications

1. APCAs occur in >80% of patients with autoimmune pernicious anemia; 50% have antibodies to intrinsic factor.
2. Occasionally, APCAs are present in the following conditions:
   a. Gastric ulcer
   b. Gastric cancer
   c. Atrophic gastritis
   d. Thyroid disease
   e. Diabetes mellitus

Interfering Factors

APCAs are present in many healthy adults >60 years of age.

Patient Preparation

1. Explain test purpose and procedure.
2. Follow guidelines in Chapter 1 regarding safe, effective, informed *pretest* care.

Patient Aftercare

1. Interpret test outcomes and monitor appropriately. Detection of APCA may suggest need for more invasive testing, ie, gastric biopsy to rule out gastrointestinal disease.
2. Follow guidelines in Chapter 1 regarding safe, effective, informed *posttest* care.

ANTIGLOMERULAR BASEMENT MEMBRANE (AGBM) ANTIBODY TEST

Normal Values

Negative: <5 EU/ml by enzyme immunoassay (EIA)
Borderline: 5.1–20.0 EU/ml
Positive: 20.1–400 EU/ml

Background

Antibodies specific for renal structural components such as the glomerular basement membrane of the kidney can bind to respective tissue-fixed antigens to produce an immune response.

Explanation of Test

This test is primarily used in the differentiating glomerular nephritis induced by antiglomerular basement membrane antibodies (AGBMs), from other types of glomerular nephritis. AGBMs cause about 5% of glomerular nephritis; about two thirds of these patients may also develop pulmonary hemorrhage (Goodpasture's syndrome).

Procedure

1. Collect a 7-ml blood serum sample in a red-topped tube. Observe standard precautions.

Clinical Implications

1. AGBM antibodies are detected in the following conditions:
   a. AGBM glomerular nephritis
   b. Tubulointerstitial nephritis
   c. AGBM Goodpasture's syndrome
   d. Some patients with SLE

Patient Preparation

1. Explain test purpose and procedure.
2. Follow guidelines in Chapter 1 regarding safe, effective, informed *pretest* care.

Patient Aftercare

1. Interpret test outcomes and need for follow-up testing and treatments that involve immunosuppressants and plasmapheresis, which are effective if treatment is started before renal failure is well advanced.
2. Follow guidelines in Chapter 1 regarding safe, effective, informed *posttest* care.

ACETYLCHOLINE RECEPTOR (AChR) BINDING ANTIBODY TEST

Normal Values

Negative for AChR or ≤0.02 nmol/L by RIA

Background

Acetylcholine receptor antibodies (AChRs) appear in myasthenia gravis (MG). It is believed that this disease involves destruction by the muscle cells of acetylcholine receptors bound by antibodies at the skeletal muscle motor endplate.

Explanation of Test

This measurement is considered to be the first-order test for MG in symptomatic patients. It also helps in managing response to immunosuppressive therapy. Second- and third-order tests for modulating and blocking antibodies, respectively, are ordered to confirm the diagnosis of acquired MG, distinguish acquired disease from congenital disease, and monitor the serologic process in the course of MG.

Procedure

1. Collect a 7-ml blood serum sample in a red-topped tube. Observe standard precautions.

Clinical Implications

1. AChR antibodies are found in ~ 90% of persons with generalized MG, 70% of persons with ocular MG, and 80% of persons in remission. These findings confirm the autoimmune nature of the disease.
2. Patients who have only eye symptoms tend to have lower titers than those with generalized myasthenia symptoms.

Interfering Factors

Positive results can be found in patients with Lambert-Eaton myasthenic syndrome (LES) or autoimmune liver disease.

Patient Preparation

1. Explain test purpose. Assess for history of immunosuppressive drug treatment. Detection of acetylcholine receptor binding antibody is infrequent in such cases.
2. Follow guidelines in Chapter 1 regarding safe, effective, informed *pretest* care.

Patient Aftercare

1. Interpret test outcomes and possible need for other testing. Other tests now available to aid in the serologic diagnosis of MG include acetylcholine receptor blocking antibodies, acetylcholine receptor modulating antibody, and striational antibodies. These are ordered according to presentation of neurologic symptoms. All of these antibodies are less frequently detected in the early stages of MG (within 1 year of onset) and in patients treated with immunosuppressive drugs. None are found in cases of congenital MG.
2. Follow guidelines in Chapter 1 regarding safe, effective, informed *posttest* care.

IgE ANTIBODY, SINGLE ALLERGEN ●

Normal Values

Based on fluorescence enzyme immunoassay (FEIA), the fluorescence is proportional to the amount of specific IgE present in the patient's sample.

Class	Interpretation
0	Negative
1	Equivocal
2	Positive
3	Positive
4	Strongly positive
5	Strongly positive
6	Strongly positive

Background

A large number of substances have been found to have allergic potential. Measurements of IgE antibodies are useful to establish the presence of allergic diseases and to define the allergen specificity of immediate hypersensitivity reactions. The patient's serum should first be screened with a selected panel of five allergens and then followed, if appropriate, by an extended panel of additional allergens.

Explanation of Test

This study tests for reactions to certain respiratory and food allergy stimulants. The FEIA tests measure the increase and quantity of allergen-specific immunoglobulin-E antibodies and diagnoses an allergy to a specific allergen (eg, molds, weeds, foods, insects). These measurements are used in persons, especially children, with extrinsic asthma, hay fever, and atopic eczema and are an accurate and convenient alternative to skin testing. Although more expensive, they do not cause hypersensitivity reactions.

Additional antigens are continually being added; up-to-date information should be sought. Examples of categories that can be tested for include grasses, trees, molds, venoms, weeds, animal dander, foods, house dust, mites, antibiotics, and insects.

Procedure

1. Collect a 7-ml blood serum sample in a red-topped tube. Observe standard precautions.
2. Spin down and separate at least 0.5 ml serum for each group of five allergens.

Clinical Implications

1. Positive results greater than or equal to class 2 are strongly associated with allergic symptoms on exposure to allergen.

Patient Preparation

1. Explain test purpose and procedure.
2. Follow guidelines in Chapter 1 regarding safe, effective, informed *pretest* care.

Patient Aftercare

1. Interpret test outcomes and counsel appropriately regarding results and need for other tests.
2. Follow guidelines in Chapter 1 regarding safe, effective, informed *posttest* care.

LATEX ALLERGY TESTING (LATEX-SPECIFIC IgE)

Normal Values:

Negative: <0.35 or 0 IU/ml based on EIA microplate assay
1: Equivocal
2 or 3: Positive
4, 5, or 6: Strongly positive

Background

Latex-containing medical devices include gloves, catheters, and bandages, among many others. Millions of people, especially those in the health care profession, are susceptible to allergic reactions ranging from mild to severe when exposed to such products. It is recommended that patients at risk for latex allergy be tested before undergoing medical procedures that would expose them to latex. High-risk groups include health care workers, workers with industrial exposure to latex, children with spina bifida or urologic abnormalities due to high exposure to latex, and people who have undergone multiple surgeries.

Explanation of Test

A latex-specific IgE test has been on the market for some time and has been evaluated in clinically defined populations. The method for testing is an EIA in which the color reaction measured is directly related to the amount of IgE specific for the test allergen in the sample.

Procedure

1. Collect a 7-ml blood serum sample in a red-topped tube. Observe standard precautions.

Clinical Implications

1. Positive results are strongly associated with a latex allergy.
2. In studies comparing latex-specific IgE results with clinical history, symptoms, and other confirmatory tests, the sensitivity has been >90% and the specificity >80%.

Patient Preparation

1. Explain test purpose and procedure. Positive history for latex may include the following factors:
   a. Swelling or itching from latex exposure
   b. Hand eczema
   c. Previously unexplained anaphylaxis
   d. Oral itching from cross-reactive foods (eg, banana, kiwi, avocado, chestnuts)
   e. Multiple surgical procedures in infancy.
2. Follow guidelines in Chapter 1 regarding safe, effective, informed *pretest* care.

Patient Aftercare

1. Interpret test outcomes based on patient's clinical history (ie, latex exposure and laboratory reference values). If negative by this test procedure yet symptomatic or if positive for this test, refer patient to an allergist.
2. Follow guidelines in Chapter 1 regarding safe, effective, informed *posttest* care.

CARDIOLIPIN ANTIBODIES, IgG AND IgM ●

Normal Values
Negative by EIA
If positive, results are titered

Background
Antiphospholipid antibodies react with most negatively charged phospholipids, including cardiolipin. Additionally, antiphospholipid antibodies are known to prolong in vitro phospholipid-dependent coagulation tests and have been historically referred to as the "lupus anticoagulant."

Explanation of Test
The test most commonly assesses risk of thrombosis in the presence of SLE.

Procedure
1. Collect a 7-ml blood serum sample in a red-topped tube. Observe standard precautions.

Clinical Implications
1. Cardiolipin antibodies (aCL) are frequently found in SLE and other autoimmune diseases. Elevated levels of aCL antibodies appear to be associated with venous or arterial thrombosis, thrombocytopenia, and recurrent fetal loss. The term "antiphospholipid syndrome" describes patients who present with these features in association with aCL antibodies or the lupus anticoagulant.
2. Patients with current or prior syphilis infections may have a false-positive result without the risk of thrombosis.
3. Anticardiolipin antibodies can be transient during many infections. Repeat the test after 6 months. The β_2-glycoprotein test is still for research use only but should prove to be a more specific assay because it eliminates phospholipid cross-reactivity.

Patient Preparation
1. Explain test purpose and procedure.
2. Follow guidelines in Chapter 1 regarding safe, effective, informed *pretest* care.

Patient Aftercare
1. Interpret test outcomes in light of the patient's history, physical findings, and other diagnostic procedures and results. If clinical findings suggest the presence of antiphospholipid antibodies and the absence of anticardiolipin antibodies, some recommend testing for the lupus anticoagulant to confirm the negative result. A patient is considered positive for antiphospholipid antibodies if one or both of the tests are positive.
2. Follow guidelines in Chapter 1 regarding safe, effective, informed *posttest* care.

ANTI-INSULIN ANTIBODY TEST

Normal Values
<3% binding of the patient's serum with labeled beef, human and pork insulin when performed by RIA

Background
Persons with diabetes may form antibodies to the insulin they take and require larger doses because insulin is not available for glucose metabolism when it is partially complexed with these antibodies. Insulin antibodies are immunoglobulins called anti-insulin AB; they act as insulin-transporting proteins. The most common type of anti-insulin AB is IgG, but it is found in all five classes of immunoglobulins in insulin-treated patients. These immunoglobulins, especially IgE, may be responsible for allergic manifestations; IgM may cause insulin resistance.

Explanation of Test
This insulin antibody level provides information for determining the most appropriate treatment for certain diabetic patients. It may focus the reason for allergic manifestations. It can identify a state of insulin resistance, in which the daily insulin requirement exceeds 200 U for >2 days, and may be associated with elevated anti-insulin antibody titers and insulin-binding capacity.

Procedure
1. Collect a 7-ml blood serum sample in a red-topped tube from a fasting patient. Observe standard precautions.

Clinical Implications
1. Anti-insulin antibody elevations are associated with insulin resistance and allergies to insulin.

Patient Preparation
1. Explain purpose of test. Fasting is required. Check with individual laboratory for time frames.
2. Follow guidelines in Chapter 1 regarding safe, effective, informed *pretest* care.

Patient Aftercare
1. Interpret test outcomes. Based on antibody levels present and clinical findings, the dosage of insulin is changed to reduce or prevent further allergic manifestations and/or insulin resistance.
2. Follow guidelines in Chapter 1 regarding safe, effective, informed *posttest* care.

GLIADIN, IgG, AND IgA ANTIBODIES ●

Normal Values
Values are given for ≥2 years of age
Negative: <25 U/ml
Weakly positive: 25-50 U/ml
Positive: >50 U/ml

Background

Antibodies to gliadin (wheat protein) have been shown conclusively to be the toxic agent in celiac disease. Originally, a series of multiple intestinal biopsies were required to diagnose celiac and related intestinal diseases. More recently, serologic testing has been strongly suggested for screening patients with suspected gluten-sensitive enteropathy as well as for monitoring dietary compliance.

Celiac disease usually begins in infancy soon after introduction of cereals to the diet, but symptoms may disappear spontaneously in later childhood, despite continued signs of malabsorption. Strict avoidance of gluten in the diet is recommended to control the disease.

Explanation of Test

Both IgG and IgA gliadin antibodies are detected in sera of patients with gluten-sensitive enteropathy. IgG antigliadin antibodies seem more sensitive but are less specific than the IgA class antibodies. The best strategy for at-risk populations includes testing for both classes of gliadin antibodies.

Procedure

1. Collect a 7-ml blood serum sample in a red-topped tube. Observe standard precautions.

Clinical Implications

1. The gliadin antibody assay has a sensitivity of 95% for active, untreated celiac patients when both IgG and IgA are used. The test has an overall specificity of 90%.
2. A negative IgA result in an untreated patient does not rule out gluten-sensitive enteropathy, especially when associated with elevated levels of IgG gliadin antibodies.
3. A significant portion of celiac patients are IgA deficient, which can serve as an explanation for this occurrence.
4. In treated patients known to express IgA antibodies, the IgA gliadin antibody level represents a better indicator of dietary compliance than the IgG level.
5. False-positive results (high antibody levels without the corresponding histologic features) are possible; other gastrointestinal disorders, especially Crohn's disease, postinfection malabsorption, and food protein intolerance (eg, cow's milk), are known to induce circulating antigliadin antibodies.
6. Results of this assay should be used in conjunction with clinical findings and other serologic tests.

Patient Preparation

1. Explain test purpose and procedure.
2. Follow guidelines in Chapter 1 regarding safe, effective, informed *pretest* care.

Patient Aftercare

1. Interpret test outcome in light of patient's dietary history, including related clinical, laboratory, and histologic data. Positive results are possible in patients with other gastrointestinal disorders.

2. Follow guidelines in Chapter 1 regarding safe, effective, informed *posttest* care.

CYTOPLASMIC NEUTROPHIL ANTIBODIES (ANCA)

Normal Values
Negative for ANCAs by indirect immunofluorescence testing (IFA). If positive for cANCA, results are quantitated. If positive for pANCA, "myeloperoxidase antibody" (MPO) testing is performed. Positive results are quantitated. Not all specimens positive for pANCA are MPO-positive.

Background
There are two types of cytoplasmic neutrophil antibodies distinguished by different immunofluorescent staining patterns using human neutrophil substrates:

1. cANCAs produce a diffuse cytoplasmic staining of neutrophils and monocytes and are specific for proteinase 3. cANCA is found in the sera of patients with Wegner's granulomatosis (WG).

2. pANCAs produce a perinuclear staining of neutrophils and are specific for other neutrophil enzymes including myeloperoxidase (MPO), elastase, and lactoferrin. pANCA specific for MPO is found in the sera of patients with systemic vasculitis, most of whom have renal involvement characterized by pauci-immune necrotizing glomerulonephritis.

Explanation of Test
Tests for ANCA are performed by an indirect immunofluorescent technique. Slides prepared from neutrophils are used as a substrate to bind ANCA so that it can be detected microscopically. Depending on the pattern of staining, as mentioned previously, two types of ANCAs exist: cANCA and pANCA.

Procedure
1. Collect a 7-ml blood serum sample in a red-topped tube. Observe standard precautions.

Clinical Implications
1. In patients with active generalized WG (pulmonary and/or renal involvement), the frequency of positive cANCA results approaches 85%. A negative test for cANCA does not rule out WG; however, false-positive results are rare.

2. In patients with known WG, rising titers of cANCA suggest relapse, and failing titers suggest successful treatment.

3. In patients with active renal disease, a positive pANCA suggests the presence of antibodies to MPO and pauci-immune necrotizing glomerulonephritis.

4. Results of tests for ANCA should be considered along with other clinical, laboratory, and histopathologic data in establishing the diagnosis of WG or systemic vasculitis.

Patient Preparation
1. Explain test purpose and procedure.
2. Follow guidelines in Chapter 1 regarding safe, effective, informed *pretest* care.

Patient Aftercare
1. Interpret test outcomes in light of the patient's history, including other clinical, laboratory, and histopathologic data. Positive ANCA results (pANCA and, rarely, cANCA) may occur in patients with diseases other than WG or vasculitis, including Goodpasture's syndrome and SLE.
2. Follow guidelines in Chapter 1 regarding safe, effective, informed *posttest* care.

ANTISPERM ANTIBODY TEST

Normal Values
Reported as percentage of sperm binding by immunobead technique; >20% binding is usually required to lower patient's fertility. Significance of percentage of binding is inversely related to patient's sperm count, antibody class involved, and site of sperm binding (sperm head, midpiece, or tail).

Background
The majority of infertile males have blocking of the efferent testicular ducts. It is likely that, similar to vasectomy, reabsorption of sperm from blocked ducts results in the formation of autoantibodies to sperm.

Explanation of Test
This test detects sperm antibodies as part of infertility investigation. Antibodies directed toward various sperm antigens can produce reduced male fertility. However, the precise nature of the immune response against sperm antigens and the particular type of antibody responsible is unknown.

Procedure
A semen test sample is preferred for values. If semen procurement presents a problem for a male patient, a blood serum sample can be tested. For females, blood serum is preferred because of the difficulty of cervical mucus collection.

Blood: Collect a 5-ml blood serum sample in a red-topped tube. Spin down and send 2.0 ml of serum to laboratory frozen in plastic vial or dry ice.
Semen: Collect contents of semen ejaculate. Send specimen to laboratory frozen in plastic vial on dry ice.
Cervical mucus: Collect 1.0 ml of cervical mucus. Send specimen to laboratory frozen in plastic vial on dry ice.

Clinical Implications
1. Antisperm antibodies are associated with the following conditions:
    a. Blocked testicular efferent ducts and the resultent resorption of sperm can produce antibodies.

b. After vasectomy, antibodies and probable cellular immunity to sperm develop in most males as a result of the interaction of sperm antigens with the immune system.

c. In some studies, ~ 75% of women with primary infertility had sperm agglutinins. However, 11% to 15% of pregnant women had the same sperm antibody titers.

Clinical Alert

The potential adverse consequences of an immune sperm response to sperm includes possible systemic effects in other organ systems and possible infertility after vasectomy reversal.

Patient Preparation

1. Explain test purpose and procedure. See details under Procedure for "Specimen Required." Patient should be advised of the need for repeat testing.

2. Follow guidelines in Chapter 1 regarding safe, effective, informed *pretest* care.

Patient Aftercare

1. Interpret test results and counsel appropriately. It may be necessary to repeat this procedure on different sample types (eg, semen, blood) to establish a possible cause for infertility.

2. Follow guidelines in Chapter 1 regarding safe, effective, informed *posttest* care.

ALZHEIMER'S DISEASE (AD) MARKERS: Tau/AB$_{42}$ ●

Reference Values

High Tau is consistent with Alzheimer's disease (AD); high AB$_{42}$ is not consistent with AD. An interpretation is included with test results.

Background

The microtubule-associated protein Tau is the major component of the neurofibrillary tangles in AD. Neurofibrillary tangles are considered a pathologic hallmark of AD. Concentration of brain tangles has been shown to correlate with the degree of dementia. High levels of Tau in cerebral spinal fluid (CSF) correlate strongly with the probability of AD.

The AB$_{42}$ peptide is produced following metabolism of the β-amyloid precursor protein. This peptide is now widely acknowledged as the key peptide deposited in amyloid plaques. The deposition of amyloid in plaques is an accepted measure of AD pathology. CSF levels of AB$_{42}$ are reduced in AD patients, possibly because the AB$_{42}$ is deposited in plaques rather than remaining in solution. High levels in CSF indicate that AD is not likely and that other causes of dementia should be explored.

Explanation of Test

Correlating Tau and AB_{42} results rule in or rule out AD with >95% specificity and 60% sensitivity in persons ≥60 years of age who have dementia. The test methodology is ELISA, and units are numerically reported in picograms per milliliter (pg/ml). An example of a high level of Tau is 900 pg/ml; an example of a low level of AB_{42} is 200 pg/ml.

Procedure

1. Collect a minimum 2-ml sample of spinal fluid in a sterile CSF collection tube. Discard the first milliliter of fluid as well as any blood-contaminated specimen. Keep the spinal fluid refrigerated, not frozen, during shipment and until the test can be performed.

Patient Preparation

1. Explain the test purpose and procedure necessary to obtain an adequate spinal fluid specimen (see Chap. 4 for protocols).
2. Follow guidelines in Chapter 1 regarding safe, effective, informed *pretest* care.

Patient Aftercare

1. Interpret test outcomes and counsel appropriately. As a result of performing this procedure, the diagnosis and understanding of Alzheimer's Disease may become clearer, and appropriate counseling and support to the patient and family may be provided with a higher degree of confidence. Measurement of these markers may help select patients for clinical trials and in identifying patients who may benefit from therapy.

● BLOOD BANKING OR IMMUNOHEMATOLOGY TESTS

These tests are done to select blood components that will have acceptable survival when transfused and to prevent possible transplant and transfusion reactions; to identify potential problems, such as hemolytic disease of newborns; need for intrauterine transfusion and to determine parentage. Immunohematology testing identifies highly reactive antigens on blood cells and their antibodies, possibly present in serum.

DONATED BLOOD TESTING AND BLOOD PROCESSING   ●

Testing of Blood Recipient and Donor Blood

All donated blood, as it is processed, must undergo several measurements. These include tests for the following factors:

1. ABO groups	6. Hepatitis C virus
2. Rh type	(anti-HCV)
3. Antibody screen	7. Syphilis (VDRL)
4. Hepatitis B surface antigen	8. HIV-1 and HIV-2
(HBsAg)	9. HTLV-I and HTLV-II
5. Hepatitis B core antigen (HBcAg)	10. HIV antigen (HIV-1-Ag)

Required testing for whole-blood or red blood cell recipients include the following:

1. ABO group
2. Rh type
3. Antibody screen
4. Crossmatch for compatibility between donor's cells and recipient's serum

Even though no crossmatch is needed for plasma administration, compatible ABO typing should be done. Routinely, no crossmatch is needed for platelet administration; compatible ABO and Rh typing should be done. If a patient becomes refractory, HLA-matched platelets may be administered. Granulocytes should be tested for HLA compatibility. Molecules described as Class I HLA gene products are found on the surface of platelets and most nucleated cells of the body. As a result of previous transfusions or pregnancy, some patients develop antibodies against these antigens and, if given incompatible blood, may have a transfusion reaction. Other donated blood testing and processing considerations regarding autologous and directed donations, cytomegalovirus tests, and blood product irradiation are presented in the following list.

1. *Autologous donations* are blood products donated by patients for their own use (ie, blood donor and recipient are the same person). Many patients opt to donate their own blood prior to scheduled surgery because of the concern regarding transfusion-transmitted diseases.
   The following are some general guidelines for autologous blood donation.
   a. There is no age limit if donor is healthy.
   b. There are no weight requirements. The volume of blood collected must comply with established weight provisions.
   c. Pregnant women can donate.
   d. Hematocrit should be ≥33%. If <33%, the patient's physician must approve the phlebotomy, usually in consultation with the blood bank medical director.
   e. Normally, phlebotomy can be done at 3-day intervals; the final phlebotomy can be done at least 72 hours before the time of the scheduled surgery. Iron supplements may be prescribed to maintain adequate hemoglobin levels.
2. *Allogeneic donations* are blood products donated by one individual for use by other individuals (ie, blood donor and blood recipient are not the same person).
3. *Directed donations* are those in which recipients choose those who donate blood for their transfusions. Laws in several states declare that this request must be honored in nonemergency situations. Standards and testing

procedures must be identical to those required for an allogeneic blood donor. (Autologous donors do not need to adhere to the same criteria as do allogeneic blood donors.)

4. *Cytomegalovirus (CMV) testing* is done for patients at risk for transfusion-associated CMV infections. These types of CMV infections were first seen as a mononucleosis syndrome after cardiopulmonary bypass surgery and were thought to be related to the use of fresh blood during the surgery. Clinical symptoms of transfusion-transmitted CMV infections include pneumonitis, hepatitis, retinitis, and disseminated infection. They generally occur in immunosuppressed patients such as premature infants weighing <1200 g at birth, bone marrow and organ transplant patients, and certain immunocompromised oncology patients. Therefore, to prevent these infections, CMV antibody testing is done. Patients at risk should receive CMV-seronegative blood and blood products. CMV in blood is associated with leukocytes. Leukocyte reduction using highly efficient leukocyte-reduction filters also appears to be an effective way of reducing CMV infection.

5. *Irradiation of blood products* is sometimes done prior to transfusion for certain immunosuppressed patients. Graft-versus-host disease (GVHD) is a rare complication that follows transfusion in severely immunosuppressed patients. GVHD occurs if donor lymphocytes from blood or blood products engraft and multiply in a severely immunodeficient recipient. The engrafted lymphocytes react against host (recipient) tissues. Clinical symptoms include skin rash, fever, diarrhea, hepatitis, bone marrow suppression, and infection which frequently leads to death. GVHD can be prevented by irradiating blood products with a minimum dose (cesium-137) of 2.5 cGy in the center of the container and a minimum dose of 1.5 cGy delivered to all other parts of the component. This practice renders the T lymphocytes in a unit of blood incapable of replication without affecting platelets or granulocytes. Irradiation does affect the red cell membrane, causing it to "leak" potassium. All irradiated red cells are given a 28-day "outdate" or may keep their original "outdate" of <28 days.

6. *Leukocyte reduction of blood products:* Leukocytes in blood products have long been known to be associated with nonhemolytic febrile transfusion reactions, possibly due more to cytokines produced by the leukocytes than the leukocytes themselves. Leukocyte reduction may reduce the number of these reactions. It may also decrease the possibility of alloimmunization to the HLA antigens on the leukocytes. Removing leukocytes effectively reduces the danger of transfusion-transmitted CMV infection.

BLOOD GROUPS (ABO GROUPS) ●

Normal Values

A

B

AB

O

Antigen Present on Red Blood Cell	Antibodies Present in Serum	Major Blood Group Designation	Distribution in the United States
None	Anti-A, Anti-B	O (universal donor* for red blood cells)	O (46%)
A	Anti-B	A	A (41%)
B	Anti-A	B	B (9%)
AB	None	AB (universal recipient† for red blood cells)	AB (4%)

*Called universal donor because no antigens are present on red blood cells; therefore, the person is able to donate to all blood groups.
†Called universal recipient because no serum antibodies are present; therefore, the person is able to receive blood from all blood groups.

Background

Human blood is grouped according to the presence or absence of specific blood group antigens (ABO). These antigens, found on the surface of red blood cells, can induce the body to produce antibodies. More than 300 distinct antigens have been identified. Compatibility of the ABO group is the foundation for all other pretransfusion testing.

Explanation of Test

All blood donors and potential blood recipients must be tested for blood type to prevent transfusion with incompatible blood products. Specifically linked sugars determine the antigenic activities named A and B. One sugar, *N*-acetylgalactosamine, gives the molecule A activity; another sugar, galactose, determines B activity. The backbone molecule, without galactose or *N*-acetylgalactosamine, has antigenic activity termed H. This H substance, as well as H gene activity, is essential for the function of the ABO antigens. The following chart lists the blood groups and their ABO antigens.

Blood Group	ABO Antigen
A	A
B	B
AB	A and B
O	Neither

In general, patients are transfused with blood of their own ABO group because antibodies against the other blood antigens may be present in their blood serum. These antibodies are designated anti-A or anti-B, depending on the antigen they act against. Under normal conditions, a person's blood serum does not contain the antibody specifically able to destroy its antigen. For example, a person with antigen A will not have anti-A antibodies in the serum; however, anti-B antibodies may be present. Therefore, antigen and antibody testing is necessary to confirm ABO grouping.

> ### Clinical Alert
>
> A transfusion reaction can be extremely serious and potentially fatal. Therefore, the blood group must be determined in vitro before any blood is transfused to an individual. Before blood administration, two health care professionals (ie, physicians or nurses) must check the recipient's blood group and type with the donor group and type to assure compatibility.

NOTE: *A blood group change or suppression may be induced by cancer, leukemia, or infection.*

Procedure

1. Collect a 7-ml venous clotted blood sample in a red-topped tube. Observe standard precautions. Do not use SST tubes (cell barrier tube).

Patient Preparation

1. Explain test purpose and procedure. The following are conditions that at some point may require transfusion:
   a. Malignant tumors (leukemias)
   b. Cardiac surgical procedures
   c. Surgical hip procedures
   d. Anemias
   e. Certain obstetrical or gynecological procedures or complications
   f. Bone and joint diseases
   g. Lung disease
   h. Kidney disease or genitourinary system surgical procedures
   i. Massive trauma
   j. Liver disease
   k. Certain blood dyscrasias
2. Follow guidelines in Chapter 1 regarding safe, effective, informed *pretest* care.

Patient Aftercare

1. Inform patient of blood group and interpret meaning. Rh type may have implications for the pregnant woman and fetus.

Incidence and Frequency of Blood Group and Rh Type		
Group and Type	*Incidence*	*Frequency of Occurrence (%)*
O-positive	1 in 3	37.4
O-negative	1 in 15	6.6
A-positive	1 in 3	35.7
A-negative	1 in 16	6.3
B-positive	1 in 12	8.5
B-negative	1 in 67	1.5
AB-positive	1 in 29	3.4
AB-negative	1 in 167	0.6

2. Follow guidelines in Chapter 1 regarding safe, effective, informed *posttest* care.

Rh TYPING

Normal Values: Incidence
Caucasian
  85% Rh-positive (have the Rh antigen)
  15% Rh-negative (lack the Rh antigen)
African American
  90% Rh-positive (have the Rh antigen)
  10% Rh-negative (lack the Rh antigen)

Background
Human blood is classified as Rh-positive or Rh-negative. This relates to the presence or the absence of the D antigen on the red cell membrane. The D antigen (now called Rh_1 [D]) is, after the A and B antigens, the next most important antigen in transfusion practice.

Explanation of Test
The Rh system is composed of antigens tested for in conjunction with the ABO group. Rh_1 (D) factor is often the only factor tested for. When this factor is absent, further typing is then done to identify any of the less common Rh antigens present before the person is identified as "Rh-negative." Rh-negative individuals may develop antibodies against Rh-positive antigens if they are challenged through a transfusion of Rh-positive blood or through a fetomaternal bleed from an Rh-positive fetus.

Need for Blood Rh Typing
Blood Rh typing must be done for the following reasons:

1. Rh-positive blood administered to an Rh-negative person may sensitize the person to form anti-D (Rh_1).
2. Rh_1 (D)–positive blood administered to a recipient having serum anti-D (Rh_1) could be fatal.

Comparison of Terms Used in Rh System Nomenclatures	
Weiner	*Fisher-Race*
Rh_1	D
Rh_2	C
Rh_3	E
Rh_4	c
Rh_5	e
Rh_6	f (ce)
Rh_{12}	G

3. RhIG (Rh immunoglobin) candidates must be identified. Rh immunoglobulin is a concentrated solution of IgG anti-D (Rh_1) derived from human plasma. A 1-ml dose of RhIG contains 300 µg and is sufficient to counteract the immunizing effects of 15 ml of packed red cells or 30 ml of whole blood.

    a. Rh-negative pregnant women with Rh-positive partners may carry Rh-positive fetuses. Fetal cells may cross the placenta to the mother and cause production of antibodies in the maternal blood. The maternal antibody, in turn, may cross through the placenta into the fetal circulation and cause destruction of fetal blood cells. This condition, called *hemolytic disease of the newborn* (formerly called erythroblastosis fetalis), may cause reactions that range from anemia (slight or severe) to fetal death in utero. This condition can be prevented if an Rh-negative pregnant woman receives an RhIG dose antepartum at 28 weeks' gestation and a postpartum injection of RhIG shortly after delivery of an Rh-D (Rh_1)–positive infant. Postpartum Rh immunization can occur despite an injection of RhIG if >30 ml of fetal blood enters the maternal circulation. The American Association of Blood Banks recommends that a postpartum blood specimen of all Rh-D (Rh_1)–negative women (ie, those at risk of immunization) be examined to detect a fetal maternal hemorrhage of >30 ml.

    b. Rh typing must also be done for patients who have had abortions, miscarriages, accidents, and amniocentesis.

Clinical Implications

1. The significance of Rh antigens is based on their capacity to immunize as a result of receiving a transfusion or becoming pregnant. The Rh_1 (D) antigen is by far the most antigenic; the other Rh antigens are much less likely to produce isoimmunization. The following general conditions must be met for immunization to Rh antigens to occur:

    a. The Rh blood antigen must be absent in the immunized person.

    b. The Rh blood antigen must be present in the immunizing blood.

    c. The blood antigen must be of sufficient antigenic strength to produce a reaction.

    d. The amount of incompatible blood must be large enough to induce antibody formation.

    e. Factors other than Rh_1 (D) may induce formation of antibodies in Rh-positive persons if the preceding conditions are met.

2. Antibodies for Rh_2 (C) are frequently found together with anti-Rh_1 (D) antibodies in the Rh-negative pregnant woman whose fetus or child is type Rh-positive and possesses both antigens.

3. With exceedingly rare exceptions, Rh antibodies do not form unless preceded by antigenic stimulation, as occurs with the following conditions:

    a. Pregnancy and abortions

    b. Blood transfusions

    c. Deliberate immunization, most commonly of repeated intravenous injections of blood for the purpose of harvesting a given Rh antibody

Patient Preparation
1. Explain purpose and procedure of Rh typing.
2. Follow guidelines in Chapter 1 regarding safe, effective, informed *pretest* care.

Patient Aftercare
1. Interpret test outcome. Inform and counsel patient regarding Rh type. Women of childbearing age may need special consideration. See page 660 for incidences of Rh types.
2. Follow guidelines in Chapter 1 regarding safe, effective, informed *posttest* care.

Rh ANTIBODY TITER TEST

Normal Values
Negative is 0 (no antibody detected)

Explanation of Test
This antibody study determines the Rh-antibody level in an Rh negative or pregnant woman whose partner is Rh-positive. If the Rh-negative woman is carrying an Rh-positive fetus, the antigen from the fetal blood cells causes antibody production in the mother's serum. The firstborn child usually shows no ill effects; however, with subsequent pregnancies, the mother's serum antibodies increase and eventually destroy the fetal red blood cells, causing hemolytic disease of the newborn.

Procedure
1. Obtain a 10-ml venous blood sample (plasma or serum) from the mother using a yellow-topped (ACD) and clotted blood (not SST) tube. Observe standard precautions.

Clinical Implications
Some institutions have established a critical titer for anti-D below which hemolytic disease of the newborn is considered unlikely. No further investigations are undertaken unless the critical titer level is reached.

Patient Preparation
1. Explain test purpose and procedure.
2. Follow guidelines in Chapter 1 regarding safe, effective, informed *pretest* care.

Patient Aftercare
1. Interpret test outcome and counsel appropriately.
2. Follow guidelines in Chapter 1 regarding safe, effective, informed *posttest* care.

ROSETTE TEST, FETAL RED CELLS (FETAL-MATERNAL BLEED) ●

Normal Values
Negative for fetal blood loss
No Rh-positive fetal red blood cells detected in maternal blood

Explanation of Test
This qualitative test detects Rh-positive fetal cells in the Rh-negative maternal circulation. The detection of fetal erythrocytes is important when it is suspected that a severe fetal red cell loss has occurred and when serious risk of the mother becoming immunized against the fetal red cell groups is anticipated. In these instances, the mother's blood sample should be collected immediately after delivery to be examined for fetal cells. This test can be performed only if mother is Rh-negative and newborn is known to be Rh-positive. The Rosette test is 97% accurate for detecting a fetomaternal bleed that exceeds 30 ml of whole blood.

Procedure
1. A 7-ml venous blood EDTA sample is obtained from the mother shortly after delivery. This test is performed and examined for rosettes or mixed field agglutinates. Following manufacturer's guidelines, the presence of rosettes above a predetermined number indicates a fetal bleed that exceeds 30 ml of whole blood.

Clinical Implications
1. When the test sample contains few or no Rh_1–positive fetal cells, rosetting or agglutination is absent, and the fetomaternal bleed is <30 ml, one dose of parenteral Rh immune globulin (RhIG) will prevent immunization. If the fetal blood loss into the maternal circulation exceeds 30 ml, a quantitative or semi-quantitative test (ie, Kleihauer-Betke) must be performed to calculate the amount of RhIG to administer.

Patient Preparation
1. Explain test purpose and procedure.
2. Follow guidelines in Chapter 1 regarding safe, effective, informed *pretest* care.

Patient Aftercare
1. Interpret test outcome. Counsel patient regarding RhIG administration and follow-up maternal testing.
2. Follow guidelines in Chapter 1 regarding safe, effective, informed *posttest* care.

KLEIHAUER-BETKE TEST (FETAL HEMOGLOBIN STAIN) ●

Normal Values
Negative: no fetal cells in maternal circulation

Explanation of Test

The Kleihauer-Betke test is a semi-quantitative test to determine the amount of fetomaternal hemorrhage in an Rh_1–negative mother and the amount of RhIG necessary to prevent antibody production. The test is done after full-term delivery if newborn anemia is present or when the mother is Rh-negative or weak-negative D. The test is also performed on mothers after invasive procedures (eg, amniocentesis), miscarriages, or traumas.

Procedure

1. A 7-ml maternal venous blood EDTA sample is obtained immediately after delivery, invasive procedure (eg, amniocentesis), miscarriage, or trauma. The specimen should be examined immediately or refrigerated until it can be examined.

Clinical Implications

1. Results indicate moderate to great fetomaternal hemorrhage (50%–90% of fetal red blood cells contain HgF).
2. With full-term delivery, newborn red blood cells must be Rh-D–positive for the Rh-D–negative mother to be a candidate for RhIG.

Patient Preparation

1. Explain test purpose and procedure.
2. Follow guidelines in Chapter 1 regarding safe, effective, informed *pretest* care.

Patient Aftercare

1. Interpret test outcomes and counsel parents appropriately regarding fetal bleed and administration of RhIG to suppress the immunization of fetal red cells or whole-blood hemorrhage (Table 8-5). The calculated dose is as follows:

$$\text{Vials of RhIG} = \frac{\text{ml of fetal blood}}{30}.$$

Many recommend doubling the calculated dose of RhIG. The method of calculating fetal blood is not entirely accurate. The results of undertreatment are serious but the effects of overtreatment are minor.
2. Follow guidelines in Chapter 1 regarding safe, effective, informed *posttest* care.

CROSSMATCH (COMPATIBILITY TEST) ●

Normal Values

Compatibility: no cell clumping or hemolysis, and absence of agglutination when serum and cells are appropriately mixed and incubated. The major crossmatch shows compatibility between recipient serum and donor cells.

Background

The primary purpose of the major crossmatch, or compatibility test, is to prevent a possible transfusion reaction.

TABLE 8-5
Recommendations for Dose of RhIG in Massive Fetomaternal Blood Based on the Acid Elution Test

| Fetal cells (%) | Fetomaternal Hemorrhage Volume (ml whole blood) | | Vials of RhIG to Inject |
	Average	Range*	
0.3–0.5	20	<50	2
0.6–0.8	35	15–80	3
0.9–1.1	50	22–110	4
1.2–1.4	65	30–140	5
1.5–2.0	88	37–200	6
2.1–2.5	115	52–250	6

*The range provides for the poor precision of the acid separation elution test. These recommendations are based upon one vial needed for each 15 ml of red blood cells or 30 ml of whole blood.

Explanation of Test

Major crossmatch detects antibodies in the recipient's serum that may damage or destroy the cells in the blood donor (Table 8-6). The type and screen determines the ABO and Rh-D type as well as the presence or absence of unexpected antibodies from the recipient. The type and screen is a safe alternative for the routine type and crossmatch ordered preoperatively for cases that may, but usually do not, require transfusion (eg, hysterectomy, cholecystectomy). If blood is needed, a major crossmatch must be done prior to transfusion.

Clinical Alert

Even the most carefully performed crossmatch will not detect all possible incompatible sources.

Procedure

1. Obtain a 10-ml venous blood sample. Observe standard precautions.

Clinical Implications

1. Crossmatch incompatibility implies that recipient cannot receive the incompatible unit of blood because antibodies are present.
2. A *transfusion reaction* occurs when incompatible blood is transfused, specifically if antibodies in the recipient's serum cause rapid red blood cell destruction in the proposed donor.

TABLE 8-6
Antibodies Found in Crossmatching

Blood Grouping System	Antibody	Description
Rh-hr	Anti-D	Rh1 May cause severe hemolytic disease of newborn
	Anti-C	Rh2 Often found with anti-D,- Ce(rh$_i$) or -C^w
	Anti-E	Rh3 Often found with anti-c
	Anti-c	Rh4 Often found with anti-E
	Anti-e	Rh5 Often found with anti-C
	Anti-C^w	Rh8
	Anti-V	Rh10 Alternative antigen names: ce^s, hr^v
Kell	Anti-K	K1 Strongly immunogenic; some non–red cell immune Occasional Kell system antibodies may not react
	Anti-k	K2 Antigen may be depressed by the presence of Kp^a
	Anti-Kp^a	K3 Few non–red cell immune
	Anti-Kp^b	K4
	Anti-Js^a	K6 Few non–red cell immune
	Anti-Js^b	K7
Duffy	Anti-Fy^a	Some antibodies exhibit dosage; quite common and may cause HDN and HTRs
	Anti-Fy^b	Some antibodies may bind complement
Kidd	Anti-Jk^a	Antibodies may exhibit dosage May cause severe delayed hemolytic transfusion reactions
	Anti-Jk^b	Antibody titers may drop rapidly below detectable levels Antibodies may require anti-C3 for detection
Lutheran	Anti-Lu^a Anti-Lu^b	Antibody gives mixed-field–like agglutination
MN	Anti-M	Common antibody Seldom clinically significant or implicated in HDN; may be pH-dependent or exhibit dosage
	Anti-N	Rare antibody Formaldehyde-induced anti-N commonly found in dialysis patients

(continued)

TABLE 8-6 *(Continued)*

Blood Grouping System	Antibody	Description
	Anti-S	Antibody may be enhanced if incubated below 37°C before AHG.
	Anti-s	
	Anti-U	Rarely found in S-, s-patients
Lewis	Anti-Le^a	Frequently found in serum of pregnant women
	Anti-Le^b	Neutralized by soluble antigen
	-Le^bh	Anti-Le^b often found with anti-Le^a
	-Le^bL	Anti-Le^b usually made by Le (a− −b− −) individuals
P	Anti-P₁	Antigen strength variable; neutralized by soluble antigen
	Anti-P	Biphasic hemolytic IgG autoantibody in PCH
		Alloantibody is usually potent IgM hemolysin
	Anti-pp₁ᵖᵏ(Tjᵃ)	Have caused hemolytic transfusion reactions and occasionally HDN
Xg	Anti-Xgᵃ	X-linked
Colton	Anti-Coᵃ	Rare antibodies
	Anti-Coᵇ	
Dombrock	Anti-Doᵃ	Incidence of Doᵃ lower in African Americans, Native Americans, and Asians
	Anti-Doᵇ	Infrequently reported antibodies
Diego	Anti-Diᵃ	Diᵃ antigen frequently higher in Asians and Native Americans
	Anti-Diᵇ	
Wright	Anti-Wrᵃ	IgM and IgG forms of antibody reported
		Frequently occurring antibody
Vel	Anti-Vel	Antibodies usually IgM;
		Antigen strength variable
		Binds complement
Sdᵃ	Anti-Sdᵃ	Antigen weaker during pregnancy
		Wide variation of antigen expression
		Agglutinates have refractile, mixed-field appearance
HLA-associated	Anti-Bgᵃ	Antigen strength variable
	-Bgᵇ	Antibodies often found in multitransfused multiparous patients
	-Bgᶜ	Antibodies characteristically weakly reactive
		Bg/HLA associations:
		Bgᵃ/HLA-B7
		Bgᵇ/HLA-B17
		Bgᶜ/HLA-A28

TABLE 8-6 *(Continued)*

Blood Grouping System	Antibody	Description
Cartwright	Anti-Yt^a	Antibody not uncommon in Yt (a−) individuals
	Anti-Yt^b	Rare antibody usually found in combination with other antibodies
HTLA	Anti	
	-Ch^a	Antigen strength variable
	-Kn^a	Antibodies characteristically weakly reactive
	-McC^a	
	-Yk^a	
	-Cs^a	
	-Gy^a	
	-Hy	
	-JMH	
	Anti-I	Most frequently detected cold autoagglutination
		Anti-I in CHD has wide thermal range, high titer
		Binds complement
		Seen as alloantibody in i adults
	Anti-i	Antibody seen in serum of patients with infectious mononucleosis
		Rare cause of CHD
		Antigen very weakly expressed on the cells of most adults

CHD, Cold Hemagglutin Disease; HTR, Hemalytic Transfusion Reaction; PCH, Paroxysmal Hemoglobinuria.

a. Certain antibodies, although not causing immediate red cell destruction and transfusion reaction, may nevertheless reduce the the normal life span of transfused incompatible cells; this may necessitate subsequent transfusions.

b. The patient will derive the most benefit from red cells that survive longest.

Clinical Alert

1. The most common cause of hemolytic transfusion reaction is the administration of incompatible blood to the recipient because of faulty matching in the laboratory, improper patient identification, and/or incorrect labeling of donor blood. If a transfusion reaction is suspected, discontinue the transfusion and notify the blood bank and attending physician immediately.

(continued)

(Clinical Alert continued)

2. Assess for the following symptoms of transfusion reaction:
   a. Fever
   b. Chills
   c. Chest, abdomen, or flank pain
   d. Hypotension or hypertension
   e. Nausea
   f. Dyspnea
   g. Shock
   h. Oliguria
   i. Back pain
   j. Feeling of heat along vein being transfused
   k. Constricting chest and lumbar back muscles
   l. Facial flushing
   m. Hemoglobinuria
   n. Oozing blood from wounds
   o. Anemia
   p. Allergic reactions such as local erythema, hives, and itching
3. After massive blood transfusions, perform the following tests:
   a. Hypocalcemia
   b. Potassium intoxication
   c. Increased blood ammonia
   d. Increased oxygen affinity
   e. Hypothermia (from blood)
   f. Hemosiderosis
4. Document transfusion reaction signs and symptoms; notify the blood bank of reaction, and carry out follow-up interventions.

3. The probable benefits of each blood transfusion must be weighed against the risks, which include the following:
   a. Hemolytic transfusion reactions due to infusion of incompatible blood (can be fatal)
   b. Febrile or allergic reactions
   c. Transmission of infectious disease (eg, hepatitis)
   d. Stimulation of antibody production (could complicate later transfusions or childbearing)

Patient Preparation

1. Explain purpose and procedure of crossmatching.
2. Follow guidelines in Chapter 1 regarding safe, effective, informed *pretest* care.

Patient Aftercare

1. Interpret test outcome and counsel patient regarding potential transfusion reactions.

2. Follow guidelines in Chapter 1 regarding safe, effective, informed *posttest* care.

COOMBS' ANTIGLOBULIN TEST   ●

Normal Values
Direct Coombs' test: negative for red blood cells
Indirect Coombs' test: negative for serum

Explanation of Test
The indirect Coombs' test detects antibodies that react only through a potentiating medium. The direct Coombs' test detects antigen-antibody complexes on the red blood cell membrane in vivo as well as red blood cell sensitization. It is diagnostic for the following conditions:

1. Hemolytic disease of the newborn in which the red cells of the infant are sensitized and exhibit antigen-antibody complexes in vivo
2. Acquired hemolytic anemia in which an antibody is produced that coats the patient's own cells (auto-sensitization in vivo)
3. Transfusion reaction in which the patient may have received incompatible blood which in turn has sensitized the donor's and possibly the patient's own red cells
4. Red blood cell sensitization caused by drugs

The Indirect Coombs' test detects serum antibodies, reveals maternal anti-Rh antibodies during pregnancy, and can detect incompatibilities not found by other methods.

Procedure
1. Obtain a 10-ml venous blood sample. Observe standard precautions.

Clinical Implications
1. The *direct Coombs' test is positive* (1+ to 4+) in the presence of the following conditions:
  a. Transfusion reactions
  b. Autoimmune hemolytic anemia (most cases)
  c. Cephalothin therapy (75% of cases)
  d. Drugs such as α-methyldopa (Aldomet), penicillin, insulin
  e. Hemolytic disease of newborn
  f. Paroxysmal cold hemoglobinuria
2. The *direct Coombs' test is negative* in nonautoimmune hemolytic anemias.
3. The *indirect Coombs' test is positive* (1+ to 4+) in the presence of specific antibodies, usually from a previous transfusion or pregnancy, or nonspecific antibodies, as in cold agglutinants.

Interfering Factors

A number of drugs may cause the direct Coombs' test to be positive.

> **Clinical Alert**
>
> Antibody identification is performed when the antibody screen or direct antiglobulin tests produce positive results and unexpected blood group antibodies need to be classified. Antibody identification tests are an important part of pretransfusion testing so that the appropriate antigen-negative blood can be transfused. These tests are also helpful for diagnosing hemolytic disease of the newborn and autoimmune hemolytic anemia. A 7-ml venous blood sample with added EDTA and 20 ml of clotted blood are studied. Notify the laboratory of diagnosis, history of recent and past transfusions, pregnancy, and any drug therapy.

Patient Preparation

1. Explain purpose and procedure of test.
2. Follow guidelines in Chapter 1 regarding safe, effective, informed *pretest* care.

Patient Aftercare

1. Interpret test outcome and counsel appropriately. Hemolytic disease of newborn can occur when the mother is Rh-negative and the fetus is Rh-positive. Diagnosis is derived from the following information: mother is Rh-negative, newborn is Rh-positive, and the direct Coombs' test is positive. Newborn jaundice results from Rh incompatibility, but more often, the jaundice results from an ABO incompatibility.
2. Follow guidelines in Chapter 1 regarding safe, effective, informed *posttest* care.

TYPES OF TRANSFUSION REACTIONS

ACUTE HEMOLYTIC TRANSFUSION REACTION (HTR) HTR reaction is triggered by an antigen-antibody reaction and activates the complement and coagulation systems. These are most always due to ABO incompatibilty because of misidentification resulting in the patient receiving incompatible blood. Symptoms include fever, chills, backache, vague uneasiness, and red urine. HTR reactions are potentially fatal.

BACTERIAL CONTAMINATION Bacteria may enter the blood during phlebotomy. These microbes will multiply faster in components stored at room temperature than in refrigerated components. Although rare, bacteria in blood or its components can cause a septic transfusion reaction. Symptoms include high fever, shock, hemoglobinuria, DIC, and renal failure. Such reactions can be fatal.

CUTANEOUS HYPERSENSITIVITY REACTIONS Urticarial reactions are very common, second in frequency only to febrile nonhemolytic reactions, and are usually characterized by erythema, hives, and itching. Allergy to some soluble substance in donor plasma is suspected.

NONCARDIOGENIC PULMONARY REACTIONS (NPR) Transfusion-related acute lung injury (TRALI) should be considered whenever a transfusion recipient experiences acute respiratory insufficiency and/or x-ray films show findings consistent with pulmonary edema without evidence of cardiac failure. These are possibly reactions between the donor's leukocyte antibodies and the recipient's leukocytes. TRALI produces white cell aggregates that become trapped in the pulmonary microcirculation. The findings on chest x-ray films are typical of acute pulmonary edema. If subsequent transfusions are needed, leukocyte-reduced red cells may prevent NPR reactions.

FEBRILE NONHEMOLYTIC (FNH) REACTION FNH reactions are defined as a temperature increase of $\geq 1°C$. They are seldom dangerous and may be caused by an antibody-antigen reaction.

ANAPHYLACTIC REACTIONS Anaphylactic reactions occur after infusion of as little as a few milliliters of blood or plasma. Anaphylaxis is characterized by coughing, bronchospams, respiratory distress, vascular instability, nausea, abdominal cramps, vomiting, diarrhea, shock, and loss of consciousness. Some reactions occur in IgA-deficient patients who have developed anti-IgA antibodies after immunization through previous transfusion or pregnancy.

CICRULATORY OVERLOAD Rapid increases in blood volume are not tolerated well by patients with compromised cardiac or pulmonary function. Symptoms of circulatory overload include coughing, cyanosis, orthopnea, difficulty breathing, and a rapid increase in systolic blood pressure.

LEUKOAGGLUTININ TEST

Normal Values
Negative for leukoagglutinins

Background
Leukoagglutinins are antibodies that react with white blood cells and sometimes cause febrile, nonhemolytic transfusion reactions. Patients who exhibit this type of transfusion reaction should receive leukocyte-poor blood for any subsequent transfusions.

Explanation of Test
This study is done when a blood reaction occurs even though compatible blood has been given. The donor plasma contains an antibody that reacts with recipient white cells to produce an acute clinical syndrome of fever, dyspnea,

cough, pulmonary infiltrates, and in more severe cases, cyanosis and hypertension. Patients immunized by previous transfusions, pregnancy, or during allografts often experience these febrile, nonhemolytic transfusion reactions because of incompatible transfused leukocytes. This type of reaction must be confirmed (as compared to hemolytic reactions) before additional transfusions can be safely administered.

Procedure
1. Obtain a 10-ml venous blood sample. Observe standard precautions.

Clinical Implications
1. Agglutinating antibodies may appear in the donor's plasma.
2. When the agglutinating antibody appears in the recipient's plasma, febrile reactions are common; however, pulmonary manifestations do not occur.
3. Febrile reactions are more common in pregnant women and in individuals with a history of multiple transfusions.

> **Clinical Alert**
>
> 1. Febrile reactions can be prevented by separating out white cells from the donor blood prior to transfusion.
> 2. Patients whose blood contains leukoagglutinins should be instructed that they generally need to be transfused with leukocyte-reduced blood to minimize these reactions.

Patient Preparation
1. Explain test purpose and procedure.
2. Follow guidelines in Chapter 1 regarding safe, effective, informed *pretest* care.

Patient Aftercare
1. Interpret test outcome and counsel patient regarding future transfusion precautions.
2. Follow guidelines in Chapter 1 regarding safe, effective, informed *posttest* care.

PLATELET ANTIBODY DETECTION TESTS

Normal Values
PLAI (negative platelet hyperlysibility): negative
ALTP (negative drug-dependent platelet antibodies): negative
PAIgG (platelet-associated IgG antibody): negative

Explanation of Test
Platelet antibody detection studies are used to diagnose posttransfusion purpura, alloimmune neonatal thrombocytopenic purpura, idiopathic thrombocy-

topenia purpura, paroxysmal hemoglobinuria, and drug-induced immunologic thrombocytopenia.

Procedure
1. A 10-ml to 30-ml venous blood sample is required.
   30 ml of venous blood when platelet count is 50,000–100,000/mm³
   20 ml of venous blood when platelet count is 100,000–150,000/mm³
   10 ml of venous blood when platelet count is >150,000/mm³

Interfering Factors
Alloantibodies formed in response to previous blood transfusions during pregnancies may produce positive reactions. Such antibodies are usually specific for human leukocyte antigens (HLA) found in platelets and other cells. Whenever possible, obtain samples for platelet antibody testing before transfusing.

Clinical Implications
1. Antibodies to platelet antigens are of two types: autoantibodies develop in response to one's own platelets as in idiopathic thrombocytopenia purpura, and alloantibodies develop following exposure to foreign platelets during transfusion.
2. Antiplatelet antibody, usually having anti-PLAI specificity, occurs in posttransfusion purpura.
3. A persistent or rising antibody titer during pregnancy is associated with neonatal thrombocytopenia.
4. PLAI incompatibility between mother and fetus appears to account for >60% of alloimmune neonatal thrombocytopenic purpura. A finding of a PLAI-negative mother and a PLAI-positive father provides presumptive diagnostic evidence.
5. Platelet-associated IgG antibody (PAIgG) is present in 95% of both acute and chronic cases of idiopathic (autoimmune) thrombocytopenic purpura. Patients responding to steroid therapy or undergoing spontaneous remission show increased circulatory times that correlate with decreased PAIgG levels.
6. The platelet hyperlysibility assay measures the sensitivity of platelets to lysis. This test is positive in and specific for paroxysmal hemoglobinuria.
7. In drug-induced immunologic thrombocytopenia, antibodies that react only in the presence of the inciting drug can be detected. Quinidine, quinine, chlordiazepoxide, sulfa drugs, and diphenylhydantoin most commonly cause this type of thrombocytopenia. Gold-dependent antibodies and heparin-dependent platelet IgG antibodies can be detected by direct assay. Approximately 1% of persons receiving gold therapy develop thrombocytopenia as a side-effect. Thrombocytopenia is also a well-known side-effect of heparin.

NOTE: *Platelet compatibility typing is done to ensure that hemostatically stable platelets can be transfused (eg, for aplastic anemia and malignant* *disorders). This is important because most patients repeatedly transfused with platelets from random donors become partially or totally refractory to further platelet transfusion because of alloimmunization. Platelet typing also provides diagnostic evidence of posttransfusion purpura. Platelets are routinely typed for PLAI, HLH-A2, and PLEI. Those matched for HLA antigens generally produce satisfactory posttransfusion improvement. A standard platelet count performed 1 hour after the end of a fresh platelet concentrate transfusion is a sensitive indicator for the presence or absence of clinically important antibodies against HLA antigens.*

Patient Preparation
1. Explain test purpose and procedure.
2. Follow guidelines in Chapter 1 regarding safe, effective, informed *pretest* care.

Patient Aftercare
1. Interpret test outcomes. Appropriately counsel and monitor patient for bleeding tendencies. Assess for prescribed medications as cause of purpura.
2. Follow guidelines in Chapter 1 regarding safe, effective, informed *posttest* care.

HUMAN LEUKOCYTE ANTIGEN (HLA) TEST ●

Normal Values
Requires clinical correlation

Background
The major histocompatibility antigens of humans belong to the HLA system. They are present on all nucleated cells but can be detected most easily on lymphocytes. Each antigen results from a gene that shares a locus on the chromosome with another gene, one paternal and one maternal (two alleles). More than 27 of these antigens have been identified. The HLA complex, located in the short arm of chromosome 6, is a major histocompatibility complex that is responsible for many important immune functions in humans.

Explanation of Test
This test determines the leukocyte antigens present on human cell surfaces. When tissue or organ transplants are contemplated, HLA typing identifies the degree of histocompatibility between donor and recipient. By matching donors and potential recipients with compatible lymphocytes and similar HLA types, it is possible to prolong transplant survival and to reduce rejection episodes. The HLA also aids in diagnosis of parentage as well as certain rheumatoid diseases, particularly ankylosing spondylitis. HLA-B27, one of the HLA antigens, is found

in 90% of patients with ankylosing spondylitis. Generally, the presence of a certain HLA antigen may be associated with increased susceptibility to a specific disease; however, it does not mandate that that person will develop the disease.

Procedure

1. Obtain a 10- to 24-ml heparinized venous blood sample. Observe standard precautions. The patient's HLA type is determined by testing the patient's lymphocytes against a panel of defined HLA antisera directed against the currently recognized HLA antigens. The HLA antigens are identified by letter and number. When viable human lymphocytes are incubated with a known HLA cytotoxic antibody, an antigen-antibody complex is formed on a cell surface. The addition of serum that contains complement kills the cells, which are then recognized as possessing a defined HLA antigen.
2. Label carefully with patient name, date, and special laboratory number. Include diagnosis and history.

Clinical Implications

1. Particular HLA antigens are associated with certain disease states:
   a. Ankylosing spondylitis (HLA-B27)
   b. Multiple sclerosis (HLA-B27 + Dw2 + A3 + B18)
   c. Myasthenia gravis (HLA-B8)
   d. Psoriasis (HLA-A13 + B17)
   e. Reiter's syndrome (B27)
   f. Juvenile insulin-dependent diabetes (Bw15 + B8)
   g. Acute anterior uveitis (B27)
   h. Graves' disease (B27)
   i. Juvenile rheumatoid arthritis (B27)
   j. Celiac disease (B8)
   k. Autoimmune chronic active hepatitis (B8)
2. Four groups of cell surface antigens (HLA-A, HLA-B, HLA-C, and HLA-D) constitute the strongest barriers to tissue transplantation.
3. In parentage determination, if a reputed father presents a phenotype (genotype completely determined by heredity; two haplotypes or gene clusters, one from father and one from mother) with no haplotype or antigen pair identical with one of the child's, he is excluded as the supposed father. If one of the reputed father's haplotypes (gene clusters) is the same as one of the child's, he *may be* the father. The chances of his being accurately identified as the father increase in direct proportion to the rarity of the presenting haplotype in the general population. Put another way, if the haplotype is very common, there is an increased probability that another man with the same haplotype also could be the father. When the frequency of the haplotype is known, the probability that the nonexcluded man is the father can be calculated. However, the degree of certainty diminishes as the incidence of the haplotype increases.

Patient Preparation

1. Explain test purpose and procedure.
2. Follow guidelines in Chapter 1 regarding safe, effective, informed *pretest* care.

Patient Aftercare

1. Interpret test outcomes and counsel appropriately. HLA testing is best used as a diagnostic adjunct and should not be considered as diagnostic by itself. Explain the need for possible further testing.
2. Follow guidelines in Chapter 1 regarding safe, effective, informed *posttest* care.

●TUMOR MARKERS

Background

Tumor markers include genetic markers (abnormal chromosomes or oncogenes), oncogene receptors, enzymes, hormones, hormone receptors, oncofetal antigens, glycoproteins, tumor antigens on cell surfaces, and substances produced in response to tumor growth (eg, cell reactive protein, circulating immune complexes, prostate-specific antigen).

Physical examination and standard radiologic techniques can usually detect tumors as small as 1 cm in volume. A tumor mass of this size has completed 30 doublings (two thirds of its growth) and contains 1 billion (10^9) cells. Certain tumor antigens, hormones, oncofetal proteins, and enzymes are secreted into the bloodstream by malignant cells.

Malignant tumor cells are produced when DNA is damaged by some form of carcinogen, virus, radiation, or chemical causing the process of mitosis to go out of control. These growing, changed (mutant) cells express oncogenes. These oncogenes are capable of inducing or transforming cells into cancer cells or tumors.

Tumor cells capable of forming metastases are likely to invade blood vessel walls; be released into the bloodstream, regional lymphatics, or interstitial stoma; and eventually spread to other organs. Tumor testing has focused on identifying certain tumor-related substances that might allow early detection of malignancy, determination of prognosis, and evaluation of tumor burden (ie, size, location, encroachment upon other tissues or organs).

Explanation of Test

Tumor markers (other than those identified in Table 8–7) are used and developed to obtain greater sensitivity and specificity in determining tumor activity. In general, these markers lack specificity for cancer; none is pathognomonic for any one type of neoplasm. Diagnosis still derives from comprehensive patient history, physical examination, and other diagnostic procedures. Tumor marker

TABLE 8-7
Tumor Markers

Tumor markers are substances produced and secreted by tumor cells and found in serum of persons with cancer. This table includes tumor-specific or tumor-associated antigens (proteins and oncofetal antigens), enzymes, hormones, cytokines. Refer to Chapter 6 and to other tests in Chapter 8 for complete listings of normal values, clinical implications, and safe, effective, informed patient preparation and aftercare.

Name of Test Clinical Marker in Current Use and Selected Normal Values	Type of Cancer in Which Tumor Marker May Be Found	Conditions Other Than Cancer That Are Associated With Abnormal Values
ENZYMES		
1. Prostatic acid phosphatase (PAP). Increased values due to increased metabolism and catabolism of cancer cells—levels increase with stage of cancer and age of individual. Not recommended for screening prostate cancer because it is not significantly increased until the tumor has metastasized. PSA preferred screening marker. NL <4. Adult: 0–3.1 mg/ml Child: 8.1–12.6 U/ml Newborn: 10.4–16.4 U/ml	1. a) Carcinoma of prostate with the following elevation: carcinoma with no metastasis 10%–20%; metastasis with one 20%–40%; metastases with bone involvement 70%–90% (usually osteoblastic) b) In three fourths of patients, arises in posterior lobe of prostate c) Used to monitor therapy with antineoplastic drugs d) Leukemia (hairy-cell) e) Cancer metastatic to bone (osteoblastic lesions)	1. a) Noncancer prostatic condition, prostate palpation, hyperplasia, infection of prostate following cystostomy, prostate surgery, and chronic prostatitis b) Other—Gaucher's disease (lipid storage disease), Nieman-Pick disease, Paget's disease, osteoporosis, renal osteopathy, hepatic cirrhosis, pulmonary embolism and hyperparathyroidism
2. Lactate dehydrogenase (LDH); increased isoenzymes I and II. Total LDH: 166–280 U/L.	2. a) Neuroblastomic carcinoma of testes. Elevated in 60% of those with stage 3 testicular cancer—serial LDH may help to detect recurrence of cancer b) Ewing's sarcoma	2. Cellular injury/hemolysis, myocardial infarction, hepatic diseases (see Cardiac Enzyme Tests)

(continued)

TABLE 8-7 *(Continued)*

Name of Test Clinical Marker in Current Use and Selected Normal Values	Type of Cancer in Which Tumor Marker May Be Found	Conditions Other Than Cancer That Are Associated With Abnormal Values
	c) Acute lymphocytic leukemia d) Non-Hodgkin's lymphoma e) LD-1 increased in germ cell tumors, LD-3 in leukemia, LD-5 in breast, lung, stomach, and colon f) Elevated in metastatic carcinoma	
3. Neuron-specific enolase (NSE): normal staining. Produced by neurons and neuroendocrine cells of the central and peripheral nervous system.	3. NSE increases: a) Neuroblastomas b) APUD system tumor—small cell lung cancers, pancreatic islet cell, medullary thyroid carcinoma c) Wilms' tumor and pheochromocytoma	
4. Alkaline phosphatase (ALP) originates in osteoblasts, lining of hepatobiliary tree and intestinal tract and placenta Adults (20–60): 35–85 µ/mL Elderly: slightly higher Child (<2 y): 85–235 µ/ml Young persons (2–21 y): 30–200 U/ml Isoenzymes offer greater specificity.	4. Increased in osteosarcoma, hepatocellular, metastatic to liver, primary or secondary bone tumors, liver and bone leukemia, lymphoma	4. Increased in Paget's disease, nonmalignant liver disease, normal pregnancy, healing fractures, hyperparathyroidism, osteomalacia and rickets, sprue, and malabsorption. Decreased in hypoparathyroidism, malnutrition, scurvy, pernicious anemia
5. Other enzymes: gammaglutamyl transpeptidase (GGT): muramidase, creatinine, phosphokinase isoenzyme BB, beta-Glucormidase, terminal	5. CPK-BB increased in prostate, lung (small cell), bladder, and gastrointestinal tract cancer; amylase increased in lung and ovarian cancer	5. CPK-BB is increased in cardiac muscle and skeletal muscle injury and brain and CNS diseases; Reye's syndrome, hypothyroid GGT increased in liver with CPK-disease, alcohol

680

deoxynucleotidyl transferase, ribonuclease, histaminase (medullary cancer of thyroid), amylase, and cystine aminopeptidase

HORMONES

1. Human chorionic gonadotropin (hCG) produced by placental syncytiotrophoblast; not usually found in sera of healthy, nonpregnant persons
   <2 ng/ml

2. Calcitonin (CT): malignant C-cell tumor produces increased CT levels. Calcitonin is a circulating peptide hormone produced by perifollicular C cells of thyroid gland.
   Ranges very with method.
   Serum:
     Adult: <150 pg/ml
   Plasma:
     Man: <19 pg/ml
     Woman: <14 pg/ml

3. Other Hormones: ACTH (lung—oat cell), PTH (lung—epidermoid), insulin (lung), glucagon (pancreas), gastrin

---

1. Increased in gestational trophoblastic tumors, seminomatous and nonseminomatous testes cancer, ovarian tumors, pancreatic islet-cell cancer, liver (21%), stomach (22%), and less valuable with lung and lymphoproliferative disease; useful to monitor testicular tumors

2. Increased in metastatic breast (greatly elevated), limited in primary small-tumor-burden breast cancer as levels lower, lung, pancreas, hepatoma, renal cell carcinoid, and skeletal metastases

---

abuse, and antiepileptic medications
Amylase increased in pancreatic, diabetic, ketoacidosis, and intestinal obstruction

1. Increased in gestational trophoblastic neoplasms (hydatiform mole); neoplasm of stomach, colon, pancreas, lungs, and liver; multiple pregnancy
   Decreased in ectopic pregnancy and abortion

2. Increased in Zollinger-Ellison syndrome, pernicious anemia, chronic renal failure, pseudohypoparathyroidism, apudomas, alcoholic cirrhosis, Paget's disease, pregnancy and benign breast or ovarian disease
   Decrease with therapy and a rise after therapy suggests progressive disease

TABLE 8-7 (*Continued*)

Name of Test Clinical Marker in Current Use and Selected Normal Values	Type of Cancer in Which Tumor Marker May Be Found	Conditions Other Than Cancer That Are Associated With Abnormal Values
(stomach and other carcinomas), prostaglandins and erythropoietin (kidney)		
ONCOFETAL ANTIGENS		
1. Alpha-fetoprotein (AFP) is a glycoprotein produced by fetal liver, yolk sac, and intestinal epithelium. Disappears from blood soon after birth and is not present in healthy individuals <15 μg/L	1. Increased in primary hepatocellular cancer, embryonal cell (nonseminomatous germ cell) testicular tumors, yolk sac ovarian tumors, teratocarcinoma, gastric, pancreatic, colonic, breast, renal, and lung	1. Increased in fetal distress and death, neural tube defects, viral hepatitis, primary biliary cirrhosis, partial hepatectomy, ataxic telangiectasia, Wiskott-Aldrich syndrome, multiple pregnancy, and abortion
2. Carcinoembryonic Antigen (CEA). Initially isolated in endodermally derived adenocarcinoma and fetal gastrointestinal tissue. <5.0 ng/L up to 10 ng/ml in smokers	2. Increased in colon (especially metastatic or recurrence), pancreas, lung, stomach, metastatic breast, ovary, bladder, limbs, neuroblastoma, leukemia, thyroid, and osteogenic carcinoma. Useful to monitor therapy with antineoplastic drugs and following surgery of neoplasm of breast, gastrointestinal tract, lung, and colorectal; FDA approved for colorectal cancer.	2. Increased in inflammatory bowel disease, rectal polyps, active ulcerative colitis, pancreatitis, alcoholic cirrhosis, peptic ulcers, cholecystitis, chronic renal failure, pulmonary emphysema, bronchitis, pulmonary infections, and fibrocystic breast disease; most levels decline with remission of disease
PROTEINS		

1. CA 15-3 antigen (breast-cystic fluid protein [BCFP]; used in conjunction with CEA)
    <30 U/ml
	1. Greatly increased in metastatic breast; limited in small-tumor-burden breast cancer
	    Decrease with therapy and increased rise after therapy suggests progressive disease
	    Increased in pancreas, lung, colorectal, ovarian, and liver cancer
		1. Increased in benign breast or ovarian disease

Tumor marker	Clinical significance	Other conditions
2. β₂-Microglobulin (β_2M) (HLA antigen system) 4–12 mg/nl	2. Increased in multiple myeloma, other B-cell neoplasms, lung cancer, hepatoma, breast cancer	2. Increased in ankylosing spondylitis and Reiters syndrome
3. Prostate-specific antigen (PSA)—more sensitive than PAP—correlates with stage of disease Males: 80% <4.0 µg/L	3. Increased in prostate cancer (the higher the level, the greater the tumor burden; successful surgery, chemotherapy, or radiation causes marked reduction in levels PSA screening for prostate cancer recommended only for men >50 y Useful for monitoring and staging prostate cancer PSA not significantly increased until tumor has grown out of prostate gland	3. Increased in benign prostatic hypertrophy, prostate surgery, and prostatitis
4. CA 19-9 carbohydrate antigen <70 U/ml and occurs in serum and tissue	4. Increased in pancreas, hepatobiliary cancer, lung cancer; primarily mild elevation—gastric and colorectal cancer	4. Increased in pancreatitis, cholecystitis, cirrhosis, gallstones, and cystic fibrosis (minimal elevations)
5. CA 125 (ovarian cancer) (glycoprotein antigen) and serum carbohydrate antigen <34 U/ml	5. Increased in epithelial ovary, fallopian tube, endometrium, endocervix, pancreas, and liver Less increased in colon, breast, lung, and gastrointestinal Ovarian and endometrial monitoring	5. Increased in pregnancy, endometriosis, pelvic inflammatory disease, menstruation, acute and chronic hepatitis, ascites, peritonitis, pancreatitis, gastrointestinal disease, Meig's syndrome, pleural effusion, and pulmonary disease
6. CA50 <17 U/ml	6. Increased in gastrointestinal and pancreatic cancer	
7. CA 72-4 TAG (a micin-like hormone adenocarcinoma associated antigen) <4.0 ng/ml	7. Used in gastric carcinoma monitoring Increased in ovarian cancer	
8. C549 (acidic glycoprotein) <15.5 U/ml (results correlate with those using CA 15-3)	8. Used in monitoring breast cancer Increased in ovarian, prostate, and lung cancer	

TABLE 8-7 *(Continued)*

Name of Test Clinical Marker in Current Use and Selected Normal Values	Type of Cancer in Which Tumor Marker May Be Found	Conditions Other Than Cancer That Are Associated With Abnormal Values
9. Tissue polypeptide antigen (TPA) 80–100 U/L in serum—may also be detected in urine, washings and effusions	9. Increased in gastrointestinal, genitourinary tract, breast, lung, thyroid	9. Increased in hepatitis, cholangitis, cirrhosis, pneumonia, and urinary tract infections
10. Immunoglobulins: monoclonal proteins (M proteins), immunoglobulins produced by B lymphocytes Absent. Refer to serum protein electrophoresis (SPEP) or urine protein electrophoresis (UPEP)	10. Multiple myeloma, macroglobulinemia, amyloidosis, B-cell lymphoma, multiple solid tumors	10. Cold agglutinin disease, Sjogren's syndrome, Gaucher's disease, lichen myxedematosus, cirrosis, renal failure, and sarcoid
11. Tumor-antigen 4 (TA-4) ≤ 2.6ng/ml	11. Squamous cancer: lung and cervix. elevations correlate with stage of cancer, especially abnormal	
12. Other antigens: colon mucoprotein antigen (CMA), colon-specific antigen (CSA), zino glycinate marker (ZGM—colon), pancreatic oncofetal antigen (POA), S-100 protein (malignant melanoma), sialoglycoprotein (wide variety of cancers), B-protein (wide variety of antigens), and "Tennessee" antigen glycoprotein (wide variety of cancers).		
CYTOKINES		
1. Interleukin (also known as IL-2) T-cell growth factor I; formed from T-helper cells and activated B cells; results highly variable	1. Leukemias	1. HIV infections

studies do not replace biopsy and pathologic tissue examination and are not ideal for screening for specific cancers, making a diagnosis, or predicting programs for symptomatic patients, but they are effective for tumor staging, monitoring, response to therapy, detecting disease recurrence, and assessing therapeutic response. The role of the clinical laboratory in relation to tumor markers remains controversial due to cost, low sensitivity, specificity of the markers, and need to use a combination of markers and diagnostic tools for accurate medical diagnosis. Because of this, the U.S. Food and Drug Administration (FDA) has approved only a few tumor markers for clinical use; these include α-fetoprotein, carcinoembryonic antigen (CEA), estrogen receptors, ovarian CA (CA125), progesterone receptor, prostate-specific antigen (PSA), and soluble interleukin-2 (IL-2) receptor. Table 8-7 displays tumor markers in current use.

Procedure

Most tumor marker tests involve obtaining either venous plasma or serum; some may require fasting. It is important to follow the specific directions from the laboratory or cancer center involved in the testing procedure, including factors that interfere with test results.

Pretest Care

1. Explain purpose and procedure of test.
2. Alleviate any fears the patient may have related to cancer test results. Tests for cancer are always anxiety provoking.
3. Follow guidelines in Chapter 1 regarding safe, effective, informed *pretest* care.

Posttest Care

1. Interpret test results using the latest knowledge in the field, recognizing that test values, significance, and specificity of tests are continually changing with technology. Generally, tumor markers are not helpful in predicting the site of origin or in recommending therapy for adenocarcinomas.
2. Provide consultation if test results reveal cancer.
3. Provide support through follow-up testing in stages of illness and in forming a therapeutic plan for treating the disease.
4. Follow guidelines in Chapter 1 regarding safe, effective, informed *posttest* care.

BIBLIOGRAPHY

Bader TF: Viral Hepatitis Practical Evaluation and Treatment. Seattle, WA, Hogrete and Huber Publishers, 1997

Bartlett, JG: 1998–1999 Guide to Medical Care of Patients With HIV Infection, 8th ed. Baltimore, Williams and Wilkins, 1998–1999

Brooks MJ, Maxson CJ, Rubin W: The infectious etiology of peptic ulcer disease: diagnosis and implications for therapy. Primary Care 23(3): 443–453, 1996

Coates TJ, Makadon HG: Can theory help in HIV prevention. In HIV Prevention: Looking Back, Looking Ahead. Center for AIDS Prevention Studies (CAPS), University of California, San Francisco, and Harvard AIDS Institute, August, 1995

Cutler AF: Testing for *Helicobacter pylori* in clinical practice. Am J Med 100(Suppl 5A): 5A-355–5A-395, 1996

Damato JJ, O'Bryan B: Resolution of indeterminate HIV-I test data using the Department of Defense HIV-1 testing program. Lab Med 22(2): 107–113, 1994

Diagnostic Product Corporation (DPC), 5700 West 96th Street, Los Angeles, CA 90045; telephone contact, October 9, 1997, to obtain reference value for ALaSTAT Latex Allergen EIA procedure by editor

Emmons W: Accuracy of oral specimen testing for human immunodeficiency virus. Am J Med 102(Suppl 4-A): 15–20, 1997

Fix AD: Tick bites and Lyme disease in an endemic setting: problematic use of serologic testing and prophylactic antibiotic therapy. JAMA 279(3): 206–210, 1998

Frank S, Esch JF, Margeson NE et al: Mandatory HIV testing of newborns: the impact on women. Am J Nurs 98(18), 1998

Frizzeau J: Antinuclear antibody testing. Am J Nurs 97(12): 14–16, 1997

George R, Fitchen JH: Future applications of oral fluid specimen technology. Am J Med 102(Suppl 4-A): 21–25, 1997

Henry JB (ed): Todd, Sanford, Davidsohn's Clinical Diagnosis and Management by Laboratory Methods, 19th ed. Philadelphia, WB Saunders, 1996

INOVA Diagnostic: Technical bulletin and notice announcing availability of anti-neutrophil cytoplasmic antibody (ANCA) IFA Kit, July, 1996.

Institute of Medicine: The Hidden Epidemic: Confronting Sexually Transmitted Diseases. Washington, DC: National Press, 1997

Jackson M, Rymer TE: Viral hepatitis, anatomy of a diagnosis. Am J Nurs 43–48, 1994

Leavelle, DE (ed): Interpretive Handbook—Interpretive data for diagnostic laboratory tests. Rochester, MN, Mayo Medical Laboratories, 1997

Litvak JE, Seigel JE, Pauker SG, Lallemant M, Fineberg HG, Weinstein MC: Whose blood is safer? the effect of the stage of the epidemic on screening for HIV. Med Decis Making 17(4): 455–463, 1997

Mainous AG, Hagen MD: Public awareness of prostate cancer and the prostate-specific antigen test. Cancer Pract 2(3): 217–221, 1994

Malamud D, Tabak L: Saliva as a diagnostic fluid. Ann N Y Acad Sci 6(94): 1993

Marchione M: Urine test provides option for HIV screening. Milwaukee Journal/Sentinel, June 7, Section 5B, 1998

Mauriuz P, Bosler EM, Luft BJ: Toxoplasma pneumonia. Semin Respir Infect 12(1): 40–43, 1997

Moder, KG: Concise review for primary care physicians—use and interpretation of rheumatologic tests: a guide for clinicians. Mayo Clin Proc 71: 391–396, 1996

Mahamad D: Oral diagnostic testing for detecting human immunodeficiency virus-1 antibodies: a technology whose time has come. Am J Med 102(Suppl 4-A): 9–14, 1997

Nerblum DR, Boynton RF: Evaluation and treatment of chronic hepatitis C infection. Primary Care 23(3): 535–547, 1996

Nymox Corporation: Accurate Test for Alzheimer's Disease Announced Also Helps Physicians Quickly Rule out AD [news release]. Rockville, MD, Nymox Corporation, July 29, 1996

Sheehan C: Clinical Immunology, Principles and Laboratory Diagnosis, 2nd ed. Philadelphia: Lippincott, 1997

Strickland GT, Karp AC, Mathews A, Rena CA: Utilization and cost of serologic tests for Lyme disease in Maryland. J Infect Dis 176: 819–821, 1997

Turgeon ML: Immunology and Serology in Laboratory Medicine, 2nd ed. St. Louis: CV Mosby, 1995

U.S. Centers for Disease Control and Prevention: HIV/AIDS Prevention "Facts About the Human Immunodeficiency Virus and its Transmission." Rockville, MD, U.S. Centers for Disease Control and Prevention, July 1997

U.S. Centers for Disease Control and Prevention: Update: "The Role of STD Detection and Treatment in HIV Prevention." Rockville, MD, U.S. Centers for Disease Control and Prevention, July 1998

U.S. Centers for Disease Control and Prevention: HIV Prevention Through Early Detection and Treatment of Other Sexually Transmitted Diseases—United States Recommendations of the Advisory Committee for HIV and STD Prevention. Rockville, MD, U.S. Centers for Disease Control and Prevention, 1998

U.S. Centers for Disease Control and Prevention: Update: Recent HIV/AIDS Treatment Advances and the Implications for Prevention. Rockville, MD, U.S. Centers for Disease Control and Prevention, June 1998

U.S. Department of Health and Human Services, Public Health Service: HIV Infection and AIDS: Are You At Risk? Washington, DC, U.S. Centers for Disease Control and Prevention and U.S. Government Printing Office, 1994, pp. 538–850

Vengelen-Tyler V: American Association of Blood Banks Technical Manual, 12th ed. Bethesda, MD, American Association of Blood Banks, 1996

Weiss J: Latex Allergy [technical report]. Los Angeles, Diagnostic Products Corporation, 1997

Wisconsin Department of Health and Family Services: Wisconsin Cancer Incidence and Mortality, 1996. Madison, WI, Wisconsin Department of Health and Family Services, Division of Health Care Financing, Bureau of Health Information, October 1998

Wisconsin State Laboratory of Hygiene: Reference Manual. Madison, WI, Wisconsin State Laboratory of Hygiene. July 1997.

Wu JT, Nakamura RM: Human Circulating Tumor Markers. Chicago, ASCP Press, 1997

Yu H, Levesque MA, Clark GM, Diamandis EP: Prognostic value of prostate-specific antigen for women with breast cancer: a large United States cohort study. Clin Cancer Res 4: 1489–1497, 1998

Zimmerman K, Ruben FL, Ahwesh FR: Hepatitis B virus infection, hepatitis B vaccine, and hepatitis B immune globulin. J Fam Pract 45(4): 295–310, 1997

U.S. Centers for Disease Control and Prevention: 1994 Revised Guidelines for the Performance of CD4+ T-cell determinations in persons with human immunodeficiency virus (HIV) Infection. Atlanta, GA, U.S. Department of Health and Human Services, Public Health Service, March 4, 1994

9

Nuclear Medicine Studies

OVERVIEW OF NUCLEAR MEDICINE STUDIES ●

Nuclear medicine is a diagnostic modality within radiology that studies the *physiology* or *function* of any organ system in the body. Other diagnostic imaging modalities in radiology, such as ultrasound, magnetic resonance imaging, computed tomography, and x-ray, generally visualize *anatomic* structures.

A pharmaceutical is labeled with a radioactive isotope to form a *radiopharmaceutical.* The radioisotope emits γ-rays. Radioisotopes are reactor produced (iodine 131), cyclotron produced (fluorine 18[F-18] for positron emission tomography [PET]), or generator produced (technetium 99m).

To visualize the function of an organ system, a radiopharmaceutical is administered. A time delay may be required, and then the organ of interest is imaged with a gamma camera. Image formation technology involves the detection with very great density of a signal (γ-rays) emanating from the radioactive isotope. There is very little signal in the image that does not come from the radiopharmaceutical. The background level of radiation within the human body is minimal and results from only a little radioactive potassium and some cesium. Routes of radiopharmaceutical administration vary with the specific study. Most commonly, a radiopharmaceutical is injected through a vein in the arm or hand. Other routes of administration include the oral, intramuscular, intrathecal, subcutaneous, or intraperitoneal.

Nuclear medicine studies are performed by certified nuclear medicine technologists, interpreted by radiologists or nuclear medicine physicians, and performed in a hospital or clinic-based nuclear medicine department.

Principles of Nuclear Medicine

The radiopharmaceutical is generally made up of 2 parts—the pharmaceutical, which is targeted to a specific organ, and the radionuclide, which emits gamma rap and allows the organ to be visualized by the gamma camera. Nuclear medicine imaging can yield quantitative as well as qualitative data. A measurement of the ejection fraction of the heart is an example of quantitative data derived from a multigated acquisition (MUGA) scan.

In general, nuclear medicine scans visualize the distribution of a particular radiopharmaceutical, with hot spots or cold spots of activity indicating an abnormality. In a *hot spot,* there is an increased area of uptake of the radiopharmaceutical in diseased tissue compared with the distribution in normal tissue. Examples of this type of uptake can be seen on bone scans. In a *cold spot,* there is an area of decreased uptake of the radiopharmaceutical compared with the distribution in normal tissue. Liver scanning and lung scanning are examples of this type of uptake.

In the nuclear medicine in vitro laboratory, radionuclides are used in numerous ways. They may be tagged to proteins and used in competitive protein-binding studies. They also may be used to label antibodies or antigens for radioimmunoassay (RIA) studies. RIA methods have a high degree of sensitivity and specificity to detect substances within the body in trace quantities—as low as 1 picogram (1 trillionth of a gram). The types of substances detected include hormones, antibiotics, carcinogens, drugs, vitamins, and immunoglobulins.

Principles of Imaging

The gamma cameras of today all have basically the same components. The camera may have 1, 2, or 3 heads, with the capability of imaging in multiple configurations. The camera is networked with a multitasking computer capable of acquiring and processing the data.

Several methods of imaging are used: dynamic, static, whole-body, and single photon emission computed tomography (SPECT). These imaging capabilities are available on all current camera systems.

Dynamic imaging allows serial display of multiple frames of data, each frame lasting 1 to 3 seconds, to visualize the blood flow associated with a particular organ. Static imaging is also known as *planar* imaging. The camera acquires 1 image at a time, covering the field of view. This image is 2-dimensional. Whole-body imaging acquires both anterior and posterior sweeps of the patient's body. This type of imaging also gives 2-dimensional information.

SPECT imaging has revolutionized the field of nuclear medicine. SPECT imaging provides 3 dimensions of data. SPECT imaging increases the specificity and sensitivity of nuclear imaging through improved resolution.

General Procedure

1. The patient may be required to follow a study-specific preparation regimen before imaging (eg, nothing by mouth, no caffeine for 24 hours, hydration, bowel preparation).
2. A radiopharmaceutical is administered through 1 of several routes: oral, intravenous, intramuscular, intrathecal, or intraperitoneal. On occasion, additional pharmaceuticals may be administered to enhance the function of the organ of interest.
3. A time delay may be necessary for the radiopharmaceutical to reach the organ of interest.
4. Imaging time depends on
   A. The specific study radiopharmaceutical used and the time that must be allowed for concentration in tissues
   B. Type of imaging equipment used
   C. Patient cooperation
   D. Additional views based on patient history and nuclear medicine protocol
   E. Patient's physical size

Benefits and Risks

Benefits and risks should be explained before testing. Patients retain the radioisotope for a relatively short period. The radioactivity decays over time. Some of the radioisotope is eliminated in urine, feces, and other body fluids.

Technetium 99m, the most commonly used radiopharmaceutical, has a radioactive half-life of 6 hours. This means that half of the dose decays in 6 hours. Other tracers such as iodine, indium, thallium, and gallium take from 13 hours to 8 days for half of the dose to decay.

BENEFITS

1. There is less radiation exposure from a nuclear medicine scan with γ-rays than from a chest radiograph with x-radiation.
2. Nuclear medicine yields functional data that are not provided by other modalities.
3. Nuclear imaging is safe, painless, and noninvasive (except for intravenous administration).
4. A nuclear medicine bone scan can detect metastases 6 to 12 months before they are detectable on a bone radiograph.

RISKS

1. A radiation exposure hazard, although minimal, always exists; toxicity, however, is nil.
2. Hematoma or infection at intravenous injection site.
3. Reactions to the radiopharmaceutical (hives, rash, itching, constriction of throat, dyspnea, bronchospasm, anaphylaxis).

Clinical Considerations

The following information should be obtained before diagnostic nuclear imaging:

1. Pregnancy (confirmed or suspected). Pregnancy is a contraindication for nuclear imaging.
2. Lactating women may be advised to stop nursing for a set period (eg, 2 to 3 days with ^{99m}Tc). Most radiopharmaceuticals are excreted in mother's milk.
3. Radiopharmaceutical uptake from a recent nuclear medicine examination could interfere with interpretation of the current study.
4. The presence of any prostheses in the body must be recorded on the patient's history, because certain devices can shield the γ-rays from imaging.
5. Current medications, treatments, and diagnostic measures (eg, telemetry, oxygen, urine collection, intravenous lines).
6. Age and current weight. This information is used to calculate the radiopharmaceutical dose to be administered. If the patient is younger than 18 years of age, notify the examining department before testing. The amount of radioactive substance administered is adjusted downward for anyone younger than 18.
7. Allergies: Past history of allergies, especially to contrast substances (eg, iodine) used in diagnostic procedures, is always determined.

Clinical Alert

The nuclear medicine department must be notified if the patient may be pregnant or is breast-feeding or is younger than 18 years of age.

Pretest Care and Standard Precautions for Nuclear Medicine Scans

1. Explain the purpose, procedure, benefits, and risks of the nuclear medicine scan.
2. Assess for allergies to substances such as iodine.
3. Inform the patient that the nuclear medicine procedure provides less radiation exposure than a chest x-ray. Reassure the patient that the scan is safe and painless.
4. Inform that patient that the procedure is performed in the nuclear medicine department. Contact the department to determine the expected scan time and scan length.
5. Have the patient appropriately dressed, usually in robes and slippers.
6. Obtain an accurate weight, because the radiopharmaceutical dose may be calculated by weight.
7. If a female patient is premenopausal, determine if the patient may be pregnant. Pregnancy is a contraindication to nuclear imaging.
8. Irradiation of the fetus should be avoided whenever possible. The radiation dose to the fetus from a nuclear scan is equal to the radiation from 1 abdominal radiograph.

> ### Clinical Alert
>
> 1. Nuclear medicine procedures are contraindicated in pregnant women. Lactating women may need to discard their breast milk for several days following the procedure.
> 2. These precautions are also to be followed for the radionuclide laboratory procedures in Part 2 and PET scans in Part 3 of this chapter.

Posttest Care and Standard Precautions for Nuclear Medicine Scans

1. Use routine disposal procedures for body fluids and excretions unless directed otherwise by the nuclear medicine department. Special considerations for disposal must be followed for therapeutic procedures.
2. Record any problems that may have occurred during the procedure.
3. Monitor the injection site for signs of bruising, hematoma, infection, discomfort, or irritation.

> ### Clinical Alert
>
> These precautions are also to be followed for the radionuclide laboratory procedures in Part 2 and PET scans in Part 3 of this chapter.

Pediatric Nuclear Medicine Considerations

Many of the nuclear medicine procedures that are performed on adults may be indicated in the pediatric patient. The procedure used on adults serves as the foundation for the pediatric procedure.

PEDIATRIC PRETEST CARE

1. Depending on hospital policy, a valid consent form may be requested to be signed by the parents or legal guardians of the patient.
2. Explain the nuclear scan purpose, procedure, benefits, and risks to the parents or legal guardians and to the patient. Reassure the patient that the test is safe and painless.
3. Assess for allergy to medications.
4. Have the patient appropriately dressed, ensuring that there are no metal objects on the patient during the procedure.
5. Obtain an accurate weight; the dose is calculated based on the patient's weight. Because pediatric patients have a different body metabolism from adults, a lower dose is given.
6. Often, immobilization techniques are used during the imaging of for pediatric patients. Wrapping an infant or small child is often necessary. Head clamps, arm boards, or sand bags may be used for patient immobilization.
7. Sedative drugs may also be administered to reduce patient motion during the examination. Disadvantages of sedation may include nausea and vomiting.
8. An intravenous line is started for administration of radiopharmaceuticals.
9. Patients should never be left unattended during the procedure.
10. Pediatric patients need constant reassurance and emotional support.
11. Patient urination is often difficult to control. A urinary catheter may be required.
12. Verify that the adolescent female patient is not pregnant.

PEDIATRIC POSTTEST CARE

1. Same as those stated for adults (see page 692).
2. Observe pediatric patients for adverse reactions to radiopharmaceuticals. Infants are more at risk for reactions.

Part One
Nuclear Medicine Scans

● CARDIAC STUDIES

MYOCARDIAL PERFUSION SCAN: REST AND STRESS ●

Normal Scan

Normal stress test: electrocardiogram and blood pressure normal
Normal myocardial perfusion under both rest and stress conditions

Explanation of Test

Technetium Tc 99m sestamibi (Cardiolite), thallium 201, and technetium Tc 99m tetrofosmin are the radioactive imaging agents available for myocardial perfusion imaging testing to diagnose ischemic heart disease and allow differentiation of ischemia and infarction. This test reveals myocardial wall defects and heart pump performance during increased oxygen demands. These scans may also be done before and after streptokinase treatment for coronary artery thrombosis and after surgery for great vessel translocation. Pediatric indications include evaluation for ventricular septal defects and congenital heart disease and postsurgical evaluation of congenital heart disease.

Thallium 201 is a physiologic analogue of potassium. The myocardial cells extract potassium, as do other muscle cells. The ^{99m}Tc sestamibi is taken up by the myocardium through passive diffusion, followed by active uptake within the mitochondria. Unlike thallium, technetium does not undergo any significant redistribution. Therefore, there are some procedural differences. Myocardial activity also depends on blood flow. Consequently, when the patient is injected during peak exercise, the normal myocardium has much greater activity than the abnormal myocardium. Cold spots indicate a decrease or absence of flow.

A completely normal myocardial perfusion study may eliminate the need for cardiac catheterization in the evaluation of chest pain and nonspecific abnormalities of the ECG. SPECT imaging can accurately localize regions of ischemia.

Administration of dipyridamole (Persantine) or adenosine is indicated in adults and children who are unable to exercise to achieve the desired cardiac stress level and maximum cardiac vasodilation. This medication has an effect similar to that of exercise on the heart. Physical stress testing may be initiated in children beginning at 4 to 5 years. Candidates for drug-induced stress testing are those with lung disease, peripheral vascular disease with claudication, amputation, spinal cord injury, multiple sclerosis, or morbid obesity. Dipyridamole stress testing is also valuable as a significant predictor of cardiovascular death, reinfarction, and risk of postoperative ischemic events and to reevaluate unstable angina.

In some nuclear medicine departments, an ejection fraction and wall motion can be assessed by computer analysis.

Myocardial Perfusion General Imaging Procedures

There are 2 phases to this scan—the rest scan and the stress scan. Either ^{99m}Tc sestamibi or ^{99m}Tc tetrofosmin may be used.

For the *rest scan,* an intravenous injection of the radioisotope is performed. A 30- to 60-minute delay is required to allow the radioisotope time to localize in the heart. SPECT imaging is then performed.

For the *stress scan,* the patient undergoes an exercise or a pharmacologic cardiac stress test. At the peak level of stress, the patient is injected with the radioisotope. SPECT imaging may begin 30 minutes after injection.

NOTE: *Myocardial perfusion imaging protocols vary among nuclear medicine departments. Some departments use a rest-stress, stress-rest, dual-isotope, or 2-day protocol, separating the phases into 2 different days.*

Pharmacologic stress tests may be performed with any of 3 routine stressing agents:

1. *Dipyridamole* is routinely infused over 4 to 6 minutes. The radiopharmaceutical is injected. Two minutes later, aminophylline, an antidote to the dipyridamole, may be administered at the cardiologist's discretion. Patient monitoring may last 20 minutes. Contraindication: Caffeine.
2. *Adenosine* is infused over 6 minutes. Three minutes into the infusion, the radiopharmaceutical is injected. The adenosine is infused for 3 additional minutes. Adenosine has an extremely short half-life; once the infusion has stopped, any symptoms will subside. Contraindications: caffeine and theophylline based drugs.
3. *Dobutamine* is infused until the predicted heart rate is achieved. The infusion protocol lasts 3 minutes at each dose increment.

Procedure

THALLIUM

1. During the cardiac stress test, the patient is monitored by a cardiologist and either a registered nurse, an electrophysiologist, or an ECG technician.
2. The patient begins walking on the treadmill.
3. When the cardiologist determines that the patient has reached 85% to 95% of maximum heart rate, an injection of radioactive thallium is administered. The patient is taken for immediate imaging.
4. SPECT imaging begins within 5 minutes of injection.
5. A second scan is acquired approximately 3 to 4 hours later, with the patient at rest, to determine redistribution of the thallium.
6. See Chapter 1 guidelines for safe, effective, informed *intratest* care.

NOTE: *Some nuclear medicine protocols may require the patient to return 24 hours later for delayed imaging.*

TECHNETIUM 99M SESTAMIBI AND ^{99M}TC TETROFOSMIN

Follow myocardial perfusion general imaging procedures on page 694.

Clinical Implications

1. A scan that is abnormal during exercise but remains normal at rest indicates transient ischemia.
2. A scan that is abnormal both at rest and under stress indicates a past infarction.
3. Hypertrophy produces an increase in uptake.
4. The progress of disease can be estimated.
5. The location and extent of myocardial disease can be assessed.
6. Specific and significant abnormalities in the stress ECG usually are indications for cardiac catheterization or further studies.

Interfering Factors

1. Inadequate cardiac stress
2. Caffeine intake
3. Injection of dipyridamole in the upright or standing position or with isometric handgrip may increase myocardial uptake.

Patient Preparation for Stress Testing

1. Explain test purpose and procedure, benefits, and risks. See standard nuclear scan *pretest* precautions on page 692.
2. Before the stress test has begun, an intravenous line is started and the patient is prepared. A resting 12-lead ECG and blood pressure measurement are performed.
3. Advise the patient that the exercise stress period will be continued for 1 to 2 minutes after injection to allow the radiopharmaceutical to be cleared during a period of maximum blood flow.
4. No discomfort is experienced during the imaging.
5. Fasting may be recommended for at least 2 hours before the stress test. Caffeine intake must be eliminated for 24 hours before the stress test.
6. For dipyridamole administration:
   A. Fasting may be required before the stress test and avoidance of any caffeine products for at least 24 hours before the test is necessary.
   B. Blood pressure, heart rate, and ECG results are monitored for any changes during dipyridamole infusion. Aminophylline may be given to reverse the effects of the dipyridamole.
7. See Chapter 1 guidelines for safe, effective, informed *pretest* care.

▶ **Clinical Alert**

1. The stress study is contraindicated on patients who
   A. Have a combination of right and left bundle branch block
   B. Have left ventricular hypertrophy
   C. Are using digitalis or quinidine
   D. Are hypokalemic (because the results are difficult to evaluate)
2. Adverse short-term effects of dipyridamole may include nausea, headache, dizziness, facial flush, angina, ST-segment depression, or ventricular arrhythmia.

Patient Aftercare

1. Observe the patient for possible effects of dipyridamole infusion.
2. Interpret test outcomes and counsel appropriately.
3. Refer to nuclear scan *posttest* precautions on page 692.
4. Follow Chapter 1 guidelines for safe, effective, informed *posttest* care.

MYOCARDIAL INFARCTION (PYP) SCAN

Normal Scan
Normal distribution of the radiopharmaceutical in sternum, ribs, and other bone structures
No myocardial uptake

Explanation of Test
Technetium Tc 99m pyrophosphate (^{99m}Tc-PYP) is the radioactive imaging agent used to demonstrate the general location, size, and extent of myocardial infarction 24 to 96 hours after suspected myocardial infarction and as an indication of myocardial necrosis, to differentiate between old and new infarcts. In some instances, the test is sensitive enough to detect an infarction 12 hours to 7 days after its occurrence. Acute infarction is associated with an area of increased radioactivity (hot spot) on the myocardial image. This test is useful when ECG and enzyme studies are not definitive.

Procedure
1. This myocardial scan involves a 4-hour delay before imaging after the intravenous injection of the radionuclide. During this waiting period, the radioactive material accumulates in the damaged heart muscle.
2. The scan takes 30 to 45 minutes, during which time the patient must lie still on a scanning table.
3. See Chapter 1 guidelines for safe, effective, informed *intratest* care.

Clinical Implications
1. A scan that is entirely normal indicates that an acute infarction is not present and the myocardium is viable.
2. Myocardial uptake of the PYP is compared with the ribs (2+) and sternum (4+). Higher uptake levels (4+) reflect greater myocardial damage.
3. Larger defects have a poorer prognosis than small defects.

Interfering Factors
False-positive infarct-avid (PYP) scans can occur in cases of chest wall trauma, recent cardioversion, and unstable angina.

Patient Preparation
1. This scan can be performed at bedside in the acute phase of infarction if the nuclear medicine department has a portable camera.
2. Explain the purpose, procedure, benefits, and risks of the nuclear scan. See standard nuclear scan *pretest* precautions on page 692.
3. Imaging must occur within a period of 12 hours to 7 days after the onset of symptoms of infarction. Otherwise, false-negative results may be reported.
4. See Chapter 1 for additional guidelines for safe, effective, informed *pretest* care.

Patient Aftercare

1. Interpret test outcome and monitor appropriately. If heart surgery is needed, counsel the patient concerning follow-up testing after surgery.
2. Refer to standard precautions and *posttest* care for nuclear scans on page 692.
3. Follow additional guidelines in Chapter 1 for safe, effective, informed *posttest* care.

MULTIGATED ACQUISITION (MUGA) SCAN: REST AND STRESS

Normal Scan

Normal myocardial wall motion and ejection fractions under conditions of stress and rest

Explanation of Test

The term *gated* refers to the synchronization of the imaging equipment and computer with the patient's ECG to evaluate left ventricular function. The primary purpose of this test is to provide an ejection fraction (the amount of blood ejected from the ventricle during a cardiac cycle).

Once injected, the distribution of the radiolabeled red blood cells (RBCs) is imaged by synchronization of the recording of cardiac images with the ECG. This technique provides a means of obtaining information about cardiac output, end-systolic volume, end-diastolic volume, ejection fraction, ejection velocity, and regional wall motion of the ventricles. Computer-aided wall motion of the ventricles can be portrayed in a cinematic mode to visualize contraction and relaxation. This scan may also be performed as a stress test. MUGA scans are not often performed on children.

Procedure for MUGA

1. This scan may be performed with or without stress.
2. A MUGA scan with the patient at rest could be performed at the bedside if necessary. The nuclear medicine department has a portable camera.
3. The patient's own RBCs are labeled with ^{99m}Tc-PYP by any of several methods. Once the blood is labeled, it is injected. In children and adults, the ^{99m}Tc-labeled RBCs are administered slowly through an intravenous line. For children younger than 3 years of age, sedation may be required for the injection and to allow the pediatric patient to hold still for the required 20 to 30 minutes. An alternative would be to perform a cardiac flow study.
4. An ECG is required, because the patient's R wave signals the computer and camera to take several image frames for each cardiac cycle.
5. The patient is imaged immediately after injection of the labeled RBCs.
6. See Chapter 1 guidelines for safe, effective, informed *intratest* care.

Clinical Implications

1. Abnormal MUGA scans are associated with
   A. Congestive cardiac failure
   B. Change in ventricular function due to infarction

C. Persistent arrhythmias from poor ventricular function
D. Regurgitation due to valvular disease
E. Ventricular aneurysm formation

Interfering Factors
If a reliable ECG cannot be obtained because of arrhythmias, the test cannot be performed.

Patient Preparation
1. Explain the purpose, procedure, benefits, and risks of the nuclear scan.
2. Follow standard precautions and *pretest* care for nuclear scans on page 692.
3. See Chapter 1 for additional guidelines for safe, effective, informed *pretest* care.

Patient Aftercare
1. Interpret MUGA outcomes and monitor appropriately for cardiac disease.
2. Refer to standard nuclear scan *posttest* precautions on page 692.
3. Follow basic Chapter 1 guidelines for safe, effective, informed *posttest* care.

CARDIAC FLOW STUDY (FIRST-PASS STUDY; SHUNT SCAN)

Normal Scan
Normal wall motion and ejection fraction
Normal pulmonary transit times and normal sequence of chamber filling

Explanation of Test
The cardiac flow study is performed to check for blood flow through the great vessels and after vessel surgery; it is useful in the determination of both right and left ventricular ejection fractions. Immediately after the injection, the camera traces the flow of the radiopharmaceutical in its "first pass" through the cardiac chambers in multiple rapid images. The first-pass study uses a jugular or antecubital vein injection of the radiopharmaceutical. A large bore needle is used.

This study is useful in examining heart chamber disorders, especially left-to-right and right-to-left shunts. Children are commonly candidates for this procedure. Indications for pediatric patients include evaluation for congenital heart disease, transposition of the great vessels, and atrial or ventricular septal defects and quantitative assessment of valvular regurgitation. In neonates, the cardiac flow study can be used in conjunction with computer software for the quantitative assessments. These quantitative values are useful in determining the degree of cardiac shunting with septal defects in the atria or ventricles.

Procedure
1. A 3-way stopcock with saline flush is used for radionuclide injection into the jugular vein or the antecubital fossa. For a shunt evaluation, the radionuclide is injected into the external jugular vein to ensure a compact

bolus. In pediatric patients it is important that the child not cry, because this disrupts the flow of the radiopharmaceutical and negates the results of the test.

2. The patient lies supine with the head slightly raised.
3. The total patient time is approximately 20 to 30 minutes; the actual imaging time is only 5 minutes.
4. A resting MUGA scan may be performed with a shunt study.
5. See Chapter 1 guidelines for safe, effective, informed *intratest* care.

Clinical Implications

1. Abnormal first-pass ejection fraction values are associated with
   A. Congestive heart failure
   B. Change in ventricular function due to infarction
   C. Persistent arrhythmias from poor ventricular function
   D. Regurgitation due to valvular disease
   E. Ventricular aneurysm formation
2. Abnormal heart shunts reveal
   A. Left-to-right shunt
   B. Right-to-left shunt
   C. Mean pulmonary transit time
   D. Tetralogy of Fallot (seen most often in children)

Interfering Factors

Inability to obtain intravenous access to the jugular vein or large bore anticubital access.

Patient Preparation

1. Explain the purpose, procedure, benefits, and risks of the nuclear scan. An intravenous line is required.
2. See Chapter 1 for additional guidelines for safe, effective, informed *pretest* care.
3. Refer to standard nuclear scan *pretest* precautions on page 692.
4. Obtain a signed, witnessed consent form if stress testing is to be done.

Patient Aftercare

1. Interpret test outcomes, monitor, and counsel appropriately.
2. Refer to standard nuclear scan *posttest* precautions on page 692.
3. Follow basic Chapter 1 guidelines for safe, effective, informed *posttest* care.

● ENDOCRINE STUDIES

THYROID SCAN ●

Normal Scan

Normal or evenly distributed concentration of radioactive iodine
Normal size, position, shape, site, weight, and function of the thyroid gland
Absence of nodules

Explanation of Test

This test systematically measures the uptake of radioactive iodine (either ^{131}I or ^{123}I) by the thyroid. Iodine (and, consequently, radioiodine) is actively transported to the thyroid gland and is incorporated into the production of thyroid hormones. The test is requested for the evaluation of thyroid size, position, and function. It is used in the differential diagnosis of masses in the neck, base of the tongue, or mediastinum. Thyroid tissue can be found in each of these 3 locations.

Benign adenomas may appear as nodules of increased uptake of iodine ("hot" nodule), or they may appear as nodules of decreased uptake ("cold" nodule). Malignant areas generally take the form of cold nodules. The most important use of thyroid scans is the functional assessment of these thyroid nodules. Pediatric indications include evaluation of neonatal hypothyroidism or thyrocarcinoma (lower incidence than adults).

A thyroid scan performed with iodine is usually acquired in conjunction with a radioactive iodine uptake study, which is usually performed at 4 to 6 hours and at 24 hours after dosing. For a complete thyroid workup, in both adults and children, thyroid hormone blood levels are usually measured, RIA blood tests are done. A thyroid ultrasound examination also may be performed.

Measurements of free serum thyroxine (free T$_4$) and free triiodothyronine (free T$_3$) by RIA are also reliable tests of thyroid function.

Procedure

1. The patient swallows radioactive iodine in a capsule or liquid form.
2. Usually, an uptake is determined at 4 to 6 hours and 24 hours after dosing. Four hours after dosing, the thyroid (neck area) is imaged.
3. Normal scan time is 45 minutes.
4. See Chapter 1 guidelines for safe, effective, informed *intratest* care.

Clinical Implications

1. Cancer of the thyroid most often manifests as a nonfunctioning cold nodule, indicated by a focal area of decreased uptake.
2. Some abnormal results are
   A. Hyperthyroidism, represented by an area of diffuse increased uptake.
   B. Hypothyroidism, represented by an area of diffuse decreased uptake.
   C. Graves' disease, represented by an area of diffuse increased uptake.
   D. Autonomous nodules, represented by focal area of increased uptake.
   E. Hashimoto's disease, represented by mottled areas of decreased uptake.
3. Imaging alone cannot definitively determine the diagnosis; uptake information is essential for a definitive diagnosis.

Interfering Factors

1. Thyroid scans need to be completed before radiographic examinations using contrast media (eg, intravenous pyelogram, cardiac catheterization, myelogram) are performed.
2. Any medication containing iodine should not be given until thyroid scans are concluded. Notify the attending physician if thyroid studies have been ordered or if there are interfering radiographs or medications.

Patient Preparation

1. Instruct the patient about nuclear scan purpose, procedure, and special restrictions. Refer to standard nuclear scan *pretest* precautions on page 692.
2. Because the thyroid gland responds to small amounts of iodine, the patient may be requested to refrain from iodine intake for at least 1 week before the test. Patients should consult with a physician. Restricted items include the following:
   A. Certain thyroid drugs
   B. Weight-control medicines
   C. Multiple vitamins
   D. Some oral contraceptives
   E. X-ray contrast materials containing iodine
   F. Cough medicine
   G. Iodine-containing foods, especially kelp and other "natural" foods
3. Alleviate any fears the patient may have about radionuclide procedures.
4. See Chapter 1 guidelines for safe, effective, informed *pretest* care.

Clinical Alert

1. Thyroid scans are contraindicated in pregnancy. Thyroid testing in pregnancy is routinely limited to blood testing.
2. This study should be completed before thyroid-blocking radiographic contrast agents are administered and before thyroid or iodine drugs are given.
3. Occasionally, tests are performed purposely with iodine or some thyroid drug in the body. In these cases, the doctor is testing the response of the thyroid to these drugs. These stimulation and suppression tests are usually done to determine the nature of a particular nodule and whether the tissue is functioning or nonfunctioning.

Patient Aftercare

1. If iodine has been administered, observe the patient for signs and symptoms of allergic reaction as needed.
2. Explain test outcomes and possible treatment.
3. Refer to standard nuclear scan *posttest* precautions on page 692.
4. Interpret test outcomes and counsel appropriately.
5. Follow Chapter 1 guidelines for safe, effective, informed, *posttest* care.

RADIOACTIVE IODINE (RAI) UPTAKE TEST ●

Normal Scan

Absorption (Uptake) by the Thyroid Gland
1% to 13% after 2 h
5% to 20% after 6 h
15% to 40% after 24 h
(Values are laboratory dependent)

Explanation of Test

This direct test of the function of the thyroid gland measures the ability of the gland to concentrate and retain iodine. When radioactive iodine is administered, it is rapidly absorbed into the bloodstream. This procedure measures the rate of accumulation, incorporation, and release of iodine by the thyroid. The rate of absorption of the radioactive iodine (which is determined by the increase in radioactivity of the thyroid gland) is a measure of the ability of the thyroid to concentrate iodide from the blood plasma. The radioactive isotopes of iodine used are ^{131}I or ^{123}I.

This procedure is indicated in the evaluation of hypothyroidism, hyperthyroidism, thyroiditis, goiter, and pituitary failure and for posttreatment evaluation. The patient who is a candidate for this test may have a lumpy or swollen neck or complain of pain in the neck; the patient may be jittery and ultrasensitive to heat or sluggish and ultrasensitive to cold. The test is more useful in the diagnosis of hyperthyroidism than in hypothyroidism.

Procedure

NOTE: *The test usually is done in conjunction with a thyroid scan and assessment of thyroid hormone blood levels (see page 700).*

1. A fasting state is preferred. A complete history and listing of all medications is a must for this test. This history should include nonprescription medications and patient dietary habits.
2. A liquid form or a tasteless capsule of radioactive iodine is administered orally.
3. Four to 6, and 24 hours later, the amount of radioactivity is measured by an uptake calculation scan of the thyroid gland. There is no pain or discomfort involved.
4. The patient must return to the laboratory at the designated time, because the exact time of measurement is crucial in determining the uptake.

Clinical Implications

▶ Clinical Alert

1. This test is contraindicated in pregnant or lactating women, in children, in infants, and in persons with iodine allergies.
2. Whenever possible, this test should be performed before any other radionuclide procedures are done, before any iodine medications are given, and before any radiographs using iodine contrast media are taken.

1. Increased uptake (eg, 20% in 1 hour, 25% in 6 hours, 45% in 24 hours) suggests hyperthyroidism but is not diagnostic for it.
2. Decreased uptake (eg, 0% in 2 hours, 3% in 6 hours, 10% in 24 hours) may be caused by hypothyroidism but is not diagnostic for it.
   A. If the administered iodine is not absorbed, as in severe diarrhea or

intestinal malabsorption syndromes, the uptake may be low even though the gland is functioning normally.
  B. Rapid diuresis during the test period may deplete the supply of iodine, causing an apparently low percentage of iodine uptake.
  C. In renal failure, the uptake may be high even though the gland is functioning normally.

Interfering Factors

1. The chemicals, drugs, and foods that interfere with the test by *lowering* the uptake are
   A. Iodized foods and iodine-containing drugs such as Lugol's solution, expectorants, cough medicines, saturated solutions of potassium iodide, and vitamin preparations that contain minerals. The duration of the effects of these substances in the body is 1 to 3 weeks.
   B. Radiographic contrast media such as iodopyracet (Diodrast), sodium diatrizoate (Hypaque, Renografin), poppy-seed oil (Lipiodol), ethiodized oil (Ethiodol), iophendylate (Pantopaque), and iopanoic acid (Telepaque). The duration of the effects of these substances is 1 week to 1 year or more; consult with the nuclear medicine laboratory for specific times.
   C. Antithyroid drugs such as propylthiouracil (PTU) and related compounds (duration, 2 to 10 days).
   D. Thyroid medications such as liothyronine sodium (Cytomel), desiccated thyroid, thyroxine (Synthroid) (duration, 1 to 2 weeks).
   E. Miscellaneous drugs—thiocyanate, perchlorate, nitrates, sulfonamides, tolbudamide (Orinase), corticosteroids, paraaminosalycilate, isoniazid, phenylbutazone (Butazolidin), thiopental (Pentothal), antihistamines, adrenocorticotripic hormone, aminosalicylic acid, cobalt, and coumarin anticoagulants. Consult with the diagnostic department for durations, which may vary.
2. The compounds and conditions that interfere by *enhancing* the uptake are
   A. Thyroid-stimulating hormone (thyrotropin)
   B. Pregnancy
   C. Cirrhosis
   D. Barbiturates
   E. Lithium carbonate
   F. Phenothiazines (duration, 1 week)
   G. Iodine-deficient diet
   H. Renal failure

Patient Preparation

1. Explain test purpose and procedure; the test takes 24 hours to complete. Assess and record pertinent dietary and medication history.
2. Advise that iodine intake is restricted for at least 1 week before testing.
3. Refer to standard nuclear scan *pretest* precautions on page 692.
4. See Chapter 1 guidelines for safe, effective, informed *pretest* care.

Patient Aftercare

1. Resume medications and normal diet.
2. Refer to standard nuclear scan *posttest* precautions on page 692.
3. Interpret test outcome and monitor appropriately.
4. Follow Chapter 1 guidelines for safe, effective, informed *posttest* care.

ADRENAL GLAND (MIBG) SCAN ●

Normal Scan

No evidence of tumors or hypersecreting hormone sites
Normal salivary glands, urinary bladder, and vague shape of liver and spleen can be seen.

Explanation of Test

The adrenal gland is divided into 2 different components: cortex and medulla. The scope of adrenal imaging is limited to the medulla. Testing can be performed in both adults and children.

The purpose of adrenal medulla imaging is to identify sites of certain tumors that produce excessive amounts of catecholamines. Pheochromocytomas develop in cells that make up the adrenergic portion of the autonomic nervous system. A large number of these well-differentiated cells are found in adrenal medullas. Adrenergic tumors have been called *paragangliomas* when they are found outside the adrenal medulla, but many practitioners refer to all neoplasms that secrete norepinephrine and epinephrine as *pheochromocytomas*. Because the only definite and effective therapy is surgery to remove the tumor, identification of the site using this test, computed tomography, and ultrasound, is an essential goal of treatment.

Procedure

1. The radionuclide iodine I 131 metaiodobenzylguanidine (MIBG) is injected intravenously.
2. Sequential images are taken at the physician's discretion, usually beginning 24 hours after injection.
3. Imaging may take 2 hours.
4. See Chapter 1 guidelines for safe, effective, informed *intratest* care.

Clinical Implications

1. Abnormal results give substance to the "rough rule of 10" for these tumors:
   - **A.** Ten percent are in children.
   - **B.** Ten percent are familial.
   - **C.** Ten percent are bilateral in the adrenal glands.
   - **D.** Ten percent are malignant.
   - **E.** Ten percent are multiple, in addition to bilateral.
   - **F.** Ten percent are extrarenal.
2. More than 90% of primary pheochromocytomas occur in the abdomen.
3. Pheochromocytomas in children often represent a familial disorder.

4. Bilateral adrenal tumors often indicate a familial disease, and vice versa.

5. Multiple extrarenal pheochromocytomas are often malignant.

6. The presence of 2 or more pheochromocytomas strongly indicates malignant disease.

Interfering Factors
Barium interferes with the test.

Patient Preparation
1. Explain nuclear scan purpose, procedure, benefits, and risks. Radiation exposure is comparable to that of a computed tomography scan of the adrenal glands or a conventional radiograph of the kidneys and adrenal glands.

2. To prevent uptake of radioactive iodine by the thyroid gland, Lugol's solution (potassium iodide) is given for 1 week before the injection.

3. Refer to standard nuclear scan *pretest* precautions on page 692.

4. See Chapter 1 guidelines for safe, effective, informed *pretest* care.

Patient Aftercare
1. Interpret test outcome and counsel appropriately about the need for possible follow-up tests. Follow-up tests include

    A. Kidney and bone scans to give further orientation to abnormalities discovered by MIBG scan

    B. Computed tomography scans if MIBG scans have failed to locate the tumor

    C. Ultrasound of the pelvis if the tumor produces urinary symptoms

2. Refer to standard nuclear scan *posttest* precautions on page 692.

3. Follow Chapter 1 guidelines for safe, effective, informed *posttest* care.

PARATHYROID SCAN   ●

Normal Scan
No areas of increased perfusion or uptake in parathyroid or thyroid

Explanation of Test
This test is done to localize parathyroid adenomas in clinically proven cases of primary hyperparathyroidism. It is helpful in demonstrating intrinsic or extrinsic parathyroid adenoma. Two tracers, TC^{99m} sestamibi and I_{123} capsules, are administered. In children, this scan is done to verify presence of the parathyroid gland after thyroidectomy.

Procedure
1. Iodine 123 is administered. Four hours later, the neck is imaged.

2. Without moving the patient, technetium 99m sestamibi is injected; after 10 minutes, additional images are acquired. Computer processing involves subtracting the technetium-visualized thyroid structures from the I_{123} accumulation in a parathyroid adenoma.

3. Total examination time is 1 hour.

4. See Chapter 1 guidelines for safe, effective, informed *intratest* care.

Interfering Factors

Recent ingestion of iodine in food or medication and recent tests with iodine content are contraindications and reduce the effectiveness of the study.

Clinical Implications

Abnormal concentrations of the radiopharmaceuticals reveal parathyroid adenoma, both intrinsic and extrinsic, but cannot differentiate between benign and malignant adenomas.

Clinical Considerations

Pregnancy is a relative contraindication. However, if primary hyperparathyroidism is suspected and surgical exploration is essential before delivery, the study may be performed.

Patient Preparation

1. Explain the purpose, procedure, benefits, and risks of the parathyroid scan.

2. Assess for the recent intake of iodine. However, this finding is not a specific contraindication to performing the study.

3. The thyroid should be carefully palpated.

4. Refer to standard nuclear scan *pretest* precautions on page 692.

5. See Chapter 1 guidelines for safe, effective, informed *pretest* care.

Patient Aftercare

1. Refer to standard nuclear scan *posttest* precautions on page 692.

2. Interpret test outcome and monitor appropriately.

3. Follow Chapter 1 guidelines for safe, effective, informed *posttest* care.

● GENITOURINARY STUDIES

RENOGRAM: KIDNEY FUNCTION AND RENAL BLOOD FLOW SCAN (WITH FUROSEMIDE OR CAPTOPRIL)

Normal Scan

Equal blood flow in right and left kidneys

In 10 minutes, 50% of the radiopharmaceutical should be excreted.

Explanation of Test

This test is performed in both adult and pediatric patients to study the function of the kidneys and to detect renal parenchymal or vascular disease or defects in excretion. The radiopharmaceutical of choice, technetium Tc 99m mertiatide (MAG-3), permits visualization of renal clearance. In pediatric patients, this procedure is done to evaluate hydronephrosis, obstruction, reduced renal function (premature neonates), renal trauma, and urinary tract infections. The renogram is ideal for pediatric evaluation because of the nontoxic nature of the radiopharmaceuticals, compared with the contrast media used in radiology procedures.

Indications

1. To detect the presence or absence of unilateral kidney disease.
2. For long-term follow-up of hydroureteronephrosis.
3. To study the hypertensive patient to evaluate for renal artery stenosis. The captopril test is a first-line study to determine a renal basis for hypertension.
4. To study the azotemic patient when urethral catheterization is contraindicated or impossible.
5. To evaluate upper urinary tract obstruction.
6. To assess renal transplant efficacy.

Procedure

1. The patient is placed in either an upright sitting or supine position for imaging; the supine position is preferred for pediatric patients.
2. The radiopharmaceutical is injected intravenously. An intravenous diuretic (furosemide [Lasix]) or angiotensin-converting enzyme (ACE) inhibitor (captopril) may also be administered during a second phase of the renogram.
3. Imaging is started immediately after injection.
4. Total examination time is approximately 45 minutes for a routine, 1-phase renogram.
5. See Chapter 1 guidelines for safe, effective, informed *intratest* care.

▶ Clinical Alert

A renogram may be performed in a pregnant woman if it is imperative that renal function be ascertained.

Clinical Implications

Abnormal distribution patterns may indicate

1. Hypertension
2. Obstruction due to stones or tumors
3. Renal failure
4. Decreased renal function
5. Diminished blood supply
6. Renal transplant evaluation
7. In pediatric patients, urinary tract infections in male neonates; the finding shifts to females after 3 months of age.

Interfering Factors

Diuretics, ACE inhibitors, and β-blockers are medications that may interfere with the test results.

Patient Preparation

1. Explain the purpose, procedure, benefits, and risks of the nuclear scan. Pediatric patients have a detectible glomerular filtration rate after 6 months of age. In the neonate, ultrasound is used in combination with nuclear medicine procedures for a more complete renal assessment. Refer to standard nuclear scan *pretest* precautions on page 692. An intravenous line is placed before imaging.
2. Unless contraindicated, the patient should be well hydrated with 2 to 3 glasses of water (10 ml per kilogram of body weight) before undergoing the scan.
3. See Chapter 1 guidelines for safe, effective, informed *pretest* care.

Patient Aftercare

1. Encourage fluids and frequent bladder emptying to promote excretion of radioactivity.
2. Interpret test outcome and counsel appropriately.
3. Refer to standard nuclear scan *posttest* precautions on page 692.
4. Follow Chapter 1 guidelines for safe, effective, informed *posttest* care.

> **Clinical Alert**
>
> 1. The test should be performed before an intravenous pyelogram.
> 2. Severe impairment of renal function or massive enlargement of the renal collecting system may impair drainage even in the absence of true obstruction.

TESTICULAR (SCROTAL) SCAN

Normal Scan

Normal blood flow to scrotal structures, with even distribution and concentration of the radiopharmaceutical

Explanation of Test

This test is performed on an emergency basis to evaluate acute, painful testicular swelling. It also is used in the differential diagnoses of torsion or acute epididymitis and in the evaluation of injury, trauma, tumors, and masses. The radiopharmaceutical technetium Tc 99m pertechnetate is injected intravenously. The images obtained differentiate lesions associated with increased perfusion from those that are primarily ischemic. In pediatric patients, the procedure is done to diagnose acute or latent testicular torsion, epididymitis, or testicular hydrocele and for evaluation of testicular masses such as abscesses and tumors.

Procedure

1. The patient lies supine under the gamma camera. The penis is gently taped to the lower abdominal wall. For proper positioning, towels may be used to support the scrotum. Lead shielding is often placed in the perineal area to reduce any background activity.

2. The radionuclide is injected intravenously. In pediatric patients, the radio-pharmaceutical should not be injected through veins in the legs because this interferes with the study.

3. Imaging is performed in 2 phases: first, as a dynamic blood flow study of the scrotum, and second, as an assessment of distribution of the radio-pharmaceutical in the scrotum.

4. Total examining time is 30 to 45 minutes.

5. See Chapter 1 guidelines for safe, effective, informed *intratest* care.

Clinical Implications

1. Abnormal concentrations reveal
  A. Tumors
  B. Hematomas
  C. Infection
  D. Torsion (with reduced blood flow). In the neonatal patient, torsion is caused primarily by developmental anomalies.
  E. Acute epididymitis

2. The nuclear scan is most specific soon after the onset of pain, before abscess is a clinical consideration.

Patient Preparation

1. Explain the purpose, procedure, benefits, and risks of the test. There is no discomfort involved in testing.

2. If the patient is a child, a parent should accompany the boy to the department.

3. The penis is taped to the lower abdominal wall.

4. Refer to standard nuclear scan *pretest* precautions, page 692.

5. See Chapter 1 guidelines for safe, effective, informed *pretest* care.

Patient Aftercare

1. Refer to standard nuclear scan *posttest* precautions, page 692.

2. Interpret test outcome and monitor appropriately.

3. Follow Chapter 1 guidelines for safe, effective, informed *posttest* care.

VESICOURETERIC REFLUX (BLADDER AND URETERS) SCAN ●

Normal Scan

Normal bladder filling without any reflux into the ureters

Explanation of Test

This procedure usually is done on pediatric patients to assess abnormal bladder filling and possible reflux into the ureter. Technetium Tc 99m pentelate (DTPA) is administered through a urinary catheter, followed by sufficient saline until the patient has an urge to urinate. The ureters and kidneys are scanned by the camera during administration to detect the reflux.

Procedure

1. The patient is placed in the supine position. A special urinary catheter kit is used, and a urinary catheter is inserted.
2. The camera is started immediately for dynamic acquisition while the radiopharmaceutical and saline are administered until the bladder is full or there is patient discomfort.
3. The catheter is removed once the imaging is completed.

Clinical Implications

Abnormal vesicoureteric reflux may be either congenital (immature development of the urinary tract) or caused by infection.

Patient Preparation

1. See standard *pretest* care for nuclear scans of pediatric patients (page 693).
2. A urinary catheter is placed with sterile saline. An absorbent, plastic-backed pad is placed under the patient to absorb any leakage of radioactive material. If a urinary catheter is contraindicated for the patient, an alternative indirect renogram method may be used.

Patient Aftercare

1. Refer to standard nuclear scan *posttest* precautions (page 695), the same as for adults.
2. Depending on cause and severity, antibiotic therapy or surgery is used to treat the condition.
3. Special handling of the patient's urine (gloves and hand washing before and after gloves are removed) is necessary for 24 hours after completion of the test.

●GASTROINTESTINAL STUDIES

HEPATOBILIARY (GALLBLADDER, BILIARY) SCAN WITH CHOLECYSTOKININ ●

Normal Scan

Rapid transit of the radionuclide through the liver cells to the biliary tract (15 to 30 minutes) with significant uptake in the normal gallbladder

Normal distribution patterns in the biliary system, from the liver, through the gallbladder, to the small intestines

Explanation of Test

This study, using technetium Tc 99m disofenin or mebrofenen, is performed to visualize the gallbladder and determine patency of the biliary system. In pediatric patients, this test is done to differentiate biliary atresia from neonatal hepatitis and to assess liver trauma, right upper quadrant pain, and congenital malformations.

A series of images traces the excretion of the radionuclide. Through computer analysis, the activity in the gallbladder is quantitated and the amount ejected (ejection fraction) is calculated.

Indications for Testing
1. To evaluate cholecystitis
2. To differentiate between obstructive and nonobstructive jaundice
3. To investigate upper abdominal pain
4. Biliary assessment after surgery
5. Evaluation of biliary atresia

Procedure
1. The radionuclide is injected intravenously. In adults and older children, cholecystokinin (CCK) may be given to stimulate gallbladder contraction. In infants, phenobarbital is given to distinguish between biliary atresia and neonatal jaundice.
2. Imaging starts immediately after injection. A series of images is taken at 5-minute intervals for as long as it takes to visualize the gallbladder and small intestine.
3. In the event of biliary obstruction, delayed views may be obtained.
4. If CCK is administered, computer-assisted quantitative measurements can determine an ejection fraction.
5. See Chapter 1 guidelines for safe, effective, informed *intratest* care.

Clinical Implications
1. Abnormal concentration patterns reveal unusual bile communications.
2. Gallbladder visualization excludes the diagnosis of acute cholecystitis with a high degree of certainty.

Interfering Factors
1. Patients with high serum bilirubin levels (>10 mg/dl) have less reliable test results.
2. Patients receiving total parenteral nutrition or with long-term fasting may not have gallbladder visualization.

Patient Preparation
1. Explain the purpose, procedure, benefits, and risks of the nuclear scan.
2. The patient should be NPO for at least 4 hours (3 to 4 hours for pediatric patients) before testing. In case of prolonged fasting (>24 hours) notify the nuclear medical department. Fasting does not apply when the indication is for biliary atresia or jaundice.
3. Discontinue opiate- or morphine-based pain medications 2 to 6 hours before the test to avoid interference with transit of the radiopharmaceutical.
4. Refer to standard nuclear scan *pretest* precautions, page 692.

5. See Chapter 1 guidelines for safe, effective, informed *pretest* care.

Patient Aftercare
1. Interpret test outcome and monitor appropriately.
2. Refer to standard nuclear scan *posttest* precautions on page 692.
3. Follow Chapter 1 guidelines for safe, effective, informed *posttest* care.

GASTROESOPHAGEAL REFLUX SCAN ●

Normal Scan
Less than 4% gastric reflux across the esophageal sphincter

Explanation of Test
This test is indicated for both adult and pediatric patients to evaluate esophageal disorders such as regurgitation and identify the cause of persistent nausea and vomiting. In infants, the study is used to distinguish between vomiting and reflux (for those with more severe symptoms). A certain amount of reflux occurs naturally in infants. If timely diagnosis and treatment of gastrointestinal reflux does not occur, additional complications may result, such as recurrent respiratory infections, apnea, or sudden infant death syndrome (SIDS).

After oral administration of the radioisotope technetium Tc 99m sulfur colloid in orange juice or scrambled eggs, the patient is immediately imaged to verify that the dose is in the stomach. Images are acquired for 2 hours. A computer analysis is used to calculate the percentage of reflux into the esophagus for each image.

Procedure
1. The patient ingests the radionuclide in orange juice or in scrambled eggs. For infants, the test usually is performed at the normal infant feeding time to determine esophageal transit. The infant drinks ^{99m}Tc-labeled sulfur colloid mixed with milk. A portion of the milk containing the radioisotope is given, and the infant is burped before the remainder is given. Then some unlabeled milk is given to clear the esophagus of the radioactive material. If a nasogastric tube is required for radiopharmaceutical administration, the nasogastric tube must be removed before the imaging occurs, to avoid a false-positive result.
2. Images are obtained for 2 hours.
3. A computer analysis generates a time-activity curve to calculate the reflux.
4. See Chapter 1 guidelines for safe, effective, informed *intratest* care.

Clinical Implications
More than 4% reflux is abnormal. The percentage of reflux is used to evaluate patients before and after surgery for gastroesophageal reflux.

> ▶ **Clinical Alert**
>
> Patients who have esophageal motor disorders, hiatal hernias, or swallowing difficulties should have an endogastric tube inserted for the procedure.

Interfering Factors
Previous upper gastrointestinal radiographic procedures may interfere with this test.

Patient Preparation
1. Explain the purpose, procedure, benefits, and risks of the nuclear scan. See standard nuclear scan *pretest* precautions on page 692.
2. See Chapter 1 guidelines for safe, effective, informed *pretest* care.
3. The patient should be fasting from midnight of the previous night until the examination.
4. Oral intake of the orange juice or scrambled eggs containing Tc-sulfur colloid.
5. Imaging is performed with the patient in a supine position.

Patient Aftercare
1. Endogastric tubes, if placed for the examination, are removed after the radiopharmaceutical is administered.
2. Refer to standard nuclear scan *posttest* precautions on page 692.
3. Interpret test outcome and monitor appropriately.
4. Follow Chapter 1 guidelines for safe, effective, informed *posttest* care.

GASTRIC EMPTYING SCAN ●

Normal Scan

Normal Half-Time Clearance Ranges
45 to 110 minutes for solids
10 to 65 minutes for liquids

Explanation of Test
Gastric emptying imaging is used in both adult and pediatric patients to assess gastric motility disorders and in patients with unexplained nausea, vomiting, diarrhea, and abdominal cramping. The emptying of food by the stomach is a complex process that is controlled by food composition (fats, carbohydrates), food form (liquid, solid), hormone secretion (gastrin, CCK), and nervous innervation. Because clearance of liquids and clearance of solids vary, the imaging procedure traces both food forms. Indications for imaging include both mechanical and nonmechanical gastric motility disorders. Mechanical disorders include peptic ulcerations, gastric surgery, trauma, and cancer. Nonmechanical disorders include diabetes, uremia, anorexia nervosa, certain drugs

(opiates), and neurologic disorders. Clearance of liquids, solids, or a combination (dual-phase examination) may be studied.

Procedure

1. The fasting patient consumes the solid phase (^{99m}Tc–sulfur colloid, usually in scrambled eggs or oatmeal) followed by the liquid phase (indium 111–DTPA in 300 ml water). For infants, the test is performed at the normal feeding time. The infant drinks ^{99m}Tc sulfur colloid mixed with milk. Older children are provided solids such as scrambled eggs mixed with ^{99m}Tc–sulfur colloid.
2. Imaging is performed immediately, with the patient in the supine position.
3. Subsequent images are obtained over the next 2 hours.
4. Computer processing is used to determine the half-time clearance for both liquid and solid phases of gastric emptying.
5. See Chapter 1 guidelines for safe, effective, informed *intratest* care.

Clinical Implications

1. *Slow or delayed* emptying is usually seen in the following conditions:
   A. Peptic ulceration
   B. Diabetes
   C. Smooth muscle disorders
   D. After radiation therapy
   E. In pediatric patients, hypomotility of the antrum portion of the stomach is the primary cause of delayed gastric emptying. However, all abnormal functions of the stomach do contribute to the delay.
2. *Accelerated* emptying is often seen in the following conditions:
   A. Zollinger-Ellison syndrome
   B. Certain malabsorption syndromes
   C. After gastric or duodenal surgery

Interfering Factors

Administration of certain medications (eg, gastrin, CCK) interferes with gastric emptying.

Patient Preparation

1. Explain the purpose, procedure, benefits, and risks of the nuclear scan.
2. The adult patient should fast for 8 hours before the test.
3. Refer to standard nuclear scan *pretest* precautions on page 692.
4. See Chapter 1 guidelines for safe, effective, informed *pretest* care.

Patient Aftercare

1. The patient may eat and drink normally.
2. Interpret test outcomes and counsel appropriately.
3. Refer to standard nuclear scan *posttest* precautions on page 692.
4. Follow Chapter 1 basic guidelines for safe, effective, informed *posttest* care.

GASTROINTESTINAL BLEEDING SCAN ●

Normal Scan
No sites of active bleeding

Explanation of Test
This test is very sensitive in the detection and location of acute gastrointestinal bleeding that occurs distal to the ligament of Treitz. (Gastroscopy is the procedure of choice for diagnosis of upper gastrointestinal bleeding.) Before this diagnostic technique was refined, barium enemas were used to identify lesions reflecting sites of bleeding, but that test was not specific and frequently missed small sites of bleeding, such as those caused by diverticular disease or angiodysplasia. This scan is also indicated for detection and localization of recent hemorrhage, both peritoneal and retroperitoneal. The radiopharmaceutical of choice for suspected active bleeding is ^{99m}Tc-labeled RBCs.

Procedure
1. Technetium 99m–labeled RBCs are injected intravenously.
2. Imaging is begun immediately after injection and continued every few minutes. Images are obtained anteriorly over the abdomen at 5-minute intervals for 60 minutes or until a bleeding site is located. If the study is negative at 1 hour, delayed images can be obtained at 2, 6, and sometimes 24 hours later, when necessary, to identify the location of difficult-to-determine bleeding sites.
3. Total examining time varies.
4. See Chapter 1 guidelines for safe, effective, informed *intratest* care.

> ### Clinical Alert
>
> 1. This test is contraindicated in patients who are hemodynamically unstable. In these instances, angiography or surgery should be the procedure of choice.
> 2. Assess the patient for signs of active bleeding during the examining period.
> 3. Recent blood transfusion may be a contraindication for this study.

Clinical Implications
Abnormal concentrations of RBCs (hot spots) are associated with active gastrointestinal bleeding sites, both peritoneal and retroperitoneal.

Interfering Factors
Presence of barium in gastrointestinal tract may obscure the site of bleeding because of the high density of barium and the inability of the technetium to penetrate the barium.

Patient Preparation

1. Explain the purpose, procedure, benefits, and risks of the gastrointestinal blood loss scan.
2. Determine whether the patient has received barium as a diagnostic agent within the last 24 hours. If the presence of barium in the gastrointestinal tract is questionable, an abdominal radiograph may be ordered.
3. Advise the patient that delayed images may be necessary. Also, if active bleeding is not seen on initial scans, additional images must be obtained for up to 24 hours after injection in a patient with clinical signs of active bleeding.
4. Refer to standard nuclear scan *pretest* precautions on page 692.
5. See Chapter 1 guidelines for safe, effective, informed *pretest* care.

Patient Aftercare

1. Refer to standard nuclear scan *posttest* precautions on page 692.
2. Interpret test outcome and monitor appropriately.
3. Follow Chapter 1 guidelines for safe, effective, informed *posttest* care.

PAROTID (SALIVARY) GLAND SCAN ●

Normal Scan

No evidence of tumor-type activity or blockage of ducts
Normal size, shape, and position of glands

Explanation of Test

This study is helpful in the evaluation of swelling masses in the parotid region. The scan is done to detect blocked ducts of the parotid and submaxillary glands, to detect tumors of parotid or salivary glands, and to diagnose Sjögren's syndrome. The radionuclide injected intravenously is ^{99m}Tc-pertechnetate. One of the limitations of the test is that it cannot furnish an exact preoperative diagnosis.

Procedure

1. The radionuclide, pertechnetate, is injected intravenously. Scanning is performed immediately. There are 3 phases to imaging: blood flow, uptake or trapping mechanism, and secreting capability.
2. Images of the gland are taken every minute for 30 minutes.
3. If a secretory function test is being performed to detect blockage of the salivary duct, three fourths of the way through the test, the patient is asked to suck on a lemon slice. If the salivary duct is normal, this causes the gland to empty. This is not done in studies undertaken for tumor detection.
4. Total test time is 45 to 60 minutes.
5. See Chapter 1 guidelines for safe, effective, informed *intratest* care.

Clinical Implications

1. The reporting of a hot nodule amidst normal tissue that accumulates the radionuclide is associated with tumors of the ducts, as in
   A. Warthin's tumor
   B. Oncocytoma
   C. Mucoepidermoid tumor
2. The reporting of a cold nodule amidst normal tissue that does not accumulate the radionuclide is associated with
   A. Benign tumors, abscesses, or cysts, which are indicated by smooth, sharply defined outlines
   B. Adenocarcinomas, which are indicated by ragged, irregular outlines
3. Diffuse decreased activity occurs in obstruction, chronic sialadenitis, or Sjögren's syndrome.
4. Diffuse increased activity occurs in acute parotitis.

Patient Preparation

1. Explain the purpose, procedure, benefits, and risks of the nuclear scan.
2. No pain or discomfort is involved.
3. Lemon may be given to the patient to stimulate parotid secretion.
4. Refer to standard nuclear scan *pretest* precautions on page 692.
5. See Chapter 1 guidelines for safe, effective, informed *pretest* care.

Patient Aftercare

1. Interpret test outcome and monitor appropriately.
2. Refer to standard nuclear scan *posttest* precautions on page 692.
3. Follow Chapter 1 guidelines for safe, effective, informed *posttest* care.

LIVER/SPLEEN SCAN AND LIVER RBC SCAN ●

Normal Scan

Normal liver size, shape, and position within the abdomen
Normal spleen size, cell function, and blood flow in the spleen
(The amount of uptake in the spleen should always be less than in the liver.)
Normally functioning liver and spleen reticuloendothelial system

Explanation of Test

This test is used to demonstrate the anatomy and size of the liver and spleen. It is helpful in determining the cause of right upper quadrant pain and in the detection of metastatic disease, cirrhosis, ascites, infarction due to trauma, and liver damage due to radiation therapy. The majority of liver and spleen scans evaluate for metastatic disease and for the differential diagnosis of jaundice.

The radioactive material, ^{99m}Tc-labeled sulfur colloid, is injected intravenously. Liver/spleen SPECT imaging is performed by which provides 3-dimensional images of radiopharmaceutical uptake. The radiopharmaceutical most specific for detection of hemangioma in the liver is ^{99m}Tc labeled to a patient's own RBCs. In many instances, ultrasound imaging replaces this test.

Procedure
1. The radiopharmaceutical is injected intravenously.
2. A SPECT study and planar images are performed.
3. The entire study usually takes 60 minutes from injection to finish.
4. See Chapter 1 guidelines for safe, effective, informed *intratest* care.

Clinical Implications
1. Abnormal liver and spleen scan patterns occur in

A. Cirrhosis	**G.** Cysts
B. Hepatitis	**H.** Perihepatic
C. Trauma	abscesses
D. Hepatomas	**I.** Hemangiomas
E. Sarcoidosis	**J.** Adenomas
F. Metastasis	**K.** Ascites

2. Abnormal splenic concentrations reveal:

A. Unusual splenic size	**E.** Tumors
B. Infarction	**F.** Metastatic spread
C. Ruptured spleen	**G.** Leukemia
D. Accessory spleen	**H.** Hodgkin's disease

3. Spleens >14 cm are abnormally enlarged; those <7 cm are abnormally small. Areas of absent radioactivity or holes in the spleen scan are associated with abnormalities that displace or destroy normal splenic pulp.
4. About 30% of persons with Hodgkin's disease with splenic involvement have a normal splenic scan.

Patient Preparation
1. Explain the purpose, procedure, benefits, and risks of the nuclear scan.
2. This test can be performed in cases of trauma or suspected ruptured spleen, at bedside or in the emergency room.
3. Refer to standard nuclear scan *pretest* precautions on page 692.
4. See Chapter 1 guidelines for safe, effective, informed *pretest* care.

Patient Aftercare
1. Refer to standard nuclear scan *posttest* precautions on page 692.
2. Interpret test outcome and monitor appropriately.
3. Follow Chapter 1 guidelines for safe, effective, informed *posttest* care.

MECKEL'S DIVERTICULUM SCAN ●

Normal Scan
Normal blood pool distribution and clearance of the radioactive tracer into the duodenum and jejunum

Explanation of Test
This test usually is done in pediatric patients diagnosed with congenital abnormality of the ileum, which sometimes continues to the umbilicus with

fistula formation. The uptake of ^{99m}Tc Pertechnetate occurs in the parietal cells of the gastric mucosa and is detected by the gamma camera. Meckel's diverticulum shows uptake in the distal portion of the ileum. This anomaly contains secretory cells similar to those of the gastric mucosa. An alternative radiopharmaceutical, ^{99m}Tc-labeled RBCs, may be considered in cases of suspected bleeding sites associated with the diverticulum.

Procedure
1. The patient lies supine and is injected with the radiopharmaceutical.
2. The camera is started immediately with a series of static images obtained at 5-minute intervals for 30 minutes.
3. Extra spot views may be requested by the physician.
4. See Chapter 1 guidelines for safe, effective, informed *intratest* care.

Clinical Implications
Abnormal results reveal rectal bleeding, the most common symptom of Meckel's diverticulum. Meckel's diverticulum can occur with or without abdominal symptoms. If it is left undetected and untreated, ulceration of the ileum may occur, and strangulation may cause intestinal obstruction.

Patient Preparation
1. See standard *pretest* care for nuclear scans of pediatric patients (page 693). Explain the purpose and procedure of the examination. Patients should be fasting. Other diagnostic procedures involving the gastrointestinal tract and medications affecting the intestines should be avoided for 2 to 3 days before the examination. This is especially true of lower and upper gastrointestinal radiographic procedures.
2. Patients are to void immediately before the examiantion.

Patient Aftercare
1. Refer to standard nuclear scan *posttest* precautions (page 692), the same as for adults. Special handling of the patient's urine (gloves and hand washing before and after glove removal) is necessary for 24 hours after test completion.

●NEUROLOGIC STUDIES

BRAIN SCAN AND CEREBRAL BLOOD FLOW SCAN ●

Normal Scan
Normal extracranial and intracranial blood flow
Normal distribution, with highest uptake in the gray matter, basal ganglia, thalamus, and peripheral cortex and less activity in the central white matter and ventricles

Explanation of Test

Brain scans provide information about regional perfusion and brain function, whereas computed tomography and magnetic resonance imaging show structural changes. Recent developments in radiopharmaceuticals and SPECT have rejuvenated brain imaging. Newer technetium complexes such as technetium Tc 99m bisicate (ECO) and technetium Tc 99m exametazine are radiopharmaceuticals that cross the blood-brain barrier. The blood-brain barrier is not a specific anatomic structure but a complex system that includes capillary endothelium with closed intracellular clefts, a small or absent extravascular fluid space between endothelium and glial sheaths, and the membrane of the neurons themselves. SPECT technology allows for 3-dimensional slices, providing depth resolution from different angles. Although PET scanning is more effective in functional diagnosis, SPECT is less expensive and more readily available. This test is indicated in both adults and children to determine brain death or the presence of encephalitis; it is also used in children with hydrocephalus, to localize epileptic foci, to assess metabolic activity, to evaluate brain tumors, and for the assessment of childhood development disorders.

Procedure

1. The radionuclide is injected intravenously. During the injection, the patient should be in a relaxed, controlled environment to minimize anxiety. In uncooperative children, sedation should not be used until after the injection, because it may affect brain activity. The patient's head must be secured during the examination.
2. Imaging may begin immediately after administration of the radiopharmaceutical or after a 1-hour delay. It takes about 1 hour to complete.
3. With the patient in the supine position, SPECT images are obtained around the circumference of the head.
4. With administration of iodoamphetamines, some departments require a dark and quiet environment.
5. See Chapter 1 guidelines for safe, effective, informed *intratest* care.

Clinical Implications

1. Abnormal radionuclide distribution patterns indicate
   - **A.** Alzheimer's disease
   - **B.** Stroke
   - **C.** Dementia
   - **D.** Seizure disorders
   - **E.** Epilepsy
   - **F.** Systemic lupus erythematosus
   - **G.** Huntington's disease
   - **H.** Parkinson's disease
   - **I.** Psychiatric diagnosis (schizophrenia)
2. The cerebral blood flow in a patient with brain death shows a very distinct image: There is a lack of tracer uptake in the anterior and middle cerebral arteries and in the cerebral hemisphere, but perfusion is present in the scalp veins.

Interfering Factors

1. Any patient motion (eg, coughing, leg movement) can alter cerebral alignment.
2. Sudden distractions or loud noises can alter the distribution of the radionuclide.

Patient Preparation

1. Explain the purpose, procedure, benefits and risks of a brain scan.
2. Refer to standard nuclear scan *pretest* precautions in page 692.
3. Because precise head alignment is crucial, advise the patient to remain quiet and still.
4. Obtain a careful neurologic history before testing.
5. See Chapter 1 guidelines for safe, effective, informed *pretest* care.

Patient Aftercare

1. Refer to standard nuclear scan *posttest* precautions on page 692.
2. Interpret test outcome and monitor appropriately.
3. Follow Chapter 1 guidelines for safe, effective, informed *posttest* care.

CISTERNOGRAPHY (CEREBROSPINAL FLUID FLOW SCAN)   ●

Normal Scan

Unobstructed flow of cerebrospinal fluid and normal reabsorption

Explanation of Test

This study, in which the radio pharmaceutical, ^{111}In DTPA is injected intrathecally during a lumbar puncture, is a sensitive indicator of altered flow and reabsorption of CSF. Congenital malformations are the most common causes of hydrocephalus in the neonate. In older patients and in cases of trauma, computed tomography or magnetic resonance imaging is often used to identify anatomic origins of obstructive hydrocephalus. In the treatment of hydrocephalus, this test aids in selection of the type of shunt and pathway and in determining the prognosis of both shunting and hydrocephalus.

Procedure

1. A sterile lumbar puncture is performed after the patient has been positioned and prepared (see Chapter 5 for lumbar puncture procedure). At this time the radionuclide is injected into the cerebrospinal circulation.
2. The patient must lie flat after the puncture; the length of time depends on the physician's order.
3. Imaging is done at 2 to 6 hours after injection and is repeated at 24 hours, 48 hours, and 72 hours if the physician so directs.
4. Examining time is 1 hour for each scan.
5. See Chapter 1 guidelines for safe, effective, informed *intratest* care.

Clinical Implications

1. Abnormal filling patterns reveal
   A. Cause of hydrocephalus (eg, trauma, inflammation, bleeding, intracranial tumor)
   B. Subdural hematoma
   C. Spinal mass lesions
   D. Posterior fossa cysts
   E. Parencephalic and subarachnoid cysts
   F. Communicating versus noncommunicating hydrocephalus
   G. Shunt patency
   H. Diagnosis and localization of rhinorrhea and otorrhea

Patient Preparation

1. Explain the purposes, procedures, benefits, and risks for both lumbar puncture and cisternography.
2. Refer to standard nuclear scan *pretest* precautions on page 692.
3. Advise the patient that it may take as long as 1 hour for each scan.
4. Because of the lumbar puncture, the patient must be taken by cart to the nuclear medicine department for the first scan.
5. See Chapter 1 guidelines for safe, effective, informed *pretest* care.

Patient Aftercare

1. Follow instructions for lumbar puncture (see Chapter 5) and standard nuclear scan *posttest* precautions on page 692.
2. Be alert to complications of lumbar puncture, such as meningitis, allergic reaction to anesthetic, bleeding into spinal canal, herniation of brain tissue, and mild to severe headache.
3. Interpret test outcome and monitor appropriately.
4. Follow Chapter 1 guidelines for safe, effective, informed *posttest* care.

● PULMONARY STUDIES

LUNG SCAN (VENTILATION AND PERFUSION SCAN)

Normal Scan

Normal, functioning lung
Normal pulmonary vascular supply
Normal gas exchange

Explanation of Test

The lung scan is performed for 3 major purposes:

1. To diagnose and locate pulmonary emboli
2. To detect the percentage of the lungs that is functioning normally

3. To assess the pulmonary vascular supply by providing an estimate of regional pulmonary blood flow

Lung scans in both adults and children are done to assess pneumonia, cystic fibrosis, cyanosis, asthma, airway obstruction, infection, inflammation, and acquired immunodeficiency syndrome (AIDS)–related pulmonary diseases. It is a simple method for monitoring the course of embolic disease, because an area of ischemia persists after apparent resolution on chest radiographs. In the case of pulmonary embolus, the blood supply beyond an embolus is restricted. Imaging results in poor or no visualization of the affected area. Assessment of the adequacy of pulmonary artery perfusion in areas of known disease can also be done reliably.

There are 2 parts to the lung scan: the ventilation ($\dot{V}$) scan and the perfusion ($\dot{Q}$) scan. The ventilation scan reveals the movement or lack of air in the lungs. An aerosol of ^{99m}Tc DTPA or xenon 133 gas demonstrates the ventilation properties of the patient's lungs. The perfusion scan demonstrates the blood supply to the tissues in the lungs.

When inhaled, the radioactive gas or aerosol follows the same pathway as the air in normal breathing. In some pathologic conditions affecting ventilation, there is significant alteration in the normal ventilation process. The $\dot{V}/\dot{Q}$ scan is significant in the diagnosis of pulmonary emboli. It is also helpful in diagnosing bronchitis, asthma, inflammatory fibrosis, pneumonia, chronic obstructive pulmonary disease, and lung cancer.

The lung perfusion study is usually performed after the ventilation scan. A macroaggregated albumin (MAA) labeled with technetium is injected intravenously, and assessment of the pulmonary vascular supply is achieved by scanning.

Certain limitations exist with these tests. With a positive chest film and a positive $\dot{V}/\dot{Q}$ scan, the differential possibilities are multiple: pneumonia, abscess, bullae, ateliosis, and carcinoma, among others. A pulmonary arteriogram is still necessary before an embolectomy can be attempted. PE is determined by a mismatch between the ventilation and perfusion images. In other words, a normal ventilation image and an abnormal perfusion image with regmental defects indicate PE.

> ▶ **Clinical Alert**
>
> Pulmonary perfusion imaging is contraindicated in patients with primary pulmonary hypertension.

Procedure

1. The patient is asked to breathe for approximately 4 minutes through a closed, nonpressurized ventilation system. During this time, a small amount of radioactive gas or aerosol is administered. It is important that the patient not swallow the radioactive aerosol during the ventilation portion of the lung scan. Doing so causes radioactive interference with the lower lobes of the lung and make an accurate diagnostic interpretation difficult. Also, take care that the patient does not aspirate the aerosol.

2. Breath-holding will be required for a brief period at some time during the scan.

3. The imaging time is 10 to 15 minutes. When the ventilation scan is performed with a lung perfusion scan (eg, in differential diagnosis of embolism), the testing time is 30 to 45 minutes.

4. The perfusion scan immediately follows the ventilation study.

5. In the pediatric patient, the number of particles given in the MAA dose is reduced because of the smaller size of the capillary beds. Use caution with MAA in patients with atrial and ventricular septal defects.

6. See Chapter 1 guidelines for safe, effective, informed *intratest* care.

Clinical Implications

1. Abnormal ventilation and perfusion patterns indicate possible

A. Tumors	**F.** Asthma
B. Emboli	**G.** Inflammatory fibrosis
C. Pneumonia	**H.** Chronic obstructive pulmonary
D. Atelectasis	disease
E. Bronchitis	**I.** Lung cancer

2. In pediatric patients, there is an increased incidence of an airway obstruction caused by mucus plugs or foreign bodies. However, pulmonary emboli do not occur in children as often as in adults.

Interfering Factors

1. False-positive scans occur in vasculitis, mitral stenosis, and pulmonary hypertension and when tumors obstruct a pulmonary artery with airway involvement.

2. During the injection of MAA, care must be taken that the patient's blood does not mix with the radiopharmaceutical in the syringe. Otherwise, "hot spots" may be seen in the lungs.

Patient Preparation

1. Explain the purpose, procedure, benefits, and risks of the test.

2. Alleviate any fears the patient may have concerning nuclear medicine procedures.

3. It is important that a recent chest radiograph be available.

4. The patient must be able to follow directions for breathing and holding the breath, including breathing through a mouthpiece or into a face mask.

5. Refer to standard nuclear scan *pretest* precautions on page 692.

6. See Chapter 1 guidelines for safe, effective, informed *pretest* care.

Patient Aftercare

1. Refer to standard nuclear scan *posttest* precautions on page 692.

2. Interpret test outcome and monitor appropriately for postprocedural signs of aspiration.

3. Follow Chapter 1 guidelines for safe, effective, informed *posttest* care.

●ORTHOPEDIC STUDIES

BONE SCAN ●

Normal Scan
Homogenous distribution of radiopharmaceutical

Explanation of Test
This test is used primarily to evaluate and monitor persons with known or suspected metastatic disease. Breast cancers, prostate cancers, lung cancers, and lymphomas tend to metastasize to bone. Bone scans visualize lesions 6 to 12 months before they appear on radiographs.

This scan may also be performed to evaluate patients with unexplained bone pain, primary bone tumors, arthritis, osteomyelitis, abnormal healing of fractures, fractures, shin splints, or compression fractures of the vertebral column; to evaluate pediatric patients with hip pain (Legg-Calve-Perthes disease); and to assess child abuse, bone growth plates, sports injuries, and stress fractures. It is also performed to determine the age and metabolic activity of traumatic injuries and infections.

Other indications are evaluation of candidates for knee and hip prostheses, diagnosis of aseptic necrosis and vascularity of the femoral head, pre and postsurgical assessment of viable bone tissue, and evaluation of prosthetic joints and internal fixation devices to rule out loosening of prothesis or infection.

The bone scan has greater sensitivity in the pediatric patient than in the adult and is used for early detection of trauma. Normally, there is increased activity in the growth plates of the long bones. The child's history is significant for correlation and diagnostic differentiation. In older children with unexplained pain, who participate in sports, stress fractures are often found in a bone scan.

A bone-seeking radiopharmaceutical is used to image the skeletal system. An example is ^{99m}Tc-labeled phosphate injected intravenously. Imaging usually begins 2 to 3 hours after injection. Abnormal pathology, such as increased blood flow to bone or increased osteocytic activity, concentrates the radiopharmaceutical at a higher or lower rate than the normal bone does. The radiopharmaceutical mimics calcium physiologically; therefore, it concentrates more heavily in areas of increased metabolic activity.

Procedure for Bone Scan
1. Radioactive ^{99m}Tc monodyphosphonate MDP is injected intravenously.
2. A 2- to 3-hour waiting period is necessary for the radiopharmaceutical to concentrate in the bone. During this time, the patient may be asked to drink 4 to 6 glasses of water.
3. Before the scan begins, the patient is asked to void, because a full bladder masks the pelvic bones.

4. The scan takes about 30 to 60 minutes to complete. The patient must be able to lie still during scanning. The table or the scanner slowly moves the patient under and over a gamma camera.
5. Additional spot views of a specific area or 3-dimensional SPECT imaging may be requested by the physician.
6. See Chapter 1 guidelines for safe, effective, informed *intratest* care.

> ▶ **Clinical Alert**
>
> For osteomyelitis, images are acquired during the injection of the radiopharmaceutical thus giving the image of the blood flow to the bone.

Interfering Factors

1. False-negative bone scans occur in multiple myeloma of the bone. When this condition is known or suspected, the bone scan is an unreliable indicator of skeletal involvement.
2. Patients with follicular thyroid cancer may harbor metastatic bone marrow disease, but these lesions are often missed by bone scans.

Clinical Implications

Abnormal concentrations indicate the following:

1. Very early bone disease and healing is detected by nuclear bone scans long before it is visible on radiographs. Radiographs are positive for bone lesions only after 30% to 50% decalcification (decrease in bone calcium) has occurred.
2. Many disorders can be detected but not differentiated by this test (eg, cancer, arthritis, benign bone tumors, fractures, osteomyelitis, Paget's disease, aseptic necrosis). The findings must be interpreted in light of the whole clinical picture, because any process inducing an increased calcium excretion rate will be reflected by an increased uptake in the bone.
3. In patients with breast cancer, the likelihood of a positive bone scan finding in the preoperative period depends on the staging of the disease, and these scans are recommended before initial therapy. *Stages 1 and 2:* 4% have a positive bone scan. *Stage 3:* 19% have a positive bone scan. Yearly bone scans should be done for follow-up.
4. Multiple myeloma is the only tumor that shows better detectibility with a plain radiograph than with a radionuclide bone scan.
5. Multiple focal areas of increased activity in the axial skeleton are commonly associated with metastatic bone disease. The reported percentage of solitary lesions due to metastasis varies on a site-by-site basis. With a single lesion in the spine or pelvis, the cause is more likely to be metastatic disease than with a single lesion occurring in the extremities or ribs.

> **Clinical Alert**
>
> 1. The "flare phenomenon" occurs in patients with metastatic disease who are receiving a new treatment. The bone scan may show increased activity or new lesions in patients with clinical improvement. This is caused by a healing response in patients with prostate or breast cancer within the first few months of starting a new treatment. These lesions should show marked improvement on scans taken 3 to 4 months later.
> 2. Radiographic correlation is necessary to rule out a benign process when solitary areas of increased or decreased uptake occur.

Patient Preparation

1. Instruct the patient about the purpose and procedure of the test. Alleviate any fears concerning the procedure. Advise the patient that frequent drinking of fluids and activity during the first 6 hours help to reduce excess radiation to the bladder and gonads.
2. The patient can be up and about during the waiting period. There are no restrictions during the day prior to imaging.
3. Remind the patient to void before the scan. If the patient is in pain or debilitated, offer assistance to the restroom.
4. A sedative should be ordered and administered to any patient who will have difficulty lying quietly during the scanning period.
5. Refer to standard nuclear scan *pretest* precautions on page 692.
6. See Chapter 1 guidelines for safe, effective, informed *pretest* care.

Patient Aftercare

1. Advise the patient to empty the bladder when imaging is completed, to decrease radiation exposure time.
2. Refer to standard nuclear scan *posttest* precautions on page 692.
3. Interpret test outcome and monitor appropriately.
4. Follow Chapter 1 guidelines for safe, effective, informed *posttest* care.

BONE MINERAL DENSITY (BONE DENSITOMETRY; OSTEOPOROSIS SCAN)

Normal Scan

Absence of osteoporosis or osteopenia
T-score: ≥1.0

Explanation of Test

Bone densitometry enables the clinician to obtain a diagnosis of osteoporosis or osteopenia, often before fractures occur, by measuring bone mineral density. No radiopharmaceuticals are used in this procedure, but special imaging techniques are used. X-ray absorptiometry for measuring bone mineral density includes these special modalities:

1. Dual-energy absorptiometry (DEXA or DXA) to measure spine, hip, and forearm density
2. Peripheral dual-energy absorptiometry (pDXA) to measure forearm density
3. Single-energy x-ray absorptiometry (SXA) to measure the heel and forearm density
4. Radiographic absorptiometry (RA) to measure the density of the phalanges

DEXA is the most common and preferred method of measuring bone mineral density because of its precision and low radiation exposure. With the use of a laser x-ray scanner and specific computer software, DEXA can assess fracture risk with relative ease and patient comfort. Fracture risk is measured in standard deviations (SD) by comparing the patient's bone mass to that of healthy 25- to 35-year-old persons. Test scores are printed out and reported with a T-score and a Z-score. The T-score is the number of SDs for the patient compared with normal young adults with mean peak bone mass. Fracture risk increases about 1.5 to 2.5 times for every SD. According to the World Health Organization, T-scores <2.5 may confirm a diagnosis of osteoporosis; scores of 2.5 to 1.0 are associated with osteopenia; and scores of ≥1.0 are considered normal. The Z-score is defined as the number of SDs for the patient compared with normal persons in the same age category. The T-score is the score most commonly reported and currently is the preferred reference point for diagnosing osteoporosis.

Procedure

1. The patient is positioned in such a way as to keep the area being scanned immobile.
2. A foam block is placed under both knees during the spine scan, a leg brace immobilizer is used during the femur scan, and an arm brace is used when scanning the forearm.
3. DEXA scans of the spine and hip take approximately 20 minutes to complete. An additional 15 minutes is needed to scan the forearm.
4. See Chapter 1 guidelines for safe, effective, informed *intratest* care.

Clinical Implications

Abnormal scans may be associated with the following:

1. Estrogen deficiency in postmenopausal women
2. Vertebral abnormalities
3. Patients with radiographic osteopenia
4. Hyperparathyroidism
5. Patients receiving long-term corticosteroid therapy

Interfering Factors

False readings may occur with the following:

1. Nuclear medicine scans within the previous 72 hours (longer for gallium or indium scans) may cause residual emission that can be misinterpreted.

2. Barium studies within the previous 7 to 10 days may interfere with the spine scan.
3. Prosthetic devices or metallic objects surgically implanted in areas of interest may interfere with the scan.

Patient Preparation

1. Explain the purpose and procedure for measuring bone density of spine, hip, forearm, heel, and phalanges. No radiopharmaceuticals are administered.
2. Patients are encouraged to wear cotton garments that are free of metal or plastic zippers or buttons.
3. Follow Chapter 1 guidelines for safe, effective, informed *pretest* care.

Patient Aftercare

1. Interpret abnormal test outcome. If needed, serial studies may be ordered to measure the effectiveness of treatment.
2. Follow Chapter 1 guidelines for safe, effective, informed *posttest* care.

> **Clinical Alert**
>
> 1. Bone densitometry tests use x-rays; the precautions outlined in Chapter 10 should be noted.
> 2. Additional means of measuring bone mineral density are
>   A. Quantitative computed tomography (QCT) to measure spine density
>   B. Peripheral quantitative computed tomography (pQCT) to measure forearm density

---

●TUMOR IMAGING STUDIES

GALLIUM (^{67}Ga) SCANS ●

Normal Scan
No evidence of tumor-type activity or infection

Explanation of Test
This scan is used to detect the presence, location, and size of lymphoma, to detect chronic infections and abscesses, to differentiate malignant from benign lesions, and to determine the extent of invasion of known malignancies. The entire body is imaged looking for lymph node involvement. In both adult and pediatric patients, these studies are used to help stage bronchogenic cancer, Hodgkin's lymphomas, and non-Hodgkin's lymphomas. Gallium scans may

also be used to record tumor regression after radiation or chemotherapy. The radionuclide used in this study is gallium citrate (^{67}Ga).

The underlying mechanism for the uptake of ^{67}Ga is not well understood. Uptake in some neoplasms may depend on the presence of transferrin receptors in tumor cells, but this is only speculation. Once gallium enters a tissue, it remains there until radioactive decay dissipates the isotope.

Procedure

1. A laxative is given the evening before the scan.
2. Laxatives, suppositories, and/or tap water enemas are often ordered before scanning. The patient may eat breakfast on the day of imaging.
3. The radionuclide is injected 24 to 96 hours before imaging.
4. The patient must lie quietly without moving during the scanning procedure. Anterior and posterior views of the entire body are taken.
5. Additional imaging may be done at 24-hour intervals to differentiate normal bowel activity from pathologic concentrations.
6. See Chapter 1 guidelines for safe, effective, informed *intratest* care.

Clinical Implications

1. Abnormal gallium concentration usually implies the existence of underlying pathology, such as
   A. Malignancy, especially lung, testes, and mesothelioma
   B. Stages of lymphoma, Hodgkin's disease, melanoma, hepatoma, soft-tissue sarcoma, primary tumor of bone or cartilage, neuroblastoma, and leukemia
   C. Abscesses
   D. Tuberculosis
   E. Thrombosis
   F. Abscessed sarcoidosis
   G. Chronic infection
   H. Interstitial pulmonary fibrosis
2. Further diagnostic studies usually are performed to distinguish benign from malignant lesions.
3. Tumor uptake of ^{67}Ga varies with tumor type, among persons with tumors of the same histologic type, and even among tumor sites of a given patient.
4. Tumor uptake of ^{67}Ga may be significantly reduced after effective treatment.
5. Although ^{111}In-labeled leukocyte imaging is more specific for acute abscess localization, gallium imaging may be used as a multipurpose screening procedure for chronic infection.

Interfering Factors

1. A negative study cannot be definitely interpreted as ruling out the presence of disease. (The rate of false-negative results in gallium studies is 40%.)
2. It is difficult to detect a single, solitary nodule (as in adenocarcinoma). Lesions smaller than 2 cm can be detectable. Tumors near the liver are difficult to detect, and interpretation of iliac nodes is difficult.

3. Because gallium does collect in the bowel, there may be an abnormal concentration in the lower abdomen. For this reason, laxatives and enemas may be ordered.
4. Degeneration or necrosis of tumor and use of antineoplastic drugs immediately before scanning cause false-negative results.

Patient Preparation

1. Explain the purpose, procedure, benefits, and risks of the gallium scan.
2. Usually, no change in eating habits is required before testing. However, some departments request that their patients eat a low-residue lunch and a clear-liquid supper the day before the examination.
3. See standard nuclear scan *pretest* precautions on page 692.
4. The usual preparation includes oral laxatives taken on the night before the first imaging session, and again on the night before each imaging session. Enemas or suppositories may also be given. These preparations clean normal gallium activity from the bowel.
5. Actual scanning time is 45 to 90 minutes per imaging session.
6. See Chapter 1 guidelines for safe, effective, informed *pretest* care.

Patient Aftercare

1. Refer to standard nuclear scan *posttest* precautions on page 692.
2. Interpret test outcome and monitor appropriately.
3. Follow Chapter 1 guidelines for safe, effective, informed *posttest* care.

> ### Clinical Alert
>
> Breast-feeding should be discontinued for at least 4 weeks after testing.

OVERVIEW OF MONOCLONAL ANTIBODY TUMOR IMAGING (ONCOSCINT, PROSTASCINT, CARCINOEMBRYONIC ANTIGEN, AND OCTREOTIDE AND PEPTIDE)

These classes of tumor imaging has revolutionized the foundation of radiopharmaceutical production. Like other radiopharmaceuticals, monoclonal antibodies (MABs) and peptide have 2 parts: a radioisotope linked to a substance specific to a target organ. In the case of MABs that substance is an antibody that has been cloned and mass-produced. Because all the daughter antibodies are identical, a high yield of very specific antibodies can be produced.

1. OncoScint MAB—This was the first monoclonal antibody radiopharmaceutical to be approved by the US Food and Drug Administration and mass-marketed. OncoScint was approved for the detection of ovarian and colon cancer. OncoScint is an anti–carcinoembryonic antigen (CEA) antibody linked to ^{111}In.
2. ProstaScint MAB—ProstaScint is a monoclonal antibody approved for the detection of lymph node metastasis from prostate cancer.

3. CEA MAB—This monoclonal antibody is similar to OncoScint in that an antibody to CEA is used. The radioisotope, however, is ^{99m}Tc-pertechnetate. This anti-CEA antibody produces a different pattern of biodistribution than OncoScint does. Each radiopharmaceutical has its own indications.
4. Octreotide-peptide—This radiopharmaceutical peptide is used for localizing neuroendocrine tumors.

ANTIBODY AND PEPTIDE TUMOR SCANS

Normal Scan
Distribution occurs in the normal liver, spleen, bone marrow, and bowel.

Explanation of Test
This test is used to detect the location and size of known extrahepatic malignancies. These scans are not screening techniques. See overview on page 732.

Procedure
1. The patient is injected with the radioisotope over a period of 5 minutes. Observe the patient for any reaction to the radiopharmaceutical.
2. Optimal whole-body images are obtained between 2 and 4 days after injection; additional images may be obtained at 24 hours and at 5 days.
3. SPECT imaging may be performed.
4. See Chapter 1 guidelines for safe, effective, informed *intratest* care.

Clinical Implications
1. Abnormal distributions are found in tumors. Any change in the distribution provides information regarding the effectiveness of surgery or therapy.
2. Abnormal results have been observed in nonspecific areas such as inflammatory bowel disease, colostomy sites, and postoperative bowel adhesions.
3. The patient's medical history should be reviewed carefully.

Interfering Factors
Radioactivity in the bowel may interfere with colorectal assessment. Follow-up imaging is useful after administration of a cathartic to clarify equivocal findings.

Patient Preparation
1. Explain the purpose, procedure, benefits, and risks of the nuclear scan.
2. Refer to standard nuclear scan *pretest* precautions on page 692.
3. An intravenous line is established before the radiopharmaceutical is injected.
4. A cathartic is required to differentiate bowel activity from abnormal pathology.

5. Follow Chapter 1 guidelines for safe, effective, informed *pretest* care.

Patient Aftercare

1. Refer to standard nuclear scan *posttest* precautions on page 692.
2. Interpret test outcome and monitor appropriately.
3. Observe the patient for 1 hour after injection of OncoScint antibody reactions (eg, chills, fever, nausea).
4. Some patients develop human anti-mouse antibody (HAMA) titers after OncoScint injection.
5. Follow Chapter 1 guidelines for safe, effective, informed *posttest* care.

> **Clinical Alert**
>
> Following Onco Scint imaging, HAMA titers may result in falsely elevated immunoassay levels for CA-125 and CEA.

IODINE 131 WHOLE-BODY (TOTAL-BODY) SCAN

Normal Scan
No functioning extrathyroid tissues outside of the thyroid gland

Explanation of Test
This study using ^{131}I can identify functioning thyroid tissue throughout the body. It is useful to determine the presence of metastatic thyroid cancer and the amount and location of residual tissue after thyroidectomy. The procedure is routinely performed in conjunction with thyroid therapy using ^{131}I for thyrocarcinoma.

Procedure
1. Radionuclide is administered orally in a capsule form.
2. Imaging takes place 24 to 72 hours after administration of the radiopharmaceutical.
3. Imaging may take as long as 2 hours to perform.
4. Sometimes, thyrotropin (TSH) is administered intravenously before the radionuclide is given. This stimulates any residual thyroid tissue and enhances ^{131}I uptake.
5. See Chapter 1 guidelines for safe, effective, informed *intratest* care.

Clinical Implications
Abnormal uptake of iodine reveals
1. Areas of extrathyroid tissue such as
   A. Stroma ovarii
   B. Substernal thyroid
   C. Sublingual thyroid

2. Residual tissue after thyroidectomy
3. Metastatic thyroid cancer

> ### Clinical Alert
>
> 1. If possible, this test should be performed before any other radionuclide procedures and before use of any iodine contrast medium, surgical preparation, or other form of iodine.
> 2. The test is most effective when endogenous TSH levels are high, so as to stimulate radionuclide uptake by metastatic neoplasms.

Patient Preparation

1. Explain the purpose, procedure, benefits, and risks of the total-body scan.
2. Advise the patient that the imaging process may take several hours. If iodine allergies are suspected, observe the patient for possible reactions.
3. Refer to standard nuclear scan *pretest* precautions on page 692.
4. See Chapter 1 guidelines for safe, effective, informed *pretest* care.

Patient Aftercare

1. Refer to standard nuclear scan *posttest* precautions on page 692.
2. Interpret test outcome and monitor appropriately.
3. Follow Chapter 1 guidelines for safe, effective, informed *posttest* care.

BREAST SCAN (SCINTIMAMMOGRAPHY)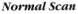

Normal Scan

Uniform distribution of radiopharmaceutical uptake in the breasts without focal points of concentration

No focal uptake in lymphatic tissue

Explanation of Test

Although x-ray mammography is the preferred examination for routine breast screening, scintimammography is often used in cases of indeterminate mammography. Other indications for performing breast imaging include follow-up to surgery, biopsy, radiation therapy, or chemotherapy. The radiopharmaceutical used for scintimammography is ^{99m}Tc miraluma. The test is more specific than x-ray mammography and may differentiate between benign and malignant lesions. The test is also used to detect any axillary lymph node involvement from breast cancer. The test decreases the number of unnecessary breast biopsies.

Procedure

1. The radiopharmaceutical is injected intravenously in the opposite arm from the breast of concern.
2. The patient lies prone on a special table with a cut out section that allows the breasts to hang through the table unobstructed.

3. The patient is also placed in the supine position with the arms raised for obtaining images of the axillary lymph nodes.
4. The total patient time is approximately 45 to 60 minutes. The actual scan time is 25 to 30 minutes.
5. An optional SPECT examination may be requested by the nuclear medicine physician. This examination may take an additional 30 to 40 minutes.
6. See Chapter 1 guidelines for safe, effective, informed *intratest* care.

Clinical Implications

1. Abnormal increased focal uptake is found in cases of a fibroadenoma and adenocarcinoma.
2. Nonuniform increased diffuse uptake of activity is associated with fibrous dysplasia, which may be unilateral or bilateral.
3. Several areas of increased focal uptake are often seen in cases of multifocal breast cancer.
4. In patients with a breast prosthesis, a focal decrease in activity is observed in relation to the size and shape of the prosthesis.
5. Axillary metastasis is detected as focal areas of increased uptake in the axillary nodes.
6. This scan is used to evaluate radiation therapy and chemotherapy.

Interfering Factors

1. There should not be any other detectable amount of radioactivity in the patient.
2. The patient should be lying supine for the injection of the radiopharmaceutical to prevent a "streaking" artifact found on the resulting image in the breast region, which corresponds to the arm that received the injection.
3. To eliminate a false-positive appearance, the patient should be injected on the side opposite a known lymphatic lesion. If the patient is known to have bilateral breast cancer, a foot vein may be used for injection.
4. Extravasation of the radiopharmaceutical can result in hot spots of radioactivity in the location of the axillary lymph nodes.

Patient Preparation

1. Explain the purpose, procedure, benefits, and risks of the nuclear scan.
2. The patient is to remove all clothing and jewelry from the waist up. The patient wears a hospital gown with the opening of the gown in the front. There are no dietary or medication restrictions.
3. See Chapter 1 guidelines for safe, effective, informed *pretest* care.
4. See standard nuclear scan *pretest* precautions on page 692.

Patient Aftercare

1. Interpret test outcome, monitor, and counsel appropriately.
2. Refer to standard nuclear scan *posttest* precautions on page 692.
3. Follow Chapter 1 guidelines for safe, effective, informed *posttest* care.

●INFLAMMATORY PROCESS IMAGING

LEUKOCYTE (WBC) SCAN (INDIUM OR CERETEC-LABELED WBCs)   ●

Normal Scan

Normal leukocyte concentration and radiopharmaceutical distribution in liver, spleen, and bone marrow

No signs of leukocyte localization outside of the reticuloendothelial system

Explanation of Test

This test, in which a sample of the patient's own white blood cells (WBCs) are isolated, labeled with indium oxine (^{111}In) or ^{99m}Tc exometazime, and reinjected, is used for localization of acute abscess formation. The study is indicated in both adults and children with signs and symptoms of a septic process, fever of unknown origin, osteomyelitis, or suspected intraabdominal abscess. It is also helpful in determining the cause of complications of surgery, injury, or inflammation of the gastrointestinal tract and pelvis. The test results are based on the fact that any collection of labeled WBCs outside the liver, spleen, and functioning bone marrow indicates an abnormal area to which the cells localize. This procedure is 90% sensitive and 90% specific for acute inflammatory disease or acute abscess formation.

Procedure

1. A venous blood sample of 60 ml is obtained for the purpose of isolating and labeling the WBCs. The laboratory process takes about 2 hours to complete. The patient's WBC count needs to be at least 4.0 so there are enough cells to label for this procedure.
2. The WBCs are labeled with radioactive ^{111}In, oxine or ^{99m}Tc exometazime and injected intravenously.
3. The patient returns for imaging at 4 hours with ceretec and 24 and/or 48 hours with indium.
4. Imaging time is about 1 hour each session.
5. See Chapter 1 guidelines for safe, effective, informed *intratest* care.

Clinical Implications

1. Abnormal concentrations indicate
   A. Acute abscess formation
   B. Acute osteomyelitis and infection of orthopedic prostheses
   C. Active inflammatory bowel disease
   D. Postsurgical abscess sites and wound infections

Interfering Factors

1. False-negative reactions are known to occur when the chemotactic function of the WBC has been altered, as in hemodialysis, hyperglycemia, hyperalimentation, steroid therapy, and long-term antibiotic therapy.

2. Gallium scans up to 1 month before the test can interfere.
3. False-positive scans occur in the presence of gastrointestinal bleeding and in upper respiratory infections and pneumonitis when patients swallow purulent sputum.

   NOTE: *See Standard Considerations, Patient Preparation, and Patient Aftercare for nuclear scans on page 692.*

> ### Clinical Alert
>
> If the patient does not have an adequate number of WBCs, additional blood may have to be drawn. Gallium imaging may be necessary if too few WBCs are present, or donor cells can be used.

Part Two

Radionuclide Laboratory Procedures (Nonradioimmunoassay Studies)

Overview of Laboratory Procedures

Very small amounts of radioactive substances may be administered to patients, and then their body fluids and glands may be examined in the laboratory for concentrations of radioactivity. Minute quantities of radioactive materials may be detected in blood, feces, urine, other body fluids, and glands.

Some procedures (eg, Schilling Test) check the ability of the body to absorb the administered radioactive compound. Others, such as blood volume determinations, test the ability of the body to localize or dilute the administered radioactive substance.

Part II of this chapter includes a sampling of tests that employ the use of radionuclides in the study of disease. Imaging may or may not be required as part of these procedures.

SCHILLING TEST ●

Normal Values

Excretion of 7% or more of the dose of cobalt-tagged vitamin B_{12} in the urine

Explanation of Test

This 24-hour urine test is used to diagnose pernicious anemia (one form of macrocytic anemia) and malabsorption syndromes. It is an indirect test of intrinsic factor deficiency. This test evaluates the body's ability to absorb vitamin B_{12} from the gastrointestinal tract and is based on the anticipated urinary excretion of radioactive vitamin B_{12}. The procedure may be done in 2 stages: stage I without intrinsic factor; stage II with intrinsic factor. The second stage is performed only when an abnormal first stage occurs.

In stage I, the fasting patient is given an oral dose of vitamin B_{12} tagged with radioactive cobalt (^{57}Co). An intramuscular injection of vitamin B_{12} is given to saturate the liver and serum protein-binding sites, which allows radioactive vitamin B_{12} to be excreted in the urine. A 24-hour urine specimen is then collected.

The amount of the excreted radioactive B_{12} is determined and expressed as a percentage of the given dose. Normal persons absorb (and therefore excrete) as much as 25% of the radioactive B_{12}. Patients with pernicious anemia absorb little of the oral dose and therefore excrete little radioactive material in the urine.

Procedure

1. The patient must fast for 12 hours before the test. (Fasting is continued for 3 hours after the vitamin B_{12} doses have been administered.)
2. A tasteless capsule of radioactive B_{12} labeled with ^{57}Co is administered orally by a nuclear medicine technologist.
3. Then a nonradioactive B_{12} injection is given intramuscularly by a registered nurse or nuclear medicine technologist.
4. All urine is collected for 24 or 48 hours after the time the patient receives the injection of vitamin B_{12}.
   A. Obtain a special 24-hour urine container from the laboratory. No preservative is required.
   B. Ensure that there is no contamination of the urine with stool.
   C. Continue collecting the urine for 24 hours (see Chapter 3).
   D. In the presence of renal disease, a 48-hour urine collection may be necessary.
5. See Chapter 1 guidelines for safe, effective, informed *intratest* care.

Clinical Implications

1. An abnormally low value (eg, <7%) or borderline (7% to 10%) allows 2 interpretations:
   A. Absence of intrinsic factor
   B. Defective absorption in the ileum
2. When the absorption of radioactive vitamin B_{12} is low from the first stage, the test must be repeated with intrinsic factor (stage II) to rule out intestinal malabsorption (confirmatory Schilling test).
   A. If urinary excretion then rises to normal levels, it indicates a lack of intrinsic factor, suggesting the diagnosis of pernicious anemia.

B. If the urinary excretion does not rise, malabsorption is considered to be the cause of the patient's anemia.

NOTE: *A dual-radionuclide test is an alternative method in which both stages are performed at the same time.*

Interfering Factors

1. Renal insufficiency may cause reduced excretion of radioactive vitamin B_{12}. If renal insufficiency is suspected, a 48- to 72-hour urine collection is advised, because eventually almost all of the absorbed material will be excreted, and urine specific gravity and volume are checked.
2. The patient should not undergo diagnostic procedures that interfere with B_{12} absorption.
3. The single most common source of error in performing the test is *incomplete collection of urine*. Some laboratories may require a 48-hour collection to allow for a small margin of error.
4. Urinary excretion of B_{12} is depressed in elderly patients, diabetics, patients with hypothyroidism, and patients with enteritis.
5. Fecal contamination in the urine leads to false results and invalidates the test.

Patient Preparation

1. Explain the purpose, procedure, benefits, and risks of the test.
2. Refer to general procedures, description of benefits, risks, clinical considerations, and standard nuclear scan *pretest* precautions on page 692.
3. A random urine sample usually is obtained before the B_{12} doses are administered.
4. Give a written reminder to the patient about fasting and collection of a 24-hour urine specimen. Water is permitted during the fasting period.
5. Food and drink are permitted 3 hours after the doses of vitamin B_{12} are given. The patient is encouraged to drink as much as can be tolerated during the entire test.
6. Be certain the patient receives the nonradioactive B_{12}. If the intramuscular dose of vitamin B_{12} is not given, the radioactive vitamin B_{12} will be found in the liver instead of the urine.
7. See Chapter 1 guidelines for safe, effective, informed *pretest* care.

> ### Clinical Alert
>
> 1. No laxatives are to be used during the test.
> 2. Bone marrow aspiration should be done before the Schilling test, because the vitamin B_{12} administered in the test destroys the diagnostic characteristics of the bone marrow.

Patient Aftercare

1. Assess for compliance with 24-hour urine collection protocols (see Chapter 3).

2. Refer to standard nuclear scan *posttest* precautions on page ● ●.

3. Interpret test outcome and monitor appropriately.

4. Follow Chapter 1 guidelines for safe, effective, informed *posttest* care.

TOTAL BLOOD VOLUME; PLASMA VOLUME; ERYTHROCYTE (RBC) VOLUME   ●

Normal Values

Total blood volume: 55 to 80 ml/kg

Erythrocyte volume: 20 to 35 ml/kg (greater in men than in women)

Plasma volume: 30 to 45 ml/kg

> **NOTE:** *Because adipose tissue has a sparser blood supply than lean tissue, the patient's body type can affect the proportion of blood volume to body weight; for this reason, test findings should always be reported in milliliters per kilogram of body weight.*

Explanation of Test

The purpose of this test is to determine circulating blood volume, to help evaluate the bleeding or debilitated patient, and to determine the origin of hypotension in the presence of anuria or oliguria when dehydration may be the cause. This determination is 1 way to monitor blood loss during surgery; it is used as a guide in replacement therapy after blood or body fluid loss and in the determination of whole-body hematocrit. The results are useful in choosing the most appropriate blood component for replacement therapy (whole blood, plasma, or packed RBCs).

Total blood volume determinations are of value in the following situations:

1. To evaluate gastrointestinal and uterine bleeding

2. To aid in the diagnosis of hypovolemic shock

3. To aid in the diagnosis of polycythemia vera

4. To determine the required blood component for replacement therapy, as in persons undergoing surgery

These tests reveal an increased or decreased volume of RBC mass. A sample of the patient's blood is mixed with a radioactive substance, incubated at room temperature, and reinjected. Another blood sample is obtained 15 minutes later. The most commonly used tracers in blood volume determinations are serum albumin tagged with ^{131}I or ^{125}I and patient or donor RBCs tagged with chromium 51. The combination of procedures (total blood volume) is the only true blood volume. Other volume studies are plasma volume and RBC volume, which may be done separately.

The plasma volume is used to establish a vascular baseline, to determine changes in plasma volume before and after surgery, and to evaluate fluid and blood replacement in patients with gastrointestinal bleeding, burns, or trauma.

The ^{51}Cr-RBC volume study is done to see what percentage of the circulating blood is composed of RBCs. This procedure is performed in connection with evaluation of RBC survival or gastrointestinal blood loss and in ferrokinetic studies.

Procedure
1. Record the patient's height and current weight.
2. Venous blood samples are obtained, and 1 blood sample is mixed with a radionuclide.
3. Fifteen to 30 minutes later, the blood radiopharmaceutical is reinjected.
4. About 15 minutes later, another venous blood sample is obtained and examined in the laboratory.
5. See Chapter 1 guidelines for safe, effective, informed *intratest* care.

Clinical Implications
1. A normal total blood volume with a decreased RBC content indicates the need for a transfusion of packed red cells.
2. Polycythemia vera may be differentiated from secondary polycythemia.
   A. Increased total blood volume due to an increased RBC mass suggests polycythemia vera. The plasma volume most often is normal.
   B. Normal or decreased total blood volume due to a decreased plasma volume suggests secondary polycythemia. The RBC most often is normal.

> **Clinical Alert**
>
> If intravenous blood component therapy is ordered for the same day, the blood volume determination should be done before the intravenous line is started.

Patient Preparation
1. Explain the purpose, procedure, benefits, and risks of the test. Blood samples and intravenous injection are part of this test. No imaging or scanning takes place.
2. The patient should be weighed just before the test if possible.
3. Refer to standard nuclear scan *pretest* precautions on page 692.
4. See Chapter 1 guidelines for safe, effective, informed *pretest* care.

Patient Aftercare
1. Refer to standard nuclear scan *posttest* precautions on page 692.
2. Interpret test outcome and monitor appropriately.
3. Follow Chapter 1 guidelines for safe, effective, informed *posttest* care.

RED BLOOD CELL (RBC) SURVIVAL TIME TEST

Normal Values
Normal half-time for survival of ^{51}Cr-labeled red blood cells is approximately 25 to 35 days.
Chromium 51 in stool: <3 ml/24 h

Explanation of Test

This blood test has its greatest use in the evaluation of known or suspected hemolytic anemia and is also indicated when the cause for anemia is obscure, to identify accessory spleens, and to determine abnormal RBC production or destruction. A sample of the patient's erythrocytes is mixed with a radioactive substance (^{51}Cr), incubated at room temperature, and reinjected. Blood specimens are drawn after 24 hours and at regular intervals for at least 3 weeks. After counting the specimens, the results are plotted and the RBC survival time is calculated. Results are based on the fact that disappearance of radioactivity from the circulation corresponds to disappearance of the RBCs, thereby determining overall erythrocyte survival.

Scanning of the spleen is often done as part of this test. The RBC survival test usually is ordered in conjunction with a blood volume determination and radionuclide iron uptake and clearance tests. When stool specimens are collected for 3 days, the test is often referred to as the "gastrointestinal blood loss test."

Procedure

1. A venous blood sample of 20 ml is obtained.
2. Ten to 30 minutes later, the blood is reinjected after being tagged with a radionuclide, ^{51}Cr.
3. Blood samples are usually obtained on the first day; again at 24, 48, 72, and 96 hours; and then at weekly intervals for 3 weeks. Time may be shortened depending on the outcome of the test. As part of this procedure, a radioactive detector may be used over the spleen, sternum, and liver to assess the relative concentrations of radioactivity in these areas. This external counting helps to determine whether the spleen is taking part in excessive sequestration of RBCs as a causative factor in anemia.
4. In some instances, a 72-hour stool collection may be ordered to detect gastrointestinal blood loss. Obtain special collection containers labeled for radiation hazard. At the end of each 24-hour collection period, the total stool is to be collected by the department of nuclear medicine. This test can be completed in 3 days.
5. See Chapter 1 guidelines for safe, effective, informed *intratest* care.

Clinical Implications

1. Shortened RBC survival may result from blood loss, hemolysis, or removal of RBCs by the spleen, as in
   - **A.** Chronic granulocytic leukemia
   - **B.** Hemolytic anemia
   - **C.** Hemoglobin C disease
   - **D.** Hereditary spherocytosis
   - **E.** Pernicious anemia
   - **F.** Megaloblastic anemia of pregnancy
   - **G.** Sickle cell anemia
   - **H.** Uremia
2. Prolonged RBC survival time may result from an abnormality in RBC production, as in thalassemia minor.

3. If hemolytic anemia is diagnosed, further studies are needed to establish whether the RBCs have intrinsic abnormalities or whether anemia results from immunologic effects of the patient's plasma.
4. Results are normal in
   A. Hemoglobin C trait
   B. Sickle cell trait
5. Half of the radioactivity in the plasma may not disappear for 7 to 8 hours.

Patient Preparation

1. Explain the purpose and procedure of the test. Emphasize that this test requires a minimum of 2 weeks of the patient's time, with trips to the diagnostic facility for venipunctures.
2. If stool collection is required, advise the patient of the importance of saving all stool and that stool must be free of urine contamination.
3. Refer to standard nuclear scan *pretest* precautions on page 692.
4. See Chapter 1 guidelines for safe, effective, informed *pretest* care.

> **Clinical Alert**
>
> 1. The test usually is contraindicated in a patient who is actively bleeding.
> 2. Record and report signs of active bleeding.
> 3. Transfusions should not be given while the test is in progress. If it is necessary to do so, notify the nuclear medicine department to terminate the test.

Patient Aftercare

1. Refer to standard nuclear scan *posttest* precautions on page 692.
2. Interpret test outcome and monitor appropriately.
3. Follow Chapter 1 guidelines for safe, effective, informed *posttest* care.

Part Three
Positron Emission Tomography

POSITRON EMISSION TOMOGRAPHY (PET) IMAGING

Normal Scan

Normal patterns of tissue metabolism based on oxygen, glucose, and fatty acid utilization and protein synthesis
Normal blood flow and tissue perfusion

Explanation of Test

PET imaging involves the combined use of positron-emitting radionuclides and emission computed tomography. PET technology generates high-resolution images of body function and metabolism. PET uses radiopharmaceuticals that are the basic elements of biologic substances. In this way, normal and abnormal biologic function of cells and organs can be determined. It produces images of molecular-level physiologic function, including glucose metabolism, oxygen utilization, blood flow, and tissue perfusion. The radiopharmaceutical dose is injected and emits radioactivity in the form of positrons, which are detected and transformed into a visual display by computer.

A broad spectrum of radiopharmaceuticals is currently used in PET imaging. A main advantage of PET derives from the positron-emitting isotopes themselves—carbon 11, nitrogen 13, and oxygen 15, which are present in organic molecules, and fluorine 18, which can be substituted for hydrogen. Typically, radionuclides used in PET imaging have very short half-lives (2 minutes to 2 hours).

Fluorine 18 is used for several purposes. Its half-life is long enough to trace biochemical reactions. It is can be used to label a glucose compound, permitting imaging of a variety of tissues. Fluorine 18 is administered primarily in a glucose form called fluorodeoxyglucose (FDG). FDG is highly sensitive. Neoplastic cells are hypermetabolic and appear to have an FDG affinity that results in high contrast. FDG has >90% specificity for myocardial viability, neoplastic processes, and infection. FDG is an outstanding tracer that can be used in many areas of the body. It is a glucose analogue and has a broad application because every cell uses glucose as fuel.

Uses of PET

Clinical PET is a useful diagnostic tool aiding diagnosis of many disease states, primarily in oncology, neurology, and cardiology. However, the technique is applicable to all parts of the body for diagnosis, disease staging, and monitoring of therapy. Unlike magnetic resonance imaging or computed tomography, PET provides physiologic, anatomic, and biochemical data.

Although PET is more sensitive than γ–SPECT, it is considerably more expensive. The use of FDG imaging with specially equipped gamma cameras has been an alternative to exclusive PET imaging systems. The patient preparation for nuclear medicine use of FDG in γ–SPECT imaging is similar to that for PET imaging of FDG. Because of the physics of [18]Fl, only multiheaded cameras can be used for γ–SPECT acquisitions. Currently, there are certain limitations with γ–SPECT imaging when compared with true PET imaging.

In oncology, FDG-PET has proved useful in several areas, including the diagnosis of pulmonary nodules, the differentiation of pancreatic cancer from mass-forming pancreatitis, and the diagnosis of breast cancer in selected cases of mammography and/or biopsy failure. PET imaging is used for the initial preoperative staging of cancer involving the lung, liver, colon, breast, head, and neck, as well as melanomas and lymphomas. For example, in lung cancer, PET is useful in determining the degree of operability. With extensive metastasis in the mediastinum, surgery is contraindicated.

In cardiology, PET has demonstrated excellent utility for measuring myocardial blood flow and perfusion and for detecting coronary artery disease. The high-energy photons of PET tracers produce high-quality images even in obese patients. In these cases, PET can provide important information for determining which patients will benefit from the more invasive procedures.

In neurology, FDG-PET imaging is a noninvasive aid in predicting prognosis and for surgical planning in epilepsy. By revealing areas of increased and decreased glucose utilization, PET helps surgeons pinpoint the surgical site. PET is being used to diagnose a wide variety of dementias, including Alzheimer's disease, which shows a distinct pattern of glucose consumption in the temporal and parietal regions of the brain. Also, distinct brain patterns can be seen in the involuntary movement disorders, such as Parkinson's disease, Huntington's disease, and Tourette's syndrome.

Procedure

1. The actual imaging time required for a single scan is 1 to 2 hours. The actual time involved with the patient may be several hours and occurs prior to and during radiopharmaceutical injection.
2. The patient is positioned on a table, then within the scanner. Before administration of the radiopharmaceutical, a background transmission scan is performed. In certain procedures, this preliminary scan is optional.
3. The radioactive drug is administered intravenously. The patient waits 30 to 45 minutes in the department, usually remaining on the table, and then the area of interest is scanned.
4. Patients undergoing PET procedures for colon cancer or kidney studies may require a urinary catheter.
5. Cardiac patients do not require fasting and glucose monitoring may be part of the patient preparation before the scan.
6. See Chapter 1 guidelines for safe, effective, informed *intratest* care.

Patient Preparation for All PET Scans

Patient preparation for FDG-PET imaging varies among institutions. However, some generalizations can be made:

1. Explain test purpose and procedure. Fasting is required for all tests (except cardiac). Sometimes fasting blood glucose levels are obtained. If blood glucose levels are too high, insulin may be ordered and administered by the physician. Caution must be taken if insulin is given, because it suppresses glucose tissue uptake. Insulin also suppresses FDG tissue uptake, which affects the quality of the resulting scan.
2. The FDG radiopharmaceutical is administered intravenously. Blood pressure is monitored.

Patient Aftercare for All PET Scans

1. Interpret test outcome and monitor appropriately for side effects.
2. Refer to standard nuclear scan *posttest* precautions on page 692.
3. Follow Chapter 1 guidelines for safe, effective, informed *posttest* care.

BRAIN IMAGING

Clinical Implications

1. *Epilepsy:* Focal areas with increased metabolism have been seen during actual episodes of epilepsy, and decreased oxygen utilization and blood flow during interictal episodes. (PET becomes an alternative to depth electrode implants.)
2. *Stroke:* An extremely complex pathophysiologic picture is being revealed, including anaerobic glycolysis, depressed oxygen utilization, and decreased blood flow.
3. *Coronary artery disease:* Excellent images of decreased myocardial blood flow and perfusion are observed.
4. *Dementia:* Decreased glucose consumption (hypometabolic activity) is revealed by PET imaging. PET is used to differentiate Alzheimer's disease from other types of dementia, such as Huntington's disease and Parkinson's disease.
5. *Schizophrenia:* Some studies using labeled glucose indicate reduced metabolic activity in the frontal region. The PET scans can also distinguish the developmental stages of cranial tumors and give information about the operability of such tumors.
6. *Brain tumors:* Data have been collected concerning oxygen use and blood flow relations for these tumors. Gliomas have relatively good perfusion compared with their decreased oxygen utilization. The high uptake of radiopharmaceutical in gliomas is reported to correlate with the tumor's histologic grade.

Interfering Factors

Excessive anxiety can alter the test results when brain function is being tested. Tranquilizers cannot be given before the test because they alter glucose metabolism.

Patient Preparation

1. Instruct the patient about the purpose, procedure, and special requirements of the PET scan (page 746). Refer to standard nuclear scan test *pretest* precautions on page 692.
2. Advise the patient that lying as still as possible during the scan is necessary. However, the patient is not to fall asleep nor count to pass the time.
3. During the scan, it is important to maintain a quiet environment.
4. See Chapter 1 guidelines for safe, effective, informed *pretest* care.

CARDIAC IMAGING ●

Clinical Implications

1. In cardiology, PET imaging provides measurements of blood flow, myocardial perfusion, and myocardial viability. These measurements are used to detect

A. Coronary artery disease, which is characterized by areas of decreased blood flow, decreased perfusion, or both.

B. Transient ischemia (both stress and rest images are performed).

2. A high rate of glucose consumption is required to meet the energy needs of the heart. Low glucose metabolism in areas of decreased blood flow indicates nonviable myocardial tissue.

Patient Preparation

1. Instruct the patient about the purpose, procedure, and special requirements of the PET scan (page 746). Refer to standard nuclear scan *pretest* precautions on page 692.

2. An intravenous line may be necessary. Cardiac patients do not require fasting and may be given glucose as part of patient preparation. Smoking and medication restrictions may be required before imaging. Consult with the referring physician or the nuclear imaging department.

3. It may be necessary to place ECG leads on the patient.

4. See Chapter 1 guidelines for safe, effective, informed *pretest* care.

TUMOR IMAGING ●

Clinical Implications

1. Measurements of glucose (FDG) metabolism are used to determine tumor growth. Because small amounts of FDG can be visualized, early tumor detection is possible before structural changes detectable by magnetic resonance imaging or computed tomography occur. Tumor grading can be assessed by the rate of increase in glucose metabolism. In cases of suspected tumor recurrence after therapy, PET differentiates any new growth from necrotic tissue.

2. PET is used to distinguish between recurrent, active tumor growth and necrotic masses in soft tissue; this differentiation is difficult to make by magnetic resonance imaging or computed tomography.

Patient Preparation

1. Explain the purpose, procedure, and special requirements of the PET scan (page 746). Refer to standard nuclear scan *pretest* precautions on page 692.

2. Usually, no special preparation is needed. Sometimes a urinary catheter may have to be inserted for colon or kidney tumor detection.

3. See Chapter 1 guidelines for safe, effective, informed *pretest* care.

BIBLIOGRAPHY ●

Arnold SE: Cardiac stress testing. Nursing '97 January: 58–61, 1997

Baum S, et al: Atlas of Nuclear Medicine Imaging. New York, Appleton & Lange, 1993

Bernier DR, Christina PE, Langa JK, et al: Nuclear Medicine Technology and Techniques, 3rd ed. St Louis, Mosby, 1994

Dawson-Hughes B, et al: Effect of calcium and vitamin D supplementation on bone density in men and women 65 years of age or older. N Engl J Med 337:670–676, 1997

Early PJ, Sodee DB: Principles and Practice of Nuclear Medicine, 2nd ed. St Louis, Mosby, 1995

Fröhlich JM, Schubergn AP, von Schulthess GK: Contrast agents and radiopharmaceuticals, in von Schulthess GK, Hennig J (eds), Functional Imaging. Philadelphia, Lippincott-Raven, 1998

Hudok CM, Gallo BM: Quick review of neurodiagnostic testing. Am J Nurs 97(7): 16CC-16FF, 1997

Kirks DR, Grissom NT (eds): Practical Pediatric Imaging. Philadelphia, Lippincott-Raven, 1998

Kumar D: PET scanning applications for treating epilepsy. Am J Nurs 98(7): 16G–17G, 1998

O'Connor MK (ed): The Mayo Clinic Manual of Nuclear Medicine. New York, Churchill Livingstone, 1996

Putnam CE, Ravin CE: Textbook of Diagnostic Imaging, 2nd ed., vols 1 and 2. Philadelphia, WB Saunders, 1994

Treves ST (ed): Pediatric Nuclear Medicine, 2nd ed. New York, Springer-Verlag, 1995

von Schulthess GK, Hennig J (eds): Functional Imaging. Philadelphia, Lippincott, 1998

Wilson MA (ed): Textbook of Nuclear Medicine. Philadelphia, Lippincott-Raven, 1998

10

X-Ray Studies

OVERVIEW OF X-RAY STUDIES ●

X-ray studies, also known as *radiographs* or *roentgenograms,* are used to examine soft and bony tissues of the body. X-rays are short-wavelength electromagnetic vibrations produced when fast-moving electrons collide with substances in their pathways. X-rays travel in straight lines at the speed of light (186,000 miles/second). When an x-ray beam passes through matter, some of its intensity is absorbed; the more dense the matter, the greater the degree of x-ray absorption. The composite image produced represents these varying degrees of tissue density in shades of black, white, and gray. Images may be captured on photographic film, displayed on a video screen, or recorded on digital media. X-rays can penetrate very dense substances to produce images or shadows that can then be recorded in a variety of formats. The basic principle of radiography is that differences in density among various body structures produce images of varying light or dark intensity, much like the negative print of a photograph. Dense structures appear white, whereas air-filled areas are black.

USE OF CONTRAST AGENTS ●

Many radiographic techniques use the natural contrasts and varying densities that exist in body tissues representing air, water (in soft tissue), fat, and bone. The lungs and gastrointestinal (GI) tract normally contain air or gases. Other body structures are encased in a fatty envelope. Bone contains naturally occurring mineral salts. However, diagnosis of certain pathologic conditions requires visualization of details that cannot be revealed through plain x-rays. In these cases, details can be highlighted by the presence of *contrast media* in the area. These contrast substances can be administered through oral, rectal, or injection administration.

The ideal contrast agent should be relatively harmless (low toxicity, nonantigenic, nonallergenic, and inert), should not interfere with any physiologic functions, and should allow high and repeated dosing at a moderate cost. A contrast medium may be classified as either *radiopaque* (not permitting the transmission of x-rays) or *radiolucent* (permitting partial transmission of x-rays). The most commonly used contrast agents are *water-insoluble* barium sulfate for GI tract evaluation and *water-soluble* iodine agents for GI examinations and intravascular procedures. Ultimately, one must always be alert to the possibility of an adverse reaction to contrast media (eg, allergic, clotting, and thrombocyte activation); consequently, emergency supplies and equipment should be readily available when using these agents.

The following contrast agents are used routinely in x-ray studies:

1. Alimentary canal water-insoluble contrast agents
   a. Barium sulfate ($BaSO_4$; eg, Polibar plus, Anatrast, Esophatrast)
2. Water-soluble agents (eg, Gastrografin, MD-Gastroview, oral Hypaque)
3. CO_2 gas (eg, calcium citrate, magnesium citrate)
4. Injectable contrast agents
   a. Nonionic iodinated contrast (low osmolar agents; eg, Optiray, Isovue, Omnipaque)

b. Ionic iodinated contrast (high osmolar agents; eg, Renovist, Hypaque, Conray)

ADVERSE REACTIONS TO CONTRAST AGENTS ●

All contrast agents have the potential for causing allergic reactions that can range from mild (eg, nausea and vomiting) to severe anaphylaxis (eg, cardiovascular collapse and central nervous system depression leading to death if untreated). Table 10–1 lists the range of possible adverse reactions to iodine contrast media. Reactions happen quickly and usually occur within minutes of administration of the contrast agent. Such reactions can occur in anyone.

Clinical Considerations When Iodine Contrast Agents Are Used

1. Know the patient's age and health status. Children and the elderly, especially those with medical problems, may be especially sensitive to contrast agents. This sensitivity may increase the chance of side-effects.
2. The presence of other medical problems may increase the risk of side-effects.
   a. Those with asthma or hay fever are at greater risk for having an allergic reaction to the contrast agent.
   b. Those with diabetes have a greater risk of developing kidney problems.
   c. Those with severe hypertension may experience a dangerous rise in blood pressure.
   d. Those with kidney and liver disease may experience exacerbation of their disease.
   e. Those with multiple myeloma may develop severe kidney problems.
   f. Those with overactive thyroid may experience a sudden increase in symptoms.
   g. Those with sickle cell disease may experience the formation of abnormal blood cells.
3. Patients who are allergic to iodine contrast media must have this information documented in their health care records. The risk of subsequent reactions increases three to four times after the first reaction; however, subsequent reactions will not necessarily be more severe than the first. The patient must be made aware of the implications of their situation. Assess for and document allergies to iodine-containing substances (eg, seafood, cabbage, kale, rape vegetables, turnips, iodine salt). Also determine each person's reactions to penicillin or to skin test for allergies as these patients have a greater chance of having a reaction.
4. Check the patient's fasting status before the x-ray procedure has begun. Except in an extreme emergency, iodine contrast media should never be administered intravenously sooner than 90 minutes after the patient has eaten. In most instances, the patient should fast the night before any x-ray procedure using an iodine contrast agent.
5. Death from an allergic reaction can occur if severe symptoms go untreated.

TABLE 10-1

Signs, Symptoms, and Incidence of Reactions to Iodine Contrast Media

Cardiovascular	Respiratory	Cutaneous	Gastrointestinal	Neurologic	Genitourinary
Pallor	Sneezing	Erythema	Nausea	Anxiety	Flank pain
Diaphoresis	Coughing	Feeling of warmth	Vomiting	Headache	Hematuria
Tachycardia	Rhinorrhea	Parotitis	Metallic taste	Dizziness	Oliguria
Bradycardia	Wheezing	Urticaria	Abdominal cramps	Agitation	Albuminuria
Palpitations	Acute asthma attack	Pruritus	Diarrhea	Vertigo	WBCs in blood
Arrhythmia	Laryngospasm	Pain at injection site	Paralytic ileus	Slurred speech	Acute renal failure
Acute pulmonary edema	Cyanosis	Angioneurotic edema		Disorientation	Uterine cramps
Shock	Laryngeal edema			Stupor	Urgency to urinate
Congestive heart failure	Apnea			Coma	
Cardiac arrest	Respiratory arrest			Convulsions	

All Iodine Contrast Reactions

	Incidence (%)
Minor reactions requiring no treatment: Sensation of heat, nausea, vomiting, local urticaria, rash, dizziness, lightheadedness, transient arrhythmia, pain at injection site, mild pallor, pruritus	1:20 (5)
Intermediate reactions that require treatment but no hospitalization and are not life-threatening: vomiting, extensive urticaria, facial edema, bronchospasm, faintness, dyspnea, mild chest pain, headache, chills and fever	1:100 (1)
Severe reactions that require hospitalization and are life-threatening: syncope, laryngeal and pulmonary edema, hypotension, convulsions, circulatory collapse, pulmonary edema, severe angina, myocardial infarction, cardiac arrhythmia, coma, respiratory arrest	1:2000 (0.05)
Cardiac arrest	1:6000 (0.017)
Death	1:40,000 (0.0025)

Staff in attendance must be qualified to administer cardiopulmonary resuscitation should it be necessary. Emergency equipment and supplies must be readily available.

6. Promptly administer antihistamines per physician's order if mild to moderate reactions to iodine contrast substances occur.

7. When coordinating x-ray testing with a contrast agent, keep in mind that studies using iodine and those using barium should be scheduled at different times.

8. Some physiologic change can be expected when an iodine contrast substance is injected, as in an intravenous pyelogram (IVP). Physiologic responses to iodine given intravenously include hypotension, tachycardia, and arrhythmias. For this reason, always check blood pressure, pulse, and respiration before and after these tests are performed.

9. If appropriate for the patient, encourage intake of large amounts of oral fluids after the test to promote frequent urination. This flushes the iodine out of the body.

10. Possible contraindications to the administration of iodine contrast substances include the following conditions:
    a. Hypersensitivity to iodine
    b. Sickle cell anemia (use may increase sickling effect)
    c. Syphilis (use may lead to nephrotic syndrome)
    d. Long-term steroid therapy (iodine substance may render part of the drug inactive)
    e. Pheochromocytoma (may produce a sudden, potentially fatal, rise in blood pressure)
    f. Hyperthyroidism
    g. Chronic obstructive pulmonary disease (COPD)
    h. Multiple myeloma
    i. Acute asthma
    j. History of renal failure
    k. Pregnancy
    l. Diabetes mellitus
    m. Severe dehydration
    n. Congestive heart failure
    o. Drug therapy known to be nephrotic (eg, cisplatin)

11. Nonionic contrast agents tend to produce fewer side-effects than do ionic materials.

12. Patients with renal failure may develop acidosis when iodine contrast is administered.

Clinical Alert

1. Careful patient preparation considers patient safety, prevents complications, and can prevent repeat procedures. Assess for the following

(continued)

(Clinical Alert continued)

risk factors associated with a higher incidence of undesirable contrast agent reactions:

a. Allergy
b. Asthma
c. Previous reactions to contrast media
d. Repeat and high dosages administered
e. Diabetes mellitus
f. Renal failure (preexisting)
g. Liver insufficiency
h. Multiple myeloma
i. Dehydration
j. Older adult (>65 years)
k. Newborns
l. History of seizures
m. Pheochromocytoma

2. No contrast agent is without risk for causing reactions. Benefit versus risk must be considered. For example, in a workup to detect cancer, the benefits of early detection far outweigh the dangers of cumulative x-radiation exposure. The patient must be informed of the risk-benefit ratio; the patient has a legal right to this knowledge.

3. Never inject iodized oils or barium into the bloodstream.

4. Contrast agent–induced acute renal insufficiency is a rare and dangerous complication that occurs 1 to 5 days following intravenous injection of a contrast medium. Dehydrated patients and those with serum creatinine levels >1.4 mg/dl are at greatest risk.

5. Special attention is necessary for diabetic patients due to their increased potential for renal failure. Diabetic persons taking the oral hypoglycemic glucophage/metformin should have this drug withheld the day of and 48 hours following the injection of iodinated contrast. In addition, advise the patient that their serum creatinine level be rechecked 24 hours after he or she has received parenteral contrast. Check with the radiology department for specific instructions.

6. Tests for thyroid function (serum tests as well as nuclear medicine studies) are adversely affected for several weeks to months following iodinated contrast injection.

7. Late reactions (2–3 days after procedure) most often occur with the use of agents such as iotrolan and iodoxane for intravascular procedures such as angiography.

Clinical Considerations When Barium Contrast Is Used

There is always some risk when introducing barium sulfate or a similar contrast agent into the GI tract.

1. Barium radiography may interfere with many other abdominal examinations. A number of studies, including other x-rays, tests using iodine, ultrasound procedures, radioisotope studies, tomograms, computed tomography, and proctoscopy, must be scheduled before barium studies. Consult with the radiography department for the proper sequencing of studies.
2. Emphasize that a laxative should be taken after a barium sulfate procedure is completed.
3. Elderly, inactive persons should be checked for stool impaction if they fail to defecate within a reasonable length of time after a barium procedure. The first sign of impaction in the elderly may be fainting.
4. Observe and record findings regarding stool color and consistency for at least 2 days to determine whether barium has been evacuated. Stools will be light in color until all barium has been expelled. Outpatients should be given a written reminder to inspect their stools for at least 2 days following barium administration.
5. If possible, avoid giving narcotics, especially codeine, when barium x-rays are ordered, because these drugs can cause constipation that can compound possible barium-associated constipation.

Clinical Alert

1. Rare instances of severe allergic reactions to barium sulfate have been reported. All patients should be questioned regarding their allergic history prior to administration of any type of contrast agent. A history of hay fever, asthma, and other allergies places the patient at higher risk for reactions to all types of contrast agents.
2. The risk of postprocedure constipation or blockage of the bowel is increased in patients with the following conditions:
   a. Cystic fibrosis
   b. Dehydration
   c. Acute ulcerative colitis
3. Barium should *not* be used for intestinal study in the following circumstances:
   a. When a bowel perforation is suspected.
   b. Following sigmoidoscopy or colonoscopy, especially if a biopsy was performed, because leakage of barium from the alimentary canal can cause peritonitis. Iodinated contrast should be used in these cases.

There are special clinical considerations for ostomy patients undergoing bowel preparation for GI studies; exam preparation and procedure should be tailored between the primary care provider and the radiology department to achieve the most optimal outcomes. In most cases, standard dietary and medication restrictions apply, but modifications involving mechanical bowel cleansing with enemas and physiologic cleansing with laxatives may be necessary.

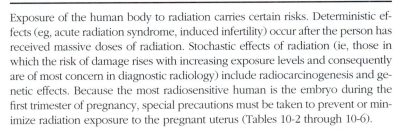

> **Clinical Alert for Patients With Ostomies**
>
> 1. Enemas and laxatives should not be given to a person with an ileostomy in preparation for x-rays or endoscopy (Chapter 12) because this puts the person at risk for dehydration and electrolyte imbalance. Conversely, a person with a sigmoid colostomy requires enemas before x-ray studies or endoscopy is performed. Consequently, it is important to identify the type of surgical procedure the patient has undergone. Moreover, not all colostomies need irrigation. For example, a person with an ascending right-sided colostomy will usually pass a liquid, pasty stool high in water content and digestive enzymes; such a patient may only require laxatives.
> 2. Notify the radiology department that the person has an ostomy.
> 3. Advise all patients to bring extra ostomy supplies and pouches for use after the procedure is completed.

See page 755 for specifics regarding barium enema preparation for patients with ostomies.

RISKS OF RADIATION ●

Exposure of the human body to radiation carries certain risks. Deterministic effects (eg, acute radiation syndrome, induced infertility) occur after the person has received massive doses of radiation. Stochastic effects of radiation (ie, those in which the risk of damage rises with increasing exposure levels and consequently are of most concern in diagnostic radiology) include radiocarcinogenesis and genetic effects. Because the most radiosensitive human is the embryo during the first trimester of pregnancy, special precautions must be taken to prevent or minimize radiation exposure to the pregnant uterus (Tables 10-2 through 10-6).

Safety Measures
Certain precautions must be taken to protect patients, medical and nursing personnel, and other clinical and technical staff from unnecessary exposure to radiation.

General Precautions
1. Staff in the radiology department should wear lead aprons (and gloves if indicated) when not within a shielded booth during x-ray exposures. Patients should be shielded appropriately insofar as the procedure allows.
2. The x-ray tube housing should be checked periodically to detect radiation leakage and to indicate when repairs or adjustments are necessary.
3. The patient's medical records should be reviewed for radiation therapy history.
4. The primary x-ray beam should pass through layers of aluminum adequate to filter out excess radiation while still providing detailed images.

TABLE 10-2
Principal Early Effects of Radiation Exposure on Humans and Approximate Minimum Radiation Dose Necessary to Produce Them

Effect	*Anatomic Site*	*Minimum Dose (Gray)*
Death	Whole body	1
Hematologic depression	Whole body	.25
Skin erythema	Small field	3
Epilation	Small field	3
Chromosome aberration	Whole body	.05
Gonadal dysfunction	Local tissue	.1

From Bushong SC: Radiologic Science for Technologists, 6th ed. St. Louis, CV Mosby, 1997.

TABLE 10-3
BEIR Committee Estimated Excess Mortality From Malignant Disease per 100,000 Persons

	Male	*Female*
Normal expectation	20,560	16,680
Excess cases		
Single exposure to 10 rad	770	810
Continuous exposure to 1 rad/y	2880	3070
Continuous exposure to 100 mrad/y	520	600

From Bushong SC: Radiologic Science for Technologists, 6th ed. St. Louis, CV Mosby, 1997.

TABLE 10-4
Relative Risk of Childhood Leukemia After Irradiation in Utero by Trimester

Time of X-Ray Examination	*Relative Risk*
First trimester	8.3
Second trimester	1.5
Third trimester	1.4
Total	1.5

From Bushong SC: Radiologic Science for Technologists, 6th ed. St. Louis, CV Mosby, 1997.

5. Fast film and high-resolution screens produce quality results. Filmless "computed radiography" may reduce radiation exposure and retakes.
6. The size or area of the x-ray must be carefully adjusted so that no more tissue than necessary is exposed to the x-radiation. Collimators (shutters),

TABLE 10-5
Summary of Effects After 10-rad in Exposure in Utero

Time of Exposure	Type of Response	Natural Occurrence	Radiation Response
0–2 w	Spontaneous abortion	25%	0.1%
2–10 w	Congenital abnormalities	5%	1%
2–15 w	Mental retardation	6%	0.5%
0–9 mo	Malignant disease	8/10,000	12/10,000
0–9 mo	Impaired growth and development	1%	Nil
0–9 mo	Genetic mutations	10%	Nil

From Bushong SC: Radiological Science for Technologists, 6th ed. St. Louis, CV Mosby, 1997.

TABLE 10-6
Representative Radiation Quantities
From Various Diagnostic X-Ray Procedures

Examination	Technique (kVp/mAs)	Entrance Skin Exposure (mrad)	Mean Marrow Dose (mrad)	Gonad Dose (mrad)
Skull	76/50	200	10	<1
Chest	110/3	10	2	<1
Cervical spine	70/40	150	10	<1
Lumbar spine	72/60	300	60	225
Abdomen	74/60	400	30	125
Pelvis	70/50	150	20	150
Extremity	60/5	50	2	<1
Head CT	125/300	3000	20	50
Pelvis CT	124/400	4000	100	3000

From Bushong SC: Radiologic Science for Technologists, 6th ed. St. Louis, CV Mosby, 1997.

cones, or lead diaphragms can assure proper sizing and x-ray exposure area.

7. The gonads should be shielded in both female and male patients of child-bearing age unless the examination involves the abdomen or gonad areas.

Precautions To Be Used With Pregnant Patients

1. Women of childbearing age who could possibly be in the first trimester of pregnancy should *not* have x-ray examinations involving the trunk or pelvic regions. A brief menstrual history should be obtained to determine if a possible pregnancy exists. If pregnancy is possible, a pregnancy test should be done before proceeding with x-ray examination.

2. All pregnant patients, regardless of trimester, should avoid radiographic, fluoroscopic, and serial film studies of the pelvic region, lumbar spine, and abdomen if at all possible.
3. Should x-ray studies be necessary for obstetric regions, repeat films should not be done.
4. If x-ray studies of nonreproductive tissues are necessary (eg, dental x-rays), the abdominal and pelvic region should be shielded with a lead apron.

Responsibilities in Ordering and Scheduling X-Ray Examinations

Correct and complete information should be entered into the computer or on the x-ray requisition. Explain to the patient the purpose and procedure of the x-ray examination. Written patient instructions may be helpful.

When a complete genitourinary-gastrointestinal (GU/GI) workup is scheduled, the sequence of x-ray procedures should follow a definite order:

First day: IVP and barium enema
Second day (or subsequent day): upper GI series

Barium studies should be scheduled after the following procedures:

1. Abdominal or pelvic ultrasound examination
2. Lumbar-sacral spine x-rays
3. Pelvic x-rays
4. Hysterosalpingogram
5. IVP

As a general rule, examinations that *do not* require contrast should *precede* examinations that *do* require contrast. All examinations that require iodine contrast should be completed before those that require barium contrast. In addition, examinations that require iodine contrast must precede nuclear medicine examinations that require radioactive iodine administration (eg, thyroid scans).

Other x-ray examinations that do not require preparation can be performed at any time. Such examinations include the following:

X-rays of the head, spine, and extremities
Noncontrast abdominal x-rays (eg, KUB, abdomen series)
Mammograms

▶ **Clinical Alert for Nursing Home Patients**

All nursing home patients should be accompanied by another adult to the x-ray testing site. If a nonfasting patient will be in the x-ray department over lunch time, the facility should send a bag lunch or money for lunch with the patient.

●PLAIN (CONVENTIONAL) X-RAYS/RADIOGRAPHY

CHEST X-RAY ●

Normal Chest X-Ray Examination

Normal-appearing and normally positioned chest, bony thorax (all bones present, aligned, symmetrical, and normally shaped), soft tissues, mediastinum, lungs, pleura, heart, and aortic arch

Explanation of Test

The chest x-ray is the most frequently requested radiograph. It is used to diagnose cancer, tuberculosis and other pulmonary diseases, and disorders of the mediastinum and bony thorax. The chest x-ray provides a record of the sequential progress or development of a disease. It can also provide valuable information about the condition of the heart, lungs, GI tract, and thyroid gland. A chest x-ray must be done after the insertion of chest tubes or subclavian catheters to determine their anatomic position as well as to detect possible pneumothorax related to the insertion procedure. In addition, the position of other devices such as nasogastric or enteric feeding tubes can be determined and adjusted if necessary.

Procedure

1. Routine chest radiography consists of two images: a frontal view (posteroanterior [PA]) and a left lateral view. Upright chest films are preferred and are of utmost importance because films taken in the supine position do not demonstrate fluid levels. This observation is especially important when testing patients on bed rest.

2. Street clothing covering the chest is removed to the waist. Only cloth or paper hospital gowns free of buttons and snaps may be worn during the x-ray. Jewelry must be removed.

3. Monitoring cables and patches should not obscure the chest area if possible.

4. The patient is instructed to take a deep breath and to exhale; then to take another deep breath and to hold it while the x-ray image is taken. After the x-ray is completed, the patient may breathe normally.

5. The procedure takes only a few minutes.

6. Follow guidelines in Chapter 1 regarding safe, effective, informed *intratest* care.

Clinical Implications

1. Abnormal chest x-ray results indicate the following lung conditions:
   a. Presence of foreign bodies
   b. Aplasia
   c. Hypoplasia
   d. Cysts

    e. Lobar pneumonia
    f. Bronchopneumonia
    g. Aspiration pneumonia
    h. Pulmonary brucellosis
    i. Viral pneumonia
    j. Lung abscess
    k. Middle lobe syndrome
    l. Pneumothorax
    m. Pleural effusion
    n. Atelectasis
    o. Pneumonitis
    p. Congenital pulmonary cysts
    q. Pulmonary tuberculosis
    r. Sarcoidosis
    s. Pneumoconiosis (eg, asbestosis)
    t. Coccidioidomycosis
    u. Westermark's sign (indicates decreased pulmonary vascularity, sometimes thought to suggest pulmonary embolus)

2. Abnormal conditions of the bony thorax include the following:
    a. Scoliosis
    b. Hemivertebrae
    c. Kyphosis
    d. Trauma
    e. Bone destruction or degeneration
    f. Osteoarthritis
    g. Osteomyelitis

3. Cardiac enlargement

Interfering Factors

An important consideration in interpreting chest radiographs is to ask whether the film was taken in full inspiration. Certain disease states do not allow the patient to fully inhale. The following conditions may alter the patient's ability to breathe properly and should be considered when evaluating radiographs:

1. Obesity
2. Severe pain
3. Congestive heart failure
4. Scarring of lung tissues

Patient Preparation

1. No special preparation is required. However, the patient should be given a brief explanation of the purpose of and procedure for the test and assured that there will be no discomfort. Screen for pregnancy status of female patients. If positive, advise the radiology department.
2. Remove all jewelry and other ornamentation in the chest area before the x-ray.

3. Remind the patient of the need to remain motionless and to follow all breathing instructions during the procedure.

4. Follow guidelines in Chapter 1 regarding safe, effective, informed *pretest* care.

> **Clinical Alert**
>
> A portable x-ray machine may be brought to the nursing unit if the patient cannot be transported. The nurse may need to assist x-ray personnel in positioning the patient and film. It is the x-ray technologist's responsibility to clear all unnecessary personnel from the radiation field before x-ray exposure.

Patient Aftercare

1. Interpret test outcomes and monitor for pulmonary disease and chest disorders. Explain changes in therapy based on chest x-ray results (eg, diuretics for pulmonary edema, endotracheal tube repositioning, starting or stopping mechanical ventilation, further testing to determine new chest infiltrates).

2. Follow guidelines in Chapter 1 regarding safe, effective, informed *posttest* care.

MAMMOGRAPHY (BREAST X-RAY)

Normal Breast X-Ray Examination

Essentially normal breast tissue: calcification, if present, should be evenly distributed; normal ducts with gradual narrowing ductal system branches

Explanation of Test

Soft-tissue mammography visualizes the breast tissue on photographic film and detects small abnormalities that could warn of cancer. Its primary use is to screen for and discover cancers that escape detection by other means such as palpation. Typically, cancers <1 cm cannot be detected by routine clinical or self-examinations. Because the average breast cancer has probably been present for some time before it reaches the clinically palpable 1-cm size, the prognosis for cure is excellent if detected in this preclinical or presymptomatic phase.

The low-energy x-ray beam used for this procedure is applied to a tightly restricted area and consequently does not produce significant radiation exposure to other areas of the body. Therefore, it is quite acceptable from a radiation safety standpoint to recommend routine screenings. Diagnosis by mammography is based on the radiographic appearance of gross anatomic structures. Benign lesions tend to push breast tissue aside as they expand, whereas malignant lesions may invade surrounding breast tissue. Although false-negative and false-positive readings can occur, mammography is highly accurate.

Most breast lumps are not malignant; many are benign cysts. For women >40 years of age, the benefits of using low-dose mammography to find early, curable cancers outweigh possible risks from radiation exposure.

Likelihood of Breast Cancer	
Age (y)	*Odds*
25	1:19,608
30	1:2525
35	1:622
40	1:217
45	1:93
50	1:50
55	1:33
60	1:24
65	1:17
70	1:14
75	1:11
80	1:10
85	1:9
≥95	1:8

National Cancer Institute

The American College of Radiology (ACR) accredits mammography services. To earn accreditation, mammograms must be performed by specially trained and credentialed radiographers and the resulting films must be interpreted by radiologists who meet criteria for continuing education in mammography. Additionally, the ACR has stringent standards for equipment, film quality, and radiation dose. Health insurers, including Medicare, require mammographic services to be performed at an ACR-accredited institution.

Indications for Mammography
1. To detect clinically nonpalpable breast cancers in women >40 years of age, younger women at high risk, or those having a history of breast cancer
2. When signs and symptoms of breast cancer are present
   a. Skin changes (eg, "orange peel" skin associated with inflammatory type cancer)
   b. Nipple or skin retraction
   c. Nipple discharge or erosion
3. Breast pain
4. "Lumpy" breast; multiple masses or nodules
5. Pendulous breasts that are difficult to examine
6. Survey of opposite breast after mastectomy
7. Patients at risk for having breast cancer (eg, family history of breast cancer)

8. Adenocarcinoma of undetermined origin
9. Previous breast biopsy
10. Tissue samples removed from the breast may be radiographed using detailed mammography techniques.
11. Follow-up studies for questionable mammographic images

> **NOTE:** *The American Cancer Society recommends a baseline mammogram for all women between 35 and 40 years of age, an annual or biannual mammogram for those 40 to 49 years of age, and a yearly mammogram for those ≥ 50 years of age.*

Procedure

1. Mammograms are performed with the person in an upright position, preferably standing. Accommodations are made for patients using wheelchairs.
2. The breast is exposed and lifted onto a film holder. The breast tissue is adjusted by hand, smoothing out all skin folds and wrinkles. A movable paddle is lowered onto the breast, rigorously compressing the breast tissue.

> **NOTE:** *Rigorous compression is a brief and uncomfortable but critical step in ensuring a high-quality mammogram.*

3. An x-ray exposure is quickly made, and the compression is immediately lifted.
4. Typically, two views (craniocaudal and mediolateral) are taken of each breast.
5. Before or following the x-ray examination, the technologist visually observes and manually palpates the breasts.
6. The complete examination takes about 30 minutes.
7. Follow guidelines in Chapter 1 regarding safe, effective, informed *intratest* care.

Clinical Alert

1. Computer-assisted diagnosis is a new detection technique. Software scans the image and notes suspicious areas that a radiologist could miss, thus acting as a second opinion.
2. Many radiologists double-read all mammograms.
3. Comparison with old mammograms is very important. Consequently, patients are advised to have all mammograms performed at the same facility or retrieve old mammograms and bring them along when having a new study performed.
4. The FDA has recently approved the use of certain Digital Mammography equipment. In this technique, x-ray film is replaced by a detector and the images are digitally captured, manipulated, and stored.

Clinical Implications

1. Abnormal mammogram findings reveal the following conditions:
   a. Breast mass
      (1) Benign breast masses (eg, cysts, fibroadenomas) are usually round and well demarcated.

(2) Malignant breast masses are usually irregularly shaped with extensions into adjacent tissue, often with an increased number of blood vessels (Fig. 10-1).

(3) When a mass is detected, additional studies are performed to help differentiate the nature of the mass. These studies may include the following:

    (a) Special x-ray magnification views of the area in question

    (b) "Spot" compression views performed using a special paddle that isolates the suspicious tissue (Fig. 10-2)

    (c) Ultrasound of the area to help differentiate a cystic (fluid-filled) mass from a solid lesion

b. Calcifications present in the malignant mass (duct carcinoma) or in adjacent tissue (lobular carcinoma) are described as innumerable punctate calcifications resembling fine grains of salt or rod-like calcifications that appear thin, branching, and curvilinear.

c. The likelihood of malignancy increases with a greater number of calcifications in a cluster. However, a cluster with as few as three calcifications, particularly if they are irregular in shape or size, can occur in cancer.

d. Typical parenchymal patterns are as follows:

N_1: normal

P_1: mild duct prominence on less than one fourth of the breast

P_2: marked duct prominence

DY: dysplasia (some diagnosticians believe that the person who exhibits dysplasia is 22 times more likely to develop breast cancer than the person with normal results)

e. Findings of breast cancer when contrast is injected are associated with extravasation of contrast, filling defects, obstruction, or irregular narrow-

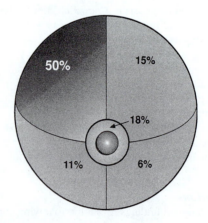

FIGURE 10-1
Half of all breast cancers develop in the upper outer section. (Source: Department of Health and Human Services, 1994)

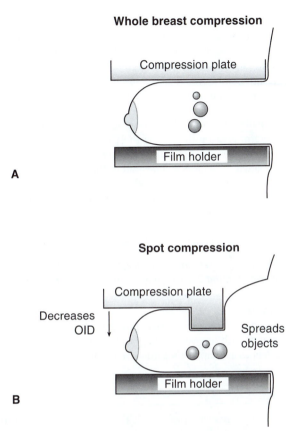

FIGURE 10-2
Examples of **(A)** Whole Breast Compression and **(B)** Spot Compression.

ing of ducts. Contrast mammography (ductogram, galactogram) is a valuable aid for diagnosing intraductal papillomas. Mammary duct injection is used when cytologic examination of breast fluid or discharge is abnormal. In contrast mammography, after careful cannulation of a discharging duct, about 1 ml of a radiopaque substance (eg, 50% sodium diatrizoate) is injected into the breast duct with a blunt, 25-gauge needle.

f. Difficult diagnoses include the following conditions:

   (1) Colloid (gelatinous or mucinous) and medullary (circumscribed) carcinomas are difficult to diagnose by mammography.

   (2) Soft tissue mammography is notoriously poor in localizing nonpalpable intraductal papillomas. Sometimes the calcifications of cancer and sclerosing adenosis may be indistinguishable, particularly if the adenosis is not bilateral.

Patient Preparation

1. Explain the purpose, procedure, benefits, and risks of mammograms. Mammography is the single best method for detecting breast cancer while it is still in a curable stage. Some discomfort is to be expected when the breast is compressed.

2. Assess pregnancy status of female patients. If positive, advise radiology department.

3. Instruct the patient not to apply deodorant, perfume, powders, or ointment to the underarm area on the day of the examination. Residue from these preparations can obscure optimal visualization.

4. Advise the patient to wear separates rather than a dress, because clothing must be removed from the upper body.

5. Suggest that patients who have painful breasts refrain from caffeinated foods and beverages (eg, coffee, tea, cola, chocolate) for 5 to 7 days before testing.

6. Follow guidelines in Chapter 1 regarding safe, effective, informed *pretest* care.

NOTE: *Patients in the reproductive age group are advised to have mammograms performed in the 2 weeks that follow their last menstrual period.*

Patient Aftercare

1. Interpret test outcomes and counsel appropriately. If a biopsy is necessary, see procedures for biopsy using x-ray technology.

2. Follow guidelines in Chapter 1 regarding safe, effective, informed *posttest* care.

Clinical Alert

1. A mammogram detects abnormalities that could warn of cancer. The actual diagnosis of cancer is made by biopsy. Only one in five biopsies test positive for cancer.

2. Several methods can be used to provide a breast tissue sample necessary for cancer diagnosis. These include stereotactic core biopsy, fine-needle biopsy, and surgical biopsy.

Procedure for Stereotactic X-Ray–Guided Core Biopsy

1. A local anesthetic and a sedative are administered.

2. The patient lies on her abdomen, allowing her breast to protrude through an opening in a special table.

3. Two stereoview mammograms are taken, allowing precise positioning of hollow-core needle.

4. The needle is inserted into the breast at precise locations using sterile lacerations. Multiple core tissue samples are taken because tumors have both benign and malignant areas.

5. The breast is cleansed, and a sterile dressing is applied.

NOTE: *A larger sample of tissue may be extracted using a special attachment called an Advanced Breast Biopsy Instrumentation (ABBI). Core biopsies may also be conducted under ultrasound guidance.*

Procedure for Needle X-Ray Localization and Surgical Biopsy

1. A local anesthetic and sedative are administered. In some instances, general anesthesia is used.
2. Using breast x-ray films as a guide, a needle that holds a fine wire is inserted into the breast tissue. When the needle point is at the tip of the x-ray–defined abnormality, the guide wire is released. It stays there until the surgeon, guided by the wire, removes it along with a specimen of the abnormal tissue.

ORTHOPEDIC X-RAY: BONES, JOINTS, AND SUPPORTING STRUCTURES

Normal Orthopedic X-Ray Examination
Normal osseous (bone) and supporting tissue structures

Explanation of Test
Orthopedic radiography examines a particular bone, group of bones, or joint. The bony or osseous system presents five functions of radiologic significance: structure support of the body, locomotion, red marrow storage, calcium storage, and protection of underlying soft tissue and organ structures. Orthopedic radiography is performed on the following structures:

1. The extremities (eg, hand, wrist, shoulder, foot, knee, hip)
2. The bony thorax (eg, ribs, sternum, clavicle)
3. The spine (eg, cervical, thoracic, lumbar, sacrum, coccyx)
4. The head and skull (eg, facial bones, mastoids, sinuses)

Optimal results from orthopedic x-ray examinations depend on proper immobilization of the area being studied. To produce a thorough image of the body part, at least two and sometimes more projections are required. These are usually taken at angles of 90 degrees to one another (eg, anteroposterior and lateral views).

To examine more complex structures such as the spine and skull, or to examine a structure in greater detail, several projections from various angles may be required.

Procedure
1. Dietary restrictions are not necessary.
2. The patient assumes the positions most favorable to capturing the best images. However, the degree of patient mobility and physical condition may also need to be considered. Typically, the anatomic structures being studied are examined from several angles and positions. This may require the

examiner to physically manipulate the body area into a position that will allow optimal visualization.

3. Jewelry, zippers, snaps, monitoring cables, and so forth interfere with proper visualization. These objects must be removed from the visual field if possible. Skull x-rays require removal of dentures and partials.

4. Surgical-type hardware used to stabilize a traumatized area must sometimes be removed. This should be done only under the direction of the attending physician.

5. Follow guidelines in Chapter 1 regarding safe, effective, informed *intratest* care.

Clinical Implications

1. Abnormal orthopedic x-ray results may reveal the following conditions:
   a. Fractures
   b. Dislocations
   c. Arthritis
   d. Osteoporosis
   e. Osteomyelitis
   f. Degenerative joint disease
   g. Hydrocephalus
   h. Sarcoma
   i. Abscess and aseptic necrosis
   j. Paget's disease
   k. Gout
   l. Acromegaly
   m. Metastatic processes
   n. Myeloma
   o. Osteochondrosis, for example,
      (1) Legg-Calvé-Perthes disease
      (2) Osgood-Schlatter disease
   p. Bone infarcts
   q. Histiocytosis X
   r. Bone tumors (benign and malignant)
   s. Foreign bodies

Interfering Factors

Radiography of the lumbosacral spine, coccyx, or pelvis must be completed before barium studies because residual barium may interfere with proper visualization. Jewelry and accessories, heavy clothing, metallic objects, zippers, buttons, snaps, cables, and other monitoring equipment and supplies can interfere with optimal views and need to be removed before the examination.

Patient Preparation

1. Explain the purpose and procedure of the test. No preparation or dietary restrictions are necessary. Screen for pregnancy status of female patients. If positive, advise the radiology department.

2. Assure the patient that the procedure in and of itself causes no pain. However, necessary manipulation of the body may cause discomfort. If appropriate, pain medication may be administered before the procedure.

3. Advise the patient that all dentures, partials, jewelry, and other ornamentation worn in the anatomic area being examined must be removed before the study. If possible, simple clothing should be worn, and the previously mentioned items should be left at home or in the patient's room.

4. Emphasize the importance of not moving during the procedure unless specifically instructed otherwise. Movement distorts or "blurs" the image and often requires repeat films.

5. Follow guidelines in Chapter 1 regarding safe, effective, informed *pretest* care.

Patient Aftercare

1. Interpret test outcomes and monitor for fractures, dislocations, and other orthopedic disorders. Counsel about need for follow-up procedures and treatment.
2. Follow guidelines in Chapter 1 regarding safe, effective, informed *posttest* care.

Clinical Alert

1. Orthopedic radiography also can provide information about soft tissue structures, such as swelling or calcifications. However, radiography alone cannot provide data about the condition of cartilage, tendons, or ligaments.
2. Portable x-ray machines can be taken to the nursing unit if the patient cannot be transported to the radiology department. Nursing personnel may need to assist in the process. The x-ray technologist is responsible for clearing all unnecessary personnel from the immediate radiation field before shooting the film.

ABDOMINAL X-RAY: PLAIN FILM OR KUB (KIDNEY, URETERS, BLADDER); SCOUT FILM; FLAT PLATE ●

Normal Abdominal X-Ray Examination

Normal abdominal structures

Explanation of Test

This radiographic study does *not* use contrast media. It is done to aid in the diagnosis of intraabdominal diseases such as nephrolithiasis, intestinal obstruction, soft tissue masses, or ruptured viscus. It may be the preliminary step in evaluating the GI tract, the gallbladder, or the urinary tract, and it is done before IVP or other renal studies. Abdominal films may provide information on the size, shape, and position of the liver, spleen, and kidneys.

Procedure

1. The patient wears a hospital gown. All metallic objects must be removed from the abdominal area.
2. The patient lies in a supine position on the x-ray table.
3. If the patient cannot sit or stand, a position lying on the left side with the right side up must be assumed.
4. Follow guidelines in Chapter 1 regarding safe, effective, informed *intratest* care.

NOTE: *An abdominal series is often performed as an aid to diagnosis of the acute abdomen. The series consists of multiple x-ray views of the abdomen performed in a number of positions, including upright and decubitus.*

Clinical Implications

1. Abnormal abdominal x-ray results reveal the following conditions:
   a. Calcium deposits in blood vessels and lymph nodes; cysts, tumors, or stones
   b. Ureters are not clearly defined, although calculi may be visualized within the ureters.
   c. The urinary bladder can often be identified by the shadow it casts, especially in the presence of high-specific-gravity urine.
   d. Abnormal kidney size, shape, and position
   e. Appendicolithiasis
   f. Foreign bodies
   g. Abnormal fluid; ascites
   h. Large tumors and masses (ovarian or uterine), if they displace normal bowel configurations
   i. Abnormal gas distribution associated with bowel perforation or obstruction
   j. Fusion anomalies
   k. Horseshoe-shaped kidneys

Interfering Factors

1. Barium may interfere with optimal visualization. Therefore, this examination should be done before barium studies.
2. A flat plate of the abdomen does not detect free air.

Patient Preparation

1. Explain the purpose and procedure of the test. Normal diet is allowed unless contraindicated. Assure the patient that the procedure in itself is not painful.
2. Remove belts, zippers, jewelry, and other ornamentation from the abdominal area.
3. Instruct the patient to remain still and to follow breathing instructions.
4. Follow guidelines in Chapter 1 regarding safe, effective, informed *pretest* care.

> ### Clinical Alert
>
> 1. Abdominal plain films are not diagnostic for certain conditions, such as esophageal varices or bleeding peptic ulcer.
> 2. A portable x-ray machine may be brought to the nursing unit if the patient cannot be moved. Assist with positioning as necessary. The x-ray technologist is responsible for clearing all unnecessary personnel from the radiation field before the x-ray is taken.

Patient Aftercare
1. Interpret test outcomes and monitor for intraabdominal disease.
2. Follow guidelines in Chapter 1 regarding safe, effective, informed *posttest* care.

DENTAL X-RAYS ●

Normal Dental X-Ray Examination
Normal mandible, maxilla, temporomandibular joints, maxillary sinuses, and primary or permanent dentition

Explanation of Test
Dental x-rays screen and diagnose causes of pain and other symptoms related to the teeth, jaws, and temporomandibular joints, and are also used as follow-up for dental therapy. Many different types of dental radiographs are available because of the complex tissue density found within the human masticatory system. The x-rays are categorized by the location at which the film is placed during the procedure. *Intraoral* refers to films taken inside the mouth; *extraoral* x-rays are taken outside the oral cavity. The most common x-rays taken are the bite wing and the periapical, both of which are intraoral. The various types of dental x-rays include the following:

Intraoral (Taken Inside the Mouth)
1. Bite wing: shows coronal portion of the tooth; also done for caries detection; shows bite correlation between upper and lower teeth
2. Peripheral: shows x-ray of the whole tooth and immediate surrounding area
3. Occlusal: shows chewing surfaces and curve of mandibular molar teeth

Extraoral (Taken Outside the Mouth)
1. Shows various projections of the skull, maxilla, sinuses, or temporomandibular joints
2. Panarex (full mouth x-ray)
3. Computed tomography
4. Arthrography of the temporomandibular joint

Procedure
1. When taking x-rays inside the mouth, the patient is seated upright and the film and holder are placed in the mouth. The patient may bite on the holder or may anchor it with a finger to keep it in place. A lead apron with a cervical collar is draped over the patient's torso and neck area.
2. Different designs of film holders facilitate proper alignment for correct x-ray tube orientation. There are also many different types of extraoral films that can be taken, each with their own procedures. For example, with the lateral skull projection, the patient sits upright and the film packet is placed on one side of the head while the x-ray source is placed on the opposite

side. In other instances, such as extraoral x-rays, the x-ray machine rotates around the face.
3. Follow guidelines in Chapter 1 regarding safe, effective, informed *intratest* care.

> ◗ **Clinical Alert**
>
> Previous extensive radiation therapy or a current state of pregnancy may present contraindications to dental x-rays. Consult the patient's physician if in doubt.

Clinical Implications
1. Abnormal dental x-ray results reveal the following conditions:
   a. Dentition
      (1) Changes in number of teeth
      (2) Changes in shape of teeth
      (3) Changes in pulp canal
      (4) Miscellaneous other tooth lesions
   b. Radiolucent lesions of the jaw
      (1) Lesions at the tooth apex
      (2) Midline tooth lesions
      (3) Lesions in place of a missing tooth
      (4) Lesions around the crown of an impacted tooth
      (5) Bubble-like radiolucencies
      (6) Other multiple but different radiolucent lesions
      (7) Lesions that destroy the cortical plate of the tooth
   c. Mixed lesions (radiopaque and radiolucent)
   d. Salivary gland lesions
   e. Soft tissue lesions
   f. Temporomandibular joint abnormalities

Interfering Factors
The following factors can interfere with proper visualization:

1. Braces and retainers
2. Partials and dentures
3. Restorations
4. Jewelry (eg, earrings)
5. Bony growths on the inside of the mandible and the midline of the hard palate (tori) or excess deposits of bone

Patient Preparation
1. Explain purpose, procedure, benefits, and risks (minimum radiation exposure). Stress the importance of holding still and breathing through the nose to lessen the gag reflex.
2. Assist the patient to rinse his or her mouth before the procedure.

3. Assess for contraindications and interfering factors.
4. Follow guidelines in Chapter 1 regarding safe, effective, informed *pretest* care.

Patient Aftercare

1. Evaluate x-ray films and explain abnormalities. Comparison with a normal x-ray film may be helpful.
2. Follow guidelines in Chapter 1 regarding safe, effective, informed *posttest* care.

● CONTRAST X-RAYS/RADIOGRAPHY

To visualize hollow internal viscera, contrast media is administered to highlight the structure. Refer to pages 752 through 757 for special care when using contrast media. Careful sequencing of multiple examinations is necessary. As a general rule the following instructions for sequencing should be followed:

1. Abdominal pelvic computed tomography (CT), ultrasound, and nuclear medicine studies should be performed before contrast studies of the intestines.
2. Examinations of the lower intestine (barium enema) should be performed 1 or 2 days before examinations of the upper intestines (UGI).
3. Examinations requiring an injection of iodinated contrast, such as an IVP, should be performed before any barium studies (eg, barium enema, UGI).
4. Consult the radiology department for specific sequencing information.
5. Special caution is needed when administering contrast agents to diabetic persons and persons with kidney problems (see p. 755).
6. Cautions on effects of concurrent use of codeine and barium contrast agents are explained on pages 756.

CONTRAST X-RAY OF THE STOMACH: GASTRIC X-RAY INCLUDING UPPER GASTROINTESTINAL EXAMINATION (UPPER GI SERIES [UGI], BARIUM SWALLOW, ESOPHAGRAM)   ●

> **NOTE:** *A video esophagram is typically performed to evaluate swallowing disorders, particularly in poststroke patients, and after head and neck surgery with plastic repair. This examination generally includes evaluation by a speech pathologist.*

Normal Upper Gastrointestinal X-Ray Examination

Normal stomach size, contour, motility, and peristaltic activity
Normal esophagus

Explanation of Test

Gastric radiography visualizes the form, position, mucosal folds, peristaltic activity, and motility of the stomach and upper GI tract. An upper GI series includes the esophagus, duodenum, and upper portion of the jejunum.

Preliminary films without the use of a contrast medium are useful in detecting perforation, presence of radiopaque foreign substances, gastric wall thickening, and displacement of the gastric air bubble, which may indicate a mass external to the stomach.

Oral contrast substances such as barium sulfate or diatrizoate meglumine (Gastrografin) highlights conditions such as hiatal hernia, pyloric stenosis, gastric diverticulitis, presence of undigested food, gastritis, congenital anomalies (eg, dextroposition, duplication), or diseases of the stomach (eg, gastric ulcer, cancer, stomach polyps).

Procedure

1. Have patient change from street clothing into a hospital gown. Jewelry and other ornamentation must be removed.
2. Instruct the patient to swallow the barium after the patient is properly positioned in front of the fluoroscopy machine. Some changes in position may be necessary during the procedure. A motorized tabletop shifts the patient from an upright to a supine position when appropriate. Fluoroscopy allows visualization and filming of actual activity taking place in real time.
3. Following fluoroscopic examination, several conventional x-ray films are taken. The patient will need to hold his or her breath during each exposure.
4. Examination time may be 20 to 45 minutes.
5. Follow guidelines in Chapter 1 regarding safe, effective, informed *intratest* care.

Clinical Implications

1. Abnormal UGI x-ray results reveal the following conditions:
   a. Congenital anomalies
   b. Gastric ulcer
   c. Carcinoma of stomach
   d. Gastric polyps
   e. Gastritis
   f. Foreign bodies
   g. Gastric diverticula
   h. Pyloric stenosis
   i. Reflux and hiatal hernia
   j. Volvulus of the stomach

   NOTE: *Normal contours may be deformed by intrinsic tumors or consistent filling defects, as well as by stenosis in conjunction with dilation.*

Interfering Factors

1. If the patient is debilitated, proper examination may be difficult; it may be impossible to adequately visualize the stomach.
2. Retained food and fluids interfere with optimal film clarity.

Patient Preparation

1. Explain purpose and procedure (consult barium contrast test precautions on pp 756 and 757). Written instructions on pretest preparation are helpful for the patient. Screen female patients for pregnancy status. If positive, inform the radiology department.
2. Complete fasting from food and fluids is required from midnight until the examination is completed. Necessary oral medications (other than glucophage/metformin) may be taken with a tiny sip of water. Inform radiology department, because pills may be visualized during the study.
3. Instruct the patient to hold still and follow breathing instructions during the procedure.
4. Follow guidelines in Chapter 1 regarding safe, effective, informed *pretest* care.

▌**Clinical Alert**
_____

1. If patient has diabetes, alert the radiology department and schedule examination for early morning. If diabetic patient is taking glucophage/metformin, special considerations may be necessary. Consult with radiology department to determine whether this medication regimen must be suspended for the day of and several days after the study.
2. Determine if patient is allergic to barium. Although rare, presence of this allergy must be communicated to the radiology department so alternate contrast can be used.
3. All female patients of reproductive age must be screened for pregnancy prior to performing this study.

Patient Aftercare

1. Pretest diet and activity may be resumed. Provide food and fluids.
2. Administer laxatives as ordered. If barium sulfate or diatrizoate meglumine has been administered, a laxative should be taken.
3. Observe and record stools for color and consistency. Monitor evacuation of barium. Counsel that follow-up procedures may be necessary.
4. Follow guidelines in Chapter 1 regarding safe, effective, informed *posttest* care.

SMALL BOWEL X-RAY; INTESTINAL RADIOGRAPHY AND FLUOROSCOPY

Normal Small Bowel X-Ray Examination

Normal small intestine contour, position, and motility

Explanation of Test

These small intestine studies, usually scheduled in conjunction with upper GI series, are done to diagnose small bowel diseases (eg, ulcerative colitis, tumors, active bleeding, obstruction). A contrast material such as barium sulfate or meglumine diatrizoate highlights Meckel's diverticulum, congenital atresia, obstruction, filling defects, regional enteritis, lymphoid hyperplasia, tuberculosis of small intestine (malabsorption syndrome), sprue, Whipple's disease, intussusception, and edema.

The mesenteric small intestine begins at the duodenojejunal valve and ends at the ileocecal valve. The mesenteric small intestine is not routinely included as part of an upper GI study.

Procedure

1. The patient must change into a hospital gown after removing street clothes and accessories. A preliminary plain-film study is done with the patient on the examining table.
2. While standing in front of the fluoroscopy machine, the patient swallows the prescribed amount of chalky contrast material.
3. After contrast material is swallowed, timed films are taken, usually every 30 minutes.
4. The examination is not complete until the ileocecal valve has filled with contrast material. This may take several minutes (for those patients with a bypass) to several hours.
5. Follow guidelines in Chapter 1 regarding safe, effective, informed *intratest* care.

Clinical Implications

1. Abnormal small bowel x-ray results indicate the following conditions:
   a. Anomalies of small intestine
   b. Errors of rotation
   c. Meckel's diverticulum
   d. Atresia
   e. Neoplasms
   f. Regional enteritis (Crohn's disease)
   g. Tuberculosis
   h. Malabsorption syndrome
   i. Intussusception
   j. Roundworms (ascariasis)
   k. Intraabdominal hernias

Interfering Factors

1. Delays in small intestine motility can be due to the following circumstances:
   a. Morphine use
   b. Severe or poorly controlled diabetes
2. Increases in motility in the small intestine can be due to the following circumstances:
   a. Fear or anxiety
   b. Excitement
   c. Nausea
   d. Pathogens
   e. Viruses
   f. Diet (eg, very high fiber)

Patient Preparation

1. Explain the purpose and procedure of the test. Refer to barium contrast test precautions (see pp. 756–757). Written reminders for pretest instructions are helpful, especially for diet limitations. Screen female patients for pregnancy status. If positive, advise the radiology department.
2. Maintain total fast from midnight until the examination is completed.
3. Do not administer laxatives or enemas to a patient with an ileostomy.
4. Instruct the patient regarding the need to hold still and to follow breathing instructions during the procedure.
5. Follow guidelines in Chapter 1 regarding safe, effective, informed *pretest* care.

Clinical Alert

1. If the patient has diabetes, alert the radiology department and schedule examination for early morning. If the diabetic patient is taking glucophage/metformin, special considerations may be necessary. Consult with the radiology department to determine whether this medication regimen must be suspended during and for several days after study.
2. Determine whether the patient is allergic to barium. Although rare, presence of this allergy must be communicated to the radiology department so alternate contrast can be used.
3. All female patients of reproductive age must be screened for pregnancy prior to performing this study.

Patient Aftercare

1. Resume pretest diet and activity. Assist patient if necessary.
2. Administer laxatives if ordered. If a barium sulfate swallow has been done, a laxative should be taken. However, do not give laxatives to a patient with an ileostomy unless specifically ordered.
3. Monitor stools for color and consistency.
4. Counsel patient about motility disorders and other small intestine abnormalities. Follow-up procedures may be necessary.
5. Follow guidelines in Chapter 1 regarding safe, effective, informed *posttest* care.

COLON X-RAY: DEFECOGRAPHY; BARIUM ENEMA; AIR-CONTRAST STUDY (EVACUATIVE PORTOGRAPHY)

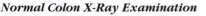

Normal Colon X-Ray Examination

Normal colon position, contour, filling, movement time, and patency

Explanation of Test

This fluoroscopic and filmed examination of the large intestine (colon) allows visualization of the position, filling, and movement of contrast medium through the colon. It can reveal the presence or absence of diseases such as diverticulitis, mass lesions, polyps, colitis, obstruction, or active bleeding. Barium or diatrizoate meglumine (Hypaque) is instilled into the large intestine through a rectal tube inserted into the colon. The radiologist, with the aid of a fluoroscope, observes the barium as it flows through the large intestine. X-ray films are taken concurrently.

For a satisfactory examination, the colon must be thoroughly cleansed of fecal matter. This is most important. Accurate identification of small polyps is possible only in a clean bowel. The presence of stool can also make the search for bleeding sources much more difficult.

If polyps are suspected, an air-contrast colon examination may be done. The procedure is basically the same as that for the barium enema; however, more complex radiographs need to be taken with the patient in several different positions. A double-contrast mixture of air and barium is instilled into the colon under fluoroscopic visualization.

Procedure

1. Initially, the patient lies on his or her back while a preliminary x-ray film is made; this step may be omitted at some institutions.
2. The patient then lies on his or her side while barium is administered by rectal enema (ie, through the rectum and up through the sigmoid, descending, transverse, and ascending colon to the ileocecal valve).
3. Following fluoroscopy, which includes several spot films, conventional x-ray films are taken. After these are completed, the patient is free to expel the barium. After evacuation, another film is made.
4. Defecography or evacuative portography are contrast-enhanced studies of the anus and rectum function during evacuation. Often used in young patients to evaluate rectoceles, rectal prolapse, or rectal intussusception, this examination requires the patient to evacuate into a specially designed commode while being evaluated fluoroscopically.
5. Follow guidelines in Chapter 1 regarding safe, effective, informed *intratest* care.

Clinical Implications

1. Abnormal colon x-ray results indicate the following conditions:

   a. Lesions or tumors (benign)   **h.** Stenosis
   b. Obstructions   **i.** Right-sided colitis
   c. Megacolon   **j.** Hernias
   d. Fistulae   **k.** Polyps
   e. Inflammatory changes   **l.** Intussusception
   f. Diverticula   **m.** Carcinoma
   g. Chronic ulcerative colitis

2. Appendix size, position, and motility can also be evaluated; however, a diagnosis of acute or chronic appendicitis *cannot* be made from x-ray findings. Instead, typical signs and symptoms of appendicitis provide the most accurate data for this diagnosis.

Interfering Factors

A poorly cleansed bowel is the most common interfering factor. Fecal matter interferes with accurate and complete visualization. Therefore, it is imperative that proper bowel cleansing be conscientiously carried out, or the procedure may need to be repeated.

Patient Preparation

Preparation involves a three-step process over a 1- to 2-day period and includes diet restrictions, physiologic cleansing of the large bowel by means of oral laxatives, and mechanical cleansing with enemas. Twelve- to 18-hour protocols are common. Follow institutional protocols.

1. Explain the purpose and procedure of the test. Patients may be apprehensive or embarrassed. Include a family member in this process if it appears likely that the patient will need assistance with preparation. Explain the need to cooperate to expedite the procedure. Emphasize that the actual time frame when the colon is full is quite brief. Screen female patients for pregnancy status. If positive, advise the radiology department.

2. A written reminder about the following may be helpful to the patient:
    a. Only a clear liquid diet should be taken before testing (according to protocols).
    b. Stool softeners, laxatives, and enemas need to be taken to assure bowel cleanliness necessary for optimal visualization. Agents such as X-Prep, citrate of magnesia, and bisacodyl assist in emptying the ascending and right-to-midtransverse colon (proximal large bowel). Enemas cleanse the left transverse, descending, sigmoid colon, and rectum. Suppositories also empty the rectum.
    c. Fasting from food and fluids is prescribed before the test. Nothing should be eaten or drunk from midnight until the test is completed. Oral medications should also be temporarily discontinued unless specifically ordered otherwise. Check with the clinician who orders the test.

3. Refer to barium contrast test precautions on pages 756 and 757.

4. Follow guidelines in Chapter 1 regarding safe, effective, informed *pretest* care.

Patient Aftercare

1. Resume pretest activity and diet. Assist the patient if necessary. This bowel examination can be very exhausting. Patients may be weak, thirsty, hungry, and tired. Provide a calm, restful environment to promote return to normal status.

2. Laxatives should be administered for at least 2 days after these studies or until stools return to normal. Instruct the patient to assess stools during this time. Stools will be light-colored until all barium has been expelled. Outpatients should be given a written reminder to inspect stools for 2 days.

3. Follow guidelines in Chapter 1 regarding safe, effective, informed *posttest* care.

Clinical Alert

1. Multiple enemas given before the procedure, especially to a person at risk for electrolyte imbalances, could induce a rather rapid hypokalemia. Enema fluid, if not expelled within a reasonable time, can be absorbed through the bowel wall and deposited into the intestinal spaces and eventually within extracellular spaces.

2. Caution should dictate administration of cathartics or enemas in the presence of acute abdominal pain, active bleeding, ulcerative colitis, or obstruction. Consult with the physician or radiology department and consider the following points:

   a. Introducing large quantities of water into the bowel of a patient with megacolon should be avoided because of the potential danger of water intoxication. In general, patients with toxic megacolon should *not* receive enemas.

   b. In the presence of colon obstruction, large volumes of water from enemas may be reabsorbed, and impaction may occur.

   c. Rectal obstruction makes it difficult or impossible to give cleansing enemas because the solution will not be able to enter the colon. Consult the physician or radiology department.

3. Strong cathartics administered in the presence of obstructive lesions or acute ulcerative colitis can present hazardous or life-threatening situations.

4. Be aware of complications that can occur when barium sulfate or other contrast media are introduced into the GI tract. For example, barium may aggravate acute ulcerative colitis or cause a progression from partial to complete obstruction. Barium also should not be given as contrast for intestinal studies when a bowel perforation is suspected, because leakage of barium through the perforation may cause peritonitis. Iodinated contrast substances should be used if perforation is suspected.

5. Determine whether patient is allergic to barium. Although rare, the presence of this allergy must be communicated to the radiology department so alternate contrast media can be used.

6. Fasting orders include oral medications except when specified otherwise.

7. If patient has diabetes, alert the radiology department and schedule examination for early morning. If diabetic patient is taking glucophage/metformin, special consideration may be necessary. Consult with the radiology department to determine whether this medication regimen must be suspended the day of and several days after the study.

8. Determine whether patient is allergic to latex. Latex products are typically used to administer the contrast agent; alternate materials must be used if patient is hypersensitive. Inform the radiology department of any known or suspected latex allergies.

9. Inform the radiology department if this procedure is to follow a sigmoidoscopy or colonoscopy, particularly if a biopsy was performed. In the case of biopsy, an iodinated contrast agent, rather than barium, is used.

Special Considerations for Children or Elderly Patients
Receiving Barium Enemas

1. Because a successful examination of the large intestine depends on the ability of the bowel to retain contrast medium during visualization and filming, special techniques are used for infants and young children or the infirm or uncooperative adult patient.

2. After inserting a small enema tip into the rectum, the infant's buttocks are gently taped together to prevent leakage of contrast material during the study.

3. For the older patient, a special retention enema tip may be used. This device resembles a regular enema tip, but it can be inflated, much like an indwelling urinary catheter, after insertion into the rectum. When the examination is done, the retention balloon is deflated and the tip removed.

Special Considerations for Barium Enema in the Presence of a Colostomy

1. See pages 756 and 757 for assessment criteria.

2. Laxatives can be taken.

3. Suppositories are of no value.

4. Follow physician's diet orders.

5. If irrigation is necessary, a preassembled colostomy irrigation kit or a soft, No.-28, standard-tip Foley catheter attached to a disposable enema bag may be used.

5. If both loops of a double-barrelled colostomy are irrigated, the irrigation solution may be expelled through the rectum as well as the stoma.

6. Advise the patient that a Foley catheter is used to introduce the barium into the stoma.

7. The patient should bring additional colostomy supplies to the radiology department for posttest use.

Aftercare for Patients With Stomas

1. Persons with descending or sigmoid colostomies may need a normal saline or tap water irrigation to wash out the barium.

2. Advise those who normally irrigate their colostomy to wear a disposable pouch for several days until all the barium has passed.

BILE DUCT X-RAY (CHOLANGIOGRAPHY, T-TUBE CHOLANGIOGRAM, OPERATIVE CHOLANGIOGRAM, PERCUTANEOUS TRANSHEPATIC CHOLANGIOGRAM) ●

Normal Bile Duct X-Ray Examination
Patent bile ducts

Explanation of Test
A cholangiogram visualizes the bile ducts by enhancing them with an iodinated contrast agent. Often performed on the post-cholecystectomy patient, the cholangiogram is used to identify intra-ductal mass lesions and calculi. A number of approaches may be used to opacify and image the bile ducts:

T-Tube Cholangiogram: Following cholecystectomy, a self-retaining T-shaped drainage tube may be inserted into the common bile duct. Prior to removal, patency is verified by injecting iodinated contrast into the T-tube to fill the biliary tree.

Cholangiogram With Stone Removal: This study combines diagnostic visualization of the bile ducts with therapeutic capture and removal of ductal calculi.

Intravenous Cholangiography: This study allows radiographic visualization of the large hepatic ducts and the common ducts by means of intravenous injection of a contrast medium. It is rarely performed.

Operative Cholangiography: Cannulation and injection of contrast medium into the exposed cystic duct or common bile duct is performed during surgery.

Percutaneous Transhepatic Cholangiography: A needle or small-diameter catheter is percutaneously introduced into the liver and the bile duct. Following injection of the contrast agent, the hepatic and common ducts should be visualized. The dilated biliary tree can be shown up to the point of obstruction, which is usually in the common duct. This procedure is frequently done for jaundiced patients whose liver cells are unable to properly transport oral or intravenous contrast agents.

Intravenous Cholecystography: Radiographic visualization of the gallbladder is performed after intravenous injection of a contrast agent.

Oral Cholecystography: Radiographic visualization of the gallbladder is performed after oral administration of an opaque medium. This test is often combined with or replaced by gallbladder sonography.

Endoscopic Retrograde Cholangiopancreatography (ERCP): This endoscopic procedure uses an injection of a contrast agent to evaluate the patency of pancreatic and common bile ducts, the duodenal papilla, and the normalcy of the gallbladder (see Chap. 12).

Procedure for T-Tube Cholangiogram

1. The patient lies on the x-ray table as an iodine contrast medium is injected into the T-tube.
2. No pain or discomfort should be felt; however, some persons may feel pressure during the injection.
3. After the procedure, the T-tube should be unclamped and allowed to drain freely unless otherwise ordered. This minimizes prolonged, irritating contact of residual contrast in the bile duct.
4. Follow guidelines in Chapter 1 regarding safe, effective, informed *intratest* care.

Clinical Implications

1. Abnormal duct and gallbladder x-ray results reveal stenosis obstruction or choledocholithiasis (bile duct calculi of the common bile duct).

Patient Preparation

1. Explain the purpose and procedure of the test. Assure the patient that the procedure is not painful, but some discomfort or pressure may be felt when

the contrast is injected. If the patient is diabetic, special precautions may be necessary (see p. 755).

2. Street clothing and accessories such as jewelry must be removed before the study. Provide a gown for patient use.

3. Stress the importance of remaining still and following breathing instructions during the procedure.

4. Refer to iodine test precautions. Assess female patients for pregnancy status. If positive, advise the radiology department.

5. Omit food and fluid before the examination. Check institutional protocols for specific dietary and fluid restrictions. A laxative may be ordered the evening before the examination.

6. Inform the patient and family that a cholangiogram can be a lengthy procedure lasting ≥2 hours.

7. Follow guidelines in Chapter 1 regarding safe, effective, informed *pretest* care.

Patient Aftercare

1. Posttest nausea, vomiting, and transient elevated temperature may occur as a reaction to the iodine contrast.

2. Document observations and notify physician if necessary.

3. Follow guidelines in Chapter 1 regarding safe, effective, informed *posttest* care.

▶ **Clinical Alert**

1. Persistent fever, especially if associated with chills, may indicate bile duct inflammation.

2. If the patient has diabetes, assess whether he or she is taking glucophage/metformin. Due to an increased risk of renal failure, this medication regimen must be discontinued the day of and several days after administration of contrast media. Consult the radiology department for specific instructions.

3. Assess patient for allergies to all substances, specifically latex, and inform the radiology department of any known or suspected sensitivities prior to study.

4. Assess whether patient is allergic to iodine. If iodine contrast sensitivities are known or suspected, inform the radiology department prior to study.

5. Monitor for hemorrhage, pneumothorax, or peritonitis after percutaneous transhepatic cholangiography. Unusual pain or tenderness, difficulty breathing, or change in vital signs may signal these complications. If these side-effects occur, take immediate action to treat.

INTRAVENOUS UROGRAPHY (IVU); EXCRETORY UROGRAPHY OR INTRAVENOUS PYELOGRAPHY (IVP); KUB X-RAYS ●

Normal KUB X-Ray Examination

Normal size, shape, and position of the kidneys, ureters, and bladder. Normal kidneys are approximately as long in dimension as three and one-half vertebral bodies. Therefore, kidney size is estimated in relation to this rule of thumb.

Normal Renal Function

1. Two to 5 minutes after the injection of contrast material, the kidney outline appears on an x-ray film. Thread-like strands of contrast material appear in the calyces.
2. When the second film is taken 5 to 7 minutes after contrast injection, the entire renal pelvis can be visualized.
3. Later films show the ureters and bladder as the contrast material makes its way into the lower urinary tract.
4. No evidence of residual urine should be found on the postvoid film.

Explanation of Test

IVU is one of the most frequently ordered tests in cases of suspected renal disease or urinary tract dysfunction.

NOTE: *IVU is indicated during the initial investigation of any suspected urologic problem, especially to diagnose kidney and ureter lesions and impaired renal function.*

An intravenous radiopaque iodine contrast substance is injected and concentrates in the urine. Following this injection, a series of x-ray films are made at predetermined intervals over the next 20 to 30 minutes. A final postvoid film is taken after the patient empties the bladder.

These films demonstrate the size, shape, and structure of the kidneys, ureters, and bladder and the degree to which the bladder can empty. Renal function is reflected by the length of time it takes the contrast material to first appear and then to be excreted by each kidney. Kidney disease, ureteral or bladder stones, and tumors can be detected with IVU.

Computed tomography also may be done in conjunction with IVU to obtain better visualization of renal lesions. This increases examination time. If kidney tomography or nephrotomograms are ordered separately, the procedure and preparation are the same as for IVU.

Procedure

1. A preliminary x-ray film is taken with the patient in a supine position to ensure that the bowel is empty and the kidney location can be visualized.
2. The intravenous contrast material is injected, usually into the antecubital vein.

3. Alert the patient that during and following the intravenous contrast injection they may experience warmth, flushing of the face, salty taste, and nausea.

   a. Should these sensations occur, instruct the patient to take slow, deep breaths. Have an emesis basin and tissue wipes available. Use standard precautions when handling secretions.

   b. Assess for other untoward signs, such as respiratory difficulty, diaphoresis, numbness, palpitations, or urticaria. Be prepared to respond with emergency drugs, equipment, and supplies. These items should be readily available whenever this procedure is performed.

4. Following injection of the contrast material, at least three x-ray films are taken at predetermined intervals.

5. After these three films are taken, instruct the patient to void before the final film is made to determine the ability of the bladder to empty.

6. Follow guidelines in Chapter 1 regarding safe, effective, informed *intratest* care.

Clinical Implications

1. Abnormal IVU findings may reveal the following conditions:
   a. Altered size, form, and position of the kidneys, ureters, and bladder
   b. Duplication of the pelvis or ureter
   c. The presence of only one kidney
   d. Hydronephrosis
   e. Supernumerary kidney
   f. Renal or ureteral calculi (stones)
   g. Tuberculosis of the urinary tract
   h. Cystic disease
   i. Tumors
   j. Degree of renal injury subsequent to trauma
   k. Prostate enlargement in males
   l. Enlarged kidneys suggesting obstruction or polycystic disease kidney
   m. Evidence of renal failure in the presence of normal-sized kidneys suggesting an acute rather than chronic disease process
   n. Irregular scarring of the renal outlines, suggesting chronic pyelonephritis

2. A time delay in radiopaque contrast visualization is indicative of renal dysfunction. No contrast visualization may indicate very poor or no renal function.

Interfering Factors

1. Feces or intestinal gas will obscure urinary tract visualization.
2. Retained barium can obscure optimal views of the kidneys. For this reason, barium tests should be scheduled after IVU when possible.

Patient Preparation

1. Explain the purpose and procedure of the test. A written reminder may be helpful to the patient. Screen patients for pregnancy status. If positive,

advise the radiology department. If patient has diabetes, special precautions may be necessary (see p. 755).

2. Observe iodine contrast test precautions. Assess for all allergies and determine prior allergic reaction to contrast substances. Many radiology departments require a recent creatinine level for all patients >40 years of age before performing this procedure in order to ensure the absence of renal insufficiency.

3. Because a relative state of dehydration is necessary for contrast material to concentrate in the urinary tract, instruct the patient to abstain from *all* food, liquid, and medication (if possible) for 12 hours before examination. Fasting after the evening meal the day before the test will meet this criteria.

NOTE: *Elderly or debilitated patients with poor renal reserves may not tolerate these dehydration protocols (fasting, laxatives, enemas). In such instances, consult with the radiologist or the patient's physician to ascertain the proper procedure. For infants and small children, fasting time usually varies from 6 to 8 hours pretest. If in doubt, verify protocols with the radiologist or attending physician.*

4. Usually, the patient is instructed to take a laxative the evening before the examination and receives an enema the morning of the test.
   a. Patients with intestinal disorders such as ulcerative colitis should be given a cathartic only when specified by the physician.
   b. Elderly patients may need assistance to the bathroom. Be alert for signs of weakness and stress.

5. Children <7 years of age should not be given pretest cathartics or enemas. Should the preliminary x-ray film show intestinal gas obscuring the kidneys, a few ounces of infant formula or carbonated beverage may relieve the concentration of gas at that particular location.

6. Evaluate stool and check for abdominal distention to evaluate for possible barium retention if it has been used in previous studies. Additional bowel preparation may be necessary.

7. Follow guidelines in Chapter 1 regarding safe, effective, informed *pretest* care.

Patient Aftercare

1. Resume prescribed diet and activity after the examination.

2. Teach and encourage the patient to drink sufficient fluids to replace those lost during the pretest phase.

3. Encourage rest, as needed, following the examination. Instruct the patient to "let their body tell them" about rest needs.

4. Observe and document mild reactions to the iodine material, which may include hives, skin rashes, nausea, or swelling of the parotid glands (iodinism). Notify the physician if the signs and symptoms persist. Oral antihistamines may relieve more severe symptoms.

5. Follow guidelines in Chapter 1 regarding safe, effective, informed *posttest* care.

Clinical Alert

1. Contraindications to an IVU or IVP include the following conditions:
   a. Hypersensitivity or allergy to iodine preparations
   b. Combined renal and hepatic disease
   c. Oliguria or anuria
   d. Renal failure: most radiology departments require recent creatinine test levels to determine whether to administer contrast materials. Generally, creatinine levels >1.5 mg/dl raise suspicion and signal the need for repeat laboratory work. A blood urea nitrogen (BUN) level >40 mg/dl also may contraindicate the use of iodine contrast.
   e. Multiple myeloma, unless the patient can be adequately hydrated during and after the study
   f. Advanced pulmonary tuberculosis
   g. Patients receiving drug therapy for chronic bronchitis, emphysema, or asthma
   h. Congestive heart failure (increased fluid load)
   i. Pheochromocytoma (increased blood pressure)
   j. Sickle cell anemia (acceleration of sickling potential, renal failure)
   k. Diabetes, especially diabetes mellitus
2. If patient has diabetes, assess whether he or she is taking glucophage/metformin. Due to an increased risk of renal failure, this medication regimen must be discontinued the day of and several days after administration of contrast media. Consult the radiology department for specific instructions.
3. Some physiologic changes can be expected after radiopaque iodine injections. Hypertension, hypotension, tachycardia, arrhythmias, or other electrocardiographic (ECG) changes may occur.
4. An iodine-based contrast medium is given with caution in the presence of hyperthyroidism, asthma, hay fever, or other allergies.
5. Observe for anaphylaxis or severe reactions to iodine, as evidenced by shock, respiratory distress, precipitous hypotension, fainting, convulsions, or actual cardiopulmonary arrest. Resuscitation supplies and equipment should be readily available.
6. In all cases except emergencies, a contrast medium should not be injected sooner than 90 minutes after eating.
7. Intravenous iodine can be highly irritating to the intimal layer of the veins and may cause painful vascular spasm. If this occurs, a 1% procaine intravenous injection may relieve vascular spasm and pain. Sometimes local vascular irritation is severe enough to induce thrombophlebitis. Warm or cold compresses to the area may relieve pain; however, these do not prevent sloughing. The attending physician should be notified. Anticoagulant therapy may need to be instituted.

(continued)

(Clinical Alert continued)

8. Local reactions to iodine may be evidenced by extensive redness, swelling, and pain at the injection site. Even a small amount of iodine contrast entering subcutaneous tissues can cause tissue sloughing, which may require skin grafting. Radiographic evidence of iodine contrast leakage within soft tissues surrounding the injection site confirms extravasation. Treatment may include a local infiltration of hyaluronidase.

9. Assess for latex allergy and inform the radiology department of any known or suspected sensitivities prior to study.

RETROGRADE PYELOGRAPHY AND OTHER TESTS TO EXAMINE THE URINARY SYSTEM ●

Normal Retrograde Pyelography Examination

Normal contour and size of ureters and kidneys

Explanation of Test

Retrograde pyelography generally confirms IVU findings and is indicated when IVU yields insufficient results because of kidney nonvisualization (congenital kidney absence), decreased renal blood flow that impairs renal function, obstruction, kidney dysfunction, presence of calculi, or patient allergy to intravenous contrast material. This x-ray examination of the upper urinary tract begins with cystoscopy to introduce ureteral catheters up to the level of the renal pelvis. Following this, iodine contrast is injected into the ureteral catheter, and x-ray films are then taken. The chief advantage of retrograde pyelography lies in the fact that the contrast substance can be indirectly injected under controlled pressure so that optimal visualization is achieved. Renal function impairment does not influence the degree of visualization.

Procedure

1. This examination is usually done in the surgical department in conjunction with cystoscopy (see Chap. 12).

2. Sedation and analgesia may precede insertion of a local anesthetic into the urethra (see Cystoscopy in Chapter 12). General anesthesia may be required if the patient is not able to fully cooperate with the procedure.

3. Follow guidelines in Chapter 1 regarding safe, effective, informed *intratest* care.

Clinical Implications

1. Urinary system x-ray results may reveal the following conditions:
   a. Intrinsic abnormality of ureters and kidney pelvis (eg, congenital defects)
   b. Extrinsic abnormality of the ureters (eg, obstructive tumor or stones)

Interfering Factors
Because barium may interfere with test results, these studies must be done before barium x-rays are performed.

Patient Preparation
1. Explain the purpose and procedure of the test. Screen female patients for pregnancy status. If positive, advise the radiology department.
2. The patient or other authorized person must sign and have witnessed a legal consent form before examination in the operating room.
3. Follow iodine contrast test precautions. A recent creatinine level may be required by the radiology department to evaluate the kidney's ability to clear the contrast.
4. Fast from food and fluids after midnight before the test.
5. Administer cathartics, suppositories, or enemas as ordered.
6. Follow guidelines in Chapter 1 regarding safe, effective, informed *pretest* care.

Patient Aftercare
1. Observe patient for signs of allergic reaction to iodine contrast.
2. Check vital signs frequently for the first 24 hours following the test. Follow institutional protocols if general anesthetics were administered.
3. Record accurate urine output and appearance for 24 hours following the procedure. Hematuria or dysuria may be common after the examination. If hematuria does not clear and dysuria persists or worsens, notify the physician. Instruct the patient to do the same.
4. Administer analgesics as necessary. Discomfort may be present immediately following the examination and may require a prescriptive analgesic (eg, codeine).
5. Follow guidelines in Chapter 1 regarding safe, effective, informed *posttest* care.

Clinical Alert

1. Renal function tests of blood and urine must be completed before this examination is done.
2. Assess whether the patient is allergic to iodine. If iodine contrast sensitivities are known or suspected, inform the radiology department prior to study.
3. Refer to Clinical Alerts posted in the text for Cytoscopy in Chapter 12.

Other Tests Used to Examine the Urinary System
Excretion Urography or Intravenous Pyelography (IVP): After injection of an intravenous contrast agent, the collecting system (ie, calyces, pelvis, and

ureter) of each kidney is progressively opacified. Radiographs are made at 5- to 15-minute intervals until the urinary bladder is visualized.

Drip Infusion Pyelography: This is a modification of conventional pyelography. An increased volume of contrast agent is administered by continuous intravenous infusion.

Cystography: The urinary bladder is opacified by means of a contrast agent instilled through a urethral catheter. After the patient voids, air may be introduced into the bladder to obtain a double-contrast study.

Retrograde Cystourethrography: After catheterization, the bladder is filled to capacity with a contrast agent, and radiography is used to visualize the bladder and urethra.

Voiding Cystourethrography: After contrast material has been instilled into the urinary bladder, films are made of the bladder and urethra during the process of voiding.

ARTHROGRAPHY (JOINT X-RAY)   ●

Normal Joint X-Ray Examination

Normal filling of encapsulated joint structures, joint space, bursae, menisci, ligaments, and articular cartilage

Explanation of Test

Arthrography involves multiple x-ray examinations of encapsulated joint structures following injection of contrast agents into the joint capsular space. Arthrography is done in cases of persistent, unexplained joint discomfort. Although the knee is the most frequently studied joint, the shoulder, hip, elbow, wrist, temporomandibular joint, and other joints may also be examined. Local anesthetics are used and aseptic conditions are observed.

Procedure

1. The patient is positioned on the examining table.
2. The skin around the joint is surgically prepared and draped.
3. A local anesthetic is injected into tissues around the joint. It is usually unnecessary to anesthetize the actual joint space.
4. If present, effusion fluids in the joint are aspirated. The contrast agents (eg, gas, water, soluble iodine) are then injected. After the needle is removed, the joint is manipulated to ensure even distribution of the contrast material. In some cases, the patient may be asked to walk or exercise the joint for a few minutes.
5. During the examination, several positions are assumed to obtain various x-ray views of the joint.
6. A special frame may be attached to the extremity to widen the joint space for a better view. Pillows and sandbags also may be used to position the joint properly.

7. Follow guidelines in Chapter 1 regarding safe, effective, informed *intratest* care.

Clinical Implications

1. Abnormal joint x-ray results reveal the following conditions:
   a. Arthritis
   b. Dislocation
   c. Ligament tears
   d. Rotator cuff rupture
   e. Synovial abnormalities
   f. Narrowing of joint space
   g. Cysts

Patient Preparation

1. Explain the purpose and procedure of the test. Advise the patient that some discomfort is normal during contrast injection and joint manipulation.
2. In most instances, a properly signed and witnessed consent form is required.
3. Refer to iodine test precautions on pages 752 through 755. Check for known allergies to iodine, other contrast substances, and latex.
4. Advise patient to bring any old (prior) x-ray films of the joint in question to the arthrogram appointment.
5. Follow guidelines in Chapter 1 regarding safe, effective, informed *pretest* care.

Patient Aftercare

1. The joint should be rested for 12 hours.
2. An elastic bandage may be applied to the knee joint for several days after the examination.
3. Ice can be applied to the area if swelling occurs. Pain can usually be controlled with a mild analgesic.
4. Cracking or clicking noises in the joint may be heard for 1 or 2 days following the test. This is normal. Notify the physician if crepitant noises persist or increased pain, swelling, or restlessness occurs.
5. Follow guidelines in Chapter 1 regarding safe, effective, informed *posttest* care.

> ### ▶ Clinical Alert
>
> If diabetic patient is taking glucophage/metformin, special considerations may be necessary. Consult with the radiology department to determine whether this medication regimen must be discontinued the day of and several days after the study.

MYELOGRAPHY (SPINE X-RAY) ●

Normal Spine X-Ray Examination
Normal lumbar, cervical, or thoracic myelogram

Explanation of Test
Myelography is a radiographic study of the spinal subarachnoid space in which iodine contrast material is introduced into that space so that the spinal cord and nerve roots are outlined and dura matter distortions can be detected.

This study is done to detect neoplasms, ruptured intravertebral disks, or extraspinal lesions such as arthritic stenosis or ankylosing spondyloses. This examination is also indicated when compression of the spinal or posterior fossa neural structure or nerve roots is suspected. The test is frequently done before surgical treatment for a ruptured vertebral disk or release of stenosis. Symptoms may include unrelieved back pain, pain radiating down the leg, absent or abnormal ankle and knee reflexes, claudication of neurospinal origin, or past history of cancer with loss of mobility or bladder control.

Myelograms fall into three categories: positive contrasts using water-soluble iodine, iodized oil contrast, and negative air contrast. Water-soluble iodine contrast is the most commonly used medium for myelograms and is often followed by CT scanning to improve visualization. In low-dose myelograms, injection of a very small amount of water-soluble contrast is immediately followed by scanning.

Procedure
1. The test is usually done in the radiography department with the patient positioned on his or her abdomen during the procedure.
2. The puncture area is prepared and draped.
3. The procedure is the same as that for lumbar puncture (see Chap. 5), except for the injection of the contrast substance and fluoroscopic x-ray films. With the use of water-soluble contrast, a narrow-bone needle (22-gauge) may be used. A lumbar puncture is done when a lumbar defect is suspected; a cervical puncture is done for a suspected cervical lesion. In children, the level at which the lumbar puncture is performed is much lower than the level in adults to avoid puncturing the spinal cord. Depending on the contrast substance used, it may be removed (oil) or left to be absorbed (water or air).
4. The table is tilted during the procedure to achieve optimal visualization. Shoulder and foot braces help maintain correct position.
5. Follow guidelines in Chapter 1 regarding safe, effective, informed *intratest* care.

Clinical Implications
1. Abnormal myelogram results reveal distorted outlines of the subarachnoid space that indicate the following conditions:
   a. Ruptured intervertebral disk
   b. Compression and stenosis of spinal cord

    c. The exact level of intravertebral tumors

    d. Spinal canal obstruction

    e. Avulsion of nerve roots

Patient Preparation

1. Explain the purpose, procedure, benefits, and risks of the test. Explain that some discomfort may be felt during the procedure. Disadvantages of water and air contrast include poor visualization and painful headache (air contrast) because of the difficulty in controlling the gas introduced into the area. Oil contrast substances can cause tissue irritation or be poorly absorbed from the subarachnoid space. Oil may remain visible on x-ray examination for up to 1 year following the original examination. For these reasons, oil and air contrast are rarely used. Refer to iodine contrast test precautions if iodine is used (see pp. 752 to 755).

2. A legal consent form must be properly signed and witnessed before the test.

3. Assess pregnancy status of female patients. Advise the radiology department if positive.

4. Explain that the examination table may be tilted during the test, but that the patient will be securely fastened and will not fall off the table.

5. Most diagnostic departments require the patient to refrain from eating for ~4 hours before testing. Clear liquids may be permitted and even encouraged to lower the incidence of headaches after the test. Check with the radiology department and physician for specific orders.

6. A myelogram usually produces some discomfort. If the patient has trouble moving, a pain reliever may be necessary to allow easier positioning and movement during the test.

7. Follow guidelines in Chapter 1 regarding safe, effective, informed *pretest* care.

Patient Aftercare

1. Bed rest is necessary for several hours after testing. If a water-soluble contrast is used, the head of the bed should be elevated at 45 degrees for 8 to 24 hours after the procedure. The patient is also advised to lie quietly. This position reduces upward dispersion of the contrast medium and keeps it out of the head, where it may cause headache. If oil contrast dye is used, the patient usually must lay prone for 2 to 4 hours and then remain on his or her back for another 2 to 4 hours. If the entire amount of oil contrast is not withdrawn at the end of the procedure, the head must be elevated to prevent the oil from flowing into the brain.

2. Encourage fluid intake to hasten absorption of residual contrast material, to replace cerebrospinal fluid, and to reduce risk of headache and unusual or metallic taste.

3. Check for bladder distention and adequate voiding, especially if metrizamide has been used.

4. Check vital signs frequently (at least every 4 hours) for the first 24 hours after the examination.

5. Follow guidelines in Chapter 1 regarding safe, effective, informed *posttest* care.

> **Clinical Alert**
>
> 1. Observe the patient for possible complications such as continued nausea and vomiting, headache, fever, seizure, paralysis of one side of the body or both arms or legs (rare), arachnoiditis (inflammation of the spinal cord coverings), change in level of consciousness, hallucinations, drowsiness, stupor, neck stiffness, and sterile meningitis reaction (severe headache, symptoms of arachnoiditis, slow-wave patterns on electroencephalogram).
> 2. Alteration of cerebrospinal fluid pressure pressure may cause an acute exacerbation of symptoms that may require immediate surgical intervention. Lumbar punctures should not be done unless absolutely necessary.
> 3. This test is to be avoided unless there is a reason to suspect a lesion. Multiple sclerosis, for example, may be worsened by this procedure.
> 4. Determine whether water-soluble, oil, or air contrast was used for the procedure, because aftercare interventions differ.
> 5. If nausea or vomiting occurs after the procedure and a water-soluble contrast has been used, do not administer phenothiazine antiemetics such as prochlorperazine (Compazine).
> 6. Assess whether the patient is allergic to latex or iodine and inform the radiology department of any known or suspected sensitivities prior to study.
> 7. If patient has diabetes, assess whether patient is taking glucophage/metformin. Due to an increased risk of renal failure, this medication regimen must be discontinued the day of and several days after administration of contrast media. Consult the radiology department for specific instructions.
> 8. Many radiology departments require the discontinuation of Coumadin therapy for several days prior to performance of a myelogram. Often, a prothrombin time is required before beginning the examination.

HYSTEROSALPINGOGRAM (UTERINE AND FALLOPIAN TUBE X-RAYS)

Normal Uterine and Fallopian Tube X-Ray Examination

Normal intrauterine cavity
Patent fallopian tubes

Explanation of Test

Hysterosalpingography involves radiographic visualization of the uterine cavity and the fallopian tubes to detect abnormalities that may be the cause of infertility or other problems. Normally, a contrast agent introduced into the uterine cavity will travel through the fallopian tubes and "spill" into the peritoneal cavity, where it will be naturally resorbed.

Procedure

1. The patient must remove all clothing and put on a hospital gown. The bladder should be emptied before the study begins.
2. The patient lies supine on the x-ray table in a lithotomy position. Preliminary pelvic x-ray films may be taken.
3. The radiologist or gynecologist introduces a speculum into the patient's vagina and inserts a cannula through the cervical canal. The iodinated contrast agent is administered into the uterus through this cannula.
4. The speculum is removed (unless it is radiolucent), and both fluoroscopic and conventional films are done.
5. Follow guidelines in Chapter 1 regarding safe, effective, informed *intratest* care.

Clinical Implications

1. Abnormal uterine and fallopian tube x-ray findings include the following conditions:
   a. Bicornuate uterus or other uterine cavity anomalies
   b. Tubal tortuosity
   c. Tubal obstruction evidenced by failure of the contrast dye to spill into the peritoneal cavity on one or both sides (bilateral tubal obstruction causes infertility)
   d. Scarring and evidence of old pelvic inflammatory disease

Patient Preparation

1. Explain test purpose and procedure. Some institutions require a properly signed and witnessed informed consent.
2. Refer to iodine contrast test precautions on pages 752 through 755.
3. Verify date of last menstrual period to ensure that the patient is not pregnant.
4. Advise patient that some discomfort may be experienced but subsides quickly.
5. Suggest that the patient bring along sanitary napkins to wear, because some spotting and contrast dye discharge may occur.
6. Follow guidelines in Chapter 1 regarding safe, effective, informed *pretest* care.

> ### ▶ Clinical Alert
>
> 1. Pregnancy and active pelvic inflammatory disease are contraindications to hysterosalpingogram.
> 2. If patient has diabetes and is taking glucophage/metformin, special considerations may be necessary. Consult with the radiology
>
> *(continued)*

(Clinical Alert continued)
department to determine whether this medication regimen must be discontinued the day of and several days after the study.
3. Assess whether patient is allergic to latex, and inform the radiology department of any known or suspected sensitivities prior to study.
4. Assess whether patient is allergic to iodine. If iodine contrast sensitivities are known or suspected, inform the radiology department prior to study.

Patient Aftercare

1. Monitor patient for discomfort and administer analgesics as ordered.
2. Instruct the patient to report heavy vaginal bleeding, abnormal discharge, unusual pain, or fever to the referring physician.
3. Interpret test outcomes and counsel about infertility problems.
4. Follow guidelines in Chapter 1 regarding safe, effective, informed *posttest* care.

ANGIOGRAPHY (DIGITAL SUBTRACTION ANGIOGRAPHY [DSA], TRANSVENOUS DIGITAL SUBTRACTION, VASCULAR X-RAY) ●

Normal Angiographic Examination

Normal carotid arteries, vertebral arteries, abdominal aorta and its branches, renal arteries, and peripheral arteries

Explanation of Test

Digital angiography is a computer-based imaging method of performing vascular studies that require catheterization of certain venous or arterial vessels. Vasculature studied includes the carotid vessels; intracranial vessels; those vessels originating from the aortic arch; abdominal vessels including the celiac, renal, and mesenteric branches; and other peripheral vessels. Digital subtraction angiography began as an intravenous technique, but because of its limitations, other methods of iodine contrast administration may be employed. Although carrying a greater complication risk, intraarterial injection can be used for detailed visceral studies. The presence of the contrast material blocks the path of x-rays and makes blood vessels visible on x-ray film. An image taken just before contrast injection is subtracted from that taken when the contrast material is actually within the vascular system. The resulting image shows only the distribution of the contrast substance. Digital subtraction is used to isolate a clinically relevant subset of information and is particularly useful in preoperative and postoperative evaluations for vascular and tumor surgery.

Visualization of the carotid and vertebral vasculature is possible in patients with a history of stroke, transient ischemic attacks, bruit, or subarachnoid hemorrhage. The procedure may be used as an adjunct to CT or magnetic resonance scanning and may be performed just before these studies in persons who have evidence of an aneurysm, vascular malformation, or hypervascular tumor.

The study names are derived from the vascular structure studied and the study method used. *Arteriography* refers to contrast agent studies of arterial vessels. Venous structures may also be visualized as these procedures progress. *Venography* is the contrast agent study of peripheral or central veins. *Lymphography* studies lymph vessels and nodes. *Angiocardiography* investigates the interior of the heart and adjacent great vessels such as the pulmonary arteries. *Aortography* refers to a contrast study of aortic segments such as the thoracic aorta (*thoracic aortography*), the abdominal aorta (*abdominal aortography*), or the lumbar aorta (*lumbar aortography*).

Types of Vascular Studies	
Name	*Structure Studied*
Arteriography	Arteries
Venography	Peripheral or ventral veins
Lymphography	Lymph vessels and nodes
Angiocardiography	Interior heart and adjacent vessels
Aortography	Thoracic, abdominal, lumbar aorta

Angiographic examinations also can be named for the route used to inject the contrast substance. For example, *renal arteriography* is performed by inserting a catheter into the abdominal aorta and then directing it into the renal artery. During *peripheral arteriography,* the contrast is injected directly into the vessel being studied (eg, femoral artery). If done through the venous route, a large bolus of contrast medium is directly injected into a peripheral vein (eg, venous aortography). X-ray films are taken to track the flow of contrast through the right side of the heart, the lungs, and the left side of the heart.

Procedure

1. Using the sterile technique, the vascular access area is cleansed, prepared, and injected with a local anesthetic. Depending on the type of study and patient factors, this is commonly the groin or the antecubital area of the arm. Standard precautions are followed.

2. The catheter containing a guide wire is advanced into the desired vessel or right atrium of the heart. The guide wire is removed, and the catheter is connected to a power injector that administers iodine under pressure in defined quantities and at prescribed intervals. X-ray images are then taken and stored on digital or film media. Therapeutic procedures such as angioplasty and stent placement may be done in concert with this examination.

3. After the procedure is terminated, the catheter is removed.

4. A dressing is placed over the insertion site, and manual pressure is applied to the puncture site for about 5 minutes or until bleeding stops. A more

permanent pressure dressing is then taped in place; this usually can be removed in 24 hours.

5. Monitor patient frequently for hemorrhage or hematoma formation.

6. Follow guidelines in Chapter 1 regarding safe, effective, informed *intratest* care.

Clinical Implications

1. Abnormal digital subtraction angiography results reveal the following conditions:

    a. Arterial stenosis

    b. Large aneurysms

    c. Intravascular or extravascular tumors or other masses

    d. Total occlusion of arteries

    e. Thoracic outlet syndrome

    f. Large or central pulmonary emboli

    g. Ulcerative plaque

    h. Tumor circulation

Interfering Factors

1. Because this examination is very sensitive to physical movement, motion artifact will produce poor images. Consequently, uncooperative or agitated patients cannot be studied. Even the act of swallowing results in unsatisfactory images. Measures to reduce swallowing, such as breath holding, using a bite block, or exhaling through a straw, do not always yield satisfactory results.

2. Vessel overlap of external and internal carotid arteries makes it almost impossible to obtain a select view of a specific carotid artery because contrast

Clinical Alert

1. These tests should be used cautiously in patients with renal insufficiency or unstable cardiac disease. Assess for contraindications to iodinated contrast drugs listed on page 754.

2. In the presence of diabetes, assess whether the patient is taking glucophage/metformin. Due to an increased risk of renal failure, this medication regimen must be discontinued the day of and several days after administration of contrast media. Consult the radiology department for specific instructions.

fills both arteries almost simultaneously.

Patient Preparation

1. Explain test purpose and procedure and document instructions given. Reinforce explanation of test benefits and risks.

2. The patient must be coherent and cooperative and able to hold his or her breath and remain absolutely still when so instructed.

3. A legal consent form must be properly signed and witnessed.

4. Refer to iodine contrast test precautions (see pp. 752 through 755).
5. Determine whether the patient has any known allergies, especially those to iodine, contrast media, or latex. See pages 752 through 755 for additional assessment criteria.
6. Assess pregnancy status of female patients. If positive, advise the radiology department.
7. Assure that preprocedure laboratory work is performed in accordance with departmental standards. This generally will include the following tests:
   a. Prothrombin time drawn on day of procedure for any patients on anticoagulation therapy (eg, Coumadin)
   b. Creatinine levels for all patients
   c. Recent prothrombin time and partial thromboplastin time (PT/PTT) and platelet count (generally within 30 days)
8. In many instances, glucagon is intravenously administered just before abdominal examinations. This serves to reduce motion artifacts by stopping peristalsis.
9. The few risks include venous thrombosis and infection. When contrast is administered through the venous route, the arteries—which are normally under higher pressure than the veins—can clear, the contrast agent through the process of normal circulation. For the same reason, there is less risk of loosening plaques.
10. No food or fluids should be taken within 2 hours before the study to minimize vomiting if an iodine contrast reaction occurs.
11. All arteries in a specific area can be visualized during one series of exposures. This overview gives the advantage of being able to evaluate the entire blood supply to a given area at one time. In contrast, during routine angiography, only one specific artery at a time can be visualized.
12. Follow guidelines in Chapter 1 regarding safe, effective, informed *pretest* care.

Patient Aftercare

1. Check vital signs frequently. Report unstable signs to the physician.
2. Observe the catheter insertion site for signs of infection, hemorrhage, or hematoma. Use sterile aseptic technique at all times. Monitor neurovascular status of the extremity. Report problems to the physician promptly.
3. Observe for allergic reactions to iodine. Mild side-effects include nausea, vomiting, dizziness, and urticaria. Also watch for other complications such as abdominal pain, hypertension, congestive heart failure, angina, myocardial infarction, and anaphylaxis. In susceptible persons, renal failure may occur because higher doses of contrast materials are given compared with conventional arteriograms. Resuscitation equipment and emergency supplies should be readily available. Immediately report these conditions to the physician.
4. Instruct the patient to increase fluid intake to at least 2000 ml during the 24 hours following the procedure to facilitate excretion of the iodine contrast substance.
5. Interpret test outcomes and monitor appropriately.
6. Follow guidelines in Chapter 1 regarding safe, effective, informed *posttest* care.

Clinical Alert

1. The catheter puncture site must be observed frequently and closely for hemorrhage or hematoma formation. These can be serious complications and require immediate attention should they occur. Many such patients received anticoagulants before the procedure.

2. Vital sign assessment, puncture site assessment, and neurovascular assessments may need to be done as frequently as every 15 minutes for the first few hours after the procedure. Neurovascular assessments include evaluation of color, motion, sensation, capillary refill time, pulse quality, and temperature (warm or cool) of the affected extremity. Compare the affected extremity with the nonaffected extremity.

3. Review the chart or question the patient or physician regarding deficits that were present before the procedure to establish baseline levels of circulatory function. Report postprocedure changes immediately.

4. If an arterial puncture was performed, the affected extremity must **not** be bent for several hours, and the patient must lie flat other than a pillow under the head. Do not raise the head of the bed or cart because this can put a strain on a femoral puncture site. The patient may turn if the affected extremity is maintained in a straight position without putting strain on the femoral puncture site. If needed, a fracture bedpan can lessen strain on a groin puncture site.

5. If bleeding or hematoma occurs, apply pressure to the site. Sometimes "sandbags" may be applied to the puncture site as a routine part of postprocedure protocols.

6. Maintain a functional intravenous access site. Usually, the patient will return to the nursing unit with an IV in place.

7. A Doppler device may reveal audible pulse sounds if pulses are nonpalpable.

8. Sudden onset of pain, numbness or tingling, greater degree of coolness, decreased or absent pulses, or blanching of extremities are always cues to notify the physician immediately. These signs can indicate arterial occlusion, which may require rapid surgical intervention.

LYMPHANGIOGRAPHY (X-RAYS OF LYMPH NODES AND VESSELS) ●

Normal Lymphangiographic Examination

Normal lymphatic vessels and nodes

Explanation of Test

Lymphangiography examines the lymphatic channels and lymph nodes by means of radiopaque iodine contrast injected into the small lymphatics of the foot. This test is commonly ordered for patients with Hodgkin's disease or cancer of the prostate to check for nodal involvement. Lymphangiography is also indicated to evaluate edema of an extremity without known cause, to determine the extent of adenopathy, to stage lymphomas, and to localize affected nodes as part of surgical or radiotherapeutic treatment.

Procedure

1. The patient is placed in the supine position on the x-ray table.
2. A blue contrast is injected intradermally between each of the first three toes of each foot to stain the lymphatic vessels.
3. After the site is infiltrated with local anesthetic, a 1- to 2-inch incision is made on the dorsum of each foot.
4. The lymphatic vessel is identified and cannulated to facilitate extremely low-pressure injection of the iodine contrast medium.
5. When the contrast medium reaches the level of the third and fourth lumbar vertebrae as seen on fluoroscopy, the injection is discontinued.
6. Abdominal, pelvic, and upper body films demonstrate the lymphatic vessels filling.
7. A second set of films is obtained 12 to 24 hours later to demonstrate filling of the lymph nodes.
8. The nodes in the inguinal, external iliac, common iliac, and periaortic areas, as well as the thoracic duct and supraclavicular nodes, can be visualized using this procedure.
9. When a lymphatic of the hand is injected, the axillary and supraclavicular nodes should be visible.
10. Because the contrast dye remains present in the nodes for 6 months to 1 year after lymphangiography, repeat studies can be done to track disease activity and to monitor treatment without the need to repeat contrast injection.
11. The patient may need to have additional films taken.
12. Follow guidelines in Chapter 1 regarding safe, effective, informed *intratest* care.

Clinical Implications

1. Abnormal lymph node and vessel x-ray results indicate the following conditions:
   a. Retroperitoneal lymphomas associated with Hodgkin's disease
   b. Metastasis to lymph nodes
   c. Abnormal lymphatic vessels

Patient Preparation

1. Explain test purpose and procedure. Obtain a signed, witnessed consent form.
2. See iodine contrast test precautions on page 754.
3. Assess pregnancy status of female patients. If positive, advise the radiology department.
4. No fasting is necessary. Usual medications can be taken.
5. Instruct the patient that he or she may feel some discomfort when the local anesthetic is injected into the feet.

6. Administer oral antihistamines per physician orders if allergy to the iodized contrast agents is suspected.
7. Follow guidelines in Chapter 1 regarding safe, effective, informed *pretest* care.

Patient Aftercare

1. Check and record the patient's temperature every 4 hours for 48 hours post-examination.
2. Provide a restful environment.
3. If ordered, elevate the legs to prevent swelling.
4. Watch for complications such as delayed wound healing, infection, leg edema, allergic dermatitis, headache, sore mouth and throat, skin rashes, transient fever, lymphangitis, and oil embolism.
5. Follow guidelines in Chapter 1 regarding safe, effective, informed *posttest* care.

> ### Clinical Alert
>
> 1. Lymphangiography is usually contraindicated in the following conditions:
>   a. Known iodine hypersensitivity
>   b. Severe pulmonary insufficiency
>   c. Cardiac disease
>   d. Advanced renal or hepatic disease
> 2. The major complication of this procedure relates to contrast media embolization into the lungs. This will diminish pulmonary function temporarily and, in some patients, may produce lipid pneumonia. The patient may require aggressive respiratory management if this complication is life-threatening.
> 3. If patient has diabetes and is taking glucophage/metformin, special considerations may be necessary. Consult with the radiology department to determine whether this medication regimen must be discontinued the day of and several days after the study.
> 4. Assess whether patient is allergic to *latex,* and inform radiology department of any known or suspected sensitivities prior to study.
> 5. Assess whether patient is allergic to *iodine.* If iodine contrast sensitivities are known or suspected, inform the radiology department prior to study.

● COMPUTED TOMOGRAPHY (CT)

Computed tomography (CT), also called CT scanning, computerized tomography, or computerized axial tomography (CAT), produces x-rays similar to those used in conventional radiography; however, CTs are taken with a special scanner system. Conventional x-rays pass through the body and produce an image of bone, soft tissues, and air on film. With CT scans, a computer provides rapid complex calculations that determine the extent to which tissues absorb multiple x-ray beams. CT is unique because it can produce cross-sectional images (ie, "slices") of anatomic structures without superimposing tissues on each other. Additionally, CT can discern the different characteristics of tissue structures within solid organs. Agents may be used for delineation of blood vessels, the opacification of certain tissue (eg, kidneys), and blood flow patterns for differentiation of hemangiomas.

The patient lies on a motorized table positioned inside a doughnut-shaped frame called the gantry. The gantry contains the x-ray tubes, which rotate around the patient during the scan. By rotating the narrow-beamed x-ray source around the patient's body, multiple attenuation readings are gathered and processed by the computer. The display, similar to a conventional radiograph, demonstrates varying densities which correspond to the absorption of x-rays by the patient's anatomy. As with traditional x-ray techniques, bones appear white, and gas and fat appear black. However, with CT, discrete differences in attenuation can be *quantified*. This means a CT scan can demonstrate minor differences in density and composition in shades of gray. A CT scan can differentiate tumors from soft tissues, air space from cerebrospinal fluid, and normal blood from clotted blood.

By interpreting the scan, structures are identified by appearance, shape, size, symmetry, and position. Usually, space-occupying lesions show characteristic displacement of surrounding viscera. Scans can be performed at different levels and planes and in different slice thicknesses to isolate small lesions. Often, hollow viscera (eg, intestines) and blood vessels need to be accentuated with the use of contrast media.

Spiral CT scanners, also known as helical CT scanners, are a modification of the conventional CT technique. A spiral scan employs a continuous, "corkscrew" scan pattern which produces a three-dimensional raw data set. This allows for three-dimensional reconstruction and CT angiography. Mobile CT scanners are available and can provide guidance during surgical and other interventional procedures.

CT scans can be performed on virtually any body part and can isolate virtually any abdominal organ. Typical CT applications include the following studies:

1. Abdomen: to include liver, pancreas, gallbladder, kidneys, adrenals, spleen, retroperitoneum, and abdominal blood vessels
2. Pelvis: to include urinary bladder, uterus, ovaries, distal colon, and prostate
3. Spine
4. Head, sinuses, orbits, mastoids, internal auditory canals, facial bones, neck
5. Chest: to include lungs, mediastinum, and heart
6. Joints and specific bones
7. CT-guided biopsy
8. Cardiac Scoring-a CT exam of the heart to assess the presence of calcifications in coronary vessels. While this procedure is not Medicare approved, it may be useful as a fee-for-service screening test to estimate the risk of cardiac disease.

COMPUTED TOMOGRAPHY (CT) OF THE HEAD AND NECK; BRAIN, EYES, AND SINUS COMPUTERIZED AXIAL TOMOGRAPHY (CAT)

Normal Computed Tomography (CT) Examination of the Head and Neck

No evidence of tumor, other pathology, or fracture

Typically, low-density tissue areas appear black, whereas higher-density tissues appear as shades of gray. The lighter the shading, the higher the density of the tissue or structure.

Explanation of Test

CT of the head is a relatively simple x-ray examination done by means of a special scanning machine to evaluate for suspected intracranial lesions (see pp. 804-805 for CT explanation). The results form a cross-sectional picture of the anatomic structure of the head that includes the internal cranial structure, brain tissue, and surrounding cerebrospinal fluid. This axial image of the head is similar to a view looking down through the top of the head.

Procedure

1. During the test, the patient must lie perfectly still on a motorized table with his or her head comfortably immobilized. The table is moved into a doughnut-shaped frame called a gantry. X-ray tubes situated within this gantry move around the patient in a circular fashion.
2. If tissue density enhancement is desired because a questionable area needs further clarification, an iodinated radiopaque contrast substance can be injected intravenously. Some patients experience nausea and vomiting after receiving this contrast agent.
3. Additional images are taken during contrast injection.
4. During and following the intravenous injection, the patient may experience warmth, flushing of the face, salty taste, or nausea. Encourage the patient to breathe deeply. An emesis basin should be readily available.
5. Watch for other untoward signs such as respiratory difficulty, diaphoresis, numbness, or palpitations.
6. Follow guidelines in Chapter 1 regarding safe, effective, informed *intratest* care.

Clinical Implications

1. Abnormal CT head and neck scan results reveal the following conditions:
    a. Bony and soft tissue tumor masses such as meningiomas, astrocytomas, angiomas, and cysts
    b. Intracranial bleeding or hematoma
    c. Aneurysm
    d. Infarction
    e. Infection
    f. Sinusitis

g. Foreign bodies

h. Multiple sclerosis

Interfering Factors

1. A false-negative CT scan can occur in the presence of hemorrhage. As hematomas age, their appearance on CT scans changes from high-intensity to low-intensity levels, partly because older hematomas become more transparent to x-rays.
2. Patient movements negatively affect image quality and accuracy.

Patient Preparation

1. Explain test purpose and procedure. Provide written instructions. Reinforce knowledge regarding possible adverse effects such as radiation exposure or allergy to iodine contrast media. The amount of x-ray exposure for this examination is about the same as that received during a routine skull x-ray.
2. Assess pregnancy status of female patients. If positive, advise the radiology department.
3. Refer to iodine contrast test precautions on page 754. A creatinine level may be required prior to the study.
4. Generally, the patient should fast 2 to 3 hours before the test if a contrast study is planned. In most cases, prescribed medications can be taken before CT studies.
5. Reassure the patient that scanning produces no greater radiation than conventional x-ray studies.
6. Check for patient allergies. Nausea and vomiting, warmth, and flushing of the face may signal a possible iodine allergy. See pages 752 through 755 for additional assessment criteria.
7. Reassure the patient who is prone to claustrophobia that claustrophobic fear of the scanner is common. Pictures of introduction to the scanner may alleviate these fears.
8. Administer analgesics and sedatives, especially to minimize pain and unnecessary movement.
9. Follow guidelines in Chapter 1 regarding safe, effective, informed *pretest* care.

Patient Aftercare

1. Determine whether an iodine contrast substance was used. If used, observe and record information about reactions if they occur. Mild reactions may include hives, skin rashes, nausea, swelling of parotid glands (iodism), or, most serious of all, anaphylaxis.
2. Notify the physician immediately if allergic reactions occur. Antihistamines may be necessary to treat symptoms.
3. Documentation should include assessment of information needs, instructions given, time examination was completed, patient response to the procedure, and allergic reactions if they occur.
4. Follow guidelines in Chapter 1 regarding safe, effective, informed *posttest* care.

> **Clinical Alert**
>
> 1. If patient has diabetes and is taking glucophage/metformin, special considerations may be necessary. Consult with the radiology department to determine whether this medication regimen must be discontinued the day of and several days after the study.
> 2. Assess whether patient is allergic to iodine or latex. If iodine contrast or latex sensitivities are known or suspected, inform the radiology department prior to study.

COMPUTED TOMOGRAPHY (CT) OF THE BODY; COMPUTERIZED AXIAL TOMOGRAPHY (CAT) BODY SCAN; CHEST, SPINE, EXTREMITIES, ABDOMEN, AND PELVIS COMPUTED TOMOGRAPHY ●

Normal Computed Tomography (CT) Examination of the Body

No apparent tumor or pathology

On CT scans, air appears black, bone appears white, and soft tissue appears in various shades of gray. Shade patterns and their correlation to different tissue densities, together with the added dimensions of depth, allow identification of normal body structures and organs.

Explanation of Test

Body CT imaging provides detailed cross-sectional images of the chest, abdomen, spine, and extremities. When used to evaluate neoplastic and inflammatory disease, CT data acquisition can be rapidly sequenced to evaluate blood flow and to determine vascularity of a mass. This technique, known as *dynamic CT scanning,* requires the administration of intravenous contrast. In addition, CT can be used to detect intervertebral disk disease, herniation, and soft tissue damage to ligaments within joint spaces.

Conventional x-ray machines produce a "flat" picture, with organs in the front of the body appearing to be superimposed over organs toward the back of the body. The result is a two-dimensional image of the three-dimensional body. CT imaging produces many cross-sectional anatomic views without superimposing structures. Spiral scanners allow CT angiography and three-dimensional reconstruction techniques.

Procedure

1. In most laboratories, CT abdominal examination is preceded by having the patient drink a special contrast preparation several minutes before the study. This contrast material outlines the bowel so that it can be more readily differentiated from other structures.
2. The patient lies supine on a motorized couch that moves into a doughnut-shaped frame called a gantry. X-ray tubes within the gantry move around

the patient as the pictures are taken. These films are concurrently projected onto a monitor screen.

3. The patient should lie without moving and be able to follow breathing instructions.

4. Should a questionable area require further clarification, iodine contrast substance is injected intravenously and more pictures are taken. Patients having pelvic CT scans are given a barium contrast enema. Furthermore, female patients undergoing pelvic CT scans may require insertion of a contrast enhanced vaginal tampon to delineate the vaginal wall. Another indication for contrast is blood vessel delineation, the opacification of well-vascularized tissue, and evaluation of blood flow patterns (as for differential diagnosis of hemangioma).

5. The patient may experience warmth, flushing of the face, salty taste, and nausea with intravenous injection of the contrast material. Slow, deep breaths may alleviate these symptoms. Have an emesis basin readily available. Watch for other untoward signs such as respiratory difficulty, heavy sweating, numbness, palpitations, or progression to an anaphylactic reaction. Resuscitation equipment and drugs should be readily available. Notify the physician immediately should any of these side-effects occur.

6. Follow guidelines in Chapter 1 regarding safe, effective, informed *intratest* care.

Clinical Implications

1. Abnormal body CT scan findings reveal the following conditions:
   a. Tumors, nodules, and cysts
   b. Ascites
   c. Abscessed or fatty liver
   d. Aneurysm of abdominal aorta
   e. Lymphoma
   f. Enlarged lymph nodes
   g. Pleural effusion
   h. Cancer of pancreas
   i. Retroperitoneal lymphadenopathy
   j. Abnormal collection of blood, fluid, or fat
   k. Skeletal bone metastasis
   l. Cirrhosis of liver
   m. Fractures
   n. Soft tissue or ligament damage

Interfering Factors

1. Retained barium can obscure organs in the upper and lower abdomen. Barium tests should be scheduled after CT scans when possible.

2. Inability of the patient to lie quietly produces less-than-optimal pictures.

Patient Preparation

1. Explain test purpose and procedure. Written explanations may be helpful. Benefits and risks of the test should be explained to the patient before the procedure.

2. Assess pregnancy status of female patients. If positive, advise the radiology department.

3. Refer to iodine and barium contrast test precautions on pages 752 through 757.

4. In most cases, usual prescribed medications can be taken prior to CT studies.

5. Inform the patient that an iodine contrast substance may be administered before and during the examination. Determine whether the patient is allergic to iodine. See pages 752 through 755 for additional assessment criteria. Pelvic CT examinations usually require both intravenous and rectal administration of contrast material. A creatinine level may be required prior to the study.

6. Abdominal cramping and diarrhea may occur; therefore, drugs such as glucagon, Lipomul, or Donnatal may be ordered to decrease these side-effects.

7. Solid foods are usually withheld on the day of the examination until after test completion. Clear liquids may be taken up to 2 hours before examination. If in doubt, check with the diagnostic department for specific protocols. A patient with diabetes may need to adjust his or her insulin dose and diet prior to the test (see Clinical Alert). For CT of the abdomen, the patient usually can take nothing by mouth.

8. Instruct the patient that he or she may experience warmth, flushing of the face, a salty metallic taste, and nausea or vomiting if intravenous iodine is administered.

9. Claustrophobic sensations while in the CT scanner are common. Show the patient a picture of the scanner before the procedure to alleviate anxiety.

10. Sedation and analgesics may help the patient lie quietly during the test to achieve optimal results.

11. Follow guidelines in Chapter 1 regarding safe, effective, informed *pretest* care.

Patient Aftercare

1. Observe and document reactions to iodine contrast material such as hives, skin rashes, nausea, swelling of parotid glands (iodism), or anaphylactic reaction.

2. Notify the physician immediately if symptoms are serious.

3. Antihistamines may relieve the more severe symptoms.

4. Document preparation and instructions given to the patient or significant others, the time the procedure was completed, patient's response to the procedure, any allergic reactions, and subsequent treatment.

5. Follow guidelines in Chapter 1 regarding safe, effective, informed *posttest* care.

> ### Clinical Alert
>
> 1. If patient has diabetes and is taking glucophage/metformin, special considerations may be necessary. Consult with the radiology department to determine whether this medication regimen must be discontinued the day of and several days after the study.
>
> *(continued)*

(Clinical Alert continued)
2. Assess whether the patient is allergic to iodine. If iodine contrast sensitivities are known or suspected, inform the radiology department prior to study.

BIBLIOGRAPHY ●

American Radiological Nurses' Association: Standards of Radiology Nursing Practice. ANA Congress of Nursing Practice, Oakville, IL 1999

Ballinger PW: Merrill's Atlas of Roentgenographic Positions and Standard Radiologic Procedures, Vols. 1–3, 7th ed. St Louis, CV Mosby, 1991

Bier V: Health Effects of Exposure to Low Levels of Imaging Radiation. Washington, DC, National Academy Press, 1990

Bontrager KL: Textbook of Radiographic Positioning and Related Anatomy, 4th ed. St. Louis, CV Mosby, 1997

Bushong SC: Radiologic Science for Technologists, 6th ed. St. Louis, CV Mosby, 1997

Cember H: Introduction to Health Physics, 3rd ed. New York, McGraw-Hill, 1996

Cochran ST: Determination of serum creatinine levels prior to administration of radiographic contrast media. JAMA 277(7): 517–518, 1997

Gignilliat J: Metformin precautions. Am J Nurs 6:17, 1996

POEMs (Patient-Oriented Evidence that Matters) [editorial]: radiological evaluation of Crohn's disease. J Fam Pract 45(6): 465–6 1997

Seeram EL: Radiation Protection. Philadelphia, Lippincott, 1997

Toole J, Good DC: Imaging in neurologic rehabilitation. New York, Demos, June 1996

Torres LS: Basic Medical Techniques and Patient Care for Radiologic Technologists, 5th ed. Philadelphia: JB Lippincott, 1997

Valdini A, Cargill L: Access and barriers to mammography in New England community health centers. J Fam Pract 45(3): 243–249, 1997

Weber ES: Questions and answers about breast cancer diagnoses. Am J Nurs 97(10): 34–38, 1997

Wentz G: Mammography for Radiologic Technologists. New York, McGraw-Hill, 1997

11

Cytologic, Histologic, and Genetic Studies

●CYTOLOGIC AND HISTOLOGIC STUDIES

OVERVIEW OF CYTOLOGIC STUDIES (CELLS) ●

Exfoliated cells in body tissues and fluid are studied to count the cells and determine the types of cells present, and to diagnose malignant and premalignant conditions. The staining technique developed by Dr. George N. Papanicolaou has been especially useful in diagnosis of malignancy and is now used routinely in the cytologic study of the female genital tract, as well as in many types of nongynecologic specimens.

Some cytologic specimens (eg, smears of the mouth, genital tract, nipple discharge) are relatively easy to obtain for study. Other samples (eg, amniotic fluid, pleural effusions, cerebrospinal fluid [CSF]) are from less accessible sources, and special techniques such as fine-needle aspiration are required for collection. Tissue (histologic) samples may be obtained by biopsy during surgery or during outpatient diagnostic procedures such as endoscopy. In all studies, the source of the sample and its method of collection must be noted so that the evaluation can be based on complete information.

Specimens for cytologic and histologic study usually consist of many different cells. Some are normally present, whereas others indicate pathologic conditions. Cells normally observed in 1 sample may, under certain conditions, be indicative of an abnormal state when observed elsewhere. All specimens are examined for the number of cells, cell distribution, surface modifications, size, shape, appearance and staining properties, functional adaptations, and inclusions. The cell nucleus is also examined. Any increases or decreases from normal values are noted.

Gynecologic specimens may be smeared and fixed in 95% alcohol. Some types of spray fixative are also available. (Gynecologic specimens collected using the ThinPrep technique are collected in special [ie, PreservCyt] solution.) Nongynecologic specimens are generally collected without preservative, and they must be handled carefully to prevent drying or degeneration. Check with your individual laboratory for collection requirements. It is important for all cytology specimens to be sent to the laboratory as soon as they are obtained to prevent disintegration of cells or any other process that could cause alteration of the material for study.

> **Clinical Alert**
>
> 1. The test is only as good as the specimen received.
> 2. Specimens collected from patients in isolation should be clearly labeled on the specimen container and requisition form with appropriate warning stickers. The specimen container should then be placed inside *two* sealed, protective biohazard bags before it is transported to the laboratory.
> 3. The US Occupational Safety and Health Administration requires that all specimens be placed in a secondary container before transportation to the laboratory. Most laboratories prefer plastic biohazard bags. Requisitions should be kept on the outside of the bag or in a separate compartment in the biohazard bag, if available.

In practice, results of cytologic studies are commonly reported as

1. Inflammatory
2. Benign
3. Atypical
4. Suspicious for malignancy
5. Positive for malignancy (in situ versus invasive)

Overview of Histologic Studies (Tissue)

Material submitted for tissue examination may be classified according to its histologic or cellular characteristics. A basic method for classifying cancers according to the histologic or cellular characteristics of the tumor is Broder's classification of malignancy:

Grade I: Tumors showing a marked tendency to differentiate; 75% or more of cells differentiated

Grade II: 75% to 50% of cells differentiated, slight to moderate dysplasia and metaplasia

Grade III: 50% to 25% of cells differentiated, marked dysplasia, marked atypical features, and cancer in situ

Grade IV: 25% to 0% of cells differentiated

The Tumor-Node-Metastasis (TNM) system is a method of identifying tumor stage according to spread of the disease. This system evolved from the work of the International Union Against Cancer and the American Joint Committee on Cancer. In addition, the TNM system further defines each specific type of cancer (eg, breast, head, neck). This staging system (Table 11-1) is employed for previously untreated and treated cancers and classifies the primary site of cancer and its extent and involvement, such as lymphatic and venous invasion.

FINE-NEEDLE ASPIRATES: CELL AND TISSUE STUDY ●

Normal Values
Negative: no abnormal cells or abnormal tissue present

Explanation of Test
Fine-needle aspiration is a method of obtaining diagnostic material for cytologic study that causes a minimal amount of trauma to the patient. Bacteriologic studies may also be done on material obtained during fine-needle aspiration. Unfixed material, left in the syringe or on a needle rinsed in sterile saline, may be taken to the microbiology department for study.

Procedure
1. Local anesthesia is used in most cases. Superficial or palpable lesions may be aspirated without radiologic aid, but nonpalpable lesions are aspirated using radiographic imaging as an aid for needle placement.
2. After the needle has been properly positioned, the plunger of the syringe is retracted to create negative pressure. The needle is moved up and down, and sometimes at several different angles. The plunger of the syringe is released, and the needle is removed.

TABLE 11-1
TNM System

Three capital letters are used to describe the extent of the cancer:
- T: Primary tumor
- N: Regional lymph nodes
- M: Distant metastasis

Lower-case letters are used to indicate the chronology of classification:
- c: Clinical-diagnostic
- p: Postsurgical treatment-pathologic
- r: Retreatment
- a: Autopsy

This classification is extended by the following designations:

T SUBCLASSES (EXTENT OF PRIMARY TUMOR)
- TX: Tumor cannot be adequately assessed
- T0: No evidence of primary tumor
- Tis: Carcinoma in situ
- T1, T2, T3, T4: Progressive increase in tumor size and involvement

N SUBCLASSES (INVOLVEMENT OF REGIONAL LYMPH NODES)
- NX: Regional lymph nodes cannot be assessed clinically
- N0: Regional lymph node metastasis
- N1, N2, N3, N4: Increasing degrees of demonstrable abnormality of regional lymph nodes

Histopathology
- GX: Grade cannot be assessed
- G1: Well-differentiated grade
- G2: Moderately well-differentiated grade
- G3: Poorly differentiated grade
- G4: Undifferentiated

METASTASIS
- MX: The minimum requirements to assess the presence of distant metastasis cannot be met
- M0: No evidence of distant metastasis
- M1: Distant metastasis present (specify sites of metastasis)

The category M1 may be subdivided according to the following notations:

Pulmonary:	PUL	Hepatic:	HEP
Osseous:	OSS	Brain:	BRA
Lymph nodes:	LYM	Skin:	SKI
Bone marrow:	MAR	Peritoneum:	PER
Pleura:	PLE	Other:	OTH

In certain sites further information regarding the primary tumor may be recorded under the following headings:

(continued)

TABLE 11-1 *(Continued)*

Lymphatic Invasion (L)
  LX: Lymphatic invasion cannot be assessed
  L0: No evidence of lymphatic invasion
  L1: Lymphatic invasion

Venous Invasion (V)
  VX: Venous invasion cannot be assessed
  V0: No venous invasion
  V1: Microscopic venous invasion
  V2: Macroscopic venous invasion

Information on residual tumor does not enter into establishing the stage of the tumor but should be recorded for use in considering additive therapy. When the cancer is treated by definitive surgical procedures, residual cancer, if any, is recorded.

Residual Tumor (R)
  RX: Residual tumor at primary site cannot be assessed
  R0: No residual tumor
  R1: Microscopic residual tumor
  R2: Macroscopic residual tumor
  M: Symbol—in parentheses indicates multiple tumors
  Y: Symbol—Y prefix indicates classification occurring with intense
     multimodality therapy
  r: Symbol—Z prefix indicates recurrent tumors after a disease-free interval

---

*Adapted from Beahrs OH, Myers MH (eds): Manual for Staging of Cancer, 4th ed. Philadelphia, JB Lippincott, 1992.

---

3. Material obtained may be expressed onto glass slides, which must be fixed immediately in 95% alcohol or spray fixative. Material may also be expressed into a fixative solution, such as 50% alcohol. Material may also be sent to the laboratory in the syringe. Check with your laboratory for specific fixation requirements.
4. See Chapter 1 guidelines for *intratest* care.

Clinical Implications
1. Abnormal results are helpful in identifying
  A. Infectious processes. The infectious agent may be seen, or characteristic cellular changes may indicate the infectious agent that is present.
  B. Benign conditions. Some characteristic cellular changes may be present, indicating the presence of a benign process.
  C. Malignant conditions, either primary or metastatic. If the disease is metastatic, the findings may be reported as consistent with the primary malignancy.

Patient Preparation
1. Explain the purpose and procedure, benefits, and risks of the test. Even though a local anesthetic is used, the procedure causes some discomfort,

and this should not be minimized. If the approach involves passing near a rib, the pain may be greater because of the sensitivity of the bone; this is not a cause for alarm. Unexpected pain may induce a vasovagal or other undesirable response. Other risks include infection and hematoma or hemorrhage, depending on the site aspirated.

2. See guidelines in Chapter 1 for safe, effective, informed *pretest* care.

Clinical Alert

Contraindications (mainly for deep-seated organs) include

1. Bleeding diathesis—anticoagulant therapy
2. Seriously impaired lung function
  A. Advanced emphysema
  B. Severe pulmonary hypertension
  C. Severe hypoxemia
3. Highly vascular lesions
4. Suspected hydatid cyst
5. Uncooperative patient

Patient Aftercare

1. Monitor for signs of inflammation and use site care infection control measures. Treat pain, which may be common in sensitive areas such as the breast, nipple, and scrotum. Monitor for specific problems, which vary depending on the site aspirated (eg, hemoptysis after a lung aspiration).
2. Counsel about follow-up procedures for infections and malignant conditions.
3. Follow guidelines in Chapter 1 for safe, effective, informed *posttest* care.

Clinical Alert

1. Traumatic complications are rare. Fine-needle aspiration of the lung infrequently results in pneumothorax. Local extension of the malignancy is a consideration, but studies have shown this to be an extremely rare occurrence.
2. A negative finding on fine-needle aspiration does not rule out the possibility that a malignancy is present. The cells aspirated may have come from a necrotic area of the tumor or a benign area adjacent to the tumor.

TISSUE BIOPSY STUDIES: OVERVIEW ●

Tissue biopsies from many body sites (ie, breast, liver, kidney, lymph nodes, skin, bone, muscle, lung, bladder, prostate, thyroid, cervix) may be examined for the presence of benign, toxic, or malignant cells and conditions. The amount of tissue obtained and submitted to the laboratory depends upon the specimen site and disease process (ie, in liver biopsy at least 2–3 liver cores >2 cm in length). These procedures may be performed in outpatient or inpatient settings. Depending upon the body site sampled, anesthetic—local or general—or conscious sedation (Appendix C) is necessary.

Tissue obtained for routine histologic and pathologic examination requires special handling, ie, place in 10% formalin or send fresh and intact. Tissue needed for frozen section examination must be delivered to the laboratory immediately with no fixative added. Tissue needed for special studies (eg, special stains for miroorganisms, hormonal studies, DNA ploidy, etc.) may need special handling. A frozen section is done upon the pathologist's recommendation. Tissue freezing (frozen section) may actually be contraindicated and not in the patient's best interest. Contact your individual laboratory for specific instructions.

BREAST BIOPSY: CELL AND TISSUE STUDY AND PROGNOSTIC MARKERS

Normal Values
Negative for malignant or other abnormal cells and tissue. Prognostic markers: Of no significance or negative.

Explanation of Test
Breast biposies are among the most common type of biopsy done. The cells and tissue obtained by breast biopsy establish the presence of breast disease, diagnose histopathology, and classify the process. It also confirms and characterizes calcifications noted in pre-biopsy mammograms. The breast tissue is examined to determine surgical margins, presence or absence of vesicular invasion, tumor type, staging, and grading. Secondary studies relevant to survival may include imaging procedures, along with the following prognostic markers:

Estrogen and progesterone receptors—These hormone receptors are indicators of prognosis and used to manage hormonal therapy in breast and endometrial cancer. Immunohistochemical (IHC) staining aids recognition of metastatic breast cancer.

DNA ploidy—This test measures cell turnover or replication; it is used to predict prognosis and shorter survival times by the presence of aneuploid (rapidly replicating cells) for certain tumor types, breast, prostate, and colon; less clear for ovarian, lung, kidney, and bladder (urine). (66% of breast cancers are aneuploid).

S phase fraction (SPF)—Low levels of SPF appear to have longer survival and reduced chance of relapse. SPF is the DNA synthesis phase obtained by a statistical method.

Cathepsin D—The presence of this lysosomal protease is estrogen related and may promote tumor spread. Prognostic significance remains ambiguous.

Epidural growth factor receptor (EGFR)—Presence is correlated with ER negatives, aneuploids, increased S-phase factors, and lymph node metastases. Increased EGFR may be associated with worse relapse free and survival time.

P 53 gene—This tumor suppression gene regulates cell cycles. Some clinicians believe that P53 gene's prognostic value is second only to lymph node status.

C-erb-B-2 (HER-2) Oncogene—High levels of this oncogene recpetor are associated with poor response to conventional chemotherapy and may be a marker for patients likely to benefit from high doses of chemotherapy.

Procedure

1. See Chapter 10 for image guided tumor localization study before biopsy.
2. Breast tissue specimens may be obtained by open surgical technique or by needly biopsy. These specimens are taken directly to the laboratory and given to the pathologist or histo-technologist.
3. See Chapter 1 guidelines for intratest care.

Clinical Implications

1. The breast tissue is examined and the extent of the tumor is determined. Resection margins are evaluated, and grade and stage of disease are identified.
2. Favorable prognostic indicators include tumor size of less than 1 cm, a low histologic grade, negative axillary lymph nodes, and positive estrogen receptors (ER), and progesterone receptors (RR).
3. Fibroplasia and firbroadenophasia are benign conditions.

Patient Preparation

1. Explain biopsy purpose and procedure. Obtain and record relevant family or personal history, prior biopsy, trauma, recent or current pregnanacy, nipple discharge, location of lump, and how lesion was detected. Informed consent is obtained.
2. Open breast biopsies are performed under lcoal or general anesthesia. Conscious sedation may be used with local anesthetics. NPO is required when general anesthesia is used.
3. Provide information and support recognizing the fear the patient experiences about the procedure.
4. See Chapter 1 guidelines for safe, effective, informed care and Tissue Biopsy Studies: Overview on p. 817.

Patient Aftercare

1. If general anesthesia is used, follow the recovery protocols. See conscious sedation precautions in Appendix C.
2. Interpret biopsy outcome and counsel appropriately about possible further testing and treatment.

LIVER BIOPSY: CELL AND TISSUE STUDY ●

Normal Values

Negative for malignant or other abnormal cells and abnormal tissue

Explanation of Test

Cellular material from the liver may be useful in evaluating the status of the liver in diffuse disorders of the parenchyma and in the diagnosis of space-occupying lesions. Liver biopsy is especially useful when the clinical findings and laboratory test results are not diagnostic (eg, an aspartate aminotransferase [AST] level 10 to 20 times less than the upper defined limit with an alkaline phosphatase [ALP] level less than 3 times the limit) and when the diagnosis or cause cannot be established by other means (enlarged liver of unknown cause or systemic disease affecting the liver, such as miliary tuberculosis). Other indications for liver biopsy include evaluation of chronic hepatitis, portal hypertension, fever of unknown origin (TB and brucellosis) and confirm alcoholic liver disease.

Procedure

1. See section on Cytologic Study of Fine-Needle Aspirates on page 814.
2. The test is done at the bedside, usually under local anesthesia. Specimens may be obtained with ultrasound or CT x-ray guidance and a tissue core biopsy needle, such as the Menghini needle, that provides histologic and cytologic material; or one may use a fine-needle aspiration needle, which obtains cytologic material only and is useful for cancer diagnosis but not other liver diseases.
3. Tissue specimens are placed in 10% formalin for fixation. Check with your laboratory for specific instructions for handling special cases (eg, liver biopsies for copper levels).
4. Cytology specimens are expressed on glass slides, which are fixed immediately in 95% alcohol or spray fixative. Material may also be expressed into an appropriate fixative, such as 50% alcohol. Needle rinses may provide helpful diagnostic material as well.
5. See Chapter 1 for safe, effective, informed *intratest* care and overview on p. 842. See Chapter 12 on endoscopic examination and liver biopsy.

Clinical Implications

Abnormalities in test results of liver biopsies may be helpful in detecting the following:

1. Benign disorders such as
   A. Metabolic disorders
      (1) Fatty metamorphosis
      (2) Hemosiderosis
      (3) Accumulation of bile (hepatitis, obstructive jaundice, malignancy)
      (4) Diabetes
   B. Hepatic cirrhosis
   C. Abscess
   D. Hepatic cysts (congenital or hydatid)
2. Malignant processes such as
   A. Primary tumors of the liver
      (1) Hepatocellular carcinoma
      (2) Cholangiocarcinoma
   B. Metastatic tumors

Interfering Factors

The reported effectiveness of liver aspirates or biopsies varies in the limited published information. Because a very small fragment of tissue, often partially destroyed, is taken in a random manner from a large organ, localized disease is easily missed.

1. False-negative results may be caused by
   A. Sampling error. Detection rate of liver metastases is approximately 50% to 70% with blind biopsy and about 85% (range, 67%–96%) with the use of ultrasound guidance. Also, many diseases produce nonspecific changes that may be spotty, healing, or minimal.
   B. Degeneration or distortion caused by faulty preparation of specimen.
2. False-positive results may be caused by misinterpretation of markedly reactive hepatocytes.

Patient Preparation

1. Explain the purpose, procedure, benefits, and risks of the test. Obtain properly signed informed consent. The procedure usually causes minimal discomfort, but only for a short while. Explain that a local anesthetic will be injected into the skin. Remember to ask whether the patient has ever had a reaction to any numbing medicines.
2. The patient should take nothing by mouth (NPO) for 4 to 6 hours before the procedure. The patient is asked to lie supine with the right arm above the head. During the biopsy, the patient should take a deep breath in, blow the air out, and then hold the breath.
3. Risks include a small but definite risk of intraabdominal bleeding and bile peritonitis. Percutaneous liver biopsy results in complications in only about 1% of cases.
4. See guidelines in Chapter 1 for safe, effective, informed *pretest* care and overview on p. 842.

> ### Clinical Alert
>
> Contraindications include
>
> 1. Bleeding diathesis—anticoagulant therapy
> 2. Highly vascular lesions
> 3. Uncooperative patient
> 4. A prothrombin time in the anticoagulant range, PTT more than 20 seconds over control
> 5. Anemia (Hgb <9.5 g/dl) or marked prolonged bleeding time
> 6. A platelet count of <50,000/mm^3
> 7. Marked ascites (risk of leakage)
> 8. Septic cholongitis

Patient Aftercare

1. Strict bed rest for at least 6 hours is usually ordered, with observation for 24 hours.
2. Assess pulse, blood pressure, and respiration every 15 minutes for the first hour, every 30 minutes for the next 2 hours, once in each of the next 4 hours, and then every 4 hours until the patient's condition is stable.

4. Notify the doctor if the blood pressure differs markedly from baseline or if the patient is in severe pain.
5. Maintain NPO status for 2 hours; previous diet can then be resumed.
6. After 6 hours, a blood specimen for hematocrit testing is usually ordered to rule out internal bleeding.
7. The patient should be warned not to cough hard or strain for 2 to 4 hours after the procedure. Heavy lifting and strenuous activities should be avoided for about 1 week.
8. Follow the guidelines in Chapter 1 and overview on p. 842 for safe, effective, informed *posttest* care.

> **Clinical Alert**
>
> The most common complications include pain, hemorrhage (cause of death from liver biopsy), peritonitis, lacerations of other organs, sepsis, and bacteremia.

RESPIRATORY TRACT: CELL AND TISSUE STUDY ●

(See also Chapter 7, under Respiratory Tract Cultures.)

Normal Values
Negative for abnormal cells or tissue

Explanation of Test
The lungs and the passages that conduct air to and from the lungs form the respiratory tract, which is divided into the upper and lower respiratory tracts. The upper respiratory tract consists of the nasal cavities, the nasopharynx, and the larynx; the lower respiratory tract consists of the trachea and the lungs. Cytologic studies of sputum and bronchial specimens are important as diagnostic aids because of the frequency of cancer of the lung and the relative inaccessibility of this organ. Also detectable are cell changes that may be related to the future development of malignant conditions and to inflammatory conditions.

Sputum is composed of mucus and cells. It is the secretion of the bronchi, lungs, and trachea and is therefore obtained from the lower respiratory tract (bronchi and lungs). Sputum is ejected through the mouth but originates in the lower respiratory tract. Saliva produced by the salivary glands in the mouth is *not* sputum. A specimen can be correctly identified as sputum in microscopic examination by the presence of dust cells (carbon dust–laden macrophages). Although the glands and secretory cells in the mucous lining of the lower respiratory tract produce up to 100 ml of fluid daily, the healthy person normally does not cough up sputum.

Procedures
PROCEDURE FOR OBTAINING SPUTUM
1. The preferred material is an early-morning specimen. Usually, 3 specimens are collected on 3 separate days.

2. The patient must inhale air to the full capacity of the lungs and then exhale the air with an expulsive deep cough.
3. The specimen should be coughed directly into a wide-mouthed, clean container containing 50% alcohol. (Some cytology laboratories prefer the specimen to be fresh if it will be delivered to the laboratory immediately.)
4. The specimen should be covered with a tight-fitting, clean lid.
5. The specimen should be labeled with the patient's name, age, date, diagnosis, and number of specimens (1, 2, or 3) and sent immediately to the laboratory.

PROCEDURE FOR OBTAINING BRONCHIAL SECRETIONS
Bronchial secretions are obtained during bronchoscopy (see Chapter 12). Diagnostic bronchoscopy involves removal of bronchial secretions and tissue for cytologic and microbiologic studies. Secretions obtained are collected in a clean container and taken to the cytology laboratory. If microbiologic studies are ordered, the container must be sterile.

PROCEDURE FOR OBTAINING BRONCHIAL BRUSHINGS
Bronchial brushings are obtained during bronchoscopy. The material collected can be smeared directly on all-frosted slides and immediately fixed, or the actual brush may be placed in a container of 50% ethyl alcohol or saline and delivered to the cytology laboratory (check with the laboratory for their preference).

PROCEDURE FOR BRONCHOPULMONARY LAVAGE
Bronchopulmonary lavage may be used to evaluate patients with interstitial lung disease. Saline is injected into the distal portions of the lung and aspirated back through the bronchoscope into a specimen container. This essentially "washes out" the alveoli. The fresh specimen should be brought directly to the laboratory. A total cell count and a differential cell count are performed to determine the relative numbers of macrophages, neutrophils, and lymphocytes.

For all procedures, see Chapter 1 guidelines for *intratest* care.

Clinical Implications
Abnormalities in sputum and bronchial specimens may sometimes be helpful in detecting the following:

1. Benign atypical changes in sputum, as in
   A. Inflammatory diseases
   B. Asthma (Curschmann's spirals and eosinophils may be found, but they are not diagnostic of the disease.)
   C. Lipid pneumonia (Lipophages may be found, but they are not diagnostic of the disease.)
   D. Asbestosis (ferruginous or asbestos bodies)
   E. Viral diseases
   F. Benign diseases of lung, such as bronchiectasis, atelectasis, emphysema, and pulmonary infarcts
2. Metaplasia (the substitution of 1 adult cell type for another); severe metaplastic changes are found in patients with
   A. History of chronic cigarette smoking

  B. Pneumonitis
  C. Pulmonary infarcts
  D. Bronchiectasis
  E. Healing abscess
  F. Tuberculosis
  G. Emphysema (Metaplasia often adjoins a carcinoma or a carcinoma in situ.)
3. Viral changes and the presence of virocytes (viral inclusions) may be seen in
  A. Viral pneumonia
  B. Acute respiratory disease caused by adenovirus
  C. Herpes simplex
  D. Measles
  E. Cytomegalic inclusion disease
  F. Varicella
4. Degenerative changes, as seen in viral diseases of the lung
5. Fungal and parasitic diseases (In parasitic diseases, ova or parasite may be seen.)
6. Tumors (benign and malignant)

Interfering Factors

1. False-negative results may be caused by
  A. Delays in preparation of the specimen, causing a deterioration of tumor cells
  B. Sampling error (Diagnostic cells may not have exfoliated into the material examined.)
2. The frequency of false-negative results is about 15%, in contrast to about 1% in studies for cervical cancer. This high incidence occurs even with careful examination of multiple deep cough specimens.

Patient Preparation

1. Explain the purpose and procedure of the test. Tell the patient **not** to drink fixative liquid in specimen container.
2. Emphasize that sputum is not saliva. If a patient is having difficulty producing sputum, a hot shower before obtaining a specimen may improve the yield.
3. Advise the patient to brush the teeth and rinse the mouth well before obtaining the sputum specimen to avoid introduction of saliva into the specimen. The specimen should be collected before the patient eats breakfast.
4. If a bronchoscopy is performed, maintain NPO for 6 hours before the procedure.
5. Manage pain with sedation as indicated.
6. Provide emotional support.
7. Instruct the patient to breathe in and out of the nose with the mouth open during the procedure. The fiberoptic bronchoscope is inserted through the nose or mouth; the rigid bronchoscope is inserted through the mouth.
8. See Chapter 1 guidelines for safe, effective, informed *pretest* care.

Selection of Medications and Media for All Respiratory Cell and Tissue Procedures

1. Mild sedative or local anesthetic (or both) may be used during bronchoscopy. Sedation is indicated for pain after bronchoscopy. See Chapter 12 for bronchoscopy care.

2. Sputum specimens are collected in a wide-mouth container; 50% alcohol may be added if transportation to the laboratory will be delayed.

3. Bronchial washings may be collected in a trap tube or wide-mouth container.

4. Bronchial brushes may be smeared directly on glass slides, which are then fixed immediately in 95% alcohol or spray fixative. Brushes may be placed in a fixative solution such as 50% alcohol.

Clinical Alert

The uncooperative patient is a contraindication.

Patient Aftercare

1. If the specimen is obtained by bronchoscopy, check the patient's blood pressure, pulse, and respirations every 15 minutes for 1 hour, then every 2 hours for 4 hours, then as ordered.

2. Assist and teach the patient to not eat or drink until the gag reflex returns.

3. Maintain bed rest and elevate the head of the bed 45 degrees.

4. Manage pain as indicated.

5. Auscultate the chest for breath sounds every 2 to 4 hours and then as ordered.

6. Perform postural drainage and oropharyngeal suctioning as ordered. (Refer to bronchoscopy care in Chapter 12.)

7. Follow guidelines in Chapter 1 for safe, effective, informed *posttest* care.

GASTROINTESTINAL TRACT: CELL AND TISSUE STUDY ●

Normal Values

Negative for abnormal cells
Squamous epithelial cells of the esophagus may be present.

Explanation of Test

Exfoliative cytology of the gastrointestinal tract is useful in the diagnosis of benign and malignant diseases. It is not, however, a specific test for these diseases. Many benign diseases, such as leukoplakia of the esophagus, esophagitis, gastritis, pernicious anemia, and granulomatous diseases, may be recognized because of their characteristic cellular changes. Response to radiation may also be noted from cytologic studies.

Procedure

1. A sedative may be given before the procedure. For esophageal studies, a nasogastric Levin tube is passed approximately 40 cm (to the cardio-esophageal junction) with the patient in a sitting position.

2. For stomach studies, a Levin tube is passed into the stomach (approximately 60 cm) with the patient in a sitting position.

3. For pancreatic and gallbladder drainage, a special double-lumen gastric tube is passed orally to 45 cm, with the patient in a sitting position. Then the patient is placed on his or her right side and the tube is passed slowly to 85 cm. It takes about 20 minutes for the tube to reach this distance. Tube location is confirmed by biopsy. Lavage with physiologic salt solution is done during all upper gastrointestinal cytology procedures.

4. Specimens can also be obtained during endoscopy procedures.

5. Material obtained with the use of brushes may be smeared directly on glass slides, which are fixed immediately in 95% alcohol or spray fixative. Brushes may also be placed in a fixative such as 50% alcohol. See Chapter 12 for endoscopic biopsy procedures. Washings must be delivered immediately to the laboratory and may need to be placed on ice. Check with your individual laboratory for specific instructions on handling of washings from the gastrointestinal tract.

Clinical Implications

1. The characteristics of benign and malignant cells of the gastrointestinal tract are the same as for cells of the rest of the body.

2. Abnormal results in cytologic studies of the esophagus may be a nonspecific aid in the diagnosis of
   A. Acute esophagitis, characterized by increased exfoliation of basal cells with inflammatory cells and polymorphonuclear leukocytes in the cytoplasm of the benign squamous cells
   B. Vitamin B_{12} and folic acid deficiencies, characterized by giant epithelial cells
   C. Malignant diseases, characterized by typical cells of esophageal malignancy

3. Abnormal results in studies of the stomach may be a nonspecific aid in the diagnosis of
   A. Pernicious anemia, characterized by giant epithelial cells. An injection of vitamin B_{12} causes these cells to disappear within 24 hours.
   B. Granulomatous inflammations seen in chronic gastritis and sarcoid of the stomach, which are characterized by granulomatous cells
   C. Gastritis, characterized by degenerative changes and an increase in the exfoliation of clusters of surface epithelial cells
   D. Malignant diseases, most of which are gastric adenocarcinomas. Lymphoma cells can be differentiated from adenocarcinoma. The Reed-Sternberg cell, a multinucleated giant cell, is the characteristic cell found along with abnormal lymphocytes in Hodgkin's disease.

4. Abnormal results in studies of the pancreas, gallbladder, and duodenum may reveal malignant cells (usually adenocarcinoma), but it is sometimes difficult to determine the exact site of the tumor.

5. Abnormal results in examination of the colon may reveal
   A. Ileitis, characterized by large, multinucleated histocytes (Bovine tuberculosis commonly manifests itself in this area.)
   B. Ulcerative colitis, characterized by hyperchromatic nuclei surrounded by a thin cytoplasmic rim
   C. Malignant cells (usually adenocarcinoma)

Interfering Factors

The barium and lubricant used in Levin tubes interferes with good results, because they distort the cells and prevent accurate evaluation.

Patient Preparation

1. The patient should be told the purpose of the test, the nature of the procedure, and to anticipate some discomfort.
2. A liquid diet usually is ordered for the 24 hours before testing. The patient is encouraged to take fluids throughout the night and in the morning before the procedure.
3. No oral barium should be administered for the preceding 24 hours.
4. Laxatives and enemas are ordered for colon cytologic studies.
5. Because insertion of the nasogastric tube can cause considerable discomfort, the patient and clinician should devise a system (eg, raising a hand) to indicate discomfort. (See gastric analysis procedure in Chapter 15.)
6. The patient should be informed that panting, mouth-breathing, or swallowing can help to ease insertion of the tube.
7. Sucking on ice chips or sipping through a straw also makes insertion of the tube easier.
8. Ballottement and massage of the abdomen are needed to release cells when a gastric wash technique is used.
9. See Chapter 1 guidelines for safe, effective, informed *pretest* care.

> **Clinical Alert**
>
> 1. The uncooperative patient is a contraindication.
> 2. Immediately remove the tube if the patient shows signs of distress: coughing, gasping, or cyanosis.

Patient Aftercare

1. Interpret test results and monitor appropriately. The patient should be given food, fluids, and rest after the tests are completed.
2. Provide rest. Patients having colon studies will be feeling quite tired.
3. Potential complications of endoscopy include respiratory distress and esophageal, gastric, or duodenal perforation. Complications of proctosigmoidoscopy include possible bowel perforation. Decreased blood pressure, pallor, diaphoresis, and bradycardia are signs of vasovagal stimulation and require immediate notification of the physician.
4. Follow Chapter 1 guidelines for safe, effective, informed *posttest* care.

PAPANICOLAOU SMEAR (PAP): CELL STUDY OF THE FEMALE GENITAL TRACT, VULVA, VAGINA, AND CERVIX ●

Normal Values
No abnormal cells, no inflammation

Hormone Function Representative Maturation Index (MI) Values: proportion of the major cell types.

Normal child:	80/20/0
Preovulatory adult:	0/40/60
Premenstrual adult:	0/70/30

Pregnant adult (2nd mo):	0/90/10
Postmenopausal adult (age 60):	65/30/5

(ie, parabasal, intermediate, and superficial)

Background

Characteristic physiologic cellular changes occur in the genital tract from birth through the postmenopausal years. Hormonal evaluation by cytologic examination should be performed only on vaginal smears taken from the lateral vaginal wall or from the vaginal fornix. Smears from the ectocervix or endocervix cannot be used for hormonal evaluation because certain conditions, such as metaplasia and cervicitis, interfere with a correct assessment. Three major cell types occur in a characteristic pattern in normal vaginal smears:

1. Superficial squamous cells (mature squamous, usually polygonal, containing a pyknotic nucleus)
2. Intermediate squamous cells (mature squamous, usually polygonal, containing a clearly structured vesicular nucleus, which may be either well preserved or peptolytically changed as a result of bacterial cytolysis)
3. Parabasal cells (immature squamous, usually round or oval, containing 1 or, rarely, >1 relatively large nucleus). These cells occur either well preserved or in proteolytic clusters as a result of degeneration or necrosis.

NOTE: *Deviation from normal physiologic cell patterns may be indicative of a pathologic condition.*

A hormonal cytologic study is valuable in the assessment of many endocrine-related conditions, especially ovarian function.

Explanation of Test

The Papanicolaou (Pap) smear is used principally for diagnosis of precancerous and cancerous conditions of the vulva, and the vagina, cervix. This test is also used for hormonal assessment and for diagnosis of inflammatory diseases. Because the Pap smear is of great importance in the early detection of cervical cancer, it is recommended that all women older than 20 years of age have the test at least once a year.

The value of the Pap smear depends on the fact that cells readily exfoliate (or can be easily stripped) from genital cancers. Cytologic study can also be used for assessing response to administered sex hormones. The microbiologic examination on cytology samples is not as accurate as bacterial culture, but it can provide valuable information.

Specimens for cytologic examination of the genital tract are usually obtained by vaginal speculum examination or by colposcopy with biopsy. Material from the cervix, endocervix, and posterior fornix is obtained for most smears. Smears for hormonal evaluation are obtained from the vagina.

Clinical Alert

Cytologic findings alone do not form the basis of a diagnosis of cancer or other diseases. Often they are used to justify further procedures, such as biopsy.

In an effort to standardize reporting of cervical-vaginal cytology specimens, the Bethesda System for reporting cervical-vaginal diagnoses was developed by a 1988 National Cancer Institute workshop and slightly modified after a second workshop in 1991. This reporting system is being adopted by numerous laboratories nationwide. The terminology of this reporting system appears in Table 11-2.

Cells are also examined for hormonal effect and organisms. Cells examined for hormonal effect may be reported on a 6-point scale.

1. Marked estrogen effect
2. Moderate estrogen effect
3. Slight estrogen effect
4. Atrophic

5. Compatible with pregnancy
6. No evaluation—specimen too bloody or inflamed or scanty

Cells can also be examined for microorganisms using routine staining techniques. These cells may be reported on a 5-point scale.

1. Normal flora
2. Scanty or absent
3. *Trichomonas*

4. *Candida*
5. Other (cocci, coccobacilli, mixed bacteria)

Note

Many new computerized technologies to aid in the manual screening of cervical-vaginal smears. The PAPNET screening system combines neural network and image processing technologies. This system can detect the presence of only a few abnormal cells, which are difficult to detect when they are scattered among hundreds of thousands of normal cells. PAPNET is being used in some places as a quality control procedure to review smears that are classified as negative after manual screening.

The AutoPap System received preliminary approval from the US Food and Drug Administration in early 1998 and is the first device of its kind to receive a recommended approval for automated initial Pap smear screening. With the AutoPap System, approximately 25% of submitted Pap smears would receive AutoPap review only and would not need to be seen by a technologist.

Cytyc has taken a different approach to create a better Pap smear: ThinPrep. The Pap smear collection device for ThinPrep is rinsed in a special solution (ie, PreservCyt) and sent to the lab. A special machine prepares a uniform monolayer Pap smear. These slides are then manually screened in the usual manner. Studies have shown that these ThinPrep smears have a higher rate of detection of biopsy-proven high-grade lesions and a lower rate of false-negative results than conventional Pap smears.

Procedure

1. The patient is usually asked to remove clothing from the waist down.
2. The patient is placed in a lithotomy position on an examining table.
3. An appropriately sized bivalve speculum, lubricated and warmed *only* with water, is gently inserted into the vagina to expose the cervix.
4. If a conventional Pap smear is being taken, the posterior fornix and external os of the cervix are scraped with a wooden spatula, a cytobrush, or a

TABLE 11-2.
The 1991 Bethesda System

ADEQUACY OF THE SPECIMEN
Satisfactory for evaluation
Satisfactory for evaluation but limited (specify reason)
Unsatisfactory for evaluation (specify reason)

GENERAL CATEGORIZATION (OPTIONAL)
Within normal limits
Benign cellular changes: See descriptive diagnosis
Epithelial cell abnormality: See descriptive diagnosis

DESCRIPTIVE DIAGNOSES
Benign cellular changes
  Infection
    Trichomonas vaginalis
    Fungal organisms morphologically consistent with *Candida* spp.
    Predominance of coccobaccilli consistent with shift in vaginal flora
    Bacteria morphologically consistent with *Actinomyces* spp.
    Other cellular changes associated with herpes simplex virus
  Reactive changes
    Reactive cellular changes associated with
      Inflammation (includes typical repair)
      Atrophy with inflammation (atrophic vaginitis)
      Radiation
      Intrauterine contraceptive device (IUD)
      Other
Epithelial cell abnormalities
  Squamous cell
    Atypical squamous cells of undetermined significance (ASC): Qualify* further
    Low-grade squamous intraepithelial lesion encompassing (LSIL): HPV† mild
      dysplasia/CIN 1
    High-grade squamous intraepithelial lesion (HSIL) encompassing moderate
      and severe dysplasia, CIS/CIN 2 and CIN 3
    Squamous cell carcinoma (SCC)
  Glandular cell
    Endometrial cells, cytologically benign, in a postmenopausal
      woman
    Atypical glandular cells of undetermined significance (AEUS): Qualify*
      further
    Endocervical adenocarcinoma
    Endometrial adenocarcinoma
    Extrauterine adenocarcinoma
    Adenocarcinoma, NOS
Other malignant neoplasms: Specify
Hormonal evaluation (applies to vaginal smears only)
  Hormonal pattern compatible with age and history

(continued)

TABLE 11-2 *(Continued)*

Hormonal pattern incompatible with age and history (specify reason)
Hormonal evaluation not possible (specify reason)

CIS, carcinoma in situ; CIN, cervical intraepithelial neoplasia (number indicates grade).
*Atypical squamous or glandular cells of undetermined significance; should be further qualified as to whether a reactive or a premalignant/malignant process is favored.
†Cellular changes of human papillomavirus (HPV)—previously termed koilocytosis, koilocytotic atypia, or condylomatous atypia—are included in the category of low-grade squamous cell intraepithelial lesion.

cytobroom. Material obtained is smeared on glass slides and placed immediately in 95% alcohol or spray fixed, before air drying can occur.

5. If a ThinPrep Pap smear is being taken, a broom-like collection device is used. Insert the central bristles of the broom into the endocervical canal deep enough to allow the short bristles to fully contact the ectocervix. Push gently and rotate the broom in a clockwise direction 5 times. Rinse the broom with a PreservCyt solution vial by pushing the broom into the bottom of the vial 10 times, forcing the bristles apart. As a final step, swirl the broom vigorously to further release material. Discard the collection device. Tighten the cap on the solution container so that the torque line on the cap passes the torque line on the vial.

6. Label the specimen properly with the patient's name and identifying number (if appropriate) and the area from which the specimen was obtained, and send it to the laboratory with a properly completed information sheet, including date of collection, patient's date of birth, last menstrual period, and pertinent clinical history.

7. Examination takes about 5 minutes.

8. See Chapter 1 guidelines for *intratest* care.

> **Clinical Alert**
>
> 1. The best time to take a Pap smear is 2 weeks after the first day of the last menstrual period and definitely not when the patient is menstruating.
> 2. Cytologic specimens should be considered infectious until fixed with a germicidal fixative. Observe standard precautions when handling specimens from all patients.

PROCEDURE FOR HORMONAL SMEARS AND MATURATION INDEX

Obtain a specimen by scraping the proximal portion of the lateral wall of the vagina, avoiding the cervical area. Otherwise the procedure is the same as for the Pap smear.

Clinical Implications

1. Abnormal cytologic responses can be classified as protective, destructive, reparative (regenerative), or neoplastic.

2. Inflammatory reactions and microbes can be identified to help in the diagnosis of vaginal diseases.

3. Precancerous and cancerous lesions of the cervix can be identified. The stages of neoplastic disease can be arbitrarily classified as dysplasia (mild, moderate, or severe), carcinoma in situ (preinvasive carcinoma), microinvasive carcinoma, or invasive carcinoma.

4. Hormonal cytology reports include several factors:

    A. *Hormonal cell pattern:* The report states that the pattern is or is not compatible with the age and menstrual history of the patient. The reason for hormone function noncompatibility is given.

    B. *Maturation index (MI):* The MI indicates the proportion of the major cell types (parabasal, intermediate, and superficial) in the sample—that is, the number of each type per 100 cells counted. It is expressed as a ratio (eg, MI = 100/0/0). See Normal Values for representative hormone function MIs.

5. The following facts should be kept in mind when hormonal cytology reports are reviewed (Table 11-3).

    A. The maturity of the epithelium cannot be expressed in degrees of estrogenic effects or estrogen deficiencies, because more than 1 hormonal stimulus is involved (estrogen, progesterone, and adrenal hormones).

    B. Surgical removal of the ovaries does not necessarily result in epithelial atrophy.

    C. Only 2 cell types can be identified with accuracy if the age and menstrual history of the patient are not known.

    (1) Abundant superficial squamous cells, indicative of unequivocal estrogenic effect

    (2) Parabasal cells, indicative of lack of cell maturation due to lack of hormone stimulation

    D. From a single specimen, it is impossible to predict whether ovulation will occur, whether it has recently occurred, or what stage of menstrual cycle the patient is in. Serial specimens must be examined to obtain these results.

    E. An intermediate cell type is always intermediate, regardless of its size.

    F. No hormonal assessment should be made without knowing the age of the patient, her menstrual history, and her history of hormone administrations.

    G. An example of a typical cytology report is on p. 833.

Clinical Alert

A cytobrush should not be used to obtain a cervical specimen from a pregnant patient.

Interfering Factors

1. Medications such as tetracycline and digitalis, which affect the squamous epithelium, alter test results.

2. The use of lubricating jelly in the vagina or recent douching interferes with test results by distorting the cells and preventing accurate evaluation.

3. The presence of infection interferes with hormonal cytology.

4. Heavy menstrual flow may make the interpretation of the results difficult and may obscure atypical cells.

A Typical Cytology Report

Cytology ID: C99-44133
Collected: 07/13/99
Received: 07/13/99
Reported:
Slides: 1

Clinical History:	LMP: n/a Previous smear: 1997 WNL
Specimen Source:	Vaginal/Cervical

Specimen Adequacy:	Satisfactory for interpretation but limited by:
	    Lack of pertinent clinical information
	    No LMP given
	    Obscuring inflammation

General Category:	BENIGN CELLULAR CHANGES
Diagnosis:	Atrophy with inflammation otherwise within normal limits
Recommedations:	Clinical correlation

Signature of Clinician

This notice should appear on all cytology reports:

The PAP smear is a screening test for cervical cancer and its precursors. Since its introduction, it has reduced the death rate from cervical cancer by more than 70%. However, the smear is not perfect. As a screening test it has an inherent false negative and false positive rate. Regular PAP smear testing should be used in conjunction with other established clinical practices in evaluating patients for cervical disease. If the results of this PAP test do not correlate with the clinical impression, or do not explain the patient's clinical signs/symmptoms, additional studies would be warranted. The PAP test is not a screening test for detecting endometrial pathology.

Name of Clinic   **Name of Director of Cytopathology**
and Clinic Director

Patient Preparation

1. Explain the test purpose and procedure.
2. Instruct the patient not to douche for 2 to 3 days before the test, because douching may remove the exfoliated cells.
3. Instruct the patient not to use vaginal medications or vaginal contraceptives during the 48 hours before examination. Intercourse is not recommended the night before the examination.
4. Have the patient empty her bladder and rectum before examination.
5. Ask the patient to give the following information:
   A. First day of last menstrual period
   B. Use of hormone therapy or birth control pills
   C. All medications taken
   D. Any radiation therapy
   E. Any other pertinent clinical history (eg, previous abnormal Pap smear)
6. Follow Chapter 1 guidelines for safe, effective, informed *pretest* care.

Clinical Alert

The only contraindication is an uncooperative patient.

TABLE 11-3.
Vaginal Cytologic Smear Findings in Gynecologic and Related Endocrinopathies

Condition	Usual Smear Types
Adrenal hyperplasia, congenital	Atrophic or atypical intermediate proliferation
Adrenogenital syndrome (hyperplasia)	Atrophic to atypical intermediate proliferation
Adrenal tumor (masculinizing)	Usually atrophic; sometimes "multihormonal" with cells from all layers
Chiari-Frommel syndrome	Markedly atrophic
Cushing's syndrome	Intermediate proliferation or atypical regressive types
Eunuchoidism, ovarian	Atrophic
Feminizing testicular syndrome	Proliferative; nuclear sex chromatin negative
Follicular cytosis	Persistently high estrogen index (EI) and karyopyknotic index (KI)
Gonadal dysgenesis	Atrophic; nuclear sex chromatin negative in 80%
Hirsutism, genetic	Normal cycling
Hypothalamic (psychogenic) amenorrhea	Most often atrophic to slight proliferation but great variation from atrophic to highly proliferative
Menopausal syndrome	At first highly proliferative, some with cycling; later, intermediate proliferation or atrophic
Ovarian tumors, feminizing	Proliferative, some with high EI and KI, occasionally regressive
Ovarian tumors, masculinizing	Variation, many atrophic, some with atypical proliferation or "multihormonal"
Precocious puberty, constitutional	Proliferative, some with high EI and KI, some with cycling
Pituitary hypogonadism	Atrophic to slight proliferation
Pseudocyesis	"Progestational" types with varying regression
Stein-Leventhal syndrome	Variation; most with intermediate proliferation, occasionally highly proliferative
Uterine defect (congenital absence or irresponsiveness)	Normal cycling

(Adapted from Keebler CM, Reagan JW (eds): Manual of Cytotechnology, 7th ed. Chicago, American Society of Clinical Pathologists, 1993.

Patient Aftercare

1. Interpret test results and counsel appropriately. Risks from the cervical-vaginal smear procedure are exceedingly rare. The patient should be asked to notify the doctor if any unusual pain or discharge occurs after the procedure.
2. Give the patient a perineal pad after the procedure to absorb any bleeding.
3. Follow Chapter 1 guidelines for safe, effective, informed *posttest* care.

ASPIRATED BREAST CYSTS AND NIPPLE DISCHARGE: CELL STUDY

Normal Values

Negative for neoplasia

Background

Nipple discharge usually is normal only during the lactation period. Any other nipple discharge is abnormal, and when it occurs the breasts should be examined for mastitis, duct papilloma, or intraductal cancer. (However, certain situations increase the possibility of finding a normal nipple discharge, such as pregnancy, perimenopausal state, and use of birth control pills.) About 3% of breast cancers and 10% of benign lesions of the breast are associated with abnormal nipple discharge.

The contents of all breast cysts obtained by needle biopsy are examined to detect malignant cells.

Procedure for Breast Cyst

The contents of the identified breast cyst are obtained by fine needle aspiration (see page 814).

Procedure

1. This procedure should be limited to patients who have no palpable masses in the breast or other evidence of breast cancer.
2. The nipple should be washed with a cotton pledget and patted dry.
3. The nipple is gently stripped, or milked, to obtain a discharge. Fluid should be expressed until a pea-sized drop appears. The patient may assist by holding a bottle of fixative beneath the breast so that the slide may be dropped in immediately.
4. The nipple discharge is spread directly on glass slides and then dropped into the fixative bottle containing 95% alcohol or spray fixed.
5. The specimen is identified with pertinent data, including from which breast it was obtained, and is sent without delay to the laboratory.
6. For all procedures, see Chapter 1 guidelines for *intratest* care.

Clinical Implications

Abnormal results are helpful in identifying

1. Benign breast conditions, such as mastitis or intraductal papilloma
2. Malignant breast conditions, such as intraductal cancer or intracystic infiltrating cancer

Interfering Factors

Use of drugs that alter hormone balance (eg, phenothiazines, digitalis, diuretics, steroids) often results in a clear nipple discharge.

Patient Preparation

1. Explain the purpose and procedure of the test.
2. The nipple should be washed with a cotton pledget and patted dry.
3. Follow guidelines in Chapter 1 for safe, effective, informed *pretest* care.

> **Clinical Alert**
>
> The only contraindication is an uncooperative patient.

Patient Aftercare

1. No special instructions are needed for aftercare, because this is not an invasive procedure. The patient should be instructed to contact the clinician if pain or discharge occurs.
2. Interpret test results and counsel appropriately.
3. Follow guidelines in Chapter 1 for safe, effective, informed *posttest* care.

> **Clinical Alert**
>
> Any discharge, regardless of color, should be reported and examined. A bloody or blood-tinged discharge is especially significant.

URINE: CELL STUDY

Normal Values

Negative
Epithelial and squamous cells are normally present in urine.
(See also Chapter 3, especially Microscopic Examination of Urine Sediment.)

Explanation of Test

Cells from the epithelial lining of the urinary tract exfoliate readily into the urine. Urine cytology is most useful in the diagnosis of cancer and inflammatory diseases of the bladder, the renal pelvis, the ureters, and the urethra. This study is also valuable in detecting cytomegalic inclusion disease and other viral diseases and in detecting bladder cancer in high-risk populations, such as workers exposed to aniline dyes, smokers, and patients previously treated for bladder cancer. A Papanicolaou stain of smears prepared from the urinary sediment, filter preparations, or cytocentrifuged smears is useful to identify abnormalities.

Procedure

1. Obtain a clean-voided urine specimen of at least 180 ml for an adult or 10 ml for a child.
2. Obtain a catheterized specimen, if possible, if cancer is suspected.
3. Deliver the specimen immediately to the cytology laboratory. Urine should

be as fresh as possible when it is examined. If a delay is expected, an equal volume of 50% alcohol may be added as a preservative.

4. Urine specimens or bladder washings are collected in wide-mouth containers; 50% alcohol may be added if laboratory transport will be delayed. Check with your laboratory for specific instructions.
5. See Chapter 1 guidelines for *intratest* care.

Clinical Implications

1. Findings possibly indicative of inflammatory conditions of the *lower* urinary tract include

   A. Epithelial hyperplasia   **C.** Abundance of red blood cells
   B. Atypical cells   **D.** Leukocytes

   NOTE: *Inflammatory conditions could be caused by benign prostatic hyperplasia, adenocarcinoma of the prostate, kidney stones, diverticula of bladder, strictures, or malformations.*

2. Findings indicative of viral disease include the following:

   A. *Cytomegalic inclusion disease:* large intranuclear inclusions

   NOTE: *Cytomegalic inclusion disease is a viral infection that usually occurs in childhood but is also seen in cancer patients treated with chemotherapy and in transplantation patients treated with immunosuppressive drugs. The renal tubular epithelium is usually involved.*

     (1) Cytomegaloviruses or salivary gland viruses are related to the herpes varicella agents.
     (2) Infected people may excrete virus in the urine or saliva for months.
     (3) About 60% to 90% of adults have experienced infection.
     (4) In closed populations (eg, institutionalized mentally disabled persons, household contacts), high infection rates may occur at an early age.

   B. *Measles:* Characteristic cytoplasmic inclusion bodies may be found in the urine before the appearance of Koplik's spots.

3. Findings possibly indicative of malacoplakia and granulomatous disease of the bladder or *upper* urinary tract include

   A. Histiocytes with multiple granules in an abundant, foamy cytoplasm
   B. Michaelis-Gutmann bodies in malacoplakia

4. Cytologic findings possibly indicative of *malignancy:* If the specimen shows evidence of any of the changes associated with malignancy, cancer of the bladder, renal pelvis, ureters, kidney, or urethra may be suspected. Metastatic tumor should be ruled out as well.

Patient Preparation

1. Patient preparation depends on the type of procedure being done. Explain the purpose, procedure, benefits, and risks to the patient.
2. If a cystoscopy is done, the patient will be given anesthesia (general, spinal, or local). Refer to Chapter 12 for cystoscopy care.
3. If a voided urine is required, instruct the patient in the procedure for collection of a clean-catch specimen.
4. See Chapter 1 guidelines for safe, effective, informed *pretest* care.

> **Clinical Alert**
>
> The only contraindication is an uncooperative patient.

Patient Aftercare

1. Interpret test results and monitor appropriately. If cystoscopy is performed gently and with adequate lubrication, the patient should experience only minimal discomfort after the procedure.
2. Aftereffects may include mild dysuria and transient hematuria, but these should disappear within 48 hours after the procedure. The patient should be able to void normally after a routine cystoscopic examination. Refer to Chapter 12 for cystoscopy care.
3. Follow Chapter 1 guidelines for safe, effective, informed *posttest* care.

CEREBROSPINAL FLUID (CSF): CELL STUDY ●

Normal Values

Total cell count, adult: 0 to 10/mm^3 (all mononuclear cells)
Total cell count, infant: 0 to 20/mm^3
Negative for neoplasia
A variety of normal cells may be seen. Large lymphocytes are most common. Small lymphocytes are also seen, as are elements of the monocytemacrophage series.
The CSF of a healthy person should be free of all pathogens.

Explanation of Test

CSF obtained by lumbar puncture is examined for the presence of abnormal cells and for an increase or decrease in the normally present cell population. Most of the usual laboratory procedures for study of CSF involve an examination of the leukocytes and a leukocyte count; chemical and microbiologic studies are also done. Cell studies of the CSF also have been used to identify neoplastic cells. These studies have been especially helpful in diagnosis and treatment of the different phases of leukemia. The nature of neoplasia is such that for tumor cells to exfoliate they must actually invade the CSF circulation and enter such areas as the ventricle wall, the choroid plexus, or the subarachnoid space.

Procedure

1. Usually, 3 to 4 specimens of at least 1 to 3 ml are obtained by lumbar puncture (see Chapter 5).
2. Generally, only 1 specimen of 1 to 3 ml goes to the cytology laboratory. Other tubes are sent to different laboratories for examination.
3. The specimen is labeled with the patient's name, date, and type of specimen.
4. The sample is sent immediately to the cytology laboratory for processing.

Clinical Alert

The laboratory should be given adequate warning that a CSF specimen is being delivered. Time is a critical factor; cells begin to disintegrate if the sample is kept at room temperature for more than 1 hour.

Clinical Implications

1. CSF abnormalities may indicate
   A. Malignant gliomas that have invaded the ventricles or cortex of the brain: leukocytes, $150/mm^3$ (The sample may be normal in 75% of patients.)
   B. Ependymoma (neoplasm of differentiated ependymal cells) and medulloblastoma (a cerebellar tumor) in children
   C. Seminoma and pineoblastoma (tumors of the pineal gland)
   D. Secondary carcinomas
      (1) Secondary carcinomas metastasizing to the central nervous system have multiple avenues to the subarachnoid space through the bloodstream.
      (2) The breast and lung are common sources of metastatic cells exfoliated in the CSF. Infiltration of acute leukemia is also common.
   E. Central nervous system leukemia
   F. Fungal forms
      (1) Congenital toxoplasmosis: leukocytes, 50 to $500/mm^3$ (mostly monocytes present)
      (2) Coccidioidomycosis: leukocytes, $200/mm^3$
   G. Various forms of meningitis
      (1) Cryptococcal meningitis: leukocytes, $800/mm^3$ (lymphocytes are more abundant than polynuclear neutrophilic leukocytes)
      (2) Tuberculous meningitis: leukocytes, 25 to $1000/mm^3$ (mostly lymphocytes present)
      (3) Acute pyogenic meningitis: leukocytes, 25 to $10,000/mm^3$ (mostly polynuclear neutrophilic leukocytes present)
   H. Meningoencephalitis (primary amebic meningoencephalitis)
      (1) Leukocytes, 400 to $21,000/mm^3$
      (2) Red blood cells are also found.
      (3) Wright's stain may reveal amebas.
   I. Hemosiderin-laden macrophages, as in subarachnoid hemorrhage
   J. Lipophages from central nervous system destructive processes
2. Characteristics of neoplastic cells
   A. Sometimes marked increase in size, most likely sarcoma and carcinoma
   B. Exfoliated cells tend to be more polymorphic as the neoplasm becomes increasingly malignant

Interfering Factors

The lumbar puncture can occasionally cause contamination of the specimen with squamous epithelial cells or spindly fibroblasts.

Patient Preparation

1. Explain the procedure to the patient (see Chapter 5). A local anesthetic will be used. Remember to ask if the patient has a history of reacting to local anesthetic. CSF is collected in tubes and delivered immediately to the laboratory. No fixative is added to the specimen. Instruct the patient that the procedure may be uncomfortable and that immobilization is extremely important. The patient should be instructed to breathe normally—not to hold the breath. Provide the patient with physical and emotional support during the procedure.
2. See guidelines in Chapter 1 for safe, effective, informed *pretest* care.

> **Clinical Alert**
>
> The only contraindication is an uncooperative patient.

Patient Aftercare

1. The patient should be placed in a supine position. Keep the head of the bed flat for 4 to 8 hours as ordered; if headache occurs, elevate the feet 10 to 15 degrees above the head. Assist and teach the patient to turn and deep breathe every 2 to 4 hours. Blood pressure, pulse, and respiration should be checked every 15 minutes for 4 times, then every hour for 4 times, then as ordered. Control pain as ordered and observe the site of puncture for redness, swelling, or drainage; and report any symptoms to physician.
2. Interpret test outcomes and monitor appropriately.
3. Follow guidelines in Chapter 1 for safe, effective, and informed *posttest* care.

EFFUSIONS (THORACENTESIS AND PARACENTESIS): CELL STUDY

Normal Values
Negative for abnormal cells

Background
Effusions are accumulations of fluids. They may be exudates, which generally accumulate as a result of inflammation (TB, abscess, pancreatitis), lung infarct or embolus, trauma, SLE, or transudates, which are fluids not associated with inflammation (ie, Cirrhosis, congestive heart failure, and nephrotic syndromes). The following is a comparison of these 2 effusions:

Exudate	Transudate
1. Accumulates in body cavities and tissues because of malignancy or inflammation	1. Accumulates in body cavities from impaired circulation
2. Associated with an inflammatory process	2. Not associated with an inflammatory process
3. Viscous; opaque to purulent	3. Highly fluid
4. High content of protein, cells, and solid materials derived from cells	4. Low content of protein (<2.5–3.0g/dL), cells, or solid materials

	derived from cells
5. May have high WBC content	5. Has low WBC content
6. Clots spontaneously (contains high concentration of fibrinogen)	6. Will not clot
7. Malignant cells as well as bacteria may be detected	7. Malignant cells may be present
8. Specific gravity >1.016	8. Specific gravity <1.016

Fluid contained in the pleural, pericardial, peritoneal, or abdominal cavity is a serous fluid. Accumulation of fluid in the peritoneal cavity is called *ascites*.

Explanation of Test
Cytologic studies of effusions (exudates or transudates) are helpful in determining the cause of these abnormal collections of fluids. The effusions are found in the pericardial sac, the pleural cavities, and the abdominal cavities. The chief problem in diagnosis is in differentiating malignant cells from reactive mesothelial cells.

Procedure
Material for cytologic examination of effusions is obtained by either thoracentesis or paracentesis. Both of these procedures involve surgical puncture of a cavity for aspiration of a fluid.

Selection of Medications and Media
Fluid may be obtained in syringes, vacuum bottles, or other containers, depending on the volume of accumulated fluid. Heparin may be added to prevent clotting. Check with your laboratory for specific instructions.

THORACENTESIS
1. Chest x-rays should be available at the patient's bedside so that the location of fluid may be determined.
2. The patient may be given a sedative.
3. The chest is exposed. The physician inserts a long thoracentesis needle with a syringe attached.
4. At least 40 ml of fluid is withdrawn. It is preferable to withdraw 300 to 1000 ml of fluid.
5. The specimen is collected in a clean container and heparin may be added, particularly if the specimen is very bloody (5 to 10 U of heparin per milliliter of fluid). Alcohol should *not* be added.
6. The specimen should be labeled with the patient's name, the date, the source of the fluid, and the diagnosis.
7. The covered specimen should be sent immediately to the laboratory. (If the specimen cannot be sent at once, it may be refrigerated.)

PARACENTESIS (ABDOMINAL)
1. The patient should be asked to void.
2. The patient is placed in the Fowler position.
3. A local anesthetic is given.

4. A no. 20 needle is introduced into the patient's abdomen and the fluid is withdrawn, 50 ml at a time, until 300 to 1000 ml has been withdrawn.
5. Follow the same procedure for collection and transport of the specimen as for thoracentesis.
6. For all procedures, see Chapter 1 guidelines for *intratest* care.

> **Clinical Alert**
>
> Paracentesis can precipitate hepatic coma in a patient with chronic liver disease. The patient must be watched constantly for indications of shock: pallor, cyanosis, or dizziness. Emergency stimulants should be ready.

Clinical Implications

1. All effusions contain some mesothelial cells. (Mesothelial cells make up the squamous layer of the epithelium covering the surface of all serous membranes.) The more chronic and irritating the condition, the more numerous and atypical are the mesothelial cells. Histiocytes and lymphocytes are common.
2. Evidence of abnormalities in serous fluids is characterized by
  A. Degenerating red blood cells, granular red cell fragments, and histiocytes containing blood. Presence of these structures means that injury to a vessel or vessels is part of the condition causing fluid to accumulate.
  B. Mucin, which is suggestive of adenocarcinoma
  C. Large numbers of polymorphonuclear leukocytes, which is indicative of an acute inflammatory process such as peritonitis
  D. Prevalence of plasma cells, which suggests the possibility of antibody formation
  E. Numerous eosinophils, which suggest parasitic infestation, Hodgkin's disease, or a hypersensitive state
  F. Presence of many reactive mesothelial cells together with hemosiderin histiocytes, which may indicate
    (1) Leaking aneurysm
    (2) Rheumatoid arthritis
    (3) Lupus erythematosus
  G. Malignant cells
3. Abnormal cells may be indicative of
  A. Malignancy (The most important criterion of cancer is the arrangement of chromatin within the nuclei.)
  B. Inflammatory conditions

Interfering Factors

Vigorous shaking and stirring of specimens causes altered results.

Patient Preparation

1. Explain the purpose of the test and the procedure. The procedure varies depending on the site of fluid accumulation. General patient preparation includes measuring blood pressure, temperature, pulse, and respirations; administering sedation as ordered; preparing local anesthetic as ordered; providing emotional support; and obtaining a signed consent form.

2. Local anesthetic and sedative may be ordered.

3. Follow guidelines in Chapter 1 for safe, effective, informed *pretest* care.

> **Clinical Alert**
>
> The only contraindication is an uncooperative patient.

Patient Aftercare

1. Monitor according to agency protocols.

2. Check blood pressure, pulse, and respiration every 15 minutes for 1 hour, then every 2 hours for 4 hours, and as ordered. Check temperature every 4 hours for 24 hours. Apply adhesive bandage or dressing to site of puncture. Check dressing every 15 to 30 minutes. Turn patient onto the unaffected side for 1 hour, then to a position of comfort. Manage pain as indicated. Measure and record the total amount of fluid removed; note its color and character.

3. See guidelines in Chapter 1 for safe, effective, informed *posttest* care.

SKIN/CUTANEOUS IMMUNOFLUORESCENCE BIOPSY: CELL STUDY

Normal Values

A descriptive interpretative report of the skin biopsy is made.

Explanation of Test

Biopsy of the skin for direct epidermal fluorescent studies is indicated in the investigation of certain disorders such as lupus erythematosus, blistering disease, and vasculitis. Skin biopsies are also used to confirm the histopathology of skin lesions, to rule out other diagnoses (ie, herpes simplex and psoriasis), and to monitor the results of treatment.

Procedure

1. A 3–6-mm punch biopsy or shave biopsy, excisional biopsy, or incisional biopsy specimen of involved or uninvolved skin is obtained. Scraping, smears and/or aspirates also may be obtained. Take care not to crush the specimen.

2. Check with your laboratory for specific guidelines for specimen handling.

3. See Chapter 1 guidelines for *intratest* care.

Clinical Implications

1. Biopsy of skin shows the lesions of discoid lupus erythematosus as a band-like immunofluorescence of immunoglobulins and complement components. Similar findings in a biopsy of normal skin are consistent with systemic lupus erythematosus and may be used to monitor the results of treatment.

2. In blistering diseases such as pemphigus and pemphigoid, where circuling antibodies may not be present, a lesion may show intercellular epidermal antibody of pemphigus or basement membrane antibody of pemphigoid.

Patient Preparation

1. Explain the purpose and procedure of the skin biopsy. Local anesthesia will be used.
2. Follow guidelines in Chapter 1 for safe, effective, informed *pretest* care and overview on p. 842.

Clinical Alert

Contraindications include

1. An uncooperative patient.
2. Bleeding diathesis tenden—anticoagulant therapy.

Patient Aftercare

1. Monitor biopsy site for infection or bleeding.
2. See Chapter 1 and overview on p. 842 guidelines for safe, effective, informed *posttest* care.

ESTROGEN/ESTRADIOL (ER), PROGESTERONE RECEPTOR (PR), AND DNA PLOIDY (TUMOR ANEUPLOIDY)

Normal Values

Estrogen Receptor (ER): Negative; ≤ 3 femtomoles/mg of protein
Progesterone Receptor (PR): Negative; ≤ 5 femtomoles/mg of protein.
DNA Index (DI): 0.9–1.0 is normal DNA ploidy (content) or the diploid state. An interpretive histogram by flow cytometry (Fc) classifies the stained nucleic as DNA diploid, DNA aneuploid, DNA tetraploid, or DNA uninterpretable.

Explanation of Test

Estrogen and progesterone receptors in the cells of breast and endometrial cancer tissues are measured to determine whether the cancer is likely to respond to endocrine therapy or to removal of the ovaries. DNA ploidy measures cell turnover (replication) in specimens identified as cancer and predict progress, shorter survival, and relapse in some patients with cancer: bladder, breast, colon, endometrial, prostate, kidney, and thyroid. The predictive value is greater for breast, prostate, and colon.

Cancers have abnormal amounts of nuclear DNA. The higher the grade of tumor cells, the more likely the DNA content will be abnormal. The determination of tumor ploidy (the number of chromosome sets in a cell (ie, diploid 2 sets, triploid 3 sets) by various methods: Flow cytometry (Fc), histograms and image analysis divide cells into triploid/diploid (slowly replicating cells) or aneuploid (rapidly replicating cells).

Procedure

1. A fresh specimen is obtained by biopsy and is delivered to histology laboratory.
2. A 1-g specimen of quickly frozen tumor is examined for saturation and expressed in a Scatchard plot. The specimen must *not* be placed in formalin. Some laboratories can perform ERA/PRA studies on paraffin-embedded tissue. Check with your laboratory for specific instructions.
3. Specimens for DNA ploidy are classified on the basis of the percentage of epithelial cells that contain diploid (2n) DNA content and nondiploid DNA (aneuploid). DNA content is calculated as the DNA index.
4. See Chapter 1 guidelines for intratest care.

Clinical Implications

1. A positive test for estrogen (ER) occurs at levels >10 femtomoles (fmol) and for progesterone (PR) binding at levels of ≥10 fmol.
2. Approximately 50% of estrogen receptor-*positive* tumors respond to anti-estrogen therapy and 60%–70% in patients with both ER and PR positive tumors.
3. Estrogen receptor-*negative* tumors rarely respond to anti-estrogen therapy.
4. The finding of positive progesterone increases the predictive value of selecting patients for hormonal therapy. There is some incidence to suggest that progesterone receptor synthesis is estrogen dependent.
5. The presence of aneuploid peaks in the replicative activity of neoplastic cells may be prognostically significant, independent of tumor grade and stage.
6. The greater the amount of cells in S phase (DNA synthesis) of the cell cycle, the more aggressive the tumor.

Patient Preparation

1. Explain purpose and procedure of testing. See Tissue Biopsy Overview and Breast Biopsy: Cells and Tissue Study Prognostic Marker on pp. 817 and 818. Obtain appropriate clinical history so that this information can be provided with the specimen.
2. See Chapter 1 for safe, effective, informed *pre-test* care.

> **Clinical Alert**
>
> Contraindications include:
>
> 1. An uncooperative patient.
> 2. Bleeding diathesis (tendency to spontaneous bleeding due to coagulation defect)—anticoagulant therapy.

Patient Aftercare

1. Interpret test results and counsel appropriately about possible treatment.
2. Follow Chapter One guidelines for safe, effective, informed *post-test* care.

● STUDIES OF INHERITED DISORDERS

OVERVIEW OF GENETIC STUDIES ●

Genetic testing determines the presence, absence, or activity of genes in cells. Genes are defined as the basic unit of heredity. Each gene has a specific place in a chromosome. With these tests, geneticists try to predict the course of a person's health state, especially if there is the possibility of deviation from normal. Basic genetic technology counts the chromosomes in a person's cells or measures the amount of specific gene blood proteins. At the other end of the spectrum, cellular DNA is assayed with molecular probes to identify a specific genetic sequence among the 3 billion base pairs of genes that make up human DNA. Many disease states reflect hereditary components even though general clinical studies usually focus on the disorder itself rather than its genetic component. This section addresses those conditions that require information about genetic components for proper diagnosis. Chromosomal studies, linkage studies, and direct detection of abnormal genes are common tests in this group.

Indications for Testing

1. *Genetic counseling:* Specific genetic diagnostic studies of biologically related family members may be necessary to determine the risks and prognosis of disease. The test results could signal those people at special risk for genetically predisposed conditions.
2. *Prenatal Care* (see Chapter 16): In some instances, psychological and medical management of a potential problem pregnancy may greatly improve the outcome. Serious fetal abnormalities sometimes cause the parents to opt for termination of the pregnancy. Others choose to sustain pregnancy despite uncertain or potentially negative outcomes.
3. *Diagnosis:* Differential and presymptomatic studies may be done to diagnose certain diseases related to chromosome or DNA disorders in the unborn, in children, or in adults and for oncogene detection in the diagnosis of cancer.

Clinical Alert

1. Tests are not performed purely for information's sake; instead, they should be ordered for those conditions for which treatment is available. The best a predictive genetic test can offer is the degree of risk for acquiring the defect.
2. All tests should be linked to genetic counseling so that patients understand the results and their implications. In many cases, it is more comforting for patients to learn that they are from a high-risk family (no test done) than to try to interpret a test result and to hear "You have the gene, but try not to let it affect your whole life."
3. The patient should be able to use test results to make informed decisions about issues such as child-bearing and medical treatment.
4. Everyone is genetically defective to some degree, but most of these defects do not impair one's ability to function normally.
5. Family history is a major tool in identifying genetic disorders. Recognize and document dysmorphic features, growth problems, developmental delays, and adult mental retardation.

OVERVIEW OF CHROMOSOMES, GENES, AND DNA ●

Genetic information is coded within deoxyribonucleic acid (DNA), which is found in the chromosomes. Chromosomes are physical structures in the cell and cell nucleus that can be directly, although not easily, observed. A chromosome is a gene holder. Each chromosome consists of many thousands of genes, which are considered to be smaller segments of DNA responsible for specific genetic traits. Genes are made up of strands of DNA.

The genes contained in the chromosomes are found in base pairs. Base pairs comprise the blueprint of coded information (genome) concerning how the individual should function, and they are present in every cell. This is why samples for DNA testing can come from anywhere in the body. These are the basic DNA concepts: DNA makes RNA; RNA makes ribosomes; ribosomes make protein; protein makes us what we are or tells us how to function. Proteins are of 6 different types: collagen, circulatory proteins (as in erythrocytes, leukocytes), transport proteins (move substances in and out of cells; eg, cholesterol), enzymes, immune system proteins (as in T cells, B cells), and hormones. There are 23 chromosome pairs in each cell. One of each pair comes from the father and the other from the mother. Twenty-two of these pairs (the autosomes) are essentially identical. The twenty-third pair consists of the sex chromosomes. Women have 2 X chromosomes (XX) and men have 1 X and 1 Y chromosome (XY). The Y chromosome contains very few genes. These differences determine male or female development.

Single abnormal genes can generate a wide range of variations that manifest themselves in a certain way.

1. *Dominant inheritance:* A single copy of an abnormal gene can produce a disorder. An affected parent has a 50% chance of transmitting this abnormal gene to any offspring. When the disorder is seen for the first time, it may be presumed that a new mutation has occurred in either the ovum or the sperm. For some conditions, manifestation of the disorder is not consistent. This leads to speculation that *one* of the parents may have the abnormal gene in question. Examples of dominant inherited disorders are Huntington's chorea and neurofibromatosis.

2. *Recessive inheritance:* Both copies of the gene must be abnormal for the problem to be apparent. If both parents carry the same recessive gene, there is a 25% chance that their child will inherit 2 copies of the abnormal gene and develop a problem. Cystic fibrosis and sickle cell disease are examples of recessive gene disorders.

3. *X-linked (sex-linked) inheritance:* Because males have only a single copy of the X chromosome genes, abnormalities of these genes will not be "covered up" by a second normal copy (as happens in females). When the female parent is a carrier, a 50% chance exists for any son to be affected by the disease or for any daughter to be a carrier of the disease. Examples of sex-linked disorders are hemophilia and Duchenne's muscular dystrophy.

4. *Multifactorial inheritance:* This causes some defects through the interactions of many genes. Often these interactions are associated with environ-

mental influences. Examples of multifactorial disorders are congenital dislocation of the hip and pyloric stenosis.

5. Genes are shared by members of a family. If 1 family member carries a gene for a disease, each of his or her parents, siblings, and offspring has a 50% chance of carrying the gene.

CHROMOSOMAL ANALYSIS   ●

Normal Values
Women: 44 autosomes + 2 X chromosomes (karyotype 46,XX)
Men: 44 autosomes + 1 X and 1 Y chromosome (karyotype 46,XY)

Background
The karyotype, a study of chromosome distribution for an individual, determines chromosome numbers and chromosome structure (Chart 11-1). Alterations in either of these can produce problems. The standard karyotype can be a diagnostic precursor to genetic counseling. Additional or missing pieces of most chromosomal material causes developmental problems. Despite much speculation, it is not known exactly how these abnormalities translate into structural or functional anomalies. Predictions almost always depend on comparisons with clinical findings from other similar cases that present the same evidence.

Explanation of Test
Standard chromosome studies can be helpful in evaluation of the following clinical situations:

1. Multiple malformations of structure and function
2. Failure to thrive
3. Mental retardation
4. Ambiguous genitalia or hypogonadism
5. Recurrent miscarriages
6. Infertility
7. Primary amenorrhea or oligomenorrhea
8. Delayed onset of puberty
9. Stillbirths or miscarriages (particularly with associated malformations)
10. Prenatal diagnosis of potential or actual abnormalities related to chromosome disorders (eg, Down syndrome, especially in mothers >35 years of age)
11. Detection of parents with chromosomal mosaicism or translocations, who may be at high risk for transmitting genetic abnormalities to their children
12. Sex determination
13. Selected cancers and leukemias in which abnormalities of the chromosomes may reveal prognosis or disease stage

Procedure
Specimens for chromosome analyses are generally obtained as follows:

1. Leukocytes from peripheral vascular blood samples are used most fre-

CHART 11-1 ▶
Definition and Nomenclature of Karyotype

BACKGROUND

The karyotype is an arrangement of the cell chromosomes into a specific order, from the largest size to the smallest, so that their number and structure can be analyzed. This is routinely done through banding, a technique that permits the appreciation of differences in structure between the different pairs. Before banding, it was often impossible to pair chromosomes correctly; instead, they were arranged in groups according to size and structure and labeled A through G. The X chromosomes were part of group C and the Y chromosomes belonged to group E. Now, they are usually placed with each other, apart from the other pairs.

The pairs of chromosomes are differentiated according to the following characteristics:

1. Their length
2. The location of the centromere, the constriction that divides chromosomes into long (q) and short (p) arms
3. Ratio of the long and short arms to each other
4. Secondary constrictions
5. Satellites, which are small variable pieces of DNA seen at the ends of the arms of some chromosomes
6. Staining or banding patterns. A variety of different stains and techniques can be used. The most common is Giemsa banding. Most of the other methods, such as centromeric or fluorescent staining, are restricted to specific situations.

NOMENCLATURE OF THE KARYOTYPE

The standard conventions for listing karyotypes is as follows:

1. The first number denotes the total number of chromosomes.
2. Second, the sex chromosome complement follows (usually XX for normal females and XY for normal males).
3. Third, the missing, extra, or abnormal chromosomes are identified.
4. The letter "p" refers to the short arm, "q" to the long arm.
5. Bands are numbered from the centromere out. As techniques evolve, these are further subdivided. For example, in the two-digit number 32, the first number (3) is the band and the second number (2) is the subdivision of that band (band 32). Decimal points indicate further division under the same system; for example (working backward), 32.41 is the first subdivision (1) of the fourth subdivision (4) of the second subdivision of the third band.
6. A 3-letter code at the end designates the banding technique. The first letter is the type of banding; the second letter denotes the general technique; the third letter indicates the stain. Probably the most common code is GTG: band type G, banding by trypsin, using Giemsa stain. Special or unusual techniques are used only in selected circumstances.

(continued)

CHART 11-1 *(continued)*

More than 80 other abbreviations can be used to label other structural findings. Some of the more common ones are mentioned in clinical implications of chromosome analyses (see page 850).

> ### Clinical Alert
>
> 1. Occasionally, it is possible to line a certain chromosomal pattern with specific genes and to then understand the clinical picture from analyzing these results. However, for the most part, the association between specific chromosomal abnormalities and specific sets of findings is not yet well understood. Interpretations from karyotype studies usually come from correlations with similar cases rather than from any theoretical considerations. Therefore, because many variables exist, predictions must be made cautiously and judiciously.
> 2. Most laboratories provide interpretations of results. However, it may be necessary to talk directly with laboratory personnel to fully understand the meaning of an unusual karyotype.

quently because they are the most easily obtained. Preparation of the cells takes at least 3 days. The time required is directly proportional to the complexity of the analytic process.

2. Bone marrow biopsies can sometimes be completed within 24 hours. However, the results are rarely as satisfactory as those obtained from leukocyte analysis. Bone marrow analysis is often done to diagnosis certain categories of leukemias.

3. Fibroblasts from skin or other surgical specimens can be grown and preserved in long-term culture mediums for future studies. Growth of a sufficient amount of the specimen for studies usually requires at least 1 week. These specimens are especially helpful in detecting mosaicism (different chromosome constitutions in different tissues).

4. Amniotic fluid obtained through amniocentesis requires at least 1 week to produce a sufficient amount of specimen for analysis. These studies are often done for prenatal detection of chromosomal abnormalities.

5. Chorionic villus sampling (CVS) can be done at earlier stages of pregnancy (about 9 weeks) than can amniocentesis. Some initial CVS studies can be done almost immediately after conception. Occasional false-positive results represent mosaicism of the placenta (the presence of several cell lines, some of which may not be found in the fetus). These studies need confirmation of findings through long-term culture.

6. Cells may be grown from fetal tissue or from early-trimester products of conception to determine causes of spontaneous abortion. Cells from the fetal surface of the placenta may be easiest to grow. However, these studies are not always successful.

7. The buccal smear, for detecting sex chromosomes, is taken from the inner cheek. However, this cell specimen is often inaccurate, especially in the newborn. It may be helpful in determining the presence or absence of the Y chromosome.

8. See Chapter 1 guidelines for *intratest* care.

Clinical Implications

Many chromosomal abnormalities can be placed into 1 of 2 classes; some examples follow:

1. *Abnormalities of number*
  A. Autosomes
    (1) Trisomy 21 (Down syndrome)
    (2) Trisomy 18
    (3) Trisomy 13
  B. Sex chromosomes
    (1) Turner syndrome (single X)
    (2) Klinefelter syndrome (XXY)
    (3) XYY
    (4) XXX
2. *Abnormalities of structure*
  A. Deletions
    (1) Cat's cry syndrome: 5p−
    (2) Missing short arm of chromosome 18: 18p−
    (3) Prader-Willi syndrome (15q− in some cases)
  B. Duplications
    (1) Extra material from the second band in the long arm of the third chromosome: 3q2 trisomy (Cornella de Lange resemblance)
  C. Translocations
    (1) Translocation of chromosomes 11 and 22: t(11;22)
  D. Isochromosomes
    (1) A single chromosome with duplication of the long arm of the X chromosome: i(Xq) (a variant of Turner syndrome)
  E. Ring chromosomes
    (1) A chromosome 13 with the ends of the long and short arms joined together, as in a ring: r(13)
  F. Mosaicism
    (1) Two cell lines, 1 normal female and the other for Turner syndrome: 46,XX/45,X

Patient Preparation for All Genetic Testing

1. Some states require procurement of an informed, signed, and witnessed consent.

2. Explain the purpose and procedure of the test together with the known risks.

3. Provide information and referrals for appropriate genetic counseling, if necessary.

4. Follow Chapter 1 guidelines for safe, effective, informed *pretest* care.

Patient Aftercare for All Genetic Testing

1. If an amniotic fluid specimen is obtained for analysis, follow the same precautions as listed in Chapter 16.
2. Provide timely information and compassionate support and guidance for parents, children, and significant others.
3. See Chapter 1 for guidelines for safe, effective, informed *posttest* care.

SPECIAL CHROMOSOMAL STUDIES

The fragile X syndrome is 1 of the most common genetic causes of mental retardation. An X-linked trait, it is most common in males. Females may carry this gene without exhibiting any of its characteristics; however, they can also be as severely affected as males. This syndrome takes its name from the small area on the long arm of the X chromosome that looks like a break in the arm (although it actually is not). The cells need to be grown in a special medium to reveal this pattern; a regular karyotype will miss it. Even with the special medium, not all cells show the characteristic. In female carriers of this trait, the syndrome becomes harder to detect as the woman ages.

Rare conditions such as excess chromosome breakage (Fanconi anemia) or abnormal centromeres (Roberts syndrome) merit special analytic processes and procedures.

DIRECT DETECTION OF ABNORMAL GENES BY DNA TESTING

Normal Values
Normal genes in chromosomes 1 through 22
X and Y chromosomes and genes normal

Background
In the past, abnormal genes were indirectly detected by the effects they produced. These effects typically presented themselves as biochemical or physical manifestations. Now, it is possible to directly detect the specific sequence of DNA that causes an abnormality to occur. This technology relies on the ability to synthesize probes (pieces of DNA with specific sequences). Such probes hybridize with (attach to) specific complementary sequences and can be labeled for ease of detection. Probes manufactured for this purpose are called *allele-specific oligonucleotides.*

Sometimes detection of abnormal genes relies on the presence of *restriction sites* (areas that have specific DNA sequences). In this case, DNA can be "chopped" into pieces by the introduction of enzymes that attack the requisite sequences. The pieces that are formed depend on the presence of restriction sites. If only a few such sites are present, the DNA pieces usually will be large. If there are only a few for a particular enzyme, they will be small.

Genes can contain several different DNA abnormalities. The bases that make up the genetic sequence may be changed. In some cases, they may be missing partially or entirely, or they may be partially duplicated. Any of these abnormalities can change the sequence at a restriction site. This means that sometimes a fragment changes in size because of a change in the DNA. When this happens, it provides a method for detecting a change in a gene. Of course, many changes that exist do not involve restriction sites and therefore cannot be detected by this method.

Explanation of Test

Genetic maps of the genetic traits for a variety of structural and functional abnormalities can be measured. The relation between genes and pathologic states is rarely simple (Chart 11-2). Almost all diseases are likely to have some genetic component. An international project Human Genome Project, is underway to identify and localize all of the genes in the human genome and is nearing completion.

CHART 11-2 ▌
Genetic Disease—What Is It?*

Genetic disease is not a collection of syndromes.

Sixty-two percent of all pregnancy losses are due to genetic errors or causes. Half of these are chromosomal errors that will not support life. First-trimester losses result from genetic causes (often before pregnancy is known).

It is estimated that every person carries at least 5 genes that could cause illness in the wrong (environmental) circumstances or could adversely affect offspring. Spina bifida, cleft lip, congenital heart disease, pyloric stenosis, and club foot are common multifunctional diseases that are affected by environment.

No more than 3% of all genetic diseases are caused by defects in a single gene (eg, sickle cell anemia), and none of these is a major killer such as heart disease or cancer. More than 360 mutations have been linked to cystic fibrosis (CF), yet it is not possible to firmly correlate the severity of the disease with the various mutations. A positive test for CF does not foretell how severe the symptoms will be. On the other hand, a negative outcome can be misleading. All DNA tests should be confirmed by biochemical studies and careful monitoring for signs and symptoms.

*Rules for what constitutes genetic disease are not clearcut. Common adult-onset diseases are probably linked to multifunctional genes *and* environment (eg, hypertension, non–insulin-dependent diabetes, cancer, stroke, major psychiatric illness).

Procedure

1. Samples or specimens of body fluids or tissues are obtained.
2. See Chapter 1 guidelines for *intratest* care.

Clinical Implications

1. Genes related to abnormal structure and function have been located in each of the chromosomes, and new ones are continually being discovered. The known numbers of gene defects related to structural and functional abnormalities for each chromosome are growing and many others are under investigation. This has led to the improved diagnoses of several types of cancerous tumors (eg, heriditary colon cancer, nonpolyp type, heriditary breast cancer, leukemia, lymphomas, heriditary thyroid cancer, and retinoblastoma.

2. Precise DNA tests can be done for some diseases. These include cystic fibrosis, cickle cell anemia, phenylketonuria, Duchennel Becker muscular dystrophy, hemophilia, thalassemia, polycystic kidneys, α-antitrypsin deficiency, paternity tests, forensic testing, and identification of microbes in infectious diseases (ie, chlamydia, cytomegalovirus, enterovirus, hepatitis B and C, herpes simplex, HIV, Lyme disease, and gonorrhea).

NOTE: *See Patient Preparation and Patient Aftercare for All Genetic Testing (page 851).*

LINKAGE STUDIES　●

Explanation of Test

Specific genes have specific locations or *loci* (singular: *locus*) on chromosomes. It is sometimes possible to track an abnormal gene that is otherwise undetectable by standard methods by observing something located nearby that is transmitted along with the abnormal gene. Chromosomes can show harmless variations (polymorphisms) of their structure. These polymorphisms can sometimes help to pinpoint the site of a particular gene on the chromosome. Other genes may be detected through their biochemical products, through physical findings, or by specific molecular probes.

Because chromosomes are specific physical structures, all genes present on a given chromosome should be transmitted as a single unit. However, because "crossing over" occurs during formation of egg and sperm cells, there is some recombination between the 2 members of any chromosome pair—a switching of material from one to another. Still, the more physically close any 2 genes are, the more likely it is that they will stay together or will be linked in transmission. Linkage studies are based on this fact. Even if a gene cannot be identified directly, it may be possible to test for another gene in close proximity and to use that gene as a marker.

To illustrate this concept, this process is like trying to trace a package on a train going from coast to coast. All the baggage cars on the line may look alike; however, if it is known that there is a distinctive caboose on this train with the package, the caboose can be tracked and linked to the baggage car with the package. Of course, at each layover the cars may be switched onto other trains or tracks. If the cars directly in front and directly in back of the 1 with the package can be identified as being the same as on the original train, it is unlikely that the package car would have been switched out by itself.

Basically, then, flanking markers, 1 on each side of the gene, reduce the likelihood of undetected crossovers that might destroy the linkage. The closer the flankers are, and the more of them there are, the better the identification process. Calculations may be complex, but they can extrapolate the odds that the gene in question can be or has been passed on to offspring.

It usually is not enough just to know that gene A is linked to gene B. The crucial question is which form of gene A is linked to which form of gene B in the person at risk. Typically, this can be determined only through studies of that particular individual. Such studies, which may need input from extended families to clarify lines of linkage, can be laborious and time consuming. Therefore, when necessary, the family unit should discuss their concerns with a medical geneticist or genetic counselor in anticipation of pregnancy or as early in the pregnancy as possible.

Procedure

1. Obtain blood samples from those individuals to be studied.
2. See Chapter 1 guidelines for *intratest* care.

Clinical Implications

1. Linkage studies are becoming more common as molecular study techniques evolve. Traditionally, these studies involved specific genes that were highly variable, such as those for the blood groups or the immune response (HLA) genes. At other times, chromosome studies were also helpful. This process has been greatly enhanced by the discovery of *restriction fragment length polymorphisms* (RFLPs), a term often found in linkage reports. Certain areas of the DNA that make up the chromosomes are highly variable in structure and form (polymorphic). These variations affect the process by which that portion of DNA is separated into pieces by different types of enzymes. The length of the DNA fragments that result (longer or shorter) depends on the sensitivity to different enzymes at different positions on the DNA strand. These can give the DNA characteristic "fingerprints" that become "markers" at different sites. Although the technology involved often differs from classic linkage studies, the results should be the same.
2. Ideally, related testing techniques (nucleic acid-based detection tests, polymerace chain reaction [PCR]) can be used to specifically detect certain gene disorders (eg, sickle cell anemia). These studies are more specific than linkage studies and may be done on 1 individual, if appropriate.

NOTE: *See Patient Preparation and Patient Aftercare for All Genetic Testing (page 851).*

BIBLIOGRAPHY

Archives of Pathology and Laboratory Medicine March, 1997 (entire issue)
ASCT Journal of Cytotechnology, 1(1): 1997 (theme issue)
ASCT Journal of Cytotechnology, 1(2): 1997 (theme issue)
Austin MR, McLenden WW: The Papanicolaou smear: Medicine's most successful cancer screening procedure is threatened (editorial). JAMA 277(9): 754–755, 1997

Beahrs OH, Myers MH (eds): Manual for Staging of Cancer, 4th ed. Philadelphia, JB Lippincott, 1992

Bibbo M (ed): Comprehensive Cytopathology, 2nd ed. Philadelphia: WB Saunders, 1997

Cervical cancer screening: Today and tomorrow. OB/GYN News and Family Practice News August(suppl), 1996

Cryer B, Lee E, Feldman M: Gastric mucosal biopsy via a nasogastric tube: a nonendoscopic method for diagnosing fundic and antral mycosal gastritis and helicobacter pylori infection in men. Gastrointestional Endoscopy 44(3):317–323

Curbow BA: Can 40 seconds of compassion reduce anxiety? Journal of Clinical Oncology 17(1): 371–379, January 1999

US Congress, Office of Technology Assessment: Cystic Fibrosis and DNA Tests: Implications of Carrier Screening. Report OTA-BA 532. Bethesda, Md, US Government Printing Office, August 1992

DeMay R: The Art and Science of Cytopathology. Chicago, ASCP Press, 1996

Goldie SJ, Weinstein MC, Kuntz KM, Freedberg KA: The costs, clinical benefits, and cost effectiveness of screening for cervical cancer in HIV-infected women. Annuals of Internal Medicine 130:97–107, January 1999

Green E: The human gemone project: Implications for clinical medicine. Oak Ridge Conference, April 23 & 24, 1999. Sponsor: American Association for Clinical Chemistry, Washington, D.C.

Holtzman MK: Promoting safe and effective genetic tests in the U.S.: Work of the Task Force on Genetic Testing. Clinical Chemistry 45(5): 725, 1999

InCyt. Cytyc Corporation Newsletter July, 1996

Jackson-Cook C, Pandya A: Strategies and Logistical Requirements for Efficient Testing in Genetic Disease. Clinics in Laboratory Medicine 15(4), December, 1995

Kadlec JV, McPherson RA: Ethical Issues in Screening and Testing for Genetic Diseases. Clinics in Laboratory Testing 15(4): 989–999, December, 1995

Keebler CM, Reagan JW (eds): Manual of Cytotechnology, 7th ed. Chicago, American Society of Clinical Pathologists, 1993

Kiechle FL: Diagnostic Molecular Pathology in the Twenty-First Century. Clinics in Laboratory Testing 16(1): 213–219, March, 1996

Koss L: Diagnostic Cytology and Its Histopathologic Bases, 4th Ed. Lippincott, 1992

Leavelle DE (ed): Mayo Medical Laboratories Interpretive Handbook. Rochester, MN, Mayo Medical Laboratories, 1997

Mayeaux EJ: A comparison of the reliability of repeat cervical smears and colposcopy in patients with abnormal cervical cytology. J Fam Pract 40(1): 1995

McCauly KM, Oi RH: Evaluating the Papanicolaou smear: Four possible colposcopic findings and corresponding management strategies, Part 2. Consultant 29(1): 36–42, 1989

Molecular Biology: Impact on Human Disease. FASEB J 6(10), 1993 (theme issue)

Papillo J, et al: Evaluation of the ThinPrep Pap test in clinical practice: A seven month, 16314 case experience in northern Vermont. Acta Cytol January/February, 1998

Pitman M, Szyfelbein W: Fine needle aspiration of the liver. Presented at the annual meeting of the American Society of Clinical Pathologists, Spring, 1995

Raab S: Atypical glandular cells of undetermined significance. Am J Clin Pathol November, 1995

Santambrogio L, et al: CT-guided fine-needle aspiration cytology of solitary pulmonary nodules. Chest 112(2): 423–425, 1997

Stellson T, Kraft AL, Elswich RK Jr: The effectiveness and safety of two cervical cytologic techniques during pregnancy. J Fam Pract 45(2): 157, 1997

The revised Bethesda System for reporting cervical/vaginal cytologic diagnoses: Report of the 1991 Bethesda workshop. Acta Cytol 36(3): 1992.

Wilkinson MM: Your role in needle biopsy of the liver. RN August 1990.

12

Endoscopic Studies

OVERVIEW OF ENDOSCOPIC STUDIES ●

Endoscopy is the general term given to all examination and inspection of body organs or cavities using endoscopes. These instruments can also provide access for certain kinds of surgical procedures or treatments. Endoscopes, known generally as *fiberoptic instruments,* are used for direct visual examination of certain internal body structures by means of a lighted lens system attached to either a rigid or flexible tube. Light travels through an optic fiber by means of multiple reflections. Fiberoptic instruments, composed of fiber bundle systems, redirect and transmit light around twists and bends in cavities and hollow organs of the body. An image fiber and a light fiber allow visualization at the distal tip of the scope. Separate ports allow instillation of drugs, lavage, suction, and insertion of a laser, brushes, forceps, or other instruments used for excision, sampling, or other diagnostic and therapeutic procedures. The flexible fiberoptic scope can be inserted into orifices or other areas of the body not easily accessible or directly visualized by rigid scopes or other means. Procedures are done for diagnosis of pathologic conditions or for therapy, such as removal of tissue or of foreign objects conscious sedation and local or general anesthetics may be used. Biopsy tissue is submitted to the laboratory for histologic examination.

Clinical Alert

The risks of endoscopic examination include local irritation and inflammation, infection, bleeding, and hemorrhage, and perforation. Infection is the most common complication.

Endoscopically related bacteremia infections may result from tissue manipulation, blood stream invasion by pathogens, or by a contaminated endoscope, usually due to improper cleansing and disinfection. It is important that strict infection control guidelines be follwed by persons who clean and disinfect the endoscopes. After endoscopic procedures, assess for fever, elevated white blood cells, signs of blood stream infection, and signs of sepsis (rigors and hypotension, hypo- or hyperthermia). Maintain a log of all endoscopic procedures in the clinic, including patient name, type of procedure, date and time of procedure, and the serial number of the scope used in each procedure. This record allows for tracing an infection back to the specific instrument. All infections suspected to have been caused by a contaminated instrument should be reported to the appropriate infection control and risk management departments for investigation.

Clinical Alert

Observe standard precautions and latex precautions for all endoscopic procedures. See Appendices A and B.

MEDIASTINOSCOPY

Normal Endoscopic Examination
No evidence of disease
Normal lymph glands

Explanation of Test
This examination, performed under general anesthesia, requires insertion of a lighted mirror-lens instrument, similar to a bronchoscope, through an incision at the base of the anterior neck, to examine and biopsy mediastinal lymph nodes. Because these nodes receive lymphatic drainage from the lungs, mediastinal biopsy specimens can allow identification of diseases such as carcinoma, granulomatous infection, sarcoidosis, coccidioidomycosis, or histoplasmosis. Mediastinoscopy has virtually replaced scalene fat pad biopsy for suspicious nodes on the right side of the mediastinum. It is the routine method of establishing tissue diagnosis and staging of lung cancer and for evaluating the extent of lung tumor metastasis. Nodes on the left side of the chest are usually biopsied through left anterior thoracotomy (mediastinoscopy) or occasionally by scalene fat pad biopsy.

Procedure

1. Mediastinoscopy is considered a surgical procedure and is usually performed under general anesthesia in a hospital.
2. The biopsy is done through a suprasternal incision in the neck.
3. Follow guidelines in Chapter 1 for safe, effective, informed *intratest* care.

Clinical Implications

1. Abnormal findings may include the following conditions:
   a. Sarcoidosis
   b. Tuberculosis
   c. Histoplasmosis
   d. Hodgkin's disease
   e. Granulomatous infections and inflammatory processes
   f. Carcinomatous lesions
   g. Coccidioidomycosis
   h. *Pneumocystis carinii* infection
2. Results assist in defining the extent of metastatic process.

Patient Preparation

1. Explain purpose, procedure, benefits, and risks of the test.
2. A legal surgical consent form must be appropriately signed and witnessed preoperatively (see Chap. 1).
3. Preoperative care is the same as that for any patient undergoing general anesthesia and surgery.
4. The patient must fast for 8 or more hours before the test.
5. Follow guidelines in Chapter 1 for safe, effective, informed *pretest* care.

Patient Aftercare

Care is the same as for any patient who has had surgery under general anesthesia.

1. Evaluate breathing and lung sounds; check wound for bleeding and hematoma.
2. Instruct patient to call physician if problems occur; mediastinoscopy is often done as an ambulatory surgical procedure.
3. Interpret test outcomes and monitor appropriately.
4. Follow guidelines in Chapter 1 for safe, effective, informed *posttest* care.

Clinical Alert

1. Previous mediastinoscopy contraindicates repeat examination because adhesions make satisfactory dissection of nodes extremely difficult or impossible.
2. Complications can result from the risks associated with general anesthesia or from preexisting conditions.

BRONCHOSCOPY ●

Normal Brochoscopic Examination

Normal trachea, bronchi, nasopharynx, pharynx, and select bronchioles (conventional bronchoscopy cannot visualize alveolar structures)

Explanation of Test

This test permits visualization of the trachea, bronchi, and select bronchioles. There are two types of bronchoscopy: flexible fiberoptic, which is almost always used for diagnostic purposes, and rigid, which is less frequently used. This procedure is done to diagnose tumors, coin lesions, or granulomatous lesions; to find hemorrhage sites; to evaluate trauma or nerve paralysis; to obtain biopsy specimens; to take brushings for cytologic examinations; to improve drainage of secretions; to identify inflammatory infiltrates; to lavage; and to remove foreign bodies. Bronchoscopy can determine resectability of a lesion as well as provide the means to diagnose bronchogenic carcinoma. A transbronchial needle biopsy may be performed during this procedure, thus obviating the need for diagnostic open-lung biopsy. A flexible needle is passed through the trachea or bronchus and is used to aspirate cells from the lung. This procedure is performed on patients with suspected sarcoidosis or pulmonary infection.

Indications

Diagnostic

Staging of bronchogenic carcinoma

Differential diagnosis in recurrent unresolved pneumonia

Evaluation of cavitary lesions, mediastinal masses, and interstitial lung disease

Localization of bleeding

Evaluate immunocompromised patients (eg, HIV, bone marrow or lung transplant patients)

Differentiate rejection from infection in lung transplantation

Assess airway damage in thoracic trauma

Evaluate underlying etiology of nonspecific symptoms of pulmonary disease such as chronic cough (>6 months), hemoptysis, or unilateral wheezing

Therapeutic

Removal of a mucous plug

Removal of an aspirated foreign body

Brachytherapy (radioactive treatment of malignant endobrachial tumors)

Placement of a stent to maintain airway patency

Drainage of lung abscess

Decompression of bronchogenic cysts

Laser photoresection of endobrachial lesions

Bronchoalveolar lavage to remove intraalveolar proteinaceous material

Alternative for difficult endotracheal intubations

Control bleeding in the presence of massive hemoptysis

The examination is usually done under local anesthesia combined with some form of sedation in an outpatient setting, diagnostic center, or operating room. It also can be done in a critical care unit, in which case the patient may be unresponsive or ventilator dependent.

Procedure

1. Topical anesthetic (eg, 4% lidocaine) is sprayed and swabbed onto the back of the nose, the tongue, the pharynx, and the epiglottis. An antisialagogue (eg, atropine) is also given to reduce secretions. If the patient has a history of bronchospasms, a bronchodilator (eg, albuterol) is administered via a hand-held nebulizer.

2. The flexible or rigid bronchoscope is inserted carefully through the mouth or nose into the pharynx and the trachea. The scope also can be inserted through an endotracheal tube or tracheostomy. Suctioning, oxygen delivery, and biopsies are accomplished through bronchoscope ports designed for these purposes.

3. Because of sedation, usually with diazepam (Valium), midazolam (Versed), or meperidine (Demerol), the patient is usually comfortable. However, when the bronchoscope is advanced, some patients may feel as if they cannot breathe or are suffocating.

    NOTE: *Morphine sulfate is contraindicated in patients who have problems with bronchospasm or asthma because it can cause bronchospasm. Analgesics, barbiturates, tranquilizers-sedatives, and atropine may be ordered and administered 30 minutes to 1 hour before bronchoscopy. The patient should be as relaxed as possible before and during the procedure but also needs to know that anxiety is normal. The patient may need additional intravenous sedatives during the procedure. Refer to intravenous conscious sedation precautions in Appendix C.*

4. Arterial blood gas measurement during and after bronchoscopy may be ordered, and arterial blood oxygen may remain altered for several hours after the procedure. Sputum specimens taken during and after bronchoscopy may be sent for cytologic examination or culture and sensitivity testing. These specimens must be handled and preserved according to institutional protocols (see Chap. 14).

5. Continuous pulse oximetry readings are routinely monitored and indicate levels of oxygen saturation before, during, and after the procedure.

6. The right lung, by convention, is normally examined before the left lung.

7. Bronchoscopic procedures include any one or a combination of the following
    a. Bronchial washings for cytology and staining for fungi and mycobacteria
    b. Bronchoalveolar lavage (BAL) for infectious (eg, *Pneumocystis carinii, Histoplasma, Mycoplasma*) and noninfectious (eg, alveolar proteinosis, eosinophilic granuloma) diseases
    c. Bronchial brushings of both visible and peripheral (under fluoroscopy) endobronchial lesions and/or transbronchial biopsies, both visible and peripheral

8. Follow guidelines in Chapter 1 for safe, effective, informed *intratest* care.

Clinical Implications

1. Abnormalities revealed through bronchoscopy include the following conditions:
   a. Abscesses
   b. Bronchitis
   c. Carcinoma (occurs in the right lung more often than the left)
   d. Tumors (usually appear more often in larger bronchi)
   e. Tuberculosis
   f. Alveolitis
   g. Evidence of surgical nonresectability (eg, involvement of tracheal wall by tumor growth, immobility of a main-stem bronchus, widening and fixation of the carina)
   h. *Pneumocystis carinii* infection
   i. Inflammatory processes
   j. Cytomegalic virus infection
   k. Aspergillosis
   l. Idiopathic nonspecific pulmonary fibrosis
   m. *Cryptococcus neoformans* infection
   n. Coccidioidomycosis
   o. Histoplasmosis
   p. Blastomycosis
   q. Phycomycosis

Clinical Considerations

The following data must be available before the procedure: history and physical examination, recent chest x-ray film, recent arterial blood gas values, and, if the patient is >40 years of age or has heart disease, electrocardiogram (ECG). Appropriate blood work, urinalysis, pulmonary function tests, and sputum studies (especially for acid-fast bacilli) must be done as well. Bronchoscopy is often done as an ambulatory surgical procedure.

Patient Preparation

1. Reinforce information related to the purpose, procedure, benefits, and risks of the test.
2. Emphasize that pain is not usually experienced because lungs do not have pain fibers.
3. Explain that the local anesthetic may taste bitter, but numbness will occur in a few minutes. Feelings of a thickened tongue and the sensation of something in the back of the throat that cannot be coughed out or swallowed are not unusual. These sensations will pass within a few hours following the procedure as the anesthetic wears off.

4. An informed consent form must be properly signed and witnessed (see Chap. 1).

5. The patient must fast for at least 6 hours before the procedure to reduce the risk of aspiration. Gag, cough, and swallowing reflexes will be blocked during and for a few hours after surgery.

6. Wigs, nail polish, makeup, dentures, jewelry, and contact lenses must be removed before the examination.

7. Use of relaxation techniques may help the patient relax and breathe more normally during the procedure. The more relaxed the patient is, the easier it is to complete the procedure.

8. Follow guidelines in Chapter 1 for safe, effective, informed *pretest* care.

Patient Aftercare

1. Usually, the patient has fasted for least 2 hours before the procedure. Be certain that swallow, gag, and cough reflexes are present before allowing food or liquids to be ingested orally.

2. Provide gargles to relieve mild pharyngitis. Monitor ECG, blood pressure, temperature, pulse, pulse oximeter readings, skin and nail bed color, lung sounds, and respiratory rate and patterns according to institution protocols. Document observations.

3. Oxygen by mask or nasal cannula may be ordered. Humidified oxygen at specific concentrations up to 100% by mask may be necessary.

4. A chest x-ray film may be ordered to check for pneumothorax or to evaluate the lungs.

5. Sputum specimens may be ordered. These must be preserved in the proper medium or solution.

6. The head of the bed may be elevated for comfort.

7. Interpret test outcomes and monitor appropriately.

8. Refer to intravenous sedation precautions in Appendix C.

9. Follow guidelines in Chapter 1 for safe, effective, informed *posttest* care.

NOTE: *Follow-up procedures may be necessary. Computed tomography (CT)-guided fine-needle cytology aspiration may be done when bronchoscopy is not diagnostic.*

Contraindications to Bronchoscopy

1. Contraindications to bronchoscopy include the following conditions:
   a. Severe hypoxemia
   b. Severe hypocapnia (carbon dioxide retention)
   c. Certain cardiac arrhythmias, cardiac states
   d. History of being hepatitis B carrier
   e. Bleeding or coagulation disorders
   f. Severe tracheal stenosis

Clinical Alert

1. Observe for possible complications, which may include the following conditions:
   a. Shock
   b. Cardiac arrhythmias
   c. Hypoxemia
   d. Partial or complete laryngospasm (inspiratory stridor) produces a "crowing" sound; it may be necessary to intubate
   e. Bronchospasm (pallor and increasing dyspnea are signs)
   f. Infection or gram-negative bacterial sepsis
   g. Pneumothorax
   h. Respiratory failure
   i. Bleeding following biopsy (rare, but can occur if there is excessive friability of airways or massive lesions, or if patient is uremic or has a hematologic disorder)
   j. Anaphylactic reactions to drugs
   k. Seizures
   l. Febrile state
   m. Hypoxia, respiratory distress
   n. Empyema
   o. Aspiration

Special Pediatric Considerations

Bronchoscopy instruments can decrease an already small airway lumen even more by causing inflammation and edema. Consequently, a child can rapidly become hypoxic and desaturate oxygen very quickly. Resuscitation, oxygen administration equipment, and drugs must be readily accessible when this procedure is performed on a child. Close monitoring of respiratory and cardiac status is imperative after the procedure. The same precautions and treatment apply to the pediatric patient as for the adult. Most children suffer cardiac arrest because of **respiratory problems,** not cardiac problems.

THORACOSCOPY

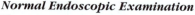

Normal Endoscopic Examination

Thoracic cavity and tissues normal and free of disease

Explanation of Test

Thoracoscopy is an examination of the thoracic cavity using an endoscope. Video-assisted thoracoscopy is a recent addition to the procedures available for diagnosing intrathoracic diseases. This procedure is making a comeback because it can be used as a diagnostic device when other methods of diagnosis fail to present adequate and accurate findings. Moreover, the discomfort and many of the risks associated with traditional diagnostic thoracotomy procedures are reduced with thoracoscopy versus other procedures. Thoracoscopy allows visualization of the parietal and visceral pleura, pleural spaces, thoracic walls, mediastinum, and pericardium without the need for more extensive procedures. It can be used to perform laser procedures; to assess tumor growth, pleural effusion, emphysema, inflammatory processes, and conditions predisposing to pneumothorax; and to perform biopsies of pleura, mediastinal lymph nodes, and lungs.

Procedure

1. Thoracoscopy is considered an operative procedure. The patient's state of health, the particular positioning needed, and the procedure itself determine the need for either local or general anesthesia.
2. Admission is frequently scheduled the morning of the procedure. Many patients are discharged the following day, provided the lung has reexpanded properly and chest tubes have been removed.
3. Follow guidelines in Chapter 1 for safe, effective, informed *intratest* care.

Clinical Implications

1. Abnormal findings can include the following conditions:
   a. Carcinoma or metastasis of carcinoma
   b. Empyema
   c. Pleural effusion
   d. Conditions predisposing to pneumothorax or ulcers
   e. Inflammatory processes
   f. Bleeding sites
   g. Tuberculosis, coccidioidomycosis, or histoplasmosis

Patient Preparation

1. Reinforce and explain the purpose, procedure, benefits, and risks of the examination, and describe what the patient will experience.
2. A surgical consent form must be appropriately signed and witnessed before the procedure begins (see Chap. 1).
3. Required blood tests, urinalysis, recent chest x-ray film, and ECG (for certain individuals) must be completed and reviewed prior to the procedure.
4. The patient must fast for 8 hours before the procedure.
5. An intravenous line must be inserted for the administration of intraoperative intravenous fluids and intravenous medication.
6. Skin preparation and correct positioning are done in the operating room.
7. After the thoracoscopy is completed, a chest tube is placed and connected to negative suction or sometimes to gravity drainage.
8. Follow guidelines in Chapter 1 for safe, effective, informed *pretest* care.

Patient Aftercare

1. A postoperative chest x-ray film is taken to check for abnormal air or fluid in the chest cavity.

2. Monitor vital signs, amount and color of chest tube drainage, fluctuation of fluid in the chest tube, bubbling in the chest bottle, and respiratory status, including arterial blood gases. Promptly report abnormalities to the physician.

3. Administer pain medication as necessary. Encourage relaxation exercises as a means to lessen the perception of pain. Monitor quality and rate of respirations. Be alert to the possibility of respiratory depression related to narcotic administration or intrathecal narcotics.

4. Encourage frequent coughing and deep breathing. Assist the patient in splinting the incision during coughing and deep breathing to lessen discomfort. Promote leg exercises while in bed and assist with frequent ambulation if permitted.

5. Use open-ended questions to provide the patient with an opportunity to express concerns.

6. Document care accurately.

7. Interpret test outcomes and monitor appropriately.

8. Follow guidelines in Chapter 1 for safe, effective, informed *posttest* care. Provide written discharge instructions.

Clinical Alert

1. **Do not clamp chest tubes unless specifically ordered to do so.** Clamping chest tubes may cause a tension pneumothorax. Sudden onset of sharp pain, dyspnea, uneven chest wall movement, tachycardia, anxiety, and cyanosis may indicate pneumothorax. Notify the physician immediately.

2. Possible complications include the following:
   a. Respiratory distress/hypoxia
   b. Infection
   c. Hemorrhage (watch for unusually large outputs of blood in a relatively short period of time into the chest bottle and notify physician immediately)
   d. Empyema
   e. Atelectasis
   f. Aspiration

ESOPHAGOGASTRODUODENOSCOPY (EGD); UPPER GASTROINTESTINAL STUDY (UGI); ENDOSCOPY; GASTROSCOPY

Normal Endoscopic Examination

Upper gastrointestinal tract within normal limits

Explanation of Test

Endoscopy is a general term for visual inspection of any body cavity with an endoscope. Endoscopic examination of the upper gastrointestinal tract (mouth to upper jejunum) is referred to when the following examinations are ordered: panendoscopy, esophagoscopy, gastroscopy, duodenoscopy, esophagogastroscopy, or esophagogastroduodenoscopy.

EGD allows visualization of the interior lumen of the upper gastrointestinal tract with a fiberoptic instrument designed for that purpose. Esophagogastroduodenoscopy is indicated for patients with dysphagia and weight loss, especially those with moderate-to-heavy alcohol and tobacco consumption. This examination can determine the cause of upper gastrointestinal tract bleeding, confirm suspicious x-ray findings, establish a diagnosis for a symptomatic patient with negative x-ray reports, permit biopsy of upper gastrointestinal tract lesions, and confirm hiatal hernia or esophagitis. It can also differentiate benign from malignant gastric ulcers; be used as a follow-up examination for gastrectomy or other gastrointestinal disturbances; and allow for diagnostic evaluation of masses, strictures, and mucosal abnormalities.

Procedure

1. This examination is usually performed in a gastrointestinal laboratory, in the operating room, or in critical care settings.
2. A topical spray is used to anesthetize the patient's throat.
3. An intravenous tranquilizer is often given prior to initiation of the procedure. The patient becomes relaxed and somewhat sleepy. A mouthpiece is inserted to prevent the patient from biting the endoscope and to prevent injury to the patient's teeth, tongue, or other oral structures.
4. The endoscope is gently inserted through the mouthpiece into the esophagus and is advanced slowly into the stomach and duodenum. Air is insufflated through the scope to distend the area being examined so that optimal visualization of the mucosa is possible. Tissue biopsy specimens and brushings for cytology may be obtained. Photos may be taken to provide a permanent record of observations.
5. Sensations of pressure or bloating are normal, but the patient should not experience actual pain.
6. Immediately after the examination is completed, the patient is asked to relax and to remain lying on his or her side for a short period of time.

Clinical Implications

1. Abnormal results may indicate the following conditions:
   a. Hemorrhagic areas or erosion of an artery or vein
   b. Hiatal hernia
   c. Esophagitis, gastritis
   d. Neoplastic tissue
   e. Gastric ulcers (benign or malignant)

Patient Preparation

1. Explain the purpose and procedure of the examination, the sensations that may be experienced, and the benefits and risks of the test. Refer to intravenous conscious sedation precautions in Appendix C. Reassure the patient

that the endoscope is thinner than most food swallowed. Inform the patient that they may be quite sleepy during the EGD and may not recall much of the experience.

2. Instruct the patient to fast for 8 hours before the examination. In the hospital, this restriction usually begins at midnight the day of the procedure. Written instructions about fasting reinforce verbal instructions. A permit must be signed and properly witnessed (see Chap. 1).

3. Oral hygiene needs to be done before the procedure. Assist patient with oral care as necessary.

4. Encourage the patient to urinate and to defecate if possible before the examination.

5. Follow guidelines in Chapter 1 for safe, effective, informed *pretest* care.

Patient Aftercare

1. No food or liquids are permitted for 2 hours following the procedure, or longer if the patient cannot swallow.

2. Be certain the patient can swallow properly before offering liquids or food.

3. Check blood pressure, pulse, and respirations every 30 minutes for 2 hours.

4. A side-lying position with the side rails up and bed flat should be maintained until the sedative has worn off (usually about 2 hours). This position usually prevents aspiration in case of emesis.

5. Encourage the patient to belch to expel air inserted into the stomach during the examination.

6. The patient should not experience discomfort or side-effects once the sedative has worn off. Occasionally, the patient may complain of a slight sore throat. Sucking on lozenges after swallowing reflexes return may be helpful if these are permitted.

7. Interpret test outcomes and monitor appropriately.

8. Follow guidelines in Chapter 1 for safe, effective, informed *posttest* care. Provide written discharge instructions.

Clinical Alert

1. Complications are rare; however, the following complications can occur:
   a. Perforation
   b. Bleeding or hemorrhage
   c. Local irritation
   d. Drug reactions
   e. Complications from unrelated diseases such as myocardial infarction or cerebrovascular accident
   f. Aspiration (bile aspiration can be a very serious complication)
   g. Death is very rare

ESOPHAGEAL MANOMETRY ●

Normal Manometric Examination
Normal esophageal and stomach pressure readings
Normal contractions
No acid reflux

Explanation of Test
This procedure tests the esophagus for normal contractile activity and effectiveness of swallowing by measurement of intraluminal pressures and acid sensors. The test consists of recording pressures simultaneously at various levels within the esophagus and evaluating the esophagus and upper and lower esophageal sphincters.

Indications for Testing
1. Abnormal esophageal muscle function
2. Difficulty swallowing (dysphagia)
3. Heartburn
4. Chest pain of unknown cause
5. Regurgitation
6. Vomiting
7. Esophagitis

Other tests often done in conjunction with manometry include acid reflux tests and the Bernstein test (discussed later). These procedures are useful for evaluating heartburn, esophagitis, and chest pain of undetermined cause.

Procedure
1. A topical anesthetic is swabbed on the tissues lining the nasal passage.
2. With the patient in a sitting position, a No. 8–lumen manometric catheter is passed through the nose and connected to an infusion pump, transducer, and recorder.
3. After the tube is passed through the nose, the patient lies supine for the remainder of the test.
4. Small amounts of water are swallowed, and pressure readings are taken.
5. *Acid reflux test:* a second catheter is passed alongside the one already in place. This tube is actually a probe that is sensitive to acid. When the valve at the esophagogastric junction is not functioning properly, acid from the stomach backs up into the esophagus. The probe in the esophagus senses this acid.
6. *Bernstein test:* evaluates for acid reflux by means of a nasogastric tube passed to a point 5 cm above the gastroesophageal junction. Concentrations of hydrochloric acid (0.1 normal HCl) is infused for 10 minutes into the esophagus to reproduce symptoms of heartburn or chest discomfort. In the first 5 minutes of testing, 0.9% sodium chloride is infused as a control. Testing takes about 15 minutes. The patient may lie down or sit up.

7. Follow guidelines in Chapter 1 for safe, effective, informed *pretest* care.

Clinical Implications
1. Abnormal results reveal the following conditions:
   a. Achalasia (failure of muscles, such as sphincters, to relax)
   b. Esophageal spasm
   c. Acid reflux

Patient Preparation
1. Explain the purpose, procedure, benefits, and risks of the test.
2. The patient should fast for 6 hours prior to testing.
3. If the patient is diabetic, notify the testing department. Check with the patient's physician regarding insulin dosage, resumption of diet, and blood sugar testing.
4. Follow guidelines in Chapter 1 regarding safe, effective, informed *pretest* care.

Patient Aftercare
1. Advise the patient that a sore throat and nasal passage irritation is common for 24 hours after the examination. Sensations of heartburn may also persist. Administer antacids if ordered.
2. Observe for or instruct patient to watch for nasal bleeding, gastrointestinal bleeding, or unusual pain.
3. Interpret test outcomes and counsel appropriately.
4. Follow guidelines in Chapter 1 for safe, effective, informed *posttest* care. Provide written discharge instructions.

ENDOSCOPIC RETROGRADE CHOLANGIOPANCREATOGRAPHY (ERCP) AND MANOMETRY ●

Normal Endoscopic Examination
Normal appearance and patent pancreatic ducts, hepatic ducts, common bile ducts, duodenal papilla (ampulla of Vater), and gallbladder
Manometry: normal pressure readings of bile and pancreatic ducts and sphincter of Oddi

Explanation of Test
This examination of the hepatobiliary system is done through a side-viewing flexible fiberoptic endoscope by instillation of contrast medium into the duodenal papilla, or ampulla of Vater. It is used to evaluate jaundice, pancreatitis, persistent abdominal pain, pancreatic tumors, common duct stones, extrahepatic and intrahepatic biliary tract disease, malformation, and strictures and as a follow-up study in confirmed or suspected cases of pancreatic disease.

ERCP manometry can be done to obtain pressure readings in the bile duct, pancreatic duct, and sphincter of Oddi at the papilla. Measurements are obtained using a catheter that is inserted into the endoscope and placed within the sphincter zone.

Procedure

1. If barium x-rays have been done prior to ERCP, a flat plate of the abdomen (KUB) should be done to check for barium. If barium is present, it will obscure views during ERCP. Screen for chest pain, shortness of breath, myocardial infarct, epigastric pain, bleeding, and acute infections (including active hepatitis or pancreatitis). Debilitated patients may be more prone to complications. Fever or flu-like symptoms may necessitate postponement of the procedure.

2. The patient gargles with or has his or her throat sprayed with a topical anesthetic.

3. An intravenous line is started and used for administration of sedatives such as meperidine, diazepam, or midazolam, as well as intravenous fluids and blood, if needed. A very ill patient often needs only a small dose of sedation. Resuscitation equipment must be available.

4. The patient assumes the left lateral position with the knees flexed while the endoscope is inserted, via a mouthpiece, through the esophagus to the duodenum. The mouthpiece also prevents the patient from biting down on the instrument and injuring his or her mouth or lips. At this point, the patient assumes a prone position with the left arm positioned behind them.

5. Simethicone may be instilled to reduce bubbles from bile secretions. Glucagon or anticholinergic agents may be given intravenously to relax the duodenum so that the papilla can be cannulated. (Atropine increases the heart rate.)

6. A catheter is passed into the ampulla of Vater, and contrast dye is instilled through the cannula to outline the pancreatic and common bile ducts. Fluoroscopy and x-rays are done at this time.

7. Biopsy specimens or cytology brushings can be taken before the endoscope is removed.

8. The patient's vital signs, ECG, and oxygen saturation (pulse oximetry) should be monitored frequently throughout the procedure.

9. Monitor for side-effects and drug allergy reactions (eg, diaphoresis, pallor, restlessness, hypotension).

10. Follow guidelines in Chapter 1 for safe, effective, informed *intra-test* care.

Clinical Implications

1. Abnormal results reveal stones, stenosis, and other abnormalities that are indicative of the following conditions:
   a. Biliary cirrhosis
   b. Primary sclerosing cholangitis
   c. Cancer of bile ducts

    d. Pancreatic cysts
    e. Pseudocysts
    f. Pancreatic tumors
    g. Cancer of head of pancreas
    h. Chronic pancreatitis
    i. Pancreatic fibrosis
    j. Cancer of duodenal papilla
    k. Papillary stenosis

Clinical Alert

Contraindications include acute pancreatitis, pancreatic pseudocysts, strictures or obstructions within the esophagus or duodenum, cholangitis, infectious disease, and cardiopulmonary disease.

Patient Preparation

1. Explain the purpose, procedure, benefits, and risks of the test. If done as an outpatient procedure, the patient should arrange for a ride home and should leave all valuables at home. Blood work, urinalysis, x-ray films, and scans should be reviewed and charted before the procedure. Record baseline vital signs.
2. A permit must be signed and properly witnessed (see Chap. 1).
3. The patient should fast for 12 hours before ERCP.
4. Inform the patient that she or he:
    a. Should swallow when requested to do so (to prevent damage to the oral pharynx)
    b. May experience a choking sensation
    c. Will have to lie quietly while x-rays are taken
    d. Should breathe deeply to relieve gagging
    e. Will be suctioned to clear secretions
5. Refer to conscious sedation precautions in Appendix C.
6. Follow guidelines in Chapter 1 for safe, effective, informed *pretest* care.

Patient Aftercare

1. Check vital signs, including temperature, according to institutional protocols.
2. Do not give food or fluids for at least 2 hours after the procedure or until the gag reflex returns and the patient can swallow properly.
3. Observe the patient for signs of complications such as infection, urinary retention, cholangitis, or pancreatitis. Check for temperature elevation, which may be the first sign of inflammation. Monitor WBCs and assess for signs of sepsis.
4. Infection may result from obstructed and infected biliary systems and/or contaminated endoscopes used during the procedure. See Clinical Alert on page 875.
5. Monitor for respiratory and central nervous system depression from nar-

cotics (naloxone may be used to reverse narcotic effects and flumazenil is used for reversing diazepam-like drugs).

6. Explain that some abdominal discomfort may be experienced for several hours after the procedure.

7. Drowsiness may last up to 24 hours. During this time, the patient should not perform any tasks that require mental alertness and legal documents should not be signed.

8. A sore throat can be relieved by gargles, ice chips, fluids, or lozenges if permitted.

9. Notify physician of any of the following signs or symptoms:
   a. Prolonged, sharp abdominal pain; abnormal weakness; faintness
   b. Fever
   c. Nausea or vomiting

10. Interpret test outcomes and counsel appropriately.

11. Follow guidelines in Chapter 1 for safe, effective, informed *posttest* care. Provide written discharge instructions.

COLPOSCOPY ●

Normal Colposcopic Examination
Normal vagina, cervix, and genital areas

Explanation of Test
Colposcopy permits examination of the vagina and cervix with the colposcope, an instrument with a magnifying lens. The colposcope is also used to examine male genital lesions suspected in sexually transmitted diseases, condylomata, or human papillomavirus. Indications for this procedure in women include abnormal Papanicolaou (Pap) smear results and/or other cervical lesions. This examination aids in the diagnosis of benign and precancerous lesions, leukoplakia, and other cancerous lesions. Biopsy specimens and cell scrapings are obtained under direct visualization. Colposcopy is also valuable for assessing women with a history of exposure to diethylstilbestrol.

Advantages of colposcopy include the following:

1. Lesions can be localized and their extent determined.
2. Inflammatory processes can be differentiated from neoplasia.
3. Invasive or noninvasive disease processes can be differentiated.

Colposcopy *cannot* readily detect endocervical lesions. Cervicitis and other changes can produce abnormal findings. When combined with findings from Pap smears, colposcopy can be a means of enhancing diagnostic accuracy. See Tables 12-1 and 12-2 regarding correlation of findings and advantages and disadvantages of Pap smears and colposcopy. See Chapter 11, page 826, for Pap smear procedure.

Whitish areas of epithelium (leukoplakia), mosaic staining patterns, irregular blood vasculature, hyperkeratosis, and other abnormal-appearing tissues can be seen using colposcopy. Leukoplakia vulvae is a precancerous condition

TABLE 12-1
Correlation of Colposcopic and Histologic Findings

Colposcopic Term	*Colposcopic Appearance*	*Histologic Correlate*
Original squamous epithelium	Smooth, pink; indefinitely outlined vessels; no change after application of acetic acid	Squamous epithelium
Columnar epithelium	Grapelike structures after application of acetic acid	Columnar epithelium
Transformation zone	Tongues of squamous metaplasia; gland openings; nabothian cysts	Metaplastic squamous epithelium
White epithelium	White, sharp-bordered lesion visible only after application of acetic acid; no vessels visible	From minimal dysplasia to carcinoma in situ
Punctation	Sharp-bordered lesion; red stippling; epithelium whiter after application of acetic acid	From minimal dysplasia to carcinoma in situ
Mosaic	Sharp-bordered lesion, mosaic pattern; epithelium whiter after application of acetic acid	From minimal dysplasia to carcinoma in situ
Hyperkeratosis	White patch; rough surface; already visible before application of acetic acid	Usually hyperkeratosis or parakeratosis; seldom carcinoma in situ or invasive disease
Atypical vessel	Horizontal vessels running parallel to surface; constrictions and dilatations of vessels; atypical branching, winding course	From carcinoma in situ to invasive carcinoma

characterized by white to grayish infiltrated patches on the vulvar mucosa. The colposcope has a definite advantage for detecting atypical epithelium, designated in the literature as *basal cell activity.* Atypical epithelium cannot be called benign and yet does not fulfill all criteria for carcinoma in situ. Its early detection promotes cancer prophylaxis.

Patients receiving colposcopy may often be spared having to undergo surgical conization (the removal of a cone of tissue from the cervix).

Another gynecology (GYN) procedure, a hysteroscopy, can be done to determine the cause of abnormal uterine bleeding, size and shape of uterine cavity, lo-

TABLE 12-2
Pros and Cons of Colposcopy and Cytology

Advantages	Disadvantages
COLPOSCOPY	
Localizes lesion	Inadequate for detection of endocervical lesions
Evaluates extent of lesion	More intensive training is necessary
Differentiates between inflammatory atypia and neoplasia	Cervicitis and regenerative changes may produce abnormal findings
Differentiates between invasive and noninvasive cervical lesions	
Enables to follow-up	
CYTOLOGY	
Ideal for mass screening	Cannot localize lesion
Economical	Inflammation, atrophic changes, or folic acid deficiency may produce suspicious changes
Specimen can be obtained by most health care personnel	Many steps between patient and cytopathologist allow misdiagnosis
Detects lesion in endocervical canal	Value of single smear is limited
Detects endocervical and endometrial carcinoma	False-negative rate is 5%–10%
High correlation with biopsy material (>90%)	

cation of misplaced IUD, and uterine abnormalities. A hysteroscopy is performed early in the menstrual cycle in a physician's office. A local anesthetic is usually administered into cervix and paracervical area before insertion of the hysteroscope.

Procedure

1. With the patient in the lithotomy position, the vagina and cervix are exposed with a speculum after the internal and external genitalia have been carefully examined. A Pap smear is obtained at this time. No part of the colposcope is inserted into the vagina.
2. The cervix and vagina are then swabbed with 3% acetic acid as needed during the procedure to improve visibility of epithelial tissues (it precipitates nuclear proteins within the cells). The cervical mucus must be completely removed. Do not use cotton-wool swabs because fibers left on the cervix may interfere with proper visualization.
3. Actual visualization with the colposcope begins with a field of white light and lower magnification to focus on sites of white epithelium or irregular cervical contours. The light is then switched to a green filter for magnification of vascular changes.

   a. Suspicious lesions are diagramed, and photographs are taken for the permanent health care record.
   b. The transformation zone and squamocolumnar junction (where the squamous epithelium meets the columnar epithelium of the cervix) are areas where many women exhibit atypical cells. It is imperative that these zones be visualized completely, especially in older women, because of changes associated with aging.
4. Biopsy specimens of the lesions are obtained using a fine biopsy forceps. Some patients note discomfort at this time.
   a. Endocervical curettage *must* be performed prior to colposcope-directed biopsy so that epithelial fragments dislodged during colposcopy do not cause false-positive results in the endocervical curettage. Endocervical curettage biopsy samples should be placed in formalin.
   b. Sterile saline or sterile water should be used to rinse acetic acid from the vaginal area to prevent burning or irritation. Bleeding can be stopped by applying toughened silver nitrate cautery sticks or ferric subsulfate (Monsel's solution).
5. A small amount of vaginal bleeding or cramping for a few hours is not abnormal.
6. A paracervical block may be necessary in patients who are extremely anxious.
7. Follow guidelines in Chapter 1 for safe, effective, informed *intratest* care.

Clinical Implications
1. Abnormal lesions or unusual epithelial patterns include the following:
   a. Leukoplakia
   b. Abnormal blood vessels
   c. Slight, moderate, or marked dysplasia
   d. Punctuation (ie, sharp borders, red stippling, epithelium whiter with acetic acid)
   e. Mosaic pattern (ie, sharp borders, mosaic pattern, epithelium whiter with acetic acid)
   f. Hyperkeratosis (ie, white, rough, visible without acetic acid)

Patient Preparation
1. Explain test purpose and procedure.
2. Follow guidelines in Chapter 1 for safe, effective, informed *pretest* care.

Clinical Alert

1. Patients may experience a vasovagal response. Watch for bradycardia and hypotension and treat accordingly. Have the patient sit for a short while before standing.
2. Antiinflammatory agents such as ibuprofen may relieve cramping.

(Clinical Alert continued)

3. Cervical scars from previous events may prevent satisfactory visualization.

4. Complications may include heavy bleeding, infection, or pelvic inflammatory disease.

5. Development of cervical changes and potential cervical carcinoma poses a greater risk for these patients. An annual Pap smear is mandatory for those who have undergone colposcopy.

Patient Aftercare

1. Instruct the patient to abstain from sexual intercourse and to not insert anything into the vagina for 2 to 7 days (per physician's orders) after the procedure.

2. If specimens were taken, slight vaginal bleeding may occur. Excessive bleeding, pain, fever, or abnormal vaginal discharge should be reported immediately.

3. Interpret test outcomes and counsel appropriately regarding follow-up treatment.

4. Follow guidelines in Chapter 1 regarding safe, effective, informed *posttest* care. Provide written discharge instructions.

CERVICOGRAPHY

Cervicography may be done in conjunction with colposcopy or by itself. A photographic method records an image of the entire cervix. The patient assumes a lithotomy position and the cervix is exposed using a speculum. After the cervical mucus is removed, 5% acetic acid is swabbed on the area for a few minutes. Photographs of the cervix are taken with a specially designed 35-mm camera. Next, aqueous iodine is swabbed on the cervix, and another picture is taken. Finally, an endocervical smear is taken and transferred onto a slide for later evaluation. The patient should be told that brown vaginal discharge (from the iodine) for a few days is not unusual.

The photographs are processed into slides (cervigrams) which allow the entire cervix to be visible on one slide. The cervigram can provide evidence for colposcopic consultations. Moreover, the cervigram can be done in conjunction with a routine gynecologic examination. It has been shown to be more sensitive than the Pap smear for the early detection of cervical intraepithelial neoplasia and invasive cervical cancer.

FLEXIBLE PROCTOSCOPY; SIGMOIDOSCOPY; PROCTOSIGMOIDOSCOPY

Normal Endoscopic Examination
Normal anal, cervical, rectal, and sigmoid colon mucosa

Explanation of Test

These tests involve the examination of an ~25-cm area of the rectum, anal canal, and sigmoid colon with a proctosigmoidoscope. Rigid scopes are not as commonly used since the advent of flexible fiberoptic instruments. Flexible proctosigmoidoscopes are tubes that usually measure 60 cm in length and incorporate a lighted lens system for illuminating the rectum and sigmoid. Their main use is for the detection and diagnosis of cancers and other abnormalities such as diverticula in this area of the gastrointestinal tract. These examinations should be routine (every 3–5 years) for cancer screening of individuals >50 years of age. These tests can also evaluate hemorrhoids, polyps, blood or mucus in the stool, unexplained anemia, and other bowel conditions.

Procedure

1. For rigid proctoscopy, the patient assumes the knee-to-chest position. When the flexible proctoscope is used, the patient must be in the left lateral position. The proctoscope or sigmoidoscope is carefully inserted into the rectum.
2. The examination can be done with the patient in bed or positioned on a special tilt-table.
3. The patient may feel a very strong urge to defecate and may experience a feeling of bloating or cramping. These sensations are normal.
4. Follow guidelines in Chapter 1 for safe, effective, informed *intratest* care.

Clinical Implications

1. Examination may reveal the following: edematous, red, or denuded mucosa; granularity; friability; ulcers; polyps; cysts; thickened areas; changes in vascular pattern; pseudomembranes; spontaneous bleeding; or normal mucosa. These findings may help to confirm or to rule out the following conditions:

   a. Inflammatory bowel disease
      (1) Chronic ulcerative colitis
      (2) Crohn's disease
      (3) Proctitis (acute and chronic)
      (4) Pseudomembranous colitis
      (5) Antibiotic-associated colitis
   c. Cancer and tumors
      (1) Adenocarcinoma
      (2) Carcinoids
      (3) Other tumors such as lipomas

   b. Polyps
      (1) Adenomatous
      (2) Familial
      (3) Diminutive
   d. Anal and perianal conditions
      (1) Hemorrhoids
      (2) Abscesses and fistulas
      (3) Strictures and stenoses
      (4) Rectal prolapse
      (5) Fissures
      (6) Contractures

Patient Preparation

1. Explain the test purpose and procedure.
2. There is no need for the patient to fast. However, a restricted diet such as

clear liquids the evening before the test may be prescribed. Diabetic patients may need to check with their physician regarding diet and insulin regimens.

3. Laxatives and enemas may be taken the night before the examination. Enemas or a rectal laxative suppository may be administered the morning of the procedure. For patients of all ages, one or two phosphate ("Fleet") enemas are frequently ordered to be performed ~1 to 2 hours before the examination. This is considered ample preparation by many endoscopy departments.

4. Follow guidelines in Chapter 1 for safe, effective, informed *pretest* care.

Clinical Alert

1. Patients with acute symptoms, particularly those with suspected ulcerative or granulomatous colitis, should be examined *without* any preparation (ie, without enemas, laxatives, or suppositories).
2. Perforation of the intestinal wall can be an infrequent complication of these tests.
3. Notify the patient's physician prior to administering laxatives or enemas to a pregnant woman.
4. Notify physician immediately of any instance of decreased blood pressure, diaphoresis, or bradycardia.

Patient Aftercare

1. Interpret test outcomes. Monitor and counsel appropriately.
2. Follow guidelines in Chapter 1 for safe, effective, informed *posttest* care. Provide written discharge instructions.

COLONOSCOPY

Normal Colonoscopic Examination
Normal large intestine mucosa

Explanation of Test
Colonoscopy visualizes, examines, and photographs the large intestine with a flexible fiberoptic or video colonoscope inserted through the anus and advanced to the ileocecal valve. Air introduced through an accessory channel of the colonoscope distends the intestinal walls to enhance visualization. This technique can differentiate inflammatory disease from neoplastic disease and can evaluate polypoid lesions that are beyond the reach of the sigmoidoscope. Suture lines and anastomoses can be checked. Polyps, foreign bodies, and biopsy specimens can be removed via the colonoscope. Photographs of the large intestine lumen can also be taken. Before colonoscopy was available, major abdominal surgery was the only way to remove polyps or suspicious tis-

sue to determine malignancy or nonmalignancy. Periodic colonoscopy is a valuable adjunct to the follow-up of persons with previous polyps, colon cancer, family history of colon cancer, or high risk factors. It is also helpful in locating the source of lower gastrointestinal bleeding.

Clinical Implications

1. Abnormal findings may reveal the following conditions:
   a. Polyps
   b. Tumors (benign or malignant)
   c. Areas of ulceration
   d. Inflammation
   e. Colitis, diverticula
   f. Bleeding sites
   g. Strictures
   h. Discovery and removal of foreign bodies

Procedure

1. A clear-liquid diet is usually ordered for 48 to 72 hours before the examination. The patient must fast for 8 hours before the procedure. Laxatives may be ordered to be taken for 1 to 3 days before the test; enemas may be ordered to be given the night before the test. To be effective, a purgative must produce fluid diarrhea. This shows that unaltered small intestinal contents are emerging and colonic residue has been cleared. Enemas must be repeated until solid matter is no longer expelled (clear liquid returns). Soapsuds enemas are contraindicated because they cause increased mucus secretion as a result of irritant stimulation.

2. Another common form of bowel preparation involves the ingestion of an oral saline iso-osmotic and isotonic (with respect to bowel contents) laxative. This washout solution may contain a number of salts, such as potassium chloride, sodium chloride, bicarbonate; an additive, such as polyethylene glycol; and distilled or deionized water. The glycol acts as an osmotic agent so there is no net ion absorption or loss; water and electrolyte balances should not change significantly. The patient drinks 3 to 6 L of the prescribed solution over a 2- to 3.5-hour period. The typical volume taken is 1 gallon (~4 liters), and this volume of fluid can be administered by nasogastric tube if necessary. This laxative acts quickly. Initial results can be expected in 30 minutes to 1 hour. Ingestion of the washout solution continues until feces expelled are nothing but clear liquid. The physician should be notified prior to administering >6 L of this solution. No special diet, laxative, or enemas are required with this method. Patients with congestive heart failure or renal failure may be at risk for fluid volume overload if this preparation is used. See Patient Preparation for other preparation measures.

3. The colonoscopy is done using conscious sedation with combinations of medications such as meperidine (Demerol), diazepam (Valium), or midazolam (Versed). The patient should be responsive enough to inform the doctor of any subjective reactions during the examination.

4. Occasionally, intravenous anticholinergic agents and glucagon may be used to relax bowel spasms.

5. The patient assumes the left-sided or Sims' position and is draped properly. A well-lubricated colonoscope is inserted ~12 cm into the bowel. The patient should take deep breaths through the mouth during this time. Air is then introduced into the bowel through a special port on the colonoscope to aid viewing. As the colonoscope advances, the patient may need to be repositioned several times to aid in proper visualization of the colon. Sensations of pressure, mild pain, or cramping are not unusual.

6. The best views are obtained during withdrawal of the colonoscope. Therefore, a more detailed examination is usually performed during withdrawal than during advancement.

7. Follow guidelines in Chapter 1 for safe, effective, informed *intratest* care.

Clinical Considerations

1. Keep colon electrolyte lavage preparations refrigerated; however, the patient may drink the solution at room temperature. Use within 48 hours of preparation, and discard unused portions.

2. Prior to testing, a complete blood count, prothrombin time, platelet count, and thromboplastin times results should be reviewed and charted.

3. Preparation for patients with a colostomy or who are paralyzed is the same whether or not the patient is taking aspirin or any blood thinners.

4. Persons with known heart disease should receive prescribed antibiotics before testing.

5. Patients should not mix or drink anything with the washout preparation. Do not add ice or glucose to the solution.

6. Diabetic persons are usually advised not to take insulin before the procedure but are to bring insulin with them to the clinic.

Patient Preparation

1. Explain the purpose, procedure, benefits, and risks of the test. When ordered, before the examination, one 12-ounce glass of liquid preparation is to be taken every 10 minutes. (Each gallon holds 10.7 12-ounce (360 ml) glasses.) The entire gallon should be taken in 2 hours, if possible. Timing is important. Slower drinking does not clean the colon properly. Some patients will receive another type of preparation when ordered (eg, Propulcid capsules and liquid Fleet laxatives).

2. Some patients will be on a clear-liquid diet for 72 hours before the test, then fasting, except for medications, after a clear-liquid supper the evening before the test. No solid food, milk, or milk products are permitted. Strained fruit juices without pulp (eg, apple, white grape), lemonade, Hi-C drink water, clear liquid, Gatorade, Kool-Aid, Jell-o, popsicles, and hard candy are permitted, but no red or purple fluids are allowed.

3. Administer purgatives and cleaning enemas as ordered. Preparation is complete when fecal discharge is clear. If returns are not clear after 4 L of solution have been ingested, continue until returns are clear, up to 6 L total (see previous note under Procedure).

4. A legal consent form must be signed and properly witnessed (see Chap. 1) after patient has received proper instruction about the test.
5. Iron preparations should be discontinued 3 or 4 days before the examination because iron residues produce an inky, black, sticky stool that interferes with visualization, and the stool can be viscous and difficult to clear. Aspirin and aspirin-containing products should also be discontinued 1 week before the examination because they may cause bleeding problems or localized hemorrhages.
6. Some protocols call for a functional intravenous line to be in place.
7. Persons with valvular heart disease need antibiotics before the test. Usually, heart or blood pressure medicine can be taken 1 hour before the test.
8. Take baseline vital signs.
9. Follow guidelines in Chapter 1 for safe, effective, informed *pretest* care.

Patient Aftercare

1. The patient should remain fasting for 2 hours after the examination.
2. Stools should be observed for visible blood. The patient should be instructed to report abdominal pain or other unusual symptoms, because perforation and hemorrhage are possible complications.
3. Vital signs should be checked frequently for 2 hours after the procedure.
4. The most frequent adverse reactions to oral purgatives include nausea, vomiting, bloating, rectal irritation, chills, and feelings of weakness.
5. The patient may expel large amounts of flatus after the procedure.
6. Interpret test outcomes and counsel appropriately.
7. Follow guidelines in Chapter 1 for safe, effective, informed *posttest* care. Provide written discharge instructions.

Clinical Alert

1. Solid food should never be taken within 2 hours before the oral cleansing regimen is begun.
2. Orally administered colon lavage is contraindicated in the following conditions:

(continued)

PERITONEOSCOPY; LAPAROSCOPY; PELVISCOPY ●

Normal Endoscopic Examination

Gynecologic examination: normal size, shape, and appearance of uterus, fallopian tubes, and ovaries

(Clinical Alert continued)

    a. Actual or suspected ulcers

    b. Gastric outlet obstruction

    c. Weight <20 kg

    d. Toxic colitis

    e. Megacolon

3. Relative contraindications for colonoscopy include the following conditions:

    a. Perforating disease of the colon

    b. Peritonitis

    c. Radiation enteritis

    d. Recent abdominal or bowel surgery

    e. Acute conditions of the anus and rectum

    f. Serious cardiac or respiratory problems (eg, recent myocardial infarction)

    g. Situations in which the bowel cannot be adequately prepared for the procedure (ie, fulminant granulomatous or irradiation colitis)

4. Observe for the following possible complications:

    a. Perforations of the bowel

    b. Hypotensive episodes

    c. Cardiac or respiratory arrest, which can be provoked by the combination of oversedation and intense vagal stimulus from instrumentation

    d. Hemorrhage, especially if polypectomy has been performed

    e. Death (extremely rare)

5. If colon preparations are administered by lavage to an unconscious patient or to a patient with impaired gag reflexes, observe for aspiration or regurgitation, especially if a nasogastric tube is in place. Keep the head of the bed elevated. If this is not possible, position the patient on his or her side. Have continuous suction equipment and supplies readily available.

6. No barium studies should be done during the preparation phase for colonoscopy.

7. Signs of bowel perforation include malaise, rectal bleeding, abdominal pain, distention, and fever.

8. Bloating, nausea, and occasional vomiting after oral laxatives is common. Advise patient to adhere to instructions if at all possible.

Intraabdominal examination: normal liver, gallbladder, spleen, and greater curvature of the stomach

Explanation of Test

These examinations of the intraabdominal and pelvic cavities are performed using a laparoscope or pelviscope inserted through a slit in the anterior abdominal wall. The pelvic organs, as well as abdominal organs such as the greater curvature of the stomach or the liver, can be viewed. The different types of examinations include peritoneoscopy, and laparoscopy (intraabdominal) and pelviscopy (gynecologic). These procedures are frequently performed under general anesthesia in a surgical setting; however, many are also done with local anesthesia.

Peritoneoscopy is most commonly done to evaluate liver disease and to obtain biopsy specimens when the liver is too small, when previous liver biopsy proves inadequate, when contraindications to percutaneous liver biopsy exist (eg, ascites), when there is unexplained portal hypertension or liver function abnormalities, and when the liver cannot be properly palpated for doing a conventional liver biopsy. It does away with the need to do a blind liver biopsy. Other indications for peritoneoscopy include unexplained ascites, staging of lymphomas or staging and follow-up of ovarian cancer, or abdominal masses. Sometimes patients with advanced chest, gastric, pancreatic, endometrial, or rectal tumors are evaluated by peritoneoscopy before surgical intervention is attempted.

Gynecologic laparoscopy and pelviscopy are used to diagnose cysts, adhesions, fibroids, malignancies, inflammatory processes, or infections in persons with pelvic and abdominal pain. Evaluation of the fallopian tubes can be done for infertile patients. These procedures also provide a means to release adhesions, to obtain biopsy specimens, to do select operative procedures such as tubal ligations, or to perform laser treatments for endometriosis. Gynecologic laparoscopy or pelviscopy is commonly performed under general anesthesia as a same-day surgical procedure.

These techniques can frequently replace laparotomy. They are less stressful to the patient, require only small incisions, can be done in shorter periods of time, can be done using local, spinal, or general anesthetics, reduce potential for formation of adhesions, and hasten healing and recovery time.

Pelviscopy differs from laparoscopy in two major respects—*endocoagulation* as a method for controlling bleeding and *endoligation* as a technique that permits suturing using extracorporeal (outside the body) or intracorporeal (inside the body) ligating and suturing methods by means of special instruments.

The pelviscope is angled at 30 degrees for better visualization. A videocamera attachment offers the physician a choice of viewing the process on a video screen instead of through the scope. Printouts and videotapes of the pelviscopy can be produced. Thus, pelviscopy is both a diagnostic and an operative modality.

Procedure

1. The patient is supine during all procedures except gynecologic laparoscopy, in which case the patient is placed in a lithotomy position.
2. The skin is cleansed and, if the procedure is to be performed under local anesthesia, a local anesthetic is injected into areas where the scope will be

introduced. Otherwise, the patient is prepped as for an abdominal procedure under general anesthesia. A sterile field is maintained.

3. An intravenous line is placed so that medications may be given intravenously as needed.

4. An indwelling catheter is placed into the bladder to reduce the risk of bladder perforation.

5. A small incision is made near the umbilicus through which a trocar is introduced, followed by passage of the pelviscope or laparoscope. Sometimes, more than one puncture site will be made so that accessory instruments can be used during the procedure. Carbon dioxide introduced into the peritoneal cavity causes the omentum to rise away from the organs and allows for better visualization. A few stitches or SteriStrips are usually needed to close the incisions. Adhesive bandages are applied as dressings.

6. Follow guidelines in Chapter 1 for safe, effective, informed *intratest* care.

Clinical Implications

1. Abnormal findings can reveal the following conditions:
   a. Endometriosis
   b. Ovarian cysts
   c. Pelvic inflammatory disease
   d. Metastasis stage of cancer
   e. Uterine fibroids
   f. Abscesses
   g. Tumors (benign and malignant)
   h. Enlarged fallopian tubes (hydrosalpinx)
   i. Ectopic pregnancy
   j. Infection
   k. Adhesions or scar tissue
   l. Ascites
   m. Cirrhosis
   n. Liver nodules (often an indication of cancer)
   o. Engorged peritoneal vasculature (correlates with portal hypertension)

Clinical Alert

1. These procedures may be contraindicated in persons known to have the following conditions:
   a. Advanced abdominal wall cancer
   b. Severe respiratory or cardiovascular disease
   c. Intestinal obstruction
   d. Palpable abdominal mass
   e. Large abdominal hernia

(continued)

(Clinical Alert continued)
   f. Chronic tuberculosis
   g. History of peritonitis
2. Possible complications include the following:
   a. Bleeding may occur from the puncture injury
   b. Misplacement of gas
   c. Thermal burns
3. The endoscopy should be aborted in favor of a laparotomy in the event of uncontrolled bleeding or suspected malignancy.

Patient Preparation

1. Laboratory tests and other appropriate diagnostic modalities need to be completed prior to these endoscopies.
2. Bowel preparation may include an enema or suppository.
3. Explain the test purpose and procedure and the type of anesthesia chosen (general, spinal, or local), as well as postoperative expectations such as activity, deep breathing, and shoulder pain.
4. A legal permit must be properly signed and witnessed (see Chap. 1).
5. Sensitivity to cultural, sexual, and modesty issues are an important part of psychological support.
6. Follow guidelines in Chapter 1 for safe, effective, informed *pretest* care.

Patient Aftercare

1. Check blood pressure frequently according to institutional policies.
2. Observe for infection, hemorrhage, and bowel or bladder perforation.
3. Advise the patient that shoulder and abdominal discomfort may be present for 1 to 2 days because of residual carbon dioxide gas in the abdominal cavity. This can be controlled with mild oral analgesics. Sitting or resting in a semi-Fowler's position can also alleviate discomfort.
4. If the patient has had a general or spinal anesthetic, follow the usual cautions and protocols for the care of any person having undergone those types of anesthesia.
5. Interpret test outcomes and counsel appropriately.
6. Follow guidelines in Chapter 1 for safe, effective, informed *posttest* care. Provide written discharge instructions.

CYSTOSCOPY (CYSTOURETHROSCOPY)

Normal Cystoscopic Examination
Normal structure and function of the interior bladder, urethra, ureteral orifices, and male prostatic urethra

Explanation of Test
These examinations are used to diagnose and treat disorders of the lower urinary tract. They provide views of the interior bladder, urethra, male prostatic urethra,

and ureteral orifices through tubular, lighted, telescopic lens instruments called cystoscopes or cystourethroscopes. These scopes come in many sizes and variations as well as in flexible fiberoptic instruments. Urethroscopy is an important part of this examination because it allows visualization of the male prostate gland.

Cystoscopy is the most common of all urologic diagnostic procedures. It may be indicated in the following conditions:

1. Unexplained hematuria (gross or microscopic)
2. Recurrent or chronic urinary tract infection
3. Infection resistant to medical treatment
4. Unexplained urinary symptoms such as dysuria, frequency, urgency, hesitancy, intermittency, straining, incontinence, enuresis, or retention
5. Bladder tumors (benign and malignant)
6. Pediatric considerations include the above and the following:
   a. Posterior urethral valves, ureteroceles in females, and other congenital anomalies.
   b. Complete workup of children with daytime incontinence usually done in conjunction with urodynamic studies
   c. Remove foreign objects and stents placed in previous surgeries.

Because intravenous pyelogram (IVP) does not allow proper visualization of the area from the neck of the bladder to the end of the urethra, cystoscopy makes it possible to diagnose and to treat abnormalities in this area.

Cystoscopy may be used to perform meatotomy and to crush and retrieve small stones and other foreign bodies from the urethra, ureter, and bladder. Biopsy specimens can be obtained. Bladder tumors can be fulgurated and strictures can be dilated through the cystoscope. In conjunction with cystoscopy, ureteroscopy can be done to determine the cause of hematuria, to detect tumors and stones, and to manipulate stones.

Procedure

1. The examination can be performed in an operating room designed for that purpose or in the urologist's office. The patient's age, state of health, and extent of surgical procedure necessary determine the setting. Pediatric cystoscopy is done in the operating room under general anesthetic.
2. The external genitalia are prepped with an antiseptic solution such as povidone-iodine after the patient is placed in the lithotomy position with his or her legs in stirrups. The patient is properly grounded, padded, and draped.
3. A local anesthetic jelly is instilled into the urethra. For males, the anesthetic is retained in the urethra by a clamp applied near the end of the penis. For best results, the local anesthetic should be administered 5 to 10 minutes before passage of the cystoscope.
4. The scope is connected to an irrigation system, and fluid is infused into the bladder throughout the procedure. Solutions used are nonconductive and retain clarity during the procedure (eg, glycine, sterile water). This solution also distends the bladder to allow better visualization. The infusion is stopped and the bladder drained when it becomes filled with 300 to 500 ml of fluid.

NOTE: *During transurethral resection procedures, venous sinuses may be opened, and irrigation fluid may enter the circulatory system, causing water intoxication. Therefore, isotonic solutions such as sorbitol, mannitol, or glycine must be used.*

5. Should blood or other matter be present in the bladder, the fiberoptic cystoscope will not provide as clear a view as a rigid cystoscope because it is more difficult to flush.
6. Institutional policies dictate general perioperative care and procedures. Follow guidelines in Chapter 1 regarding safe, effective, informed *intratest* care.

Clinical Implications

1. Abnormal conditions revealed by cystoscopy include the following:
   a. Prostatic hyperplasia or hypertrophy
   b. Cancer of the bladder
   c. Bladder stones
   d. Urethral strictures or abnormalities
   e. Prostatitis
   f. Ureteral reflux (shown on cystogram)
   g. Vesical neck stenosis
   h. Urinary fistulas
   i. Ureterocele
   j. Diverticula
   k. Abnormally small or large bladder capacity
   l. Polyps

Patient Preparation

1. Explain the purpose and procedure of the test. Special sensitivity to and concern for cultural, social, sexual, and modesty issues are an important part of psychological support. Emphasize that there is little pain or discomfort from cystoscopy; however, a strong desire to void may be experienced.
2. Bowel preparation and other laboratory and diagnostic tests may be necessary if extensive procedures are planned.
3. If cystoscopy is performed in the hospital, a properly signed and witnessed surgical permit must be obtained (see Chap. 1).
4. At times, the patient may take a full liquid breakfast. Liquids may be encouraged until the time of the examination to promote urine formation if the procedure is a simple cystoscopy done under local anesthesia. Fasting guidelines are followed when spinal or general anesthesia is planned.
5. Sometimes an intravenous line may be started for the administration of intravenous conscious sedative medications such as diazepam (Valium) or midazolam (Versed) to relax the patient. Amnesia may be a side-effect. Younger men may experience more pain and discomfort than older men. Women usually require less sedation because the female urethra is shorter. The patient should be instructed to relax the abdominal muscles to lessen discomfort. See Appendix C regarding intravenous conscious sedation precautions.
6. Follow guidelines in Chapter 1 regarding safe, effective, informed *pretest* care.

Patient Aftercare

1. After cystoscopy, voiding patterns and bladder emptying should be monitored. Check vital signs as necessary.

2. The intake of fluids should be encouraged.

3. Clots may form and may cause difficulty in voiding.

4. Report unusual bleeding or difficult urination to the physician promptly.

5. Urinary frequency, dysuria, pink-to-light-red urine, and urethral burning are common after cystoscopy.

6. Antibiotics may be prescribed before and after cystoscopy to prevent infection.

7. The potential for gram-negative shock is always present with urologic procedures because the urethra is such a vascular organ that any break in the tissues can allow bacteria to enter the bloodstream directly. Onset of symptoms can be rapid and may actually begin during the procedure if it is fairly lengthy. Observe for and *promptly* report chills, fever, increasing tachycardia, hypotension, and back pain to the physician. Blood cultures are usually ordered, followed by an aggressive regimen of antibiotic therapy.

8. Ureteral catheters may be left in place to facilitate urinary drainage, especially if there is concern about edema.

9. Routine catheter care is necessary for retention or ureteral catheters. Follow institutional protocols. The patient may need instructions if discharged with catheter in place.

10. Interpret test outcomes and counsel appropriately.

11. Follow guidelines in Chapter 1 for safe, effective, informed *posttest* care. Provide written discharge instructions.

Clinical Alert

1. If urethral dilatation has been part of the procedure, the patient is advised to rest and to increase fluid intake.

2. Evaluate and instruct the patient to watch for edema. Edema may cause urinary retention, hesitancy, weak urinary stream, or urinary dribbling any time within several days after the procedure. Warm Sitz baths and mild analgesics may be helpful; however, an indwelling catheter may sometimes be necessary for relief.

●URODYNAMIC STUDIES

CYSTOMETROGRAM (CMG); URETHRAL PRESSURE PROFILE (UPP); RECTAL ELECTROMYOGRAM (EMG); CYSTOURETHROGRAM ●

Normal Urodynamic Examination

Normal bladder sensations of fullness, heat, and cold.

Adult: Normal bladder capacity of 400 to 500 ml, residual urine less than 30 ml, first desire to void is at 175 to 250 ml, fullness felt at 350 to 450 ml, stream is strong and uninterrupted.

Pediatric: Bladder capacity varies with age. Compliant bladder: Stretches to capacity without pressure increase. Bladder stability: No involuntary contractions.

Explanation of Test

These tests evaluate bladder, urethral, and sphincter function, identify abnormal voiding patterns and consist of two main components: the cystometrogram (CMG) and the sphincterelectromyogram (EMG). The combined measurement of the CMG and the EMG provides information about how the bladder adapts to being filled as well as how it reacts to the filling itself. These studies are indicated in an incontinent persons and when there is evidence of neurological disease, spinal cord injury, or specific neuropathies such as those found in multiple sclerosis, diabetes, and tabes dorsalis.

Procedures

CYSTOMETROGRAM (CMG) PROCEDURE

1. The patient voids and urine flow rate, voiding pressure, and amount of urine voided are recorded.
2. A non-latex double lumen catheter is inserted into the bladder. Adhesive patch electrodes are placed parallel on each side of the anus. Residual urine is measured. The catheter is then connected to the cystometer. (A cystometer evaluates the neuromuscular mechanism of the bladder by measuring bladder capacity and pressure.) The bladder is gradually filled with sterile saline or sterile water or carbon dioxide gas in predetermined increments and pressure readings are taken at these increments. Water or saline offer a more physiologic result and is less irritating.
3. During the CMG, observations are made about the patient's perception of heat and cold, bladder fullness, urge to void, and ability to inhibit voiding when bladder contractions occur.
4. When the bladder is completely emptied of fluid, the catheter and patch electrodes are removed.
5. Cholinergic and/or anticholinergic drugs (eg, methantheline bromide (Banthine, atropine), or bethanechol chloride (Urecholine) may be injected to determine their effects upon bladder function.
6. The cystometric study may be performed as a control, followed by repeat study 20 to 30 minutes after injection of the drugs.
7. A change in posture from supine to standing or walking may be required during the examination.
8. Sleep studies may be performed in conjunction with an electroencephalogram to evaluate persons having nocturnal incontinence (see Chap. 15 for EEG study.)
9. Pediatric CMGs: The bladder is filled until the pressures reach 40 to 60 cm of water, the child voids around the catheter or until the child seems very uncomfortable. In the older child, questions are asked about bladder fullness, when they would normally void, and are asked to hold urine until extreme urgency ensues. Patents may void on the table with the catheter in place, or they may void in a special container which measures urine flow, voiding pressure, and length of time to void. These pressures are depicted on a graph.

RECTAL ELECTROMYOGRAPHIC (EMG) PROCEDURE

1. The EMG monitors the pelvic floor muscles responsible for hoding urine in the bladder. Electrodes are applied close to the anus, and a ground is attached to the thigh.
2. A needle electrode may be introduced into the periurethral striated muscle.
3. These electrodes record electromyographic activity during voiding and produce a simultaneous recording of urine flow rate. (See Chap. 15 for EMG study.)
4. Pediatric rectal EMG: Patch electrodes record the coordination of the external sphincter and the pelvic floor muscles response to filling and the abillity to inhibit bladder contractions. If the child voids of the table, it will demonstrate that the sphincter relaxes during voiding (which is normal).

URETHRAL PRESSURE PROFILE (UPP) PROCEDURE

1. A special catheter, connected to a transducer, is slowly withdrawn, and the pressures along the urethra are recorded.
2. Pediatric UPP: This profile assesses the functional urethral length as well as general competency of the urethra and sphincter. The same double lumen catheter is used which has pre-marked lines on it for both the CMG and the UPP. As the catheter is slowly withdrawn the pressures are noted at the pre-marked spots.

CYSTOURETHROGRAM PROCEDURE

1. This study evaluates bladder wall and urethral abnormalities and tumors. It can be used to assess reflux, stress incontinence in women, and to identify urine extravasation following trauma.
2. An x-ray contrast medium is instilled into the bladder through a catheter until the bladder is filled. The catheter is clamped and x-rays are done with the patient assuming several different positions.
3. After the catheter is removed, more x-rays are taken as the patient voids and the contrast material passes through the urethra (voiding cystourethrogram).
4. Pediatric cystourethrogram: Rarely are voiding cystourethrograms (VCUG) done at the same time as EMGs. VCUGs are done in children to assess vesicle urethral reflux, to identify structural abnormalities, to evaluate for voiding dysfunction, and are usually done as part of the workup before considering EMG.
5. See Chapter 1 guidelines for safe, effective, informed *intra-test* care for all procedures.

Clinical Alert

In children, the bladder is filled at 10% of what the bladder is expected to hold at a specific age (ex: age capacity [in ounces] plus two ounces).

Clinical Implications

1. Abnormal results reveal motor and sensory defects, altered pressures and/or bladder capacity, and inappropriate or absent contractions of the pelvic floor muscles and internal sphincter during voiding.

   a. Bladder noncompliance: During filling, the bladder is stiff, does not stretch as expected, and can possibly compromise kidney function over time. A large capacity low pressure bladder (high compliance) may indicate chronic over-distention from infrequent voiding habits.

   b. Bladder instability (hyperreflexia): During filling, the bladder contracts involuntarily; this occurs when the pressures go up and down in a wave-like pattern during filling, due to over-activity of involuntary contractions. The unstable bladder may be asymptomatic, may times no contractions are felt, but commonly patients have frequency, urgency, and incontinence.

   c. The most common cause of incontinence is a vesical-sphincter dyssynergia (disturbance of muscular coordination). This dyssynergia is thought to be responsible for incomplete emptying of the bladder, inappropriate voiding, perineal dampness, and predisposition to urinary tract infections.

   d. Detrusor hyperreflexia: The patient cannot suppress voiding on command due to upper or lower motor neuron lesions, as in cerebrovascular aneurysm, Parkinson's disease, multiple sclerosis, cervical spondylosis, and spinal cord injury above the conus medullaris.

   e. Detrusor areflexia occurs when the detrusor reflex cannot be evoked because the peripheral innervation of the detrusor muscle has been interrupted and results in difficulty in initiating voiding without a residual volume being present in the bladder. The cause may be associated with trauma, spinal arachnoiditis, spinal cord birth defects, diabetic neuropathy, or anticholinergic effects of phenothiazides. In postmenopausal women, the urethral pressure profile may be altered because the mucosal sphincter is deprived of estrogen.

   f. Urethrovesical hyperreflexia is caused by benign prostatic hypertrophy and stress urge incontinence.

Patient Preparation

1. Explain the purpose and procedure of the bladder funcion test, often done before and after certain types of spinal surgery. Be sensitive to the patient's potential anxiety and embarrassment.

2. For accurate results the patient must be relaxed and cooperative. For children, a favorite toy or book may provide security. Sedation is not given because patient participation is necessary to verify sensations and perceptions. However, the patient must avoid movement during the examination unless instructed otherwise.

3. The test and filling fo the bladder continue until the patient either leaks or voids around the catheter.

4. See Chapter 1 guidelines for safe, effective, informed *pre-test* care.

Patient Aftercare

1. Encourage the patient to increase oral fluid intake to dilute the urine and to minimize bladder sensitivity.
2. Explain that some minor discomfort or burning may be noted, especially if carbon dioxide is used, but it will lessen and disappear with time.
3. Interpret test outcomes and counsel appropriately.
4. Follow Chapter 1 guidelines for safe, effective, informed *posttest* care. Provide written discharge instructions.

Clinical Alert

1. Certain patients with cervical cord lesions may exhibit an autonomic reflex that produces an elevated blood pressure, severe headache, lower pulse rate, flushing, and diaphoresis. Propantheline bromide (Pro-Banthine) alleviates these symptoms.
2. Careful use of sterile technique reduces the incidence of urinary tract infections. Preprocedural urinary tract infections can lead to sepsis as a result of bacterial spread into the bloodstream.

ARTHROSCOPY

Normal Arthroscopic Examination

Normal joint: normal vasculature and color of the synovium, capsule, menisci, ligaments, and articular cartilage

Explanation of Test

Arthroscopy is a visual examination of a joint by means of a fiberoptic endoscope system. The examination is frequently associated with a surgical procedure It is most commonly done for the diagnosis of athletic injuries and for the differential diagnosis of acute or chronic joint disorders. For example, degenerative processes can be accurately differentiated from injuries. Postoperative rehabilitation programs can be initiated to shorten recovery periods. Arthroscopy can also assess response to treatment or identify whether other corrective procedures are indicated.

Although the knee is the joint most frequently examined, the shoulder, ankle, hip, elbow, wrist and metacarpophalangeal joints can also be explored. Calcium deposits, biopsy specimens, bone spurs, torn meniscus or cartilage, and scar tissue can be removed during the procedure. Currently, many of these procedures are performed in an ambulatory surgical setting.

Procedure

1. The examination is usually performed under general anesthesia for the following reasons:
   a. The joint is very painful.
   b. Definitive treatment or surgical intervention can be done at the same time if within the realm of arthroscopic surgery.

    c. An inflated tourniquet may be used during part of the procedure to minimize bleeding at the site.

    d. Complete muscle relaxation permits a thorough examination and eliminates the risk of inadvertent patient movement while the arthroscope is in the joint.

2. The surgical site is draped and prepped according to institutional protocols. Proper monitoring equipment is attached to the patient.

3. A tourniquet is applied to the appropriate area of the extremity after it is exsanguinated by the use of an elastic bandage or elevation. Some surgeons choose not to inflate the tourniquet unless bleeding cannot be controlled by irrigation.

4. The joint is aspirated with a 15- or 16-gauge needle. A specimen of aspirate may be sent to the laboratory. The joint is then injected with 75 to 100 ml of normal saline or lactated Ringer's solution to distend the joint before the arthroscope is inserted. Additional puncture sites allow manipulation of accessory instruments. The wound is irrigated with an appropriate solution throughout the procedure.

5. Joint washings are collected and examined for loose bodies or cartilage fragments.

6. All parts of the joint are carefully examined. Photographs or videotapes of the procedure may be taken. The physician may choose to perform surgical interventions for problems that can be corrected via arthroscopy.

7. As the arthroscope, accessory pieces, and irrigating needles are slowly withdrawn, the joint is compressed to squeeze out excess irrigation fluid.

8. Steroids or local anesthetics may be injected into the joint for postoperative pain control and reduction of inflammation. The wounds are closed with sutures or adhesive strips, and small dressings are applied to the wound or wounds (eg, two to three small incisions for the knee joint). Compressive dressings and splints or immobilizers may then be applied to the extremity.

9. Follow guidelines in Chapter 1 for safe, effective, informed *intratest* care.

Clinical Implications

1. Abnormal results reveal the following conditions:

    a. Torn or displaced meniscus or cartilage (symptoms relate to clicking, locking, and/or swelling of the joint)

    b. Trapped synovium

    c. Loose fragments of joint contents

    d. Torn or ruptured ligaments

    e. Necrosis

    f. Nerve entrapment

    g. Fractures or nonunion of fractures

    h. Ganglions

    i. Infections

    j. Osteochondritis dissecans: inflammation of bone or cartilage occurs when a cartilage fragment and underlying bone detach from the articular surface (common in the knee)

k. Chronic inflammatory arthritis

l. Secondary osteoarthritis caused by injury, metabolic disorders, and wearing away of weight-bearing joints

m. Chondromalacia of femoral condyle (wearing down of back of kneecap, often producing a grinding sensation)

Patient Preparation

1. History and physical examination, requisite laboratory work, x-ray films, and other preoperative requirements should be completed, reviewed, and documented on the patient's record.

2. Explain the purpose and procedure of the test. The patient should fast from midnight before the examination unless otherwise ordered (eg, if scheduled late in the day, a liquid breakfast may be permitted).

3. A properly signed and witnessed permit must be completed. See Chapter 1.

4. Peripheral pulses are checked. The surgical site is prepped, positioned, and draped according to institutional protocols. An intravenous line is started.

5. Crutch walking should be taught prior to the procedure if its necessity is anticipated postoperatively.

6. Follow guidelines in Chapter 1 for safe, effective, informed *pretest* care.

Patient Aftercare

1. Assess vital signs, bleeding, neurologic status, and circulatory status of the affected extremity (eg, color, pulse, temperature, capillary refill times, sensation, and motion).

2. Apply ice immediately and, if ordered, elevate the extremity to minimize swelling and pain. Dressing changes and suture removal are performed at the physician's discretion. The dressing is kept clean and dry. Notify the physician of unusual bleeding or swelling.

3. Appropriate pain medication should be administered.

4. The patient can usually be ambulatory after recovery from the anesthetic. Crutches may be used. Degree of weight-bearing and joint motion is at the discretion of the physician; however, patient should be cautioned to avoid excessive joint use for at least 24 to 48 hours.

5. Exercises and physical therapy may be ordered postoperatively. These are designed to strengthen and maximize use of the joint.

6. If the patient is discharged the same day as the procedure, arrangements for transportation by another person must be made preoperatively. The patient should not drive for at least 24 hours.

7. The patient should consume no alcohol for 24 hours after the procedure. Progress diet from fluid to solid foods as tolerated.

8. Instruct the patient to report altered sensation, numbness, tingling, coldness, duskiness (ie, bluish color), swelling, bleeding, or abnormal pain to the physician immediately.

9. Interpret test outcomes and counsel appropriately.

10. Follow guidelines in Chapter 1 for safe, effective, informed *posttest* care. Provide written discharge instructions.

Clinical Alert

1. Arthroscopy is usually contraindicated if ankylosis or fibrosis is present because it is very difficult to maneuver the examining instrument in this type of joint.

2. For knee arthroscopy, the posterior approach is not used because of the neurovascular structures present in that area.

3. Do not place pillows under the knee; flexion contractures can occur as a result. If the patient's *entire* leg is ordered to be elevated, make sure the knee is not flexed. Pad pressure points such as the heel.

4. If there is risk of sepsis or if sepsis is present in any part of the body, the procedure should not be done.

5. Arthroscopy is usually not done <7 to 10 days after arthrography, because chemical synovitis caused by a contrast medium can adversely affect the visual examination. However, it may be necessary to perform arthroscopy if the patient is experiencing severe pain. In this case, the joint must be thoroughly irrigated to remove contrast medium.

6. Be alert for signs of thrombophlebitis postoperatively. Instruct patient to watch for calf tenderness, pain, and heat and to report these symptoms to the physician immediately. *Warn the patient not to massage the affected area.*

7. Other complications may include hemarthrosis, adhesions, neurovascular injury, pulmonary embolus, effusion, scarring, and compartmental syndrome as a result of swelling. Compartmental syndrome is a musculoskeletal complication that occurs most commonly in the forearm or leg. The compartment of fascia surrounding muscles does not expand when bleeding or edema occurs. Consequently, the neurovascular status of the extremity may be severely compromised. This presents an emergency situation that usually requires surgical intervention to release pressure. Assess the neurovascular status of an affected extremity frequently for 24 hours after the procedure.

SINUS ENDOSCOPY

Normal Sinus Endoscopy Examination
Normal sinuses or resolution of sinus disease

Explanation of Test
This examination visualizes the anterior ethmoid, middle turbinate region, and middle meatus sinus areas. Although the purpose of sinus endoscopy is primarily to relieve infectious and other symptoms and to alter structural abnormalities in these areas, it can also be a valuable diagnostic tool. Retained secretions may contribute to chronic recurrent sinus infections which may lead

to systemic infections, cyst formation, or mucoceles that can erode sinus walls into areas of the eyeball, eye orbit, or brain.

Patients having recurrent episodes of acute or chronic sinusitis that are not responsive to antibiotic and/or allergy therapy are candidates for sinus endoscopy as both a diagnostic and therapeutic modality.

Procedure

Sinus endoscopy may be performed as an outpatient or office procedure. Normally, the diagnostic procedure is performed in the office. More extensive examination and operative procedures normally require outpatient admission to a health care facility or special diagnostic center.

1. A cocaine solution of select concentration is usually sprayed into the nares to produce local anesthesia. The endoscope is introduced to permit visualization of the nasal interior; the sinus cavities are *not* opened. Some patients become very talkative and euphoric as a response to cocaine.
2. Sinus computed axial tomography (CT, CAT) scans and magnetic resonance imaging (MRI) may be necessary adjuncts to this procedure to permit visualization of areas not accessible through endoscopy.
3. Treatment for underlying disease or malformations is performed using local or general anesthesia and intravenous sedation. Diagnostic and surgical techniques vary according to preoperative findings.
4. Endoscopes using a fiberoptic light delivery system are the mainstay of visualization for diagnosis and laser treatment.
5. Follow guidelines in Chapter 1 for safe, effective, informed *intratest* care.

Clinical Implications

1. Abnormalities that may be revealed include the following conditions:
   a. Chronic sinusitis (edematous or polypoid mucosa)
   b. Cysts
   c. Mucocele
   d. Sinus erosion
   e. Anatomical deformities or obstructions
   f. Pathologic sinus discharge (infectious process)
   g. Enlarged middle turbinates

Patient Preparation

1. Explain test purpose, benefits, risks, and procedure. (Steps 2 through 6 refer to treatment modalities.) The procedure may take place in the office or outpatient hospital setting.
2. A properly signed and witnessed surgical consent form (see Chapter 1), appropriate laboratory and diagnostic test results, history and physical examination, current drug therapies, and allergies must be reviewed and documented in the health care record prior to the procedure.

3. Preprocedure preparation may require the patient to:
   a. Be processed through preadmission testing if procedure will be done in a hospital surgical setting
   b. Fast from midnight the day of the procedure
   c. Remove facial prostheses, dentures, hairpieces, and jewelry before the procedure
   d. Have an intravenous line placed
   e. Arrange transportation home when discharged
4. In the surgical suite, the patient assumes a supine position. The face and throat are prepped according to established protocols, and the area is properly draped. Eye pads taped in place protect the eyes from injury. Other positioning and pressure point padding is done as necessary.
5. Intravenous sedation is administered as needed. The nose is sprayed with a topical anesthetic, and a small amount of 1% lidocaine with 1:200,000 aqueous epinephrine is injected into the appropriate areas (unless contraindicated because of allergy or for other reasons) to provide anesthesia and control of bleeding. Refer to Appendix C for intravenous conscious sedation precautions.
6. At the end of the procedure, a 10-ml syringe is filled with antibiotic ointment. A small catheter attached to the syringe tip allows ointment to be directed to the appropriate areas. A small (2-×-2 inches) "mustache dressing" taped to the end of the nose collects secretions and blood. Usually, this dressing can be changed as needed. Nasal packing may be inserted into the nares.
7. Follow guidelines in Chapter 1 for safe, effective, informed *pretest* care.

Patient Aftercare

1. Oral fluids are encouraged after nausea or vomiting has resolved; the patient may experience nausea or vomiting if blood is swallowed, because blood is irritating to the gastrointestinal system.
2. Postprocedural instructions may include the following:
   a. Take prescribed medications as ordered (usually a broad-spectrum antibiotic and pain medication). Soothing gargles may be ordered.
   b. Report excessive bleeding or sinus discharge, unusual pain, fever, nausea or vomiting, or visual problems immediately. Provide patient with phone numbers of hospital and physician and instruct him or her to contact the physician (or the outpatient surgical department or emergency department if unable to reach physician) in the event of an emergency. This process may differ according to various health insurance regulations and protocols.
   c. The patient should not drive or sign legal documents for 24 hours because of the effects of anesthetics and sedation.
3. If the patient has received intravenous sedation, follow the usual cautions involved in the care of any person having this type of sedation. The patient who has received conscious sedation may require closer monitoring, positioning on the side to prevent aspiration, and a longer recovery time than those who receive lacal anesthesia.
4. Interpret test outcomes and counsel appropriately. Numbness of the face may continue for several weeks.

5. Follow guidelines in Chapter 1 for safe, effective, informed *posttest* care. Provide written discharge instructions.

Clinical Alert

1. Sinuses are poorly visualized through routine sinus x-ray films.

2. If sinus problems appear to be related to dental problems, the patient should see a dentist or oral surgeon before sinus endoscopy is performed.

3. Severe nasal-septal deviation must be corrected prior to endoscopy.

4. Potential complications include periorbital bleeding, cerebrospinal fluid leak, cellulitis, visual disturbances, and subcutaneous orbital emphysema.

5. Direct trauma to the nasofrontal duct is associated with increased risk of postoperative stenosis.

BIBLIOGRAPHY ●

Brunner LS, Suddarth DS: The Lippincott Manual of Nursing Practice, 8th ed. Philadelphia, Lippincott, 1996

Clinical News Infection Control, TB and the link to bronchoscopies. AJN 98(4): 9, April 1998 (From) Source: JAMA: 278–1077, 1093–1095, 1111 (editorial), October 1, 1997.

Favaro MS, Pugliese G: Infections transmitted by endoscopy: An international problem. American Journal of Infection Control 24: 343–345, October 1996

Finkelmeier BA: Cardiothoracic Surgical Nursing. Philadelphia, Lippincott, 1995

Finkelstein LE: Infection risks from contaminated endoscopes. AJN 97(2): 56, Feb. 1997

Forsch R: Best bowel prep for flexible sigmoidoscopy. The J of Fam Prac 45(2): 98–106, August 1997

Goroll AH, May LA, Mulley AG Jr (eds): Primary Care Medicine: Office Evaluation and Management of the Adult Patient, 3rd ed. Philadelphia, Lippincott, 1995

Lanser K: Bronchoscopy in respiratory tract disease (review). Internist 22(6): 564–568, 1995

Larson K: Bronchoscopy in respiratory tract diseases (review). Internist 23(6): 564–568, 1995

Lefton HB, Pelchman J, Harnatz A: Colon cancer screening and the evaluation and follow-up of colonic polyps. Primary Care 23(3): 515–523, Sept. 1996

Muller AD & Sonnenberg A: Protection by endoscopy against death from colorectal cancer. Archives of Internal Medicine, 155: 1741–1748, 1995

Norris TE: Esophagogastroduodenoscopy. Primary Care 24(2): 327–340, June 1997

Pierzchajlo K, Ackerman RJ and Vogel RL: Esophagogastroduodenoscopy performed by a family physician, a case series of 793 procedures. J Fam Prac 46(1): 41–46, Jan. 1998

Pierzchajlo K, Ackerman RJ & Vogel RL: Colonoscopy performed by a family physician. The J of Fam Prac 44(5): 473–478, May 1997

Raju T, Steel R, & Ahnja S: Complications of urological laparoscopy. J Urology 156: 6469–6471, August, 1996

Sharma VK et al: Best bowel prep for flexible sigmoidoscopy. Am J Gastroenterology 92: 809–811, 1997

Thompson JM, McFarland GK, Hersch JE, Tucker SG: Clinical Nursing, 3rd ed. St. Louis, Mosby, 1998

13

Ultrasound Studies

Ultrasonography is a noninvasive procedure for visualizing soft tissue structures of the body by recording the reflection of inaudible sound waves directed into the tissues. This diagnostic procedure, which requires very little patient preparation, is now used in many branches of medicine for accurate diagnosis of certain pathologic conditions (Chart 13-1). It may be used diagnostically with the obstetric, gynecologic, or cardiac patient and in patients with abnormal conditions of the kidney, pancreas, gallbladder, lymph nodes, liver, spleen, thyroid, or peripheral blood vessels. Frequently, it is used in conjunction with radiology or nuclear medicine scans. The procedure is relatively quick (often requiring only a few minutes to an hour) and causes little discomfort. No harmful effects have yet been established at the low intensities that are used (<100 mW/cm^2). However, as with any diagnostic procedure, ultrasound should not be used frivolously. The terms *ultrasound* and *sonogram* are used interchangeably.

Principles and Technique

Ultrasound uses high-frequency sound waves to produce an "echo map" that characterizes the position, size, form, and nature of soft tissue organs. Echoes of varying strength are produced by different types of tissues and are displayed as a visual pattern after computer processing of the echo information. The capability of acquiring real-time images means that ultrasound can readily demonstrate motion, as in the fetus or the heart. Ultrasound, however, cannot appropriately image air-filled structures such as the lungs.

Doppler Method

A phenomenon that accompanies movement, the *Doppler effect,* can be combined with diagnostic ultrasound imaging to produce *duplex scans.* Duplex scans provide anatomic visualization of blood vessels and a graphic representation of blood flow characteristics. Flow direction, velocity, and the presence of flow disturbances can readily be assessed. *Color Doppler* imaging provides a color-coded depiction of selected blood flow parameters. The newest technology (known as *color Doppler energy, power Doppler,* or *color angio*) is sensitive to very low blood velocity states. These techniques establish the patency of a given blood vessel and are useful in investigating perfusion to an organ or mass. They are also helpful in evaluating complications in transplanted organs.

Procedure

1. A gel or lubricant is applied to the skin over the area to be examined to conduct the sound waves.
2. An operator, known as a *sonographer,* holds a microphone-like device called a *transducer.* The transducer is moved over a specific body part, producing a display that is viewed on the monitor.
3. Sonography of structures in the abdominal region often require the patient to control breathing patterns. Deep inspiration and exhalation may be used.
4. Selected images are recorded for documentation purposes.
5. The examination causes no physical pain. However, in certain applications,

CHART 13-1 ▶
Uses of Ultrasound

Obstetrical ultrasound: Commonly performed to evaluate fetal health, size, and number of fetuses, level of amniotic fluid, and maternal and placental anatomy.

Abdominal ultrasound: Used to characterize soft tissue organs, including
Hepatobiliary: to evaluate organ size and presence of masses, calculi, or diffuse parenchymal conditions. Doppler ultrasound is helpful in demonstrating signs of portal hypertension.
Pancreas: to detect pathologic states such as tumor involvement, pseudocysts, and inflammatory processes.
Kidneys: to diagnose cysts, masses, hydronephrosis, and certain diffuse conditions. Doppler evaluation of the renal vessels and parenchyma is commonly used to evaluate transplanted kidneys and in the staging of known renal cell carcinoma.
Aorta and other large abdominal vessels: to detect aneurysms, the presence of clots or tumors, and other defects.
Spleen and lymph nodes: to evaluate organ size and pathologic states such as lymphoma and metastatic spread of known cancers.
Additional structures: to demonstrate suspected ascites, abscesses, retroperitoneal tumors, and signs of appendicitis.

Pelvic ultrasound: Gynecologic scan is done to evaluate the urinary bladder, uterus, and ovaries. Is used to monitor follicle development during infertility treatments and also as a guide for oocyte retrieval.

Male reproductive organs sonogram: Used to evaluate scrotal masses and swelling and combined with Doppler examination of the penis to detect physiologic causes for male impotence. Transrectal ultrasound is an accepted method of screening for prostatic disease.

Head and neck sonograms: Used to evaluate pathologies in the following structures:
Thyroid and parathyroid: for differentiating cysts from solid tumors.
Carotid and vertebral arteries: to demonstrate vessel patency and flow patterns.
Eye: to assist ophthalmologist in the removal of foreign bodies and in the evaluation of the eye's structure.
Neonatal brain: to diagnose cerebral hemorrhage and other intracranial pathologies.
Adult cerebral blood flow: by using a method known as transcranial Doppler, the larger blood vessels within the brain may be interrogated to rule out vascular disturbances.

Breast sonograms: Performed to differentiate cysts from solid lesions and to guide cyst aspirations and needle biopsies.

(continued)

CHART 13-1 *(continued)*

Extremities sonograms: Used to evaluate arterial and venous blood flow and to characterize soft tissue masses such as Baker's cysts. Sonography is often used to evaluate the pediatric hip for dislocations or other structural deformities.

Invasive procedures: Serve as a guide for diagnostic procedures, such as amniocentesis, thoracentesis, and biopsy.

Heart sonograms: Performed to evaluate the cardiac structure and blood flow through chambers and valves.

---

pressure may be applied to the transducer, causing some degree of discomfort. Long examinations may leave the patient feeling tired.

6. Tests usually take 20 to 45 minutes. This is the actual procedure time and does not include waiting and preparation times.

7. Some examinations require the patient to fast or to have a filled urinary bladder. Each examining department determines its own guidelines for patient preparation.

Advances in technology have allowed the development of very small, high-resolution transducers. Catheter-sized transducers are used to visualize blood vessels "from the inside out" during angiographic procedures. Small transducers passed through the esophagus permit exquisite visualization of the heart during transesophageal echocardiography (TEE). Slim transducers are introduced into the vagina to visualize gynecologic anatomy. Transrectal visualization of the prostate gland is an accepted method of screening for disease in that organ. Of course, before introduction into the body, these small transducers are properly cleansed and/or draped.

Benefits and Risks of Ultrasound Studies

1. It is a noninvasive procedure with no radiation risk for patient or examiner.

2. It requires little, if any, patient preparation and aftercare (Chart 13-2).

3. As far as is known, the examination can be repeated as often as necessary without being injurious to patient. No harmful cumulative effect has been seen.

4. Because ultrasound studies demonstrate structure rather than function, they may be useful for patients whose organ function is impaired.

5. Ultrasound is useful in the detection and examination of moving parts, such as the heart.

6. It does not require the injection of contrast materials or isotopes or ingestion of opaque materials.

Disadvantages of Ultrasound Studies

1. An extremely skilled examiner is required to operate the transducer. The scans should be read immediately and interpreted for adequacy. If the scans are not satisfactory, the examination must be repeated.

CHART 13-2
Patient Preparation for Ultrasound Studies*

EXAMINATION (TYPE OF SONOGRAM)	NPO 8 HR BEFORE STUDY	NO SMOKING 2 HR BEFORE STUDY	FULL BLADDER	NO PREPARATION	FLEET ENEMA
Obstetric (fetal age)			×		
Fetal Doppler echocardiogram			×		
Pelvic/Gynecologic			×	× (transvaginal)	
Renal			×	×	
Urinary bladder			×		
Hepatobiliary	× (last meal preferably low-fat)				
Abdominal aorta	× (last meal preferably low-fat)				
Breast				×	
Prostate					×

(continued)

CHART 13-2 *(continued)*
Patient Preparation for Ultrasound Studies*

EXAMINATION (TYPE OF SONOGRAM)	NPO 8 HR BEFORE STUDY	NO SMOKING 2 HR BEFORE STUDY	FULL BLADDER	NO PREPARATION	FLEET ENEMA
Scrotal				X	
Eye and Orbit				X	
Thyroid				X	
Carotid (cerebrovascular)		X			
Lower extremity arterial and upper extremity arterial		X			
Ankle brachial index		X			
Lower extremity venous and upper extremity venous		X			
Doppler echocardiogram					
Transesophageal echocardiogram	X				X

*Always consult with the laboratory for specific instructions. X means yes.

2. Air-filled structures (eg, lungs) cannot be studied by ultrasonography.
3. Certain patients (eg, restless children, extremely obese patients) cannot be studied adequately unless they are specially prepared.

Difficult-to-Study Patients

The following general categories of patients may provide some difficulties in ultrasound studies:

1. *Postoperative patients and those with abdominal scars:* The area surrounding an incision is to be avoided whenever possible. If a scan must be performed over an incision, the dressing must be removed and a sterile coupling agent and probe must be employed.
2. *Children and agitated adults:* Because the procedure requires the patient to remain still, some patients may need to be sedated so that their movements do not cause artifacts.
3. *Obese patients:* Certain patients cannot be studied adequately in any case. For example, it may be difficult to obtain an accurate scan on a very obese patient, owing to alteration of the sound beam by fatty tissue. There is no preparation that would help here.

Interfering Factors

1. Barium has an adverse effect on the quality of abdominal studies, so sonograms should be scheduled before barium studies are done.
2. If the patient has a large amount of gas in the bowel, the examination may be rescheduled, because air (bowel gas) is a very strong reflector of sound and does not permit accurate visualization.

● OBSTETRIC AND GYNECOLOGIC SONOGRAMS

OBSTETRIC SONOGRAM ●

Normal Sonogram

Normal image of placental position, size, and structure
Normal fetal position and size with evidence of fetal movement, cardiac activity, and breathing activity
Adequate amniotic fluid volume
Normal fetal intracranial, thoracic, and abdominopelvic anatomy; 4 limbs visualized

Explanation of Test

Ultrasound studies of the obstetric patient are valuable in (1) confirming pregnancy; (2) facilitating amniocentesis by locating a suitable pool of amniotic fluid; (3) determining fetal age; (4) confirming multiple pregnancy; (5) ascertaining whether fetal growth is normal, through sequential studies; (6) determining fetal viability; (7) localizing the placenta; (8) confirming masses associated with pregnancy; and (9) identifying postmature pregnancy (increased amount of amniotic fluid and degree of placental calcification). A pregnancy can be dated with considerable accuracy if 1 sonogram is done at 20 weeks and a follow-up scan is done at 32 weeks. This validation is most important when early delivery is anticipated and prematurity is to be avoided. Conditions in which determination of pregnancy duration is useful include maternal diabetes, Rh immunization, preterm labor, and any medical condition that is worsening with the progress of labor (Tables 13-1, 13-2, and 13-3).

The pregnant uterus is ideal for echographic evaluation because the amniotic fluid–filled uterus provides strong transmitting interfaces between the fluid, the placenta, and the fetus. Ultrasonography has become the method of choice for evaluating the fetus and placenta, eliminating the need for the potentially injurious radiographic studies that were used previously.

Procedure

1. The pregnant woman lies on her back with her abdomen exposed during the test. This may cause some shortness of breath and supine hypotensive syndrome, which can be relieved by elevating the upper body or turning the patient onto her side.
2. *Transabdominal scan:* In the second trimester, the examination usually is performed while the patient has a full bladder. Exceptions are made when the scan is performed to locate the placenta before amniocentesis, for evaluation of an incompetent cervix, or during labor and delivery. A full bladder allows the examiner to assess the true position of the placenta, repositions the uterus and cervix for better visibility, serves as a reference point, and acts as a sonic window to the pelvic organs.
3. A coupling agent (special transmission gel, lotion, or mineral oil) is applied liberally to the skin to prevent air from absorbing sound waves. The sonographer slowly moves the transducer over the entire abdomen to obtain a picture of the uterine contents.
4. *Endovaginal (transvaginal) scan:* During the first trimester, some laboratories use a transvaginal approach when performing obstetric sonograms. This method does not require a full bladder. A slim transducer, properly covered and lubricated, is gently introduced into the vagina. Because the sound waves do not need to traverse abdominal tissue, exquisite image detail is produced. Check with your laboratory to determine the approach to be used.
5. The examining time is about 30 to 60 minutes.
6. For all procedures, see Chapter 1 guidelines for *intratest* care.

Clinical Implications

1. During the *first trimester,* the following information can be obtained:
   A. Number, size, and location of gestational sacs
   B. Presence or absence of fetal cardiac activity and body movement
   C. Presence or absence of uterine abnormalities (eg, bicornuate uterus, fibroids) or adnexal masses (eg, ovarian cyst, ectopic pregnancy)

TABLE 13-1
Major Uses of Obstetric Ultrasound—Levels I and II*

INDICATIONS DURING FIRST TRIMESTER	INDICATIONS DURING SECOND TRIMESTER
Confirm pregnancy	Establish or confirm dates[†]
Confirm viability	If no fetal heart tones
Rule out ectopic pregnancy	Clarify discrepancy between
Confirm gestational age[†]	dates and size
Birth control pill use	If large for dates, rule out
Irregular menses	Poor estimate of dates
No dates	Molar pregnancy
Postpartum pregnancy	Multiple gestation
Previous complicated pregnancy	Leiomyomata
Caesarean delivery	Polyhydramnios
Rh incompatibility	Congenital anomalies
Diabetes mellitus	If small for dates, rule out
Fetal growth retardation	Poor estimate of dates
Clarify discrepancy between	Fetal growth retardation
dates and size	Congenital anomalies
If large for dates, rule out	Oligohydramnios
Leiomyomata	If history of bleeding, rule out
Bicornuate uterus	total placenta previa
Adnexal mass	If Rh incompatibility, rule out fetal
Multiple gestation	hydrops
Poor estimate of dates	
Missed abortion	
Blighted ovum	

**INDICATIONS DURING
THIRD TRIMESTER**

If no fetal heart tones	Poor estimate of dates[‡]
Clarify discrepancy between	Determine fetal position—
dates and size	rule out
If large for dates, rule out	Breech
Macrosomia (diabetes	Transverse lie
mellitus)	If history of bleeding, rule out
Multiple gestation	Placenta previa
Polyhydramnios	Abruptio placentae
Congenital anomalies	Determine fetal lung maturity
Poor estimate of dates*	Amniocentesis for lecithin/
If small for dates, rule out	sphingomyelin ratio
Fetal growth retardation	Placental maturity (grade 0–3)
Oligohydramnios	
Congenital anomalies	

T[†]Accuracy ± 3 days
[‡]Accuracy ± 1 to 1.5 days
*Ultrasound is a diagnostic tool for assessment of fetal age, health, and growth. Level I ultrasound is performed to assess gestational age, number of fetuses, fetal viability, and the placenta. Level II ultrasound is used for assessment of specific congenital anomalies or abnormalities. (See also Fetal Echocardiography, page 915.)

D. Pregnancy dating (eg, biparietal diameter, crown-rump length)

E. Presence and location of an intrauterine device

2. During the *second* and *third trimesters,* ultrasound can be performed to obtain the following information:

   A. Fetal viability, number, position, gestational age, growth pattern, and structural abnormalities

   B. Amniotic fluid volume

   C. Placental location, maturity, and abnormalities

   D. Uterine fibroids and anomalies

   E. Adnexal masses

   F. Early diagnosis of fetal structural abnormalities makes the following choices possible:

   (1) Intrauterine surgery or other prenatal therapy if possible

   (2) Discontinuation of pregnancy

   (3) Preparation of the family for care of a child with a disorder or planning of other options.

3. *Fetal viability:* Fetal heart activity can be demonstrated as early as 5 weeks of gestation in most cases. This information is helpful in establishing dates and in the management of vaginal bleeding. Molar pregnancies and incomplete, complete, and missed abortions can be differentiated.

4. *Gestational age:* Indications for gestational age evaluation include uncertain dates for the last menstrual period, recent discontinuation of oral hormonal suppression of ovulation, bleeding episode during the first trimester, amenorrhea of at least 3 months' duration, uterine size that does not agree with dates, previous cesarean birth, and other high-risk conditions.

5. *Fetal growth:* The conditions that serve as indicators for ultrasound assessment of fetal growth include poor maternal weight gain or pattern of weight gain, previous intrauterine growth retardation (IUGR), chronic infection, ingestion of drugs such as anticonvulsants or heroin, maternal diabetes, pregnancy-induced or other hypertension, multiple pregnancy, and other medical or surgical complications. Serial evaluation of biparietal diameter and limb length can help differentiate between wrong dates and IUGR. Doppler evaluation of the umbilical artery, uterine artery, and fetal aorta can also assist in the detection of IUGR. IUGR can be symmetric (the fetus is small in all measurements) or asymmetric (head and body growth vary). Symmetric IUGR may be caused by low genetic growth potential, intrauterine infection, maternal undernutrition, heavy smoking by the mother, or chromosomal aberration. Asymmetric IUGR may reflect placental insufficiency secondary to hypertension, cardiovascular disease, or renal disease. Depending on the probable cause, the therapy varies.

6. *Fetal anatomy:* Depending on the gestational age, the following structures may be identified: intracranial anatomy, neck, spine, heart, stomach, small

text continues on page 913

TABLE 13-2
Measurements Timetable

Parameter	Advantages	Disadvantages	When to Use	Predictive Accuracy (±2 Standard Deviations [SD])
Embryonic heart rate (EHR) before 9.2 wk after last menstrual period (LMP)	High accuracy, easy; predictive of first-trimester outcome	Not available after 9.2 wk, after LMP; requires M-mode	5–9.2 wk after LMP	±6 d ±0.8 d ±10.0% AA
3-D biparietal diameter correction—average, 3 cranial diameters	High accuracy in late pregnancy; encourages close neurologic observation	Requires 3 cranial measurements	Use when head shape or molding affects cranial measurements	±1 wk ±0.9 wk ±3.6% AA
Fractional spine (FSL); 7 thoracolumbar vertebral spaces and bodies	Easy when fetus in prone position	Relatively low accuracy; fetal position can make measurements impossible	15 wk after LMP to term	±3.5 wk ±3.4 wk ±1.3 % AA

Bernes M. Diagnostic medical sonography, a guide to clinical practice. In Allen M, Kawamura DM, Craig M et al (eds): Obstetrics and Gynecology. Philadelphia, JB Lippincott, p. 368, 1997.

TABLE 13-3
Accuracy of Obstetric Measurements

Parameter	Advantages	Disadvantages	When to Use	Predictive Accuracy (± 2 Standard Deviations [SD])
Gestational sac diameter (GSD)	Easiest measurement early in gestation	High variability of measurements, low accuracy	Before 8 wk after LMP	±2 wk ±0.9 wk ±11.5% AA
Crown–rump length (CRL)	Highest accuracy early in gestation; easy to obtain	Not available after first trimester	5–15 wk after LMP	±3–5 d ±0.7 wk ±3.2% AA
Transverse head circumference (THC)	Requires only 2 measurements; accepted as standard	Does not reflect vertical cranial diameter molding	12 wk after LMP to term if cranial shape is normal	±1.0 wk ±1.0 wk ±3.7% AA
Biparietal diameter (BPD)	Easy to obtain; low interoperator error	Affected by cranial shape and molding	9–33 wk after LMP if cranial shape is normal	±2 wk ±1.2 wk ±4.3% AA
Binocular distance (BiOD)	Occasionally easy when fetus faces up and BPD is difficult	Relatively low accuracy; fetal position can make measurements impossible	15–30 wk after LMP	±3.3 wk ±1.7 wk ±6.6% AA
Cerebellum (CERB)	Encourages close neurologic observation	Relatively low accuracy; difficult to obtain early or late in gestation	18–35 wk after LMP	±3 wk ±2.7 wk ±6.5% AA
Abdominal circumference (AC)	Important for fetal weight and health	Interoperator variability and fetal position may affect accuracy	12 wk after LMP to term	±3.5 wk ±1.8 wk ±5.9% AA

(continued)

TABLE 13-3 *(Continued)*

Parameter	Advantages	Disadvantages	When to Use	Predictive Accuracy (± 2 SD ±%AA)
Femoral length (FemL)	Relatively easy to obtain	Fetal motion may make measurements difficult	14 wk after LMP to term	±3.4 wk ±1.7 wk ±6.2% AA
Humeral length (HumL)	Relatively easy to obtain	Fetal motion may make measurements difficult	14 wk after LMP to term	±3.8 wk ±1.8 wk ±6.4% AA
Last normal menstrual period (LNMP) by menstrual history	Often the only independent date available for a pregnancy	Very low accuracy; often unknown or unreliable	When available, use only for comparable ages	±4.0 wk ±4.9 wk ±33.7% AA

Bernes M. Diagnostic medical sonography, a guide to clinical practice. In Allen M, Kawamura DM, Craig M et al (eds): Obstetrics and Gynecology. Philadelphia, JB Lippincott, p. 368, 1997.

bowel, liver, kidneys, bladder, and extremities. Structural defects may be identified before delivery. The following are examples of structural defects that may be diagnosed by ultrasound: hydrocephaly, anencephaly, and myelomeningocele are often associated with polyhydramnios. Potter's syndrome (renal agenesis) is associated with oligohydramniosis. These can be diagnosed before 20 weeks of gestation, as can skeletal defects (dwarfism, achondroplasia, osteogenesis imperfecta) and diaphragmatic hernias. Other structural anomalies that can be diagnosed by ultrasound are pleural effusion (after 20 weeks), intestinal atresias or obstructions (early pregnancy to second trimester), hydronephrosis and bladder outlet obstruction (second trimester to term with fetal surgery available). Two-dimensional studies of the heart, together with echocardiography, allow diagnosis of congenital cardiac lesions and prenatal treatment of cardiac arrhythmias.

7. *Detection of fetal death:* Inability to visualize the fetal heart beating and separation of bones in the fetal head are signs of death. With real-time scanning, the absence of cardiac motion for 3 minutes is diagnostic of fetal demise.

8. *Placental position and function:* The site of implantation (eg, anterior, posterior, fundal, in lower segment) can be described, as can location of the placenta on the other side of midline. The pattern of uterine and placental growth and the fullness of the bladder influence the apparent location of the placenta. For example, when ultrasound scanning is done in the second trimester, the placenta seems to be overlying the os in 15% to 20% of all pregnancies. At term, however, the evidence of placenta previa is only 0.5%. Therefore, the diagnosis of placenta previa can seldom be confirmed until the third trimester. Placenta abruptio (premature separation of placenta) can also be identified.

9. *Fetal well-being:* The following physiologic measurements can be accomplished with ultrasound: heart rate and regularity, fetal breathing movements, urine production (after serial measurements of bladder volume), fetal limb and head movements, and analysis of vascular wave forms from fetal circulation. Fetal breathing movements are decreased with maternal smoking and alcohol use and increased with hyperglycemia. Fetal limb and head movements serve as an index of neurologic development. Identification of amniotic fluid pockets is also used to evaluate fetal status. A pocket of amniotic fluid measuring at least 1 cm is associated with normal fetal status. The presence of 1 pocket measuring <1 cm or the absence of a pocket is abnormal; it is associated with increased risk of perinatal death.

10. *Assessment of multiple pregnancy:* Two or more gestational sacs, each containing an embryo, may be seen after 6 weeks. Of twin pregnancies diagnosed in the first trimester, only about 30% will deliver twins, owing to loss or absorption of 1 fetus. Of value is assessment of the relative fetal growth of twins when IUGR or twin-to-twin transfusion is sus-

pected. One cannot unequivocally diagnose whether twins are monozygotes or heterozygotes with ultrasound alone unless fetuses of opposite sex are evident. Routine ultrasound cannot totally be relied on to exclude the possibility of triplets or quadruplets, instead of only twins.

11. If the fetal position and amniotic fluid volumes are favorable, fetal sex can be determined by visualization of the genitalia. It must be cautioned, however, that sex determination is not the purpose of obstetric sonography.

Interfering Factors

1. Artifacts can be produced when the transducer is moved out of contact with the skin. This can be resolved by adding more coupling agent to the skin and repeating the scan.

2. Artifacts (reverberation) may be produced by echoes emanating from the same surface several times. This can be avoided by careful positioning of the transducer.

3. A posterior placental site may be difficult to identify because of the angulation of the reflecting surface or insufficient penetration of the sound beam due to the patient's size.

Patient Preparation

1. A brief explanation of the procedure to be performed is given, emphasizing that it is not uncomfortable or painful and that it does not involve ionizing radiation that might be harmful to the mother or fetus. The studies can be repeated without harm, but the procedure is being studied carefully to determine whether there are any long-term adverse side effects. Benefits of the procedure should be explained.

2. Most studies are performed via a transabdominal approach with a full bladder. The patient is asked to drink 5 or 6 glasses of fluid (water or juice) approximately 1 to 2 hours before the examination. If she is unable to do so, intravenous fluids may be administered. She is asked to refrain from voiding until the examination is complete. Tell the patient that she will have a strong urge to void during the examination. Discomfort caused by pressure applied over a full bladder may be experienced. If the bladder is not sufficiently filled, three to four 8-oz glasses of water should be ingested, with rescanning done 30 to 45 minutes later.

3. Some laboratories use a transvaginal (endovaginal) approach during the first trimester of pregnancy. No patient preparation is required for this method. Contact the laboratory performing the study to determine the method to be used.

4. Explain that a liberal coating of coupling agent must be applied to the skin so that there is no air between the skin and the transducer and to allow for easy movement of the transducer over the skin. A sensation of warmth or wetness may be felt. Although the acoustic couplant does not stain, advise the patient not to wear good clothing for the examination.

5. The woman may face the screen, and the sonographer may explain the images in basic terms. In some institutions, the father is encouraged to observe the testing. A photograph or videotape for the family to keep is sometimes provided.

6. See Chapter 1 guidelines for safe, effective, informed pretest care.

Clinical Alert

1. A full bladder may not be needed or desired for patients in the late stages of pregnancy or active labor. However, if a full bladder is required and the woman has not been instructed to report with a full bladder, at least another hour of waiting time may be needed before the examination can begin.

2. A transvaginal (endovaginal) scan does not require the patient to have a full bladder. Contact the laboratory to determine method to be used.

3. Endovaginal studies typically involve the use of a latex condom to sheath the transducer before it is inserted into the vaginal vault. Contact the laboratory if the patient has a known or suspected latex sensitivity.

4. Fetal age determinations are most accurate during the crown-rump stage in the first trimester. The next most accurate time for age estimation is during the second trimester. Sonographic dating during the third trimester has a large margin of error (up to ± 3 weeks).

FETAL ECHOCARDIOGRAPHY (FETAL DOPPLER) ●

Normal Sonogram

Normal structure of heart and great vessels

Normal heart rate and rhythm, with proper hemodynamic flow through heart and great valves

Explanation of Test

This procedure is performed after the detection of a potential cardiac abnormality during an obstetric sonogram. Not a screening procedure, fetal echocardiograms are most commonly performed in specialized laboratories or teaching hospitals. The heart is imaged in numerous planes, using Doppler and M-mode tracings (see Heart Sonogram, page 943), similar to an electrocardiogram. Valves and other cardiac structures are measured, and blood velocities and volumes are calculated.

Procedure

1. The fetal echocardiogram is performed in the same manner as a routine obstetric scan and requires similar patient preparation. The pregnant patient lies on her back with the abdomen exposed. Couplant is applied to the skin, and a transducer is moved across the abdomen. Unless combined with an obstetric sonogram, the fetal echocardiogram does not require the mother to have a full bladder.
2. For all procedures, see Chapter 1 guidelines for *intratest* care.

Clinical Implications

Abnormalities detected during fetal echocardiography include

1. Cardiac arrhythmias
2. Septal defects, including tetralogy of Fallot
3. Hypoplastic heart syndrome
4. Valvular abnormalities, including Ebstein's anomaly
5. Cardiac tumors
6. Vessel abnormalities, including coarctation of the aorta, transposition, and truncus arteriosus

Interfering Factors

Same as for obstetric sonogram.

Patient Preparation

Same as for obstetric sonogram.

Patient Aftercare

Same as for obstetric sonogram.

PELVIC GYNECOLOGIC (GYN) SONOGRAM; PELVIC (UTERINE MASS) ULTRASOUND DIAGNOSIS; INTRAUTERINE DEVICE (IUD) LOCALIZATION ●

Normal Sonogram

Normal pattern image of bladder, uterus, fallopian tubes, and vagina

Explanation of Test

This pelvic ultrasound study examines the area from the umbilicus to the pubic bone in women. It may be used in the evaluation of pelvic masses, to determine the position of an intrauterine contraceptive device (IUD), to evaluate postmenopausal bleeding, or to aid in the diagnosis of cysts and tumors. Information can be provided on the size, location, and structure of masses. The examination cannot provide a definitive diagnosis of pathology but can be used as an adjunct procedure when the diagnosis is not readily apparent. It is also used in treatment planning and follow-up radiation therapy for gynecologic cancer. Additionally, follicle development after infertility treatment can be monitored.

This test may be performed via a transvaginal (endovaginal) or transabdominal approach. With the transvaginal method, a slim, covered, lubricated transducer is gently introduced into the vagina. A full bladder is not required. Because the sound waves do not need to traverse abdominal tissue, exquisite image detail is produced. This approach is most advantageous for examining the obese patient, the patient with a retroverted uterus, or the patient who has difficulty maintaining bladder distention. The transvaginal method is the approach of choice in monitoring follicular size during fertility workups and during aspiration of follicles for in vitro fertilization.

For pelvic sonograms using the transabdominal approach, a full bladder is necessary. The distended bladder serves 4 purposes. It acts as a "window" for transmission of the ultrasound beam; it pushes the uterus away from the pubic symphysis, thereby providing a less obstructed view; it pushes the bowel out of the pelvis; and it may be used as a reference for comparison in evaluating the internal characteristics of a mass under study.

Procedure

TRANSABDOMINAL METHOD

1. The patient lies on the back on the examining table during the test.
2. A coupling agent is applied to the area under study.
3. The active face of the transducer is placed in contact with patient's skin and swept across the area being studied.
4. Examination time is about 30 minutes.

TRANSVAGINAL (ENDOVAGINAL) METHOD

1. The patient lies on an examining table with hips slightly elevated in a modified lithotomy position. The patient is draped.
2. A slim vaginal transducer, protected by a condom or sterile sheath, is lubricated and introduced into the vagina. Some laboratories prefer that the patient insert the transducer herself. A depth of <8 cm is all that is usually required.
3. Scans are performed by using a slight rotation or movement of the handle and by varying the degree of transducer insertion. Typically, the transducer is inserted only a few inches into the vaginal vault.
4. Examination time is about 15 to 30 minutes.
5. For all procedures, see Chapter 1 guidelines for *intratest* care.

Clinical Implications

1. Uterine abnormalities such as fibroids, intrauterine fluid collections, and variations in structure such as bicornuate uterus can be detected. Uterine

and cervical carcinomas may be visualized, although definitive diagnosis of cancer cannot be made by sonography alone.

2. Very small adnexal masses may not be demonstrated by ultrasound studies. Masses identified on ultrasound may be evaluated in terms of size and consistency.

3. *Cysts*

   A. Ovarian cysts (the most common ovarian mass detected by ultrasound) appear as smoothly outlined, well-defined masses. Cysts cannot be confirmed as either malignant or benign, but ultrasound studies can increase the suspicion that a particular mass is malignant.

   B. A corpus luteum cyst is a single, simple cyst commonly visualized in early pregnancy.

   C. Theca-lutein cysts are associated with hydatidiform mole, choriocarcinoma, or multiple pregnancy.

   D. Because normal ovaries often have numerous visible small cysts, the diagnosis of polycystic ovaries is difficult to make on the basis of ultrasound alone.

   E. Dermoid cysts or benign ovarian teratomas may be found in young adult women and have an extremely variable appearance. Because of their echogenicity, they are often missed on ultrasound. The only initial clue may be an indentation of the urinary bladder. When a dermoid cyst is suspected on ultrasound, a pelvic radiograph should be obtained.

4. Solid ovarian tumors such as fibromas, fibrosarcomas, Brenner's tumors, dysgerminomas, and malignant teratomas are not distinguishable by diagnostic ultrasound. Ultrasound documents the presence of a solid lesion but can go no further in narrowing the diagnosis.

5. Metastatic tumors of the ovary are common and may be solid or cystic in ultrasonic appearance. They are variable in size and are usually bilateral. Because ascites is often present, the pelvis and remainder of the abdomen should be scanned for fluid.

6. *Pelvic inflammatory disease:* Ultrasound differentiation between pelvic inflammatory disease and endometriosis is difficult. Evaluation of laboratory results and the clinical history leads to correct diagnosis. Other entities that may have similar ultrasonic presentations include appendicitis with rupture into the pelvis, chronic ectopic pregnancy, posttraumic hemorrhage into the pelvis, and pelvic abscesses from various causes (eg, Crohn's disease, diverticulitis).

7. *Bladder distortion:* Any distortion of the bladder raises the possibility of an adjacent mass. Tumor, infection, and hemorrhage are the major causes of increased thickness of the urinary bladder wall. Masses such as calculi and catheters may be seen within the bladder lumen. Urinary bladder calculi are highly echogenic. A urinary bladder diverticulum appears as a cystic mass adjacent to the urinary bladder. It may be mistaken for a cystic mass arising from some other pelvic structure, so attempts are made to demonstrate its communication to the bladder.

8. Ultrasound studies can help to determine whether a pelvic mass is mobile.

9. Solid pelvic masses such as fibroids and malignant tumors may be differentiated from cystic masses, which show sound patterns similar to those of the bladder.
10. Lesions may be shown to have metastasized.
11. Studies may aid in the planning of tumor radiation therapy.
12. The position of an IUD may be determined.

Interfering Factors

1. Results may be only fair, may vary with the patient's habits and preparation (as described in Clinical Implications), and can be used only in conjunction with other studies. However, masses 1 cm and smaller can be seen with high-resolution equipment.
2. The success of a transabdominal scan depends on full bladder distention.

Patient Preparation

1. Explain the purpose and procedure of the test. Fasting is not required.
2. For transabdominal scans, have the patient drink 4 glasses of water or other liquid 1 hour before the examination. Advise the patient not to void until the test is over.
3. If a transvaginal (endovaginal) approach is to be used, no patient preparation is required. Contact the laboratory performing the study to determine method to be used.
4. Explain that a liberal coating of coupling agent must be applied to the skin so that there is no air between the skin and the transducer and to allow for easy movement of the transducer over the skin. A sensation of warmth or wetness may be felt. Although the acoustic couplant does not stain, advise the patient not to wear good clothing for the examination.
5. If a transvaginal (endovaginal) approach is to be used, determine whether the patient has a latex sensitivity and communicate such sensitivities to the examining laboratory. See latex precautions in Appendix B.
6. Reassure the patient that she will have no pain or discomfort.
7. See Chapter 1 guidelines regarding safe, effective, informed *pretest* care.

Clinical Alert

1. If the patient is taking nothing by mouth (NPO) or in certain emergency situations, the patient may be catheterized and the bladder filled via the catheter.
2. Endovaginal studies, when indicated, typically involve the use of a latex condom to sheath the transducer before it is inserted into the vaginal vault. Contact the laboratory if the patient has a known or suspected latex sensitivity. See Appendix B regarding latex precautions.

Patient Aftercare

1. Interpret test outcomes and counsel appropriately.
2. Follow Chapter 1 guidelines for safe, effective, informed *posttest* care.

● ABDOMINAL SONOGRAMS

KIDNEY (RENAL) SONOGRAM ●

Normal Sonogram
Normal pattern image indicating normal size and position of kidneys

Explanation of Test
This noninvasive test is used to visualize kidney parenchyma and associated structures, including renal blood vessels. This procedure is often performed after an intravenous pyelogram (IVP) to define and characterize mass lesions or the cause of a nonvisualized kidney. Because no contrast medium is administered, renal ultrasound is valuable for visualizing the kidneys of patients with iodine hypersensitivities. This procedure is also helpful in monitoring the status of a transplanted kidney, guiding stent and biopsy needle placement, and evaluating the progression of chronic conditions.

Procedure
1. The patient lies quietly on an examining table. Scans are often performed with the patient in the decubitus position.
2. Warm oil or gel is applied to the patient's skin.
3. For visualization of the upper parts of the kidney, the patient must inspire as deeply as possible.
4. The total study time varies from 15 to 30 minutes.
5. For all procedures, see Chapter 1 guidelines for *intratest* care.

Clinical Implications
1. Abnormal pattern readings reveal
   A. Cysts
   B. Solid masses
   C. Hydronephrosis
   D. Obstruction of ureters
   E. Calculi
2. Results provide information on the size, site, and internal structure of a nonfunctioning kidney.
3. Results differentiate between bilateral hydronephrosis, polycystic kidneys, and the small, end-stage kidneys of glomerulonephritis or pyelonephritis.
4. Results may be used to monitor kidney development in children with congenital hydronephrosis. This approach is safer than repeated IVP studies.
5. Perirenal fluid collections such as those associated with complications of transplantation may be detected. These collections include abscesses, hematomas, urinomas, and lymphoceles.
6. Solid lesions may be differentiated from cystic lesions.
7. The spread of cancerous conditions from the kidney into the renal vein or inferior vena cava can be detected.
8. If ultrasound is combined with Doppler evaluation, the patency and flow characteristics of the renal vessels may be scrutinized.

Interfering Factors

1. Retained barium from radiology studies causes poor results.
2. Obesity adversely affects tissue visualization.

Patient Preparation

1. Explain the purpose and procedure of the test.
2. Assure the patient that there is no pain involved; the only discomfort is that caused by lying quietly for a long period.
3. Explain that a liberal coating of coupling agent must be applied to the skin so that there is no air between the skin and the transducer and to allow for easy movement of the transducer over the skin. A sensation of warmth or wetness may be felt. Although the acoustic couplant does not stain, advise the patient not to wear good clothing for the examination.
4. Explain that the patient will be instructed to control breathing patterns while the images are being made.
5. Fasting usually is not necessary but may be required in certain laboratories. Check with your ultrasound department for guidelines.
6. See Chapter 1 guidelines for safe, effective, informed *pretest* care.

Patient Aftercare

1. Interpret test outcomes and counsel appropriately.
2. Follow Chapter 1 guidelines for safe, effective, informed *posttest* care.

Clinical Alert

1. Scans cannot be done over open wounds or dressings.
2. This examination must be performed before radiographic studies involving barium. If such scheduling is not possible, at least 24 hours must elapse between the barium procedure and the renal echogram.
3. Biopsies are often done with ultrasound as a guide. If a biopsy is to be done, a surgical permit must be signed by the patient.

URINARY BLADDER SONOGRAM

Normal Sonogram

Normal pattern image of the exact dimensions and contour of the bladder and little residual volume

Explanation of Test

This examination is done as part of the investigation of possible bladder tumor and provides a simple method of estimating postvoid residual urine volume. This test reduces the need for urinary catheterization and the risk of subsequent urinary tract infection.

Procedure

1. The patient, with bladder fully distended, is instructed to lie on the back on an examination table.

2. A coupling agent is applied to the anterior pelvic region to allow maximum penetration of the ultrasound beam.
3. The active face of the transducer is placed in contact with the patient's skin and swept across the area being studied.
4. Typically, when the full-bladder scans are completed, the patient is instructed to void. Additional images are then taken to check for residual volume.
5. Total examination time is about 20 to 30 minutes.
6. For all procedures, see Chapter 1 guidelines for *intratest* care.

Clinical Implications
Abnormal results reveal the following:
   A. Tumors of bladder
   B. Cancerous extension to urinary bladder
   C. Thickening of bladder wall
   D. Masses posterior to bladder
   E. Ureterocele

Interfering Factors
1. Residual barium from previous radiology studies affects test results.
2. Overlying gas or fat tissue affects test results.

Patient Preparation
1. Explain the purpose and procedure of the test.
2. The bladder should be full at the beginning, then emptied to complete the examination.
3. Assure the patient that there is no pain involved. Some discomfort may be experienced from maintaining a full urinary bladder.
4. Explain that a liberal coating of coupling agent must be applied to the skin so that there is no air between the skin and the transducer and to allow for easy movement of the transducer over the skin. A sensation of warmth or wetness may be felt. Although the acoustic couplant does not stain, advise the patient not to wear good clothing for the examination.
5. See Chapter 1 guidelines for safe, effective, informed *pretest* care.

Patient Aftercare
1. Patient may return to normal routines.
2. Interpret test outcomes and counsel about bladder abnormalities.
3. Follow Chapter 1 guidelines regarding safe, effective, informed *posttest* care.

HEPATOBILIARY SONOGRAMS; GALLBLADDER (GB) ULTRASOUND; LIVER ULTRASOUND ●

Normal Sonogram
Normal size, position, and configuration of the gallbladder and bile ducts
Normal adjacent liver tissue

Explanation of Test

These tests are helpful in differentiating hepatic disease from biliary obstruction. Unlike the oral cholecystogram, this procedure allows visualization of the gallbladder and ducts in patients with impaired liver function. Stones and evidence of cholecystitis are readily visualized. This procedure is indicated as an initial study for persons with right upper quadrant pain. It is also useful as a guide for biopsy or other interventional procedures.

Procedure

1. The patient is asked to lie quietly on an examination table. Scans usually are performed with the patient in the supine and decubitus positions.
2. The skin is covered with a layer of coupling gel, oil, or lotion.
3. The patient will be asked to regulate breathing patterns as instructed during the examination.
4. Total examination time is about 20 to 30 minutes.
5. For all procedures, see Chapter 1 guidelines for *intratest* care.

Clinical Implications

1. *Gallbladder* abnormal patterns reveal
   A. Size variations
   B. Thickened wall, indicative of cholecystitis, adenomyomatosis, or tumor and commonly seen as a manifestation of cholecystopathy in patients with the acquired immunodeficiency syndrome (AIDS)
   C. Benign and malignant lesions such as polyps

   NOTE: *Results of sonograms alone cannot differentiate cancers from benign processes.*

   D. Gallstones
2. *Bile duct* abnormalities reveal
   A. Dilation of ducts
   B. Duct obstruction by calculi, tumor, or parasites
   C. Congenital abnormalities such as choledochal cysts
3. Adjacent liver pathologies may include
   A. Parenchymal disease such as cirrhosis
   B. Masses, including cysts, solid lesions, and metastatic tumors

   NOTE: *Results of sonograms alone cannot differentiate cancers from benign processes.*

4. If combined with Doppler evaluation, portal hypertension and hepatofugal flow can be detected.

Interfering Factors

1. Intestinal gas overlying the area of interest interferes with sonographic visualization.
2. Barium from recent radiographic studies compromises the study.
3. Obesity adversely affects tissue visualization.

Patient Preparation

1. Explain the purpose and procedure of the test.
2. Instruct the patient to remain NPO at least 8 hours before the examination to fully dilate the gallbladder and improve anatomic visualization. Some laboratories prefer that the last meal before the study contain low quantities of fat.
3. Assure the patient that there is no pain involved. However, the patient may feel uncomfortable lying quietly for a long period.
4. Explain that a liberal coating of coupling agent must be applied to the skin so that there is no air between the skin and the transducer and to allow for easy movement of the transducer over the skin. A sensation of warmth or wetness may be felt. Although the acoustic couplant does not stain, advise the patient not to wear good clothing for the examination.
5. Explain that the patient will be instructed to control breathing patterns while the images are being made.
6. See Chapter 1 guidelines for safe, effective, informed *pretest* care.

Patient Aftercare

1. Interpret test outcomes and counsel appropriately.
2. Follow Chapter 1 guidelines for safe, effective, informed *posttest* care.

> **Clinical Alert**
>
> 1. Scans cannot be done over open wounds or through dressings.
> 2. This examination must be performed before radiographic studies involving barium. If such scheduling is not possible, at least 24 hours must elapse between the barium procedure and the sonogram.
> 3. The gallbladder's ability to contract may be tested by administering a fatty substance and rescanning.

ABDOMINAL AORTA SONOGRAM

Normal Sonogram

Normal pattern image showing regular contour and diameter of the aorta
The walls strongly reflect echoes, whereas the blood-filled lumen is echo free.

Explanation of Test

This noninvasive ultrasound examination is used to evaluate the abdominal aorta and its major tributaries for structural abnormalities such as aneurysms and the presence of thrombus. Many laboratories include Doppler evaluations to characterize blood flow through the vessels. Typically, the path of the abdominal aorta is traced from its most proximal portion to the region of its bifurcation into the iliac arteries.

Procedure

1. The patient is asked to lie quietly on an examination table. Scans are generally performed with the patient in the supine and decubitus positions.

2. The skis is covered with a layer of coupling gel, oil, or lotion.
3. The patient will be asked to regulate breathing patterns as instructed during the examination.
4. Total examination time is about 30 minutes.
5. For all procedures, see Chapter 1 guidelines for *intratest* care.

Clinical Implications

1. The typical abnormal pattern reveals aortic aneurysms with or without thrombus. Intimal dissections and leaks also may be detected.
2. Para-aortic lymphadenopathy may be visualized.

Interfering Factors

1. Intestinal gas overlying the area of interest interferes with sonographic visualization.
2. Barium from recent radiographic studies compromises the study.
3. Obesity adversely affects tissue visualization.

Patient Preparation

1. Explain the purpose and procedure of the test.
2. Instruct the patient to remain NPO for at least 8 hours before the examination to fully dilate the gallbladder and improve anatomic visualization of all structures.
3. Assure the patient that there is no pain involved. However, the patient may feel uncomfortable lying quietly for a long period.
4. Explain that a liberal coating of coupling agent must be applied to the skin so that there is no air between the skin and the transducer and to allow for easy movement of the transducer over the skin. A sensation of warmth or wetness may be felt. Although the acoustic couplant does not stain, advise the patient not to wear good clothing for the examination.
5. Explain that the patient will be instructed to control breathing patterns while the images are being made.
6. See Chapter 1 guidelines for safe, effective, informed *pretest* care.

> ### Clinical Alert
>
> 1. Scans cannot be done over open wounds or through dressings.
> 2. This examination must be performed before radiographic studies involving barium. If such scheduling is not possible, at least 24 hours must elapse between the barium procedure and the sonogram.

Patient Aftercare

1. The patient may resume normal diet and fluids.
2. Interpret test outcomes and counsel appropriately.
3. Follow Chapter 1 guidelines for safe, effective, informed *posttest* care.

ABDOMINAL ULTRASOUND ●

Normal Sonogram
Normal size, position, and appearance of the liver, gallbladder, bile ducts, pancreas, kidneys, adrenals, and spleen, as well as the abdominal aorta and inferior vena cava and their major tributaries

Explanation of Test
This noninvasive procedure visualizes all solid organs of the upper abdomen including the liver, gallbladder, bile ducts, pancreas, kidneys, spleen, and large abdominal blood vessels. Some diagnostic laboratories may perform organ-specific studies, such as renal or hepatobiliary ultrasound, together with abdominal ultrasound. This study is valuable in detecting a variety of pathologies, including fluid collections, masses, infections, and obstructions.

Procedure
1. The patient is asked to lie quietly on an examination table. Scans are generally performed with the patient in the supine and decubitus positions.
2. The skin is covered with a layer of coupling gel, oil, or lotion.
3. The patient will be asked to regulate breathing patterns as instructed during the examination.
4. Total examination time is about 30 to 60 minutes.
5. For all procedures, see Chapter 1 guidelines for *intratest* care.

Clinical Implications
1. *Liver* abnormalities reveal
   A. Cysts, abscesses, tumors, and metastases

   NOTE: *The results of sonograms alone cannot differentiate malignant from benign conditions.*

   B. Parenchymal disease (eg, cirrhosis)
   C. Variations in portal venous flow
2. *Gallbladder* and *bile duct* abnormalities reveal
   A. Duct dilation or obstruction
   B. Gallstones
   C. Cholecystitis
   D. Tumors

   NOTE: *The results of sonograms alone cannot differentiate malignant from benign conditions.*

3. *Pancreas* abnormalities reveal
   A. Pancreatitis
   B. Pseudocyst
   C. Cysts and tumors, including adenocarcinoma

   NOTE: *The results of sonograms alone cannot differentiate malignant from benign conditions.*

4. *Kidney* abnormalities reveal
   A. Hydronephrosis
   B. Cysts, tumors, abscesses

   NOTE: *The results of sonograms alone cannot differentiate malignant from benign conditions.*

   C. Abnormal size, number, location of kidneys
   D. Calculi
   E. Perirenal fluid collections
5. *Adrenal* abnormalities reveal
   A. Pheochromocytoma
   B. Adrenal hemorrhage
   C. Metastases
6. *Spleen* abnormalities reveal
   A. Splenomegaly
   B. Evidence of lymphatic disease, lymph node enlargement
   C. Evidence of trauma
7. *Vascular* abnormalities in the upper abdomen reveal
   A. Aneurysm
   B. Thrombi
   C. Abnormal blood flow patterns
8. *Miscellaneous* pathologies include
   A. Ascites
   B. Mesenteric or omental cysts or tumors
   C. Congenital absence or malplacement of organs
   D. Retroperitoneal tumors
   E. Hematomas

Interfering Factors
1. Intestinal gas overlying the area of interest interferes with sonographic visualization.
2. Barium from recent radiology studies compromises the study.
3. Obesity adversely affects tissue visualization.

Patient Preparation
1. Explain test purpose and procedure.
2. Instruct the patient to remain NPO for a minimum of 8 hours before the examination to fully dilate the gallbladder and improve anatomic visualization of all structures. Some laboratories prefer that the last meal before the study contain low quantities of fat.
3. Assure the patient that there is no pain involved. However, the patient may feel uncomfortable lying quietly for a long period.
4. Explain that a liberal coating of coupling agent must be applied to the skin so that there is no air between the skin and the transducer and to allow for easy movement of the transducer over the skin. A sensation of warmth or wetness may be felt. Although the acoustic couplant does not stain, advise the patient not to wear good clothing for the examination.

5. Explain that the patient will be instructed to control breathing patterns while the images are being made.
6. See Chapter 1 guidelines for safe, effective, informed care.

> **Clinical Alert**
>
> 1. Scans cannot be done over open wounds or through dressings.
> 2. This examination must be performed before radiographic studies involving barium. If such scheduling is not possible, at least 24 hours must elapse between the barium procedure and the sonogram.

Patient Aftercare
1. Normal diet and fluids are resumed.
2. Interpret test outcomes and counsel appropriately.
3. Follow Chapter 1 guidelines for safe, effective, informed *posttest* care.

●OTHER BODY STRUCTURE SONOGRAMS

BREAST SONOGRAM ●

Normal Sonogram
Symmetric echo pattern in both breasts, including subcutaneous, mammary, and retromammary layers

Explanation of Test
Ultrasound mammography is useful for differentiating cystic, solid, and complex lesions; in the diagnosis of disease in women with very dense breasts; and in the follow-up care of women with fibrocystic breast disease. It is recommended as the initial method of examination in a young woman with a palpable mass and in a pregnant woman with a newly palpable mass. The pregnant patient presents a dilemma, because malignancies in pregnancy grow rapidly and the increased glandular tissue causes difficulties in mammography. Ultrasound may be used to evaluate women who have silicone prostheses in their breasts. The prosthesis is readily penetrated by the ultrasound beam, and tissues behind the prosthesis can be examined. Such prostheses are known to obscure masses on physical examination; they also absorb x-ray beams, obscuring portions of the breast parenchyma.

Breast sonography is a valuable guide during breast biopsies and needle localization procedures. Although not optimal, sonographic visualization of the breast is an alternative for women who refuse to have a radiographic mammogram and for those who should not be exposed to radiation.

Two types of breast sonography are performed. Most commonly, a hand-held transducer is slowly moved across the breast tissue, as in most other forms of sonography. A few institutions perform breast sonography by using a dedicated (automated) breast sonography apparatus. These units consist of a special examination table that houses an ultrasound machine within a tank of treated water. The patient lies on the table with the breast suspended within the water tank during the study. Either form of sonography is capable of producing detailed images of the soft tissue contents of the breast.

Procedure

1. The patient is asked to lie on an examining table.
2. A coupling medium, usually a gel, is applied to the exposed breast to promote the transmission of sound.
3. In most laboratories, a handheld transducer is slowly moved across the breast. In some, an automated breast scanner is used. The automated examination requires the patient to assume a position with the breast immersed in a tank of water. The tank contains transducers that are moved by remote control to image the breast.
4. Total examining time is 15 minutes.
5. For all procedures, see Chapter 1 guidelines for *intratest* care.

Clinical Implications

1. Unusual and distinctive echo patterns indicate the presence of
   A. Cysts
   B. Benign solid growths
   C. Malignant tumors
   D. Tumor metastasis to muscles and lymph nodes
   E. Ductal ectasia
   F. Enlarged lymph nodes

Interfering Factors for Automated Scanners

1. Women with back problems and those with limited flexibility may have difficulty maintaining the positions necessary for the procedure.
2. Although the tank is built to accommodate breasts of most sizes, 1% of breasts are too large to examine by this method.

Patient Preparation

1. Explain the purpose and procedure of the examination. There is no discomfort involved. Many diagnostic departments show the patient a videotape that explains the test.
2. On the day of examination, the patient should wear a 2-piece outfit, because the garments on the torso are removed before the examination.
3. Explain that a liberal coating of a coupling agent must be applied to the skin so that there is no air between the skin and transducer and to allow for easy movement of the transducer over the skin. A sensation of warmth

or wetness may be felt. Although the acoustic couplant does not stain, advise the patient not to wear good clothing for the examination.

4. See Chapter 1 guidelines for safe, effective, informed *pretest* care.

> **Clinical Alert**
>
> 1. If the breast sonogram is to be performed on the same day as a radiographic mammogram, advise the patient not to apply any powders, lotions, or other cosmetics to the upper body on the day of the examination.
> 2. If the breast sonogram is to be used for guidance during a biopsy, make certain that a signed informed consent is secured.

Patient Aftercare

1. The breasts are cleaned and dried and the patient is advised to contact her referring clinician for outcomes.
2. Answer the patient's questions regarding procedures.
3. Follow Chapter 1 guidelines for safe, effective, informed *posttest* care.

PROSTATE SONOGRAM

Normal Sonogram

Normal size, volume, shape, location, and echo texture of prostate and adjacent structures

Explanation of Test

This study is used to visualize the prostate gland, typically in response to an elevated concentration of prostate-specific antigen (PSA) on a blood test or as a complement to a digital rectal examination. Ultrasound of the prostate is also used as a guidance mechanism for biopsy procedures and to assist in placement of radiation "seeds." Carcinoma of the prostate is the second most common cause of cancer-related death in American men.

The patient typically is instructed to prepare by administering a Fleet enema before the procedure. The patient usually is examined with the use of a small endorectal transducer that is inserted while the patient is in a left lateral decubitus position with the knees flexed toward the chest. Multiple images of the prostate, rectal walls, prostatic urethra, and ejaculatory ducts are taken. Prostatic volumes are calculated from 2-dimensional measurements. If indicated, Doppler evaluation is used to assess blood flow through the prostate or any mass that might be detected.

Procedure

1. The patient is asked to void and to remove clothing from the waist down.
2. The patient is positioned on an examination table in the left lateral decubitus position, with his knees flexed toward the chest. The patient is draped.

3. A digital rectal examination usually precedes insertion of the rectal transducer.
4. A slim endorectal transducer, lubricated and sheathed with a condom, is carefully inserted a few centimeters into the rectum.
5. Scans are performed by using a slight rotation of the probe handle. Total examination time is about 15 to 30 minutes.
6. For all procedures, see Chapter 1 guidelines for *intratest* care.

Clinical Implications
Abnormalities that may be detected include
1. Prostatic enlargement—increased volume measurements may indicate
   A. Benign prostatic hypertrophy (BPH)
   B. Space-occupying lesion (tumor, cyst, abscess)
2. Prostatic calcifications
3. Prostatitis
4. Prostate cancer, classically seen as a low-level echo structure within the outer gland (peripheral and central zones)

Interfering Factors
Excess fecal matter in the rectum compromises the study.

Patient Preparation
1. Explain the purpose and procedure of the test.
2. Assure the patient that no pain is involved. However, a sensation of fullness within the rectum is to be expected. Because the transducer is typically draped within a condom, check for latex sensitivities.
3. Many laboratories require administration of a Fleet enema about 1 hour before the study.
4. Advise the patient to empty the bladder immediately before the study.
5. See Chapter 1 guidelines for safe, effective, informed *pretest* care.

> **Clinical Alert**
>
> 1. If the prostate examination is performed in conjunction with a prostatic biopsy, be certain to obtain a signed informed consent.
> 2. If the patient is latex sensitive, contact the laboratory.

Patient Aftercare
1. Interpret test outcomes and counsel about any identified prostatic abnormalities.
2. Follow Chapter 1 guidelines for safe, effective, informed *posttest* care.

SCROTAL SONOGRAM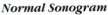

Normal Sonogram
Normal scrotal structure, testicles, epididymis, and spermatic cord

Explanation of Test

This noninvasive ultrasound study is useful in diagnosing testicular masses, hydroceles, spermatoceles, and diffuse processes. Doppler ultrasound or color flow Doppler evaluation is helpful in demonstrating the presence of torsion of the testes.

Procedure

1. The patient lies on his back. The penis is gently retracted, and the scrotum is supported on a rolled towel.
2. After an acoustic gel is applied to the skin, the transducer is repeatedly passed over the scrotum. Sonographic images are generated.
3. Total examination time is about 30 minutes.
4. Color Doppler studies are used to assess presence, absence (as in torsion), or increase (as in infection and certain neoplasms) of blood flow in the testicle.
5. For all procedures, see Chapter 1 guidelines for *intratest* care.

Clinical Implications

1. Abnormal results are associated with
   A. Abscess
   B. Infarcted testes (torsion)
   C. Tumor (primary and metastatic)
   D. Hydrocele
   E. Spermatocele
   F. Adherent scrotal hernia
   G. Cryptorchism
   H. Epididymitis (chronic or acute)
   I. Hematoma (associated with trauma)
   J. Tuberculosis infection (associated with AIDS)

Patient Preparation

1. Explain the purpose and procedure of the test.
2. Assure the patient that there is no pain involved.
3. Explain that a liberal coating of coupling media must be applied to the scrotum. A sensation of warmth or wetness may be felt. Although the acoustic couplant does not stain, advise the patient not to wear good clothing for the examination.
4. See Chapter 1 guidelines regarding safe, effective, informed *pretest* care.

Patient Aftercare

1. Interpret test outcomes and counsel appropriately.
2. Follow Chapter 1 guidelines for safe, effective, informed *posttest* care.

EYE AND ORBIT SONOGRAMS ●

Normal Sonogram

Pattern image indicating normal soft tissue of eye and retrobulbar orbital areas, retina, choroid, and orbital fat

Explanation of Test

Ultrasound can be used to describe both normal and abnormal tissues of the eye when no alternative visualization is possible because of opacities caused by inflammation or hemorrhage. This information is valuable in the management of eyes with large corneal leukomas or conjunctival flaps and in the evaluation of eyes for keratoprosthesis. Orbital lesions can be detected and distinguished from inflammatory and congestive causes of exophthalmus with a high degree of reliability. An extensive preoperative evaluation before vitrectomy or surgery for vitreous hemorrhages is also done. In this case, the vitreous cavity is examined to rule out retinal and choroidal detachments and to detect and localize vitreoretinal adhesions and intraocular foreign bodies. Also, persons who are to have intraocular lens implants after removal of cataracts must be measured for the exact length of the eye (within 0.1 mm).

Procedure

A small, very-high-frequency transducer is placed on the eye directly or is positioned over a water standoff pad placed onto the eye surface. Multiple images and measurements are taken.

1. The eye area is anesthetized by instilling eye drops.
2. The patient is asked to fix the gaze and hold very still.
3. A probe is gently placed on the corneal surface.
4. If a lesion in the eye is detected, as much as 30 minutes may be required to accurately differentiate the pathologic process.
5. Orbital examination can be done in 8 to 10 minutes.
6. For all procedures, see Chapter 1 guidelines for *intratest* care.

Clinical Implications

1. Abnormal patterns are seen in
   A. Alkali burns with corneal flattening and loss of anterior chamber
   B. Detached retina
   C. Keratoprosthesis
   D. Extraocular thickening in thyroid eye disease
   E. Pupillary membranes
   F. Cyclotic membranes
   G. Vitreous opacities
   H. Orbital mass lesions
   I. Inflammatory conditions
   J. Vascular malformations
   K. Foreign bodies
2. Abnormal patterns are also seen in tumors of various types based on specific ultrasonic patterns:
   A. Solid tumors (eg, meningioma, glioma, neurofibroma)
   B. Cystic tumors (eg, mucocele, dermoid, cavernous hemangioma)
   C. Angiomatous tumors (eg, diffuse hemangioma)
   D. Lymphangioma
   E. Infiltrative tumors (eg, metastatic lymphoma, pseudotumor)

Interfering Factors

If at some time the vitreous humor in a particular patient has been replaced by a gas, no result can be obtained.

Patient Preparation

1. Explain the purpose and procedure of the test.
2. Topical anesthetic drops are instilled into the eyes before the examination is performed; this usually is done in the examining department.
3. See Chapter 1 guidelines for safe, effective, informed *pretest* care.

Patient Aftercare

1. Instruct the patient to refrain from rubbing the eyes until the effects of anesthetic have disappeared. This type of friction could cause corneal abrasions.
2. Advise the patient that minor discomfort and blurred vision may be experienced for a short time.
3. Follow Chapter 1 guidelines for safe, effective, informed *posttest* care.

> **Clinical Alert**
>
> When a ruptured globe is suspected, ophthalmic ultrasound should not be performed. Excessive pressure applied to the globe may cause expulsion of the contents and increases the risk of introduction of bacteria.

THYROID SONOGRAM (NECK ULTRASOUND)

Normal Sonogram

Normal, homogenous pattern of the thyroid and adjacent structures, including strap muscles and blood vessels

Explanation of Test

This ultrasound study is used to evaluate a neck mass or to determine the size of the thyroid and reveal the depth and dimension of thyroid goiters and nodules. The response of a mass in the thyroid to suppressive therapy can be monitored by successive examinations. Theoretically, this technique offers the possibility of a good estimation of thyroid weight—information that is important in radioiodine therapy for Graves' disease.

The examination is easy to do, is done before surgery, and gives 85% accuracy. Often, these studies are done in conjunction with radioactive iodine uptake tests. With pregnant patients, ultrasound studies are the method of choice, because radioactive iodine is harmful to the developing fetus.

Procedure

1. The patient lies on the back on the examining table, with the neck hyperextended.

2. A pillow is placed under the shoulders for comfort and to bring the transducer into better contact with the thyroid.

3. An acoustic couplant (gel, lotion, or oil) is applied to the patient's neck. This affords good contact between the transducer and the patient's skin and allows the transducer to be moved easily across the neck's surface.

4. An alternate procedure involves separation of the neck surface from the transducer by a gel-filled pad that permits proper transmission of the ultrasound waves through the thyroid.

5. Examination time is about 30 minutes.

6. For all procedures, see Chapter 1 guidelines for *intratest* care.

Clinical Implications

1. An abnormal pattern may consist of a cystic, complex, or solid echo pattern.

2. Solitary "cold" nodules identified on radioisotope scans may appear as echo-free cysts on ultrasound. Most often, cysts are benign. Solid-appearing lesions may represent benign adenomas or malignant tumors. A biopsy is the only definitive method to determine the nature of such tumors.

3. Overall gland enlargement is indicative of goiter or thyroiditis.

4. Sonographic studies of the neck may also reveal parathyroid lesions or evidence of changed lymph nodes.

5. Certain congenital deformities related to the embryologic development of neck structures may be detected, most commonly thyroglossal duct cyst, brachial cleft cyst, or cystic hygroma.

Interfering Factors

1. Nodules <1 cm in diameter may escape detection.

2. Cysts not originating in the thyroid may show the same ultrasound characteristics as thyroid cysts.

3. Lesions >4 cm in diameter frequently contain areas of cystic or hemorrhagic degeneration and give a mixed echogram that is difficult to correlate with specific disease.

Patient Preparation

1. Explain the purpose and procedure of the test.

2. Assure the patient that there is no pain involved. However, the patient may feel uncomfortable maintaining the neck in position during the examination.

3. Explain that a liberal coating of coupling agent must be applied to the skin so that there is no air between the skin and the transducer and to allow for easy movement of the transducer over the skin. A sensation of warmth or wetness may be felt. Although the acoustic couplant does not stain, advise the patient not to wear good clothing for the examination.

4. Advise the patient to refrain from wearing necklaces to the laboratory.

5. See Chapter 1 guidelines for safe, effective, informed *pretest* care.

> ### Clinical Alert
>
> Thyroid or neck biopsies are often performed with ultrasound guidance. If a biopsy is performed, a witnessed, informed consent must be signed in advance by the patient.

Patient Aftercare

1. Interpret test outcomes and counsel about follow-up treatment for thyroid or neck abnormalities.
2. Follow Chapter 1 guidelines regarding safe, effective, informed *posttest* care.

● VASCULAR ULTRASOUND STUDIES (DUPLEX SCANS)

OVERVIEW OF DUPLEX SCANS ●

The combination of anatomic imaging of blood vessels and hemodynamic information provided by Doppler ultrasound results in duplex scans. These non-invasive studies can be performed on literally any area of human anatomy. Blood velocity is detected by positioning the Doppler sample gate within the lumen of the desired vessel. The resultant *spectral trace* (Fig. 13-1) also provides information as to the direction, phase, pulsatile rhythm, and resistivity of flow. *Antegrade* flow is demonstrated above the baseline. *Retrograde* flow (ie, flow in the direction opposite the expected) is demonstrated by a spectral trace below the baseline. Flow that is antegrade through all phases (systole as well as diastole) demonstrates a *low-resistive* profile, which is normally associated with many visceral blood vessels (eg, renal artery, internal carotid artery). High resistance, or *triphasic,* flow is typically associated with peripheral arteries (eg, femoral artery, brachial artery) and shows a forward-backward-forward pattern in each cycle. *Spectral broadening* occurs when the sample contains blood cells moving at many velocities; this is generally associated with a flow disturbance. Mathematical ratios that contrast peak or mean velocities at various stages in the cycle can give further clues as to the integrity of the vascular system examined. Color Doppler ultrasound generally is used to code flow velocities and direction with color and can readily differentiate the patency of vessels.

CEREBROVASCULAR ULTRASOUND (CAROTID AND VERTEBRAL ARTERIES) DUPLEX SCANS ●

Normal Duplex Scan

Normal vascular anatomy and course of common carotid artery, internal and external carotids, and vertebral arteries

No evidence of stenosis or occlusion; normal flow patterns

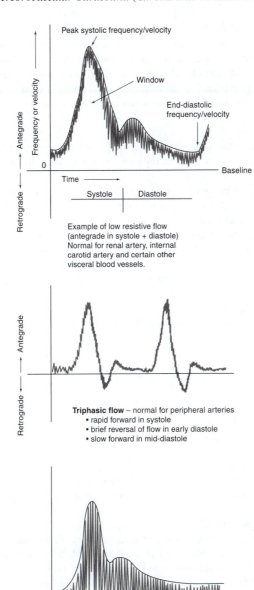

FIGURE 13-1

Blood velocity tracings show direction, phasicity, pulsatility, and resistivity of flow.

Explanation of Test

Carotid duplex scans examine the major extracranial arteries supplying the brain to gain information about cerebrovascular blood flow. Carotid scans are used in the evaluation of ischemia, headache, dizziness, hemiparesis, paresthesias, and speech and visual disturbances. Testing is commonly performed before major cardiovascular surgery and as a follow-up to many surgeries.

Procedure

1. The patient usually is asked to lie on the examining table with the neck slightly extended. The head typically is turned away from the side being examined.
2. Acoustic coupling gel is applied to the neck area to enhance the transmission of sound. During Doppler evaluation, an audible signal, representing blood flow, can be heard.
3. A handheld transducer is gently moved up and down the neck while images of appropriate blood vessels are made. Both sides of the neck are examined, resulting in an examination time of 30 to 60 minutes.
4. For all procedures, see Chapter 1 guidelines for *intratest* care.

Clinical Implications

Abnormal images and Doppler signals may provide evidence of the following:

1. Plaque
2. Stenosis
3. Occlusion
4. Dissection
5. Aneurysm
6. Carotid body tumor
7. Arteritis

Interfering Factors

1. Severe obesity compromises examination quality.
2. Cardiac arrhythmias and disease may cause changes in hemodynamic patterns.

Patient Preparation

1. Explain the test purpose and procedure. Patient should refrain from smoking or consuming caffeine for at least 2 hours before the study. Assure the patient that no radiation is employed, typically no contrast medium is injected, and no pain is involved. Some slight discomfort may be experienced from lying with head extended.
2. Advise the patient that a liberal coating of coupling gel must be applied to the skin to promote sound transmission. A sensation of warmth or wetness may be felt during application. Although the acoustic couplant does not stain, advise the patient not to wear good clothing for the examination. Necklaces and earrings must be removed before the study.
3. See Chapter 1 guidelines for safe, effective, informed *pretest* care.

Patient Aftercare

1. Remind the patient to remove any residual gel from the skin.
2. Interpret test outcomes, provide support, and counsel appropriately should an abnormality be detected. Monitor and counsel for arterial disease.
3. See Chapter 1 guidelines for safe, effective, informed *posttest* care.

PERIPHERAL ARTERIAL DOPPLER STUDIES; LOWER EXTREMITY ARTERIAL (LEA) AND UPPER EXTREMITY ARTERIAL (UEA) DUPLEX SCANS ●

Normal Duplex Scans

Normal arterial anatomy of the extremity
Normal triphasic blood flow and flow velocities
No evidence of plaques or other pathologic processes

Explanation of Test

Peripheral arterial studies visualize and document the arterial blood flow in the extremities. Duplex ultrasound scans can determine the presence, amount, and location of plaques and are helpful in assessing the cause of claudication. Graft patency and condition may also be evaluated. Some institutions also incorporate *segmental blood pressure* readings into these examinations. Flow characteristics of upper versus lower extremities can be contrasted by calculating a mathematical ratio between pressures (see Ankle-Brachial Index and Segmental Pressures, page 940).

Procedure

1. The patient usually is asked to lie on the examining table with the leg or arm turned out slightly and the knee or elbow partially bent.
2. Acoustic coupling gel is applied to the leg from groin down or to the arm from the shoulder down to enhance the transmission of sound. During Doppler evaluation, an audible signal, representing blood flow, can be heard.
3. A handheld transducer is gently moved up and down the limb while images of appropriate blood vessels are made. Both sides are examined, resulting in an examination time of about 60 minutes.
4. For all procedures, see Chapter 1 guidelines for *intratest* care.

Clinical Implications

Abnormal tracings and Doppler signals may provide evidence of the following (see Fig. 13-1):

1. Plaque or calcification (particularly in the diabetic patient)
2. Stenosis (hemodynamically significant lesions produce >50% stenosis)
3. Occlusion
4. Arteritis
5. Aneurysm

6. Pseudoaneurysm
7. Graft diameter reduction

Interfering Factors
1. Severe obesity compromises examination quality.
2. Cardiac arrhythmias and disease may cause changes in hemodynamic patterns.

Patient Preparation
1. Explain the test purpose and procedure. Instruct the patient to refrain from smoking or consuming caffeine for at least 2 hours before the test. Assure the patient that no radiation is employed, typically no contrast medium is injected, and no pain is involved. Some slight discomfort may be experienced from lying with the extremity extended or if segmental blood pressures are taken.
2. Advise the patient that a liberal coating of coupling gel must be applied to the skin to promote sound transmission. A sensation of warmth or wetness may be felt during application. Although the acoustic couplant does not stain, advise the patient not to wear good clothing for the examination.
3. See Chapter 1 guidelines for safe, effective, informed *pretest* care.

Patient Aftercare
1. Remind the patient to remove any residual gel from the skin.
2. Interpret test outcomes, provide support, and counsel appropriately should an abnormality be detected. Monitor and counsel for arterial disease.
3. See Chapter 1 guidelines for safe, effective, informed *posttest* care.

ANKLE-BRACHIAL INDEX (ABI) AND SEGMENTAL PRESSURES ●

Normal Index and Pressures
An ABI ≥1.0 is considered normal when a normal multiphasic waveform is present.

A difference of 20 mmHg between the right and left brachial pressures may indicate proximal arterial obstruction on the side with reduced pressure.

The gradual pressure drop, as measured from upper thigh or arm to ankle or wrist, should not exceed 20 mm Hg between any 2 segments.

Explanation of Test
In some laboratories, as an adjunct to duplex scanning, blood pressures throughout the extremities are measured and contrasted. In the typical 4-cuff technique, pneumatic cuffs are applied to the upper thigh, the lower thigh, the upper calf, and the area just above the ankle. Additionally, cuffs are applied to the upper arms to determine brachial pressures. Segmental pressures provide physiologic information that can confirm a vascular cause for ischemic rest pain and claudication. ABI is calculated by dividing the ankle pressure (in mmHg) by the brachial pressure.

Procedure
1. The patient is asked to lie on a table with the extremity extended.
2. Pneumatic cuffs (usually 4) are placed at intervals along the extremity.
3. A flow-sensing device (often a continuous-wave Doppler device) is placed

distal to a cuff. The cuff is inflated (often automatically) to suprasystolic values and slowly deflated until flow resumes. The pressure at which flow resumes is recorded.

4. This technique is repeated, distal to each cuff, until the entire extremity has been evaluated. Brachial pressures are measured as well.

5. Both extremities are examined. Total examination time (for pressures only) is generally <15 minutes.

6. For all procedures, see Chapter 1 guidelines for *intratest* care.

Clinical Implications

1. Asymmetry in brachial pressure of >10 mm Hg is suspicious for arterial disease.

2. An ABI of <1.0 is suspicious for disease. The lower the numeric value for this index, the more severe the disease may be (eg, an ABI of <0.25 is associated with impending tissue loss).

3. Generally speaking, pressure gradients between successive segments on the same extremity should vary by <20 mg Hg. Variations that exceed this value suggest significant disease (occlusion or stenosis).

4. A difference of ≥20 mm Hg between similar segments on opposite sides may suggest obstructive vascular disease.

Clinical Alert

1. Segmental pressures are a screening tool that cannot distinguish stenosis from total occlusion and cannot be specific in determining the exact location of disease.

2. Vessel calcifications (commonly seen in the diabetic patient) can falsely elevate systolic pressures.

Interfering Factors

1. Severe obesity compromises examination quality.

2. Cardiac arrhythmias and disease may cause changes in hemodynamic patterns.

Patient Preparation

1. Explain the test purpose and procedure. Instruct the patient to refrain from smoking or consuming caffeine for at least 2 hours before the study. Assure patient that no radiation is employed, typically no contrast medium is injected, and no pain is involved. Some discomfort may be experienced from lying with the extremity extended or when pneumatic cuffs are inflated.

2. See Chapter 1 guidelines for safe, effective, informed *pretest* care.

Patient Aftercare

1. Interpret test outcomes, provide support, and counsel appropriately should an abnormality be detected. Monitor and counsel for arterial disease.

2. See Chapter 1 guidelines for safe, effective, informed *posttest* care.

PERIPHERAL VENOUS DOPPLER STUDIES; LOWER EXTREMITY VENOUS (LEV) AND UPPER EXTREMITY VENOUS (UEV) DUPLEX SCANS ●

Normal Duplex Scan

Normal venous anatomy of the extremity

Spontaneous phasic flow pattern (rises and falls with respiration)

Normal venous augmentation (exhibits increased flow proximal to the site of venous compression)

Competent, intact valves, with no evidence of thrombi

Explanation of Test

This procedure examines venous blood flow in the selected extremity (upper or lower). It is most commonly used to assess deep venous thrombosis and can also be used to "map" veins to be harvested and used for grafts. This examination has replaced contrast venography in many institutions.

Procedure

1. The patient usually is asked to lie on the examining table with the leg or arm turned out slightly and the knee or elbow partially bent.
2. Acoustic coupling gel is applied to the leg from the groin down or to the arm from the shoulder area down to enhance the transmission of sound. During Doppler evaluation, an audible signal, representing blood flow, can be heard.
3. A handheld transducer is gently moved up and down the limb while images of appropriate blood vessels are made. At intervals, gentle compression is applied to the vessel. Both sides are examined, resulting in an examination time of about 30 minutes.
4. For all procedures, see Chapter 1 guidelines for *intratest* care.

Clinical Implications

Abnormal images and Doppler signals may provide evidence of the following:

1. Acute or chronic deep venous thrombosis
2. Occlusive venous disease
3. Valvular incompetence

Interfering Factors

1. Severe obesity compromises examination quality.
2. Cardiac arrhythmias and disease may cause changes in hemodynamic patterns.

Patient Preparation

1. Explain the test purpose and procedure. Instruct the patient to refrain from smoking for at least 2 hours before the study. Assure the patient that no radiation is employed, typically no contrast medium is injected, and no pain

is involved. Some slight discomfort may be experienced from lying with the extremity extended or when compression is applied.

2. Advise the patient that a liberal coating of coupling gel must be applied to the skin to promote sound transmission. A sensation of warmth or wetness may be felt during application. Although the acoustic couplant does not stain, advise the patient not to wear good clothing for the examination.

3. See Chapter 1 guidelines for safe, effective, informed *pretest* care.

Patient Aftercare

1. Remind the patient to remove any residual gel from the skin.

2. Interpret test outcomes, provide support, and counsel appropriately should an abnormality be detected. Monitor and counsel for venous disease.

3. See Chapter 1 guidelines for safe, effective, informed *posttest* care.

● HEART ULTRASOUND STUDIES

HEART SONOGRAM (ECHOCARDIOGRAM; DOPPLER ECHOCARDIOGRAPHY) ●

Normal Sonogram

Normal position, size, and movement of heart valves and chamber walls as visualized in 2-D, M-mode, and Doppler mode

Color M-mode and color Doppler assessments of heart structures within normal limits

Explanation of Test

This noninvasive technique for examining the heart can provide information about its position and size, movements of the valves and chambers, and velocity of blood flow. Echoes from pulsed high-frequency sound waves are used to locate and study the movements and dimensions of cardiac structures. Because the heart is a blood-filled organ, sound can be transmitted through it readily to the opposite wall and to the heart-lung interface. This test is commonly used to determine biologic and prosthetic valve dysfunction, to evaluate a pericardial effusion, to evaluate the velocity and direction of blood flow, to furnish direction for further diagnostic study, and to monitor cardiac patients over an extended period. One of the advantages of this diagnostic technique is that it can be performed at the bedside with mobile equipment or done in the laboratory.

The various modes of echocardiography are capable of providing a great range of information concerning cardiac structure and function. The following are common types of echocardiograms:

Two-dimensional (2-D): used to produce gray-scale, cross-sectional images of the heart's anatomy

M-mode: used to generate depictions of rapidly moving structures such as valves and for standardized dimensional measurements

Continuous-wave Doppler and pulsed-wave Doppler: used to determine velocity of blood flow

Color 2-D: used for identifying areas of disturbed or eccentric blood flow

Color M-mode: used for evaluating movement of cardiac structures

Specialized types of echocardiography include the following

Stress echocardiography: This is used to provide information relating to the function of heart structures during high cardiac output states. A treadmill or upright bicycle may be used, or the heart can be stressed by an infusion of dobutamine.

Transesophageal echocardiography (TEE): A miniature ultrasound transducer is placed at the end of a tube inserted into the esophagus so as to provide a closer view of cardiac structures without interference from superficial chest tissues (see page 945).

Fetal echocardiography: This is performed through the pregnant woman's abdomen when there is a question of congenital cardiac defect (see page 906).

Contrast echocardiography: A liquid containing nontoxic microbubbles is injected into a vein to opacify cardiac structures.

These special techniques may require a signed, informed consent before performance and involve more complicated procedures. Check with the individual laboratory for specific guides and protocols.

Procedure

1. A specific diagnosis should accompany the request for the test (eg, "rule out pericardial effusion," "determine severity of mitral stenosis"). If a stress echocardiogram is ordered, the patient's ability to perform exercise must be indicated.
2. The patient lies on the examining table in a slight side-lying position.
3. The skin surface over the chest is lubricated with acoustic gel to permit maximum penetration of the ultrasound beam. The transducer is held over various regions of the chest and upper abdomen to obtain the appropriate views of the heart.
4. There is no pain or discomfort involved. Leads may be attached for a simultaneous electrocardiogram reading during the ultrasound procedure.
5. Examination time is 30 to 45 minutes.
6. For all procedures, see Chapter 1 guidelines for *intratest* care.

Clinical Implications

Abnormal values help to diagnose

1. Acquired cardiac disease:
   A. Valvular disease, stenosis, prolapse, and regurgitation
   B. Cardiomyopathies
   C. Evidence of coronary artery disease

D. Pericardial disease, including effusion, tamponade, and pericarditis
E. Endocarditis
F. Cardiac neoplasm
G. Intracardiac thrombi
2. Prosthetic valve function
3. Congenital heart disease

Interfering Factors
1. Dysrhythmias interfere with the test.
2. Hyperinflation of the lungs with mechanical ventilation, especially with positive end-expiratory pressure (PEEP) of >10 cm H_2O, precludes adequate ultrasound imaging of the heart.
3. False-negative and false-positive diagnoses have been identified (especially in M-mode echocardiograms), including diagnoses of pleural effusion, dilated descending aorta, pericardial fat pad, tumors encasing the heart, clotted blood, and loculated effusions.
4. Doppler study results can vary greatly if the transducer position does not provide satisfactory angles for the beam.

Patient Preparation
1. Explain the purpose and procedure of the test.
2. Assure the patient that no pain is involved. However, some discomfort may be felt from lying quietly for a long period.
3. Explain that a liberal coating of coupling agent must be applied to the skin so that there is no air between the skin and the transducer and to permit easy movement of the transducer over the skin. A sensation of warmth or wetness may be felt. Although the acoustic couplant does not stain, advise the patient not to wear good clothing for the examination.
4. See Chapter 1 guidelines for safe, effective, informed *pretest* care.

> ▶ **Clinical Alert**
>
> Certain specialized echocardiographic procedures, such as stress echocardiography and TEE, may require individualized patient preparation. Check with the laboratory to determine specific protocols and preparation.

Patient Aftercare
1. Interpret test outcomes and counsel appropriately about cardiac disorders.
2. Follow Chapter 1 guidelines for safe, effective, informed *posttest* care.

TRANSESOPHAGEAL ECHOCARDIOGRAM (TEE)

Normal Sonogram
Normal position, size, and function of heart valves and heart chambers

Explanation of Test

This test permits optimal ultrasonic visualization of the heart when traditional transthoracic (noninvasive) echocardiography fails or proves inconclusive. A miniaturized high-frequency ultrasound transducer is mounted on an endoscope and coupled with an ultrasound instrument to display and record ultrasound images from the heart. Endoscope controls allow remote manipulation of the transducer tip. Various images of heart anatomy can be displayed by rotating the tip of the instrument and by varying the depth of insertion into the esophagus.

Indications for TEE include situations in which transthoracic echocardiography has not been satisfactory (eg, obesity, trauma to the chest wall, chronic obstructive pulmonary disease) or the results of traditional transthoracic echocardiography do not agree or correlate with other clinical findings.

Procedure

1. A topical anesthetic is applied to the pharynx. A bite block is inserted into the mouth. This reduces the risk of damage to the patient's teeth and oral structures and accidental damage to the endoscope.
2. The patient assumes a left lateral decubitus position while the lubricated endoscopic instrument is inserted to a depth of 30 to 50 cm. The patient is asked to swallow to facilitate advancement of the device.
3. Manipulation of the ultrasound transducer provides a number of image planes.

   NOTE: *A variety of medications may be used during this procedure. Generally, these drugs are intended to sedate, anesthetize, reduce secretions, and serve as contrast agents for the ultrasound.*

4. For all procedures, see Chapter 1 guidelines for *intratest* care.

Clinical Implications

Abnormal TEE findings include

1. Heart valve diseases
2. Pericardial effusion
3. Congenital heart disease
4. Aortic dissection
5. Left ventricular dysfunction
6. Endocarditis
7. Intracardiac tumors or thrombi

Patient Preparation

1. Explain the purpose and procedure and the benefits and risks of the test.
2. The patient must remain NPO for at least 4 to 8 hours before the procedure to reduce the risk of aspiration. Pretest medications such as analgesics or sedatives may be ordered. Check with the laboratory or physician for specific instructions.

3. Obtain baseline vital signs.

4. Establish an intravenous access line to administer medications or contrast agents.

5. Remove dentures and any loose objects from patient's mouth.

6. See Chapter 1 guidelines for safe, effective, informed *pretest* care.

Patient Aftercare

1. Interpret test results; monitor vital signs and level of consciousness (if the patient is sedated). Ensure patent airway.

2. Position the patient on the side, if sedated, to prevent risk of aspiration.

3. Ascertain return of swallowing, coughing, and gag reflexes before allowing patient to take oral food or fluids. Generally, the patient should remain NPO for at least 1 hour after the test.

4. Follow Chapter 1 guidelines for safe, effective, informed *posttest* care.

> ### Clinical Alert
>
> Swallowing reflexes may be diminished for several hours because of the effects of the topical anesthetic.

BIBLIOGRAPHY

Berman MC: Diagnostic Medical Sonography: Obstetrics and Gynecology. Philadelphia, Lippincott-Raven Publishers, 1997

Craig M: Diagnostic Medical Sonography: Echocardiography. Philadelphia, Lippincott-Raven Publishers, 1998

D'Cruz IA: Echocardiographic Anatomy. Stamford, CT, Appleton & Lange, 1996

Goldberg BB: An Atlas of Ultrasound Color Flow Imaging. Boston Blackwell Science, 1998

Hickey J: Ultrasound Review of Obstetrics and Gynecology. Philadelphia, Lippincott-Raven, 1996

Kawamura DM: Diagnostic Medical Sonography: Abdomen and Superficial Structures. Philadelphia, Lippincott-Raven Publishers, 1997

Kurtz AB: Ultrasound: The Requisites. St. Louis, Mosby, 1996

McMillan D: Imaging in Ophthalmological Diagnosis. St. Louis, CV Mosby, 1996

Rudolphi DM: Duplex scanning. Am Nurs J 90(4):123–124, 1990

Rumak CM: Diagnostic Ultrasound, Vols 1 and 2. St. Louis, CV Mosby, 1997

Specht NT: Practical Guide to Diagnostic Imaging. St. Louis, Mosby, 1997

Von Schultess GK, Hennig J (eds): Function Imaging. Philadelphia, Lippincott-Raven Publishers, 1998

Zagzebski JA: Essentials of Ultrasound Physics. St. Louis, Mosby, 1996

14

Pulmonary Function and Blood Gas Studies

Pulmonary Physiology

There are 3 aspects of pulmonary function: perfusion, diffusion, and ventilation. *Perfusion* relates to blood flow through pulmonary vessels; *diffusion* refers to movement of oxygen and carbon dioxide across alveolar capillary membranes; *ventilation* relates to air exchange between alveolar spaces and the atmosphere.

During breathing, the lung-thorax system acts as a bellows to provide air to the alveoli for adequate gas exchange to take place. Like a spring or rubber band, the lung tissue also possesses the property of elasticity. When the inspiratory muscles contract, the thorax and lungs expand; when the same muscles relax and the force is removed, the thorax and lungs return to their resting position. Also, when the thorax and lungs expand, the alveolar pressure is lowered below atmospheric pressure. This permits air to flow into the trachea, bronchi, bronchioles, and alveoli. Expiration is mainly passive. It occurs because the thorax and lungs recoil to their resting position: the alveolar pressure increases above atmospheric pressure, and air flows out through the respiratory tract. The major function of the lung is to provide adequate ventilation to meet the metabolic demands of the body during rest and during exercise. The primary purpose of pulmonary blood flow is to conduct mixed venous blood through the capillaries of the alveoli so that oxygen (O_2) can be taken up by the blood and carbon dioxide (CO_2) can be removed from the blood.

Purpose of Tests

Pulmonary function tests determine the presence, nature, and extent of pulmonary dysfunction caused by obstruction, restriction, or both. When ventilation is disturbed by an increase in airway resistance, the ventilatory defect is called an *obstructive* ventilatory impairment. When ventilation is disturbed by a limitation in chest wall excursion, the defect is referred to as a *restrictive* ventilatory impairment. When ventilation is altered by both increased airway resistance and limited chest wall excursion, the defect is termed a *combined* or *mixed* defect. Table 14-1 presents the conditions that affect ventilation.

Pulmonary function studies may reveal locations of abnormalities in the airways, alveoli, and pulmonary vascular bed early in the course of a disease, when the physical examination and radiographic studies still appear normal.

Indications for Tests

1. Early detection of pulmonary or cardiogenic pulmonary disease
2. Differential diagnosis of dyspnea
3. Presurgical assessment (eg, ability to tolerate intraoperative anesthetics, especially during thoracic procedures)
4. Evaluation of risk factors for other diagnostic procedures
5. Detection of early respiratory failure
6. Monitoring progress of bronchopulmonary disease
7. Periodic evaluation of workers exposed to materials harmful to the respiratory system

TABLE 14-1
Conditions That Affect Ventilation

Examples	*Causes*
RESTRICTIVE VENTILATORY IMPAIRMENTS*	
Chest wall disease	Injury, kyphoscoliosis, spondylitis, muscular dystrophy, other neuromuscular diseases
Extrathoracic conditions	Obesity, peritonitis, ascites, pregnancy
Interstitial lung disease	Interstitial pneumonitis, fibrosis, pneumoconioses (eg, asbestosis, silicosis), granulomatosis, edema, sarcoidosis
Pleural disease	Pneumothorax, hemothorax, pleural effusion, fibrothorax
Space-occupying lesions	Tumors, cysts abscesses
OBSTRUCTIVE VENTILATORY IMPAIRMENTS†	
Peripheral airway disease	Bronchitis, bronchiectasis, bronchiolitis, bronchial asthma, cystic, fibrosis
Pulmonary parenchymal disease	Emphysema
Upper airway disease	Pharyngeal, tracheal or laryngeal tumors, edema, infections, foreign bodies, collapsed airway, stenosis
MIXED-DEFECT VENTILATORY IMPAIRMENTS‡	
Pulmonary congestion	Both increased airway resistance and limited expansion of chest cavity and/or chest wall; obstruction caused by bronchial edema, compression of respiratory airway owing to increased interstitial (and intravenous fluid) pressure; restriction caused by impaired elasticity, anatomic deformity (eg, kyphosis, lordosis, scoliosis)

*Characterized by interference with chest wall or lung movement, "stiff lung", and an actual reduction in the volume of air that can be inspired.
†Characterized by the need for increased effort to produce airflow; respiratory muscles must work harder to overcome obstructive forces during breathing; prolonged and impaired airflow during expiration; airway resistance increases and lungs become very compliant.
‡Combined or mixed; exhibits components of both obstructive and restrictive ventilatory impairments.

8. Epidemiologic studies of selected populations to determine risks for or causes of pulmonary diseases

9. Workers' compensation claims

10. Monitoring after pharmacologic or surgical intervention

Classification of Tests

Pulmonary function tests evaluate the ventilatory system and alveoli in an indirect, overlapping way. The patient's age, height, weight, ethnicity, and gender are recorded before testing because they are the basis for calculating predicted values.

Pulmonary function tests are generally divided into 3 categories:

1. *Airway flow rates* typically include measurements of instantaneous or average airflow rates during a maximal forced exhalation to assess airway patency and resistance. These tests also assess responses to inhaled bronchodilators or bronchial provocations.

2. *Lung volumes and capacities* measure the various "air-containing compartments" of the lung to assess air trapping (hyperinflation, overdistention) or reduction in volume. These measurements also help to differentiate obstructive from restrictive ventilatory impairments.

3. *Gas exchange (diffusion capacity)* measures the rate of gas transfer across the alveolar capillary membranes to assess the diffusion process. It can also monitor for side effects of drugs, such as bleomycin (antineoplastic) or amiodarone (antiarrhythmic), which can cause interstitial pneumonitis or pulmonary fibrosis. Diffusion capacity in the absence of lung disease (eg, anemia) can also be evaluated.

SYMBOLS AND ABBREVIATIONS ●

Pulmonary function studies and blood gas analyses measure quantities of gas mixtures and their components, blood and its constituents, and various factors affecting these quantities. The symbols and abbreviations given here are based on standards developed by American physiologists. Familiarity with the major and secondary symbols facilitates interpretation of any combination of these symbols (see Charts 14-1, 14-2, 14-3, and 14-4).

● PULMONARY FUNCTION TESTS

SPIROMETRY ●

Lung capacities, volumes, and flow rates are clinically measured by a *spirometer*. The electrical recording of the amounts of gas breathed in and out produces a *spirogram*. Spirometers can be grouped into 2 major categories: the

CHART 14-1 ▶
Gas Volumes: Symbols and Abbreviations

Large capital letters denote primary symbols for gases.

V = Gas volume

$\dot{V}$ = Gas volume per unit time (the dot over the symbol indicates the factor per unit time, as in flow)

P = Gas pressure or partial pressure of a gas in a gas mixture (exhaled air) or in a liquid (blood)

F = Fractional concentration of a gas

Small capital letters indicate the type of gas measured in relation to respiratory tract location or function.

A = Alveolar gas

D = Dead space gas

E = Expired gas

I = Inspired gas

T = Tidal gas

Chemical symbols for gases may be placed after the small capital letters previously listed.

O_2 = Oxygen

CO = Carbon monoxide

CO_2 = Carbon dioxide

N_2 = Nitrogen

COMBINATIONS OF SYMBOLS
The following are some examples of the ways these symbols may be combined:

F_{ICO_2} = Fractional concentration of inspired oxygen

V_T = Tidal volume

V_E = Volume of expired gas

P_{ACO_2} = Partial pressure of carbon dioxide in alveolar gas

BLOOD GAS SYMBOLS
Large capital letters are used as primary symbols for blood determinations.

C = Concentration of a gas in blood

S = Percent saturation of hemoglobin

Q = Volume of blood

$\dot{Q}$ = Volume of blood per unit time (blood flow)

To indicate whether blood is capillary, venous, or arterial, *lower case letters* are used.

v = Venous blood

a = Arterial blood

c = Capillary blood

s = Shunted blood

CHART 14-2 ▶
Combinations of Symbols and Abbreviations

Blood gas symbols may be combined in the following ways:

P_{O_2}	= Oxygen tension or partial pressure of oxygen
Pa_{O_2}	= Arterial oxygen tension or partial pressure of oxygen in arterial blood
PA_{O_2}	= Alveolar oxygen tension or partial pressure of oxygen in the alveoli
P_{CO_2}	= Carbon dioxide tension or partial pressure of carbon dioxide
Pa_{CO_2}	= Partial pressure of carbon dioxide in arterial blood
Pv_{CO_2}	= Partial pressure of carbon dioxide in venous blood
pH	= Hydronium ion concentration
pHa	= Hydronium ion concentration in arterial blood
S_{O_2}	= Oxygen saturation
Sa_{O_2}	= Percent saturation of oxygen in arterial blood as measured by hemoximetry (direct method)
Sp_{O_2}	= Percent saturation of oxygen in arterial blood as determined by pulse oximetry (indirect method)
Sv_{O_2}	= Percent saturation of oxygen in venous blood
T_{CO_2}	= Total carbon dioxide content

---

mechanical or volume-displacement types (water-filled, dry-rolling seal, wedge, or bellows) and the electronic or flow-sensing types (pneumotachometer or hot-wire anemometer).

The water-seal spirometer has been the basic tool for many years. It consists of a bell suspended in a sleeve of water (Fig. 14-1). The bell rises and falls in response to inhalation and exhalation through a tube connected to the spirometer. The proportional movements of the bell are recorded, either on a kymograph (a rotating drum on which a tracing is made with a stylus) or by an electrical potentiometer.

Flow-sensing or electronic spirometers have also become very popular. The most common type consists of a pressure-differential pneumotachometer that measures a pressure drop as air moves across a resistive element. The greater the air flow, the greater the pressure difference on one side of the resistive element compared with the other side.

Measured (actual) spirometry values are compared with predicted values by means of regression equations using age, height, weight, ethnicity, and gender and are expressed as a percentage of the predicted value. Typically, a value >80% of predicted is considered to be within normal limits.

Spirometry determines the effectiveness of the various mechanical forces involved in lung and chest wall movement. The values obtained provide quantitative information about the degree of obstruction to air flow or the degree of restriction of inspired air (Figs. 14-2 and 14-3).

CHART 14-3 ▌
Lung Volume Symbols: Pulmonary Function Terminology

This list indicates terms used in measuring lung volumes and the units that
express these measurements.

FVC	=	*Forced vital capacity:* maximum amount of air that can be exhaled forcibly and completely after a maximal inspiration (liters)
FEV_t	=	Forced expiratory volume at specific time intervals (eg, 1, 2, and/or 3 seconds): volume of air expired during the first, second, third, etc. second of FVC maneuver (liters)
FEV_t/FVC	=	Ratio of a timed forced expiratory volume to the forced vital capacity (eg, FEV_1/FVC) (percent)
$FEF_{200-1200}$	=	*Forced expiratory flow* between 200 ml and 1200 ml: average flow of expired air measured after the first 200 ml and average during the next 1000 ml of the FVC maneuver (liters/second)
FEF_{25-75}	=	*Forced expiratory flow* between 25% and 75%: average flow of expired air measured between 25% and 75% of the FVC maneuver (liters/second)
PEFR	=	*Peak expiratory flow rate:* maximum flow of expired air attained during an FVC maneuver (liters/second or liters/minute)
PIFR	=	*Peak inspiratory flow rate:* maximum flow of inspired air achieved during a forced maximal inspiration (liters/second or liters/minute)
FEF_{25}	=	Forced instantaneous expiratory flow rate at 25% of lung volume achieved during an FVC maneuver (liters/second or liters/minute)
FEF_{50}	=	Forced instantaneous expiratory flow rate at 50% of lung volume achieved during an FVC maneuver (liters/second or liters/minute)
FEF_{75}	=	Forced instantaneous expiratory flow rate at 75% of lung volume achieved during an FVC maneuver (liters/second or liters/minute)
FIVC	=	*Forced inspiratory vital capacity:* maximum amount of air that can be inhaled forcibly and completely after a maximal expiration (liters)
FRC	=	*Functional residual capacity:* volume of air remaining in the lung at the end of a normal expiration (eg, end-tidal expiration) (liters)
IC	=	*Inspiratory capacity:* maximum amount of air that can be inspired from end-tidal expiration (liters)
IRV	=	*Inspiratory reserve volume:* maximum amount of air that can be inspired from end-tidal inspiration (liters)

(continued)

CHART 14-3 *(continued)*

ERV	=	*Expiratory reserve volume:* maximum amount of air that can be expired from end-tidal expiration (liters)
RV	=	*Residual volume:* volume of gas left in the lung after a maximal expiration (liters)
VC	=	*Vital capacity:* maximum volume of air that can be expired after a maximal inspiration (liters)
TLC	=	*Total lung capacity:* volume of gas contained in the lungs after a maximal inspiration (liters)
DLCO	=	Carbon monoxide diffusing capacity of the lung: rate of diffusion of carbon monoxide across the alveolar capillary membrane (ie, rate of gas transfer across the alveolar capillary membrane) (milliliters/minute per millimeter of mercury)
DL/VA	=	Carbon monoxide diffusing capacity per liter of alveolar volume (milliliters/minute per millimeter of mercury per liter of alveolar volume)
CV	=	*Closing volume:* volume at which the lower lung zones cease to ventilate, presumably as a result of airway closure (percent of vital capacity)
MVV	=	*Maximum voluntary ventilation:* maximum number of liters of air a patient can breathe per minute by a voluntary effort (liters/minute)
VISOV̇	=	*Volume of isoflow:* volume for which flow is the same with air and with helium during an FVC maneuver (percent)

Procedure for Spirometry

The following procedure applies generally to spirometry measurements such as FVC, FEV_1, FEV_2, FEV_3, FEV_t/FVC, $FEF_{200-1200}$, and FEF_{25-75} (see definitions in Chart 14-3).

1. The patient may sit or stand.
2. The patient is fitted with a mouthpiece connected to the spirometer and a nose clip that closes the nares so that only mouth breathing is possible.
3. The patient is then asked to inhale maximally, hold the breath momentarily, and then exhale forcibly and completely.
4. Between brief rest periods, the preceding step is repeated twice. In this way, a minimum of 3 tracings are obtained. The 2 best tracings should come within 5% of each other.
5. The entire procedure takes about 15 to 20 minutes.
6. See Chapter 1 guidelines for *intratest* care.

CHART 14-4 ▶
Miscellaneous Symbols

This list shows some of the other symbols found in this chapter.

f	=	Frequency (of breathing)
C_L	=	Compliance of the lung
D	=	Diffusing capacity
COHb	=	Carboxyhemoglobin
DLO_2	=	Oxygen diffusing capacity of the lung (milliliters/minute per milliliter of mercury)
$A–aDO_2$	=	Alveolar-to-arterial oxygen gradient
BSA	=	Body surface area (square meters)
H_2CO_3	=	Carbonic acid
HCO_3^-	=	Bicarbonate ion
TGV	=	Thoracic gas volume (also expressed as V_{TG})
Raw	=	Airway resistance
Gaw	=	Airway conductance
sGaw	=	Specific airway conductance
F–V	=	Flow-volume
V–T	=	Volume-time

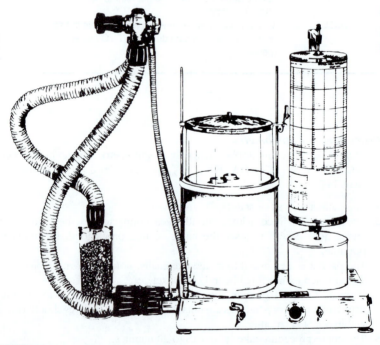

FIGURE 14-1

The Collins Stead-Wells spirometer. (Courtesy of Warren E. Collins, Inc., Braintree, MA)

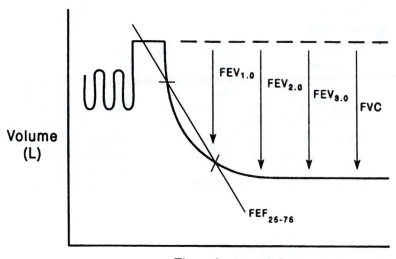

FIGURE 14-2

Typical volume-time spirogram illustrating the measurements of FVC, FEV_1, FEV_2, FEV_3, and FEF_{25-75} (see text for further explanation).

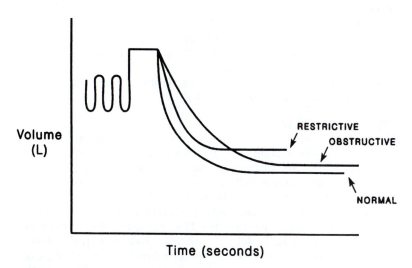

FIGURE 14-3

Examples of normal, obstructive, and restrictive volume-time spirograms.

> **Clinical Alert**
>
> 1. Before testing, assess the patient's ability to comply with breathing requirements.
> 2. The patient may experience lightheadedness, shortness of breath, or other slight discomforts. These symptoms are generally transitory. An appropriate rest period is usually all that is needed. If symptoms persist, testing is terminated.
> 3. Rarely, momentary loss of consciousness (caused by anoxia during forced expiration) may occur. Follow established protocols for testing this.
> 4. Assess for contraindications such as pain or altered mental status.

● AIRWAY FLOW RATES

Airway flow rates provide information about the severity of airway obstruction and serve as an index of dynamic function. The lung volume at which the flow rates are measured is useful for identifying a central or peripheral location of airway obstruction.

VOLUME-TIME SPIROGRAM (V-T TRACING) ●

Normal Values
FVC: 80% of predicted value
FEV_t: FEV_1, FEV_2, and FEV_3 >80% of predicted value
FEV_t/FVC: FEV_1, 80%–85% of FVC; FEV_2, 90%–94% of FVC; and FEV_3, 95%–97% of FVC
Predicted values based on the patient's age, height, ethnicity, and gender are calculated from a nomogram (Fig. 14-4).

Explanation of Test
The forced expiratory maneuver (spirometry) is useful to quantify the extent and severity of airway obstruction. The maximum amount of air that can be exhaled rapidly and forcibly, after a maximal deep inspiration, is corrected for body temperature, pressure, and saturation (BTPS) and recorded as the forced vital capacity (FVC), expressed in liters.

The forced expiratory volumes exhaled within 1, 2, or 3 seconds are sometimes referred to as *timed vital capacities* (FEV_1, FEV_2, and FEV_3, respectively). These measurements are useful for evaluating a patient's response to bronchodilators. Generally, if the FEV_1 is <80% of predicted and/or the FEF_{25-75} (see Chart 14-3) is <60% of predicted, a bronchodilator such as albuterol sulfate (Proventil) or ipratropium bromide (Atrovent) is administered with a handheld nebulizer and the spirometry is repeated. Recently, a combination of albuterol and ipratropium (combivent) has been introduced in which studies have shown to demonstrate a better bronchodilator response than either alone. See Figure 14–2 for an example of a volume-time spirogram (V-T). An increase in these values of 20% or more above the prebronchodilator level suggests a significant response to the bronchodilator and is consistent with a diagnosis of reversible obstructive airway disease (eg, asthma). Persons with emphysema typically do not demonstrate this type of response to bronchodilators.

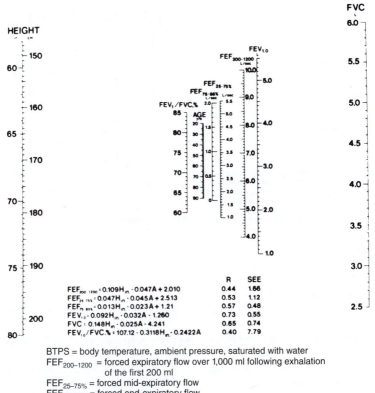

$FEF_{200-1200} = 0.109H_{in} \cdot 0.047A + 2.010$ R 0.44   SEE 1.66
$FEF_{25-75\%} = 0.047H_{in} \cdot 0.045A + 2.513$ 0.53   1.12
$FEF_{75-85\%} = 0.013H_{in} \cdot 0.023A + 1.21$ 0.57   0.48
$FEV_{1.0} = 0.092H_{in} \cdot 0.032A - 1.260$ 0.73   0.55
$FVC = 0.148H_{in} \cdot 0.025A - 4.241$ 0.65   0.74
$FEV_{1.0}/FVC.\% = 107.12 \cdot 0.3118H_{in} \cdot 0.2422A$ 0.40   7.79

BTPS = body temperature, ambient pressure, saturated with water
$FEF_{200-1200}$ = forced expiratory flow over 1,000 ml following exhalation of the first 200 ml
$FEF_{25-75\%}$ = forced mid-expiratory flow
$FEF_{75-85\%}$ = forced end-expiratory flow
$FEV_{1.0}$ = one-second forced expiratory volume
FVC = forced vital capacity

FIGURE 14-4

This is an example of a typical nomogram for determining various predicted expiratory flow rates in normal males *(A)* and normal females *(B)*. The values are determined by laying a ruler across the height scale and age scale (corresponding to the patient's height and age) and then reading the values where the ruler crosses the other scales. When the test site has computer equipment, the values are computed electronically. Values obtained include the FVC, $FEV_{1.0}$, FEF_{25-75}, and $FEF_{200-1200}$.

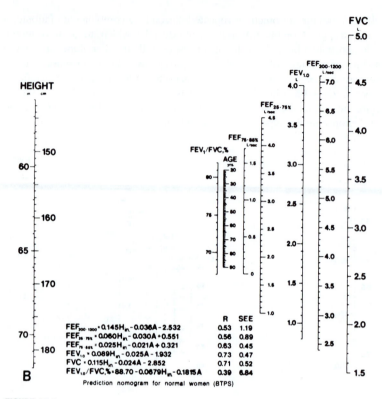

FIGURE 14-4

(Continued)

Procedure

1. The patient is asked to exhale forcibly and rapidly after a maximal air inspiration.
2. The measurements are obtained from spirometry tracings (see Spirometry, page 951).
3. Bronchodilators are administered with a handheld nebulizer, and spirometry is repeated.

Clinical Implications

1. Abnormal configurations of V-T spirograms are shown in Figure 14-3.
2. With obstructive ventilatory impairments such as asthma, airway collapse occurs during forced expiratory effort. This leads to decreases in airway flow rates and also, in the more severe forms, to apparent loss of volumes.
3. Decreased values occur in chronic lung diseases that cause trapping of air (emphysema), chronic bronchitis, or asthma.
4. With restrictive ventilatory impairments, the FVC is reduced; however, flow rates can be normal or elevated.

Patient Preparation

1. Explain the purpose and procedure of the spirometry test (see page 951). Emphasize that this is a noninvasive test; however, it does require cooperation and effort.
2. Withhold bronchodilators for 4 to 6 hours before the study, if tolerated.
3. Assess for interfering factors and contraindications such as pain or physical or mental impairment.
4. Follow guidelines in Chapter 1 for safe, effective, informed *pretest* care.

Patient Aftercare

1. Evaluate complaints of fatigue, shortness of breath, or chest discomfort or pain. Monitor and provide rest as necessary.
2. Assess patient and test outcomes and monitor appropriately for signs of asthma, emphysema, and other chronic lung diseases.
3. Follow guidelines in Chapter 1 for safe, effective, informed, *posttest* care.

FLOW-VOLUME LOOPS (F-V LOOPS)

Normal Values

Qualitative: A "scooped-out," concave appearance of the expiratory portion of the F-V loop is characteristic of obstructive ventilatory impairment. This contrasts with the normal F-V loop, which may actually be somewhat convex on the descending portion of the expiratory limb. The restrictive F-V loop looks similar in configuration to the normal loop except for being smaller.

Explanation of Test

This test provides both a graphic analysis and a quantitative measurement of flow rates for any lung volume. It evaluates the dynamics of both large and medium-sized (central) airways and is also helpful in ruling out small peripheral airway obstruction. Values obtained include FVC, FEV_1, FEF_{25-75}, PEFR, PIFR, FEF_{25}, FEF_{50}, and FEF_{75} (see definitions in Chart 14-3). See Fig. 14-5 for an example of a flow-volume (F-V) loop.

Procedure

The procedure is the same as for spirometry except for the addition of a maximal forced inspiration at the end of the forced expiratory maneuver.

Clinical Implications

Abnormal configurations of F-V loops are shown in Fig. 14-6). Such findings indicate

1. Obstructive ventilatory impairments:
    A. Small airway obstructive disease (eg, bronchitis, asthma)
    B. Large airway obstructive disease (eg, tumors of the trachea and bronchioles)
2. Restrictive ventilatory impairments (eg, interstitial pulmonary fibroses, obesity)

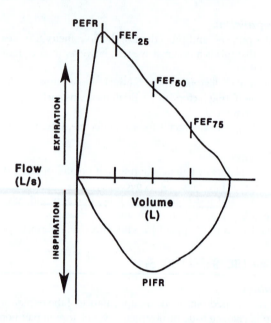

FIGURE 14-5
Typical flow-volume loop illustrating the measurements of PEFR, PIFR, FEF_{25}, FEF_{50}, and FEF_{75} (see text for further explanation).

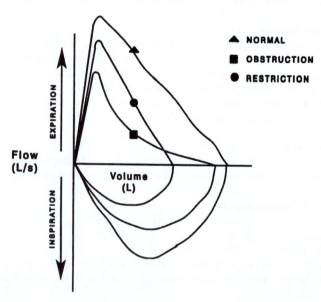

FIGURE 14-6
Examples of a normal, obstructive, and restrictive flow-volume loop.

Patient Preparation
1. Explain the purpose and procedure of the spirometry test. Explain that the patient will be asked to perform a maximal forced inspiration in addition to the forced expirations.
2. A light meal may be eaten before the test. However, no caffeine should be taken before testing.
3. Follow Chapter 1 guidelines for safe, effective, informed *pretest* care.

Patient Aftercare
1. See Chapter 1 guidelines for safe, effective, informed *posttest* care.
2. See aftercare guidelines for volume-time spirogram (page 958).
3. Evaluate for dizziness, shortness of breath, chest discomfort. Usually these symptoms are transitory and subside after a short rest. If symptoms persist, use established follow-up protocols.

PEAK INSPIRATORY FLOW RATE (PIFR) ●

Normal Values
Approximately 300 L/min
Predicted values are based on age, sex, and height.

Explanation of Test
The peak inspiratory flow rate (PIFR) measurement identifies reduced breathing on inspiration and is totally dependent on the effort the patient makes to inspire. The PIFR is the maximum flow of air achieved during a forced maximal inspiration. (See Indications for Tests, page 949.)

Procedure
1. The PIFR is obtained from the F-V loop procedure by using the spirometer with a special X-Y recorder (see Fig. 14-5).
2. The patient is instructed to inspire maximally, exhale forcibly and completely, and then inspire forcibly and completely.
3. PIFR can also be measured with a handheld peak flow meter.

Clinical Implications
1. PIFR is *reduced* in neuromuscular disorders, with weakness or poor effort, and in extrathoracic airway obstruction (ie, substernal thyroid, tracheal stenosis, and laryngeal paralysis).
2. The PIFR is altered in upper airway obstruction.

Interfering Factors
Poor patient effort compromises the test.

Patient Preparation
1. Explain the purpose and procedure of the spirometry test. Assess the patient's ability to comply.
2. Follow Chapter 1 guidelines for safe, effective, informed, *pretest* care.

Patient Aftercare

1. See Chapter 1 guidelines for safe, effective, informed *posttest* care.
2. See aftercare guidelines for volume-time spirogram (page 958).

PEAK EXPIRATORY FLOW RATE (PEFR) ●

Normal Values

Approximately 450 L/min
Predicted values are based on age, sex, and height.

Explanation of Test

The peak expiratory flow rate (PEFR) measurement is used as an index of large airway function. It is the maximum flow of expired air attained during a forced expiratory maneuver. (See Indications for Tests, page 949.)

Procedure

1. The PEFR is obtained from the F-V loop procedure by using the spirometer with an X-Y special recorder (see Fig. 14-5).
2. The patient is asked to inspire maximally, exhale forcibly and completely, and then to inspire forcibly and completely.

Clinical Implications

1. The PEFR usually is *decreased* in obstructive disease (eg, emphysema), during acute exacerbations of asthma, and in upper airway obstruction (eg, tracheal stenosis).
2. The PEFR usually is *normal* in restrictive lung disease but is reduced in severe restrictive situations.

Interfering Factors

Poor patient effort compromises the test.

Patient Preparation

1. Explain the purpose and procedure of the spirometry test. Assess the patient's ability to comply.
2. See Chapter 1 guidelines for safe, effective, informed *pretest* care guidelines.

Patient Aftercare

1. See Chapter 1 guidelines for safe, effective, informed, *posttest* care.
2. See aftercare for volume-time spirogram (page 958).

● LUNG VOLUMES AND CAPACITIES

Lung volumes can be considered as basic subdivisions of the lung (not actual anatomic subdivisions). They may be subdivided as follows:

1. Total lung capacity (TLC)
2. Tidal volume (VT)
3. Inspiratory capacity (IC)
4. Inspiratory reserve volume (IRV)
5. Residual volume (RV)
6. Functional residual capacity (FRC)
7. Expiratory reserve volume (ERV)
8. Vital capacity (VC)

Combinations of 2 or more volumes are termed *capacities*. These volumes and capacities are shown graphically in Figure 14-7. Also shown are the values found in normal adult men. Measurement of these values can provide information about the degree of air-trapping or hyperinflation.

FUNCTIONAL RESIDUAL CAPACITY (FRC) ●

Normal Values
Approximately 2.50–3.50 L
Predicted values are based on age, height, weight, ethnicity, and gender.
The observed value should be 75% to 125% of the predicted value.

Explanation of Test
Functional residual capacity (FRC) is used to evaluate both restrictive and obstructive lung defects. Changes in the elastic properties of the lungs are re-

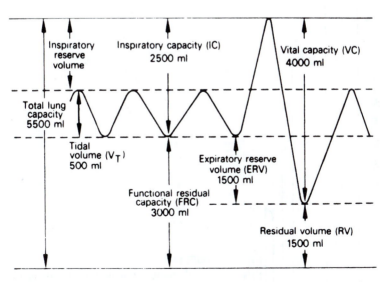

FIGURE 14-7
Subdivisions of lung volume in the normal adult. (Geschickter CF: The Lung in Health and Disease. Philadelphia, JB Lippincott, 1973).

flected in the FRC. The FRC is the volume of gas contained in the lungs at the end of a normal quiet expiration.

Procedure

1. After being fitted with nose clips, the patient is instructed to breathe through the mouthpiece on the lung volume apparatus.
2. There are 2 methods, depending on the instrument used:
   A. The patient breathes 100% oxygen (O_2) until the alveolar nitrogen content ($\%N_2A$) reaches approximately 1.5% to 2.0%. Calculation of the FRC is based on the fact that 79% of the air in the lung is N_2; the volume of N_2 that was "washed out" of the lungs by the pure O_2 is collected and measured. V_E is the total volume of expired gas.

   Nitrogen washout or open-circuit technique:

$$FRC = \frac{Final\ \%N_2 \times V_E}{\%N_2A}$$

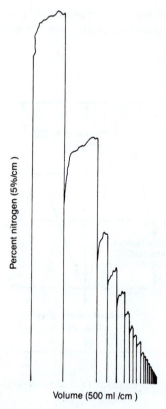

Percent nitrogen (5%/cm)

Volume (500 ml /cm)

FIGURE 14-8

Typical tracing of a multiple breath nitrogen workout curve for determining FRC. The patient breathes 100% oxygen until alveolar nitrogen reaches 1.5-2.0%.

B. The patient rebreathes a mixture of room air with 10% to 12% helium (He) until equilibrium is reached.

Helium dilution or closed-circuit technique:

$$FRC = \frac{\text{Initial \%He} - \text{Final \%He}}{\text{Final \%He}} \times \text{Initial volume}$$

3. Results are recorded either by an X-Y recorder on semilog paper (Fig. 14-8) or by a respirometer on a kymograph drum.
4. The test should be performed a second time. Results for FRC should vary by not more than 5% to 10%.
5. See Chapter 1 guidelines for *intratest* care.

Clinical Implications
1. A value <75% of predicted is consistent with restrictive ventilatory impairment.
2. A value >125% of predicted demonstrates air-trapping (hyperinflation), consistent with obstructive airway disease (eg, emphysema, asthma, bronchiolar obstruction).

Patient Preparation
1. Explain the purpose and procedure of the test. Explain that this is a noninvasive test requiring patient cooperation. Assess the patient's ability to comply.
2. Record the patient's age, gender, weight, and height.
3. Follow Chapter 1 guidelines for safe, effective, informed *pretest* care.

Patient Aftercare
1. Explain test outcomes; allow the patient to rest if necessary.
2. See Chapter 1 for safe, effective, informed *posttest* care guidelines.

RESIDUAL VOLUME (RV) ●

Normal Values
Approximately 1200–1500 ml
Predicted values are based on age, gender, and height.

Explanation of Test
Residual volume (RV) can be helpful to distinguish between restrictive and obstructive ventilatory defects. It is the volume of gas remaining in the lungs after a maximal exhalation. Because the lungs cannot be completely emptied (ie, a maximal expiratory effort cannot expel all of the gas), RV is the only lung volume that cannot be measured directly from the spirometer. It is calculated mathematically by subtracting the expiratory reserve volume (ERV) from the FRC (see Fig. 14-7).

Procedure
The RV is determined indirectly from other tests. There is no actual procedure.

Clinical Implications

1. An increase in the RV (>125% of predicted) indicates that, despite a maximal expiratory effort, the lungs still contain an abnormally large amount of gas (air-trapping). This type of change occurs in young asthmatics and usually is reversible. In emphysema, the condition is permanent.
2. Increased RV is characteristic of emphysema, chronic air-trapping, and chronic bronchial obstruction.
3. The RV and the FRC usually increase together, but not always.
4. The RV sometimes decreases in diseases that occlude many alveoli.
5. An RV <75% of predicted is consistent with restrictive disorders (eg, interstitial pulmonary fibrosis).

Interfering Factors

Residual volume normally increases with age.

Patient Preparation

1. Explain the purpose of the test and how the results are calculated.
2. See Chapter 1 guidelines for safe, effective, informed *pretest* care.

Patient Aftercare

1. Interpret test results and monitor as necessary.
2. Follow Chapter 1 guidelines for safe, effective, informed *posttest* care.

EXPIRATORY RESERVE VOLUME (ERV)

Normal Values

Approximately 1200–1500 ml
Predicted values are based on age, height, and gender.

Explanation of Test

Expiratory reserve volume (ERV) is the largest volume of gas that can be exhaled from end-tidal expiration. This measurement identifies lung or chest wall restriction. The ERV can be estimated mathematically by subtracting the inspiratory capacity (IC) from the vital capacity (VC). The ERV accounts for approximately 25% of the VC and can vary greatly in patients of comparable age and height (see Fig. 14-7).

Procedure

1. Record the patient's age and height.
2. Have the patient breathe normally into a spirometer for several breaths and then exhale maximally from the end-tidal expiratory level.
3. Results are recorded on graph paper (spirogram).
4. Repeat this maneuver until 2 values are within 5% of one another.

Clinical Implications

1. A decreased ERV indicates a chest wall restriction resulting from nonpulmonary causes.
2. Decreased values are associated with an elevated diaphragm (eg, massive

obesity, ascites, pregnancy). Decreased values also occur with massive enlargement of the heart, pleural effusion, kyphoscoliosis, or thoracoplasty.

3. Decreases in ERV also are seen in obstruction resulting from an increase in the RV impinging on the ERV.

Patient Preparation

1. Explain the purpose and procedure of the spirometry test. Inform the patient that the test is noninvasive. Assess the patient's ability to comply with test procedures.

2. Follow Chapter 1 guidelines for safe, effective, informed *pretest* care.

Patient Aftercare

1. Interpret test outcomes and counsel about respiratory abnormalities.

2. Follow Chapter 1 guidelines for safe, effective, informed *posttest* care.

INSPIRATORY CAPACITY (IC)

Normal Values

Approximately 2500–3600 ml
Predicted values are based on age, height, and gender.

Explanation of Test

Inspiratory capacity (IC) measures the largest volume of air that can be inhaled from the end-tidal expiratory level. This measurement is used to identify lung or chest wall restrictions. Mathematically, the IC is the sum of the tidal volume (VT) and the inspiratory reserve volume (IRV) (see Fig. 14-7).

Procedure

1. Record the age, gender, and height of the patient.

2. The patient breathes normally into a spirometer for several breaths and then inhales maximally, expanding the lungs as much as possible from end-tidal expiration. Normal breathing is then resumed.

3. Step 2 is usually repeated 2 or more times until the 2 best values are within 5% of each other. The largest inspired volume value is selected.

Clinical Implications

1. Changes in the IC usually parallel increases or decreases in the vital capacity (VC).

2. Decreases in IC can be related to either restrictive or obstructive ventilatory impairments.

Patient Preparation

1. Instruct the patient about the purpose and procedure of the test and the need for patient cooperation.

2. Follow Chapter 1 guidelines for safe, effective, informed *pretest* care.

Patient Aftercare

See Chapter 1 guidelines for safe, effective, informed *posttest* care.

VITAL CAPACITY (VC) ●

Normal Values
Approximately 3.00–5.00 L
Predicted values are based on age, gender, height, and ethnicity.

Explanation of Test
Measurement of the vital capacity (VC) identifies defects of lung or chest wall restriction. The VC is the largest volume of gas that can be expelled from the lungs after the lungs are first filled to the maximum extent and then slowly emptied to the maximum extent. Mathematically, it is the sum of the IC and the ERV (see Fig. 14-7).

Procedure
1. While breathing into a spirometer with nose clips, the patient inhales as deeply as possible and then exhales completely, with no forced or rapid effort.
2. Results are recorded on graph paper.
3. The procedure should be repeated at least twice. The VC measurements should be within 5% of each other.

Clinical Implications
1. A reduced VC is defined as a value <80% of predicted.
2. The VC can be lower than expected in either a restrictive or an obstructive disorder.
3. A decreased VC can be related to depression of the respiratory center in the brain, neuromuscular diseases, pleural effusion, pneumothorax, pregnancy, ascites, limitations of thoracic movement, scleroderma, kyphoscoliosis, or tumors.

Interfering Factors
1. The VC increases with physical fitness and greater height.
2. The VC decreases with age (after age 30 years).
3. The VC is generally less in women than in men of the same age and height.
4. The VC is decreased by approximately 15% in African Americans and by 20% to 25% in Asians, compared with Caucasians of the same age, height, and gender.
5. Inadequate patient effort causes lower VC values.

Patient Preparation
1. Explain the purpose and procedure of the test and need for patient cooperation. Assess for interfering factors.
2. Follow Chapter 1 guidelines for safe, effective, informed *pretest* care.

Patient Aftercare
1. See Chapter 1 for safe, effective, informed *posttest* care guidelines.

2. Interpret outcomes, monitor patient signs and symptoms, and follow up if necessary.

TOTAL LUNG CAPACITY (TLC)

Normal Values
Approximately 4.00–6.00 L
Predicted values are based on age, height, gender, and ethnicity.

Explanation of Test
Total lung capacity (TLC) is used mainly to evaluate obstructive defects and to differentiate restrictive from obstructive pulmonary disease. It measures the volume of gas contained in the lungs at the end of a maximal inspiration. Mathematically, it is the sum of the VC and the RV, or the sum of the primary lung volumes (see Fig. 14-7). This value is calculated indirectly from other tests.

Procedure
1. The patient is instructed to breathe normally into a spirometer and then to inspire maximally and exhale maximally. The total amount of air exhaled is the VC.
2. The TLC is derived by the following formula: TLC = VC + RV.

Clinical Implications
1. An obstructive impairment is characterized by an *increased* TLC. However, a normal or increased TLC does not mean that ventilation or the surface area for diffusion is normal. The TLC may be normal or increased in bronchiolar obstruction with hyperinflation and in emphysema.
2. The TLC is *decreased* in edema, atelectasis, neoplasms, pulmonary congestion, pneumothorax, or thoracic restriction.
3. A *decreased* TLC is the hallmark of a *restrictive* ventilatory impairment.

Patient Preparation
1. Explain the purpose and procedure of the spirometry test. Even though it is noninvasive, it does require patient effort and cooperation.
2. Follow Chapter 1 guidelines for safe, effective, informed *pretest* care.

Patient Aftercare
1. Interpret outcomes and monitor for complaints of nausea, lightheadedness, or chest pain.
2. See Chapter 1 guidelines for safe, effective, informed *posttest* care.

GAS EXCHANGE (DIFFUSING CAPACITY)

The diffusing capacity measurement determines the rate of gas transfer across the alveolar capillary membranes.

CARBON MONOXIDE DIFFUSING CAPACITY (DLCO) ●

Normal Values

Approximately 25 ml/min per millimeter of mercury

Predicted values are based on the patient's height in centimeters (H), age in years (A), and gender:

DLCO in men = 0.0984(H) − 0.177(A) + 19.93

DLCO in women = 0.1118(H) − 0.117(A) + 7.72

Background

Carbon monoxide (CO) combines with hemoglobin about 210 times more readily than does O_2. If there is a normal amount of hemoglobin in the blood, the only other significant limiting factor to CO uptake is the state of the alveolar capillary membranes. Normally, the amount of CO in the blood is insufficient to affect the test.

Two categories of factors determine the rate of gas (CO) transfer across the lung. The physical determinants are CO driving pressure, surface area, thickness of capillary walls, and diffusion coefficient for CO. The chemical determinants are red blood cell volume and reaction rate with hemoglobin.

Explanation of Test

This test is used to diagnose pulmonary vascular disease, emphysema, and pulmonary fibrosis and to evaluate the extent of functional pulmonary capillary bed in contact with functional alveoli. The alveolar volume (VA) can also be determined. The DLCO measures the diffusing capacity of the lungs for CO. The DLO_2 is obtained by multiplying the DLCO by 1.23.

Procedure

1. Record the patient's age, height, weight, and gender.
2. Two techniques are used by laboratories:
   A. *Single-breath or breath-holding technique:* The patient is instructed to exhale to residual volume, then maximally inhale a diffusion gas mixture (eg, 10% He and 0.3% CO in room air), hold the breath for 10 to 12 seconds, and then exhale. A sample of alveolar gas is collected after washout of dead space volume.

$$DLCO_{SB} = \frac{VA \times 60}{(PB - PH_2O) \times t} \, ln \, \frac{FACO_0}{FACO_t}$$

where

$FACO_B$ = initial alveolar CO concentration at the beginning of breath-holding time

$FACO_E$ = alveolar CO concentration at end of breath-holding time

VA = alveolar volume

60 = conversion factor (seconds to 1 minute)

t = breath-holding time in seconds

PB = barometric pressure in mm Hg

PH_2O = water vapor pressure in mm Hg

ln = natural logarithm

B. *Steady-state technique:* The patient is asked to breathe from a bag containing 0.1% to 0.2% CO for several minutes. During the final 2 minutes, the exhaled air is collected and then analyzed for O_2, CO_2, and CO concentrations. An arterial blood gas sample is also drawn during the final 2 minutes of the procedure.

$$\text{DLCO}_{ss} = \frac{\dot{V}CO}{PACO}$$

where

$\dot{V}CO$ = milliliters of CO transferred per minute (adjusted for STPD)
PACO = partial pressure of CO in the alveoli

3. See Chapter 1 guidelines for intratest care.

Clinical Implications

1. *Decreased* values are associated with
   A. Multiple pulmonary emboli
   B. Emphysema
   C. Lung resection
   D. Pulmonary fibroses:
      (1) Sarcoidosis
      (2) Systemic lupus erythematosus
      (3) Asbestosis
      (4) Pneumonia
   E. Anemia
   F. Increased levels of carboxyhemoglobin (COHb)
   G. Pulmonary resection
   H. Scleroderma
2. *Increased* values are observed in polycythemia, left-to-right shunts, pulmonary hemorrhage, and exercise.
3. The value is relatively *normal* in chronic bronchitis.

Interfering Factors

Exercise (with an increased cardiac output) and polycythemia increase the value. Because increased levels of COHb (as seen in smokers) and anemia decrease the value, the D_LCO is corrected for COHb levels >10% and hemoglobin (Hb) values <8 g per 100 ml of blood.

Patient Preparation

1. Explain the purpose and procedure. Assess for interfering factors and explain that this noninvasive test requires patient cooperation. Assess the patient's ability to comply.
2. Follow Chapter 1 guidelines for safe, effective, informed *pretest* care.

Patient Aftercare

1. Explain test outcomes and possible need for follow-up testing to monitor course of therapy (eg, anti-inflammatory drugs, bronchodilators, some antiarrhythmics, antineoplastics).
2. See Chapter 1 for safe, effective, informed *posttest* care guidelines.

MAXIMUM VOLUNTARY VENTILATION (MVV) ●

Normal Values

Approximately 160–180 L/min

Predicted values are based on the patient's age in years (A), height in inches (H), and gender (a healthy person may vary by as much as 25% to 35% from mean group values):

MVV in men = 3.03(H) − 0.816(A) − 37.9

MVV in women = 2.14(H) − 0.685(A) − 4.87

Explanation of Test

Maximum voluntary ventilation (MVV) measures several physiologic phenomena occurring at the same time, including thoracic cage compliance, lung compliance, airway resistance, and available muscle force. It is the number of liters of air that the patient can breathe per minute with maximal voluntary effort.

Procedure

1. The patient breathes into a spirometer as deeply and rapidly as possible for 10 to 15 seconds. Usually, the frequency reaches 40 to 70 breaths per minute and the tidal volumes are about 50% of VC (Fig. 14-9).
2. Actual values are extrapolated from the 10- to 15-second time interval to a 1-minute time period.
3. Typically, the maneuver is performed twice. The largest value is reported.

Interfering Factors

Poor patient effort can be ruled out by using the following formula to predict the MVV of the patient: Predicted MVV = 35 × FEV_1. This is a useful check to determine whether the recorded MVV is indicative of adequate patient effort. Low values can be related to patient effort and not to pathophysiology.

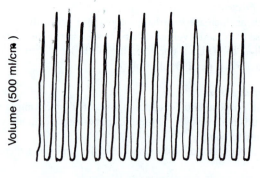

Time (2 sec/cm)

FIGURE 14-9

Maximum voluntary ventilation. Patient breathes into a spirometer as deeply and rapidly as possible for 10 to 15 seconds.

Clinical Implications

1. Obstructive ventilatory impairments of moderate to severe degree, abnormal neuromuscular control, and poor patient effort are causes of low values.
2. In restrictive disease, the value is usually normal; however, in more severe forms, MVV may be decreased.

Patient Preparation

1. Explain the purpose and procedure of the test. Explain that it is a noninvasive test that requires patient cooperation. Assess the patient's ability to comply.
2. Record the patient's age, height, and gender.
3. Follow Chapter 1 guidelines for safe, effective, informed *pretest* care.

Patient Aftercare

1. Explain test outcome and possible need for follow-up testing and treatment.
2. See Chapter 1 regarding safe, effective, informed *posttest* care guidelines.

MAXIMAL RESPIRATORY PRESSURES (MRP) ●

Normal Values

Maximal expiratory pressure (MEP): approximately 100–250 cm H_2O
Maximal inspiratory pressure (MIP): approximately 40–125 cm H_2O
Predicted values are based on the patient's age in years (A) and gender:

MEP in men = $268 - 1.03(A)$
MIP in men = $143 - 0.55(A)$
MEP in women = $170 - 0.53(A)$
MIP in women = $104 - 0.51(A)$

Explanation of Test

The maximal respiratory pressure (MRP) measurements assess ventilatory muscle strength in persons with neuromuscular disorders such as poliomyelitis, emphysema, and pulmonary fibroses. The maximal expiratory pressure (MEP) is the greatest pressure that can be generated at or near total lung capacity after a maximal inspiration, whereas the maximal inspiratory pressure (MIP) is measured at or near the residual volume after a maximal expiration.

Procedure

1. The patient, in a seated position and wearing a nose clip, is instructed to inspire maximally and then place the mouthpiece of the handheld pressure manometer into the mouth and perform a forced expiration. This maximal sustained (1 to 3 seconds) pressure against the internal occlusion of the manometer is recorded as the MEP.
2. This same procedure is repeated to obtain the MIP, except that this time the patient fully exhales before placing the mouthpiece of the manometer in the mouth. The patient then inspires forcefully, and the maximal sustained (1 to 3 seconds) pressure is recorded.

3. Each procedure is repeated, and the best of 3 measurements is recorded for each.
4. See Chapter 1 guidelines for *intratest* care.

Interfering Factors

The MIP and MEP measurements depend on patient effort; low values may be caused by poor effort rather than loss of respiratory muscle strength. If the patient does not inspire or expire maximally before performing the pressure measurement, the value may be low. Also, sustained efforts longer than 3 seconds should be avoided, because they can cause a decrease in cardiac output as a result of increased intrathoracic pressures.

Clinical Implications

1. *Decreases in both MEP and MIP* are seen in neuromuscular disorders (eg, myasthenia gravis, poliomyelitis).
2. *Decreased MEP* is common in both severe obstructive disease (eg, emphysema) and severe restrictive ventilatory impairment (eg, interstitial pulmonary fibrosis).
3. *Decreased MIP* is observed in patients with chest wall abnormalities (eg, kyphoscoliosis) and in hyperinflation (eg, emphysema).

Patient Preparation

1. Explain the purpose and procedure of the test. Explain that it is a noninvasive, effort-dependent maneuver that requires patient cooperation.
2. Record the patient's age and sex.
3. Follow Chapter 1 guidelines for safe, effective, informed *pretest* care.

Patient Aftercare

1. Explain test outcomes and possible need for follow-up testing and treatment.
2. See Chapter 1 guidelines for safe, effective, informed *posttest* care.

CLOSING VOLUME (CV)

Normal Values
Average is 10% to 20% of VC.
Predicted values are derived from mathematical regression equations and are based on the patient's age in years (A) and gender:
CV in men = $0.562 + 0.357(A) \pm 4.15$
CV in women = $2.812 + 0.293(A) \pm 4.90$

Explanation of Test
In a healthy person, the concentration of alveolar nitrogen, after a single breath of 100% O_2, rapidly increases near the end of expiration. This rise is caused by closure of the small airways in the bases of the lung. The point at which this closure occurs is called the *closing volume* (CV).

CV is used as an index of pathologic changes occurring within the small airways (those <2 mm in diameter). The conventional pulmonary function tests are not sensitive enough to make this determination. This test relies on the fact that the upper lung zones contain a proportionately larger residual volume of gas than the lower lung zones do; there is a gradient of intrapleural pressure from the top to the bottom of the lung. Additionally, the uniformity of gas distribution within the lungs can be measured.

Procedure

1. The patient is asked to exhale completely, to inhale 100% O_2 and then to exhale completely at the rate of approximately 0.5 L/second.
2. During exhalation, both the expired volume and percentage of alveolar nitrogen are monitored simultaneously on an X-Y recorder. A sudden increase in nitrogen represents the closing volume (Fig. 14-10).

Clinical Implications

1. Values are *increased* for those conditions in which the airways are narrowed (eg, bronchitis, early airway obstruction, chronic smokers, old age).
2. A change in the *slope* of the nitrogen curve of >2% is indicative of maldistribution of inspired air (ie, uneven alveolar ventilation).

Interfering Factors

1. The CV increases with age.
2. Patients in congestive heart failure may show an increased CV.

Patient Preparation

1. Explain the purpose and procedure of the test. Explain that this is a noninvasive test that requires patient cooperation. Assess the patient's ability to

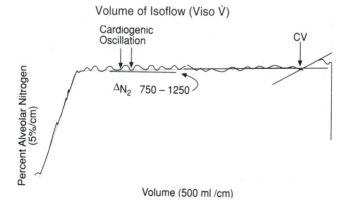

FIGURE 14-10

Typical single-breath nitrogen washout curve for determination of closing volume (CV). The patient inspires 100% oxygen to total lung capacity and then exhales slowly (0.5 LPS) until the lung is empty (i.e. reaches residual volume). The change in the slope of the curve over 1 liter (ΔN_2 750-1250) is an index of the evenness of alveolar ventilation.

comply with breathing requirements and instructions. Assess for interfering factors.

2. Follow Chapter 1 guidelines for safe, effective, informed *pretest* care.

Patient Aftercare

1. Explain the meaning of test outcomes and possible need for follow-up testing and treatment for early small airway disease. Congestive heart failure, with subsequent edema, may also contribute to decreasing patency of the small airways.

2. See Chapter 1 for safe, effective, informed *posttest* care guidelines.

VOLUME OF ISOFLOW (VisoV̇) ●

Normal Values

Average is 10% to 25% of VC.
Values cover a wide range based on age in years (A):
VisoV̇ = 0.450(A) + 4.69

Explanation of Test

This test is designed to detect pathologic changes occurring in the small airways and may be more sensitive than conventional pulmonary function tests. Helium has the unique property of lowering gas density. Therefore, after the patient breathes a helium-oxygen gas mixture, the effects of convective acceleration and turbulence are negated. Any abnormality observed in the F-V loop, then, results from an increase in resistance to (nonturbulent) laminar flow, which indicates small airway abnormalities or lung disease.

Procedure

1. The patient is fitted with nose clips and a baseline F-V loop is recorded on the spirometer with an X-Y recorder.

2. The patient breathes a mixture of 80% He and 20% O_2 for several breaths and then performs another F-V loop maneuver; this is the HeliOx F-V loop.

3. The F-V loop tracings are superimposed, and the volume of isoflow is measured at the point at which the 2 loops intersect.

Clinical Implications

An *increased* volume of isoflow is consistent with early small airway obstruction (eg, asthma).

Patient Preparation

1. Explain the purpose and procedure of the test.

2. Follow guidelines in Chapter 1 regarding safe, effective, *pretest* care.

Patient Aftercare

1. Interpret test outcomes and possible need for follow-up testing and treatment.

2. See Chapter 1 for safe, effective, informed *posttest* care guidelines.

BODY PLETHYSMOGRAPHY ●

Normal Values

V_{TG} = approximately 2.50–3.50 L

Predicted values are based on the patient's age in years (A), height in centimeters (H), weight in kilograms (W), and gender:

V_{TG} in men = 0.052(H) − 5.16(W)

V_{TG} in women = 0.0469(H) − 4.85(W)

C_L = 0.2 L/cm H_2O

Raw = 0.6 − 2.4 L/s/cm H_2O

Gaw = 0.42 − 1.67 L/s/cm H_2O

sGaw = 0.10 − 0.15 L/s/cm H_2O

Explanation of Test

This test measures several parameters. Thoracic gas volume (V_{TG}) comprises all the air contained within the thorax, whether or not it is in ventilatory communication with the rest of the lung. Compliance of the lung (C_L) is an indication of its elasticity, and airway resistance (Raw) is a measurement of the resistance to air flow in the tracheobronchial tree. Airway conductance (Gaw), the reciprocal of airway resistance, is the flow generated per unit of pressure. The specific airway conductance (sGaw) relates to conductance per liter of lung volume.

The measurement of V_{TG} via body plethysmography is an application of Boyles' law, which states that, for a gas at constant temperature, pressure and volume vary inversely ($P_1V_1 = P_2V_2$). Therefore,

$$V_{TG} = \frac{P_1}{\Delta P / \Delta V}$$

$$C_L = \frac{\Delta V}{\Delta P}$$

$$Raw = \frac{P_{atm} - P_{alv}}{\text{Flow rate in L/sec}}$$

$$Gaw = \frac{1}{Raw}$$

$$sGaw = \frac{Gaw}{V_{TG}}$$

where

P_{atm} = atmospheric pressure

P_{alv} = alveolar pressure

ΔP = change in pressure (in cm H_2O)

ΔV = change in volume (in liters)

Raw increases with decreased lung volumes and decreases with higher lung volumes in a nonlinear, hyperbolic fashion. To provide a volume-standardized Raw measurement, Gaw and sGaw are typically calculated.

Procedure

1. The patient sits in the plethysmograph (body box), is fitted with nose clips, and breathes through a mouthpiece connected to a transducer.
2. Once the body box door is secured, the test is delayed for a few minutes, to allow the box pressure to stabilize.
3. The patient is then instructed to perform a panting maneuver while holding the cheeks rigid and the glottis open against a closed shutter located within the transducer assembly. Box and mouth pressures are recorded on the oscilloscope to provide data for V_{TG}.
4. Next, the patient is told to breathe rapidly and shallowly. Box pressure changes versus flow are recorded on the oscilloscope to provide data for Raw.
5. To determine C_L, a balloon catheter must be passed through the nose into the patient's esophagus. The inflated balloon is connected to a transducer, and the patient is instructed to breathe normally. A recording of the changes in intraesophageal pressure during normal respiration (which mimic changes in intrapleural pressure) provides data for C_L.
6. See Chapter 1 guidelines for *intratest* test.

Clinical Implications

1. An *increased* V_{TG} demonstrates air-trapping, consistent with obstructive pulmonary disease.
2. An *increased Raw* demonstrates increased resistance to air flow through the tracheobronchial tree; this is seen in asthma, emphysema, bronchitis, and other forms of obstruction. The Raw distinguishes between restrictive and obstructive ventilatory defects.
3. An *increase* in C_L (ie, lung is more distensible) is seen in obstructive diseases.
4. A *decrease* in C_L (ie, lung is more stiff) is seen in fibrotic diseases, restrictive diseases, pneumonia, congestion, and atelectasis.

Patient Preparation

1. Record the patient's age, height, weight, and gender.
2. Explain the purpose and procedure of the test and instruct and demonstrate the actual maneuvers that will be necessary. Assess for compliance with procedure.
3. Assure the patient that although the chamber is airtight, the test only takes a few minutes. A technician will be in constant attendance to open the door should that be necessary. Assess for ability to comply with test requirements and instructions. Tactfully assess for predisposition to claustrophobia, panic attacks, or other similar responses.
4. Follow Chapter 1 guidelines for safe, effective, informed *pretest* care.

Patient Aftercare

1. Allow the patient time to rest quietly if necessary.
2. Explain the meaning of test outcomes.
3. See Chapter 1 for safe, effective, informed *posttest* care guidelines.

BRONCHIAL PROVOCATION ●

Normal Values

Positive response to inhaled antigen: >20% decrease in FEV_1 from baseline
Negative response: <20% decrease in FEV_1 from baseline

Explanation of Test

Bronchial provocation challenge testing is performed in patients with normal pulmonary function tests who have suspected underlying bronchial hyperreactivity. Additionally, the asthmatic patient is more sensitive to the bronchoconstrictive effects of cholinergic agents (eg, methacholine chloride) than is the healthy person. Airway resistance tests are sensitive monitors of response to bronchoconstrictive agents.

Clinical Implications

A positive response to methacholine or histamine is consistent with bronchial hyperreactivity. Approximately 5% to 10% of asthmatic persons do not respond to the methacholine challenge test.

Procedure

1. The patient performs an FVC maneuver, and the baseline FEV_1 is measured and recorded.
2. The patient then inhales increasing concentrations of methacholine chloride (0.075 to 25.00 mg/ml) by nebulizer. The FVC maneuver is repeated after each successive concentration is inhaled. A 20% reduction in the FEV_1 is considered a positive response.
3. When or if a decrease of >20% from baseline is reached, an inhaled bronchodilator is administered.
4. If a patient goes through all dilution ratios and a 20% reduction in the FEV_1 is not reached, the test is considered negative.
5. If the methacholine causes no change, histamine testing may be ordered.
6. See Chapter 1 for guidelines for *intratest* care.

Patient Preparation

1. Explain the purpose and procedure of the test and the need for patient cooperation. Assess the patient's ability to comply.
2. Withhold bronchodilators for 8 hours and antihistamines for 48 hours before testing, if tolerated.
3. Follow Chapter 1 guidelines for safe, effective, informed *pretest* care.

> **Clinical Alert**
>
> 1. Inhalation of methacholine can cause bronchospasm, chest pain, shortness of breath, and general discomfort.
> 2. These effects can be reversed with a bronchodilator.

Patient Aftercare

1. Explain the meaning of test outcomes.
2. If the test is positive, advise the patient to avoid antigens that may be causing hypersensitivity reaction and bronchospasms.
3. See Chapter 1 guidelines for safe, effective, informed *posttest* care.

CARBON DIOXIDE (CO_2) RESPONSE ●

Normal Values

The act of breathing in successively greater concentrations of CO_2 should result in an increase in minute volume ($\dot{V}E$), when compared with the $\dot{V}E$ during breathing of room air alone. (Room air contains 0.03% CO_2.) In the healthy person there is a linear increase in $\dot{V}E$ of 3 L/min for every 1 mm Hg increase in the partial pressure of CO_2 (PCO_2).

Explanation of Test

This test evaluates the respiratory response to increasing concentrations of inspired CO_2. As alveolar levels of CO_2 increase, so does arterial CO_2. The central chemoreceptors respond by initiating impulses to the respiratory control centers. In the healthy person, this causes the rate and depth of breathing to increase.

Procedure

1. $\dot{V}E$ is determined while the patient breathes room air for several minutes into an instrument (eg, spirometer) that records the frequency of breathing (f) and the tidal volume (VT). The minute volume is then mathematically calculated: $\dot{V}E = f \times VT$.
2. Next, the patient breathes a gas mixture of 2% CO_2 in room air for 5 minutes. During the last 2 minutes, f and VT are recorded and the $\dot{V}E$ is calculated.
3. The patient then breathes gas mixtures of 4% CO_2 and 6% in room air. Mixtures can be increased to as much as 8% CO_2. The entire process is repeated with each successive concentration.
4. A graph is then constructed to plot the changes in $\dot{V}E$ against the concentration of inspired CO_2 ($FICO_2$).
5. See Chapter 1 guidelines for *intratest* care.

Clinical Implications

Lack of response to increasing inspired CO_2 concentrations suggests a disturbance in the normal physiologic pathway of ventilatory changes to hypercapnia. This may result from ingestion of central nervous system depressants (eg, anesthetics, barbiturates, narcotics) or from airflow obstruction (eg, chronic obstructive pulmonary disease [COPD]).

Patient Preparation

1. Explain the purpose and procedure of the test and need for patient cooperation. Assess the patient's ability to comply.
2. Follow Chapter 1 guidelines for safe, effective, informed *pretest* care.

Patient Aftercare

1. Interpret the test outcome and advise that pharmacologic intervention may be necessary to sensitize the chemoreceptors.
2. See Chapter 1 guidelines regarding safe, effective, *posttest* care.

EXERCISE STRESS TESTING

Normal Values

The normal response to graded exercise is an increase in ventilation and cardiac output such that alveolar and arterial gases are maintained at optimal levels to meet metabolic demands. Measurement of the patient's ventilatory and alveolar-arterial gas responses is the primary objective of a pulmonary exercise stress test.

No significant or abnormal changes in the electrocardiographic (ECG) complex, arterial blood pressures, air flow patterns during inspiration and expiration, arterial blood gases and chemistry, or hemodynamic pressures should occur.

Normal Ventilatory and Arterial Blood Gas Responses to Graded Exercise

Value	Change
O_2 consumption ($\dot{V}O_2$)	Increase
CO_2 production ($\dot{V}CO_2$)	Increase
Ventilatory equivalents for O_2 and CO_2	No change
Respiratory exchange ratio (RER)	Increase
Minute ventilation ($\dot{V}_E$)	Increase
Blood lactate	Increase
V_D/V_T ratio	Decrease
A-aDO_2	Slight increase
Arterial blood gas tensions (eg, PaO_2, $PaCO_2$)	No change
Bicarbonate concentration (HCO_3^-)	Decrease
Oxygen saturation (SaO_2)	No change

Background

Respiratory disease reduces the ability to perform exercise. Dynamic exercise that involves large muscle groups produces increases in metabolic O_2 consumption and CO_2 production. This increase in metabolic demand leads to stresses on other mechanisms taking part in O_2 and CO_2 transport. Exercise testing measures the functional reserves of these mechanisms by testing under load. Analysis of bronchogenic and cardiovascular disorders includes procedures that measure respiratory outcomes and blood gas values during exercise. Ventilation and gas exchange are altered during exercise in healthy persons; however, specific abnormalities are noted in the presence of cardiovascular or respiratory impairment. Exercise tests are valuable for assessing the severity and type of impairment in existing or undiagnosed conditions.

Explanation of Test

Exercise testing is done to evaluate fitness, functional capacity, and other limiting factors in persons with obstructive or restrictive diseases. The efficiency of the cardiopulmonary system may be altered during exercise; exercise testing assesses ventilation, gas exchange, and cardiovascular function during increased demands. Dyspnea on exertion due to cardiovascular causes can be differentiated from that due to respiratory causes. Precise information about mechanisms that influence O_2 and CO_2 transport during exercise can be obtained by using a staged approach.

An exercise test can detect or exclude many conditions, even though the response may be nonspecific. For example, if the patient complains of severe shortness of breath despite a normal exercise response, a psychogenic cause is likely. However, a few conditions exhibit diagnostic responses (eg, exercise-induced asthma, myocardial ischemia). These tests can also reveal the degree of impairment in conditions affecting the respiratory and circulatory systems and may uncover unsuspected abnormalities.

The majority of clinical problems can be assessed during the simple procedures included in stage 1 and should be done before more complex tests. Abnormal results indicate that more precise information is required through stage 2 protocols. If stage 3 protocols are implemented, arterial blood analysis is necessary. In 75% of cases, stage 1 is sufficient. Oxygen titration can be done during graded exercise to determine the oxygen needs for improving exercise tolerance and increasing functional capacity.

Clinical Alert

1. *Absolute contraindications* to exercise testing include
   A. Acute febrile illness
   B. Pulmonary edema
   C. Systolic blood pressure >250 mm Hg
   D. Diastolic blood pressure >120 mm Hg
   E. Uncontrolled hypertension
   F. Uncontrolled asthma
   G. Unstable angina
2. *Relative contraindications* to exercise testing include
   A. Recent myocardial infarction (<4 weeks)
   B. Resting tachycardia (>120 bpm)
   C. Epilepsy
   D. Respiratory failure
   E. Resting ECG abnormalities

Procedure

1. *Stage 1*
   A. Blood pressure readings, ECG analysis, and ventilation are recorded during incremental cycle ergometry or treadmill walking.
   B. Measurements are made at the end of each minute. The test continues until maximum allowed symptoms occur (ie, to a symptom-limited maximum). O_2 uptake and CO_2 output are measured if possible.
   C. Total examination time is approximately 30 minutes.
2. *Stage 2*
   A. More complex analytic methods are required.
   B. Exercise builds to a steady state, usually 3 to 5 minutes for each workload.
   C. In addition to stage 1 measurements, mixed venous CO_2 tension is determined by means of rebreathing techniques.
3. *Stage 3*
   A. Blood gas sampling and analysis are required.
   B. An indwelling catheter is inserted into the brachial or radial artery.
   C. In addition to stage 2 tests, measurements for cardiac output, alveolar ventilation, ratio of dead space to tidal volume (VD/VT), alveolar-arterial O_2 tension difference (A-aDo$_2$), venous admixture ratio, and lactate concentration are determined.
4. See Chapter 1 guidelines for *intratest* care.

Clinical Implications

Altered values may reveal

1. Cardiac dysrhythmias or ischemia
2. Degree of functional impairment caused by obstructive or restrictive ventilatory disease
3. Hypoventilation
4. Workload level at which metabolic acidosis (lactic acidosis) occurs

Interfering Factors

1. The exercise tolerance of any person is affected by the degree of impairment related to
   A. Mechanical factors
   B. Ventilatory efficiency
   C. Gas exchange factors
   D. Cardiac status
   E. Physical condition
   F. Sensitivity of the respiratory control mechanism
2. Obese persons have a higher than normal oxygen consumption at any given work rate, even though muscular and work efficiency values are normal.

Patient Preparation

1. Explain the purpose and procedure for exercise stress testing, and assess for contraindications, interfering factors, and ability to comply.
2. Follow Chapter 1 guidelines for safe, effective, informed *pretest* care.

Patient Aftercare

1. Explain the meaning of test outcomes and possible need for lifestyle changes.
2. See Chapter 1 for safe, effective, informed *posttest* care guidelines.

● ARTERIAL BLOOD GASES (ABGs)

OVERVIEW OF ARTERIAL BLOOD GAS TESTS ●

Measurements of arterial blood gases (ABGs) are obtained to assess adequacy of oxygenation and ventilation, to evaluate acid-base status by measuring the respiratory and nonrespiratory components, and to monitor effectiveness of therapy. They are also used to monitor critically ill patients, to establish baseline values in the perioperative and postoperative period, to detect and treat electrolyte imbalances, to titrate appropriate oxygen flow rates, to qualify a patient for use of oxygen at home, and in conjunction with pulmonary function testing.

Reasons for using *arterial* rather than *venous* blood to measure blood gases include the following:

1. Arterial blood provides a better way to sample a mixture of blood from various parts of the body.
   A. Venous blood from an extremity gives information mostly about that extremity. The metabolism in the extremity can differ from the metabolism in the body as a whole. This difference is accentuated in the following instances:
      (1) In shock states, when the extremity is cold or underperfused;
      (2) During local exercise of the extremity, as in opening and closing a fist;
      (3) If the extremity is infected.
   B. Blood from a central venous catheter usually is an incomplete mix of venous blood from various parts of the body. For a sample to be completely mixed, the blood would have to be obtained from the right ventricle or pulmonary artery.
2. Arterial blood measurements indicate how well the lungs are oxygenating blood.
   A. If it is known that the arterial O_2 concentration is normal (indicating that the lungs are functioning normally) but the mixed venous O_2 concentration is low, it can be inferred that the heart and circulation are failing.
   B. Oxygen measurements of central venous catheter blood reveal tissue oxygenation but do not separate contributions of the heart from those of the lungs. If central venous catheter blood has a low O_2 concentration, it means either that the lungs have not oxygenated the arterial blood well or that the heart is not circulating the blood effectively. In the latter case, the body tissues must take on more than the normal

amount of O_2 from each cardiac cycle because the blood is flowing slowly and permits this to occur; this produces a low venous O_2 concentration.

3. Arterial samples provide information about the ability of the lungs to regulate acid-base balance through retention or release of CO_2. Effectiveness of the kidneys in maintaining appropriate bicarbonate levels also can be gauged.

NOTE: *Arterial puncture sites must satisfy the following requirements: (1) available collateral blood flow; (2) superficial or easily accessible location; and (3) relatively nonsensitive periarterial tissues.*

The radial artery is usually the site of choice, but brachial and femoral arteries can also be used. Samples can be drawn from direct arterial sticks or from indwelling arterial lines.

Clinical Alert

1. Before obtaining an arterial blood sample, assess for the following contraindications to an arterial stick or indwelling line:
   A. Absent palpable radial artery pulse
   B. Negative modified Allen's test, indicating obstruction in the ulnar artery (ie, compromised collateral circulation)—do not attempt to use radial artery for blood sample
   C. Cellulitis or infection in the area
   D. Arteriovenous fistula or shunt
   E. Severe thrombocytopenia
   F. Prolonged prothrombin or partial thromboplastin time (relative contraindication)
2. A Doppler probe or finger-pulse transducer may be used to assess circulation. This may be especially helpful with dark-skinned or uncooperative patients.
3. Before obtaining an arterial blood sample, record the most recent hemoglobin concentration (Hb), the mode and flow of oxygen therapy, and the temperature. If the patient has recently undergone suctioning or placed on mechanical ventilation, or if the inspired oxygen concentration has been changed, wait at least 15 minutes before drawing the sample. This waiting period allows circulating blood levels to return to baseline. Hyperthermia and hypothermia also influence oxygen release from hemoglobin at the tissue level.

Procedure for Obtaining Arterial Blood Sample
1. *Observe universal precautions and follow agency protocols.*
2. The patient assumes a sitting or supine position.
3. Perform the modified Allen's test to assess collateral circulation before performing a radial puncture, as follows: use pressure to obliterate both

radial and ulnar pulses, make the hand blanch, then release pressure over only the ulnar artery. In a positive test, flushing is immediately noted; the radial artery may then be used for puncture. If collateral circulation from the ulnar artery is inadequate (negative test), another site must be chosen.

4. Elevate the patient's wrist with a small pillow, and ask the patient to extend the fingers downward (this flexes the wrist and positions the radial artery closer to the surface).

5. Palpate the artery and maneuver the patient's hand back and forth until a satisfactory pulse is felt.

6. Swab the area liberally with an antiseptic agent (eg, an agent with an iodine base).

7. Optional: After assessing for allergy, inject the area with a small amount (≤ 0.25 ml) of 1% plain lidocaine (Xylocaine) if necessary to anesthetize site. This allows for a second attempt without undue pain.

8. Prepare a 20- or 21-gauge needle on a preheparinized self-filling syringe, puncture the artery, and collect a 3- to 5-ml sample. During the procedure, if the patient feels a dull or sharp pain radiating up the arm, withdraw the needle slightly and reposition it. If repositioning does not alleviate the pain, the needle should be withdrawn completely.

9. Withdraw the needle and place a 4×4-inch absorbent bandage over the puncture site. Maintain pressure over the site with 2 fingers for a minimum of 2 minutes or until no bleeding is evident; it may be necessary to use a pressure dressing, secured to the site with elastic tape, for several hours.

10. Meanwhile, all air bubbles in the blood sample must be expelled as quickly as possible. Air in the sample changes ABG values. The syringe should then be capped and gently rotated to mix heparin with the blood.

11. Label the sample with patient's name, identification number, date, time, mode of O_2 therapy, and flow rate.

12. Place the sample on ice and transfer it to the laboratory. This prevents alterations in gas tensions resulting from metabolic processes that continue after blood is drawn.

13. See Chapter 1 guidelines for *intratest* care.

Patient Preparation
1. Explain the purpose and procedure for obtaining an arterial blood sample.
2. If the patient is apprehensive, explain that a local anesthetic can be used.

Patient Aftercare
1. Evaluate color, motion, sensation, degree of warmth, capillary refill time, and quality of pulse in the affected extremity or at the puncture site.
2. Monitor puncture site and dressing for arterial bleeding for several hours. No vigorous activity of the extremity should be undertaken for 24 hours.

Clinical Alert

1. Some patients experience lightheadedness, nausea, or vasovagal syncope during arterial puncture. Respond according to established protocols.
2. ABG measurements do not indicate the degree of an abnormality. For this reason, the vital signs and mental function of the patient must be used as guides to determine adequacy of tissue oxygenation.
3. Pressure must be applied to the arterial puncture site, and the site must be watched carefully for bleeding for several hours. Instruct the patient to report any bleeding from the site.
4. Information for the laboratory should include the fraction of inspired oxygen (FIO_2), which is .21 for room air, and the time when the sample was obtained. Do not use blood for ABG measurements if sample is >3 hours old.
5. In the clinical setting (eg, perioperative or intensive care environment), ABG studies usually include the following: pH, PCO_2, SaO_2, CO_2 content, O_2 content, PO_2, base excess or deficit, HCO_3^-, hemoglobin, hematocrit, CO, Na^+, and K^+ (Chart 14-5).

CHART 14–5 ▶
Normal Values for Commonly Ordered Arterial Blood Gas Studies

pHa	=	7.35–7.45
$PaCO_2$	=	35–45 mm Hg
SaO_2	=	95% or higher
CO_2 content	=	23–30 mmol/L
O_2 content	=	15–22 vol%
PaO_2	=	80 mm Hg or greater
Base excess	=	>3 mEq/L
Base deficit	=	<3 mEq/L
HCO_3^-	=	24–28 mEq/L
Hb	=	12–16 g/dl (women); 13.5–17.5 g/dl (men)
Hct	=	37%–47% (women); 40%–54% (men)
COHb	=	<2%
$[NA^+]$	=	135–148 mmol/L
$[K^+]$	=	3.5–5 mEq/L

ALVEOLAR-TO-ARTERIAL OXYGEN GRADIENT ($A-aDO_2$); ARTERIAL-TO-ALVEOLAR OXYGEN RATIO (a/A RATIO) ●

Normal Values

$A-aDO_2$ = <10 mm Hg at rest (room air)
$A-aDO_2$ = 20–30 mm Hg at maximum exercise (room air)
a/A ratio = 75%

Explanation of Test

This test gives an approximation of the partial pressure of O_2 the alveoli and arteries. It identifies the cause of hypoxemia and intrapulmonary shunting as either (1) ventilated alveoli but no perfusion, (2) unventilated alveoli with perfusion, or (3) collapse of both alveoli and capillaries.

Procedure

An arterial blood sample is obtained and analyzed. This gives the *arterial* partial pressures of oxygen (PaO_2) and of carbon dioxide ($PaCO_2$). The barometric pressure (PB) and water vapor pressure (PH_2O) are also known, as is the fractional concentration of inspired oxygen (FIO_2), which is .21 for room air. From these, the *alveolar* oxygen tension (PAO_2), the arterial-to-alveolar oxygen ratio (a/A ratio), and the alveolar-to-arterial difference for PO_2 ($A-aDO_2$) are derived by solving the following mathematical formulas:

$$PAO_2 = FIO_2 (PB - PH_2O) - 1.25 (PaCO_2)$$

$$\text{a/A ratio} = \frac{PaO_2}{PAO_2}$$

$$A\text{-}aDO_2 = PAO_2 - PaO_2$$

Clinical Implications

1. *Increased* values may be caused by
   A. Mucus plugs
   B. Bronchospasm
   C. Airway collapse, as seen in
      (1) Asthma
      (2) Bronchitis
      (3) Emphysema
2. Hypoxemia (increased $A-aDO_2$) is caused by
   A. Atrial septal defects
   B. Pneumothorax
   C. Atelectasis
   D. Emboli
   E. Edema

Interfering Factors

Values increase with age and increasing O_2 concentration.

Patient Preparation

1. Explain the purpose, benefits, and risks of arterial blood sampling (see page 987).
2. Follow Chapter 1 guidelines for safe, effective, informed *pretest* care.

Patient Aftercare

1. Interpret test outcome and assess, monitor, and intervene appropriately for hypoxemia and ventilatory disturbances.

2. Frequently observe the puncture site for bleeding (see page 991).

3. See Chapter 1 guidelines for safe, effective, informed *posttest* care.

PARTIAL PRESSURE OF CARBON DIOXIDE (Pco$_2$)

Normal Values
Paco$_2$ (arterial blood): 35–45 mm Hg
Pvco$_2$ (venous blood): 41–51 mm Hg
Ten percent of CO$_2$ is carried in plasma and 90% in red blood cells.

Explanation of Test
This test measures the pressure or tension exerted by dissolved CO$_2$ in the blood and is proportional to the partial pressure of CO$_2$ in the alveolar air. The test is commonly used to detect a respiratory abnormality and to determine the alkalinity or acidity of the blood. To maintain CO$_2$ within normal limits, the rate and depth of respiration vary automatically with changes in metabolism. This test is an index of the effectiveness of alveolar ventilation; it is the most physiologically reflective blood gas measurement. An arterial sample directly reflects how well air is exchanged with blood in the lungs.

CO$_2$ tension in the blood and in cerebrospinal fluid is the major chemical factor regulating alveolar ventilation. When the CO$_2$ tension in arterial blood (Paco$_2$) rises from 40 to 45 mm Hg, it causes a 3-fold increase in alveolar ventilation. A Paco$_2$ of 63 mm Hg increases alveolar ventilation 10-fold. When the Fico$_2$ is >0.05 (5%), the lungs can no longer be ventilated fast enough to prevent a dangerous rise of CO$_2$ concentration in tissue fluids. Any further increase in CO$_2$ begins to depress the respiratory center, causing a progressive decline in respiratory activity rather than an increase.

Procedure
1. Obtain an arterial blood sample (or venous sample if requested) according to protocols. See page 991 for arterial blood sample specimen collection and Chapter 2 for venous blood sample specimen collection.

2. A small amount of this blood is introduced into a blood gas analyzing machine, and the CO$_2$ tension is measured by a silver–silver chloride electrode.

Clinical Implications
1. A *rise* in Paco$_2$ (hypercapnia) usually is associated with hypoventilation (CO$_2$ retention); a *decrease* is associated with hyperventilation ("blowing off" CO$_2$). A reduction in Paco$_2$, through its effect on plasma bicarbonate concentration, decreases renal bicarbonate reabsorption. For each 1mmHg decrease in the Paco$_2$, the plasma bicarbonate will decrease by aproximately 1mEq/L. Because HCO$_3^-$ and Paco$_2$ bear this close mathematical relationship, and this ratio, in turn, defends the hydrogen ion concentration, the outcome is that the steady-state Paco$_2$ in simple metabolic acidosis is equal to the last 2 digits of the arterial pH (pHa). Also, addition of 15 to the bicarbonate level equals the last 2 digits of the pHa. Failure of the Paco$_2$ to achieve predicted levels defines the presence of superimposed respiratory acidosis on alkalosis.

2. Causes of *decreased* $Paco_2$ include
   A. Hypoxia
   B. Nervousness
   C. Anxiety
   D. Pulmonary emboli
   E. Pregnancy
   F. Pain
   G. Other cause of hyperventilation
3. Causes of *increased* $Paco_2$ include
   A. Obstructive lung disease
      (1) Chronic bronchitis
      (2) Emphysema
   B. Reduced function of respiratory center
      (1) Overreaction
      (2) Head trauma
      (3) Anesthesia
   C. Other, less common causes of hypoventilation (eg, Pickwickian syndrome)

Clinical Alert

Increased $Paco_2$ may occur, even with normal lungs, if the respiratory center is depressed. Always check laboratory reports for abnormal values. When interpreting laboratory reports, remember that $Paco_2$ is a gas and is regulated by the lungs, not the kidneys.

Patient Preparation

1. Explain the purpose, benefits, and risks of the invasive arterial blood sampling procedure. Assess the patient's ability to cooperate.
2. Follow Chapter 1 guidelines for safe, effective, informed *pretest* care.

Patient Aftercare

1. Interpret the test outcome. Assess, monitor, and intervene appropriately for hypoxemia and ventilatory disturbances.
2. See Chapter 1 guidelines for safe, effective, informed *posttest* care.

OXYGEN SATURATION (So_2)

Normal Values

Sao_2 (arterial blood): $\geq 95\%$
Svo_2 (mixed venous blood): 70%-75%
Sao_2 (arterial) in a newborn infant: 40%–90%
Values decrease with age.

Explanation of Test

This measurement is a ratio between the actual O_2 content of the hemoglobin and the potential maximum O_2 carrying capacity of the hemoglobin. The So_2

is a percentage indicating the relationship between O_2 and hemoglobin; it does not indicate the O_2 content. The maximum amount of O_2 that can be combined with hemoglobin is called the *oxygen capacity*. The combined measurements of So_2, Po_2, and hemoglobin (Hb) indicate the amount of O_2 available to tissues (tissue oxygenation). Pulse oximetry (Spo_2) is a noninvasive technique that permits continuous real-time monitoring and trending of arterial oxygen saturation. However, it cannot differentiate carboxyhemoglobin (COHb). As a result, the Spo_2 is generally higher than the Sao_2 by the amount of COHb.

Procedure

1. Obtain an arterial blood sample (see page 987 for arterial and Chapter 2 for venous). Two methods are used for determining So_2:
    A. *Direct method:* The blood sample is introduced into hemoximeter, a spectrophotometric device for direct determination of So_2.
    B. *Calculated method:* So_2 is calculated from oxygen content (the volume of O_2 actually combined with hemoglobin) and oxygen capacity (the volume of O_2 to which hemoglobin could combine). Both of these values are expressed as volume percentages (vol%), or milliliters per deciliter of blood. The formula is as follows:

$$So_2 = 100 \times \frac{O_2 \text{ content}}{O_2 \text{ capacity}}$$

The O_2 content of the blood sample (see page 994) is measured both before and after exposure to the atmosphere.
2. *Pulse oximetry:* A small, clip-like sensor is placed on a digit over the fingernail (or toenail, if necessary). The instrument, using transmitted light waves (in the infrared spectrum and sensors, determines So_2 noninvasively.

Limitations

1. So_2 measures only the percentage of oxygen being carried by hemoglobin; it does not reveal the actual amount of oxygen available to the tissues (oxygen content).
2. Pulse oximetry equipment evaluates pulsatile blood flow. Many factors can interfere with the ability to measure flow:
    A. Digit motion
    B. A decrease in blood flow to the digit (eg, cool extremity, decreased peripheral pulses, vasoconstriction, nailbed thickening, ambient light, digit malformation, vasoconstrictive drugs, localized obstruction)
    C. Decreased hemoglobin (anemia) or abnormal hemoglobin (COHb)

Interfering Factors

Recent smoking or exposure to close second-hand smoke or to CO can increase the level of COHb, as can use of certain paint and varnish-type stripping agents, especially when they are applied in closed or poorly ventilated areas. The effect is to decrease the Sao_2 with little or no affect on the Pao_2.

Clinical Implications

1. Abnormal results occur in pulmonary diseases involving cyanosis and erythrocytosis.
2. Abnormal results occur with venous-to-arterial shunts.
3. Values are abnormal in Rh incompatibility caused by blocking antibodies.
4. Values usually are normal in polycythemic vera.
5. Values are decreased in ventilation-perfusion mismatching.

Patient Preparation

1. Explain the purpose, benefits, and risks of invasive arterial blood sampling. Assess the patient's ability to comply with the procedure.
2. Follow Chapter 1 guidelines for safe, effective, informed *pretest* care.

Patient Aftercare

1. Interpret test outcomes. Assess, monitor, and intervene appropriately for bleeding at puncture site and for hypoxemia or other respiratory dysfunctions.
2. See Chapter 1 guidelines for safe, effective, informed *posttest* care.

OXYGEN (O_2) CONTENT (Co_2) ●

Normal Values

Cao_2 (arterial blood): 15–22 mol% (15–22 ml/dl of blood)
Cvo_2 (venous blood): 11–16 mol% (11–16 ml/dl of blood)

Explanation of Test

The actual amount of O_2 in the blood is termed the *oxygen content* (Co_2). Blood can contain less O_2 than it is capable of carrying. About 98% of all O_2 delivered to the tissues is transported in chemical combination with hemoglobin. One gram of hemoglobin is capable of combining with 1.34 ml of O_2, whereas 100 ml of blood plasma can carry a maximum of only 0.3 ml of O_2 (under normoxic conditions or atmospheric conditions). The Co_2 measurement is determined mathematically.

Procedure

1. An arterial or venous blood sample is obtained.
2. The So_2, Po_2, and hemoglobin concentration (Hb) are measured.
3. The formulas for calculating O_2 content are as follows:

$$Cao_2 = 1.34(Sao_2 \times Hb) + 0.003(Pao_2)$$

$$Cvo_2 = 1.34(Svo_2 \times Hb) + 0.003(Pvo_2)$$

Note: 0.003 = Bunsen solubility for oxygen in the blood.

Clinical Implications

Decreased Cao_2 is associated with

1. COPD
2. Postoperative respiratory complications
3. Flail chest

4. Kyphoscoliosis
5. Neuromuscular impairment
6. Obesity-caused hypoventilation
7. Anemia

Patient Preparation
1. Explain the purpose, benefits, and risks of invasive arterial blood sampling (see page 987).
2. Follow Chapter 1 guidelines for safe, effective, informed *pretest* care.

Patient Aftercare
1. Interpret test outcome. Assess, monitor, and intervene appropriately for bleeding at the puncture site and for hypoxemia or ventilatory disturbances.
2. See Chapter 1 guidelines for safe, effective, informed *posttest* care.

PARTIAL PRESSURE OF OXYGEN (Po₂) ●

Normal Values
Pao₂ (arterial blood): ≥80 mm Hg
Pvo₂ (venous blood): 30–40 mm Hg

Background
Oxygen is carried in the blood in 2 forms: dissolved in plasma ($<2\%$) and combined with hemoglobin (98%). The partial pressure of a gas determines the force it exerts in attempting to diffuse through the pulmonary membrane. The Po₂ reflects the amount of O_2 passing from the pulmonary alveoli into the blood; it is directly influenced by the fraction of inspired oxygen (Fio₂).

Explanation of Test
This test measures the pressure exerted by the O_2 dissolved in the plasma. It evaluates the ability of the lungs to oxygenate the blood and is used to assess the effectiveness of oxygen therapy. The Po₂ indicates the ability of the lungs to diffuse O_2 across the alveolar membrane into the circulating blood.

Procedure
1. An arterial (or venous, if requested) blood sample is obtained (see page 987 for arterial and Chapter 2 for venous).
2. A small amount of this blood is introduced into a blood gas analyzing machine, and the O_2 tension is measured with a polargraphic electrode (developed by Leland Clark, sometimes referred to as the Clark electrode).

Clinical Implications
1. *Increased* Pao₂ is associated with
   A. Polycythemia
   B. Increased Fio₂
   C. Hyperventilation
2. *Decreased* Pao₂ is associated with
   A. Anemias
   B. Cardiac decompensation
   C. Insufficient atmospheric O_2

    D. Intracardiac shunts
    E. COPD
    F. Restrictive pulmonary disease
    G. Hypoventilation caused by neuromuscular disease
3. *Decreased* PaO_2 with normal or decreased $PaCO_2$ is associated with
    A. Diffuse interstitial pulmonary infiltration
    B. Pulmonary edema
    C. Pulmonary embolism
    D. Postoperative extracorporeal circulation

> **Clinical Alert**
>
> In persons with COPD, ventilatory efforts are stimulated by the hypoxic state (whereas for a healthy person the respiratory stimulus is the buildup of CO_2). Although supplemental oxygen increases the PaO_2 in such patients, it can also result in less effective breathing, because ventilatory efforts are no longer stimulated. The administration of oxygen "knocks out" this hypoxic drive and CO_2 retention results.

Patient Preparation
1. Explain the purpose, benefits, risks of arterial blood sampling. Assess the patient's level of cooperation and understanding.
2. Follow guidelines in Chapter 1 for safe, effective, informed *pretest* care.

Patient Aftercare
1. Interpret the test outcome. Assess, monitor, and intervene appropriately for bleeding at the puncture site and for respiratory or ventilatory disturbances.
2. See Chapter 1 guidelines for safe, effective, informed *posttest* care.

CARBON DIOXIDE (CO_2) CONTENT
(TOTAL CARBON DIOXIDE [TCO_2])

Normal Values
23–30 mmol/L

Background
In normal blood plasma, >95% of the total CO_2 content (TCO_2) is contributed by bicarbonate ion (HCO_3^-), which is regulated by the *kidneys*. The other 5% is contributed by the dissolved CO_2 gas and by carbonic acid (H_2CO_3). Dissolved CO_2 gas, which is regulated by the *lungs,* therefore contributes little to the TCO_2, and the TCO_2 gives little information about the lungs.

    The HCO_3^- in the extracellular spaces exists first as CO_2, then as H_2CO_3; later, much of it is changed to sodium bicarbonate ($NaHCO_3$) by the buffers in the plasma and erythrocytes.

Explanation of Test

This test is a general measure of the alkalinity or acidity of venous, arterial, or capillary blood. This test measures the CO_2 contributions from dissolved CO_2 gas, total H_2CO_3, HCO_3^-, and carbaminohemoglobin (CO_2HHb).

Procedure

1. A venous or arterial blood sample of 6 ml is collected in a heparinized syringe.
2. If the collected blood sample cannot be studied immediately, the syringe should be placed in an iced container.
3. $TCO_2 = HCO_3^- + H_2CO_3$

Clinical Implications

1. *Increased* TCO_2 occurs in
   A. Severe vomiting
   B. Emphysema
   C. Aldosteronism
   D. Use of mercurial diuretics
2. *Decreased* TCO_2 occurs in
   A. Severe diarrhea
   B. Starvation
   C. Acute renal failure
   D. Salicylate toxicity
   E. Diabetic acidosis
   F. Use of chlorothiazide diuretics

NOTE: *In diabetic acidosis, the supply of ketoacids exceeds the demands of the cell. Blood plasma acids rise. Blood plasma HCO_3^- decreases because it is used to neutralize these excess acids.*

Table 14-2 presents the changes in pH, HCO_3^-, and PaO_2 that occur in various ventilatory disturbances and acid-base imbalances.

> ### Clinical Alert
>
> 1. A double use of the term *CO_2* is one of the main reasons why understanding of acid-base problems may be difficult. Use the terms *CO_2 content* and *CO_2 gas* to avoid confusion. Remember the following:
>   A. *CO_2 content* (ie, TCO_2) is mainly bicarbonate and a base. It is a solution and is regulated by the kidneys.
>   B. *CO_2 gas* is mainly acid. It is regulated by the lungs.
> 2. The panic value for CO_2 content is 6.0 mmol/L or less; it usually is associated with severe metabolic acidosis, with the pH often <7.1. *This is a life-threatening situation.*

TABLE 14-2
Summary of Ventilatory and Acid-Base Changes in Four Underlying Conditions of Acid-Base Imbalance*

Form of Disturbance†	pHa‡	Bicarbonate $(HCO_3{}^-)^s$	$PaCO_2{}^{\parallel}$	Occurrence
RESPIRATORY ACIDOSIS				
Acute: caused by decreased alveolar ventilation and retention of CO_2	Decrease	Normal	Increase	*Depression of respiratory centers* Drug overdose Barbiturate toxicity Use of anesthetics *Interference with mechanical function of the thoracic cage* Deformity of thoracic cage Kyphoscoliosis *Airway obstruction* Extrathoracic tumors Asthma Bronchitis Emphysema *Circulatory disorders* Congestive heart failure Shock
Chronic: compensated via renal reabsorption of the bicarbonate ion	Normal	Increase	Increase	

RESPIRATORY ALKALOSIS				
Acute: caused by increased alveolar ventilation and excessive blowing off of CO_2 and water	Increase	Normal	Decrease	*Hyperventilation* *Hysteria* *Lack of oxygen* *Toxic stimulation of the respiratory centers* High fever Cerebral hemorrhage Excessive artificial respiration Salicylates
Chronic: compensated via glomerular filtration of the bicarbonate ion	Normal	Decrease	Decrease	
NONRESPIRATORY OR METABOLIC ACIDOSIS				
Acute: caused by accumulation of fixed body acids or loss of bicarbonate from the extracellular fluid	Decrease	Decrease	Normal	*Acid gain* Renal failure Diabetic ketoacidosis Lactic acidosis Anaerobic metabolism *Hypoxia* Base loss Diarrhea Renal tubular acidosis
Chronic: compensated via *hyperventilation* through stimulation of central chemoreceptors	Normal	Decrease	Decrease	

(continued)

TABLE 14-2 *(Continued)*

Form of Disturbance†	pHa‡	Bicarbonate (HCO$_3^-$)§	PaCO$_2$‖	Occurrence
NONRESPIRATORY OR METABOLIC ALKALOSIS				
Acute: caused by loss of fixed body acids or gain in bicarbonate in extracellular fluid	Increase	Increase	Normal	Acid loss Loss of gastric juice Vomiting *Potassium or chloride depletion* *Base gain* Excessive bicarbonate or lactate administration
Chronic: compensated via *hypoventilation*	Normal	Increase	Increase	

*Although these four basic imbalances occur individually, a combination of two or more is observed more frequently. These disturbances may have an antagonistic or a synergistic effect on each other.

†Uncompensated disturbances are referred to as *acute* and compensated ones as *chronic.* Compensation occurs via the mechanism not involved. Compensation is most efficient in respiratory acidoses.

§The degree of hypoventilation is precisely related to the degree of hypobicarbonatemia. For each 1 mEq/L fall in bicarbonate, PCO$_2$ falls by 1 to 1.3 mm Hg. A close mathematical relationship prevails between bicarbonate and PCO$_2$; their ratio defines the prevailing hydrogen ion concentration. For this reason, the steady-state PCO$_2$ in simple metabolic acidosis is equal to the last 2 digits of the pH. Failure of the PCO$_2$ to reach predicted levels defines the presence of superimposed respiratory acidosis or alkalosis.

‖Decreases in PaO$_2$ are interpreted separately and are referred to as *hypoxemia.*

‡Acid-base disturbances force kidney and lungs to compensate for changes in pH. Hyperventilation or hypoventilation can restore pH to normal within 15 minutes; the kidney, however, can take 2 to 3 days to compensate.

Interfering Factors
A number of drugs cause either increased or decreased Tco_2.

Patient Preparation
1. Explain the purpose, benefits, and risks of arterial blood sampling. Assess the patient's ability to comply with the procedure.
2. Follow guidelines in Chapter 1 for safe, effective, informed *pretest* care.

Patient Aftercare
1. Interpret test outcomes. Assess, monitor, and intervene appropriately for acid-base imbalances.
2. Monitor and intervene for bleeding at the puncture site and for respiratory or ventilatory disturbances.
3. See Chapter 1 guidelines for safe, effective, informed *posttest* care.

BLOOD pH ●

Normal Values
pHa (arterial blood): 7.35–7.45
pHv (venous blood): 7.31–7.41

Background
The pH is the negative logarithm of the hydrogen ion concentration in the blood. The sources of hydrogen ions are volatile acids, which can vary between a liquid and a gaseous state, and nonvolatile acids, which cannot be volatilized but remain fixed (eg, dietary acids, lactic acids, ketoacids).

> **NOTE:** *A pH value of 7 is neutral; acidity increases as the pH falls from 7 to 1, and alkalinity increases as the pH rises from 7 to 14. Limits of pH compatible with life fall within the range of 6.9 to 7.8.*

Explanation of Test
Blood pH measures the body's chemical balance and represents a ratio of acids to bases. It is also an indicator of the degree to which the body is adjusting to dysfunctions by means of its buffering systems. It is one of the best ways to determine whether the body is too acid or too alkaline and is an indicator of the patient's metabolic and respiratory status. The acid-base balance in the extracellular fluid is extremely delicate and intricate and must be kept within the very narrow range of 7.35 to 7.45 (slightly alkaline). Values <7.35 indicate an *acid state*, whereas pH values >7.45 indicate an *alkaline state*.

Procedure
1. An arterial (or venous if requested) blood sample is obtained.
2. The pH can be determined by either of 2 methods.
   - **A.** *Direct method:* A small amount of blood is analyzed by a blood gas machine; the pH is measured by a modified Severinghaus electrode.
   - **B.** *Indirect method:* The Henderson-Hasselbalch equation for the pH of a

buffer system is solved. In this equation, pK is the negative logarithm of the acid dissociation constant (the pH at which the associated and unassociated forms of an acid exist in equal concentrations). [A⁻] is the concentration of the ionized form (in this case HCO_3^-, the major blood base), and [HA] is the concentration of the free acid (in this case H_2CO_3, the major blood acid), in milliequivalents per liter.

$$pH = pK + \log \frac{[A^-]}{[HA]}$$

$$pH = pK + \log \frac{[HCO_3^-]}{[H_2CO_3]}$$

$$pH = 6.1 + \log \frac{[HCO_3^-]}{0.03(PaCO_2)}$$

Clinical Implications

1. Generally speaking, the pH is *decreased* in acidemia (acidosis) because of increased formation of acids, and pH is *increased* in alkalemia (alkalosis) because of a loss of acids.
2. When interpreting an acid-base abnormality, certain steps should be followed:
   A. Check the pH to determine whether an acid or an alkaline state exists.
   B. Check the PCO_2 to determine whether a respiratory acidosis or alkalosis is present. (PCO_2 is the *breathing* component.)
   C. Check the HCO_3^- concentration to determine whether a metabolic acidosis or alkalosis is present. (HCO_3^- is the *renal* component.)
3. See Table 14-2 for a more complete explanation of the changes occurring in acute and chronic respiratory and metabolic acidosis and alkalosis.
4. Metabolic acidemia (acidosis) occurs in
   A. Renal failure
   B. Ketoacidosis in diabetes and starvation
   C. Lactic acidosis
   D. Strenuous exercise
   E. Severe diarrhea
5. Metabolic alkalemia (alkalosis) occurs in
   a. Hypokalemia
   B. Hypochloremia
   C. Gastric suction or vomiting
   D. Massive doses of steroids
   E. Sodium bicarbonate administration
   F. Aspirin intoxication
6. Respiratory alkalemia (alkalosis) occurs in
   A. Acute pulmonary disease
   B. Myocardial infarction
   C. Chronic and acute heart failure
   D. Adult cystic fibrosis

E. Third trimester of pregnancy and during labor and delivery

F. Anxiety, neuroses, psychoses

G. Pain

H. Central nervous system diseases

I. Anemia

J. Carbon monoxide poisoning

K. Acute pulmonary embolus

L. Shock

7. Respiratory acidemia (acidosis) occurs in

A. Acute or chronic respiratory failure

B. Ventilatory failure

C. Neuromuscular depression

D. Obesity

E. Pulmonary edema

F. Cardiopulmonary arrest

Interfering Factors

Clinical Alert

1. *Ventilatory failure is a medical emergency. Aggressive and supportive measures must be taken immediately.*

2. Rate and depth of respirations may give a clue to blood pH.

A. Acidosis usually *increases* respirations; this is the body's way of adjusting once the state is established.

B. Alkalosis usually *decreases* respirations; this is the body's way of adjusting once the state is established.

3. Respiratory alkalosis may reflect hyperventilation in response to treatment for hypoxemia; however, correction of hypoxemia is essential.

4. Metabolic alkalosis, which is compensated through hypoventilation, may produce hypoxemia.

A number of drugs may alter the components of acid-base balance. See Appendix J.

Patient Preparation

1. Explain the purpose, benefits, and risks of invasive blood sampling.

2. Follow guidelines in Chapter 1 for safe, effective, informed *pretest* care.

Patient Aftercare

1. Interpret test outcome. Assess, monitor, and intervene appropriately for metabolic and respiratory acidosis and alkalosis (see Table 14-2).

2. Frequently observe the arterial puncture site for bleeding (see page 987). Be prepared to initiate proper interventions in the event of life-threatening situations.

3. See Chapter 1 guidelines for safe, effective, informed *posttest* care.

BASE EXCESS OR DEFICIT ●

Normal Values
Normal values are between ± 3 mEq/L or mmol/L.
A positive value indicates a base excess (ie, nonvolatile acid deficit).
A negative value indicates a base deficit (ie, nonvolatile acid excess).

Explanation of Test
This test quantifies the patient's total base excess or deficit so that clinical treatment of acid-base disturbances (specifically those that are nonrespiratory in nature) can be initiated. It is also referred to as the *whole blood buffer base* and is the sum of the concentration of buffer anions (in milliequivalents per liter) contained in whole blood. These buffer anions are the bicarbonate ion (HCO_3^-) present in plasma erythrocytes, and the hemoglobin, plasma proteins, and phosphates in plasma and red blood cells.

The total quantity of buffer anions is 45 to 50 mEq/L, or about twice that of HCO_3^- alone (24 to 28 mEq/L). Therefore, the quantity of HCO_3^- ions accounts for only about half of the total buffering capacity of the blood. The base excess or deficit measurement provides a more complete picture of the buffering that is taking place and is a critical index of nonrespiratory versus respiratory changes in acid-base balance.

Procedure
Calculation is made from the measurements of pH, $Paco_2$, and the hematocrit. These values are plotted on a nomogram, and the base excess or deficit is read.

Clinical Implications
1. A *negative* value (lower than −3 mEq/L) reflects a nonrespiratory or metabolic disturbance or true base deficit, or a nonvolatile acid accumulation caused by
   A. Dietary intake of organic and inorganic acids
   B. Lactic acid
   C. Ketoacidosis
2. A *positive* value (higher than +3 mEq/L) reflects a nonvolatile acid deficit or true base excess.

ANION GAP (AG) ●

Normal Values
Normal values are between 12 ± 4 mEq/L or mmol/L.
If potassium concentration is used in the calculation, the normal value is 16 ± 4 mEq/L or mmol/L.

Explanation of Test
This test measures the difference between the sum of the sodium (Na^+) and potassium (K^+) ion concentrations (the measured cations) and the sum of the chloride (Cl^-) and bicarbonate (HCO_3^-) concentrations (the measured anions).

This difference reflects the concentrations of other anions that are present in the extracellular fluid but are not routinely measured, the components of which include phosphates, sulfates, ketone bodies, lactic acid, and proteins. Increased amounts of these unmeasured anions are produced in the acidotic state.

Primary *hypobicarbonatemia* is brought about by any combination of 3 mechanisms: (1) overproduction of acids, which causes replacement of $NaHCO_3$ by the Na^+ salt of the offending acid (eg, lactate replaces HCO_3^- in lactic acidosis); (2) loss of $NaHCO_3$ through diarrhea along with renal retention of dietary NaCl, which causes hyperchloremic metabolic acidosis; and (3) generalized renal failure or specific forms of renal tubular acidosis, which cause retention of acids that are normally produced by intermediary metabolism or by urinary excretion of alkali. (Refer to Table 14-3.)

Hyperbicarbonatemia with sustained increases in HCO_3^- levels is brought about by a source of *new* alkali or by the presence of factors that stimulate renal retention of excess HCO_3^-. These mechanisms include excessive gastrointestinal loss of acid, exogenous alkali in persons whose kidneys avidly retain $NaHCO_3$, and renal synthesis of HCO_3^- in excess of daily consumption. Other pathophysiologic factors that affect renal reabsorption of >25 mEq/L of HCO_3^- and contribute to sustained hyperbicarbonatemia include extracellular fluid volume contraction, hypercapnia, hypokalemia, hyperaldosteronemia, and hypoparathyroidism. (Refer to Table 14-4.)

Procedure

This measurement is obtained by calculating the difference between the measured serum cation concentrations (either with or without K^+) and the measured serum anion concentrations:

$$AG = ([Na^+] + [K^+]) - ([Cl^-] + [HCO_3^-])$$

or

$$AG = [Na^+] - ([Cl^-] + [HCO_3^-])$$

TABLE 14-3
Subclassification of Anion Gap Metabolic Acidosis (Hypobicarbonatemia) into High- and Low-Potassium Forms*

High-Potassium Form	*Low-Potassium Form*
Acidifying agents	Diarrhea
Mineralocorticoid deficiency	Ureteral sigmoidostomy and malfunctioning
Renal diseases such as systemic lupus erythematosus, interstitial nephritis, amyloidosis, hydronephrosis, sickle cell nephropathy	Ileostomy
	Renal tubular acidosis, both proximal and distal
Early nonspecific renal failure	

*All metabolic acidoses can be classified on the basis of how they affect the anion gap.

TABLE 14-4
Classification of Anion Gap Metabolic Alkalosis (Hyperbicarbonatemia) on the Basis of Urinary Excretion

Saline-Responsive Urinary Chloride Excretion of <10 mEq/d	*Saline-Unresponsive Chloride Excretion of <10 mEq/d*
EXCESS BODY BICARBONATE CONTENT	
Renal alkalosis	Renal alkalosis—normotensive conditions
Diuretic therapy	Bartter's syndrome
Poorly reabsorbable anion therapy, (eg, carbenicillin, penicillin, sulfate, phospate)	Severe potassium depletion
	Refeeding alkalosis
Gastrointestinal alkalosis	Hypercalcemia and hypopara-thyroidism
Gastric alkalosis	
Intestinal alkalosis (eg, chloride diarrhea	Hypertensive conditions—endogenous mineralocorticoids
Exogenous alkali	Primary aldosteronism
Baking soda	Hyperreninism
Sodium citrate, lactate, gluconate, acetate	Adrenal enzyme deficiency: 11- and 17-hydroxylase
Transfusions	Liddle syndrome
Antacids	Exogenous mineralocorticoids
	Licorice
	Carbenoxolone
	Chewing tobacco

NORMAL BODY BICARBONATE CONTENT
Contraction alkalosis—urinary loss of NaCl and water without bicarbonate loss causes extracellular fluid contraction around an unchanged body content of alkali, resulting in hyperbicarbonatemia (especially important in persons with edema and persons who have excess body stores of water, sodium, bicarbonate, and chloride)

Clinical Implications

1. An anion gap (AG) occurs in acidosis that is caused by excess metabolic acids and excess serum chloride levels. If there is no change in sodium content, anions such as phosphates, sulfates, and organic acids increase the AG because they replace bicarbonate.

2. *Increased* AG is associated with an increase in metabolic acid when there is excessive production of metabolic acids, as in
   A. Alcoholic ketoacidosis
   B. Diabetic ketoacidosis
   C. Fasting and starvation
   D. Ketogenic diets
   E. Lactic acidosis
   F. Poisoning by salicylate, ethylene glycol (antifreeze), methanol, or propyl alcohol

3. *Increased* AG is also associated with decreased loss of metabolic acids, as

in renal failure. In the absence of renal failure or intoxication with drugs or toxins, an increase in AG is assumed to be caused by ketoacidosis or lactate accumulation.

4. Increased bicarbonate loss with a *normal* AG is associated with
   A. Decreased renal losses, as in
      (1) Renal tubular acidosis
      (2) Use of acetazolamide
   B. Increased chloride levels, as in
      (1) Altered chloride reabsorption by the kidney
      (2) Parenteral hyperalimentation
      (3) Administration of sodium chloride and ammonium chloride
   C. Loss of intestinal secretions, as in
      (1) Diarrhea
      (2) Intestinal suction or fistula
      (3) Biliary fistula
5. *Low* AG is associated with
   A. Multiple myeloma
   B. Hyponatremia caused by viscous serum
   C. Bromide ingestion (hyperchloremia)

> **Clinical Alert**
>
> 1. Interpret test outcomes and assess and monitor appropriately for acid-base disturbances.
> 2. The AG may provide evidence of a mixed rather than a simple acid-base disturbance.
> 3. Lactic acidosis should be considered in any metabolic acidosis with increased AG of >15 mEq/L.

LACTIC ACID

Normal Values
In venous blood: 0.5–2.2 mEq/L
In arterial blood: 0.5–1.6 mEq/L

Background
Lactate is a product of carbohydrate metabolism. Lactic acid is produced during periods of anaerobic metabolism when cells do not receive adequate oxygen to allow conversion of fuel sources to CO_2 and water. Lactic acid accumulates because of excess production of lactate and decreased removal of lactic acid from blood by the liver.

Explanation of Test
This measurement contributes to the knowledge of acid-base volume and is used to detect lactic acidosis in persons with underlying risk factors such as cardiovascular or renal disease that predispose them to this imbalance. Lactate is

elevated in a variety of conditions in which hypoxia occurs and in liver disease. Lactic acidosis can occur in both diabetics and nondiabetics. It is often fatal.

Procedure

A venous or arterial blood sample of at least 4 ml is obtained. The specimen must be brought to the laboratory immediately.

Clinical Implications

1. Values are *increased* in
   A. Lactic acidosis
   B. Cardiac failure
   C. Pulmonary failure
   D. Hemorrhage
   E. Diabetes
   F. Shock
   G. Liver disease
2. Lactic acidosis can be distinguished from ketoacidosis by the absence of severe ketosis and hyperglycemia in this state.

Interfering Factors

Lactic acid levels normally rise during strenuous exercise, when blood flow and oxygen cannot keep pace with the increased needs of exercising muscle.

Clinical Alert

An unexplained decrease in pH associated with a hypoxia-producing condition is reason to suspect lactic acidosis.

Patient Preparation

1. Explain the purpose and procedure of arterial blood sampling. Assess patient cooperation.
2. Follow guidelines in Chapter 1 for safe, effective, informed *pretest* care.

Patient Aftercare

1. Frequently observe the puncture site for bleeding. Manual pressure and a pressure dressing should be applied to the puncture site if necessary.
2. Base *posttest* assessments on patient outcomes; monitor and intervene appropriately for ventilatory and acid-base disturbances and hypoxemia.
3. Follow guidelines in Chapter 1 for safe, effective, informed *posttest* care.

BIBLIOGRAPHY ●

American Thoracic Society: Single breath carbon monoxide diffusing capacity (transfer factor): Recommendations for a standard technique. Am J Respir Crit Care Med 152: 2185–2198, 1995

American Thoracic Society: Standardization of spirometry: 1994 update. Am J Respir Crit Care Med 152:1107–1136, 1995

American Thoracic Society: Lung function testing: Selection of reference values and interpretive strategies. Am Rev Respir Dis 144: 1202–1218, 1991

Anderson S: Six easy steps to interpreting blood gases. Am J Nurs August: 42–45, 1991

Carroll P: Pulse oximetry at your fingertips. RN February: 22–26, 1997

Cherniack RM: Pulmonary Function Testing. Philadelphia, WB Saunders, 1992

Dunning MB: Respiratory physiology, in Raff H (ed), Physiology Secrets. Philadelphia, Hanly & Balfus, 1999

Erbis R, Schaberg T, Loddenkemper R: Lung function tests in patients with idiopathic pulmonary fibrosis. Chest 111(1): 5–57, 1997

Kassier JP, Green HL II: Current therapy in adult medicine, 4th ed. St. Louis, CV Mosby, 1997

Kirkland SH, Winterbauer RH: Pulmonary function tests and idiopathic pulmonary fibrosis: Simple may be better. Chest 111(1): 7–8, 1997

Ladebauche P: Peak flow meters: Child's play. Office Nurse 9(2): 22–28, 1996

Madama VC: Pulmonary function testing and cardiopulmonary stress testing, 2nd ed. Albany, NY, Delmar Publishers, 1998

McArdle WD, Katch FI, Katch VL: Essentials of Exercise Physiology. Philadelphia, Lea & Febiger, 1994

Ruppel G: Manual of Pulmonary Function Testing, 7th ed. St. Louis, CV Mosby, 1997

Shapiro BA, Peruzzi WT, Templin RK: Clinical Application of Blood Gases, 5th ed. St. Louis, Mosby, 1994

Social Security Administration: A guide to pulmonary function studies under the Social Security Disability program. Pittsburgh, Government Printing Office, 1998

Stiesmeyer JK: A four-step approach to pulmonary assessment. Am J Nurs August: 22–28, 1993

Wasserman K, Hansen JE, Sue DY, Whipp BJ, Casaburi R: Principles of Exercise Testing and Interpretation, 2nd ed. Philadelphia, Lea & Febiger, 1994

Zavala DC: Manual on Exercise Testing: A Training Handbook, 3rd ed. Iowa City: University of Iowa Publishers, 1993

15

Special Systems, Organ Functions and Postmortem Studies

These special studies have been selected for discussion because of their great diagnostic value in identifying diseases and disorders of certain organs and systems. Tests after death serve to identify previously undiagnosed disease; evaluate accuracy of predeath diagnosis; provide information about sudden, suspicious, or unexplained deaths; assist in organ donation and postmortem legal investigations; and promote quality control in health care settings.

● BRAIN AND NERVOUS SYSTEM

ELECTROENCEPHALOGRAPHY (EEG) ●

Normal EEG

Normal, symmetric patterns of electrical brain activity
Range of alpha: 8–11 Hz (cycles per second)

Explanation of Test

The EEG measures and records electrical impulses from the brain cortex. It is used to investigate causes of seizures, to diagnose epilepsy, and to evaluate brain tumors, brain abscesses, subdural hematomas, cerebral infarcts, and intracranial hemorrhages, among other conditions. It can be a tool for diagnosing narcolepsy, Alzheimer's disease, and certain psychoses. It is common practice to consider the EEG pattern, along with other clinical procedures, drug levels, body temperature, and thorough neurologic examinations, to establish electrocerebral silence, otherwise known as "brain death." The American Electroneurodiagnostic Society sets guidelines for obtaining these recordings. When an electrocerebral silence pattern is recorded in the absence of any hope for neurologic recovery, the patient may be declared brain dead despite cardiovascular and respiratory support.

Procedure

1. An EEG can be done at any time. Scalp hair should be recently washed.
2. Electrodes containing conduction gel are fastened to the scalp with a special skin glue or paste. Seventeen to 21 electrodes are used according to an internationally accepted measurement known as the *10–20 System.* This system correlates electrode placement with anatomic brain structure (see Fig. 15-6 on p. 1062).
3. The patient is placed in a recumbent position, instructed to keep his or her eyes closed, and encouraged to sleep during the test (resting EEG). (Seizure activating procedure [see numbers 4 to 6]).
4. Prior to beginning the EEG, some patients may be instructed to breathe deeply through the mouth 20 times per minute for 3 minutes. This hyperventilation may cause dizziness or numbness in the hands or feet but is nothing to be alarmed about. This activating breathing procedure induces

alkalosis, which causes vasoconstriction, which in turn may activate a seizure pattern.

5. A light flashing at frequencies of 1 to 30 times per second may be placed close to the face. This technique, called *photic stimulation,* may cause an abnormal EEG pattern not normally recorded.

6. Certain persons may be intentionally sleep deprived before the test to promote sleep during the test. An oral medication to promote sleep (Voludna chloral hydrate) is usually administered. The sleep state is valuable for revealing abnormalities, especially different forms of epilepsy. Recordings are made while the patient is falling asleep, during sleep, and while the patient is waking.

7. After the EEG, electrodes, glue, and paste are removed. The patient may then wash his or her hair.

8. Follow guidelines in Chapter 1 for safe, effective, informed *intratest* care.

Clinical Implications

1. Abnormal EEG pattern readings reveal seizure activity (eg, grand mal epilepsy, petit mal epilepsy) if recorded during a seizure. If a patient suspected of having epilepsy shows a normal EEG, the test may have to be repeated using sleep deprivation or special electrodes. The EEG may also be abnormal during other types of seizure activity (eg, focal [psychomotor], infantile myoclonic, or Jacksonian seizures); between seizures, 20% of patients with petit mal epilepsy and 40% with grand mal epilepsy show a normal EEG pattern, and the diagnosis of epilepsy can be made only by correlating the clinical history with the EEG abnormality, if one exists.

2. An EEG may often be normal in the presence of cerebral pathology. However, most brain abscesses and glioblastomas produce EEG abnormalities.

3. Electroencephalographic changes due to cerebrovascular accidents depend on the size and location of the infarcts or hemorrhages.

4. Following a head injury, a series of EEGs may be helpful in predicting the likelihood of posttraumatic epilepsy, especially if a previous EEG is available for comparison.

5. In cases of dementia, the EEG may be normal or abnormal.

6. In early stages of metabolic disease, the EEG is normal; in the later stages, it is abnormal.

7. The EEG is abnormal in most diseases or injuries that alter the level of consciousness. The more profound the change in consciousness, the more abnormal the EEG pattern usually is.

Interfering Factors

1. Sedative drugs, mild hypoglycemia, or stimulants can alter normal EEG tracings.

2. Oily hair, hair spray, and other hair care products interfere with the placement of EEG patches and the procurement of accurate EEG tracings.

3. Artifacts can appear in technically well-done EEGs. Eye and body move-

ments cause changes in brain wave patterns and must be noted so that they are not interpreted as abnormal brain waves.

Patient Preparation

1. Explain test purpose and procedure to allay patient fears and concerns. Emphasize that the EEG is not painful, that it is not a test of thinking or intelligence, that no electrical impulses pass through the body, and that it is *not* a form of shock therapy. The transmitted impulses are magnified at least 1 million times and transcribed to permanent hard copy for further study.
2. Food may be given if the patient is to be sleep deprived. However, no coffee, tea, or cola is permitted within 12 hours of the test. Emphasize that food should be eaten to prevent hypoglycemia.
3. Smoking is usually allowed, but not encouraged, before the test.
4. Hair should be washed and thoroughly rinsed with clear water the evening before the EEG so that EEG patches will remain firmly in place during the test. Do not apply conditioners or oils after shampooing.
5. If a sleep study is ordered, the adult patient should sleep as little as possible the night before (ie, stay up past midnight) so that sleep can occur during the test.
6. If a sleep-deprivation study is ordered for a child, call the EEG department for special instructions.
7. Follow guidelines in Chapter 1 regarding safe, effective, informed *pretest* care.

Patient Aftercare

1. The hair should be washed after the test. Application of oil to the adhesive before shampooing can ease its removal.
2. If a sedative was given during the test, allow the patient to rest posttest. Put bedside rails in the raised position for safety.
3. Skin irritation from the electrodes usually disappears within a few hours.
4. Interpret test results and monitor appropriately. If repeat testing is necessary, provide explanations and support to the patient.
5. Follow guidelines in Chapter 1 for safe, effective, informed *posttest* care.

EVOKED RESPONSES/POTENTIALS: BRAIN STEM AUDITORY EVOKED RESPONSE (BAER); VISUAL EVOKED RESPONSE (VER); SOMATOSENSORY EVOKED RESPONSE (SSER) ●

These tests use conventional EEG recording techniques with specific electrode site placement for each procedure and include computer data processing to evaluate electrophysiologic integrity of the auditory, visual, and sensory pathways.

Normal Potentials, Brain Stem Auditory Evoked Response (BAER), and Visual Evoked Response (VER)

Absolute latency, measured in milliseconds (msec), of the first five waveforms at a sound stimulation rate of 11 clicks/second

Wave	Mean ± Standard Deviation (SD)
I	1.7 ± 0.15
II	2.8 ± 0.17
III	3.9 ± 0.19
IV	5.1 ± 0.24
V	5.7 ± 0.25

Normal Visual Evoked Response (VER)

Absolute latency, measured in milliseconds of the first major positive peak (P_{100})

Wave	Mean ± SD	Range
P_{100}	102.3 ± 5.1	89–114

Normal Somatosensory Evoked Response (SSER)

Absolute latency of major waveforms, measured in milliseconds at a stimulation rate of 5 impulses/second (see table of contents)

Wave	Mean ± SD
EP	9.7 ± 0.7
A	11.8 ± 0.7
B	13.7 ± 0.8
II	11.3 ± 0.8
III	13.9 ± 0.9
N_2	19.1 ± 0.8
P_2	22.0 ± 1.2

Explanation of Tests

BRAIN STEM AUDITORY EVOKED RESPONSE

This study allows evaluation of suspected peripheral hearing loss, cerebellopontine angle lesions, brain stem tumors, infarcts, multiple sclerosis, and comatose states. Special stimulating techniques permit recording of signals generated by subcortical structures in the auditory pathway. Stimulation of either ear evokes potentials that can reveal lesions in the brain stem involving the auditory pathway without affecting hearing. Evoked potentials of this type are also used to evaluate hearing in infants, children, and adults through *electrical response audiometry.*

VISUAL EVOKED RESPONSE

This test of visual pathway function is valuable for diagnosing lesions involving the optic nerves and optic tracts, multiple sclerosis, and other disorders. Visual stimulation excites retinal pathways and initiates impulses that are conducted through the central visual path to the primary visual cortex. Fibers from this area project to the secondary visual cortical areas on the brain's occipital convexity. Through this path, a visual stimulus to the eyes causes an electrical response in the occipital regions, which can be recorded with electrodes placed along the vertex and the occipital lobes.

SOMATOSENSORY EVOKED RESPONSE

This test assesses spinal cord lesions, stroke, and numbness and weakness of the extremities. It studies impulse conduction through the somatosensory pathway. Electrical stimuli are applied to the median nerve in the wrist or peroneal nerve near the knee at a level near that which produces thumb or foot twitches. The milliseconds it takes for the current to travel along the nerve to the cortex of the brain is then measured. Somatosensory evoked responses can also be used to monitor sensory pathway conduction during surgery for scoliosis or spinal cord decompression and/or ischemia. Loss of the sensory potential can signal impending cord damage.

Procedures

1. *Brain stem auditory evoked responses* are obtained through electrodes placed on the vertex of the scalp and on each earlobe. Stimuli in the form of clicking noises or tone bursts are delivered to one ear through earphones. Because sound waves delivered to one ear can be heard by the opposite ear, a continuous masking noise is simultaneously delivered to the opposite ear.
2. Electrodes used in *visually evoked response* are placed on the scalp along the vertex and occipital lobes. The patient is asked to watch a checkerboard pattern flash for several minutes, first with one eye, then with the other, while brain waves are recorded.
3. *Somatosensory evoked responses* are recorded through several pairs of electrodes. Electrical stimuli are applied to the median nerve at the wrist or to the peroneal nerve at the knee. Scalp electrodes placed over the sensory cortex of the opposite hemisphere of the brain pick up the signals and measure, in milliseconds, the time it takes for the current to travel along the nerve to the cortex of the brain.
4. Follow guidelines in Chapter 1 for safe, effective, informed *intratest* care.

Clinical Implications

1. Abnormal BAERs are associated with the following conditions:
   a. Acoustic neuroma
   b. Cerebrovascular accidents
   c. Multiple sclerosis
   d. Lesions affecting any part of the auditory nerve or brain stem area
2. Abnormal VERs are associated with the following conditions:
   a. Demyelinating disorders such as multiple sclerosis
   b. Lesions of the optic nerves and eye (prechiasma defects)
   c. Lesions of the optic tract and visual cortex (postchiasma defects)

    d. Abnormal visual evoked potentials may also be found in persons without a history of retrobulbar neuritis, optic atrophy, or visual field defects. However, many patients with proven damage to the postchiasma visual path and known visual field defects may have normal visual evoked potentials.

3. Abnormal SSERs are associated with the following conditions:
    a. Spinal cord lesions
    b. Cerebrovascular accidents
    c. Multiple sclerosis
    d. Cervical myelopathy accident

Interfering Factors

Some difficulty in interpreting brain stem evoked potentials may arise in persons with peripheral hearing defects that alter evoked potential results.

Patient Preparation

1. Explain the test purpose and procedure.
2. Hair should be washed and rinsed before testing. Instruct patient **not** to apply any other hair preparations.
3. Follow guidelines in Chapter 1 for safe, effective, informed *pretest* care.

Patient Aftercare

1. The patient may wash his or her hair (assist if necessary). Remove gel from other skin areas.
2. Interpret test results and monitor appropriately for neurologic problems.
3. Follow guidelines in Chapter 1 for safe, effective, informed *posttest* care.

COGNITIVE TESTS: EVENT-RELATED POTENTIALS (ERPs)   ●

Normal Event-Related Potentials (ERPs)

No shift of P_3 components to longer latencies
ERP: absolute latency of P_3 waveform

Wave	Mean ± SD
P_3	294 ± 21 msec

Explanation of Test

Event-related potentials are used as objective measures of mental function in neurologic diseases that produce cognitive defects. These measurements use the method of auditory evoked response testing (see p. 1013), in which sound stimuli are transmitted through earphones. A rare tone is associated with a prominent endogenous P_3 component that reflects the differential cognitive processing of that tone. Although a systematic neurologic increase in P_3 component latency occurs as a function of increasing age in normal persons, in many instances of neurologic diseases associated with dementia, the latency of the P_3 component has been reported to substantially exceed the normal age-matched value.

This test is useful in evaluating persons with dementia or decreased mental functioning. It is also helpful in differentiating persons with real organic brain defects affecting cognitive function from those who are unable to interact with the examiner because of motor or language defects or those unwilling to cooperate because of problems such as depression or schizophrenia.

Procedure
1. The procedure is the same as that for auditory brain stem responses (see p. 1013).
2. Patients are asked to count the occurrences of audible rare tones they hear through the ear phones.
3. Follow guidelines in Chapter 1 for safe, effective, informed *intratest* care.

Interfering Factors
Latency of P_3 component normally increases with age.

Clinical Implications
1. An increased or abnormal P_3 latency is associated with neurologic diseases producing dementia such as the following:
   a. Alzheimer's disease
   b. Metabolic encephalopathy such as that associated with hypothyroidism or alcoholism with severe electrolyte disturbances
   c. Brain tumor
   d. Hydrocephalus

Patient Preparation
1. Explain the purpose and procedure of the test.
2. Follow guidelines in Chapter 1 regarding safe, effective, informed *pretest* care.

Patient Aftercare
1. Interpret test results and monitor appropriately for neurologic disease.
2. Follow guidelines in Chapter 1 for safe, effective, informed *posttest* care.

BRAIN MAPPING: COMPUTED TOPOGRAPHY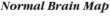

Normal Brain Map
Normal frequency signals and evoked responses presented as a color-coded map of electrical brain activity

Explanation of Test
Brain mapping uses traditional EEG data and specialized computer digitization to display the diagnostic information as a topographic map of the brain

and spinal cord. The computer analyzes EEG signals for amplitude and distribution of alpha, beta, theta, and delta frequencies and displays the analysis as a color map. Specific and/or *minute* abnormalities are enhanced and allow comparison with normal data. This methodology is used for assessing cognitive function and for evaluating patients with migraine headaches, trauma, or episodes of vertigo or dizziness. Persons who lose periods of time and select patients with generalized seizures, dementia of organic origin, ischemic abnormalities, or certain psychiatric disorders are also candidates for this testing. With this procedure, it is possible to localize a specific area of the brain which may otherwise show up as a generalized area of deficit in the conventional EEG. Children or adults who demonstrate hyperactivity, dyslexia, dementia, or Alzheimer's disease may benefit from evaluation through brain mapping.

Procedure

1. The patient should be rested and awake for the test so that no sleep signals appear as indicators of beta activity.
2. After the skin of the scalp is cleansed with an abrasive solution, 42 electrodes are placed at designated areas on the scalp and are held in place with adhesive or paste formulated for this purpose.
3. The patient is placed in a recumbent position and instructed to keep his or her eyes closed and to refrain from any movement.
4. Follow guidelines in Chapter 1 for safe, effective, informed *intratest* care.

Clinical Implications

1. Abnormal brain maps can pinpoint the following conditions:
   a. Areas of focal seizure discharge in persons who experience generalized seizures
   b. Areas of focal irritation in persons with migraine
   c. Areas of ischemia
   d. Areas of dysfunction in states of dementia
   e. Areas of possible brain abnormalities associated with schizophrenia or other psychotic states

Interfering Factors

1. Tranquilizers may alter results.
2. Unwashed hair or the use of hair preparations can interfere with electrode placement.
3. Eye and body movements cause changes in signals and wave patterns.

Patient Preparation

1. Explain the test purpose and procedure. There are no known risks. Emphasize the fact that electrical impulses pass from the patient to the machine and not the opposite.
2. Food and fluids can be taken prior to testing. However, no coffee, tea, or caffeinated drinks should be ingested for at least 8 hours before the test.

3. Hair must be recently washed.
4. Tranquilizers should not be taken prior to testing (check with physician). Other prescribed medications such as antihypertensives and insulin may be taken. If in doubt, contact the testing laboratory for guidelines.
5. Follow guidelines in Chapter 1 for safe, effective, informed *pretest* care.

Patient Aftercare
1. Remove the conduction gel and encourage the patient to wash his or her hair. Provide supplies if possible.
2. Interpret test results and monitor appropriately for seizure activity and other neurologic manifestations.
3. Follow guidelines in Chapter 1 for safe, effective, informed *posttest* care.

ELECTROMYOGRAPHY (EMG); ELECTROMYONEUROGRAM (EMNG) ●

Normal EMG and EMNG
Nerve conduction: normal
Muscle action potential: normal
> On insertion
> At rest
> During minimum voluntary muscle contraction
> During maximum voluntary muscle contraction

Explanation of Test
Electromyoneurography combines electromyography and electroneurography. These studies, done to detect neuromuscular abnormalities, measure nerve conduction and electrical properties of skeletal muscles. Together with evaluation of range of motion, motor power, sensory defects, and reflexes, these tests can differentiate between neuropathy and myopathy. The electromyogram can define the site and cause of muscle disorders such as myasthenia gravis, muscular dystrophy, and myotonia; inflammatory muscle disorders such as polymyositis; and lesions that involve the motor neurons in the anterior horn of the spinal cord. EMG can also localize the site of peripheral nerve disorders such as radiculopathy and axonopathy. Skin and needle electrodes measure and record electrical activity. Electrical sound equivalents are amplified and recorded on tape for later studies.

Procedure
1. The test is done in a copper-lined room to screen out outside interference.
2. The patient may lie down or sit during the test.
3. A surface disk or lead strap is applied to the skin around the wrist or ankle to ground the patient. The muscles and nerves examined are chosen according to the patient's signs and symptoms, history, and physical condition (select nerves innervate specific muscles).

4. The patient is encouraged to relax (the examiner may massage certain muscles to get the patient to relax) or to contract certain muscles (eg, to point to toes) at specific times during the test.
5. Testing is divided into two parts. The first test determines *nerve conduction*.
   a. Metal surface electrodes are coated with electrode paste and firmly placed over a specific nerve area. Electrical current (maximum, 100 mAmp for 1 msec) is passed through the area and causes sensations, similar to shock from carpeting or static electricity or the equivalent of an AA battery, that are directly proportional to the time the current is applied. Patients with mild forms of neuromuscular disorders may feel mild discomfort, whereas those with polyneuropathies may experience moderate discomfort.
   b. The amplitude wave is read on an oscilloscope and recorded on magnetic tape for later studies.
   c. Electrical current leaves no mark but can cause unusual sensations that are not usually considered unpleasant. How fast and how well a nerve transmits messages can be measured. Nerves in the face, arms, or legs are appropriate for testing in this way.
6. The second test determines *muscle potential*.
   a. A monopolar electrode (a 1.25- to 7.5-cm-long small-gauge needle) is inserted and incrementally advanced into the muscle. The examiner may manipulate the needle without actually removing it to see if readings change, or the needle may be placed in another muscle area.
   b. The electrode usually causes no pain unless the tip is near a terminal nerve. Ten or more needle insertions may be necessary. The needle electrode detects electricity normally present in muscle.
   c. The examiner observes the oscilloscope for normal wave forms and listens for normal quiet sounds at rest. A "machine-gun popping" sound or a rattling sound like hail on a tin roof is normally heard when the patient contracts the muscles.
   d. If the patient complains of pain, the examiner must remove the needle because the pain stimulus yields false results.
   e. Total examining time is 45 to 60 minutes if testing is confined to a single extremity; testing may take up to 3 hours for more than one extremity. There is no completely "routine" EMG. The length of the test depends on the clinical problem.
7. Follow guidelines in Chapter 1 regarding safe, effective, informed *intratest* care.

Clinical Implications

1. Abnormal neuromuscular activity occurs in diseases or disturbances of striated muscle fibers or cell membranes in the following categories:
   a. Muscle fiber disorders (eg, muscular dystrophy)
   b. Cell membrane hyperirritability; myotonia and myotic disorders (eg, polymyositis, hypocalcemia, thyrotoxicosis, tetanus, rabies)

   c. Myasthenia (muscle weakness states) caused by the following conditions:

      (1) Myasthenia gravis

      (2) Cancer due to nonpituitary adrenocorticotropic hormone (ACTH) secretion by the tumor

         (a) Bronchial cancer

         (b) Sarcoid

      (3) Deficiencies

         (a) Familial hypokalemia

         (b) McArdle's phosphorylase

      (4) Hyperadrenocorticism

      (5) Acetylcholine blocking agents

         (a) Curare

         (b) Botulin

         (c) Kanamycin

         (d) Snake venom

2. Disorders or diseases of lower motor neurons

   a. Lesions involving motor neuron on anterior horn of spinal cord (myelopathy)

      (1) Tumor

      (2) Trauma

      (3) Syringomyelia

      (4) Juvenile muscular dystrophy

      (5) Congenital amyotonia

      (6) Anterior poliomyelitis

      (7) Amyotrophic lateral sclerosis

      (8) Peroneal muscular atrophy

   b. Lesions involving the nerve root (radiculopathy)

      (1) Guillain-Barré syndrome

      (2) Entrapment of the nerve root

         (a) Tumor

         (b) Trauma

         (c) Herniated disk

         (d) Hypertrophic spurs

         (e) Spinal stenosis

   c. Damage or disease to peripheral or axial nerves

      (1) Entrapment of the nerve

         (a) Carpal or tarsal tunnel syndrome

         (b) Facial, ulnar, radial, or peroneal palsy

         (c) Neuralgia paresthetica

      (2) Endocrine

         (a) Hypothyroidism

         (b) Diabetes

      (3) Toxic

         (a) Heavy metals

         (b) Solvents

(c) Antiamebicides
(d) Chemotherapy
(e) Antibiotics

d. Early peripheral nerve degeneration and regeneration

Interfering Factors

1. Conduction can vary with age and normally decreases with increasing age.
2. Pain can yield false results.
3. Electrical activity from extraneous persons and objects can produce false results as a result of movement.
4. The test is ineffective in the presence of edema, hemorrhage, or thick subcutaneous fat.

Patient Preparation

1. Explain the test purpose and procedure. There is a risk of hematoma if the patient is on anticoagulant therapy.
2. Sedation or analgesia may be ordered.
3. Follow guidelines in Chapter 1 for safe, effective, informed *pretest* care.

Patient Aftercare

1. If the patient experiences pain, provide pain relief through appropriate interventions. Obtain an order for an analgesic if necessary.
2. Promote rest and relaxation.
3. Interpret test results and monitor appropriately for nerve and muscle disease. Provide assistance as necessary.
4. Follow guidelines in Chapter 1 for safe, effective, informed *posttest* care.

> **Clinical Alert**
>
> 1. When ordering the test, the more information that is known, the more precise the interpretation of findings will be.
> 2. Enzyme levels that reflect muscle activity (eg, Aspartate Amino Transferase, Lactate Dehydrogenase, Creatine Phosphokinase) must be determined before actual testing, because the EMG causes elevation of these enzymes for up to 10 days postprocedure.
> 3. Although rare, hematomas may form at needle insertion sites. Take measures, such as application of pressure to the site, to control bleeding. Notify the physician. Ascertain whether the patient is taking anticoagulants or aspirin-like drugs.

ELECTRONYSTAGMOGRAM (ENG)   ●

Normal ENG

Vestibular-ocular reflex: normal nystagmus accompanying head turning is expected

Explanation of Test

This study aids in the differential diagnosis of lesions in the brain stem and cerebellum. It can confirm the causes of unilateral hearing loss of unknown origin, vertigo, or ringing in the ears. Evaluation of the vestibular system and the muscles controlling eye movement is based on measurements of the nystagmus cycle. In health, the vestibular system maintains visual fixation during head movements by means of *nystagmus,* the involuntary back and forth eye movement caused by initiation of the vestibular-ocular reflex.

Procedure

1. The test is usually done in a darkened room with the patient sitting or lying.
2. If ear wax is present, it should be removed prior to testing.
3. Five electrodes are taped at designated positions around the eye.
4. During the study, the patient is asked to look at different objects, to open and close his or her eyes, and to change head position.
5. Toward the end of the test, air is gently blown into each external ear canal, first on the affected side. Water may also be instilled into the ears during the test to record eye movement in response to various stimuli.
6. Follow guidelines in Chapter 1 for safe, effective, informed *intratest* care.

Clinical Implications

1. Prolonged nystagmus and postural instability following a head turn is abnormal and can be caused by lesions of the vestibular or ocular system, as in the following conditions:
   a. Cerebellum disease
   b. Brain stem lesion
   c. Peripheral lesion occurring in the elderly; head trauma; middle ear disorders
   d. Congenital disorders

Interfering Factors

1. Test results are altered by the inability of the patient to cooperate, poor eyesight, blinking of the eyes, or poorly applied electrodes.
2. The patient's anxiety or medications such as central nervous system depressants, stimulants, or antivertigo agents can cause false-positive test results.

Patient Preparation

1. Explain the test purpose and procedure. No pain or known risks are associated with the test. The procedures to stimulate involuntary rapid eye movement are uncomfortable.
2. The patient must remove makeup.
3. The patient must abstain from all caffeinated and alcoholic beverages for at least 48 hours. Heavy meals should be avoided prior to testing.

4. In most cases, medications such as tranquilizers, stimulants, or antivertigo agents should be withheld for 5 days before the test. If in doubt, consult the clinician who ordered the test.

5. Follow guidelines in Chapter 1 for safe, effective, informed *pretest* care.

> **Clinical Alert**
>
> **1.** The test is contraindicated in persons who have pacemakers.
> **2.** Water irrigation of the ear canal should not be done when there is a perforated eardrum. Instead, a finger cot may be inserted into the ear canal to protect the middle ear.

Patient Aftercare

1. Allow the patient to rest as necessary.

2. If present, nausea, vertigo, and weakness may require treatment and medication. Check with the clinician who ordered the test.

3. Interpret test results and monitor appropriately for brain disease, which may manifest as loss of balance, or middle ear disease, which may cause spasmodic eye movement, vertigo, or hearing loss.

4. Follow guidelines in Chapter 1 for safe, effective, informed *posttest* care.

● HEART

ELECTROCARDIOGRAPHY (ECG OR EKG), WITH BRIEF DESCRIPTION OF VECTOR CARDIOGRAM ●

Normal ECG or EKG

Normal positive and negative deflections in an ECG recording

Normal cardiac cycle components (one normal cardiac cycle is represented by the P wave, QRS complex, and T wave; additionally, a U wave may be observed. This cycle is repeated continuously and rhythmically)

The P wave indicates atrial depolarization; QRS complex indicates ventricular depolarization; T wave indicates ventricular repolarization/resting stage between beats; and U wave indicates nonspecific recovery afterpotentials (Fig. 15-1).

Waves

Capital letters refer to relatively large waves (>5 mm), and small letters refer to relatively small waves (<5 mm).

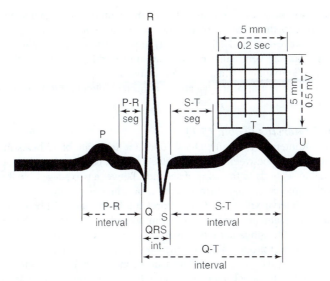

FIGURE 15-1

Commonly measured complex components. (From Smeltzer, Brunner, and Suddarth's *Textbook of Medical-Surgical Nursing*, 8th ed. Philadelphia: Lippincott-Raven Publishers, 1996).

1. The *P wave* is normally upright; it represents *atrial* depolarization and indicates electrical activity associated with the original impulse which travels from the sinus node through the atrial sinus. If P waves are present; are of normal size, shape, and deflection; have normal conduction intervals to the ventricles; and demonstrate rhythmic timing variances between cardiac cycles, it can be assumed that the stimulus began in the sinoatrial node.

2. The T_a or T_p designation is used to differentiate atrial repolarization, which ordinarily is obscured by the QRS complex, from the more conventional T wave, which signifies ventricular repolarization (see number 8).

3. The Q(q) wave is the first downward/negative deflection in the QRS complex; it results from ventricular depolarization. The Q(q) wave may not always be apparent.

4. The R(r′) wave is the first upright/positive deflection after the P wave (or in the QRS complex); it results from ventricular depolarization.

5. The S(s′) wave is the downward/negative deflection that follows the R wave.

6. The Q and S waves are negative deflections that do not normally rise above the baseline.

7. The T wave is a deflection produced by ventricular repolarization. There is a pause after the QRS complex, and then a T wave appears. The T wave

is a period of no cardiac activity before the ventricles are again stimulated. It represents the recovery phase after ventricular contraction.

8. The U wave is a deflection (usually positive) following the T wave. It represents late ventricular repolarization of Purkinje's fibers or the intraventricular papillary muscles. This wave may or may not be present on an EKG. If it appears, it may be abnormal, depending on its configuration.

Normal Intervals (Table 15-1)

1. The R-R interval (normally 0.83 second at a heart rate of 72 beats/minute) is the distance between two successive R waves. In normal rhythms, the interval, in seconds or fractions of seconds, between two successive R waves divided into 60 seconds provides the heart rate per minute.

2. The P-P interval (normally 0.83 second at a heart rate of 72 beats/minute) will be the same as the R-R interval in normal sinus rhythm. The responsiveness of the sinus node to physiologic activity (eg, exercise, rest, respiratory cycling) produces a rhythmic variance in P-P intervals.

3. The PR interval (~0.16 second) measures conduction tone and includes the time it takes for atrial depolarization and normal conduction delay in the atrioventricular node to occur. It terminates with the onset of ventricular depolarization. It is the period from the start of the P wave to the beginning of the QRS complex. This interval represents the time it takes for the impulse to traverse the atria, proceed through the atrioventricular node, and reach the ventricles and initiate ventricular depolarization.

4. The QRS interval (normally 0.12 second) represents ventricular depolarization time and tracks the electrical impulse as it travels from the atrioventricular node through the bundle branches to the Purkinje fibers and into the myocardial cells. Normal waves consist of an initial downward deflection (Q wave), a large upward deflection (R wave), and a second downward deflection (S wave). It is measured from the onset of the Q wave (or R if no Q is visible) to the termination of the S wave.

Normal Segments and Junctions

1. The PR segment is normally isoelectric and is the portion of the ECG tracing from the end of the P wave to the onset of the QRS complex.

2. The J junction (or J point) is the point at which the QRS complex ends and the ST segment begins.

3. The ST segment is that part of the ECG from the J point to the onset of the T wave. Elevation or depression is determined by comparing its location with the portion of the baseline between the end of the T wave and the beginning of the P wave or relating it to the PR segment. This segment represents the period between the completion of depolarization and onset of repolarization (ie, recovery) of the ventricular muscles.

4. The TP segment (~0.25 second) is the portion of the ECG record between the end of the T wave and the beginning of the next P wave. It is usually isoelectric.

TABLE 15-1
Normal Measurements and Ranges of Components of P–Q–R–S–T–U Cycle*

	P Wave		PR Interval		Q Wave Q% of R	
	Amplitude	Width			WIDTH	DEPTH
	MAXIMUM	MAXIMUM	0.12 SEC–0.20 SEC		Less than 0.04 sec	QR ratio
	2.5 mm	0.10 sec				
L₁						15% of R wave
L₂						20% of R wave
L₃					Up to 0.08 sec	25% of R wave
AVR					Up to 0.08 sec	
AVL					Less than 0.04 sec	25% of R wave
AVF						
V₁					Up to 0.08 sec	
V₂						
V₃					Less than 0.04 sec	
V₄						
V₅						
V₆						

*For practical purposes, these are the upper and lower limits of the normal ECG. However, there are "gray zones," and variation from these limits may not necessarily imply abnormality.

continued

TABLE 15-1   *(Continued)*
Normal Measurements and Ranges of Components of P–Q–R–S–T–U Cycle*

	QRS Interval	R-Wave Amplitude	ST Segment	T-Wave Amplitude	U-Wave Amplitude/Width
	0.10 sec	Maximum to minimum	1 mm	1 mm–5 mm	1.5 mm 0.24 sec
		5 mm–16 mm	Above or below		
L₁			1 mm elevation		
L₂					
L₃		↓		↓	
AVR		Less than +4 mm		Except in this lead (T is neg)	
AVL		5 mm–13 mm Transverse heart	1 mm elevation		
AVF		5 mm–21 mm Vertical heart		↓	
V₁	↓	5 mm–27 mm	1 mm–2 mm depression	13 mm	
V₂	0.11 sec				
V₃	0.11 sec				
V₄			2 mm–4 mm elevation		
V₅					
V₆	↓	↓		↓	↓ ↓

(Ritota MC: Diagnostic Electrocardiography, 2nd ed. Philadelphia, JB Lippincott, 1977)

Normal Voltage Measurements

1. Voltage from the top of the R wave to the bottom of the S wave is 1 mV. Voltage of the P wave is ~0.1 to 0.3 mV. Voltage of the T wave is ~0.2 to 0.3 mV. Upright deflection voltage is measured from the upper part of the baseline to the peak of the wave.
2. Negative deflection voltage is measured from the lower portion of the baseline to the nadir of the wave.

Explanation of Test

An ECG records the electrical impulses that stimulate the heart to contract. It also records dysfunctions that influence the conduction ability of the myocardium. The ECG is helpful in diagnosing and monitoring the origins of pathologic rhythms; myocardial ischemia; myocardial infarction; atrial and ventricular hypertrophy; atrial, atrioventricular, and ventricular conduction delays; and pericarditis. It can be helpful in diagnosing systemic diseases that affect the heart; determining cardiac drug effects (especially digitalis and antiarrhythmic agents); evaluating disturbances in electrolyte balance (especially potassium and calcium); and analyzing cardiac pacemaker or implanted defibrillator functions.

An ECG provides a continuous picture of electrical activity during a complete cycle. Heart cells are charged or polarized in the resting state, but they depolarize and contract when electrically stimulated. The intracellular body fluids are excellent conductors of electrical current and are an important component of this process. When the depolarization (stimulation) process sweeps in a wave across the cells of the myocardium, the electrical current generated is conducted to the body's surface, where it is detected by special electrodes placed on the patient's limbs and chest. An ECG tracing shows the voltage of the waves and the time duration of waves and intervals. By studying the amplitude of the waves and measuring the duration of the waves and intervals, disorders of impulse formation and conduction can be diagnosed (see Fig. 15-1).

Recording the Electrical Impulses

1. Because cardiac electrical forces extend in several directions at the same time, a comprehensive view of heart activity is possible only if the flow of current in several different planes is recorded.
2. For a 12-lead ECG, 12 leads are simultaneously used to present this comprehensive picture:
   a. Limb leads (I, II, III, AVL, AVF, AVR) record events in the frontal plane of the heart.
   b. Chest leads (V_1, V_2, V_3, V_4, V_5, and V_6) record a horizontal view of the heart's electrical activity.
3. Occasionally, an esophageal lead, which is swallowed or placed in the esophagus, can supply additional information. This type of lead is frequently used during surgical procedures.

ECG Versus Vectorcardiogram

The vectorcardiogram, like the ECG, records the electrical forces of the heart. The major difference between these two methods is the way in which these forces are displayed. A vectorcardiogram records a *three-dimensional* display of the heart's electrical activity, whereas the ECG is a *single-plane* representation. The following are the three planes of the vectorcardiogram:

1. Frontal plane (combines the Y and X axes)
2. Sagittal plane (combines the Y and Z axes)
3. Horizontal plane (combines the X and Z axes)

The following table compares ECG and vectorcardiograms (Fig. 15-2).

ECG	Vectorcardiogram
Records electrical forces as positive or negative deflections on a scale	Depicts electrical forces as vector loops, which show the *direction* of electrical flow
Records activity in the frontal and horizontal planes	Records activity in the frontal, horizontal and sagittal planes
	The term *vector* indicates the directional flow of electrical activity

Procedure

The following steps apply to both the ECG and the vectorcardiogram:

1. The patient usually assumes a supine position; however, recordings can be taken during exercise.

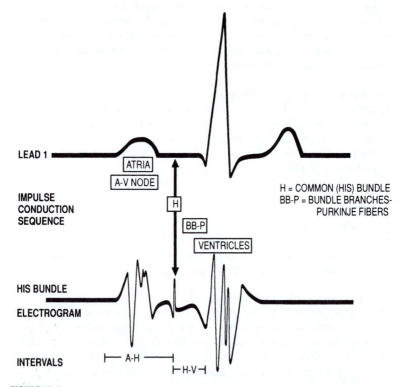

FIGURE 15-2

His bundle electrogram. Note electrophysiologic events are presented in relation to the surface electrocardiogram. (After Phillips, R.E., Feeney, M.K.: The Cardiac Rhythms, 3rd ed. Philadelphia: WB Saunders, 1990.)

2. The skin sites are prepared and, if necessary, shaved, and electrodes are placed on each of the four extremities and on specific chest sites. The right leg is the ground (Fig. 15-3).
3. All 12 leads can be recorded simultaneously by newer ECG machines.
4. A rhythm strip is a 2-minute recording from a single lead, usually lead II. It is frequently used to evaluate dysrhythmias.
5. Follow guidelines in Chapter 1 for safe, effective, informed *intratest* care.

Clinical Implications of ECG

1. The ECG does not depict the actual mechanical state of the heart or functional status of the valves.
2. An ECG may be normal in the presence of heart disease unless the pathologic process disturbs the electrical forces. It cannot predict future cardiac events.

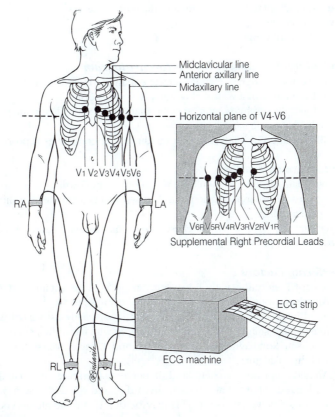

FIGURE 15-3

ECG electrode placement. (From Smeltzer, Brunner, and Suddarth's Textbook of Basic Nursing, 8th ed. Philadelphia: Lippincott-Raven Publishers, 1996.)

3. An ECG should be interpreted and treatment ordered within the context of a comprehensive clinical picture.
4. ECG abnormalities are categorized according to five general areas:
   a. Heart rate
   b. Heart rhythm
   c. Axis or position of the heart
   d. Hypertrophy
   e. Infarction/ischemia
5. Typical abnormalities include the following:
   a. Pathologic rhythms
   b. Conduction system disturbances
   c. Myocardial ischemia
   d. Myocardial infarction
   e. Hypertrophy of the heart
   f. Pulmonary infarction
   g. Altered potassium, calcium, and magnesium levels
   h. Pericarditis
   i. Effects of drugs

Clinical Implications of the Vectorcardiogram
1. The vectorcardiogram is more sensitive than the ECG for diagnosing myocardial infarction; it is probably not any more specific.
2. Vectorcardiography is more specific than the ECG in determining hypertrophy or ventricular dilatation.
3. Differentiation of intraventricular conduction abnormalities is possible.

Clinical Considerations
1. Chest pain, if present, should be noted on the ECG strip.
2. The presence of a pacemaker and the use of a magnet in testing should be documented.
3. Marking the position on the chest wall in ink ensures a reproducible precordial lead placement.

Interfering Factors
1. Race: ST elevation with T wave inversion is more common in African Americans, but disappears with maximal exercise effort.
2. Food intake: high carbohydrate content is especially associated with an intracellular shift of potassium in association with intracellular glucose metabolism. Nondiagnostic ST depression and T wave inversion is evident with hypokalemia.
3. Anxiety: episodic anxiety and hyperventilation are associated with prolonged PR interval, sinus tachycardia, and ST depression with or without T wave inversion. This may be due to autonomic nervous system imbalances.
4. Deep respiration: the position of the heart in the chest shifts more vertically with deep inspiration and more horizontally with deep expiration.

5. Exercise/movement: strenuous exercise before the test can produce misleading results. Muscle twitching can also alter the tracing.

6. Position of heart within the thoracic cage: there may be an anatomic cardiac rotation in both horizontal and frontal planes.

7. Position of precordial leads: inaccurate placement of the bipolar chest leads and the transposition of right and left arm and left leg electrodes will affect test results. In normal persons, lead reversal produces the typical ECG findings of dextrocardia in frontal plane leads and can mimic a myocardial infarction pattern.

8. A leftward shift in the QRS axis occurs with excess body weight, ascites, and pregnancy.

9. Age: at birth and during infancy, the right ventricle is hypertrophied because the fetal right ventricle performs more work than the left ventricle. T wave inversion in leads V_1–V_3 persists into the second decade of life and into the third decade in black persons.

10. Gender: women exhibit slight ST segment depression.

11. Chest configuration and dextrocardia: in this congenital anomaly in which the heart is transposed to the right side of the chest, the precordial leads must also be placed over the right side of the chest.

12. Severe drug overdose, especially with barbiturates, and many other medications can influence ECG configuration.

13. The serious effects of electrolyte imbalances show up on the ECG as follows:

    a. Increased Ca^{2+}: shortened QT; less frequently, prolonged PR interval and QRS complex

    b. Decreased Ca^{2+}: prolonged QT

    c. Alterations in K^+ may produce cardiac arrhythmias.

Patient Preparation

1. Explain the test purpose, procedure, and interfering factors. Emphasize that ECG is painless and does not deliver electrical current to the body. A resting ECG is no more than a 1-minute record of the heart's electrical activity.

2. The patient should completely relax to ensure a satisfactory tracing.

3. Ideally, the person should rest for 15 minutes prior to ECG recording. Heavy meals and smoking should be avoided for at least 30 minutes prior to the ECG, and longer if possible.

4. Follow guidelines in Chapter 1 for safe, effective, informed *pretest* care.

Patient Aftercare

1. Recognize the limitations of an ECG. A normal ECG does not rule out coronary artery disease or areas of cardiac ischemia. Conversely, an abnormal ECG in and of itself does not always signify heart disease.

2. Interpret test results and counsel and monitor the patient appropriately. A resting ECG is usually normal for those patients who experience only angina. It can provide evidence of prior heart damage. The ECG is one

diagnostic tool within a repertoire of diagnostic modalities and should be viewed as such. The presence or absence of heart disease should not be presumed solely upon the basis of the ECG.

3. Follow guidelines in Chapter 1 for safe, effective, informed *posttest* care.

Clinical Alert

1. When an ECG shows changes that indicate ischemia, injury, or infarction, these changes must be reported and acted on immediately. The goal of diagnosis and treatment is to increase myocardial blood supply and reduce oxygen demand.
   a. When ECG changes represent stages of ischemia, injury, or necrosis and symptoms of possible myocardial infarction appear, the primary concern is balancing myocardial oxygen supply and demand as follows:
      (1) Nitroglycerin dilates blood vessels.
      (2) Narcotics relieve pain and anxiety.
      (3) Calcium channel blockers relieve coronary spasm.
      (4) Oxygen increases O_2 supply available to the myocardium.
      (5) Beta-blocking drugs slow rapid heart rates.
      (6) Antiarrhythmic agents correct abnormal rhythms.
      (7) Frequent reassurances alleviate patient anxiety.
   b. Monitoring for cardiac rhythm disturbances is an essential component of care. Potentially lethal dysrhythmias, especially ventricular tachyarrhythmias, require immediate intervention and may signal the need for possible cardiopulmonary resuscitation.
2. Serious diagnostic errors can be made if the ECG is not interpreted in the broader context of the patient's history, signs, and symptoms.
3. The electrical axis is not synonymous with the anatomic position of the heart.

SIGNAL-AVERAGED ELECTROCARDIOGRAM (SAE) ●

Normal SAE
Normal QRS complexes and ST segments

Explanation of Test
The signal-averaged ECG (SAE) is a noninvasive tool for identifying patients at risk for malignant ventricular dysrhythmias particularly after myocardial infarction. During the later phase of the QRS complex and ST segment, the myocardium produces high-frequency, low-amplitude signals termed *late potentials*. These late potentials correlate with delayed activation of certain areas within the myocardium, a condition that predisposes to reentrant forms of ventricular tachycardia.

Indications

SAEs are performed to evaluate the etiology of ventricular dysrhythmias or as a precursor to electrophysiology studies. Disorders that may produce regions of delayed myocardial conduction include myocardial infarction, nonischemic dilated cardiomyopathy, left ventricular aneurysm, and some forms of healed ventricular incisions (ie, scar from tetralogy of Fallot surgical intervention).

Procedure

1. The SAE, which is a modification of the conventional ECG, uses computerized techniques to provide signal averaging, amplification, and filtering of electrical potentials. Electrodes are placed on the abdomen and anterior and posterior thorax. The signals received are converted to a digital signal. A typical QRS complex is used as a template against which subsequent cardiac cycles are compared. Typically, several hundred beats are averaged to analyze for late potentials. Data collection usually takes about 20 minutes. Optimal recordings require the patient to be in a comfortable position and to remain quiet, proper application of electrodes, and elimination of interference from other electrical equipment.
2. Follow guidelines in Chapter 1 for safe, effective, informed *intratest* care.

Clinical Implications

1. SAE provides predictive values for potential ventricular tachycardias in patients who have a history of myocardial infarction or coronary artery disease.
2. Late potentials are stronger predictors of sudden death or sustained ventricular tachycardias than are ventricular dysrhythmias from a Holter monitor recording.
3. Evidence shows that late potentials associated with ventricular tachycardias are abolished following successful surgical intervention.
4. Patients who experience late potentials have a 17% incidence of sustained ventricular tachycardia or sudden death versus a 1% incidence in patients without late potentials. The incidence is even greater in the presence of decreased ejection fractions.
5. SAE may explain the cause of syncope subsequently identified as ventricular tachycardia during EP study.

Interfering Factors

1. Increased time is required for recording beats in the presence of slow heart rates or frequent ventricular ectopics. Patient movement, talking, and restlessness also delays data procurement.
2. Bundle branch block can interfere with impulse averaging.
3. SAE does not provide information about antiarrhythmic drug effectiveness.
4. Late potentials do not occur in every patient with ventricular tachycardia.
5. Ventricular pacing prolongs ventricular activation time and obscures late potentials. Conversely, atrial pacing, even at rapid rates, does not alter ventricular late potentials.

Patient Preparation

1. Explain test purpose, procedure, benefits, and risks. Caution patient to remain still and quiet during testing.
2. Follow guidelines in Chapter 1 for safe, effective, informed *pretest* care.

Patient Aftercare

1. Interpret test results and monitor appropriately when late potentials are identified.
2. Follow guidelines in Chapter 1 for safe, effective, informed *posttest* care.

HOLTER CONTINUOUS ECG MONITORING ●

Normal Holter ECG

Normal sinus rhythm

Explanation of Test

Holter monitoring is a method of continuously recording the ECG on magnetic tape for prolonged (24 hours) periods of time. The tape recorder is a battery-powered device with very slow (3.75 inches/minute) tape speeds and is encased and worn on a strap over the shoulder or around the waist, similar to a small purse. Two ECG channels recorded simultaneously present graphic records of electrical conduction activities. The Holter recorder is equipped with a digital clock that is synchronized to the tape recorder to allow for accurate time marking. The patient also uses a diary to enter any symptoms experienced during monitoring, along with the activity status and the time of noted symptoms. When a symptom is felt, the patient pushes an event-marker button on the recorder to mark one of the channels for event recognition during playback and evaluation.

A 24-hour recording contains >100,000 cardiac cycles. Playback and tape analysis are done at 60, 120, or 180 times real time. The tape may be rapidly analyzed by computers that provide summaries of heart rates, frequency and type of arrhythmias, coupling intervals, and other variations. Another method of tape scanning superimposes each QRS complex on the preceding QRS complex. This makes variations in QRS contours apparent. With either scanning method, segments of the recording can be reproduced on ECG paper. The diary the patient keeps is also used to analyze correlations between symptoms and ECG findings.

Indications for Holter Monitoring

1. To document suspected rhythm disturbances. The recording, along with the patient's diary, allows correlation of rhythm disturbances with symptoms such as syncope, palpitations, chest pain, lightheadedness, or unexplained dyspnea. If these symptoms have no obvious cause, a Holter recording can detect unsuspected arrhythmias such as supraventricular and ventricular

tachycardias, bradycardia-tachycardia associated with sick sinus syndrome, and other ventricular and supraventricular arrhythmias.
2. To record the onset and termination of a rhythmic disturbance which may provide insights into electrophysiologic mechanisms responsible for the arrhythmia
3. To check pacemaker and automatic implantable defibrillator functional status
4. To track drug and treatment effectiveness

Procedure
1. The patient assumes a supine position.
2. The skin is prepared, shaved (if necessary), cleansed with alcohol, and rubbed with gauze or similar rough material to ensure proper electrode contact and adhesion.
3. Two electrodes for each channel and one ground electrode are positioned over selected bony prominences. Two negative electrodes are placed on the manubrium. The corresponding positive electrodes are placed in the V_1 and V_5 positions.
4. Leads and cables are secured, and the recorder is activated and calibrated. The patient is then free to pursue normal activities except for bathing.
5. After the predetermined (24 to 48 hours) time has elapsed, the recorder and electrodes are removed.
6. The tape is scanned and interpreted, and a written summary of findings is submitted to the physician.
7. Follow guidelines in Chapter 1 for safe, effective, informed *intratest* care.

Interfering Factors
1. Incomplete diary or event marker not pushed during symptom episodes.

   NOTE: *The patient may not always be aware of existing cardiac events.*

2. Mechanical interferences (eg, scratching, friction) can alter the recording.

Clinical Implications
1. Abnormal results show evidence of rhythm disturbances such as:
   a. Tachycardias (atrial and ventricular)
   b. Bradycardia
   c. Premature atrial or ventricular beats
   d. Heart blocks
   e. Junctional rhythms
   f. Atrial flutter or fibrillation
   g. Other ventricular and supraventricular rhythm disturbances
2. Hypoxic/ischemic changes

> **Clinical Alert**
>
> Advise the patient to take only sponge baths while wearing the Holter monitor.

Patient Preparation

1. Explain test purpose and benefits and the procedure for keeping a diary of events.
2. Explain that the patient may experience itching at the electrode site, but caution against removing or readjusting electrodes in any manner.
3. Follow guidelines in Chapter 1 for safe, effective, informed *pretest* care.

Patient Aftercare

1. Interpret test results. Counsel and monitor appropriately for symptoms of cardiac arrhythmias and other related conditions. Review treatment guidelines.
2. Follow guidelines in Chapter 1 for safe, effective, informed *posttest* care.

STRESS TEST/EXERCISE TESTING
(GRADED EXERCISE TOLERANCE TEST) ●

Normal Stress Test

Negative when the patient does not exhibit significant symptoms, arrhythmias, or other ECG abnormalities at 85% of maximum heart rate predicted for age and gender

Explanation of Test

This test measures the efficiency of the heart during a dynamic exercise stress period on a motor-driven treadmill or ergometer. It is valuable for diagnosing ischemic heart disease and investigating physiologic mechanisms underlying cardiac symptoms such as angina, dysrhythmias, inordinate blood pressure elevations, and functionally incompetent heart valves. Exercise testing can also measure functional capacity for work, sports, or participation in rehabilitation programs, and it can be a predictor of potential response to medical or surgical treatment. Additionally, upper limits of physiologically responsive pacemakers can be evaluated.

Systolic blood pressure normally increases with exercise, and diastolic pressure normally remains essentially unchanged. Stress exercise testing takes place under controlled conditions that include low temperatures (20°C) and lower humidity.

Procedure

There are many different types of stress tests. Most include the following steps:

1. Recording electrodes are placed on the patient's chest (see description of ECG) and attached to a monitor. A blood pressure recording device is also placed appropriately.

2. As the patient walks on a motor-driven treadmill, or pedals an ergometer if walking is not possible, computerized ECG and heart monitoring devices record performance. The patient walks at progressively greater speeds and higher levels of elevation to increase both heart rate and workload.

3. The initial or resting ECG, heart rate, and blood pressure are recorded. The patient is asked to report any symptoms such as chest pain or shortness of breath experienced during the test. Normal persons are symptom-free at submaximal efforts; however, at peak or maximal efforts, symptoms expected in normal persons include exhaustion, fatigue, and sometimes nausea or dizziness.

4. The patient undergoes stress testing in stages. Each stage consists of a predetermined treadmill speed (in miles per hour) and a treadmill grade elevation (in percent grade).

5. The ECG, heart rate, and blood pressure are continually monitored for abnormalities and any unusual symptoms such as intolerable dyspnea, chest pain, or severe cramping (claudication) in the legs.

6. Vital signs, together with other abnormalities and complaints, are recorded at 1- to 3-minute intervals for 6 to 8 minutes posttest as the patient rests. The test is terminated if ECG abnormalities, fatigue, weakness, abnormal blood pressure changes, or other intolerable symptoms occur during the test.

7. Common criteria for terminating a test include the following:
   a. Achieving maximum possible performance
   b. Emerging signs or symptoms that indicate an existing disease process
   c. Recording a predetermined endpoint, such as 85% of age-related maximal heart rate, arbitrary work load (one that raises heart rate to 150 beats/minute), or diagnostic ECG changes

8. Total examination time is about 30 minutes; however, the patient should plan to be in the laboratory for 1 to 1.5 hours.

9. Follow guidelines in Chapter 1 for safe, effective, informed *intratest* care.

Clinical Implications

1. Abnormal responses to exercise testing include the following:
   a. Alterations in blood pressure, such as:
      (1) Failure of systolic pressure to rise
      (2) Progressive fall in systolic pressure
      (3) Elevation of diastolic blood pressure
   b. Alterations in heart rate, such as:
      (1) Tachycardia above that which is predetermined.
      (2) Bradycardia
   c. Changes in ECG, such as:
      (1) Repression or elevation of ST segments caused by ischemia
      (2) Dysrhythmias, ventricular tachycardia, multifocal premature ventricular contractions, atrial tachycardia, second- or third-degree atrioventricular block
      (3) Pacemaker failure to perform within set rate limits

d. Ventricular or supraventricular ectopies are considered abnormal responses not necessarily ischemic in origin.

e. Ischemic ST-segment depression ≥0.2 mm or elevation ≥1 mm is the most common abnormality. Men aged 40 to 59 years who develop ST depression during exercise that is not present at rest have five times the risk of developing overt coronary heart disease than men without this ST depression.

f. Unusual symptoms such as:
  (1) Anginal pain
  (2) Severe breathlessness
  (3) Faintness, dizziness, lightheadedness, confusion
  (4) Claudication, leg pain

g. Unusual signs such as:
  (1) Cyanosis, pallor, skin mottling
  (2) Cold sweats, piloerection
  (3) Ataxia, glassy stare
  (4) Gallop heart sounds
  (5) Valvular regurgitation

Interfering Factors

Common causes of false-positive exercise ECG responses include the following:

1. Left ventricular hypertrophy
2. Digitalis toxicity
3. ST segment abnormality at rest
4. Hypertension
5. Valvular heart disease
6. Left bundle branch block
7. Anemia
8. Hypoxia
9. Vasoregulatory asthenia
10. Lown-Ganong-Levine syndrome
11. "Panic" or anxiety attack
12. Wolff-Parkinson-White syndrome

Patient Preparation

1. Explain the test purpose and procedure. No food, coffee, or cigarettes are allowed 2 hours prior to testing. Water may be taken.
2. A legal consent form must be signed by the patient or patient's designee.
3. The patient should wear flat walking shoes or tennis shoes (no slippers). Men should wear gym shorts or light, loose-fitting trousers. Women should wear a bra, a short-sleeved blouse that buttons in front, and slacks, shorts, or pajama pants (no one-piece undergarments, pantyhose, or slips).
4. Certain medications should be withheld or discontinued before testing. β-Adrenergic blocking agents (eg, propranolol) should have dosage reduced or be tapered off gradually. The physician should write orders regarding management of the patient's drug regimen well before the test.

5. Follow guidelines in Chapter 1 regarding safe, effective, informed *pretest* care.

Patient Aftercare

1. Interpret test results and monitor appropriately for abnormal responses to exercise. Report significant events or symptoms without delay.
2. The patient should not be discharged until acceptable levels for vital signs and ECG monitoring have been met.
3. Follow guidelines in Chapter 1 for safe, effective, informed *posttest* care.

> **Clinical Alert**
>
> Stress exercise testing can be risky for patients with recent onset of chest pain associated with significantly elevated blood pressures or with frequent attacks of angina. Testing may require a 4- to 6-week delay in these situations.

CARDIAC CATHETERIZATION AND ANGIOGRAPHY
(ANGIOCARDIOGRAPHY, CORONARY ARTERIOGRAPHY)

Normal Cardiac Catheterization

Normal heart values, chamber size, and patent coronary arteries
Normal wall and valve motion
Normal cardiac output (CO): 4–8 L/minute
Normal percentage of oxygen content (15–22 vol. %) and oxygen saturation (95%–100% of capacity, or 0.95–1.00)

Normal Cardiac Volumes

End-diastolic volume (EDV): 50–90 ml/m^2
End-systolic volume (ESV): 25 ml/m^2
Stroke volume (SV): 45 ± 12 ml/m^2
Ejection fraction (EF): 0.67 ± 0.07

Normal Hemodynamic Pressures (mm Hg)		
	Average	*Range*
Right atrium		
A wave	6	2–7
U wave	5	2–7
Mean	3	1–5
Right ventricle		
Peak systolic	25	15–30
End diastolic	4	1–7

(continued)

Normal Hemodynamic Pressures (mm Hg) *(Continued)*		
PAP		
Peak systolic	25	15–30
End diastolic	9	4–12
Mean	5	9–19
PCWP	9	4–12
Left atrium		
A wave	10	4–16
U wave	12	6–21
Mean	8	2–12
Left ventricle		
Peak systolic	130	90–140
End diastolic	8	5–12
Complete aortic		
Peak systolic	130	90–140
End diastolic	70	60–90
Mean	85	70–105

Explanation of Test

This method is chosen to study and diagnose defects of the chambers of the heart, the heart valves, and certain blood vessels by means of inserting arterial and venous catheters which can carry contrast material into the right and left sides of the heart. As these catheters are introduced and advanced toward the heart, fluoroscopy and high-speed x-ray pictures projected onto monitors show actual heart function and motion. Injected contrast medium provides a visual definition of cardiac structures. Coronary artery patency and circulation is filmed as well. The patient's heart rate, rhythm, and pressures are monitored continuously.

Coronary arteriograms are useful for evaluating abnormal stress tests, diagnosing heart disease, assessing the complications of a myocardial infarction, diagnosing congenital abnormalities, identifying cardiac structure and function, and measuring hemodynamic pressures within heart chambers and great vessels. They are used to measure cardiac output using contrast dilution, thermodilution, and Fick method and to obtain cardiac blood samples for measuring oxygen content and oxygen saturation.

Cardiac catheterization combined with angiography is indicated for patients who exhibit angina, chest pain, syncope, valve problems, ischemic heart disease, cholesteremia, symptoms with history of familial heart disease, abnormal resting or exercise ECGs; and recurring cardiac symptoms postrevascularization. Other indications include young patients with a history of coronary insufficiency or ventricular aneurysm and patients who experience coronary neurosis and need assurance that their cardiac status is normal. This test can be performed during the acute stage of myocardial infarction, and if necessary, surgical intervention can be accomplished without significant delay. Although cardiac catheterization poses some risk, it is a highly accurate diagnostic resource.

Procedure

1. The test is normally done in a special, darkened procedure room.
2. To decrease anxiety, explain the procedure and provide information about sensations the patient may experience.
   a. For right-heart catheterization, the medial cubital, brachial, or femoral vein is used. The catheter is threaded through the vena cava to the right atrium, through the tricuspid valve and right ventricle, to the pulmonary artery. Pressure measurements and O_2 saturations are taken from these areas as the catheter is manipulated.

   NOTE: *If left-to-right shunt is suspected, blood samples are also obtained from the superior and inferior vena cava.*

   b. For left-heart catheterization procedure, the patient is heparinized. The catheter is threaded through the femoral or brachial artery and on through the aortic valve to the left ventricle. Again, pressure readings are taken. Introduction of contrast material, if done, provides data about left ventricular contractility, contour size, and presence of mitral regurgitation.

   NOTE: *Left atrial function and measurements are usually calculated from other measurements. If direct measurements are necessary, a transseptal approach must be done by advancing the catheter through the saphenous leg vein into the right atrium and then passing a needle through the catheter to puncture the atrial septum so that direct pressure readings may be obtained. The patient may be asked to exercise during the procedure to evaluate consistent changes; atrial pacing may be done during the procedure to incrementally stress and rest the heart for those patients unable to move normally (eg, paraplegic patient).*

   Sterile surgical conditions are observed. The skin is prepared with an antiseptic solution scrub. A local anesthetic is injected into the catheter insertion site area (eg, groin [femoral artery], antecubital [brachial artery]). Small incisions may be made to facilitate insertion. Once inserted, the catheters are gently advanced to the heart and great vessels.
3. The patient lies on a special x-ray table, and the ECG is monitored continuously. Intravenous sedation may be used if necessary. During the procedure, the patient is placed in several different positions. The patient may be asked to exercise to evaluate heart changes associated with activity. Atrial pacing can also be done as part of the procedure in persons who cannot walk (eg, paraplegics) or use a treadmill. In these instances, there is a sequence of events that stress the heart followed by a rest period; then measurements are taken. The heart is paced again, followed by another rest period.
4. Sometimes the patient can watch the procedure on a television monitor if it happens to be positioned properly.
5. After x-ray films have been taken from all angles, the catheters are removed, and manual pressure is applied to the site for 20 to 30 minutes. A sterile pressure bandage may be applied for several additional hours. Some facilities no longer use pressure bandages. Skin incisions are closed with

sutures. Less pressure and less time may be required for venous sites. Protamine sulfate may be given to reverse the effects of heparinization.

6. Reassure the patient frequently.

7. Follow guidelines in Chapter 1 for safe, effective, informed *intratest* care.

Clinical Implications

1. Abnormal results include the following:
   a. Altered hemodynamic pressures
   b. Injected contrast agent reveals altered ventricular structure and dynamics or occluded coronary arteries
   c. Blood gas analysis confirms cardiac, circulatory, or pulmonary problems

2. Abnormal hemodynamic pressures indicate the following conditions:
   a. Valve stenosis or insufficiency
   b. Left and/or right ventricular failure
   c. Idiopathic hypertrophic subaortic stenosis (IHS)
   d. Rheumatic fever sequelae
   e. Cardiomyopathies

3. Abnormal blood gas results indicate the following conditions:
   a. Congenital or acquired circulatory shunting
   b. Septal defects
   c. Other cardiac and pulmonary defects or pathology

4. When a contrast agent is injected into the ventricles, abnormalities of size, function, structure, ejection fractions, aneurysms, leaks, stenosis, and altered contractility can be detected.

5. When contrast is injected into coronary arteries, occluded vessels and circulatory function can be recorded.

Patient Preparation

1. Explain the test purpose, procedure, benefits, and risks. A legal permit must be signed before the examination. Always check for allergies, especially to iodine and contrast media. Extensive teaching may be necessary.

2. The patient should fast for 6 to 8 hours before the procedure. Routine, scheduled medications such as cardiac drugs or insulin may be given prior to the procedure unless directed otherwise. Anticoagulants should be discontinued at least 1 to 2 days before the procedure.

3. Analgesics, sedatives, or tranquilizers may be given prior to the procedure.

4. The patient should void before the procedure.

5. The patient may wear dentures; jewelry and other accessories must be removed.

6. Instruct the patient regarding the need to do deep breathing and coughing during the test, and inform them that they may feel certain sensations.
   a. Catheter insertion via antecubital or groin sites may produce significant pressure sensations when the sheath, through which the catheter is inserted and advanced, is introduced.
   b. A slight shock or "funny bone" sensation may be felt if the nerve adjacent to the artery is touched. A tiny "bump" in the neck may be felt as the catheter is inserted into the heart. Normally, pain is not felt.

c. When the contrast agent is injected into the catheter, a pumping sensation with feelings of palpitations and hot flashes may last 30 to 60 seconds. Skin vessels vasodilate and blood rises to the skin surface for a short time.

d. Patients may experience nausea, vomiting, headache, and cough.

e. Angina may occur with exercise or with the contrast agent injection. Nitroglycerin or narcotics may be given.

7. Follow guidelines in Chapter 1 for safe, effective, informed *pretest* care.

Patient Aftercare

1. Bed rest is usually maintained for 6 to 12 hours after the test, based on the nature of the procedure, physician's protocols, and patient status. The patient is usually not permitted to raise his or her head more than 30 degrees during this time because greater angles put strain on the insertion site. Conversely, movement of the uninvolved extremities should be promoted.

2. Check vital signs frequently according to institution protocols. At the same time, check catheter insertion site for hematomas, swelling, bleeding, or bruits. Normal or other mechanical pressure to the catheter insertion site may be necessary if bleeding or hematoma develops. A bruised appearance around the site is normal. Swelling or lumps should be promptly reported to physician. Neurovascular checks should be done along with assessment of vital signs in bilateral extremities and results compared. Assess color, motion, sensation, capillary refill times, temperature, and pulse quality. Report significant changes immediately.

3. Prophylactic antibiotics may be administered.

4. Encourage fluid intake. Unless contraindicated, an intravenous infusion site may be maintained while the patient is on bed rest in the event that rapid intravenous access is needed.

5. Keep the affected extremity extended, not elevated or flexed. Immobilize the legs with sandbags if necessary. Apply ice packs and/or sandbags to the catheter site, if ordered. Prescribed analgesics can be administered for pain or discomfort.

6. Sutures, if used, are removed per the physician's instructions.

7. Interpret test results and monitor appropriately for cardiac, circulatory, neurovascular, and pulmonary problems.

8. Follow guidelines in Chapter 1 for safe, effective, informed *posttest* care.

Clinical Alert

1. This procedure is contraindicated in patients with gross cardiomegaly.

2. Complications include the following:

   a. Dysrhythmias

   b. Allergic reactions to contrast agent (evidenced by urticaria, pruritus, conjunctivitis, or anaphylaxis)

(continued)

(Clinical Alert continued)
- **c.** Thrombophlebitis
- **d.** Insertion site infection
- **e.** Pneumothorax
- **f.** Hemopericardium
- **g.** Embolism
- **h.** Liver lacerations, especially in infants and children
- **i.** Excessive bleeding at the catheter site

3. Notify attending physician immediately if increased bleeding, hematoma, dramatic fall or elevation in blood pressure, or decreased peripheral circulation and abnormal or changed neurovascular findings are noted. Rapid treatment may prevent more severe complications.

4. The following equipment should always be available to treat complications of angiography:
- **a.** Resuscitation equipment
- **b.** DC defibrillator
- **c.** External pacemaker
- **d.** EEG monitor
- **e.** Emergency drugs

ELECTROPHYSIOLOGY (EP) STUDIES; HIS BUNDLE PROCEDURE ●

Normal EP/His Bundle Procedure
Normal conduction intervals, refractory periods and recovery times
Controlled, induced arrhythmias

Explanation of Test
Electrophysiology studies are accomplished through an invasive test for diagnosis and treatment of ventricular and supraventricular arrhythmias. It is similar to cardiac catheterization, the difference being that an EP study measures cardiac electrical conduction system activity through solid electrode catheters instead of the open-lumen catheters used to measure circulatory system pressures. These electrode catheters are almost always inserted into veins because of the greater risk they pose in the arterial system (spasms, occlusion). Using fluoroscopy as a visual guide, the catheters are advanced into the right atrium and right ventricle. An x-ray monitor tracks the catheter location, and a physiologic monitor shows ECG rhythms as well as intracardiac catheter electrograms.

An EP study is highly useful for diagnosing diseases of the cardiac conduction system and provides indications for optimal treatment. In addition to measuring baseline values, the electrode catheters are used to pace the heart in an attempt to induce the same arrhythmia causing the problem. When the patient is on antiarrhythmic drugs, the EP study can determine how well the medication is working by how easily the arrhythmia can be induced. This is in contrast to the trial-and-error method, in which there is no way to know that a particular drug is ineffective until that drug has failed to resolve the problem, frequently over a significant period of time.

EP is indicated to differentiate disorders of impulse formation (supraventricular versus ventricular rhythms). Electrophysiology studies also provide diagnostic insight into the etiology and mechanism of conduction disorders. EP studies are often part of the workup for syncope, sick sinus syndrome, or tachyarrhythmias. Finally, EP studies are indicated for testing the effectiveness of antiarrhythmic drugs. Each antiarrhythmic drug has certain effects that must be anticipated during the loading phase (eg, hypotension with quinidine and procainamide, abdominal cramping with quinidine, venous pain with phenytoin). A state of "happy drunkenness" may also occur. Intravenous saline is normally used to support blood pressure in the event hypotension occurs.

Procedure

1. The room is usually darkened.
2. To decrease anxiety, the patient is kept informed of what is being done as the procedure evolves.
3. The patient is positioned on an x-ray table, and ECG leads are attached to specific locations.
4. Sterile, aseptic surgical conditions are maintained. Usually one or two sites are chosen and prepared for catheter insertion (right and/or left antecubital area, right and/or left groin). The sites chosen depend on where in the heart the catheters have to be placed and the patency and size of the patient's veins. The insertion site is injected with local anesthetic prior to catheter insertion.
5. As the catheters are advanced toward the desired location, baseline information is recorded. Sometimes cardiac pacing may be necessary; for example, measuring sinus node recovery times requires pacing the atrium until the sinus is fatigued and then measuring the time the sinus takes to recover.
6. After baseline values have been determined, pacing can be used to induce arrhythmias. If a sustained arrhythmia is induced, an attempt may be made to terminate the arrhythmia through pacing. Should the patient lose consciousness, an external cardioverter/defibrillator can be used to terminate the arrhythmia.
7. A continuous, quiet conversation is held to assess the patient's level of consciousness.
8. After the procedure, catheters are removed, and a sterile pressure bandage is applied to the catheter insertion site. Manual pressure on the site may be necessary if bleeding occurs.

Clinical Implications

1. Abnormal EP results will reveal the following conditions:
   a. Conduction intervals longer or shorter than normal
   b. Refractory periods longer than normal

   c. Prolonged recovery times

   d. Induced dysrhythmia in a normal subject

2. Abnormal results indicate the following conditions:

   a. Long atrial His (AH) bundle intervals indicate disease in the atrioventricular node if sympathetic and vagal influences on the AV node have been eliminated.

   b. Long ventricular His (VH) bundle intervals indicate disease in the His-Purkinje system.

   c. Prolonged sinus node recovery times indicate sinus node dysfunction such as sick sinus syndrome.

   d. Prolonged sinoatrial conduction times can indicate sinus exit block.

   e. A wide or split His bundle deflection indicates a His bundle lesion.

   f. Induction of a sustained ventricular and supraventricular tachycardia confirms the diagnosis of recurrent ventricular tachycardia.

Patient Preparation

1. Explain the test purpose, procedure, benefits, and risks. Describing possible physical sensations that may be felt helps to reduce patient anxiety. These sensations may include the following:

   a. The sensation of a bug crawling in the arm and neck as the catheter is advanced

   b. Palpitations or racing heart during pacing

   c. Lightheadedness or dizziness (these must be reported when felt)

2. Obtain a legal, signed permit before the procedure.

3. Blood samples for potassium levels, and other drug levels if the effectiveness of a drug is to be determined, may be drawn.

4. A standard 12-lead EKG should be performed before testing.

5. Nothing should be consumed for at least 3 hours before testing.

6. Analgesics, sedatives, or tranquilizers are usually withheld before the procedure.

7. The patient should void before the procedure is initiated.

8. The patient may wear dentures.

9. Follow guidelines in Chapter 1 for safe, effective, informed *pretest* care.

Patient Aftercare

1. The patient remains on flat bed rest for 4 to 8 hours postprocedure and is not to flex or bend the extremity used for the catheter insertion because this may lead to bleeding or vascular occlusion. A pillow may be placed under the head.

2. Check vital signs, neurovascular status of extremity used, and insertion site for swelling, bleeding, hematoma, or bruit every 15 minutes for 4 hours, 30 minutes for 2 hours, and every hour for 2 hours postprocedure, or according to institutional protocols. Neurovascular checks include assessing for pulses, color, motion, sensation, temperature, and capillary refill times.

3. Keep the affected extremity extended, not elevated or flexed, to decrease discomfort and risk of bleeding. Prescribed analgesics can be administered.

4. Range of motion exercise of uninvolved limbs should be encouraged.

5. If an electrode catheter is left in place for sequential studies, it is sutured in place and covered with sterile dressings. Care for the site using sterile, aseptic technique.

6. Interpret test results and monitor ECG and other parameters appropriately. Stress the importance of compliance with prescribed therapies including drugs.

7. Follow guidelines in Chapter 1 regarding safe, effective, informed *posttest* care.

Clinical Alert

1. Relative contraindications to EP: although an acute myocardial infarction may limit detailed and prolonged EP procedures, brief but clinically useful procedures can be performed in this situation.

2. Complications can include the following conditions:
   a. Rapid, dramatic hemorrhage at the catheter insertion site (apply manual pressure to the site and notify the physician immediately)
   b. Thrombosis at the puncture site; thromboembolism
   c. Phlebitis
   d. Hemopericardium
   e. Atrial fibrillation (usually transient)
   f. Ventricular fibrillation or ventricular ectopy

3. Notify the attending physician of bleeding, hypotension, altered neurovascular status, decrease in distal perfusion, or life-threatening arrhythmias. Be aware of drug studies performed and monitor for effects of that drug. Have cardiopulmonary resuscitation equipment and drugs readily available for emergency use.

TRANSESOPHAGEAL ECHOCARDIOGRAPHY (TEE) ●

Normal TEE

Normal position, size, and function of heart valves and heart chambers

Explanation of Test

This test permits optimal ultrasonic visualization of the heart when traditional transthoracic (noninvasive) echocardiography fails or proves inconclusive. A miniaturized high-frequency ultrasound transducer is mounted on an endoscope and coupled with an ultrasound instrument to display and record ultrasound images from the heart. Endoscope controls allow remote manipulation of the transducer tip. Various images of heart anatomy can be displayed by rotating the tip of the instrument and by varying the depth of insertion into the esophagus. Indications for TEE include the following:

1. To assess function of prosthetic valves, diagnose endocarditis, evaluate valvular regurgitation and congenital abnormalities, and examine the aorta for dissecting aneurysms

2. To monitor left ventricular wall motion intraoperatively
3. Situations in which a transthoracic echocardiogram has not been satisfactory (eg, obesity, chest wall trauma, chronic obstructive pulmonary disease)
4. When results of traditional transthoracic echocardiography do not agree or correlate with other clinical findings

Procedure

1. Explain test purpose, procedure, benefits, and risks.
2. Apply a topical anesthetic to the pharynx. Insert a bite block into the mouth to reduce the risk of damage to the teeth and other oral structures as well as the endoscope itself (see Chap. 12).
3. The patient assumes a left lateral decubitus position before the lubricated endoscopic instrument is inserted to a depth of 30 to 50 cm. The patient may be asked to swallow so that the scope advances more easily.
4. Manipulation of the ultrasound transducer allows a number of image planes to be visualized.
5. Follow guidelines in Chapter 1 for safe, effective, informed *intratest* care.

Clinical Implications

1. Abnormal TEE findings may reveal the following conditions:
   a. Heart valve diseases
   b. Pericardial effusion
   c. Congenital heart disease
   d. Endocarditis
   e. Intracardiac tumors or thrombi
   f. Left ventricular dysfunction

Patient Preparation

1. Explain test purpose, procedure, benefits, and risks.
2. The patient must fast from food and fluids at least 8 hours prior to the procedure to reduce the risk of aspiration. Premedications such as analgesics or sedatives may be ordered. Prescribed oral medications may be taken with small sips of water (see Appendix C for conscious sedation precautions).
3. Follow guidelines in Chapter 1 for safe, effective, informed *pretest* care.

Patient Aftercare

1. Interpret test results. Monitor vital signs and level of consciousness (if sedated). Ensure patent airway at all times.
2. Position patient on his or her side if sedated to prevent risk of aspiration.
3. Evaluate return of swallow, cough, and gag reflexes before introducing food or fluids orally.
4. Follow guidelines in Chapter 1 for safe, effective, informed *posttest* care.

> **Clinical Alert**
>
> Swallowing reflexes may be diminished for several hours because of topical anesthetic effects. Ingesting food or fluids may result in aspiration if these reflexes are not intact.

● OTHER ORGANS AND BODY FUNCTIONS

MAGNETIC RESONANCE IMAGING (MRI); MAGNETIC RESONANCE ANGIOGRAPHY (MRA); MAGNETIC RESONANCE SPECTROSCOPY (MRS) ●

Normal MRI, MRA, and MRS

Soft tissue structures: normal brain, spinal cord, subarachnoid spaces, fat, muscles, tendons, ligaments, nerves, blood vessels, marrow of limbs and joints, heart, abdomen, and pelvis

Blood vessels: normal size, anatomy, and hemodynamics

Explanation of Test

Magnetic resonance is a diagnostic modality that employs a superconducting magnet and frequency signals (RF) to cause hydrogen nuclei to emit their own signal; computers use these signals to construct detailed, sectional images of the body. Unlike computed tomography (CT), no ionizing radiation is used. Additionally, the ability of magnetic resonance to discern anatomy is more closely linked to the molecular nature of tissue. For example, MR spectroscopy provides information about the chemical composition of tissue and is commonly used to evaluate brain function. Special techniques primarily based on the magnetic reactions of hydrogen nuclei can influence the MR signal to enhance certain types of tissue (eg, fat is accentuated in T_1-weighted images, cerebrospinal fluid and other pure fluids are highlighted in T_2-weighted images). Computer reconstruction techniques allow images to be produced in any plane as well as in the three-dimensional views.

During the procedure, the patient lies on specially designed couch which is moved either into a narrow, closed, high-magnet scanner, or into an open, low-magnet scanner (Figs. 15-4 and 15-5). For certain procedures, surface coils are placed over the body area to be imaged. During the test, loud, rhythmic knocking sounds are produced; less noise is associated with the open-design scanner. To relieve patient anxiety and the potential for claustrophobia, some laboratories provide music for relaxation. Two-way communication systems and pulse oximeters are commonly used to monitor patient responses to the procedure. Magnetic resonance applications are continually evolving and improving. In general, the most common MR applications include the following:

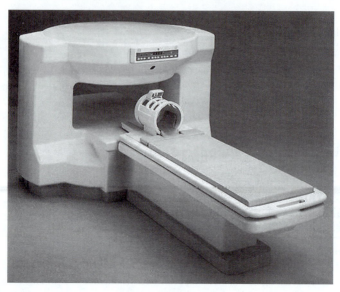

FIGURE 15-4
Open MRI. (From General Electric Medical Systems).

MR of the brain provides exquisite visualization of the soft tissue structures of the brain. Although bony anatomy is seen using MRI, CT is the test of choice to evaluate bone lesions and fractures.

MR of the spine provides excellent views of the spinal cord and subarach-noid space without intrathecal contrast injection.

MR of limbs and joints accurately demonstrates fat, muscles, tendons, liga-ments, nerves, blood vessels, and bone marrow. If the anatomic region of

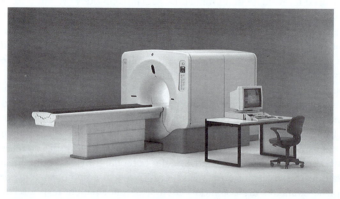

FIGURE 15-5
Closed MRI. (From General Electric Medical Systems).

interest is a small area, a surface coil, which produces the RF signal, is placed directly on the skin overlying the part to be examined.

MR of the heart (cardiac MRI) allows visualization of the structures of the heart, including valves and coronary vessels. Image acquisition is synchronized to the ECG—a process known as "gating"—to help eliminate motion artifacts.

MR of the abdomen and pelvis visualizes soft tissue organs, particularly the liver, pancreas, spleen, adrenals, kidneys, blood vessels, and reproductive organs.

MR angiography provides both anatomic and hemodynamic information in 2-dimensional and 3-dimensional representations (likened to noninvasive angiography). MRI angiography is becoming more common and is used to evaluate known vascular lesions.

Magnetic resonance spectroscopy uses a conventional MR scanner to detect chemicals in all body tissues to evaluate tumors, muscle disease, or ischemic heart disease; to differentiate causes of coma; to rule out Alzheimer's disease; to monitor cancer treatment; to differentiate the diagnosis of multiple sclerosis, human immunodeficiency virus (HIV) infection, and adrenoleukodystrophy; to prepare for temporal lobe epilepsy surgery; and to assess the extent of stroke and head injury.

Intravenous MR contrast agents, all primarily containing water-soluble gadolinium complex (most commonly gadolinium-50-DTPA or -DOTA) or other metals such as manganese (Mn-DPDP), and iron (Mion, USP10) are often used in evaluating the central nervous system. These agents have been approved as safe for patients, including those <2 years of age. Gadolinium presents with very low toxicity and fewer side-effects than traditional x-ray contrast agents because of its rapid renal clearance. Other agents used include gadodiamide (nonionic) and gadopentetate, which are used for body scanning. MR contrast agents have lower toxicity and fewer side-effects than x-ray contrast agents. However, since these MR contrast agents are primarily excreted via the kidneys, *renal failure is a contraindication* for use. Other potential contraindications include pregnancy, allergies or asthma, anemia or hypotension, epilepsy, and sickle cell disease.

Clinical Alert

1. Adverse effects of Gd-DOTA include vomiting, sensations of local warmth or coldness, headache, dizziness, urticaria, paresthesias, unusual mouth sensations, and respiratory problems.
2. MR contrast agents allow for better basic contrast and tissue signals; most abnormal tissues show regions of increased T_1 and T_2 (relaxation time, RF signals) regardless of the nature of tumors, edema, hemorrhage, inflammation, and necrosis.

> ### Clinical Alert
>
> Usually, no special dietary restrictions or preparations are necessary prior to MRI, unless conscious sedation is to be used. However, numerous safety factors must be considered.
>
> 1. Absolute contraindications to MRI include the following conditions:
>   a. Implanted devices, including pacemakers, cochlear implants, certain prosthetic devices (consult with MR laboratory for specific information), implanted drug infusion pumps, neurostimulators, bone growth stimulators, certain intrauterine contraceptive devices
>   b. Internal metallic objects such as bullets or shrapnel and surgical clips, pins, plates, screws, metal sutures, or wire mesh.
> 2. MRI is generally not advised for pregnant patients (increase in amniotic fluid temperature may be harmful) or individuals with epilepsy. All patients having an MRI need to remove hearing aids, dentures, jewelry, hair pins, wigs, hairpieces, and other accessories.
> 3. Patients unable to remain still or who are claustrophobic may require intravenous conscious sedation prior to MRI.
> 4. Certain types of eye makeup and permanent eye liners which contain metallic fragments sometimes cause discomfort during MRI. Assess for these cosmetic enhancements.
> 5. A thorough patient history is mandatory prior to any MR study. Commonly, radiology services perform conventional x-ray imaging to confirm or rule out the presence of metallic fragments prior to MR imaging.

General Procedure

1. The patient is placed supine on a movable examination couch after a thorough medical history is obtained.
2. Sedation may be necessary if the patient is claustrophobic or restless. Earplugs may reduce discomfort from noises generated by the scanner. Earphones with music are another option. A two-way communication system between the patient and the operator allows continual monitoring and vocal feedback, and somewhat reduces the patient's sense of isolation. Many MR laboratories routinely use a pulse oximeter to monitor the patient during the study.
3. For examining many superficial structures (eg, knee, neck, shoulder, breast), a surface coil is applied over the skin. Improved images of the prostate or reproductive organs can be obtained by using a transrectal coil.
4. Once the patient is positioned and instructed to remain still, the couch is moved into the scanner.

NOTE: *The closed-gantry design is narrow and may upset some individuals. Reassure patients that there is sufficient air to breathe and that they will be monitored and given voice contact during the entire procedure.*

5. In some instances, a noniodinated contrast is injected into a vein for better anatomic visualization. For abdominal or pelvic scans, glucagon may be administered to reduce bowel peristalsis.
6. Examination time varies and averages between 30 and 90 minutes.
7. Follow guidelines in Chapter 1 for safe, effective, informed *intratest* care.

> ### Clinical Alert
>
> The open MR imaging system uses only a fraction of the traditional high-field magnets (eg, 0.2–0.3 Tesla compared with 1.0–1.5 Tesla). This results in a slimmer profile and much less intimidating appearance for the magnet. Although extremely appealing in certain instances, the open-designed magnet is currently not the best choice for all MRI imaging. Certain types of studies can only be performed with a high-field magnet. Some scans performed on an open-design low-field magnet must be repeated.

Advantages of Open MRI
May not need to sedate the claustrophobic patient
Suitable for the extremely obese patient
Enhances patient comfort—because of the low magnetic field, another person may stay with the patient (especially useful with children or confused patients)
Kinematic studies of joints (eg, shoulders) are possible
Improved accessibility to the patient allows open MRI to be used as a guide for interventional and select surgical procedures (eg, biopsies)
The open head coil features a unique mirror which allows patient to see outside the magnet during the procedure
Less noise

See Figures 15-4 and 15-5 to compare open- and closed-design MR imaging systems.

Interfering Factors

1. Respiratory motion causes severe artifacts with abdominal and thoracic imaging.
2. Morbidly obese persons may not fit into the gantry opening or surface coil configurations.

Clinical Implications

1. MRI and MRS of the brain demonstrate the following conditions:
  a. White matter disease (eg, multiple sclerosis)
  b. Infectious disorders affecting the brain (eg, acquired immunodeficiency syndrome [AIDS])
  c. Neoplasms
  d. Ischemias, cerebrovascular accident
  e. Aneurysms/hemorrhage

2. MRI and MRS of the spine demonstrate the following conditions:
  a. Disc herniation or degeneration
  b. Neoplasm (primary and metastases)
  c. Inflammatory disease
  d. Demyelinating disease
  e. Congenital abnormalities

3. MRI of the heart demonstrates the following conditions:
  a. Abnormal chamber size or myocardial thickness
  b. Cardiac tumors
  c. Congenital heart disorders
  d. Pericarditis
  e. Graft patency
  f. Thrombic disorders
  g. Aortic dissection or aneurysm
  h. Cardiac ischemia

4. MRI and MRS of the limbs and joints demonstrate the following conditions:
  a. Neoplasms of soft tissue and bone
  b. Ligament or tendon damage
  c. Osteonecrosis
  d. Bone marrow disorders
  e. Muscle fatigue
  f. Changes in blood flow
    (1) Atherosclerosis
    (2) Aneurysm
    (3) Thrombus
    (4) Embolism
    (5) Bypass grafts
    (6) Endocarditis
    (7) Shunt placement

5. MRI of the abdomen and pelvis demonstrates the following conditions:
  a. Neoplasms (especially useful in staging tumors)
  b. Retroperitoneal structures
  c. Status of renal transplants

6. MRI angiography demonstrates the following conditions:
  a. Aneurysms
  b. Stenosis or occlusions
  c. Graft patency
  d. Vascular malformations

Patient Preparation

1. Explain the test purpose, procedure, benefits, and risks. Safety concerns for the patient and staff during MRI procedures are based on interaction of strong magnetic fields with body tissues and metallic objects. These potential hazards are mainly due to projectiles (metallic objects can be displaced, giving rise to potentially dangerous projectiles); torquing of metallic objects (implanted surgical clips and other metallic structures or implants can be torqued or twisted within the body when exposed to strong magnetic fields); local heating (exposure to radiofrequency [RF] pulses can cause heating of tissues or metallic objects within the patient's body; for this reason, pregnant women are not routinely scanned because an increase in the temperature of amniotic fluid or fetus may be harmful); interference with electromechanical implants (electronic device implants are at risk for damage from both magnetic fields and the RF pulses; consequently, patients with cardiac pacemakers, implanted drug infusion pumps, cochlear implants and similar devices should not be exposed to MR procedures); and allergic reactions to MR contrast agents.

> ### Clinical Alert
>
> In the event of respiratory/cardiac arrest, the patient must be removed from the scanning room prior to resuscitation. Most general hospital equipment (eg, oxygen tanks, intravenous pumps, monitors) are not permitted in the MR suite.

2. Assess for contraindications to testing. Obtain a relevant history regarding any implanted devices such as heart valves, surgical and aneurysm clips, plates, internal orthopedic screws and rods, and pacemakers, among other objects.
3. The following materials must be removed prior to the procedure: removable dental bridges and oral appliances, credit cards, keys, hair clips, shoes, belts, jewelry, clothing with metal fasteners, wigs, hairpieces, and removable prostheses.
4. Claustrophobic feelings can be avoided if the patient keeps his or her eyes closed during the test. Recommend that the patient not eat a large meal within 1 hour of testing to reduce physiologic demands and possible emesis while in the scanner.
5. Encourage the patient to relax and instruct him or her to remain as motionless as possible during testing. Reassure the patient that this is a painless procedure.
6. Patients having blood flow testing should abstain from alcohol, nicotine, caffeine, and prescription drugs for iron. Fast for 2 hours prior to testing to avoid unexpected blood vessel vasoconstrictions or dilation. No smoking is permitted before the test. Promote rest in the supine position for 10 minutes before the test.

7. Fasting or drinking only clear liquids may be necessary for several hours prior to an abdominal pelvic MR.
8. Follow guidelines in Chapter 1 for safe, effective, informed *pretest* care.

Patient Aftercare

1. Interpret test results. Counsel and monitor appropriately for side-effects of the MR contrast agent. Common side-effects include coldness at the injection site, dizziness, and headache. Treatment is usually not needed unless symptoms are bothersome or prolonged. Rare side-effects include convulsions, irregular or rapid heart rate, itching and watery eyes, skin rash or hives, facial swelling, thickening of tongue, fatigue or weakness, wheezing, chest tightness, and difficulty breathing. Alert the physician if any of these occur and initiate treatment as indicated.
2. Assess the contrast dye injection site for signs of inflammation, bruising, irritation, or infection.
3. Follow guidelines in Chapter 1 for safe, effective, informed *posttest* care.

Special Pediatric Considerations for MR Testing

Pediatric cautions related to MR testing include the following considerations:

1. Age, ability to understand and cooperate, physical condition, and reasons for testing
2. MRI body imaging: most of the adult guidelines apply. Sedatives, tranquilizers, or modified restraints may be necessary if the child is uncooperative or fearful.
3. MRI for blood flow studies in extremities: simple restraints may be used to restrict motion of arms or legs. No tranquilizers or sedatives may be used because blood flow will be affected.
4. Also see Cautions (pp. 1053, 1054, and 1057).

SLEEP STUDIES ●

Excessive daytime sleepiness (hypersomnolence) is a classic symptom of inadequate nocturnal sleep which manifests itself pathologically in various ways. Typically, much of the daytime sleepiness in today's society is a result of irregular sleep patterns and times (eg, shift workers), lack of adequate sleep, poor nutrition, and certain medications. Sleep disorders are grouped into four major categories:

1. Dyssomnias
2. Parasomnias
3. Medical/psychiatric
4. Others

The dyssomnias are those sleep disorders associated with too little or too much sleep as a result of problems initiating or maintaining sleep states or exhibiting excessive sleepiness states. Examples include sleep apnea (an intrinsic sleep disorder), periodic limb movement disorder, narcolepsy, and restless-leg syndrome. Parasomnias include arousal disorders, sleep-wake transition disorders, nightmares, sleep paralysis, and other rapid eye movement (REM) disorders. Dementia, Parkinson's disease, anxiety, and mood and panic disorders are the most common forms of medical/psychiatric sleep disorders. The "others" category includes "short" and "long" sleepers, pregnancy-associated sleep disorder, and sleep choking syndrome. These disorders are diagnosed using polysomnograph methodology (eg, EEG, EMG, EOG).

A "short sleeper," also referred to as a "healthy" hyposomniac, sleeps substantially less in a 24-hour period than is expected (sleep duration of <5 hours in a 24-hour period before age 60 years). A "long sleeper," also referred to as a "healthy" hypersomniac, consistently sleeps more in a 24-hour period than is expected (sleep duration of >10 hours in a 24-hour period). People with "sleep choking syndrome" awaken suddenly with a feeling of shortness of breath and a choking sensation. The etiology of this disorder is unknown, but it is more prevalent in early to middle adulthood in persons with obsessive-compulsive anxiety disorders.

The solution to the problem relates to reversing pathologic sleep patterns to more normal status by means of various interventions.

TERM	*EEG DEFINITION*
Sleep onset	Transition from wakefulness to sleepfulness; usually takes at least 10 minutes (ie, nREM stage I)
Stage I nREM	Occurs at sleep onset, consists of low-voltage EEG with mainly theta and alpha activity; 4%–5% of sleep
Stage II nREM	Follows stage I; low-voltage EEG with sleep spindles and K complexes; 45%–55% of sleep
Stage III nREM	Consists of 20%–50% high-amplitude delta waves, referred to as delta or slow wave sleep; 4%–6% of sleep
Stage IV nREM	Consists of >50% of high-amplitude delta waves and is also called slow wave sleep; 12%–15% of sleep
Stage REM	Low-voltage, mixed frequency, nonalpha activity with rapid eye movements, called paradoxical sleep; 20%–25% of sleep
Sleep offset	Transition from sleepfulness to wakefulness, alpha and beta activity, also called awakening

Sleep staging is done in 30-second epochs.

Use of Tests

Sleep studies, or polysomnography (PSG), can be divided into two types: full PSG, or 16-channel recording, and screening PSG, or 4-channel recording. Full PSG can be used to diagnose any of the previously described sleep disorders, whereas the 4-channel limited PSG is reserved for sleep disorders involving breathing (eg, sleep apnea).

Classification of Tests

The full PSG includes the following tests:

1. Electroencephalogram (EEG): at least 2 channels are recorded to determine sleep onset, sleep stages, and sleep offset.
2. Electrooculogram (EOG): documents both slow rolling and rapid eye movements seen at sleep onset and in REM sleep, respectively.
3. Electromyogram (EMG): the chin EMG is used as a criterion for REM sleep; the leg EMG is used to evaluate periodic leg movements or leg jerks.
4. Electrocardiogram (ECG): monitors heart rate and rhythm.
5. Chest impedance: monitors respiratory effort by use of cardiopneumotachographs, strain gauges, or piezoelectric crystal belts.
6. Airflow monitors: thermistors or thermocouples are used to monitor oral/nasal airflow.
7. Capnography end-tidal CO_2 (ETCO$_2$): continuous monitoring of carbon dioxide.
8. Pulse oximetry (SpO$_2$): continuous monitoring of arterial oxygen saturation by noninvasive means.
9. Snoring sensor: microphone placed just below the jaw and lateral to the trachea.
10. pH meter: pH probe is placed in the lower third of the esophagus transnasally to monitor episodes of gastric reflux.
11. Audio/video recordings: documents restless sleep, sleep walking, sleep talking, and night terrors, among other conditions.

The 4-channel limited PSG includes the following tests:

1. Electrocardiogram (ECG)
2. Chest impedance
3. Airflow monitoring
4. Pulse oximetry

POLYSOMNOGRAPHY (PSG)   ●

Normal PSG

Electroencephalogram (EEG): normal sleep onset time, sleep stages, and sleep offset (going from sleepfulness to wakefulness [ie, awakening])

Airflow monitors: evidence of sustained airflow throughout the night

Electrooculogram (EOG): normal slow, rolling movements at sleep onset; rapid eye movement during REM sleep

Capnography end-tidal CO_2 (ETCO$_2$): normocapnic (35–45 mm Hg during the awake state, increasing a couple of mm Hg during sleep)

Electromyogram (EMG): absence of periodic leg movements or jerks

Pulse oximetry (SpO$_2$): >90%

Snoring sensor: absence of abnormal patterns of snoring

Electrocardiogram (ECG): absence of rhythmic disturbances, bradycardias, or tachycardias

Audio/video recordings: absence of restless sleep, sleep walking, sleep talking, and night terrors, among other conditions

Chest impedance: evidence of sustained respiratory effort throughout night

Respiratory disturbance index (RDI): <5 apneas/hypopneas per hour

Oxygen desaturation index (ODI): <5 times per hour (SpO$_2$ <90%)

Explanation of Test

The PSG determines underlying sleep disorder pathology, provides qualitative and quantitative measurements associated with the disorder, and provides information upon which to base the proper course of treatment. PSG is indicated for persons complaining of daytime sleepiness, fatigue, unable to stay on task, falling asleep at inappropriate times, insomnia, nocturnal awakenings, waking with gasping or choking feelings, witnessed sleep-related apneas, abnormal snoring patterns, and any other unexplained symptoms associated with disruption of normal sleeping patterns that have persisted for 6 to 12 months.

Procedure

1. The patient is instructed to keep a sleep log for 1 to 2 weeks prior to the polysomnogram (PSG).
2. The day of the study, caffeinated beverages, alcohol, and sedatives are not permitted.
3. Extra time is needed to set up and attach equipment to the patient. Typically, the PSG is recorded during the patient's normal sleep time; however, partial or extended periods of sleep deprivation may be necessary if seizure activity is suspected.
4. The sleep technologist records the patient's history and factors such as age, height, weight, current medications, visual problems, and history of seizures, head injuries, headaches, or strokes. The sleep log is reviewed, and a bedtime questionnaire is completed. The patient wears normal bedtime attire.
5. The following list identifies the monitoring equipment used:

2 Sets of scalp electrodes to monitor sleep stages (EEG)

1 Electrode to the outer canthus of each eye (EOG)

1 Electrode to the chin (submental)

Electrodes to the legs (anterior tibialis; EMG)

ECG leads for heart rhythms and rates

Impedance monitor (respiratory effort)

Oral/nasal thermistor between nose and upper lip (air flow)

Pulse oximeter (SaO$_2$; O$_2$ sensor)

> **NOTE:** *If seizures are a factor, up to 16 additional scalp electrodes are applied according to the International 10–20 System of Electrode Placement. The International 10–20 System of Electrode Placement is the conventional system (established in 1958) used to identify and place scalp surface electrodes for the recording of brain electrical potentials. The 10–20 System nomenclature is used because the majority of the electrodes are spaced ei-*

ther 10% or 20% between specific skull landmarks (eg, the nasion or inion; Fig. 15-6) or in relation to the circumference of the head.

6. After application, all electrode leads are interfaced with a "jack box," which contains the preamplifiers and impedance meter. From the jack box, signals are sent through additional amplifiers and filters, and finally to a multi-channel recorder or polygraph. The polygraph can provide a hard copy recording of all channels and signals can be computer processed and displayed on a monitor. Electrode connections are subsequently tested for integrity and adjustments made before the patient retires.

7. During the recording, both audio and infrared camera video recordings are made.

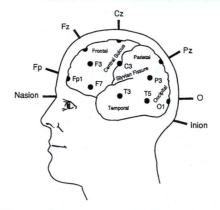

ANATOMICAL NAME	Left Hemisphere	Right Hemisphere	Midline
FRONTAL POLAR	Fp1	Fp2	FPZ
MID-FRONTAL			Fz
FRONTAL	F3	F4	
INFERIOR FRONTAL	F7	F8	
MID-TEMPORAL	T3	T4	
POSTERIOR-TEMPORAL	T5	T6	
VERTEX			Cz
CENTRAL	C3	C4	
MID-PARIETAL			Pz
PARIETAL	P3	P4	
OCCIPITAL	O1	O2	

FIGURE 15-6

Descriptive anatomical nomenclature. Also, lobes of brain with electrode placement, by convention odd numbers are used on the left side and even on the right side of the head. International 10-20 System of Electrode Placement. Source: Basic EEG for PSG Technologists, Polysomnography Curriculum, California College for Health Sciences, National City, CA.

8. A bedside commode is provided because the leads are relatively short.
9. When the test is completed and equipment removed from the patient, another questionnaire is completed and scored related to the patient's sleep experience during the test.
10. Follow guidelines in Chapter 1 for safe, effective, informed *intratest* care.

> ### Clinical Alert
>
> A home sleep study is an alternative for patients who have trouble falling asleep in a sleep laboratory. Sensors are applied in the clinic and the patient is shown how to attach the mobile monitoring unit.

Interfering Factors

1. Caffeinated beverages and alcohol can delay sleep onset or exacerbate some types of sleep disorders.
2. Sedatives (hypnotics) shorten sleep onset and reduce nocturnal awakenings, which may skew the results of the PSG.
3. Changes in daily routine on the day of the sleep study may cause false-positive or false-negative results.
4. During the PSG, environmental noise, lights, and temperature may have an adverse effect on the patient's ability to fall asleep.

Clinical Implications

1. Abnormal EEG recordings indicate problems with either sleep architecture (eg, sleep onset, stages, offset) or seizure disorders.
2. Abnormal leg EMG is consistent with movement disorders (eg, restless-leg syndrome, nocturnal myoclonus, leg jerks).
3. A respiratory sleep index (RDI) of >5 indicates sleep-disordered breathing. Obstructive sleep apnea (OSA) is characterized by absence of airflow for >10 seconds despite continued respiratory effort (eg, thoracic breathing or snoring accompanied by periods of apnea). Central sleep apnea (CSA) is characterized by absence of both airflow and respiratory effort; airflow ceases because respiratory effort is absent. Mixed sleep apnea (MSA) generally begins as a central apnea and becomes obstructive apnea. Sleep apnea has been linked with cardiac arrest, strokes, pulmonary hypertension, brain stem lesions, and head trauma.
4. An ODI (oxygen desaturation index) of >5 is associated with oxygen desaturation, which generally occurs with an apneic event but can also occur with hypoventilation.

Patient Preparation

1. Explain test purpose and procedure. These tests are done when signs and symptoms have persisted for at least 6 to 12 months. Caution the patient not to change his or her daily routine the day before the test.

2. Reassure the patient that lead wires, monitors, and sensors will not interfere with changes of position during sleep.
3. Record the patient's age, height, weight, and gender. A brief history and pre- and post-bedtime questionnaires are taken.
4. The patient should prepare for sleep at the normal time according to routine.
5. Follow guidelines in Chapter 1 for safe, effective, informed *pretest* care.

Patient Aftercare

1. Patient may resume usual activities and routines.
2. Interpret test outcomes and monitor appropriately. If test results indicate obstructive sleep apnea syndrome (OSA), explain possible need for further treatment.
3. Follow guidelines in Chapter 1 for safe, effective, informed *posttest* care.

SLEEPINESS TESTS, MULTIPLE SLEEP LATENCY TEST (MSLT); MAINTENANCE OF WAKEFULNESS TEST (MWT) ●

The multiple sleep latency test (MSLT) is used as an objective measure of excessive daytime sleepiness and determines its severity. Typically, the MSLT is administered the morning following a sleep study. An alternative to this test is the maintenance of wakefulness test (MWT), which measures the ability of an individual to stay awake rather than to fall asleep. Both the MSLT and MWT are used to diagnose narcolepsy and to evaluate the effectiveness of pharmacologic interventions in the treatment of daytime hypersomnolence. Indications for these tests include falling asleep at inappropriate times, daytime hypersomnolence, suspected narcolepsy, and evaluation of drug effectiveness in treating various sleep disorders.

Classification of Tests

The MSLT includes the following tests:

1. EEG: at least 2 channels are recorded to determine sleep onset, sleep stages, and sleep offset.
2. EOG: to document both slow and rapid eye movements present at sleep onset and during REM sleep, respectively.
3. EMG: the chin EMG is used as a criterion for REM sleep.
4. ECG: to monitor heart rate and rhythm.

The MWT includes the following tests:

1. Electromyogram (EMG): the chin EMG is used as a criterion for REM sleep.
2. Electrocardiogram (ECG): to monitor heart rate and rhythm.

Normal Sleepiness Test

Mean sleep latency >10 minutes

Explanation of Test

The MSLT is an objective measure of a patient's sleepiness and is done to evaluate the severity of daytime sleepiness, to diagnose narcolepsy or falling asleep at inappropriate times, and to evaluate effectiveness of drug therapy for daytime hypersomnolence. The MSLT is administered after a sleep study to rule out any sleep-related pathology which might affect the results and to assess the quality of sleep. An alternative to the MSLT is the MWT, which measures the ability of a person to stay awake rather than to fall asleep.

Procedure

1. Typically, the MSLT is administered the morning following a sleep study. Following the sleep study, the patient dresses, eats, (avoiding caffeine), and reports back to the sleep laboratory.
2. The electrodes are reapplied if necessary (see Polysomnography [PSG] for electrode sites and interfaces, p. 1062).
3. The first nap will begin 1.5 to 2 hours after morning awakening with a minimum of four additional naps at 2-hour intervals throughout the day.
4. The nap is terminated after 20 minutes, unless the patient falls asleep, in which case the recording is continued for 15 minutes after sleep onset.

   NOTE: *The term "nap" indicates a short intentional or unintentional episode of subjective sleep taken during habitual wakefulness, whereas the term "falling asleep" or "sleep onset" is defined objectively by electroencephalographic recordings (EEG) (ie, stage 1 of NREM sleep).*

5. Between naps, the patient must remain awake and is encouraged to move around.
6. Following the naps, all equipment is disconnected and the patient is discharged.
7. The technologist then scores the MSLT and PSG test results.
8. Follow guidelines in Chapter 1 for safe, effective, informed *intratest* care.

Interfering Factors

Caffeinated beverages can delay sleep, whereas sedatives (hypnotics) shorten sleep onset. Additionally, sleep deprivation may result in a false-positive MSLT result. During naps, environmental noise, lights, and temperature can have an adverse effect on the patient's ability to fall asleep.

Clinical Implications

1. An average sleep onset of 6 to 9 minutes is considered a "gray area" diagnostically, because these tests are done in a laboratory setting and not in the patient's home environment. Reevaluation may be necessary if the patient complains and symptoms persist.
2. An average sleep onset of <5 minutes and two or more REM periods in the five to six naps is diagnostic for narcolepsy. This indicates a disturbance of the normal sleep architecture pattern, although the REM periods are not unlike nocturnal REM periods. These REM episodes, however, occur prematurely in the sleep cycle and are termed sleep-onset REM (SOREM).

Patient Preparation

1. Explain MSLT test purpose and procedure. Remind the patient not to change daily routines the day of testing.

2. Reassure the patient that lead wires, monitors, and sensors will not interfere with sleep.
3. Record the patient's age, height, weight, and gender.
4. No alcohol or caffeinated beverages should be consumed the day of the test.
5. Standard sleep questionnaires or scales (eg, Epworth Scale, Stanford Scale) may be administered and evaluated (see Appendix I for examples).
6. Follow guidelines in Chapter 1 regarding safe, effective, informed *pretest* care.

Patient Aftercare
1. Explain test outcome and possible need for follow-up testing.
2. Follow guidelines in Chapter 1 for safe, effective, informed *posttest* care.

NASAL CONTINUOUS POSITIVE AIRWAY PRESSURE (nCPAP) TITRATION ●

Normal Titration
EEG: normal time to sleep onset, sleep stages, and sleep offset
Chest impedance: evidence of continuous respiratory effort throughout the night
EOG: normal slow, rolling movements at sleep onset and rapid eye movement during REM sleep
Airflow monitors: evidence of continuous airflow throughout night
EMG: submental chin placement used as a criterion for REM sleep
Capnography end-tidal CO_2 (ETCO$_2$): normocapnic (35–45 mm Hg during wakefulness which may increase a couple of mm Hg during sleep)
ECG: absence of rhythmic disturbances or bradycardias/tachycardias
Pulse oximetry (SpO$_2$): >90%
Respiratory disturbance index (RDI): <5 apneas/hypopneas per hour
Oxygen desaturation index (ODI): <5 times per hour (SaO$_2$ <90%)

Explanation of Test
Following the diagnosis of obstructive sleep apnea (OSA), this test is done before treatment is begun. The nCPAP machine supplies air under pressure, acting as a pneumatic splint that keeps the upper airway open during sleep. The pressure required depends on the severity of the OSA and can vary; therefore, the patient is typically required to return to the sleep laboratory on a second night to repeat the sleep study (PSG) while wearing an nCPAP mask. Positive airway pressures are increased until the apneas "break." This procedure is referred to as nCPAP titration. Under some circumstances (eg, severe sleep apnea), titration can be done on the same night as the PSG. In that case, it is termed a "split-night study." The nCPAP machine provides continuous positive pressure during both inspiration and expiration. Conversely, bilevel positive airway pressure (nBiPAP) uses two separate pressures: one during inspiration and a lower pressure during expiration. In cases in which nCPAP is not well tolerated, nBiPAP may be a better alternative. An nCPAP unit may be used in the home and preset to the test pressures that ameliorated the apneas.

Procedure

1. On the day of the titration, the patient is instructed to avoid caffeinated beverages, alcohol, and sedatives, and to keep a sleep log.
2. Sufficient time is allowed before testing to be attached to the monitoring devices and other equipment, including the nCPAP machine. A brief orientation to nCPAP should take place prior to the actual day of titration to relieve the patient's anxiety.
3. The sleep technologist takes a brief patient history. The sleep log is reviewed, and a bedtime questionnaire is completed (see Appendix I). The patient then prepares for sleep.
4. The technologist applies the electrodes, monitors, sensors, and microphone, and interfaces these with the other electronic devices (see Polysomnography [PSG], p. 1062).
5. The patient is fitted with an nCPAP mask and assured that it can be easily removed in case of discomfort, shortness of breath, or claustrophobia.
6. A bedside commode is placed because the leads are relatively short.
7. CPAP pressures are adjusted throughout the sleep period, beginning with 3 to 5 cm H_2O and increasing in 2.5-cm H_2O increments until the apneas "break." Time increments can vary from 15 minutes to 2 hours per pressure setting. Decisions are based on protocols being used, severity of sleep apnea, and patient tolerance for testing. If nBiPAP is being performed, inspiratory and expiratory pressures are adjusted separately, keeping the inspiratory pressure at least 2 to 4 cm H_2O above the expiratory pressure.
8. After the test, the equipment is removed and the patient completes another questionnaire, which the sleep technologist evaluates and scores.
9. Follow guidelines in Chapter 1 for safe, effective, informed *intratest* care.

Interfering Factors

1. Caffeinated beverages and alcohol can delay sleep onset or exacerbate obstructive sleep apnea (OSA), which may interfere with determining optimal pressure settings.
2. Changes in the patient's daily routine on the day of titration can alter results.
3. Patients with a deviated nasal septum or chronic sinusitis may have problems tolerating the nCPAP. The use of nCPAP is contraindicated in persons with severe bullous emphysema or chronic perforated tympanic membrane.
4. Skin irritations from tight-fitting masks (especially on the bridge of the nose), nasal congestion, and headaches are occasional complaints with the use of nCPAP.
5. The benefit of nCPAP to patients with central sleep apnea has not been well documented.

Clinical Implications

1. An RDI >5 indicates OSA, which is characterized by the absence of airflow for >10 seconds in the presence of continued respiratory effort. nCPAP used in treating OSA has been shown to be clinically beneficial.

2. Following even short-term nCPAP use there is documented evidence of rapid symptomatic improvement, with restoration of nocturnal sleep and subsequent improvement in lessening of daytime sleepiness and improving quality of life.

Patient Preparation

1. Explain test purpose and nCPAP titration procedure.
2. Reassure patients that the mask can easily be removed if anxiety or claustrophobia develops.
3. Record the patient's age, height, weight, and gender. A brief history is taken, and pre- and post-bedtime questionnaires are filled out.
4. Patient prepares for sleep at the normal time in the usual manner.
5. Follow guidelines in Chapter 1 for safe, effective, informed *pretest* care.

Patient Aftercare

1. Explain test outcome and possible need for follow-up testing and treatment. Depending on the test outcome, an nCPAP unit may be ordered for home use.
2. Follow guidelines in Chapter 1 for safe, effective, informed *posttest* care.

GASTRIC ANALYSIS (TUBE GASTRIC ANALYSIS); GASTRIC FLUIDS ●

Normal Gastric Analysis

Fluid: clear or opalescent; no food, blood, drugs, or bile present in sample
pH: 1.5–2.5
Culture: negative for mycobacterial organisms
Fasting specimen total acidity: <2 mEq or mmol/L
Basal acid output (BAO) without stimulation: 0–5 mmol/hour
Maximal acid output (MAC) or normal secretory ability when using a gastric stimulant such as histamine or betazole hydrochloride intramuscularly or phentogastrin subcutaneously: 10–20 mEq or mmol/hour

Explanation of Test

This test examines stomach contents for abnormal substances and also measures gastric acidity. It aids in diagnosing ulcers, obstructions, pernicious anemia, or carcinoma of the stomach. It can determine the cause of gastrointestinal bleeding as well as the effectiveness of medical or surgical therapies. Examinations of gastric washings (eg, tuberculosis studies) can identify mycobacterial infection when previous sputum tests have been negative.

Procedure

1. Fasting gastric analysis specimens can be collected during endoscopy (see Chap. 12) or through a nasogastric (NG) tube inserted for the test. Follow NG tube institutional protocols.

2. Initial gastric acid is aspirated through the NG tube with a syringe, tested for pH, and discarded. If no acid is present, reposition the NG tube and obtain another specimen.

3. Specimens are normally collected via continuous intermittent low suction over 1 to 2 hours at 15-minute intervals, depending on the type of gastric stimulant given. Each specimen is placed in a separate specimen cup and labeled BAO or MAO, along with patient's name, date, and time collected.

4. The NG tube is removed after all specimens are collected.

5. Documentation includes date and time; type of procedure; type and size of tubes used; number of specimens collected; appearance, consistency, and measured volumes of gastric fluid obtained; the patient's response to testing; complications; interventions; and other pertinent information.

6. Follow guidelines in Chapter 1 for safe, effective, informed *intratest* care.

Clinical Implications

1. *Decreased levels* of gastric acid (hyposecretion and hypochlorhydria) occur in the following conditions:
   a. Pernicious anemia
   b. Gastric malignancy
   c. Atrophic gastritis
   d. Adrenal insufficiency
   e. Vitiligo
   f. Rheumatoid arthritis
   g. Thyroid toxicosis
   h. Chronic renal failure
   i. Post-vagotomy

2. *Increased levels* of gastric acid (hypersecretion and hyperchlorhydria) occur in the following conditions:
   a. Peptic or duodenal ulcer
   b. Zollinger-Ellison syndrome
   c. Hyperplasia and hyperfunction of antral gastric cells
   d. Post–small intestine resection

Interfering Factors

1. Lubricants or barium from previous tests present in the sample affects the result.

2. Medications such as antacids or histamine blockers, foods, and smoking alter gastric secretions.

3. Gastric secretions are altered in patients with diabetes who use insulin or in those who have had a surgical vagotomy.

4. Elderly patients have lower levels of gastric hydrochloric acid.

Patient Preparation

1. Assess for contraindications to the procedure, including carcinoid syndrome, congestive heart failure, recent myocardial infarction, or hypertension. The use of histamine may exacerbate these conditions.

2. Explain test purpose and procedure. Inform patient that there may be some discomfort when the nasogastric tube is inserted and that a gastric stimulant may be injected. Devise a method of communication for the patient prior to insertion of nasogastric tube (eg, raise index finger to indicate "wait" before proceeding). Explain that panting, mouth breathing, and swallowing facilitate tube insertion.

3. Record baseline vital signs. Remove dentures prior to test.

4. Fast from food, fluids, smoking, and gum chewing for at least 8 to 12 hours prior to testing.

5. Restrict or withhold anticholinergic agents, cholinergic agents, adrenergic blockers, antacids, steroids, alcohol, and caffeine for at least 24 hours before testing. Check with the clinician well before the procedure.

6. Follow guidelines in Chapter 1 for safe, effective, informed *pretest* care.

> ### Clinical Alert
>
> 1. If histamine is injected, the patient may experience flushing, dizziness, headache, faintness, and numbness of the extremities and abdomen during or immediately after testing. These symptoms must be reported immediately. Have epinephrine easily available.
>
> 2. Specimens for acid-fast bacillus (AFB) and tuberculosis (TB) cultures must be warm and should be taken to the laboratory immediately. Laboratory personnel should be alerted.

Patient Aftercare

1. Monitor vital signs. Observe for possible drug side-effects, gastrointestinal bleeding, or respiratory distress (gastrointestinal bleeding may signal perforation).

2. Provide nasal and oral care after tube removal. Allow patient to rest. Provide food or fluids as tolerated and ordered. If a local anesthetic was used on the throat, assess for return of gag and swallow reflexes before allowing patient to drink or eat (usually 2 hours postadministration).

3. Interpret test outcomes. Counsel patient regarding possible lifestyle alterations such as smoking cessation, restricted alcohol intake, dietary changes, stress reduction, medication, medical treatment, or surgical intervention.

4. Follow guidelines in Chapter 1 for *pre, intra,* and *posttest* care.

DNA TYPING OR FINGERPRINTING ●

Normal Values
Specific and unique to each person

Background
Deoxyribonucleic acid (DNA) is a complex, high-molecular-weight protein composed of deoxyribose, phosphoric acid, and four bases (adenine, quanine, thymine, cytosine). These six substances are arranged in two long chains that twist

around each other to form a double helix. The complementary components on each of these two chains link together between the chains. The nucleic acid component is present in the cell nuclei chromosomes and forms the chemical foundation for heredity. It carries the genetic material for every living organism except RNA viruses. DNA provides the actual code for individual genetic characteristics through a specific sequence, or "blueprint," that is unique to that person alone.

Explanation

DNA testing is used to establish identity (ie, military and disaster casualties), to determine parentage (ie, infant abductions), and during immigration disputes and during criminal investigations (ie, murder, sexual abuse, rape) through a process termed *restriction fragment length polymorphism (RFLP)*. This process allows evaluation of different DNA tissue samples from several sources to determine matching patterns, similar to comparing bar codes.

Procedure

1. DNA can be extracted from any tissue that contains nucleated cells (eg, skin, saliva, hair shafts, semen).
2. DNA samples are processed until DNA fragments can be visually represented on x-ray film. These films are called "autoradiographs" or "autorads." At this point, the fragments somewhat resemble bar codes.
3. The autorads are compared for matching or nonmatching characteristics among several samples. If a match between two or more different autorads is found, there exists a high probability that the different samples come from the same source or person.

Clinical Implications

1. Identity is confirmed when there are matching patterns in certain areas of the autorads. Adhere to caution when collecting and storing DNA specimens to prevent contamination and to preserve the specimens which may have crucial legal implications.
2. In parentage studies, even though each person has a unique DNA profile, matching characteristics in certain areas of autorads that come from two different individuals can indicate a parent-child relationship.
3. In criminal cases, matching DNA characteristics associated with tissue samples retrieved from both victim and suspect *may* establish the suspect's presence at the crime scene. A nonmatch definitively disproves that the different samples came from the same person.

Interfering Factors

1. Insufficient amount of DNA
2. DNA tissue sample deterioration/degradation
3. Lack of material database to conduct effective sample comparison

POSTMORTEM TESTS ●

It is the basic civil right of deceased human beings to have competent medical investigations of their deaths. This is particularly true in today's environment of social ills, drug use, crime, and violence among all sociocultural and political classes. Any death has potential civil, legal, criminal, or economic implications for the deceased, the family and significant others, and for society as a whole.

As with establishing a medical diagnosis for a living person, the medical process is similarly executed in developing a postmortem diagnosis. A history is taken, consisting of past medical history, risk factors, and death interpretation; a physical examination is performed (ie, autopsy); and laboratory tests are interpreted (tissue, organ, postmortem blood, and other body fluids such as vitreous fluids, urine, bile, or gastric contents).

Death Investigation

All deaths, whether from a natural sequence of events, during medical treatment, in unexplained circumstances, or criminally related, need to be investigated regarding *cause* and *manner* of death so that the legal death certificate may be accurately completed, signed, and recorded. Deaths can be defined as *natural* or *medical/legal.*

Natural Death	Medical/Legal Death
Cessation of cardiorespiratory function due to a medical disease process (eg, metastatic cancer, cerebrovascular accident) or natural progression of life events (ie, "old age")	Results from some "unnatural" (unexpected, unusual, or suspicious) event such as homicide, suicide, or accident; this situation is specifically governed by legal statutes and requires that a coroner, medical examiner, and law enforcement officials be involved

Death Interpretation

The process of postmortem interpretation follows a certain sequence. First, the history portion of the investigation is obtained. In natural death without autopsy, the medical history, diagnostic tests prior to death, clinical record, and knowledge about lifestyle can provide reasonably sufficient information to arrive at conclusions regarding cause and manner of death. Only autopsy, however, can definitively confirm these suspicions.

Clinical Alert

Postmortem examination falls under the domain of the physician pathologist. In criminal cases, forensic pathologists who have specialized knowledge, skills, and the latest investigative techniques at their disposal should perform the autopsy.

Medical/legal death investigation first focuses on the death scene. Interviews lay the groundwork for the investigation. Evaluation of the site of death involves a detailed examination of blood stains, disrupted environment, position of body, and signs of struggle or injury manifested by fluids leaking from

CHART 15-1 ▶
Time of Death

Although time of death is usually not a major issue, determination of time of death is important in both natural deaths (for insurance and other death benefits) and unnatural deaths, either witnessed or when body parts have been intentionally altered to conceal an individual's distinguishing features. Time of death estimate is based upon presence of the following:

Rigor mortis: stiffening of body as pH changes and lack of adenosine triphosphate in muscles; rigidity appears anywhere from instantly to 6–12 hours after death

Livor mortis: reddish-purple color caused by settling of blood in dependent body parts due to gravity; onset immediate, sometimes beginning before death (maximum in 8–12 hours)

Algor mortis: cooling of body; body temperature is subject to interpretation, based on cocaine use, presence of infection or fever before death, death scene, heat absorption, amount and type of clothing, size of body, activity just before death, and decomposition

Decomposition: processes occur due to chemical breakdown of cells and organs due to intracellular enzymes and putrefaction due to bacterial action

Gastric Emptying: food in stomach; digestion and stomach emptying varies in both life and death

Chemical Changes: potassium in vitreous fluid of the eye; as the time since death becomes greater, so does the concentration of potassium increase

Insect Activity: flies and other insects are associated with decomposed bodies; any attempt to fix time of death using insect evidence should be done only with the aid of an entomologist

Clinical Alert

1. Time of death is expressed as an estimate of the time range during which death could have occurred and varies according to cooling of body, color change, decomposition of stomach contents, clinical changes, and insect activity.
2. There is no single accurate marker of time of death.
3. When the time interval between actual death and the initial death investigation is months or years, body changes may be quite variable and can include saponification of subcutaneous tissue (changes due to prolonged exposure to moisture taking several months); mummification (drying process due to lack of moisture; occurs quickly in hot, dry climate, exposure to air, dying of thirst); skeletization (takes months to years). Examination of bones may yield general knowledge of deceased (eg, estimate of age, stature, race, gender).

body orifices, eyes, ears, nose, or mouth. Color changes and rigidity can be beneficial in establishing time frames for events (Chart 15-1).

The second part of the death interpretation process involves the autopsy itself. The autopsy consists of a detailed, comprehensive examination of both external and internal body features and organs.

Clinical Alert

In the case of a medical/legal autopsy, samples of organs and specimen sections (slides) should be retained for 3 to 5 years pending outcomes of litigation and legal system appeals. Photographs should accompany reports and should be archived.

The third step in death interpretation includes collection of blood, bile, urine, and ocular fluids (if available) for analysis. Blood toxicology studies must be performed at a state-certified laboratory. Blood samples are the *only* life/death determinants; urine samples provide information about levels of substances excreted, but they do not provide blood level values of these same substances. Typical blood toxicology screens include the following tests:

No. 1. Alcohol screens determine levels of various alcohols.

No. 2. Acid-neutral screens detect barbiturates and salicylates.

No. 3. Basic screens detect tranquilizers, synthetic narcotics, local anesthetics, antihistamines, antidepressants, and alkaloids.

No. 4. Higher volatile screens use gas chromatography to detect substances such as toluene, benzene, trichloroethane, and trichloroethylene.

No. 5. Cannabis screens detect the presence of cannabis (marijuana).

All of these screens serve a purpose in cases that involve accidents and work-related deaths.

After the life events and scene investigation, the autopsy, and the laboratory tests are complete, data from all sources are scrutinized and analyzed. Findings and conclusions are then documented and certified on the death certificate, which then becomes a matter of public record. Findings may then be

---

Clinical Alert

Some examiners may be reluctant to include HIV-positive information in public record autopsy reports out of compassion for the decedent's family. However, certain states require that every autopsy done through the medical examiner's office include an HIV test. As with other issues of confidentiality, the applicable laws must be obeyed; however, the pathologist must make every effort to protect the patient's and family's right to privacy to the degree that the law will allow.

shared with the decedent's immediate family or may become part of a court deposition process.

NOTE: *If the HIV status of decedent is not directly related to the cause of death, the decedent's HIV status need not be recorded.*

AUTOPSY

Normal Values
External and internal findings: within normal limits or demonstrate significant pathology related to cause of death
Gross and microscopic findings: within normal limits or abnormalities related to cause of death
No drugs or alcohol present

Explanation of Test
An autopsy is an investigation of the cause and manner of death by direct examination of the body. Cause of death is the disease or injury that, through its physiologic effects, results in the actual death of the individual. Manner of death is the type of event that led to death and is categorized as natural, homicidal, suicidal, accidental, pending, or undetermined. Interpretation of physical findings results in setting forth an opinion regarding the probable cause of death. Prior to autopsy, as much pertinent information as possible is gathered about the deceased. Available medical records are reviewed thoroughly. In cases of medical/legal death investigation, not only the medical and social background but also the terminal events and circumstances of death, including the environment, presence of drugs and alcohol, and the exact condition and position of the body are thoroughly investigated.

General Procedure
1. Standard precautions are observed throughout. The body is identified and "tagged" (usually on the great toe) with the decedent's name (if available), gender, age, and a number. The body is then weighed and measured.
2. The head and chest are photographed and marked with an identification number. This step occurs in nonhospital, non–clinical institution deaths (eg, deaths at home, work, school, industry, roadway, whenever foul play is suspected, and whenever a 911 call results in law enforcement officers at the death scene).
3. Information about clothing and valuables is described and recorded. When the body is found by someone other than a family member (eg, at work, road accident), these items are removed, inventoried, and given to family or the law enforcement agency.
4. Fingerprints are made (of the fingertips in children) only in criminal cases.
5. The body is cleansed. In trauma cases or unusual death findings, the face is photographed again if blood, dirt, and other materials were present initially.
6. An external examination is performed on the entire body. The location

and description of all identifying marks, scars, tattoos, incisions, injuries, and other significant findings are recorded on a body diagram.

7. When foul play is suspected, all injuries are photographed in at least two views: one showing the location of the injury on the body and the other providing a close-up view of the injury.

8. In some instances, x-rays films may be necessary to verify gross anatomic deformities, injuries (cervical spine and skull fracture), or pathologies that may provide clues regarding the cause of death. Radiography tracks the trajectory of bullets and other projectiles through the entire body or just through a specific area and may also be performed on exhumed organs. In some instances bodies may be completely unrecognizable (eg, putrefied beyond recognition). X-ray studies can determine age and can establish a victim's identity by comparing bone and dental detail to previous x-ray films and dental x-rays of the victim.

9. The autopsy proceeds in an orderly manner, observing universal precautions. Descriptions of color and distinguishing features of the hair and eyes and appearance of the nose, ears, mouth, teeth, face, head, neck, genitalia, torso, and extremities are documented in detail. The front, side, and back of the body are examined in detail. Injuries, wounds, bruises, contusions, and lacerations are described, mapped, and detailed. Descriptions of size, depth, location, and presence of foreign objects or materials at or near the injured areas, as well as fluids draining from body orifices and wounds, are entered into the report. Internal examination includes a complete head and pelvic dissection with removal of all organs from the skull, neck, abdomen, and pelvis. Specific organs are subjected to gross examination that includes measurement of size and estimated weight. Once this is done, organ sections are prepared for microscopic slides to be examined later. The slides are saved for evidence. Virtually any part of the body can be microscopically examined. The brain and the neck organs are always removed and examined. As part of this examination, the dura matter is removed to permit visualization of the skull and calvarium.

10. Blood and fluid specimens are withdrawn by syringe from the heart, aorta, eyes (vitreous fluid), gallbladder (bile), and bladder (urine). These specimens are refrigerated until examined and can be saved for an indefinite period. In the instance of trauma, blood samples can be retrieved from the pulmonary trunk or the chest. If clots are present and syringe sampling cannot be done, pericardial tapping is an alternative method of procuring a blood sample.

11. Sometimes it is necessary to collect specimens for culture. Most internal organs of previously uninfected persons remain sterile for about 20 hours after death.

Protocols for Retrieving Postmortem Cultures
Follow standard precautions. See Appendix A.
Use sterile instruments and gloves when obtaining specimens for culture.
Cleanse the area with a povidone-iodine 5-minute scrub followed by a 70% alcohol 5-minute scrub.

For sample collection, either aspirate body fluid samples and transfer them to a sterile tube or swab the area with sterile swabs.

Obtain blood culture specimens from the right ventricle of the heart.

Collect peritoneal fluid immediately after entering the peritoneal cavity.

Collect bladder urine directly from the bladder with a syringe and needle.

Sample pericardial or pleural cavity fluid on a swab or with a syringe and needle.

Sear the external surface of an abscess to dryness with a red hot spatula; collect pus via syringe and needle (if possible) or use a swab.

13. The organs are returned to the body after examination is completed.

> **Clinical Alert**
>
> **1.** Organs and tissues for transplant are procured prior to and during autopsy.
> **2.** A special consent form must be signed by a responsible adult and witnessed by a professional.
> **3.** Life-saving organs (eg, kidneys, lungs, heart, pancreas, liver, intestines) are harvested prior to autopsy.
> **4.** Other tissues and organs are harvested simultaneously with autopsy procedures or after autopsy: Eyes, bones, connective tissues, joints, ligament, heart valves, and veins.
> **5.** A request for organ donation is made in any hospital or medical examiner death (in many states), and the request and answer report are documented in the deceased person's chart/record.

14. The body is released immediately to the funeral home for burial or cremation per family wishes. If there are legal questions, the body may be kept for some time (eg, months).

> **Clinical Alert**
>
> **1.** If an external examination is done in lieu of an autopsy, collect blood from the subclavian vessel and vitreous humor from the eyes.
> **2.** Do not use plastic envelopes for storing biologic samples such as tissue and hair or foreign objects such as bullets. Plastic captures moisture and promotes fungal growth. Instead, place objects in clean paper envelopes. Label each item properly and store appropriately.

Clinical Implications

Causes of death are categorized as natural and unnatural.

NATURAL CAUSES

Cardiovascular

1. The most common cardiovascular disease causes and contributing factors of sudden death are myocardial infarction, ventricular tachycardias and fibrillation, hypertensive cardiovascular disease, strenuous activity during extremes of heat or cold weather, drug use, and anorexia nervosa.

Brain
2. The most common brain disease or brain injury–related causes of sudden death include poorly controlled epilepsy or seizure disorders complicated by cardiac arrest related to O_2 deprivation, brain hemorrhage, primary brain tumors, aneurysms, and head trauma.

Respiratory
3. The most common respiratory causes of sudden death are epiglottitis, pulmonary thrombosis/embolus, status asthmaticus, aspiration of food/gastric contents/blood, cavernous TB, premature birth, fulminating pneumonia, and chest trauma.

Gastrointestinal
4. The most common gastrointestinal causes of sudden death are trauma, peritonitis, massive splenic enlargement or rupture, ingested caustic substances, liver or pancreatic diseases, and diabetes mellitus in the presence of diabetic coma (diagnosed by elevated glucose in vitreous of eye).

Other
5. Other causes of sudden death include tubal pregnancy rupture leading to massive hemorrhage, HIV infection, chronic illness in bedridden persons with septic decubitus ulcers, malnutrition, dehydration, environmental causes (eg, Legionnaires' disease, hantavirus).

UNNATURAL CAUSES
6. The most common unnatural causes of sudden death are trauma due to body wounds, cuts, lacerations, traumatic amputations, self-inflicted and self-defense wounds, asphyxia, motor vehicle/cycle accidents, and airplane crashes.
7. Other unnatural causes of sudden death include sudden infant death syndrome (SIDS), which is the unexpected death of an apparently healthy infant. Postmortem examination may not reveal the cause of death. Neonaticide refers to the deliberate killing of an infant within 24 hours of birth; infanticide indicates murder of a child. Additional unnatural causes of sudden death include fire or smoke inhalation, drowning, electrocution, hyperthermia (heat), hypothermia (cold), and embolism. Homicide may be associated with rape, criminal abortion, drug overdose, drug abuse, and drug-related or alcohol-related deaths (Chart 15-2).

Family Preparation
1. Explain rationale for postdeath procedures (Chart 15-3). Concern and respect for the deceased and significant others can reduce anxiety and objections to or misinterpretations of after-death testing. Obtain a signed, witnessed consent form for autopsy.

CHART 15-2 ▶
Special Criminologic Postmortem Procedures

GUNSHOT WOUND PROCEDURE
Mandatory x-ray of all gunshot wounds, including entrance/exit; locate bullet/fragments. *Note:* copper- and aluminum-jacket bullets remain in the body. Aluminum jackets are difficult to visualize on x-ray films, especially when lodged in bone. Photograph entry/exit; cleanse wound; repeat photograph.

BLUNT FORCE INJURY PROCEDURE
X-ray affected areas. X-ray hands and forearms for "defense wounds." Photograph the wounds in original condition after cleansing. Use rape kit if possible rape is suspected (both male and female) or when the nature of the injury suggests uncontrolled rage (hammer, axe, stab wounds).

SHARP WOUND PROCEDURE
X-ray wound sites. Photograph wounds in original condition after cleansing, after approximating wound margins. Check for "defense wounds" on hands and arms. Trace wounds on clear plastic sheet (optional). Save and photograph severed cartilage.

DRUG OVERDOSE PROCEDURE
Photograph evidence suggesting drug abuse, such as injection sites on body; presence of drug paraphernalia or drugs, and drug residue on lips, face, teeth, oral cavity, tongue, nose, or hands. Assess mouth area and body for bite marks and "fall" injuries (suggests seizure activity associated with drug ingestion). Check lymph nodes, spleen, liver (abnormal in intravenous drug abuser).

SPECIAL BATTERY PROCEDURE
If sexual assault is suspected, the following are done *in order:* body supine (face up), obtain scalp and pubic hair, oral samples, semen from inner thighs. Body prone (face down), obtain anal specimen first, then vaginal specimen. Collect fingernail evidence. Collect 25 pubic hairs from entire vulvar area. Collect 25 head hairs from affected area. Obtain oral, anal, cervical, and other specimens suspected of containing semen.

CHILD ABUSE/SIDS PROCEDURE
X-ray and photograph entire body. Perform external examination of conjunctival petechiae, fingertip bruises, torso and shoulders (front/back), frenulum, and back; posterior thighs and buttocks may be incised (from buckles or other sharp objects). Perform internal examination for hematomas (due to direct injury); if present and *no* evidence of head trauma, remove

(continued)

CHART 15-2 *(continued)*

eyes and examine retina (shows characteristic signs in presence of sudden infant death syndrome). Document recent or healed fractures and estimated time of injury. Reexamine and rephotograph the following day to delineate bruises not previously evident.

> ▶ **Clinical Alert**
>
> 1. Observe standard precautions during these procedures. Risk of disease transmission, hepatitis, and HIV exposure is high.
> 2. Sketch, measure, and mark wounds on diagram in both inches and centimeters (U.S. residents relate to inches more accurately). Projectile (bullet) caliber is estimated as small, medium, or large.
> 3. Procure toxicologic specimens if indicated. Specimens for toxicologic analysis include the following:
>   a. All ocular fluid from both eyes
>   b. Blood-sodium fluoride preservative (50 ml)
>   c. Blood-sodium fluoride preservative (retainer tube) (10 ml)
>   d. Liver (3 g)
>   e. Bile (10 ml)
>   f. Urine (50 ml)
>   g. Stomach and small bowel contents
> 4. Store specimens and fragments in paper envelopes or bags; *never* use plastic, which allows mold and fungus to grow.
> 5. Route specimens and reports to appropriate department or individual.

2. Consider cultural habits and practices. Human responses and practices surrounding the death of a loved one vary among societies, religions, cultures, and races. In this light, postmortem examination may be offensive to some groups.
3. Assure the family that nothing will be done without their permission except where required by law.
4. If fear of mutilation or delay in release of body for burial are concerns, provide clear and concise information to help with decision making. In the case of religious dilemmas, facilitate counsel and communication between clergy and other appropriate individuals or agencies.
5. Conflict can occur when statutory authority is at odds with family wishes. Explanations may help.

Family Aftercare

Interpret postmortem test results and counsel families appropriately about organs procured for donation (as appropriate).

CHART 15-3
Information for Families Regarding an Autopsy

Autopsies are frequently mandatory procedures, especially in sudden, suspicious, or unexplained deaths.

Investigate accident and work-related deaths serve the following functions:

Serve as quality control indicators to confirm predeath diagnoses and to assess effectiveness of drug therapy, diagnostic procedures, surgical techniques, gene therapy, and other diagnostic and treatment modalities

Identify, track, and monitor disease prevalence, incidence, trends, or association with certain life-style, environmental, or occupational influences

Information gathered from autopsy findings provides a framework for developing better and more sophisticated treatments for disease and illness control or eradication

Consent from family is required unless autopsy is ordered by the coroner or medical examiner

Should family members be undecided regarding autopsy:

They may wish to consider it as an option when no firm medical diagnosis has been established

To answer questions about an unexpected or mysterious death due to apparent natural causes

If there are hereditary, genetic, or contagious diseases

When the cause of death could affect insurance settlements and other legal matters

When death occurs in the presence of unexpected medical or obstetric complications

During the use of experimental drug therapies

If death is a result of certain dental, invasive, surgical, or diagnostic procedures

When the death does not come under the jurisdiction of the medical examiner

BIBLIOGRAPHY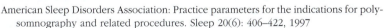

American Sleep Disorders Association: Practice parameters for the indications for polysomnography and related procedures. Sleep 20(6): 406–422, 1997

American Sleep Disorders Association: The indications for polysomnography and related procedures. Sleep 20(6): 423–487, 1997

American Sleep Disorders Association: The International Classification of Sleep Disorders, ASDA, Rochester, 1998

Bach M: Electroencephalogram (EEG). In Von Schulthess GK, Hennig J (eds): Functional Imaging, pp. 391–408. Philadelphia, Lippincott-Raven, 1998

Bontrager KL: Textbook of Radiographic Positioning and Related Anatomy, 4th ed. St. Louis, Mosby, 1997

Chediak AD: Pathogenesis of obstructive sleep apnea. Resp Care 43(4): 265–276, 1998

Cryer B, Lee E, Feldman M, New methods, new materials. Gastrointestinal Endoscopy 44(3): 317–323, 1996

Frizell J: Cerebral angiography. AJN 98(9): 16ii–16jj, September 1998

Frizell J: Transesophageal echocardiography. AJN 97(9): 17–18, September 1997

Guyton AC, Hall JE: Textbook of Medical Physiology. Philadelphia, WB Saunders, 1997, pp. 27–32, 763–764

Haubuck WS, Schaffner F, Berk JE: Gastroenterology, 5th ed., vol. 1. Philadelphia, WB Saunders, 1995, pp. 370–371

Higgins CB, Hricak H, Helms CA: Magnetic Resonance Imaging of the Body, 3rd ed. Philadelphia, Lippincott-Raven, 1997, pp. 153–169, 1448–1449

Jabobs DS, Demott UR, Grady HJ: Laboratory Test Handbook, 4th ed. Cleveland, Lexi Comp Inc., 1996

Kahn MG: On Call Cardiology. Philadelphia, WB Saunders, 1997, pp. 47–52

Kruger MM, Roth T, Dement WC: Principles and Practice of Sleep Medicine, 2nd ed. Philadelphia WB Saunders, 1994

Lufkin RB: The MRI Manual, 2nd ed. St. Louis, Mosby, 1997

Montes P: Managing outpatient cardiac catheterization. AJN 97(8): 34–37, August 1997

Moser W: Magnetic Resonance Spectroscopy May Help Battle Heart Disease. Advance for Radiologic Science Professionals, June 2, 1997, pp. 19–26

Murphy KJ: Adverse reactions to gadolinium contrast media: a review of 36 cases. AJR Am J Roentgenol 167(4): 847–849, 1996

Plankey ED, Knohf J: Prep talk: What patients need to know about magnetic resonance imaging. Am J Nurs 90(1): 27–28, 1990

Trenko LA: Understanding diagnostic cardiac catheterization. AJN 97(2): 16K–16R, February 1997

Van Riper S, Van Riper J: Cardiac Diagnostic Tests. Philadelphia, WB Saunders, 1997, pp. 33–44, 87–92, 159–163, 219–244, 265–313

Wirth CV, Mittleman RE, Rao VJ: Atlas of Forensic Pathology. Chicago, ASCP Press, 1998

16

Prenatal Diagnosis and Tests of Fetal Well-Being

OVERVIEW OF PRENATAL DIAGNOSIS ●

Fetal well-being depends on maternal health. Many routine prenatal tests assess maternal health and well-being. Prenatal testing usually includes a complete blood count or hemoglobin and hematocrit, Rh type and ABO blood group, red cell antibody screening, rubella immunity status, glucose challenge testing (see Chapter 6), urinalysis, maternal serum α-fetoprotein (MS-AFP) or maternal triple screen, hepatitis B testing, culture for sexually transmitted diseases, the Venereal Disease Research Laboratory (VDRL) test, and surveillance for group B streptococci. Screening for human immunodeficiency virus (HIV) infection is recommended for all pregnant women to improve the care of HIV-positive women and to identify infants at risk; perinatal transmission is the primary route of HIV infection in children.

Tests in this chapter monitor the status of the maternal-fetal unit, identify the fetus at risk for intrauterine asphyxia, aid in the early diagnosis of infection, and identify genetic and biochemical disorders and major anomalies. Tests are also performed to predict normal fetal outcome or to identify the fetus at risk for asphyxia during labor.

MATERNAL TRIPLE SCREEN ●

These tests are offered to pregnant women to identify risks for chromosome disorders such as Down syndrome (trisomy 21); major birth defects, including open neural tube defects such as spina bifida; placental insufficiency; and oligohydramnios. The evaluation consists of 3 separate blood protein tests done on maternal serum between 14 and 19 weeks of gestation: MS-AFP is decreased in Down syndrome and neural tube defects, estriol (E_3) in Down syndrome, and β-human chorionic gonadotropin (hCG) in Down syndrome. Results are reported as "multiples of the median" (MoM).

The maternal triple screen is a screening test; therefore, an abnormal (positive) result is not diagnostic, and further testing with ultrasound, amniocentesis, and genetic counseling is indicated. The markers can be positive in normal variations such as multiple births or miscalculated gestational age.

Ultrasound testing is a method of assessing fetal well-being that has become a diagnostic tool for assessment of fetal age, health, growth, and identification of anomalies. Level I ultrasound assesses gestational age, number of fetuses, fetal death, and the condition of the placenta. Level II ultrasound assesses specific congenital anomalies or abnormalities. In some diagnostic centers, fetal echocardiography is also available. Color-enhanced Doppler sonography is used to measure the velocity and direction of blood flow in fetal and uterine anatomy, to provide information about placental function, and as an especially good predictor of outcome for fetuses that are small for gestational age (see Chapter 13).

Although magnetic resonance imaging (MRI) is used at some prenatal centers, it is still under investigation for diagnostic evaluation in pregnancy, especially in the final trimester (see Chapter 15). Some of the advantages of MRI during pregnancy are that it is a noninvasive technique, it permits easy differentiation between fat and soft tissue, it does not require a full bladder, and it can show the entire fetus in 1 scan. Currently, MRI confirms fetal abnormalities found by ultrasound and can be used for pelvimetry, placental localization, and determination of size. MRI is especially useful for definition of maternal anatomy in cases of suspected intra-abdominal or retroperitoneal disease.

Also under investigation is the combined use of a blood test for pregnancy-associated plasma protein A (PAPPA), which is increased in Down pregnancy, and ultrasound measurement of neck membrane thickness, which is increased in Down syndrome.

MATERNAL SERUM α-FETOPROTEIN (MS-AFP) ●

Normal Values
25 ng/ml
At 15 to 18 wk gestation: 10–150 ng/ml or 0.4–2.5 MoM

Explanation of Test
AFP, a product of the fetal liver, is normally found in fetal serum, maternal serum, and amniotic fluid. Maternal serum AFP (MS-AFP) testing is routinely offered between 15 and 18 weeks of gestation to all pregnant women as a screen for neural tube defects; only 5% to 10% of neural tube defects occur in families with previous occurrences.

Procedure
1. Obtain a 10-ml venous blood sample (red top tube). Observe standard precautions.
2. Plan the first screening at 15 to 18 weeks. If the result is normal, no further screening is necessary. If MS-AFP is low, consider ultrasound studies to determine exact fetal age. A second screening may be done after an initial elevated MS-AFP. If the result is normal, no further screening is necessary.

Clinical Implications
Abnormal levels should be followed by ultrasound and amniocentesis.
1. *Elevated* MS-AFP can indicate
   A. Neural tube defects of spina bifida (a vertebral gap) or anencephaly (>2.5 MoM)
   B. Underestimation of gestational age
   C. Multiple gestation (>4.5 MoM)
   D. Threatened abortion
   E. Other congenital abnormalities
2. *Elevated* MS-AFP early in pregnancy is associated with
   A. Congenital nephrosis
   B. Duodenal atresia
   C. Umbilical hernia or protrusion
   D. Sacrococcygeal teratoma
3. *Elevated* MS-AFP in the third trimester is associated with
   A. Esophageal atresia

   B. Fetal teratoma
   C. Hydroencephaly
   D. Rh isoimmunization
   E. Gastrointestinal tract obstruction
4. *Low* MS-AFP is associated with
   A. Long-standing fetal death
   B. Down syndrome (trisomy 21)
   C. Other chromosome abnormalities (trisomy 13, trisomy 18)
   D. Hydatidiform mole
   E. Pseudopregnancy

Interfering Factors

1. Obesity causes low MS-AFP.
2. Race is a factor: MS-AFP levels are 10% to 15% higher in blacks and are lower in Asians.
3. Insulin-dependent diabetes results in low MS-AFP.

> ### Clinical Alert
>
> **1.** The incidence of neural tube defect is 1 per 1000 births in the United States, 1 per 5000 in England.
> **2.** Knowledge of the precise gestational age is paramount for the accuracy of this test.
> **3.** If the MS-AFP is elevated and no fetal defect is demonstrated (ie, by ultrasound or amniocentesis), then the pregnancy is at an increased risk (eg, premature birth, low-weight infant, fetal death).

Patient Preparation

1. Explain the reason for testing the mother's blood.
2. See Chapter 1 guidelines for safe, effective, informed *pretest* care.

Patient Aftercare

1. Interpret test outcomes and counsel appropriately. Explain possible need for further testing (eg, ultrasound, amniocentesis).
2. Follow Chapter 1 guidelines for safe, effective, informed *posttest* care.

HORMONE TESTING

Normally, the amounts of all steroid hormones increase as pregnancy progresses. The maternal unit responds to altered hormone levels even before the growing uterus is apparent. Serial testing may be done to monitor rising levels of a particular hormone over a period of time. Decreasing levels indicate that the maternal-placental-fetal unit is not functioning normally. Biochemical analyses of several hormones can be used to monitor changes in the status of the maternal-fetal unit (see Chapters 3 and 6).

1. In early pregnancy, hCG in maternal blood provides evidence of a viable pregnancy. The hCG in maternal serum is measured as a sensitive pregnancy test (the hCG level doubles every 48 hours during early pregnancy). Also, it is used to monitor the success of in vitro fertilization or insemination, to diagnose trophoblastic tumor, to diagnose ectopic pregnancy (indicated by decrease in hCG over a 48-hour period), and to screen for Down syndrome in pregnancy. For further discussion of pregnancy tests, see Chapter 6.

2. hCG, together with prolactin and luteinizing hormone (LH), prolongs the life of the corpus luteum once the ovum is fertilized. hCG stimulates the ovary for the first 6 to 8 weeks of pregnancy, before placental synthesis of progesterone begins. Its function later in pregnancy (in maternal blood) is unknown.

3. Late in pregnancy, the levels of E_3 and human placental lactogen (hPL) in maternal blood reflect fetal homeostasis. hPL is a protein hormone produced by the placenta. Testing of hPL evaluates only placental functioning. Blood testing of the mother usually begins after the 30th week and may be done weekly thereafter. A concentration of 1 μg/ml hPL may be detected at 6 to 8 weeks of gestation. The level slowly increases throughout pregnancy and reaches 7 μg/ml at term before abruptly dropping to zero after delivery. hLP functions primarily as a fail-safe mechanism to ensure nutrient supply to the fetus, for example at times of maternal starvation. However, it does not appear to be required for a successful pregnancy outcome (see Chapter 6).

ESTRIOL (E_3) ●

Normal Values

Weeks of Gestation	E_3 (ng/ml)
28–30	38–140
32	35–330
34	45–260
36	48–350
38	59–570
40	90–460

Levels peak in the middle or late afternoon.
The day-to-day variation is 12%–15%.

Background

Estriol (E_3) is the predominant estrogen in the blood and urine of pregnant women and is of fetal origin. Normal production serves as a measure of the integrity of the maternal-fetal unit and of fetal well-being.

Explanation of Test

This test is used during pregnancy to evaluate fetal disorders and is part of the maternal triple screen. Declining serial values indicate fetal distress. E_3 is decreased in Down syndrome and in trisomy 18.

Procedure

1. A 5-ml serum sample is obtained by venipuncture using a red top tube. Draw the specimen at same time of day on each visit. Observe universal precautions. Record weeks of gestation on the requisition or computer screen. Serial measurements may be recommended to establish a trend.

2. During the third trimester, 24-hour urine specimens may be collected.

Clinical Implications

1. *Decreased* E_3 is associated with risk of
   A. Growth retardation
   B. Fetal death
   C. Fetal anomalies (Down syndrome, fetal encephalopathy)
   D. Fetus past maturity
   E. Pre-eclampsia
   F. Rh immunization

2. *Decreased* E_3 also occurs in
   A. Anemia
   B. Diabetes
   C. Malnutrition
   D. Liver disease
   E. Hemoglobinopathy

Interfering Factors

Administration of radioactive isotopes within the previous 48 hours interferes with this test.

Patient Preparation

1. Explain test purpose and procedures. Serial testing may be required. See hormone testing, page 1068.

2. No fasting is necessary.

3. See Chapter 1 guidelines for safe, effective, informed *pretest* care.

Clinical Alert

1. A single determination cannot be interpreted in a meaningful fashion.

2. In some high-risk pregnancies, E_3 is not reduced.

Patient Aftercare

1. Interpret test results and monitor appropriately. Continuously low E_3 values are sometimes seen in normal pregnancy. A decreasing trend is indicative of fetal distress. Provide counseling and support.

2. Follow Chapter 1 guidelines for safe, effective, informed *posttest* care.

HUMAN PLACENTAL LACTOGEN (hPL)
(CHORIONIC SOMATOMAMMOTROPIN)

●

Normal Values
Maternal serum (5–38 wk gestation): 0.5–11.0 µg/ml
Men and nonpregnant women: nondetectible

Background
Human placental lactogen (hPL) is a growth-promoting hormone of placental origin and is similar to hCG (see Hormone Testing, page 1068).

Explanation
This test is used to evaluate placental function as an index of fetal well-being in at-risk pregnancies. Low hPL levels are associated with intrauterine growth retardation. Falling levels indicate a poor prognosis. The level of hPL correlates best with placental weight, but the clinical significance of this hormone is controversial.

Procedure
1. Obtain a serum sample of at least 1 ml in 2 separate vials (red top tube) by venipuncture. Observe standard precautions.
2. Record the week of gestation or last menstrual period (LMP) on the test requisition or computer screen. These tests are usually done as serial measurements.

Clinical Implications
1. *Normal* values are associated with normal intrauterine growth but do not ensure lack of complications.
2. *Decreased* or *falling* values are associated with
   A. Growth retardation
   B. Placental disease
   C. Fetal death
   D. Hypertensive
3. Low levels are also associated with some normal pregnancies.
4. *Increased* values are found in trophoblastic tumors.

Interfering Factors
Administration of radiopharmaceuticals 24 hours before venipuncture interferes with this test.

Patient Preparation
1. Explain the reason for testing the mother's blood.
2. See Chapter 1 guidelines for safe, effective, informed *pretest* care.

Patient Aftercare
1. Interpret test outcomes and counsel appropriately. Explain possible need for serial blood testing if results are abnormal.
2. Ultrasound studies should be used to assess any abnormal results.

FETAL FIBRONECTIN (fFN)   ●

Normal Values

Negative (<0.050 μg/ml): delivery is unlikely to occur within 14 days
Positive (≥0.050 μg/ml): delivery within 7–14 days

Background

Fetal fibronectin is abundant in amniotic fluid and may be useful in the diagnosis of ruptured membranes. The detection of fFN in vaginal secretions before membrane rupture may be a marker for impending preterm labor within the next 7 to 14 days.

Explanation of Test

This test helps to predict a preterm delivery when the presenting symptoms are questionable so that early intervention (eg, tocolytics, corticosteroids, transport to a tertiary center) can be initiated when indicated. This test is for women with intact membranes and cervical dilatation of <3 cm. fFN is secreted in early pregnancy to help attach the fertilized egg to the implantation site in the uterus, but it is not secreted after 22 weeks until near term. This test detects preterm labor from 24 until 34 weeks' gestation.

Procedure

Using a sterile speculum, obtain secretions from the cervix and vagina by rotating a sterile Dacron swab near the outside of the cervix and the posterior fornix of the vagina. Observe standard precautions. Send the specimen to laboratory. Results take 24 to 48 hours.

Clinical Implications

A level of fFN equal to or greater than a reference value (0.050 μg/ml) is considered positive and means that preterm labor is imminent.

Patient Preparation

1. Explain test purpose and procedure to the patient.
2. Refer to Chapter 1 guidelines for safe, effective, informed *pretest* care.

Patient Aftercare

1. Counsel the patient regarding test results and need for follow-up medication, tocolysis (inhibition of contractions), or preparation for probable delivery.
2. Be sure the mother knows the warning signs of preterm labor:
   A. *Uterine contractions*—a hard feeling over the entire surface of the uterus which lasts 20 seconds or longer. The contractions can be painless. If ≥4 are felt per hour, notify clinician.
   B. *Menstrual-like cramps* felt low in abdomen; may be constant or come and go.
   C. *Pelvic pressure* or a fullness in the pelvic area or back of the thighs.

D. *Backache*—a dull pain in the lower back, either constant or rhythmic, that is not relieved by changing positions

E. *Persistent diarrhea*

F. *Intestinal cramps* with or without diarrhea

G. *Vaginal discharge* that is greater than normal or changes in consistency or color (especially if it is pink, bloody, or greenish)

H. A general *feeling or sense that something is wrong*

3. Explain the possible causes and increased risks associated with preterm labor and birth:

A. Past preterm birth

B. Spontaneous abortion in second trimester

C. Uterine anomaly

D. Diethylstilbestrol exposure

E. Incompetent cervix

F. Hydramnios

G. Bleeding in second and third trimester

H. Preterm labor

I. Premature rupture of membrane

J. Multiple gestation

K. Preterm cervical dilatation of ≥2 cm (multipara) or ≥1 cm (primipara)

L. Prepregnancy weight of <115 pounds

M. Mother <15 years of age

4. Follow Chapter 1 guidelines for safe, effective, informed *posttest* care.

●TESTS TO PREDICT FETAL OUTCOME AND RISK FOR INTRAUTERINE ASPHYXIA

CONTRACTION STRESS TEST (CST) ●

Normal Values

The test result is normal (negative) if there are no late decelerations associated with at least 3 contractions within a 10-minute period.

A normal (negative) CST implies that placental support is adequate; that the fetus is probably able to tolerate the stress of labor, should it begin within 1 week; and that there is a low risk of intrauterine death due to hypoxia.

Explanation of Test

This test is done in a hospital or clinic setting to assess fetal heart rate (FHR) in response to uterine contractions via electronic fetal monitoring.

Procedure

The FHR is obtained by using an external transducer, and uterine activity is monitored by a tocodynamometer.

Clinical Implications

A positive result indicates increased risk of intrauterine death due to hypoxia. See further discussion of results and contraindications under Oxytocin Challenge Test (see below).

Patient Preparation

1. Explain the reason for testing.
2. See Chapter 1 guidelines for safe, effective, informed *pretest* care.

Patient Aftercare

1. Interpret test outcomes and counsel appropriately. Explain possible need for follow-up testing.
2. Follow Chapter 1 guidelines for safe, effective, informed *posttest* care.

OXYTOCIN CHALLENGE TEST (OCT); NIPPLE STIMULATION TEST; BREAST STIMULATION TEST (BST)

Normal Values

The test result is normal if there are no late decelerations associated with at least 3 contractions within a 10-minute period.

A normal (negative) result is reassuring; it implies that placental reserve is sufficient should labor begin within 1 week. There is a false-normal rate of 1 to 2 per 1000 pregnancies. The procedure is usually repeated weekly.

Explanation of Test

This test is performed after 28 weeks of gestation, when a nonstress test (NST) is nonreactive or a CST is either positive or unsatisfactory. Continuous external fetal monitoring is used. Because uterine contractions are associated with a reduction in uteroplacental blood flow, spontaneous, oxytocin-induced (OCT), or nipple stimulation–induced contractions with a frequency of 3 in 10 minutes may be used clinically as a standard test of fetoplacental respiratory function. Stress of this magnitude has been proven clinically to be useful in separating the fetus with suboptimal oxygen reserve from those with adequate reserve (the vast majority), and it does not significantly compromise the normal fetus.

Procedure

1. Contractions may occur spontaneously, after breast stimulation (BST), or after administration of intravenous oxytocin (OCT) to produce 3 good-quality contractions, of at least 40 seconds' duration each, within a 10-minute period.
2. The FHR is monitored for reaction to this stress.

Clinical Implications

1. The presence of consistent and persistent late decelerations with most uterine contractions, regardless of their frequency, constitutes a positive (abnormal) OCT result. This is often associated with decreased baseline FHR variability, a lack of FHR acceleration with fetal movement, and a fetus at risk for intrauterine asphyxia.

2. The results of the OCT can be categorized as follows:

    A. *Negative:* No late decelerations.

    B. *Positive:* Late decelerations follow 50% or more of contractions, even if the frequency of the contractions is <3 in 10 minutes.

    C. *Equivocal:* Intermittent, late, or variable decelerations.

    D. *Unsatisfactory:* <3 contractions within 10 minutes or a poor-quality tracing.

Patient Preparation

1. Explain purpose and procedure of the test.

2. See Chapter 1 guidelines for safe, effective, informed *pretest* care.

▶ Clinical Alert

1. With all methods of OCT/CST there is a risk of hyperstimulation, which could result in extended FHR decelerations that could be hypoxic for the fetus.

2. Contraindications for OCT/CST include

    A. Third-trimester bleeding (unexplained vaginal bleeding)

    B. Preterm labor (premature)

    C. Presence of classic uterine incision

    D. Placenta previa

Patient Aftercare

1. Interpret test outcomes and counsel accordingly about meaning of fetal heart activity and movement.

2. Follow Chapter 1 guidelines for safe, effective, informed *posttest* care.

NONSTRESS TEST (NST) ●

Normal Values

Normal (negative) result: reactive NST

American College of Obstetricians and Gynecologists (ACOG) criteria for a reactive NST (with or without stimulation): 2 or more accelerations of FHR, peaking at least 15 bpm above the baseline FHR and last at least 15 seconds from baseline to baseline, within a 20-minute period.

Explanation of Test

This test can be performed in a hospital, a clinic, or possibly a home care setting. Test results reflect the functions of the fetal brain stem, autonomic nervous system, and heart.

Clinical Implications

A nonreactive NST (positive test) consists of fewer than 2 accelerations of FHR (ACOG criteria). If the fetus does not react within the first 20 minutes, stimulation should be applied. The test is considered nonreactive if, after extension to 40 minutes, the ACOG criteria are not met. This extended testing minimizes the possibility of lack of activity due to fetal sleep. If the FHR pattern is unclear, the test is considered inconclusive or unsatisfactory.

> **Clinical Alert**
>
> 1. The NST is a screening test and can easily and safely be done once a week.
> 2. A nonreactive NST (positive test) should be followed by a CST.
> 3. Ultrasound studies and a fetal biophysical profile (FBP) may be needed after a nonreactive NST.

Interfering Factors

A false-positive result may be caused by fetal sleep, preterm gestation, smoking before the NST, congenital anomalies, or maternal use of drugs such as central nervous system depressants or β-blockers.

Procedure

1. Assess maternal vital signs, last oral intake (including medicines or street drugs), smoking history, and fetal movement history.
2. Apply the external fetal monitor with the woman positioned off her back (semi-Fowler's or side-lying position).
3. After 26 weeks of gestation, this assessment of the FHR pattern without contractions evaluates fetal oxygenation. Fetal movement may or may not be identified by the woman during the test. If gestation is <26 to 30 weeks, the fetus may not meet the criteria for a reactive NST yet still be a healthy fetus.
4. It is no longer recommended to feed the woman before this test because of the possibility of emergency delivery. Glucose does not alter the FHR pattern.

Patient Preparation

1. Explain the reason for testing and the procedure.
2. See Chapter 1 guidelines for safe, effective, informed *pretest* care.

Patient Aftercare

1. Interpret test outcome and counsel appropriately.
2. Follow Chapter 1 guidelines for safe, effective, informed *posttest* care.

FETAL ACTIVITY-ACCELERATION DETERMINATION (FAD)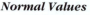

Normal Values

Normal (negative) result: reactive test.

Criteria are similar to those for NST, but fetal movement is also required: ≥3 discrete body or limb movements within 30 minutes. In a reactive test (well-oxygenated fetus), spontaneous accelerations of FHR begin at about the time of onset of fetal movement. This effect expresses the condition of the neurologic system and its effect on fetal movement and FHR.

Explanation of Test

This test often is not distinguished from NST, but it is different. In the fetal activity-acceleration determination (FAD), both acceleration of FHR and fetal movement are evaluated.

Procedure

The procedure is the same as for the NST. The woman is given a button to push when fetal movement occurs; pushing the button causes a mark to appear on the monitor strip.

Clinical Implications

1. A nonreactive FAD is ascertained in the same manner as for the NST. Results are of questionable validity before 30 weeks' gestation. Follow-up for a nonreactive test should include an ultrasound study to assess fetal movement and tone.
2. A nonreactive FAD (positive result) is associated with greater risk for hypoxia.

Clinical Alert

Fetal movement tends to decrease as gestation progresses.

Patient Preparation

1. Explain the reason for testing and fetal heart rate monitoring.
2. This test may be performed in a hospital or clinic setting.
3. Follow Chapter 1 guidelines for safe, effective, informed *pretest* care.

Patient Aftercare

1. Interpret test outcome and counsel appropriately. Explain need for possible follow-up ultrasound.
2. Follow Chapter 1 guidelines for safe, effective, informed *posttest* care.

CONTINUOUS FETAL HEART RATE (FHR) MONITORING ●

Continuous FHR monitoring is done (both before and during labor) to evaluate postterm pregnancy (>42 weeks); after a nonreactive stress or nonstress test; and in the presence of diabetes, pre-eclampsia, chronic hypertension, or intrauterine growth retardation. Normally, the rate is 100 to 150 bpm; accelerations occur with fetal movement, and a return of variable decelerations to baseline occurs with no evidence of decreasing baseline variability or increasing baseline rate.

FETAL BIOPHYSICAL PROFILE (FBP) (BIOPHYSICAL PROFILE [BPP]) ●

Normal Values

Fetal well-being score: ≥8 points, based on normal NST, normal fetal muscle tone, movement, and breathing; and normal volume of amniotic fluid.

Explanation of Test

These measurements, used in the later stages of pregnancy, assess fetal well-being. The biophysical profile (BPP or FBP) is more accurate and provides more information than the nonstress test (NST) alone. It can identify the fetus affected by hypoxia who is at risk of in utero distress or death. In high-risk pregnancies, testing usually begins by 32 to 34 weeks' gestation; those with severe complications may require earlier testing, at 26 to 28 weeks.

The FBP uses ultrasound imaging to evaluate 5 distinct parameters: (1) evidence of FHR (cardiac rate) accelerations (NST); (2) muscle tone; (3) fetal movement; (4) fetal breathing; (5) volume of amniotic fluid. Based on sonographic evidence during a typical 20- to 30-minute survey, each parameter is assigned a value of 0 to 2 points (2 is optimal). The maximum number of points obtainable is 10; a score of 10 indicates a normal test without evidence of fetal distress. Generally, a score ≥8 indicates fetal well-being.

The FBP also provides the clinician with valuable information regarding fetal size and position, number of fetuses, placental location and grade, and evidence of specific fetal activities such as micturition and eye movements. In some laboratories, Doppler examinations of the umbilical vessels assess utero-fetal blood flow. Abnormal Doppler blood flow studies (umbilical artery velocimetry) may be detected before changes in the NST, contraction stress test (CST), or FBP are detectable. Abnormal Doppler umbilical artery waveforms become indicative of acidosis, hypoxia, and intrauterine growth retardation, which result in a poor outcome.

Procedure

1. Explain the test purpose and procedure.
2. Position the patient on her back (as for an obstetric sonogram). Apply a gel (coupling agent) to the skin of the lower abdomen. Then, move the ultrasound transducer across the lower abdominal area to visualize the fetus and surrounding structures.
3. Examining time is usually 30 minutes but may vary because of fetal age or fetal state.
4. An CST or NST is also done at this time (see pages 1092 and 1093).

Clinical Implications

1. Variables that influence FBP include fetal age, fetal behavioral states, maternal or fetal infection, hypoglycemia, hyperglycemia, and postmaturity.
2. If a fetus of <36 weeks' gestation does not have stable behaviors, a longer test may be needed. Infection may cause absence of FHR reactivity and fetal breathing movements. Frequency of fetal breathing increases during maternal hyperglycemia and decreases with maternal hypoglycemia. Other variables that influence FBP include use of therapeutic or nontherapeutic chemicals. Magnesium sulfate may decrease or eliminate fetal breathing movements and decrease FHR variability. Nicotine can decrease the profile parameters, and cocaine may also decrease the FBP score.
3. When the 5 major biophysical profile parameters can be observed, the fe-

tus is considered to be free of distress. Generally, a score of 8 points indicates fetal well-being.

4. A score of 6 points is equivocal, and retesting should be done in 12 to 24 hours.

5. A score <4 indicates the potential for or the existence of fetal distress. This warrants further testing or the consideration of delivery.

> ### Clinical Alert
>
> To assess the fetal state properly, a sonographic determination of eye movement and respiration must be done. If no eye movements and no respirations are evident, the fetus is most likely asleep. On the other hand, if rapid eye movement is evident but breathing is absent, the fetus is probably in distress.

Patient Preparation
1. Explain the test purpose and procedure and include information regarding each part of the test and how it relates to fetal well-being.
2. See Chapter 1 guidelines for safe, effective, informed *pretest* care.

Patient Aftercare
1. Interpret test outcomes and counsel appropriately.
2. Follow Chapter 1 guidelines for safe, effective, informed *posttest* care.

FETOSCOPY

Normal Values
Normal fetal development; no evidence of fetal developmental defects.
Negative for hemophilia types A and B and sickle cell anemia.

Explanation of Test
Fetoscopy allows direct observation of the fetus and facilitates fetal blood or skin sampling. It provides direct visualization of the fetus in 2- to 4-cm segments so that developmental defects can be more accurately identified. The fetal blood sample allows early diagnosis of disorders such as hemophilia A and B that are not amenable to detection through other means. Fetoscopy can also be used for therapeutic interventions such as shunt placement.

Procedure
1. Obtain a properly signed and witnessed consent form.
2. Apply a local anesthetic to the mother's abdominal wall. Meperidine (Demerol), which crosses the placenta, may be given to the mother to quiet the fetus.

3. Real-time ultrasound locates the proper maternal abdominal area through which to make a small incision and then to insert the cannula and the trocar into the uterus.
4. After cannulation into the uterus, an endoscope (fetoscope), consisting of a fiberoptic light source and a self-focusing lens, is inserted and then manipulated for optimal views and fetal tissue sampling (eg, skin, blood, amniotic fluid).

Clinical Implications
Abnormal results reveal

1. Fetal malformation
2. Neural tube defects
3. Sickle cell anemia
4. Hemophilia

Clinical Alert

1. Fetoscopy poses an increased risk of spontaneous abortions (5% to 10%), preterm delivery (10%), amniotic fluid leakage (1%), and intrauterine fetal death.
2. Fetoscopy is offered only when the woman has a significant risk of producing a child with a major birth defect that can be diagnosed only by this method.

Patient Preparation

1. The woman (or couple) should receive genetic counseling and a thorough explanation of the procedure and its benefits, risks, and limitations.
2. Antibiotics may be ordered before the procedure to prevent amnionitis. Assess for possible allergies to the drug.
3. See Chapter 1 guidelines for safe, effective, informed *pretest* care.

Patient Aftercare

1. Monitor mother and fetus for several hours after the procedure. Institute proper protocols for dealing with maternal blood pressure and pulse changes, FHR abnormalities, uterine activity, vaginal bleeding, or amniotic fluid leakage. Rh-negative mothers should receive human $Rh_o(D)$ immune globulin (RhoGAM) unless the fetus is also known to be Rh-negative. Repeat ultrasound studies should be done to check amniotic fluid volume and fetal viability.
2. Instruct the patient to report any pain, bleeding, infected cannulation site, amniotic fluid leakage, or fever (amnionitis).
3. Interpret test outcomes and counsel appropriately.
4. Follow Chapter 1 guidelines for safe, effective, informed *posttest* care.

PERCUTANEOUS UMBILICAL BLOOD SAMPLING (PUBS) (CORDOCENTESIS) ●

Normal Values
No abnormalities noted (see explanation of test)

Explanation of Test
Percutaneous umbilical blood sampling (PUBS) has somewhat replaced fetoscopy because of the risk factors associated with the latter test. PUBS, for which research is ongoing, is probably a safer and easier way to sample blood from the umbilical cord of the fetus in utero. Fetal blood can be examined for hemophilias, hemoglobinopathies, fetal infections, chromosomal abnormalities, fetal distress, fetal drug levels, and other blood studies.

Procedure
Scanning with a real-time ultrasound transducer (placed into a sterile glove) is used to provide landmarks as a 20- to 25-gauge spinal needle is first inserted into the maternal abdomen and then guided into the fetal umbilical vein, 1 to 2 cm from the cord insertion site on the placenta. The fetal blood sample is aspirated into a syringe containing anticoagulant to prevent clotting of the sample.

> ### ● Clinical Alert
>
> Risks include transient fetal bradycardia, maternal infection, premature labor, and a 1% to 2% incidence of fetal loss.

Clinical Implications
1. Abnormal blood results reveal
   A. Hemoglobinopathies
   B. Hemophilia A or B, other coagulation disorders
   C. Fetal infection
   D. Chromosome abnormalities, genetic diseases
   E. Isoimmunization
   F. Metabolic disorders
   G. Fetal hypoxia

Patient Preparation
1. Explain the procedure and its purpose, benefits, and risks. Obtain a properly signed and witnessed consent form.
2. Assist with relaxation exercises during the procedure. Antibiotics may be given before the test to prevent infection.
3. See Chapter 1 guidelines for safe, effective, informed *pretest* care.

Patient Aftercare

1. Monitor maternal vital signs and perform external fetal monitoring or an NST. Observe for signs of fetal distress.
2. An ultrasound should be done 1 hour after the procedure to ensure that there is no bleeding at the puncture site.
3. Interpret test outcomes and counsel appropriately about fetal therapy (eg, red blood cell and platelet transfusion and drug treatment).
4. Follow Chapter 1 guidelines for safe, effective, informed *posttest* care.

CHORIONIC VILLUS SAMPLING (CVS)   ●

Normal Values
Negative for chromosomal and DNA abnormalities
No fetal metabolic enzyme or blood disorders

Explanation of Test
Chorionic villus sampling (CVS) can provide very early diagnosis of fetal genetic or biochemical disorders. CVS involves extraction of a small amount of tissue from the villi of the chorion frondosum. This tissue is composed of rapidly proliferating trophoblastic cells that ultimately form the placenta. Although not a part of the fetus, these villi cells are genetically identical to the fetus and are considered fetal rather than maternal in origin.

CVS differs from amniocentesis in several respects. In amniocentesis, the cells examined are desquamated fetal cells; the cells sampled in CVS divide rapidly and are easier to culture. For this reason, karyotyping (see Chapter 11) can be performed much more rapidly, and diagnostic information can be provided within 24 hours, much faster than with amniotic fluid cells. Also, CVS can be performed much earlier in pregnancy, typically at 7 to 11 gestational weeks, whereas amniocentesis usually is performed after 16 weeks' gestation, with results available several weeks later. CVS therefore has the advantage of providing first-trimester diagnosis, which is of particular value when the choice is made to abort an affected fetus, because first-trimester terminations of pregnancy are medically safer.

CVS reveals chromosome abnormalities and fetal metabolic or blood disorders. However, because CVS cannot be used to measure α_1-fetoprotein (AFP), it cannot detect neural tube defects or other disorders associated with increased AFP levels.

Indications for CVS include the following:
1. Abnormal ultrasound test
2. Fetus at risk for detectable Mendelian disorders:
   A. Tay-Sachs disease
   B. Hemoglobinopathies
   C. Cystic fibrosis
   D. Muscular dystrophy
3. Birth of previous child with evidence of chromosome abnormality

4. Parent with known structural chromosomal rearrangement
5. Diagnosis of fetal infection

Procedure (Transcervical Method)

1. The mother is positioned on her back to permit ultrasound documentation of the number of fetuses in utero and their viability and localization of trophoblastic tissue. The patient may be asked either to maintain a full bladder or to empty the bladder so as to optimize the sampling path. A bimanual pelvic examination is often performed concurrently with this preliminary ultrasound examination.
2. The patient then assumes a lithotomy position. A sterile speculum is inserted after the vagina has been cleansed with an iodine-based antiseptic.
3. A sterile flexible catheter with a stainless steel obturator is introduced into the vaginal canal and advanced through the cervical canal into the trophoblastic tissue. The catheter is visually tracked by the ultrasound device.
4. Once the catheter is in place, a syringe is attached to the end of the catheter to extract approximately 5 cc of tissue. The tissue sample is immediately examined under a low-power microscope to determine that both quantity and tissue quality are acceptable.
5. Up to 3 passes of the catheter may be made. A new, sterile catheter is used each time. After sufficient tissue has been gathered, ultrasound is again used to monitor fetal viability. The tissue sample is used for chromosome and enzyme analysis and for other tests.
6. A transabdominal method may also be used. This method is similar to amniocentesis, except that the thin-walled needle is inserted into the chorionic bed.

Clinical Implications

Abnormal CVS results indicate
1. Abnormal fetal tissue
2. Chromosome abnormalities
3. Fetal metabolic and blood disorders
4. Fetal infection

Patient Preparation

1. Genetic counseling typically precedes any CVS procedure.
2. Explain the purpose, procedure, and risks of the test.
3. A legal consent form must be signed by the mother and the father of the baby and must be properly witnessed.
4. The patient must drink four 8-oz glasses of water about 1 hour before the examination. The patient should not void until instructed to do so.
5. Obtain baseline measurements of maternal vital signs and FHR.
6. Advise the patient that she may experience cramping as the catheter passes through the cervical canal.
7. Help the patient to relax.
8. See Chapter 1 guidelines for safe, effective, informed *pretest* care.

Patient Aftercare

1. Monitor maternal vital signs and FHR every 15 minutes for the first hour after test completion.
2. Instruct the patient to notify her physician if she experiences abdominal pain, vaginal bleeding or abnormal discharge, elevated temperature, chills, or amniotic fluid leakage.
3. Interpret test outcomes and counsel appropriately. Rh-negative women usually receive RhoGAM.
4. Support the mother and significant others during decision making. Provide opportunity for questions and discussion.
5. Follow Chapter 1 guidelines for safe, effective, informed *posttest* care.

Clinical Alert

1. CVS is not considered a routine alternative to amniocentesis. The safety of the CVS procedure is related to the experience and skill of the examiner. In experienced hands, the rates of complications and fetal loss are only slightly greater than for amniocentesis. Risks include leakage of amniotic fluid, bleeding, intrauterine infection, spontaneous abortion, maternal tissue contamination of specimen, Rh isoimmunization, and fetal death (5%).
2. Transcervical CVS is difficult in patients who have a fundal placental implantation site or an extremely retroflexed or anteflexed uterus. In such patients, a transabdominal approach similar to that used for amniocentesis is employed.
3. CVS cannot detect neural tube defects or other disorders associated with abnormal maternal serum.
4. Some specialists advise that this procedure be reserved for evaluation of conditions that present relatively high genetic risks (eg, hemoglobinopathies).
5. An increased risk for severe limb deformities is associated with this procedure.

●AMNIOTIC FLUID STUDIES

OVERVIEW OF AMNIOTIC FLUID STUDIES ●

The fluid filling the amniotic sac serves several important functions. It provides a medium in which the fetus can readily move, cushions the fetus against possible injury, helps maintain an even temperature, and provides useful information concerning the health and maturity of the fetus. The origin of amniotic fluid is not completely understood. In early pregnancy, it is produced by the amniotic membrane covering the placenta and the cord. As the pregnancy progresses, it is believed to be primarily a byproduct of fetal pulmonary secretions, urine, and metabolic products from the intestinal tract.

Initially, amniotic fluid is produced from the amniotic membrane cells. Later, most of it is derived from the maternal blood. The volume increases from about 30 ml at 2 weeks' gestation to 350 ml at 20 weeks. After 20 weeks, the volume ranges from 500 to 1000 ml. The volume of amniotic fluid changes continuously because of fluid movement in both directions through the placental membrane. Later in pregnancy, the fetus contributes to amniotic fluid volumes through excretion of urine and swallowing of amniotic fluid. The fetus also absorbs up to 400 ml of amniotic fluid every 24 hours through its gastrointestinal tract, bloodstream, and umbilical artery exchanges across the placenta. Probably, some fluid also is absorbed by direct contact with the fetal surface of the placenta. Amniotic fluid contains castoff cells from the fetus and resembles extracellular fluid with suspended, undissolved material. It is slightly alkaline and contains albumin, urea, uric acid, creatinine, lecithin, sphingomyelin, bilirubin, fat, fructose, epithelial cells, leukocytic enzymes, and lanugo hair.

When amniocentesis is advised early in pregnancy (15 to 18 weeks), the purpose is to study the fetal genetic makeup and to determine developmental abnormalities. Fetal cells are separated from the amniotic fluid by centrifugation and are placed in a tissue culture medium so that they can be grown and harvested for subsequent karyotyping to identify chromosome disorders. Testing in the third trimester is done to determine fetal age and well-being, to study blood groups, or to detect amnionitis.

AMNIOCENTESIS ●

Normal Values
Normal amniotic fluid constituents and properties vary according to the age of fetus and the laboratory methods used; pH is slightly alkaline. See descriptions of individual tests.

Explanation of Test
Amniotic fluid is aspirated by means of a needle guided through the mother's abdominal and uterine walls into the amniotic sac. Amniocentesis is preferably performed after the 15th week of pregnancy. By this time, amniotic fluid levels have expanded to 150 ml, so a 10-ml specimen can be aspirated. If the purpose of amniocentesis is to ascertain fetal maturity, it should be done after the 35th week of gestation.

Amniocentesis provides a method to detect fetal abnormalities in situations in which the risk of an abnormality may be high. The test can evaluate fetal hematologic disorders, fetal infections, inborn errors of metabolism, and sex-linked disorders. It is not done to determine the sex of the fetus simply out of curiosity.

Chromosomal abnormalities and neural tube defects such as anencephaly, encephalocele, spina bifida, and myelomeningocele can be determined, as can estimates of fetal age, fetal well-being, and pulmonary maturity.

The development of significant maternal Rh antibody titers or a history of previous erythroblastosis can be an indication for amniocentesis.

High-Risk Parents Who Should Be Offered Prenatal Diagnosis

1. Women of advanced maternal age (≥35 years) who are at risk for having a child with a chromosome abnormality, especially trisomy 21. At maternal age 35 to 40 years, the risk for Down syndrome is 1% to 3%; at age 40 to 45, it is 4% to 12%; and at >45 years, the risk is 12% or greater.
2. Women who have previously borne a trisomic child or a child with another kind of chromosome abnormality
3. Parents of a child with spina bifida or anencephaly or a family history of neural tube disorders
4. Couples in which either parent is a known carrier of a balanced translocation chromosome for Down syndrome
5. Couples in which both partners are carriers for a diagnosable metabolic or structural autosomal recessive disorder. More than 70 inherited metabolic disorders can be diagnosed by amniotic fluid analysis.
6. Couples in which either partner or a previous child is affected with a diagnosable metabolic or structural dominant disorder
7. Women who are presumed carriers of a serious X-linked genetic disorder
8. Couples from families whose medical history reveals mental retardation, ambiguous genitalia, or parental exposure to toxic environmental agents (eg, drugs, irradiation, infections)
9. Couples whose personal and family medical history reveals multiple miscarriages, stillbirths, or infertility
10. Parents with anxiety about the health status of potential offspring
11. Women with abnormal ultrasound results.

Clinical Implications

1. Elevated AFP can indicate possible neural tube defects as well as multiple gestations, fetal death, abdominal wall defects, teratomas, Rh sensitization, and fetal distress.
2. Decreased AFP is associated with fetal trisomy 21 (Down Syndrome).
3. Creatinine levels are reduced in fetal prematurity. At 37 weeks of gestation, creatinine in amniotic fluid should be >2 mg/dl.
4. Increased or decreased total amniotic fluid volumes are associated with certain types of arrested fetal development.
5. Increased bilirubin levels are associated with impending fetal death. (See page •• for normal values.)
6. Amniotic fluid color changes are associated with fetal distress and other disorders such as chromosome abnormalities.
7. Sickle cell anemia and thalassemia can be detected through analysis of amniotic fibroblast DNA.
8. X-linked disorders are not routinely diagnosed in utero. However, because these disorders affect only men, the fetal sex may need to be de-

termined when the mother is a known carrier of the X-linked gene in question (eg, hemophilia, Duchenne's muscular dystrophy).

9. Screening for carrier state or affected fetus is done through chromosomal testing.

10. The presence of some of the more than 100 detectable metabolic disorders can be detected in the amniotic fluid sample. Examples include Tay-Sachs disease, Lesch-Nyhan syndrome, Hunter's syndrome, Hurler's syndrome, and various hemoglobinopathies. Hereditary metabolic disorders are caused by absence of an enzyme due to gene deletion or by alteration of the structure or synthesis of an enzyme due to gene mutation. If the enzyme in question is expressed in amniotic fluid cells, it can potentially be used for prenatal diagnosis. An unaffected fetus would have a normal enzyme concentration, a clinically normal carrier of the gene defect would have perhaps half of the normal enzyme level, and an affected fetus would have a very small amount or none of the enzyme.

11. For these disorders in which an abnormal protein is not expressed in amniotic fluid cells, other test procedures are necessary, such as *DNA restriction endonuclease analysis.*

> **Clinical Alert**
>
> The in utero diagnosis of many genetic disorders may lead the parents to consider abortion as an option for dealing with an unfavorable situation. Because this can be a very difficult and controversial choice, communication between the parents and the health care team must take place in a nonjudgmental, nonthreatening manner.

Interfering Factors

1. Fetal blood contamination can cause false-positive results for AFP.
2. False-negative and false-positive errors in karyotyping can occur.
3. Polyhydramnios may falsely lower bilirubin values as a result of dilution.
4. Hemolysis of the specimen can alter test results.
5. Oligohydramnios may falsely increase some amniotic fluid analysis values, especially bilirubin; this can lead to errors in predicting the clinical status of the fetus.

Procedure (in Combination With Ultrasound)

1. The patient is positioned on her back with her arms behind her head to prevent touching of the abdomen and the sterile field during the procedure (see Obstetric Sonogram in Chapter 13).

2. Ultrasound scanning is performed before the procedure to assess fetal number, viability, and position. An appropriate pocket of amniotic fluid is localized on the scan. The tap site should be located away from the fetus, from the site of umbilical cord insertion, and from any thick placental segments.

3. The skin is thoroughly cleansed with an appropriate antiseptic solution and properly draped with sterile drapes. A local anesthetic is slowly injected at the puncture site.

4. A 3.5-inch spinal needle (20- to 22-gauge) with stylet is then advanced through the abdominal and uterine walls into the amniotic sac but away from the fetus and, when possible, from the placenta. Continuous ultrasound surveillance is used to track the position of the fetus. Should the fetus move close to the needle, the needle is withdrawn.

5. Once the needle is properly positioned, the stylet is removed and a syringe is attached to the needle to permit aspiration of a 20- to 30-ml specimen. The first 0.5 ml of aspirated fluid is discarded to prevent contamination by maternal cells or blood.

6. After the needle is withdrawn, an adhesive bandage is placed over the puncture site. Postprocedure ultrasound scanning confirms fetal viability.

7. The amniotic fluid specimen must be placed in a sterile brown or foil-covered silicone container to protect it from light and thereby prevent breakdown of bilirubin. Label the container properly. Include the estimated weeks of gestation and the expected delivery date. Deliver the sample to the laboratory immediately.

8. The laboratory work-up for genetic diagnoses usually takes 2 to 4 weeks to complete. However, specimens obtained for determination of fetal age (eg, creatinine) take 1 to 2 hours; determinations of lecithin/sphingomyelin (L/S) ratio and phosphatidyl glycerol take 3 to 4 hours; Gram stain to rule out infection takes one-half hour, and cultures take 48 to 72 hours.

9. The procedure may have to be repeated if no amniotic fluid is obtained or if there is failure of cell growth or culture results are negative.

10. Record the type of procedure done, date, time, name of physician performing the test, maternal-fetal response, and disposition of specimen.

Patient Preparation

1. Elective genetic counseling should include a discussion of the risk of having a child with a genetic defect, and problems (eg, depression, guilt) associated with selective abortion. The father should be present and should be a partner in the decision-making process. In genetic counseling, the parents must not be coerced into undergoing abortion or sterilization; this should be an individual choice.

2. Explain test purpose, procedure, and risks; assess for contraindications.

3. A properly signed and witnessed legal consent form must be obtained.

4. Instruct the patient to empty her bladder just before the test.

5. Obtain baseline measurements of fetal and maternal vital signs. Monitor fetal signs for 15 minutes.

6. Alert the patient to the possibility that short-lived feelings of nausea, vertigo, and mild cramping may occur during the procedure. Help the patient to relax.

7. See Chapter 1 guidelines for safe, effective, informed *pretest* care.

Patient Aftercare

1. Check maternal blood pressure, pulse, respiration, and fetal heart tone every 15 minutes for the first half-hour after test completion. Palpate the uterine fundus to assess fetal and uterine activity; monitor for 20 to 30 minutes with an external fetal monitor, if one is available.
2. Position the mother on her left side to counteract supine hypotension and to increase venous return and cardiac output.
3. Instruct the patient to notify her physician if she experiences amniotic fluid loss, signs of onset of labor, redness and inflammation at the insertion site, abdominal pain, bleeding, elevated temperature, chills, unusual fetal activity, or lack of fetal movement.
4. Follow Chapter 1 guidelines for safe, effective, informed *posttest* care.

Clinical Alert

1. Fetal loss attributable to the procedure is <0.5%. Repeat amniocentesis is necessary in 0.1% of cases.
2. Fetal complications include
   A. Spontaneous abortion
   B. Injury to the fetus (fetal puncture)
   C. Hemorrhage
   D. Infection
   E. Rh sensitization if fetal blood enters the mother's circulation
3. Maternal complications include
   A. Hemorrhage
   B. Hematomas
4. This test is contraindicated in women with a history of premature labor or incompetent cervix and in the presence of placenta previa or abruptio placentae. If the amniotic fluid is bloody (blood is usually of maternal origin), and if a significant number of fetal cells (Kleihauer-Betke positive smear) are present in the amniotic fluid of an Rh-negative mother, administration of RhoGAM should be considered. Some doctors prefer to administer RhoGAM to all Rh-negative mothers after amniocentesis, unless they are already sensitized at that time.
5. Families need to know that prenatal diagnoses based on amniotic fluid assay are not infallible; sometimes, results do not reflect the true fetal status. Findings from amniocentesis cannot guarantee a normal or an abnormal child; they can only determine the relative likelihood of specific disorders within the limits of laboratory measurements. Some conditions cannot be predicted by this method, including nonspecific mental retardation, cleft lip and palate, and phenylketonuria (PKU).

(continued)

(Clinical Alert continued)

6. Accurate and optimally safe results from amniocentesis are possible only if the following protocols are observed:
   A. Gestation ≥15 weeks
   B. Ultrasound monitoring to locate suitable pools of amniotic fluid, outline the placenta, exclude the presence of a multiple pregnancy, and accurately estimate fetal maturity. These considerations are necessary to correctly interpret AFP values in amniotic fluid and maternal blood.
   C. Precise and meticulous amniocentesis technique, including use of 20- or 22-gauge needle.
   D. Maximum of 2 needle insertion attempts for a single tap.
   E. Administration of RhoGAM for the Rh-negative woman.
7. Cytogenetic analysis can produce results that are 99.8% accurate.
8. Techniques have been developed for performing amniocentesis in the presence of twin fetuses. Amniotic fluid is aspirated from one of the amniotic sacs, and a small amount of contrast material is injected into the sac. When the adjacent sac is tapped and produces clear amniotic fluid, the clinician is assured that each sac has been tapped and each fetus will be accurately assessed.
9. An anteriorly located placenta does not preclude amniocentesis. A thin portion of placenta can be traversed during amniocentesis with no apparent increase in postamniocentesis complications.

AMNIOTIC FLUID α_1-FETOPROTEIN (AFP) ●

Normal Values
12 to 16 weeks: 10 µg/ml
Normal values vary considerably according to age of fetus and laboratory methods used. Values peak at 12 to 16 gestational weeks and then gradually decline to term.

Background
α_1-Fetoprotein (AFP) is synthesized by the embryonic liver and is the major protein (glycoprotein) found in fetal serum. It resembles albumin in molecular weight, amino acid sequence, and immunologic characteristics. However, it is not normally detectable after birth. Ordinarily, high levels of fetoproteins are found in the developing fetus and low levels exist in maternal serum and amniotic fluid.

Explanation of Test
The amniotic fluid AFP test is used to diagnose fetal neural tube defects (malformations of the central nervous system); fetoprotein leaks into the amniotic fluid during such pregnancies. The causes of neural tube defects are not known; however, a genetic component is assumed because an increased risk

of recurrence exists. Neural tube defects usually exhibit polygenic (multifactional) traits. In cases of anencephaly and open spina bifida, both MS-AFP and amniotic fluid AFP concentrations are abnormal by the 18th week of gestation.

Additionally, AFP measurements have been used as indicators of fetal distress; in such cases, both amniotic fluid AFP and MS-AFP may be increased. However, final confirmation must come from further studies.

Procedure
In the laboratory, amniotic fluid is analyzed for concentration of AFP.

Clinical Implications
Increased amniotic AFP levels are associated with

1. Neural tube defects such as anencephaly (100% reliable), encephalocele, spina bifida, and myelomeningocele (90% reliable)
2. Congenital nephrosis
3. Omphalocele
4. Turner's syndrome with cystic hydromas
5. Gastrointestinal tract obstruction
6. Missed abortion
7. Fetal distress
8. Imminent or actual fetal death
9. Severe Rh immunization
10. Esophageal or duodenal atresia
11. Fetal liver necrosis secondary to herpes virus infection
12. Sacrococcygeal teratoma
13. Spontaneous abortion
14. Trisomy 13
15. Urinary obstruction (eg, fetal bladder neck obstruction with hydronephrosis)
16. Cystic fibrosis

Interfering Factors
1. Fetal blood contamination causes increased AFP.
2. Increased AFP is associated with multiple pregnancies.
3. False-positive (0.1% to 0.2%) results may be associated with fetal death, twins, or genetic anomalies, but sometimes no explanation can be given for the results.

Clinical Alert

1. Any couple who have already produced a child with a neural tube defect should be offered antenatal studies in anticipation of future pregnancies. If 1 parent has spina bifida, the pregnancy should be closely monitored.
2. High-resolution ultrasound studies must be used to confirm increased AFP levels.

Patient Preparation

1. Explain the test purpose and the meaning of positive and negative test results.
2. Provide for genetic counseling.
3. See Chapter 1 guidelines for safe, effective, informed *pretest* care.

Patient Aftercare

1. Interpret test outcomes, counsel, and monitor appropriately.
2. Follow Chapter 1 guidelines for safe, effective, informed *posttest* care.

AMNIOTIC FLUID TOTAL VOLUME   ●

Normal Values

Weeks of Gestation	Average Volume (ml)
12	approximately 50
15	350
20	450
25	750
30 to 35	1500

After 35 weeks, values decrease to 1250 ml at term.

Explanation of Test

Measurement of amniotic fluid total volume is helpful for estimating the changes in total amounts of certain substances that circulate in the amniotic fluid, including bilirubin, creatinine, and surface-active agents. Knowledge of total amniotic fluid volume is important because marked changes in the amount of amniotic fluid can decrease the predictive value of serial concentration measurements of specific substances. This measurement is most important when test results do not agree with the clinical picture.

Procedure

1. A sample of amniotic fluid is studied with the use of a solution of para-aminohippuric acid (PAH) for absorbency and dilution to calculate the probable amniotic fluid volume in milliliters.
2. Amniotic fluid total volume is corrected by multiplying the measured levels of specific substance times actual fluid volume divided by average volume (for gestation age).

Clinical Implications

1. Polyhydramnios (increased amniotic fluid, >2000 ml) is suggested by a total intrauterine volume >2 standard deviations above the mean for a given gestational age. It is estimated that 18% to 20% of fetuses in such pregnancies have congenital anomalies, the 2 most common being anencephaly and esophageal atresia (fetal swallowing is greatly impaired). The remainder have involvement secondary to Rh disease, diabetes, or other, unknown causes. Polyhydramnios is also associated with multiple births (eg, twins).

2. Oligohydramnios (reduced volume of amniotic fluid, <300 ml) is suggested by a total intrauterine volume >2 standard deviations below the mean occurring before the 25th week of gestation. A disturbance of kidney function caused by renal agenesis or kidney atresia can result in oligohydramnios (fetal urination is impaired). After 25 weeks, the suspected causes of decreased amniotic fluid volume are premature rupture of membranes, intrauterine growth retardation, and postterm pregnancy.

> ### Clinical Alert
>
> If either polyhydramnios or oligohydramnios is suspected, the fetus should be screened with ultrasound to detect physical anomalies.

Patient Preparation
1. Explain the reason for amniotic fluid testing and the meaning of results.
2. See Chapter 1 guidelines for safe, effective, informed *pretest* care.

Patient Aftercare
1. Interpret amniotic fluid test results and monitor appropriately.
2. Follow Chapter 1 guidelines for safe, effective, informed *posttest* care.

AMNIOTIC FLUID INDEX (AFI)   ●

Normal Values
At term, the AFI is usually between 8 and 18 cm. Values <5 cm indicate oligohydramnios, and those >24 cm indicate polyhydramnios.

Clinical Implications
Oligohydramnios and polyhydramnios are indicators of poor outcome in pregnancy. An amniotic fluid index (AFI) lower than the 2.5th percentile for a certain gestational age is considered to represent oligohydramnios. Oligohydramnios can indicate chronic uteroplacental insufficiency or renal anomaly. An AFI higher than the 97.5th percentile for a certain gestational age is considered to indicate polyhydramnios. Polyhydramnios is associated with upper gastrointestinal tract obstruction or malformation (eg, tracheal-esophageal fistula, hydrops fetalis).

Procedure
1. The pregnant woman lies supine with displacement of the uterus to the left. The abdomen is divided into 4 quadrants.
2. Ultrasound is used to locate the largest pocket of amniotic fluid in each of the 4 quadrants, and each pocket is measured vertically. The 4 values are added together to obtain the AFI. The advantage of this test is that serial follow-up measurements can be done.

Interfering Factors
False-positive results can occur in a severely dehydrated woman.

Patient Preparation
1. Explain the reason for the AFI procedure.
2. See Chapter 1 guidelines for safe, effective, informed *pretest* care.

Patient Aftercare
1. Explain the test results to patient. Prepare the patient for follow-up procedures or need for delivery of the infant.
2. Follow Chapter 1 guidelines for safe, effective, informed *posttest* care.

AMNIOTIC FLUID CREATININE

Normal Values
A value >2 mg/dl or >177 μmol/L indicates fetal maturity (at 37 weeks) if maternal creatine is normal.

Background
Creatinine, a byproduct of muscle metabolism found in amniotic fluid, reflects increased fetal muscle mass and the ability of the maturing kidney (ie, glomerular filtrating system) to excrete creatinine into the amniotic fluid. The amniotic fluid creatinine concentration progressively increases as pregnancy advances. The mother's blood creatinine level should be known before the amniotic fluid creatinine value is interpreted.

Explanation of Test
Creatinine indicates fetal physical maturity and correlates reasonably well with the level of lung maturity. Normal lung development is dependent on normal kidney development. As pregnancy progresses, the amniotic fluid creatinine level increases. A value of 2 mg/dl is accepted as an indicator that gestation is at 37 weeks or more. However, the use of this value alone to assess maturity is not advised for several reasons. A high creatinine concentration may reflect fetal muscle mass but not necessarily kidney maturity. For example, a large fetus of a diabetic mother may have high creatinine levels because of increased muscle mass. Conversely, a small, growth-retarded infant of a hypertensive mother may have low creatinine levels because of decreased muscle mass. Creatinine levels can be misleading if they are used without other supporting data. So long as maternal blood creatinine levels are not increased, amniotic fluid creatinine measurements have a certain degree of reliability if they are interpreted in conjunction with other maturity studies.

Procedure
1. A 0.5-ml amniotic fluid sample is necessary.
2. Protect the specimen from direct light.

3. Obtain maternal venous blood sample.

Clinical Implications

Creatinine levels lower than expected may occur in the following situations:

1. Early in the gestational cycle (not yet at 37 weeks)
2. Fetus smaller than normal (growth-retarded)
3. Fetal kidney abnormalities
4. Prematurity

Interfering Factors

Causes of elevated amniotic fluid creatinine concentrations that are not consistent with gestational age include abnormal maternal creatinine, diabetes, and pre-eclampsia.

Patient Preparation

1. Explain the purpose of the test.
2. See Chapter 1 guidelines for safe, effective, informed *pretest* care.

Patient Aftercare

1. Interpret test outcomes and counsel appropriately.
2. Follow Chapter 1 guidelines for safe, effective, informed *posttest* care.

AMNIOTIC FLUID LECITHIN/SPHINGOMYELIN RATIO
(L/S RATIO; SURFACTANT COMPONENTS)

Normal Values

A ratio of 2:1 or greater indicates pulmonary maturity.

Background

Lecithin and sphingomyelin have detergent (surfactant) ability. These substances, produced by lung tissue, stabilize the neonatal alveoli to prevent their collapse on expiration and consequent atelectasis. The amount of lecithin in amniotic fluid is less than the amount of sphingomyelin until 26 weeks of gestation; at 30 to 32 weeks gestation, the 2 lipid values are about equal. At 35 weeks, lecithin level rises abruptly, but sphingomyelin stays constant or decreases slightly. Saturated phosphatidylcholine, a subfraction of total lecithins, is a major surface-active component of lung surfactant.

Explanation of Test

The relationship between the phospholipids and the surface-active agents, lecithin and sphingomyelin, is used as an index of fetal lung maturity. If early delivery is anticipated because of conditions such as diabetes, premature rupture of membranes, maternal hypertension, placental insufficiency, or erythroblastosis (Rh disease), the lecithin/sphingomyelin (L/S) ratio can be used to predict whether the fetal lung will function properly at birth. When early delivery is necessary for fetal viability, the result may be prematurity, pulmonary immaturity, or perinatal mortality. The L/S ratio should be determined on all repeat cesarean sections before delivery to ascertain when fetal lungs are functionally mature. Sphingomyelin exhibits surface-active properties in the lung but plays no role in the surfactant system except to be used as a convenient marker.

Procedure

At least 3 ml of amniotic fluid must be withdrawn or collected from a free flow of fluid from the vagina in cases of ruptured membranes. The fluid is centrifuged and prepared for analysis, and the results are read in a reflectance densitometer. The L/S ratio is then calculated.

Clinical Implications

1. A decreased L/S ratio (<1.5:1) is often associated with pulmonary immaturity and respiratory distress syndrome (RDS).
2. An L/S ratio of >2:1 signifies fetal lung maturity. The occurrence of RDS is extremely unlikely.
3. An L/S ratio between 1.5:1 and 1.9:1 indicates possible mild-to-moderate RDS (50% risk).
4. Fetuses of women with insulin-dependent diabetes develop RDS at higher ratios. The L/S ratio should be ≥3.5:1 for these infants.

Clinical Alert

1. If the L/S ratio is <1.5:1, it is preferable to delay induced delivery until the fetal lung becomes more mature.
2. Fetal lung maturity appears to be regulated by hormonal factors, some stimulatory and others possibly inhibitory. For this reason, hormones such as betamethasone (Celestone) are given in two doses, administered 12 to 18 hours apart, if premature labor occurs.
3. Under certain stressful conditions, premature fetal lung maturation may be seen. This accelerated fetal lung maturation is thought to be a protective mechanism for the preterm fetus should delivery actually occur.
   A. Premature rupture of the membranes. Prolonged rupture of the membranes (after 72 hours) has an acute negative effect on lung maturation.
   B. Acute placental infarction
   C. Placental insufficiency
   D. Chronic abruptio placentae
   E. Renal hypertensive disease caused by degenerative forms of diabetes
   F. Cardiovascular hypertensive disease associated with drug abuse
   G. Severe pregnancy-induced hypertension
4. Delayed fetal lung maturation may be seen in the following conditions. In these instances, a higher L/S ratio (>3:5) may be necessary to ensure adequate fetal lung maturity.
   A. Infants born to mothers with insulin-dependent diabetes
   B. Infants born to mothers with nonhypertensive glomerulonephritis
   C. Hydrops fetalis
5. A *lung profile* of amniotic fluid to evaluate lung maturity looks not only for lecithin but also for 2 other phospholipids—phosphatidyl

(continued)

(Clinical Alert continued)

glycerol (PG) and phosphatidylinositol (PI). PI increases in the amniotic fluid after 26 to 30 weeks of gestation, peaks at 35 to 36 weeks, and then decreases gradually. PG appears after 35 weeks and continues to increase until term; measurements are classified as positive PG or negative PG. The lung profile is a useful adjunct in evaluating the L/S ratio. It appears that lung maturity can be confirmed in most pregnancies if PG is present (positive) in conjunction with an L/S ratio of 2:1. PG may provide stability that makes the infant less susceptible to RDS when experiencing hypoglycemia, hypoxia, or hypothermia. The PG measurement is especially useful in borderline cases and in class A, B, and C diabetes when pulmonary maturation is delayed.

Interfering Factors

1. High false-negative rates
2. Unpredictability or borderline values
3. Unpredictability of contaminated blood specimens
4. Occasional false-positive values associated with conditions such as Rh disease, diabetes, or severe birth asphyxia

Patient Preparation

1. Explain the reason for testing and the meaning of results.
2. See Chapter 1 guidelines for safe, effective, informed *pretest* care.

Patient Aftercare

1. Interpret test results and counsel appropriately.
2. Follow Chapter 1 guidelines for safe, effective, informed *posttest* care.

AMNIOTIC FLUID SHAKE TEST (FOAM STABILITY TEST) ●

Normal Values

Positive: Persistence of a foam ring for 15 minutes after shaking (at an amniotic fluid–alcohol dilution of 1:2) indicates lung maturity.

Explanation of Test

The shake test is a qualitative measurement of the amount of pulmonary surfactant contained in the amniotic fluid. It is quick and inexpensive. It is a "bedside test" of lung maturity. In an obstetric emergency, an immediate decision about delivery can be made. The advantage of this test over the L/S ratio is that a physician, technician, or nurse can perform it and the results are highly reliable. The L/S ratio usually is not determined when the shake test is positive, because the shake test also indicates fetal maturity. A table of dilutions is used to determine the stage of lung maturity.

Procedure

The test is based on the ability of amniotic fluid surfactant to form a complete ring of bubbles on the surface of the amniotic fluid in the presence of 95%

ethanol. A mixture of 95% ethanol and amniotic fluid is placed in an appropriate container and shaken for 15 seconds. A commercial kit may be used.

Clinical Implications

1. If a complete ring of foam forms and persists for 15 minutes, the test is positive.
2. If no ring of bubbles forms, the test is negative.
3. The test has a high false-negative rate but a low false-positive rate. The L/S ratio must be ≥4:1 for this test to be positive.

Interfering Factors

1. Blood or meconium contamination can alter results.
2. Contamination of glassware or reagents can alter test results.

AMNIOTIC FLUID FOAM STABILITY INDEX (FSI)

Normal Values
FSI: >.47

Explanation of Test

The foam stability index (FSI) is a modification of the shake test. It provides a functional measurement of fetal lung maturity based on the surface tension properties of surfactant phospholipids.

Procedure

A fixed amount of undiluted amniotic fluid is mixed with increasing volumes of ethanol. The sample is then shaken and observed for foam. The largest volume of ethanol in which the amniotic fluid can form and support foam is documented. This test is almost as reliable as the L/S ratio in normal pregnancies, and it seems to have a lower false-positive rate than the shake test.

Clinical Implications

FSI of ≥.48 is termed *mature;* a value of ≤.46 is termed *immature.*

Interfering Factors

1. Blood or meconium contamination can produce a false "mature" result.
2. The test is not reliable for amniotic fluid collected from the vagina.

AMNIOTIC FLUID FERN TEST

Normal Values
Positive test for presence of amniotic fluid

Background

Fern production is a result of the concentration of electrolytes, especially sodium chloride, in the cervical glands; it is under the control of estrogen.

Close to term, amniotic fluid shows a typical fern pattern similar to that seen in cervical mucus; this indicates a predominantly estrogen effect rather than progesterone.

Explanation of Test

This study differentiates urine from amniotic fluid. It is done to determine whether the fluid passed is urine or prematurely leaked amniotic fluid. This is a relatively fast and inexpensive test that can be easily done.

Procedure

1. A vaginal examination is done with the use of a sterile speculum.
2. A few drops of fluid are placed on a slide and allowed to dry.
3. A fern or "palm leaf" pattern (arborization) is sought under the microscope (See Fig. 16-1).

Clinical Implications

1. A positive test shows the fern pattern indicative of amniotic fluid.
2. A negative test shows no ferning or crystallization; this indicates little or no estrogen effect.
3. No fern pattern is seen if the specimen is urine.

Interfering Factors

Blood contaminating the specimen inhibits fern formation.

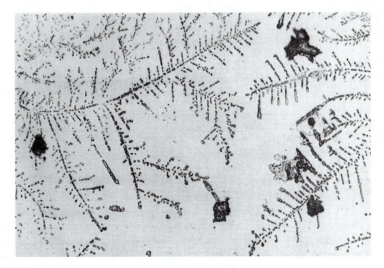

FIGURE 16-1
Amniotic fluid "ferning" as seen under microscope.

> **Clinical Alert**
>
> Urine can also be differentiated from amniotic fluid if the fluid is tested for the presence of urea, nitrogen, potassium, and creatinine and the absence of AFP.

Patient Preparation
1. Explain test purpose and procedure.
2. See Chapter 1 guidelines for safe, effective, informed *pretest* care.

Patient Aftercare
1. Interpret test results and counsel appropriately.
2. Follow Chapter 1 guidelines for safe, effective, informed *posttest* care.

AMNIOTIC FLUID COLOR ●

Normal Values
Colorless or pale straw-yellow color

Explanation of Test
Amniotic fluid specimens may vary from no color to a pale straw-yellow color. White particles of vernix caseosa from fetal skin and lanugo hair may be present. In certain disorders such as missed abortion, chromosomally abnormal fetus, and fetal anencephaly, the amniotic fluid color is altered.

Procedure
Every amniotic fluid specimen should be visually inspected for color.

Clinical Implications
1. *Yellow* amniotic fluid indicates blood incompatibility, erythroblastosis fetalis, or presence of bile pigment released by red blood cell hemolysis (fetal bilirubin).
2. *Dark yellow* aspirate indicates probable fetal involvement.
3. *Red* color indicates blood, in which case it must be determined whether the blood is from the mother or the fetus. Fetal blood in the amniotic fluid is of grave concern.
4. *Green, opaque* fluid indicates meconium contamination. The fetus passes meconium because of hyperperistalsis in response to a stressor that may be very transient or may be more serious and protracted (eg, hypoxia). A very good correlation states that the more meconium present, the more severe and immediate the stressor. Additional assessments, such as amnioscopy and amniography, must be made to determine whether the fetus is experiencing ongoing episodes of hypoxia or other stressors. Green color can also indicate erythroblastosis but is not necessarily indicative of it.

5. *Yellow-brown, opaque* fluid may indicate intrauterine death and fetal maceration (although not necessarily from erythroblastosis), oxidized hemoglobin, or maternal trauma.

Clinical Alert

1. Before the amniotic membranes have ruptured, color changes and staining can be observed through amnioscopy. During this procedure, an amnioscope is placed into the vagina and against the fetal presenting part. The amniotic fluid is then visualized through the amniotic membranes. Problems with amnioscopy include inadvertent rupture of membranes, insufficient dilatation of the cervix and consequent difficulty inserting the amnioscope, intrauterine infection, and occasional difficulty in interpreting amniotic fluid color. The test may also be difficult to perform if the patient is in active labor.

2. Meconium staining may also be observed when an amniocentesis is done. After the membranes have ruptured, meconium staining may be observed in the vaginal discharge. Once meconium staining is identified, more assessments (eg, fetal heart rate patterns) must be made before delivery is contemplated to determine whether the fetus is experiencing ongoing episodes of hypoxia.

3. The presence of meconium in the amniotic fluid is normal in breech presentations.

Patient Preparation
1. Explain the purpose of the test and the procedure if amnioscopy is done.
2. See Chapter 1 guidelines for safe, effective, informed *pretest* care.

Patient Aftercare
1. Interpret the test result, counsel, and monitor appropriately.
2. Follow Chapter 1 guidelines for safe, effective, informed *posttest* care.

AMNIOTIC FLUID BILIRUBIN OPTICAL DENSITY (OD) ●

Normal Values
OD ≤0.02 at 450 absorbances, nm wavelength by Liley method, or 0.025 mg/dl by the Diazo method, indicates maturity.

Background
Bilirubin is a pigment acquired by the amniotic fluid during its circulation through the gastrointestinal tract. Bilirubin may be found in amniotic fluid as early as the 12th week of gestation. It reaches its highest concentration between 16 and 30 weeks. As the pregnancy continues, the amount of bilirubin progressively decreases until it finally disappears near term. Bilirubin levels increase in the presence of erythroblastotic fetuses and fetuses with anencephaly or intestinal obstruction.

Explanation of Test

This measurement is used to monitor the fetal state in a Rh_o-negative pregnant woman who has a rising anti-Rh_o antibody titer. The rising titer is synonymous with Rh erythroblastosis fetalis or hemolytic disease of the newborn (HDN). This determination usually is not made before 20 to 24 weeks' gestation because no therapy is available to the fetus before that time. Close to term, the amniotic fluid bilirubin pigment concentration normally decreases in the absence of Rh sensitization.

Determination of optical density (OD) is only 1 of several laboratory methods used to measure bilirubin. The degree of hemolytic disease falls into 3 zones, using OD measurement and a wavelength (absorbance) of 450 nm (Liley's method or Diazo method).

1. If OD = 0.28 to 0.46 (zone 1, low zone, 2+ OD) at 28 to 31 weeks, the fetus will not be affected or will have very mild hemolytic disease.
2. If OD = 0.47 to 0.90 (zone 2, middle zone, 3+ OD), there is a moderate effect on the fetus. The fetal age and the trend in OD indicate the need for intrauterine transfusion and early delivery.
3. If OD = 0.91 to 1.0 (zone 3, high zone, 4+ OD), the fetus is severely affected and fetal death is a possibility. In this case, a decision concerning delivery or intrauterine transfusion, depending on the age of the fetus, should be made. After 32 to 33 weeks of gestation, early delivery and extrauterine treatment are preferred.
4. An OD <0.04 indicates fetal maturity and well-being.

Procedure

1. Five to 10 ml of amniotic fluid should be collected in a light-proof container.
2. The fluid should be sent to the laboratory immediately.
3. The specimen may be refrigerated for up to 24 hours. It can be frozen if a longer time will elapse before analysis.
4. Avoid blood in the specimen. If initial aspiration produces a bloody fluid, the needle should be repositioned to obtain a specimen free of red cells. If a blood-free specimen cannot be obtained, the specimen must be examined at once, before hemolysis occurs.

Clinical Implications

Increased OD is found in

1. Erythroblastosis fetalis
2. Other fetal hemolytic diseases
3. Maternal infectious hepatitis
4. Maternal sickle cell crisis

Interfering Factors

1. Blood, hemoglobin, or meconium in the specimen can produce inaccurate results.
2. Maternal use of steroids interferes with the test.

3. Exposure of the amniotic fluid to light compromises the test.
4. Fetal acidosis interferes with the test.

Clinical Alert

1. Difficulty in interpretation occurs frequently. Findings must be interpreted by a knowledgeable person who can recognize pitfalls. Obtain clinical information and study other laboratory data.
2. After 30 weeks' gestation, the Liley test result is usually combined with an assessment of fetal lung maturity (L/S ratio) to assist in the decision of whether to induce delivery.
3. A bilirubin level that fails to decline as expected or increases indicates that the fetal status is deteriorating.

Patient Preparation
1. Explain the test purpose and the meaning of test results.
2. See Chapter 1 guidelines for safe, effective, informed *pretest* care.

Patient Aftercare
1. Interpret test outcome, monitor, and counsel appropriately.
2. Follow Chapter 1 guidelines for safe, effective, informed *posttest* care.

AMNIOTIC FLUID AND DESATURATED PHOSPHATIDYLCHOLINE (DSPC) ●

Normal Values
A DSPC of >500 µg/dl indicates fetal maturity.

Background
Desaturated phosphatidylcholine (DSPC) is the major component (50%) of fetal pulmonary surfactant. The concentration in amniotic fluid can be measured by separating DSPC from unsaturated lecithin. Phosphatidylcholine is the second most surface-active component of surfactant.

Explanation of Test
This test is a direct measure of primary phospholipid in surfactant and is used in the assessment of fetal lung maturity.

Procedure
Amniotic fluid is obtained and examined for the primary phospholipid (DSPC).

Clinical Implications
1. Normal levels are consistent with fetal lung maturity and indicate a negligible risk of RDS.
2. Low levels are associated with immaturity and a high risk of RDS.

Interfering Factors
Results may be altered by changes in amniotic fluid volume (oligohydramnios or polyhydramnios).

Patient Preparation
1. Explain the test purpose and the amniotic fluid sampling procedure.
2. See Chapter 1 guidelines for safe, effective, informed *pretest* care.

Patient Aftercare
1. Interpret test outcomes, monitor, and counsel appropriately.
2. Follow Chapter 1 guidelines for safe, effective, informed *posttest* care.

BIBLIOGRAPHY ●

American College of Obstetricians and Gynecologists and American Academy of Pediatrics: Guidelines for Prenatal Care, 4th ed. Washington, DC, ACOG/AAP, 1997

Boland M: Overview of perinatally transmitted HIV infection. Nurs Clin North Am 31(1): 155–163, March 1996

Cunningham F, McDonald RC, Gant AF, Leveno KJ, Gilstrap LC: Williams Obstetrics, 19th ed. Norwalk, CT, Appleton & Lange, 1993

Depp R: Clinical evaluation of fetal status, in Danforth's Obstetrics and Gynecology, 7th ed. Philadelphia, JB Lippincott, 1997

Escher-Davis L: Fetal fibronectin: A biochemical marker for preterm labor. Voice. Association of Women's Health, Obstetrics & Neonatal Nurses (AWHONN) 14(3): 1–7, April 1996

Gabbe, Niebyl, Simpson (eds): Obstetrics: Normal and problem pregnancies. New York, Churchill Livingstone, 1991

Kochinour N: Normal pregnancy and prenatal care, in Danforth's Obstetrics and Gynecology, 7th ed. Philadelphia, JB Lippincott, 1997

Kuppermann M, Goldberg JD, Lease Jr RF, Washington AE: Who should be offered prenatal diagnoses? The 35-year-old question. Jounal of Public Health 89(2): 160–163, February 1999

Murray M: Antepartal and Intrapartal Fetal Monitoring, 2nd ed. Alberquerque, Learning Resources International, 461–467, 1997

Raines DA: Fetal surveillance: Issues and implications. JOGNN 25(7): 559–564, 1996

Scott, Disaia, Hammond, Spellacy (eds): Obstetrics and Gynecology, 6th ed. Philadelphia, JB Lippincott, 1990

Tietz N: Clinical Guide to Laboratory Tests, 3rd ed. Philadelphia, WB Saunders, 1995

Waller DK, Lustig LS, et al: The association between maternal serum alpha-fetoprotein and pre-term birth, small for gestational age infants, preeclampsia and placental complications. Obstet Gynecol 88(5): 816–822, November 1996

Wilkins-Huag L, Horton J, et al: Antepartum screening in office based practice: Findings from collaborative ambulatory research network. Obstet Gynecol Part I, 88(4): 483–489, October 1996

Wisconsin Association for Perinatal Care: Laboratory Testing During Pregnancy Recommendations of Perinatal Testing Committee, Madison, pp 2–32, April 1997

APPENDICES

APPENDIX A

Standard/Universal Precautions

The term *standard precautions* refers to a system of disease control which assumes that every direct contact with body fluids or tissues is infectious and that all persons exposed to these substances need to protect themselves. Standard precautions are designed to reduce the risk of transmission of microorganisms from both recognized and unrecognized sources of infection in health care facilities. Standard precautions direct safe practice and are designed to protect health care workers, patients, and others from exposure to bloodborne pathogens or other potentially infectious materials from **any** body fluid or *unfixed* human tissue from any person, *living or dead*.

Revised guidelines are based upon new information about infectious disease patterns and modes of transmission. The guidelines, designed to be more user friendly, contain two tiers of precautions. Tier **one,** *Standard Precautions,* is designed to control nosocomial infections and reduce the risk of transmission of both known and suspected infections. Tier **two,** used in addition to standard precautions, includes airborne, droplet, and contact precautions to prevent the spread of highly transmissible and virulent pathogens.

SAFE PRACTICE

When handling specimens and performing or assisting with diagnostic procedures, it is important for all health care workers to protect and *always* take care of themselves *first*. Presume that all patients have hepatitis B, human immunodeficiency virus (HIV), or other potential pathogens, and practice standard precautions consistently. Use special care when collecting, handling, packaging, transporting, storing, and receiving specimens. Initial observations and specimen handling are to be performed under a laminar flow hood, and protective clothing, glasses, and masks are to be worn. These same precautions prevail in the performance of invasive diagnostic procedures. Follow Chapter 1 guidelines for safe, effective, informed pretest, intratest, and posttest care.

Common Categories of Body Substances, and Fluids*, regardless of whether they contain visible blood	
Blood and blood products	Respiratory secretions
Urine	Semen
Vaginal secretions	Synovial fluid
Saliva	Vomitus
Pericardial fluid	Wound or ulcer drainage
Peritoneal fluid	Ascites
Pleural fluid	Amniotic fluid
Cerebrospinal fluid	All excretions except sweat
Gastric fluid	

*Standard precautions should also be used when handling amputated limbs and during removal of body parts (surgery, autopsy, or donation).

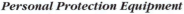

STANADARD PRECAUTION GUIDELINES AND PRACTICES FOR SPECIFIC SITUATIONS

Personal Protection Equipment

Take appropriate barrier precautions when exposure of skin and mucous membranes to blood, blood droplets, or other body fluids is anticipated.

Use protective equipment devices to protect eyes, face, head, extremities, air passages, and clothing. This equipment must always be used during invasive procedures. Ensure proper fit.

Gloves

Wear gloves when collecting and handling specimens; touching blood, urine, other body fluids, mucous membranes, or nonintact skin; or performing vascular access procedures or other invasive procedures.

Wear gloves when handling items or surfaces soiled with blood, urine, or body fluids.

Mandate wearing of gloves when the health care worker's skin is cut, abraded, or chapped; during examination of a patient's oropharynx, gastrointestinal or genitourinary tract, nonintact or abraded skin, or active bleeding wounds; and when cleaning specimen containers or engaged in decontaminating procedures.

Possible exceptions to use of gloves:

When gloves impede palpation of veins for venipuncture (eg, neonates, morbidly obese patients)

In a life-threatening situation where delay could be fatal (wash hands and wear gloves as soon as possible)

Disposable gloves must *be changed:*

When moving between patients

When moving from a contaminated to a cleaner site on a patient or on an environmental surface

When gloves are torn or punctured or their barrier function is compromised (do so as soon as feasible).

> ### Clinical Alert
>
> Gloves, barrier gowns, aprons, and masks are worn only at the site of use. They are disposed of appropriately at the site of use.

Gowns, Masks, and Eye Protection

Wearing of gowns, aprons, and/or lab coats to cover all exposed skin is necessary whenever there is a potential for splashing onto clothing.

Gowns or aprons may *not* be hung and reused.

Wear masks correctly situated over nose and chin and tied at the crown of the head and the nape of the neck. Do not hang the mask around the neck. Change the mask when it becomes moist.

Wear mask, face shields, and goggles (or prescription glasses with side shields) when contamination of eye, nose, or mouth from sepsis is most likely to occur.

Shoe covers should be worn in areas where contamination might occur (eg, operating room, obstetrics or emergency department). These are disposed of at the site of care.

Provide masks, bags, or other ventilation devices as part of emergency resuscitation equipment kept in strategic locations.

Disposal of Medical Wastes

Pour fluids "low and slow" to prevent splash, spray, or aerosol effect.

Take precautions to prevent injuries caused by needles, lancets, scalpels, and other sharp instruments and devices during and after procedures and when disposing of used needles. Do *not* recap needles under normal circumstances.

Dispose of all disposable sharp instruments in specially designed, puncture-resistant containers. Do not recap, bend, break by hand, or remove needles from disposable syringes. Use forceps or cut intravenous tubing if necessary. Use care when transferring "sharps" to another person. Use forceps or put the "sharp" in a receptacle.

Place and transport specimens in leakproof receptacles with solid, tight-fitting covers. Cap ports of containers. Before transport, contaminated materials must be decontaminated or placed in a tightly sealed bag marked with a "biohazard" tag. Biohazard symbols warn of biologic hazards and must be displayed in the presence of these hazardous biologic agents or locations.

Soiled linens and similar items must be placed in leakproof bags before transport.

Placement of Warning Tags and Signs

Properly place warning tags to prevent accidental injury or illness to clinicians who are exposed to equipment or procedures that are hazardous, unexpected, or unusual.

Require warning tags to contain a *signal word* or symbol, such as "Biohazard" or "Biochemical Material," along with the major message, such as "Blood Banking Specimen Inside." All specimens are placed in biohazard bags.

General Environmental Cautions

Use approved antimicrobial soaps between care of individual patients.

Wash hands immediately after removing gloves.

Wash hands and other skin surfaces immediately and thoroughly if contaminated with blood or other body fluids.

Consider saliva to be potentially infectious, even though it has not been implicated in HIV transmission.

Transmission of acquired immunodeficiency syndrome (AIDS) is possible from stool specimens, especially if there is a possibility of blood existing in the stool.

Health care workers with skin lesions or skin conditions should not engage in direct care until the condition clears up or does not present a risk to the patient.

Development of an HIV infection during pregnancy may put the fetus at risk for infection.

In Case of Exposure to Human Immunodeficiency Virus or Hepatitis B Virus

Identify, obtain consent, and test source of exposure (patient with HIV or hepatitis B infection). If the patient refuses consent or the outcome is positive, the clinician or health care worker *must* receive HIV antibody testing immediately.

Advise the HIV-negative worker to seek medical evaluation of any acute febrile illness that occurs within 12 weeks after exposure to HIV and be retested at 6 weeks, 12 weeks, and 6 months after exposure.

Vaccine is available at no cost to health care workers to prevent hepatitis B infection. There is *no* vaccine for HIV.

Hand Washing Protocols

Unless the situation is a true emergency, hands must *always* be washed:

Before and after care activities that involve direct contact
Before surgical or obstetric procedures
Before and after endoscopy
Before and after invasive procedures
Before direct contact with an immunocompromised patient
After contact with body fluids or tissues or with soiled equipment, supplies, or surfaces
After direct contact with patients in isolation units

For more information, refer to:

Garner, JS and the Hospital Infection Control and Practice's Advisory Committee and the Center for Disease Control and Practice: Guidelines for Isolation Precautions in Hospitals. American Journal of Infection Control 24(1):24–44, February 1996

APPENDIX B

Latex and Rubber Allergy Precautions

BACKGROUND

The rise in incidence of latex allergy may be attributed not only to increased use of latex products in patient care (especially since standard/universal precautions were mandated) but also to the manner in which raw latex is now collected and aged. Allergic reactions are caused by latex proteins retained in the finished products, which can show great variations in latex allergen levels. The greatest environmental hazard exposure is produced by latex gloves and the powder from these gloves that becomes airborne.

The US Food and Drug Administration now requires that all medical devices containing natural rubber latex that may directly or indirectly contact the patient display the following statement: "THIS PRODUCT CONTAINS NATURAL RUBBER LATEX."

As allergy to latex products becomes more prevalent, both in the health care setting and in the general environment, it becomes necessary for agencies to institute specific guidelines and protocols to maximize latex-free environments for patients and for health care personnel.

Persons at greatest risk for latex or rubber allergy include

Health care workers (an estimated 17% are affected) and 1% to 3% of the general population

Persons with spina bifida, spinal cord injury, myelodysplasia, or urogenital anomalies (up to 73% are affected)

Individuals with a personal or family history of allergies (including hay fever, bee stings, asthma, pet dander, and food or drug allergies)

Persons with a chronic illness or a history of multiple surgeries

Persons with occupational exposure (eg, rubber industry workers; 10% of those handling or manufacturing rubber are affected)

Persons with atopic dermatitis or eczema

Persons with intraoperative anaphylaxis (for unknown reason)

Increased or continued exposure increases sensitivity to latex allergens and worsens allergic reactions. Patients and health care workers can become sensitized to latex through repeated skin or mucous membrane contact or by inhaling aerosolized glove allergens.

Persons with latex allergies are more likely to react to certain foods, especially bananas, avocados, chestnuts, almonds, kiwi fruit, raw potato, tomato, peach, plum, cherry, melons, celery, apple, pear, and papaya. Latex allergy often begins with a rash on the hands (from gloves). Besides latex allergies, other glove-associated reactions may occur.

Reaction	*Signs and Symptoms*	*Causes*
Irritant contact dermatitis (nonallergic irritation)	Dry, crusty, hard bumps, sores, and horizontal cracks on skin may manifest as itchy dermatitis on the back of the hands under the gloves.	Hand washing, insufficient rinsing, scrubs, antiseptics, glove occlusion, glove powder
Delayed-type hypersensitivity; allergic contact dermatitis; chemical allergy	Red, raised, palpable area with bumps, sores, and horizontal cracks may extend up the forearm. Occurs after a sensitization period. Appears several hours after glove contact and may persist for many days.	Exposure to chemicals used in latex manufacturing, mostly thiurams
Immediate-type hypersensitivity; latex allergy; protein allergy	Wheal and flare response or itchy redness on the skin under the glove. Occurs within minutes, fades away rapidly after removal of the glove. In chronic form may mimic irritant and allergic contact dermatitis.	Exposure to proteins in latex on glove surface and/or bound to powder and suspended in the air, settled on objects, or transferred by touch
	Symptoms can include facial swelling, generalized rashes, nasal, sinus, and eye symptoms, asthma and respiratory distress. In rare cases, anaphylactic shock may occur and is life-threatening. Generalized hives, bronchospasm, hypotension, extreme facial edema and laryngeal edema, tachycardia may occur	

American Nurses Association latex allergy work place information series, Washington, DC, 1996.

LATEX ALLERGY PRECAUTIONS TO PROTECT THE PATIENT ●

Strategies and protocols include the following:

1. Identify allergic patients (those with a history of problems related to condoms, latex gloves, balloons, toys, and so on); allergy testing (see Chapter 8) may be desirable. Communicate and document data appropriately.

2. Sensitive persons should carry autoinjectable epinephrine (Epi-Pen), nonlatex gloves, and emergency medical instructions; should wear a medical alert bracelet; should avoid *all* forms of latex; and should alert clinicians, family, friends, and employers of the diagnosis and need to avoid latex.

3. *Never* wear powdered latex gloves when caring for a sensitized patient.

4. Avoid contact of latex with tissue (eg, wounds, mucous membranes, vaginal skin). *Practice proper hand washing.*

   NOTE: *Assembling and maintaining a cart with latex-free supplies and equipment may be desirable to facilitate safe patient care.*

5. Use latex-free products; examples include

   A. Gloves
   B. Endotracheal tubes
   C. Suction and wound drainage tubes and reservoir systems
   D. Catheters
   E. Blood pressure cuffs
   F. Stethoscopes

   NOTE: *If latex-free blood pressure cuffs and stethoscopes are not available, shield the patient's arm with stockinette and apply the cuff over it. Small-diameter (finger-sized) stockinette can be used to cover stethoscope tubing, leads, and so on.*

   G. Temperature probe covers, tape, dressings, "Ace" wraps
   H. Monitoring equipment and supplies (leads, pulse oximeter probes, and cables)

6. Remove rubber stoppers from vials before withdrawing or reconstituting contents. Rinse syringes with sterile water or saline before use.

7. Remove latex ports from intravenous tubing and replace with stopcocks or nonlatex plugs. Tape ports shut if no other alternative is available. Replace ports on intravenous therapy bags with nonlatex ports.

8. Keep resuscitation equipment and emergency supplies and medications readily accessible at all times in the event that anaphylaxis occurs. (*Caution: Some resuscitation supplies and equipment may contain latex.*)

9. Instruct the patient about latex-containing supplies, both medical and nonmedical, that could pose problems (see lists).

> **Clinical Alert**
>
> Symptoms of anaphylaxis include a dangerous drop in blood pressure, dyspnea, flushed facial appearance, swelling (of throat, tongue, and nose), and loss of consciousness.

Medical Supply Items That Frequently Contain Latex[1]	*Home And Community Items That Frequently Contain Latex[1]*
Anesthesia equipment/ET tubes, airways	Balloons/toys/water toys and equipment
Bandaids/tapes	Art supplies (paint, glue, rubber bands, erasers, ink), kitchen gloves, appliance cords
Bed protectors	
Blood pressure tubing/cuffs	Balls (tennis, koosh)
Bulb syringes	Carpet backing/rubber floors/cushions
Catheters (many and varied types)	Appliques (clothing); Spandex
Dressings/elastic wraps	Elastic in socks, underwear, etc.
G-tubes/drains	Condoms/diaphragms
IV access (Y-sites, tourniquets, adapters, etc.)	Crutch accessories (tips/grips)
	Dental braces, chewing gum
OR masks, hats, shoe covers	Diapers/incontinence products
Oxygen masks/cannula/resuscitation devices	Feeding nipples/pacifiers
	Handles on garden/sporting equipment
Suction equipment	Tires, hoses
Reflex hammers, syringes	

[1]NOTE: These lists are not all-inclusive. If latex content is unknown, checking with the manufacturer or supplier before use is strongly advised.

10. The Spina Bifida Association of America publishes updated lists of latex-containing products twice a year. Their address is Spina Bifida Association of America, 4590 MacArthur Boulevard NW, Suite 250, Washington, DC 20007-4226 (telephone 800-621-3141).

STRATEGIES AND PRECAUTIONS TO REDUCE THE RISK OF LATEX ALLERGIES FOR HEALTH CARE PERSONNEL ●

Latex sensitivity is a health hazard for health care workers. It is one problem with many causes. Consequently, workplace practices to reduce the incidence of exposure are absolutely necessary to maintain a safe environment for clinicians. Early identification and treatment of latex allergy are important. Allergists who specialize in treating latex allergy may recommend patch testing with glove chemical sensitizers and latex allergy testing by serum or skin prick tests. Blood tests are not as sensitive or as accurate as the skin tests.

Ways to reduce the risk of latex allergies for health care workers include the following:

Use latex-free gloves (powder-free gloves low in protein and chemical allergens) whenever possible and keep exposure to latex at a minimum.

▌ **Clinical Alert**

Simply using powder-free gloves will not solve the problem.

Wear gloves that are appropriate for the task; remove gloves at least hourly to air and dry the hands.

Wash, rinse, and dry hands thoroughly after removal of gloves or between glove changes.

Use a pH-balanced soap and avoid cutaneous contact with damaging chemicals.

Apply nonsensitizing products (outside of the workplace) to restore the skin's lipid barrier.

Wear synthetic gloves or cotton liners with latex work gloves for wet work, if possible.

Seek early medical diagnosis to prevent further allergy complications.

Advocate for and promote purchase of latex-free products that are of comparable function and quality.

Observe all latex allergy precautions that apply to patients. Natural latex is found in many consumer products, such as condoms, balloons, tires, rubber toys, nipples, and pacifiers.

Clinical Alert

Protocols for management of an allergic reaction:

Airway maintenance	Diphenhydramine
Administration of oxygen	Steroids
Volume expansion (intravenous	Epinephrine
lactated Ringer's or normal saline solution)	Aminophylline

MANDATES AND STRATEGIES FOR EMPLOYEES REGARDING LATEX OR RUBBER ALLERGY

1. Include latex allergy information as part of new-employee orientation and conduct inservice education training on this subject.

2. Occupational Safety and Health Administration "Right To Know" laws require employers to inform employees of potentially dangerous substances in the workplace on an annual basis.

3. Make available current latex allergy information in newsletters; latex allergy should be on the agenda of risk management committees.

4. Make alternative products available.

5. Establish protocols and procedures related to latex allergy to ensure a safe practice environment.

6. Protect latex-allergic workers from being required to work in latex-contaminated areas.

NOTE: *In March, 1999, the U.S. House of Representatives conducted a hearing to examine latex allergy recommendations of OSHA, CDC, and the FDA (Food and Drug Administration). A copy of the hearing materials can be obtained at the House Education and Workforce Subcommittee's website at:www.house.gov/eeo/hearings/106th/oi/oihearings.htm*

APPENDIX C

Intravenous Conscious Sedation Precautions

BACKGROUND

Increasing numbers of patients are receiving short-term intravenous sedation (often referred to as *conscious sedation*) for invasive diagnostic procedures. Even though the anesthesiologist or attending physician assumes responsibility for intravenous conscious sedation, other clinicians may administer the drugs and monitor the patient's response to these drugs. Advantages of conscious sedation include short, rapid recovery, early ambulation, patient preference for light sleep and amnesia, patient cooperation during procedure, vital reflexes remain, vital signs stable, and infrequent complications.

GUIDELINES FOR CARING FOR PATIENTS UNDERGOING INTRAVENOUS CONSCIOUS SEDATION

Patient Preparation

1. Explain the purpose of the intravenous conscious sedation before administering the medication. It is most commonly used for these diagnostic procedures: breast biopsy, bronchoscopy, ERCI, colonoscopy, gastroscopy, cardiac catherization, EP studies, and cystoscopy.

2. Assess the patient's health status, history of chronic or acute conditions, previous diagnostic test results, level of understanding, orientation, mental status, and ability to cooperate with the procedure. Screen and identify patients who are at high risk for development of complications.

3. Explain the process and procedure and what the patient may experience. Use a calm, caring manner. Normal fasting and liquid intake is required. Controversy exists about fasting time frames. Check your agency policy. For adults, fast 6 to 8 hours; clear liquids: 2 to 3 hours. For infants under 6 months, fast 4 to 6 hours (this includes milk, formula, and breast milk); clear liquids 2 hours.

4. Before beginning the procedure, establish an intravenous line and keep it open with the ordered intravenous solution. Monitor patency of the line.

5. Monitor vital signs, electrocardiogram, pulse oximetry, and patient response according to established guidelines before administering conscious sedation. Such information should be documented.

6. Provide a safe and caring environment. In anticipation of emergency situations, have resuscitation equipment and supplies readily available.

7. Follow Chapter 1 guidelines for safe, effective, informed *pretest* care.

Intratest Patient Care During Intravenous Conscious Sedation Procedure

1. Continuously assess pain or discomfort and sedation levels at frequent established intervals.
2. Administer sedation and analgesics as ordered, often in incremental doses.
3. Recognize physiologic effects of agents used for intravenous conscious sedation. These medications include the following, among others:
   - **A.** Meperidine hydrochloride (Demerol)
   - **B.** Diazepam hydrochloride (Valium)
   - **C.** Midazolam hydrochloride (Versed)
   - **D.** Lorazepam (Ativan)
   - **E.** Droperidol (Inapsine)
   - **F.** Fentanyl citrate
   - **G.** Morphine sulfate
4. Monitor the intravenous site for infiltration and for the general effects of the medication.
5. Anticipate and monitor for potential complications of intravenous conscious sedation. Arrhythmias should be promptly reported and treated if necessary. Many of these medications are respiratory depressants, mandating frequent respiratory assessments. If oxygen saturation drops below acceptable levels (90%), sedation may need to be held or reversed. Have intravenous reversal agents such as naloxone (Narcan) and flumazenil (Romazicon) readily available. Oxygen therapy may be necessary until oxygen saturation levels, vital signs, neurologic response, and cardiac rhythms are acceptable.
6. Rapidly and appropriately respond to emergencies during administration of, or recovery from, intravenous conscious sedation.
7. Document carefully and completely all observations, including medications and dosages. Record unexpected outcomes and follow-up care.
8. Follow Chapter 1 guidelines for safe, effective, informed *intratest* care.

Patient Aftercare

1. Monitor vital signs, electrocardiogram, pulse oximetry, neurologic signs, and patient response according to establish guidelines.
2. Monitor the patient after the procedure until the patient is stable and reactive to preprocedure levels.
3. Provide both verbal and written posttest instructions. Intravenous sedation may not completely wear off for several hours. Patients should *not:*
   - **A.** Drive or operate power machinery or tools for at least 24 hours.
   - **B.** Consume alcoholic beverages or make legal decisions for 24 hours.
   - **C.** Smoke—if the patient is a smoker, emphasize the risks of smoking in the postsedation state (ie, falling asleep).
   - **D.** Take tranquilizers, pain medications, or other medications that may interact with drugs used for intravenous sedation without first contacting the physician.
4. Provide instructions for posttest care and the need for contacting the physician if any unexpected outcomes should occur.
5. Evaluate the patient for readiness for discharge. Provide a safe transport or discharge in the presence of a responsible adult.
6. Follow Chapter 1 guidelines for safe, effective, informed *posttest* care.

Diazepam (Valium)	Midazolam (Versed)	Promethazine (Phenergan)	Meperidine (Demerol)	Droperidol (Inapsine)	Fentanyl (Sublimaze)
ACTION					
Central nervous system depressant, amnesic	Central nervous system depressant; 3–4 times as potent as diazepam	Antihistamine effect, sedative, antiemetic, anticholinergic	Narcotic analgesic, 50–100 mg sedative; 60–80 mg	Major tranquilizer; no analgesic properties; produces cognitive dissociation—a sense of detachment; antiemetic	Narcotic analgesic sedative
INTRAVENOUS DOSAGE GUIDELINES					
2.5-mg to 10-mg increments with or without narcotics. Wait 3 min before redosing. Onset 2–3 min. Reduce dose by one third when an opioid is being used concomitantly.	Initial dose should be as low as 0.5–1 mg over at least 2–3 min, not to exceed 5 mg. Wait at least 2 min before redosing. Give in small increments after initial dose. Onset 1–2 min; decrease dose if given with narcotic (by 25%–30% in healthy adult, by	25–50 mg, no more than 25 mg/min; decrease dose in elderly.	10-mg increments slowly. Titrate to desired effects; decrease dose in elderly or debilitated patient.	1.25–2.5 mg; decrease dose in elderly. Onset in 3–10 min. Peak action in 30 min.	0.05–2 μg/kg, titrating time to patient response. Onset of sedation is 1–3 min; onset of analgesia may not be noted for several minutes.

(continued)

(Continued) Diazepam (Valium)	Midazolam (Versed)	Promethazine (Phenergan)	Meperidine (Demerol)	Droperidol (Inapsine)	Fentanyl (Sublimaze)
	55%–60% in elderly or debilitated patient.				Causes analgesia, respiratory depression, euphoria. Use cautiously with bradycardia, seizures, lactation, cardiac arrest, or shock (rare).

PRECAUTIONS

Diazepam (Valium)	Midazolam (Versed)	Promethazine (Phenergan)	Meperidine (Demerol)	Droperidol (Inapsine)	Fentanyl (Sublimaze)
Increased effects if taking central nervous system depressants, alcohol, cimetidine, or disulfiram. Avoid in patients with renal disease.	Contraindicated in patients with narrow-angle glaucoma.	Increased effects with monoamine oxidase inhibitors, barbiturates, narcotics, hypnotics, tricyclic antidepressants, alcohol; decreased effects with oral anticoagulants and heparin. Use with great caution in children. Because of anticholinergic actions, use with caution in patients with asthma, narrow-angle glaucoma, prostatic hypertrophy, or bladder neck outlet obstruction.	Contraindicated if patient has taken a monoamine oxidase inhibitor within past 14 days; may precipitate severe and irreversible reaction and death; decrease dose if given with other narcotic, barbiturate, tranquilizer, tricyclic anti-depressant, or sedative. Use with caution in patients with supraventricular	Potentiates narcotics and other central nervous system depressants. Produces mild α-adrenergic block.	

tachycardia; may
cause increase
in ventricular
response.
Duration of
analgesic effect
is 30–60 min.
Duration of
respiratory
depression is >1 h
unless a reversal
agent is used.

APPENDIX D

Examples of Conversions to Systéme International (SI) Units

Component	System	Present Reference Intervals	Present Unit	Conversion Factor	SI Reference Intervals	SI Unit Symbol
Alanine aminotransferase (ALT)	Serum	5–40	U/L	1.00	5–40	U/L
Albumin	Serum	3.9–5.0	mg/dl	10	39–50	g/L
Alkaline phosphatase	Serum	35–110	U/L	1.00	35–110	U/L
Aspartate aminotransferase (AST)	Serum	5–40	U/L	1.00	5–40	U/L
Bilirubin	Serum					
Direct		0–0.2	mg/dl	17.10	0–4	μmol/L
Total		0.1–1.2	mg/dl	17.10	2–20	μmol/L
Calcium	Serum	8.6–10.3	mg/dl	0.2495	2.15–2.57	mmol/L
Carbon dioxide, total	Serum	22–30	mEq/L	1.00	22–30	mmol/L
Chloride	Serum	98–108	mEq/L	1.00	98–108	mmol/L
Cholesterol	Serum					
Age <29 yr		<200	mg/dl	0.02586	<5.15	mmol/L
30–39 yr		<225	mg/dl	0.02586	<5.80	mmol/L
40–49 yr		<245	mg/dl	0.02586	<6.35	mmol/L
>50 yr		<265	mg/dl	0.02586	<6.85	mmol/L
Complete blood count	Blood					
Hematocrit						
Men		42–52	%	0.01	0.42–0.52	1
Women		37–47	%	0.01	0.37–0.47	1

Red cell count								
Men		4.6–6.2 × 10⁶	/mm³	10⁶	4.6–6.2 × 10¹² /L			
Women		4.2–5.4 × 10⁶	/mm³	10⁶	4.2–5.4 × 10¹²/L			
White cell count		4.5–11.0 × 10³	/mm³	10⁶	4.5–11.0 × 10⁹/L			
Platelet count		150–300 × 10³	/mm³	10⁶	150–300 × 10⁹/L			
Cortisol	Serum							
8ᴀᴍ		5–25	µg/dl	27.59	140–690	nmol/L.		
8ᴘᴍ		3–13	µg/dl	27.59	80–360	nmol/L.		
Cortisol	Urine	20–90	µg/24 hr	2.759	55–250	nmol/24 hr		
Creatine kinase	Serum							
High CK group (black men)		50–250	U/L	1.00	50–520	U/L		
Intermediate CK group (nonblack men, black women)		35–345	U/L	1.00	35–345	U/L		
Low CK group (nonblack women)		25–145	U/L	1.00	25–145	U/L		
Creatinine kinase isoenzyme, MB fraction	Serum	>5	%	0.01	>0.05	1		
Creatinine	Serum							
Men		0.4–1.3	mg/dl	88.40	35–115	µmol/L		
Women		0.7–1.3	mg/dl	88.40				
		0.4–1.1	mg/dl	88.40				
Digoxin, therapeutic	Serum	0.5–2.0	ng/ml	1.281	0.6–2.6	nmol/L		
Erythrocyte indices	Blood							
Mean corpuscular volume (MCV)		80–100	microns³	1.00	80–100	fl.		
Mean corpuscular hemoglobin (MCH)		27–31	pg	1.00	27–31	pg		
Mean corpuscular hemoglobin concentration (MCHC)		32–36	%	0.01	0.32–0.36	1		

(continued)

Examples of Conversions to Systéme International (SI) Units (*Continued*)

Component	System	Present Reference Intervals	Present Unit	Conversion Factor	SI Reference Intervals	SI Unit Symbol
Ferritin	Serum					
Men		29–438	ng/ml	1.00	29–438	µg/L
Women		9–219	ng/ml	1.00	9–219	µg/L
Folate	Serum	2.5–20.0	ng/ml	2.266	6–46	nmol/L
Follicle-stimulating hormone (FSH)	Serum					
Children		12 or <	mIU/ml	1.00	12 or <	IU/L
Men		2.0–10.0	mIU/ml	1.00	2.0–10.0	IU/L
Women, follicular		3.2–9.0	mIU/ml	1.00	3.2–9.0	IU/L
Women, midcycle		3.2–9.0	mIU/ml	1.00	3.2–9.0	IU/L
Women, luteal		2.0–6.2	mIU/ml	1.00	2.0–6.2	IU/L
Gases, arterial	Blood					
PO_2		80–95	mm Hg	0.1333	10.7–12.7	kPa
PCO_2		37–43	mm Hg	0.1333	4.9–5.7	kPa
Glucose	Serum	62–110	mg/dl	0.05551	3.4–6.1	mmol/L
Iron	Serum	50–160	µg/dl	0.1791	9–29	µmol/L
Iron-binding capacity	Serum					
TIBC		230–410	µg/dl	0.1791	41–73	µmol/L
Saturation		15–55	%	0.01	0.15–0.55	1
Lactic dehydrogenase	Serum	120–300	U/L	1.00	120–300	U/L
Luteinizing hormone	Serum					
Men		4.9–15.0	mIU/ml	1.00	4.9–15.0	IU/L
Women, follicular		5.0–25	mIU/ml	1.00	5.0–25	IU/L

		3.1–13	mIU/ml	1.00	3.1–31	IU/L
Women, luteal						
Magnesium	Serum	1.2–1.9	mEq/L	0.4114	0.50–0.78	mmol/L
Osmolality	Serum	278–300	mOsm/kg	1.00	278–300	mmol/kg
Osmolality	Urine	None defined	mOsm/kg	1.00	None defined	mmol/kg
Phenobarbital, therapeutic	Serum	15–40	µg/ml	4.306	65–175	µmol/L
Phenytoin, therapeutic	Serum	10–20	µg/ml	3.964	40–80	µmol/L
Phosphate (phosphorus, inorganic)	Serum	2.3–4.1	mg/dl	0.3229	0.75–1.35	mmol/L
Potassium	Serum	3.7–5.1	mEq/L g/ml	1.00	3.7–5.1	mmol/L
Protein, total	Serum	6.5–8.3	g/dl	10.0	65–83	g/L
Sodium	Serum	134–142	mEq/L	1.00	134–142	mmol/L
Theophylline, therapeutic	Serum	5–20	µg/ml	5.550	28–110	µmol/L
Thyroid-stimulating hormone (TSH)	Serum	0–5	µIU/ml	1.00	0–5	mIU/L
Thyroxine	Serum	4.5–13.2	µg/dl	12.87	58–170	nmol/L
T_3-uptake ratio	Serum	0.88–1.19	1	1.00	0.88–1.19	1
Triiodothyronine (T_3)	Serum	70–235	ng/ml	0.01536	1.1–3.6	nmol/L
Triglycerides	Serum	50–200	mg/dl	0.01129	0.55–2.25	mmol/L
Urate (uric acid)	Serum					
Men		2.9–8.5	mg/dl	59.48	170–510	µmol/L
Women		2.2–6.5	mg/dl	59.48	130–390	µmol/L
Urea nitrogen	Serum	6–25	mg/dl	0.3570	2.1–8.9	mmol/L
Vitamin B_{12}	Serum	250–1000	pg/ml	0.7378	180–740	pmol/L

(Blair ER et al (eds): Damon Clinical Laboratories Handbook. Lexi-Comp, Inc., Stow OH, 1989).

APPENDIX E

Guidelines for Specimen Transport and Storage

Routines for collection and handling of specimens and reporting of specific patient information vary depending on agency protocols, the clinical setting, and specialty laboratory requirements. The primary objectives in the transport of diagnostic specimens are to maintain the sample as near to its original state as possible with minimum deterioration and to minimize hazards to specimen handlers. Specimens should be collected and transported as quickly as possible (a 2-hour time limit is recommended). For urine transport, a small amount of boric acid may be used; a holding or transport medium can be used for most other specimen types. Follow carefully the instructions for handling and transport of specimens provided on the kit or by the manufacturer.

1. When the patient delivers the specimen directly, provide a biohazard bag and include clearly written directions about specific handling precautions and specific directions for locating the physical facility.

2. Specimens may be mailed or transported to specialty laboratories located in other cities or distant areas. To avoid delays in specimen analysis, it is important to follow specific instructions for collection, packaging, labeling, and transporting of specimens. Some specimens must be received in the laboratory within an exact time frame.

   A. When packaging a specimen for shipping to a specialty laboratory, place the specimen in a securely closed, watertight container (such as a test tube, vial, or other primary container), then enclose the whole in a second, durable, watertight container (secondary container). Each set of primary and secondary containers should then be enclosed in a sturdy, strong outer shipping container (Fig. E-1).

   B. Follow appropriate labeling for etiologic agents and biomedical materials (Fig. E-2). If the package becomes damaged or leaks, the carrier is required, by federal regulations, to isolate the package and notify the Biohazards Control Office, Centers for Disease Control and Prevention, in Atlanta, Georgia. The carrier must also notify the sender; again, this special transport requirement can cause a significant delay in specimen analysis, reporting of results, and medical diagnosis and treatment of the patient's problem. Examples of specialty laboratory requirements for transporting, packaging, and mailing of specific specimens are shown in the table.

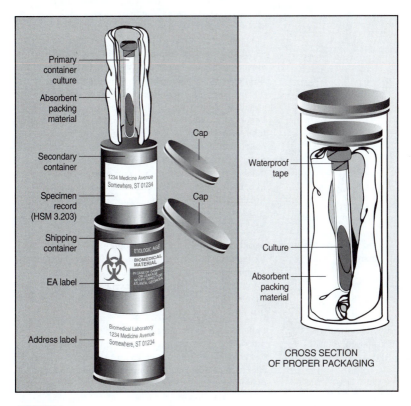

FIGURE E-1

Proper technique for packaging of biologically hazardous materials (CDC Laboratory Manual. DHEW publication No. [CDC] 74-8272, Atlanta, Centers for Disease Control, 1974)

Specimen	Cautions (also include Packaging and Mailing Instructions)
Blood for trace metals	Observe contamination control in sample collection— for example, most blood tubes are contaminated with trace metals, and all plastic syringes with black rubber seals contain aluminum, varying amounts of zinc, and all heavy metals (lead, mercury, cadmium, nickel, chromium, and others). The trace metal sample should be collected first—once the needle has punctured the rubber stopper, it is contaminated and should not be used for trace metal collection. Use alcohol swabs to cleanse sets; avoid iodine-containing disinfectants, use only stainless steel phlebotomy needles. Blood for serum testing of trace elements should be collected in a royal-blue top (sodium heparin anticoagulant) trace element blood collection tube. After collecting and centrifuging, place in a 5-ml, metal-free, screw-capped polypropylene vial; do not use a pipette to transfer serum to container. Cap vial tightly, attach specimen label, and send to lab cool or frozen. All specimens stored >48 hours should be frozen and sent on dry ice. (Keep specimen cool with *frozen* coolant April–October, *refrigerated* coolant November–March.)
Blood for photosensitive analysis	Avoid exposure to any type of light (artificial or sunlight) for any length of time. These specimens need aluminum foil wrap or brown plastic vial. Specimens for vitamin A, vitamin B_6, β-carotene, porphyrins, vitamin D, and bilirubin are examples of substances that need to be protected from light.
Routine urinalysis, random, midstream	Preferred transport container is a yellow plastic screw-top tube that contains a tablet that preserves any formed element (crystals, casts, or cells) and prevents alteration of chemical constituents caused by bacterial overgrowth. Pour urine into tube, cap tube securely, and invert to dissolve the tablet.
Urine culture	Use a culture and sensitivity (C&S) transport kit containing a sterile plastic tube and transfer device for collection. This tube contains a special urine maintenance formula that prevents rapid multiplication of the bacteria in the urine. Pour the urine specimen into the tube and seal properly.
Urine for calcium, magnesium, and oxalate	Use acid-washed plastic containers for collection and transport of specimen. If urine pH is >4 the results may be inaccurate. Do not collect urine in metal-based containers such as metal bed pans or urinals.

(continued)

(Continued)

Specimen	Cautions (also include Packaging and Mailing Instructions)
Stool	Use a special 1,000-ml container, such as Nalgeno, for total sample collection and 100-ml white polypropylene container for a portion of a large sample (aliquot) for feces collection. Each container should have a similar label affixed before it is given to the patient:

Stool Collection Container Label

Only fill to this line

Duration: ___ Random   ___ 24 hrs

               ___ 72 hrs   ___ 48 hrs

               ___ Other   _____

Is this the entire collection?

___ Yes   ___ No

Total number of containers sent: _____

Patient Name:

_____

When the container is given to the patient, provide the following instructions: test to be done, specimen requirements, diet requirements, collection and storage of specimen; two 1000 ml Nalgene™ containers provided for timed collection and one 100 ml container for a random collection specimen; information on how to obtain additional containers if necessary, and *do not* fill any container more than ¾ full (indicated line on label).

At the time that the patient returns the container to the clinic, the health care worker fills in the label with the correct information. If "Other" is checked, enter duration on line on label. If more than one container is sent, be sure to indicate total number sent on the line.

Specimen	
Stool, homogenized	For a homogenized (blended) specimen, the required mailed specimen is an 80-ml portion of homogenized feces. Homogenize and weigh according to laboratory protocol. Pour the homogenate into the container as soon as possible (to avoid settling). On the request form, indicate specimen total weight and amount of water added. Include length of period of collection on request form, also. Send the homogenized specimen

(Continued)

Specimen	Cautions (also include Packaging and Mailing Instructions)
	at the preferred transport temperature listed in agency specimen requirements protocol.
Infectious material	An "Etiologic Agent" label must be affixed to all patient specimens for transport. Body fluids have been recognized by the Centers for Disease Control and Prevention as being directly linked to the transmission of HIV (AIDS) and hepatitis B virus (HBV). Universal precautions apply to these fluids and include special handling requirements of blood, semen, blood products, vaginal secretions, cerebrospinal fluid, synovial fluid, pleural fluid, peritoneal fluid, pericardial fluid, amniotic fluid, and concentrated HIV and HBV. Also, a "Biohazard" label must be affixed to all microbiology specimens, including anaerobic and aerobic bacteria, mycobacteria, fungi, and yeast. The specimen must be sent on an agar slant tube in a special transport container (a pure culture, actively growing); do *not* send on culture plates. The outer shipping container of all etiologic agents transported via interstate traffic must be labeled as illustrated in Figure E-2.

▶ Clinical Alert

The Code of Federal Regulations governing the shipment of etiologic agents (S72.2 *Transportation of Diagnostic Specimens, Biological Products, and Other Materials; Minimum Packaging Requirements*) reads as follows:

"No person may knowingly transport or cause to be transported in interstate traffic, directly or indirectly, any material, including, but not limited to, diagnostic specimens and biological products which such persons reasonably believe may contain an etiologic agent unless such material is packaged to withstand leakage of contents, shocks, pressure changes, and other conditions incident to ordinary handling in transportation."

Specimens requiring exceptional handling	Clearly and accurately label each specimen with patient's full name, sex, birth date, identification number, time and date of specimen collection, name of practitioner ordering specimen, and signature of person collecting specimens. The test order form and sample should be checked for a match and transported in a single package.

(Continued)

Specimen	Cautions (also include Packaging and Mailing Instructions)
Frozen	If a delay of >4 days before specimen examination is expected, freezing of the specimen is preferred. Place the specimen in a plastic vial (not glass); the container should not be more than three-fourths full, to allow for expansion when frozen. Store in freezer or on dry ice until specimen is picked up by carrier or transported to the laboratory. Label vial with patient's name, date, type of specimen (eg, EDTA plasma, serum, urine).
Refrigerated (iced or cooled)	Urine, respiratory exudates, and stool or feces (transport medium is not used) must all be refrigerated before transport. Specimen that *cannot* be refrigerated before inoculation of media include spinal fluids and other body fluids, specimen for *Neisseria gonorrhoeae* isolation, and blood and wound cultures. Place specimen in the refrigerator for storage before pickup by courier. When packaging, place the specimen container in the zip-lock portion of bag and the required coolant in the outer pouch. If dry ice or a refrigerant is used, it must be placed outside the secondary container and the outer shipping container; the shock-absorbant material should be placed so that the secondary container does not become loose inside the outer shipping container as the dry ice evaporates.
Anaerobic	Aspiration with a needle and syringe, rather than a swab, is the preferred method of collection of a specimen for recovery of anaerobic bacteria; once collected, the specimen must be protected from ambient oxygen and kept from drying until it can be processed in the laboratory. Transport container for anaerobic specimen includes a. Syringe and needle for aspiration—valid *only* if specimen can be transported without delay. (This procedure is under question because of the chance of HIV transmission from needle-stick injury.) b. Tube or vials—Tube is used primarily for insertion of swab specimens; vials are used for inoculation of liquid specimen. c. Swab and plastic jacket system—plastic tube or jacket is fitted with a swab and contains either transport or prereduced medium. The culturette system also includes a vial or chamber separated by a membrane that contains chemicals that

(Continued)

Specimen	**Cautions (also include Packaging and Mailing Instructions)**
	generate CO_2 catalysts and desiccants to get rid of any residual O_2 that may get into the system.
	d. Bio-bag or plastic pouch system—a transparent plastic bag that contains a CO_2-generating system, palladium catalyst cups, and an anaerobic indicator. Bag is sealed after inoculated plates have been inserted and the CO_2-generating system is activated. The advantage of this system is that the plates can be directly observed for early growth of colonies.

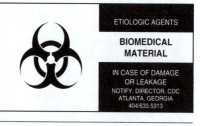

ETIOLOGIC AGENTS

BIOMEDICAL MATERIAL

IN CASE OF DAMAGE
OR LEAKAGE
NOTIFY: DIRECTOR, CDC
ATLANTA, GEORGIA
404/633.5313

NOTICE TO CARRIER

This package contains LESS THAN 50 ml of AN ETIOLOGIC AGENT, N. O. S., is packaged and labeled in accordance with the U.S. public Health Service Interstate Quarantine Regulations (42 CFR, Section 72.25(c), (1) and (4), and MEETS ALL REQUIREMENTS FOR SHIPMENT BY MAIL AND ON PASSENGER AIRCRAFT.

This shipment is EXEMPTED FROM ATA RESTRICTED ARTICLES TARIFF 6-D (see General Requirements 386 ([d] [1]) and from DOT HAZARDOUS MATERIALS REGULATIONS (see 49 CRF, Section 173, 386 [d] [3]). SHIPPERS CERTIFICATES, SHIPPING PAPERS, AND OTHER DOCUMENTATION OR LABELING ARE NOT REQUIRED.

Date   Signature of Shipper

CENTERS FOR DISEASE CONTROL
ATLANTA, GEORGIA 30333

FIGURE E-2

Etiologic agents logo and "notice to carrier" that must be affixed to the outside of any package containing potentially hazardous and infectious biologic materials. (Source: Koneman EA, Allen SD, Janda WM, Schreckenberger PC, & Winn WC: *Color Atlas and Textbook of Diagnostic Microbiology,* 5th Ed., Philadelphia, Lippincott, 1997, p. 82.)

APPENDIX F

Vitamins in Human Nutrition

Both fat-soluble and water-soluble vitamins play a variety of physiologic roles in the body. Vitamin concentrations in blood, urine, and certain body tissues can be measured and reflect the nutritional status of the patient.

Normal Values

Dietary Reference Intakes (DRIs), the most recent approach adopted by the Food and Nutrition Board, Institute of Medicine, and National Academy of Sciences, provide estimates of vitamin intake. The DRIs look beyond deficiency disease and include the role of nutrients and food components in long-term health. The DRIs consist of four reference intakes: Recommended Daily Allowances (RDAs), Tolerable Upper Intake Levels (ULs), Estimated Average Requirements (EARs), and Adequate Intake (AI). When a RDA cannot be set, an AI is given as a normal value; both are to be used as goals for the patient. Levels are given for each individual vitamin. The RDAs are the amounts of ingested vitamins needed by a healthy person to meet daily metabolic needs, allow for biologic variation, maintain normal blood serum values, prevent depletion of body stores, and preserve normal body functions.

Background

Vitamins have varying modes of action. For instance, vitamin E is an antioxidant, vitamin C is an enzyme cofactor, and vitamin A is an anti-infection agent.

Sources of *fat-soluble* vitamins include ingested (dietary) substances and biologic or intestinal microorganisms. Fat-soluble vitamins include vitamin A (known as retinol or carotene), vitamin D (calciferol), vitamin E (tocopherol), and vitamin K (consisting of phylloquinones or K_1, menaquinones or K_2, and menadiones or K_3).

The sources of *water-soluble* vitamins are dietary (ingested) substances and intestinal microorganisms. Water-soluble vitamins include ascorbic acid (vitamin C) and the B-complex vitamins, such as biotin, cobalamin (vitamin B_{12}), folate (folic acid), niacin (vitamin B_3), pyridoxine (vitamin B_6), riboflavin (vitamin B_2), thiamine (vitamin B_1), and pantothenic acid.

Explanation of Test

These tests are measurements of nutritional status. Low levels indicate recent inadequate oral intake, poor nutritional status, and/or malabsorption problems. They may not reflect tissue stores. High levels indicate excessive intake, intoxication, or absorption problems.

Procedure

Blood, urine, hair or nail samples are examined for vitamin levels. The types of specimens needed are listed in the table. Vitamins are tested by both direct and indirect methods.

Clinical Implications
Increased and decreased levels and critical ranges are shown in the table.

Interfering Factors
Factors that affect vitamin levels include age, certain drugs, various diseases, and long-term hyperalimentation.

Patient Preparation
1. Assess overall nutritional status and address potential deficiencies. Oftentimes, one deficiency is accompanied by several nutrient deficiencies.
2. Evaluate signs and symptoms of disrupted vitamin-related metabolic reactions that indicate the need for testing.
3. Cost of testing (high) and time frames for obtaining test results (slow) are issues here. Samples for vitamin tests are usually sent to specialty laboratories which increases cost and turn around time dramatically.
4. Explain the purpose of the test before collecting blood, urine, hair, or nail specimens.
5. Inform the patient that vitamins are micronutrients that can be detected in the blood and urine as an indication of overt nutritional deficiency states, toxic levels, or subclinical hypovitaminosis. The potential for toxicity from excessive intake exists.
6. See Chapter 1 guidelines for safe, effective, informed *pretest* and *intratest* care.

Patient Aftercare
1. Verify and report reference ranges (RR) and critical ranges (CR). Take appropriate action when values are too high or too low. Treat nutrient deficiencies and toxicities immediately.
2. Counsel the patient about abnormal results, follow-up tests, dietary changes, and treatment. Water-soluble vitamins are needed on a daily basis. Reference ranges vary and are method dependent. Check with your laboratory.
3. Follow Chapter 1 guidelines for safe, effective, informed *posttest* care.

Substance Tested (Specimen Needed), Reference Range (RR), and Critical Toxic Range (CR) and RDIs when available	Patient Preparation, Substance Function, and Indications for Test	Clinical Significance of Values	
		Increase	Decrease
FAT-SOLUBLE VITAMINS			
Vitamin A			
Retinol (serum) RR: 360–1200 µg/l 0.70–1.75 µmol/L CR: <10 µg/dl or <0.35 µmol/L indicates severe deficiency; >100–2000 µg/dl indicates hypervitaminosis A	Fasting. No alcohol 24 h before blood draw.	Activation of phagocytes and/or cytotoxic T-cells	Acute infections
	Prevents night blindness and other eye problems and skin disorders (acne).	Alopecia	Arthralgia (gout)
		Amenorrhea	Bile duct obstruction
	Enhances immunity, protects against pollution and cancer formation.	Arthralgia (gout)	Bitot's spots
Carotene (serum) RR: 50–300 µg/dl or 1.5–7.4 µmol/L CR: >250 µg/dl indicates carotenemia	Needed for maintenance repair of epithelial tissues.	Birth defects	Celiac disease
		Carotenodermia/aurantiasis	Cirrhosis of the liver
	Aids fat storage.	Cheilosis	Congenital obstruction of the jejunum
	Protects against colds, infections.	Chronic nephritis	Cystic fibrosis
RR: Retinyl esters <10 µg/L when selected	Acts as antioxidant (protects cells against cancer and other diseases).	Cortical hyperostoses	Duodenal bypass
		Excessive dietary or supplement intake	Fat malabsorption syndrome
			Giardiasis
Relative dose response (%): RR, >20; CR, >50 deficiency	Evaluate night blindness, malabsorption disorders, chronic nephritis, acute protein deficiency, Bitot's spots, intestinal parasites, acute infections, chronic intake of >10 mg retinol equivalent (RE).	Hepatosplenomegaly	Immunity compromised (cell-mediated response, antibody response)
		Hypercholesterolemia	Insufficient dietary intake
		Hyperlipemia	Keratinization of lung, gastrointestinal tract, and urinary epithelia
		Peeling of skin	Keratomalacia
Children show an age-related rise in serum retinol, and values lower before puberty.		Permanent learning disabilities	Measles
		Pregnancy	
		Premature epiphyseal closure	
		Pseudotumor cerebri	
		Spontaneous abortions	
		Nyctalopia (night blindness)	
		Oral contraceptives (carotene)	

(Continued)

Substance Tested (Specimen Needed), Reference Range (RR), and Critical Toxic Range (CR) and RDIs when available	Patient Preparation, Substance Function, and Indications for Test	Clinical Significance of Values	
		Increase	**Decrease**
Levels in adults increase slightly with age. Premenopausal women have slightly lower values than men. After menopause, values are similar. RDI: Men: 1000 μg/retinol equivalent (RE)/day Women: 800 μg/retinol equivalent (RE)/day		Pancreatic surgery Protein-energy malnutrition (marasmus or kwashiorkor) Perifollicular hyperkeratosis (Darier's disease) Sprue Xerophthalmia Xerosis of the conjunctiva and cornea	
Vitamin D 1, 25-dihydroxycholecalciferol, calciferol (serum) RR: 60 ng/ml Toxic: >150 ng/ml Deficient: <10 ng/ml CR: Serum calcium levels of 12–16 mg/dl (vitamin D toxicity) RDI: Adults: 10 μg/day Cholecalciferol or 400 U of vitamin D	Fasting Synthesized by skin exposure to the sunshine Required for absorption of calcium and phosphorous by the intestinal tract. Necessary for normal development of bones in children. Protects against muscle weakness, involved in regulation of heartbeat. Important in treatment of osteoporosis and hypocalcemia.	Gastrointestinal symptoms (anorexia, nausea, vomiting, constipation) Infants: "elfin facies," hypercalcemia with failure to thrive, mental retardation, stenosis of the aorta Metastatic extraosseous calcification Renal colic Supplements Williams' syndrome	Anticonvulsants Familial hypophosphatemic rickets (diabetes mellitus, Fanconi's syndrome, hypoparathyroidism, renal osteodystrophy, renal tubular growth acidosis) High phosphate or phytate intake Inadequate diet Inadequate exposure to

Vitamin E		
Vitamin E Alpha Tocopherol, TE (most active) RR (plasma): Adults: 5.5–17 mg/L Significant deficiency: <3 mg/L Significant excess: >40 mg/L NOTE: Concentration of Vitamin E in newborns is less than half that of adults. RDI: Men: 10 mg Alpha tocopherol equivalent (α-TE) Women: 8 mg/α-TE	Fasting (No alcohol 24 hours before draw) Antioxidant. Important in prevention of cancer and cardiovascular diseases. Promotes normal blood clotting, healing. Reduces wound scarring. Improves circulation necessary for tissue repair; maintains healthy nerves and muscles while strengthening capillary walls. Prevents cell damage by inhibiting the oxidation of lipids and formation of free radicals (antioxidants). Aids utilization of vitamin A. Retards aging and may prevent age spots. Evaluate premature birth weight infants, abelalhypoproteinemia, malabsorption	Low-birth-weight infants (sepsis, necrotizing enterocolitis) Vitamin E supplementation Increased bleeding tendency Impaired leukocyte formation Reduced cataract formation (with high β-carotene and ascorbic acid levels)	Menstrual problems Infertility (men and women) Biliary atresia Carotid deposits in muscle Cholestasis Dermatitis (flaky) Edema Malabsorption syndromes with steatorrhea Neurologic syndromes affecting the spinal posterior columns and the retina (abeta- or hyperlipoproteinemia), blinding loop syndrome, chronic pancreatitis, cystic fibrosis, inborn errors of metabolism, obstructive liver disease, short bowel syndrome) Premature infants (bronchopulmonary dysplasia, intraventricular

(continued from previous nutrient)

Evaluate rickets, osteomalacia, fat malabsorption; disorders of parathyroid, liver or kidney; prolonged supplement intake of 2,000 IU/d

sunlight (especially in the elderly)
Liver disease
Malabsorption syndromes
Osteomalacia (adults)
Rachitic tetany
Rickets (children)

(Continued)

Substance Tested (Specimen Needed), Reference Range (RR), and Critical Toxic Range (CR) and RDIs when available	Patient Preparation, Substance Function, and Indications for Test	Clinical Significance of Values	
		Increase	Decrease
			hemorrhage, platelet dysfunction, low retinopathy) Protein-energy malnourished children Reperfusion injury Platelet hyperaggregation, decreased erythrocyte survival and increased susceptibility to hemolysis
Vitamin K Phylloquinone (K$_1$) plants; menaquinone (K$_2$ series) bacterial; menadione (K$_2$) synthetic. RR: PIVKA 11 test (proteins induced in vitamin K absence). This test is superior. Plasma prothrombin concentration 10.5–12.5 seconds RDI: Men: 80 µg/day Women: 60–65 µg/day	Fasting. Needed for the production of prothrombin (blood clotting). Essential for bone formation and repair. Necessary for synthesis of osteocalcin (the protein in bone tissue on which calcium crystalizes). Therefore prevents osteoporosis. Plays role in converting glucose into glycogen for storage in liver.	Glucose-6-phosphate dehydrogenase deficiency Increased dietary intake or administered vitamin K preparation Low-birth-weight infants (increased menadione) Anemia with Heinz bodies Hyperbilirubinemia Kernicterus (bilirubin encephalophathy) Loss of sucking reflex Postkernicterus syndrome	Breast-fed infants (no Vitamin K received) Conditions limiting for absorption or synthesis of vitamin K Coumarin (warfarin) Excessive oral mineral oil Hypoprothrombinemia Dietary lack Lack of bile salts (external biliary fistulas, obstructive jaundice)

	Function	Considerations/Interactions	Deficiency/Conditions
	Antibiotics interfere with absorption of vitamin K.		Liver disease
			Nonabsorbable sulfonamides
			Salicylate therapy
			Megadoses of fat soluble vitamins A or E are known to antagonize vitamin K
	Evaluate renal insufficiency and chronic antibiotic treatment.		Long-term total parenteral nutrition
			Chronic fat malabsorption, pancreatic disease, gastrointestinal disease

WATER-SOLUBLE VITAMINS

Ascorbic acid

	Function	Considerations/Interactions	Deficiency/Conditions
Vitamin C, ascorbic acid	Antioxidant needed for tissue growth and repair, adrenal gland function, and healthy gums.	Decreased anticoagulant effect of heparin and warfarin (Coumarin)	Adult scurvy (acne, listlessness, deep muscle hemorrhages, swan neck hair deformity, gingivitis, perifollicular hemorrhages, hyperkeratosis, and hypochondriasis)
RR: 28–84 µmol/L plasma; 0.6–2.0 mg/dL plasma, 114–301 nmol/10^8 cells (mixed leukocytes), 20–53 µg/10^8 cells (mixed leukocytes)	Aids in production of antistress hormones and interferon; needed for metabolism of folic acid, tyrosine, and phenylalanine.	Diarrhea	Alcoholism and drug abuse
	Increases absorption of iron, reduces cholesterol levels and high blood pressure.	Overabsorption of iron	Anemia (microcytic hypochromic)
CR: <11 µmol/L plasma ascorbate, <0.2 mg/dl plasma ascorbate, <57 nmol/10^8 cells (mixed leukocytes), <10 mg/10^8 cells (mixed leukocytes).	Essential in neurotransmitter synthesis and metabolism	Supplementation (alteration of tests for diabetes and occult blood)	Burns
	Essential in the formation of collagen, promotes wound healing, protects against infection.	Nausea	Cold or heat stress
Women consistently show higher vitamin C	Enhances immunity.	Some patients with history of kidney stones are at an increased risk of oxalate stones with too much vitamin C intake	Edema, lower extremities
			Gastric ulcers
			Impaired iron absorption
			Inadequate diet (especially elderly men)

(Continued)

Substance Tested (Specimen Needed), Reference Range (RR), and Critical Toxic Range (CR) and RDIs when available	Patient Preparation, Substance Function, and Indications for Test	Clinical Significance of Values	
		Increase	Decrease
levels in tissues and fluids than men. Plasma values are the best indicator of recent dietary intake. Leukocyte vitamin C levels are indicative of cellular stores and body pool. NOTE: Salivary vitamin C levels are not consistent; urinary vitamin C levels are not useful. RDI: Adults: 60 mg/day	Evaluate scurvy, poor diet, and nephrolithiasis.		Infantile scurvy (Barlow's disease, "pithed frog" position) Inflammatory diseases, oxidative damage (proteins, DNA, human sperm DNA) Lactation Petechiae and total ecchymoses Pregnancy Risk of cancer (esophagus, oral cavity, uterine, cervix) Smokers (decreased ascorbic acid half-life) Thyrotoxicosis Toxicity from chemical carcinogens (anthracene, benzpyrene, organochloride pesticides, heavy metals, nitrosamines) Poor wound healing Bleeding gums, dyspnea, edema, and weakness

Biotin

(Plasma)
RR: 0.82–2.87 nmol/L
CR: <1.02 nmol/L deficiency
Prenatal diagnosis of multiple carboxylase deficiency (MCD) by direct analysis of amniotic fluid for methylcitric acid or 3-hydroxyisovaleric acid.
RDI: 30 µg/day

Biotin is produced by the gut flora. Aids in cell growth, fatty acid production, metabolism of fats, carbohydrates, and proteins, and utilization of other complex vitamins. Promotes healthy sweat glands, nerve tissue, and bone marrow. Needed for healthy hair and skin.

Assess for: ingestion of raw eggs, inflammatory bowel disease, alcoholism, sulfonamide therapy, depression.

Alopecia
Anorexia with nausea
Antibiotics
Biotin responsive MCD syndromes
Changes in mental status (depression)
Glossitis (magenta hue)
High fetal resorption rate
Hyperesthesia (algesia)
Immunodeficiency
Increased serum, cholesterol and bile pigments
Ingestion of large amounts of (6/d) of *raw* egg white, ingestion of raw (avidin)
Localized paresthesia
Maculosquamous dermatitis of the extremities
Myalgia
Pallor
Long-term total parenteral nutrition after gut resection, if not supplemented
High blood sugar

(Continued)

Substance Tested (Specimen Needed), Reference Range (RR), and Critical Toxic Range (CR) and RDIs when available	Patient Preparation, Substance Function, and Indications for Test	Clinical Significance of Values	
		Increase	Decrease
Cobalamin (Vitamin B₁₂) (Serum) RR: >200–800 pg/ml CR: <100 pg/ml deficiency RDI: Adults 2.4 µg/day	Overnight fast. Avoid heparin, ascorbic acid, fluoride, and alcohol before testing. Aids folic acid in formation of iron; prevents anemia. Required for proper digestion, absorption of food, synthesis of protein and metabolism of fats and carbohydrates. Prevents nerve damage, maintains fertility, production of acetylcholine (neurotransmitter that assists memory and learning). Found mostly in animal sources, so strict vegetarians may need supplements. Regional enteritis. Evaluate strict vegetarian diet spanning 20–30 y, alcoholism, after gastrectomy, and parasitic infections.	Improved mental function in elderly receiving B₁₂ supplements Toxicity to Vitamin B₁₂ has not been reported.	Deficiency caused by malabsorption—common in elderly and those with digestive disorders Alcoholism Addisonian pernicious anemia Thalassemia Diet lacking microorganisms and animal foods (sole B₁₂ sources) Distal sensory neuropathy ("glove and stockings") sensory loss Gastrectomy Gastric atrophy (superficial gastritis, hereditary—degenerative congenital) Liver disease Pigmentation of skin creases and nailbeds (brownish) Polyendocrinopathy

Pregnancy
Renal disease
Small intestine disorders (cancer, gluten-induced enteropathy—celiac disease, granulomatous lesions, intestinal resections, "stagnant bowel" syndrome, tropical sprue)
Subacute combined degeneration of the cord
Tapeworms
Tinnitus and noise-induced hearing loss
Tongue—red, smooth, shining, painful
Vegans (and their breast-fed infants)
Visual loss from optic atrophy
Zollinger-Ellison syndrome

Alcohol, alcoholics
Liver disease
Elderly
Breast-fed infants of mothers taking estrogen-progesterone contraceptives
Cervical dysplasia
Cigarette smoking

Folacin is dominant form in serum and RBC
Loss of seizure control
Acute renal failure
Active liver disease
Red blood cell hemolysis
Supplemental folate (400 μg/4 mg/d—side effects)

Fasting.
Needed for energy production and formation of red blood cells.
Strengthens immunity by aiding white blood cell functioning.
Important for healthy cell division and replication (DNA and RNA)

Folate (Folic Acid)
(pteroylglutamate, pteroyl-glutamic acid, 5-methyltetrahydrofolate)
Red blood cell folate (best indicator of status)
RR: 150–800 ng/ml whole blood, corrected to packed cell volume of 45%

Substance Tested (Specimen Needed), Reference Range (RR), and Critical Toxic Range (CR) and RDIs when available	Patient Preparation, Substance Function, and Indications for Test	Clinical Significance of Values	
		Increase	Decrease
Tissue folate depletion (serum dietary fluctuations): <160 ng/ml, <360 nmol/L RR: 3–21 ng/ml 11.33–36.25 nmol/L CR: <1.5 ng/ml deficiency Negative folate balance: <7 nmol/L, <3 ng/ml RDI: Adults: 400 µg/day Other methods (infrequently used): Deoxyuridine suppression test (DU or dUST), a functional indicator of folate status; in vitro laboratory test that defines presence of megaloblastosis and identifies which nutrient deficiency is responsible (folate or vitamin B_{12}).	synthesis). Protein metabolism. Prevention of folic acid anemia. In pregnancy, regulates embryonic and fetal nerve cell formation, Prevents premature birth. Works best when combined with Vitamins B_{12} and C. Cooking destroys folic acid. Evaluate megaloblastic anemia, cancer, inflammatory bowel disease, alcoholism, drug treatment with phenytoin, cholestyramine, sulfasalazene, oral contraceptives.		Drug therapy (phenytoin, primidone, barbiturates), methotrexate, melformin, cholestyramine, cycloserine, azothioprine, oral contraceptives, antacids) Increased requirements Hematopoiesis (thalassemia major) Increased metabolism Infancy Lactating women Malignancy (lympho-proliferative) Pregnancy HPV-16 infection Inadequate dietary intake Malabsorption syndromes (celiac disease, sprue, blind loop syndrome) Megaloblastosis Neural tube defects (spina bifida, anencephaly)

Formiminoglutamic acid (FIGLU)—after histidine loading.

Pancytopenia
Protection from malaria
Psoriasis
Renal dialysis
Scurvy
Tongue papillae atrophy (shiny, smooth)
Vitamin B_{12} deficiency
Increased mean corpuscular volume
Depression
Methotrexate-treated patients
Hyperhomocysteinemia
Long-term unsupplemented total parenteral nutrition
Rheumatoid arthritis

Riboflavin (Vitamin B_2)
(serum or plasma)
RR: 4–24 µg/dl
(urine—much more sensitive to nutritional status)
RR: 80–269 µg/g;
>40 nmol/dl erythrocyte;
>15 µg/dl erythrocyte;
<30 riboflavin per gram
Creatinine indicates deficiency:
<27 nmol/dl (erythrocyte) deficient status, <10 µg/dl (erythrocyte) deficient status.

Fasting

None

Necessary for red blood cell formation, antibody production, cell respiration, and growth
Alleviates eye fatigue and important in treatment and prevention of cataracts.
Aids metabolism of fat, carbohydrates, and protein.
With Vitamin A, maintains and improves mucous membranes in

Alcoholism
Angular stomatosis
Ariboflavinosis
Barbiturate use (long-term)
Cheilosis
Chronic diarrheas
Dyssebacia (shark skin)
Glossitis
Inadequate consumption of milk and other animal products
Irritable bowel syndrome

Substance Tested (Specimen Needed), Reference Range (RR), and Critical Toxic Range (CR) and RDIs when available	Patient Preparation, Substance Function, and Indications for Test	Clinical Significance of Values	
		Increase	Decrease
	digestive tract.		Liver disease
Erythrocyte glutathione reductase assay, expressed in activity coefficients (AC). Test cannot be used in persons with glucose-6-phosphate deficiency. AC <1.2 acceptable; AC 1.2–1.4 low; AC <1.4 deficient.-	Helps absorption of iron and B₆. Pure, uncomplicated riboflavin deficiency is rare—if seen, it is usually accompanied by multiple nutrient deficiencies		Normocytic anemia Nutritional amblyopia Oroaggulogenital syndrome Perleche (Candida albicans infection with cheilosis) Photophobia and lacrimation of eye
Flavin adenine dinucleotide (FAD) stimulation test. RR (stimulation): <20%. RDI: Men: 1.3 mg/day Women: 1.1 mg/day	Needed for metabolism of amino acid tryptophan, which is converted to niacin in the body. Easily destroyed by light, antibiotics, and alcohol. Increased need for B₂ with use of oral contraceptives or strenuous exercise. Assess poor dietary intake, as in congenital heart disease, some cancers, and excess.		Sore throat Tongue (magenta hue) Use of phenothiazine derivative
Niacin (Vitamin B₃)			
Nicotinic acid, niacinamide (urinary N′-methylnicatinamide, NMN) (24-h urine) CR: <5.8 μmol/d (deficiency); <0.8 mg/day (deficiency).	24-h urine collection Essential for proper circulation and healthy skin. Aids functioning of nervous system and metabolism of carbohydrates, fats, and protein in the production of hydrochloric acid for digestion.	Abnormal liver function Hypocholesterolemia Use as hypolipidemic drug Atrial fibrillation Cystoid maculopathy Epigastric discomfort Glucose intolerance	Alcoholics Carcinoid syndrome Casal's necklace Cirrhosis of the liver Diarrheal disease Diet lacking in niacin and tryptophan

RDI: Men: 16 mg/day
Women: 14 mg/day

Pyridoxine (Vitamin B₆)

RR (direct):
Plasma vitamin B_6:
5–24 ng/ml
Plasma pyridoxal 5 phosphate >30 nmol/L
Plasma total vitamin B_6: >40 nmol/L
Urinary 4-pyridoxic acid (4rPA) <3.0 μmol/d (useful short-term index)
Urinary total vitamin B_6 >0.5 μmol/day isoniazid, penicillamine, cycloserine)
RR (indirect):
Erythrocyte alanine transaminase index (EALT/EGPT) >1.25 (EALT is a better indicator than EAST;

Involved in normal secretion of bile and stomach fluids and synthesis of sex hormones.
Lowers cholesterol.
Helpful for schizophrenia and other mental diseases.

Evaluate antituberculosis drug therapy (isoniazid), malabsorptive disorders, and alcoholism.

Fasting or urine collection.

Needed for production of hydrochloric acid and absorption of fats and protein, sodium and potassium balance, and red blood cell formation.
Required by nervous system for normal brain function.
Tryptophen metabolism
Niacin formation
Gluconeogenesis
Synthesis of nucleic acids, RNA and DNA; activate many enzymes and aids in absorption of vitamin B_{12}.
Cancer immunity, prevents arteriosclerosis.

Mild diuretic—reduces premenstrual syndrome.
Diuretics and cortisone drugs block absorption of B_6.

Gout
Hyperglycemia
Hypotension
Pruritus
Smooth, swollen tongue
Upper body flushing.

Infants: neurologic symptoms and abdominal distress
Peripheral neuropathy; progressive sensory ataxia; lower limb impairment
Photosensitivity
Neurotoxicity

Dyssebacia
Hartnup's disease
Isoniazid therapy
Pellagra dermatosa; glossitis (scarlet, raw beef)
Gastrointestinal dysfunction
Central nervous system dysfunction
Organic psychosis
Encephalopathic syndrome

Alcoholism
Anemias
Asthma
Breast cancer
Cheilosis
Coronary heart disease
Depression and confusion
Diabetes
Drugs (iproniazid, cycloserine, penicillamine, ethinyl, estradiol, mestranol)
Glossitis
Hodgkin's disease
Impaired interleukin-2 production
Increased metabolic activity
Infants (abnormal electroencephalogram pattern, confusions)

Substance Tested (Specimen Needed), Reference Range (RR), and Critical Toxic Range (CR) and RDIs when available	Patient Preparation, Substance Function, and Indications for Test	Clinical Significance of Values	
		Increase	Decrease
standardized approach needed to compare tests).	Antidepressants, estrogen therapy, and oral contraceptives increase need for B₆.		Irritability Lymphopenia Peripheral neuropathy Premenstrual syndrome Seborrheic dermatosis Sickle cell anemia Smokers Stomatitis
Erythrocyte aspartic transaminase index (EAST/EGOT) >1.80 (valid but somewhat outdated indicator of hepatic vitamin B₆ status) 2 g L-tryptophan load; urinary xanthurenic acid >65 µmol/d; 3 g L-methionine load; urinary (24-h urines, several collected over 1–3 weeks) <350 u/mol/day RDI: Adults: 2.4 µg/day	Evaluate groups at risk, including newborn infants with low B₆, some cancers, excess alcohol.		
Thiamine (Vitamin B₁) (serum or plasma): RR: 10–64 ng/ml; 79–178 0.75–1.3 IU/gm Hgb; nmol/L (whole blood) Late changes: <50 µg/d urine with elevated blood pyruvate	Fasting Enhances circulation and blood formation, carbohydrate metabolism and production of hydrochloric acid. Optimizes cognitive activity and brain function.	Parenteral dosages High C-carbohydrate diet increases need for B₁ Thiamin is poorly absorbed in adults with folate or protein deficiency	Antibiotics, sulfa drugs, oral contraceptives Alcoholism Beriberi—dry beriberi (peripheral neurologic changes; ie, symmetric foot drop); infantile beriberi; wet beriberi

Red blood cell transketolase measurement (most reliable method)

Enzyme assays—using thiamine pyrophosphate (TPP): 79–178 nmol/L RR (stimulation): 0%–25%; deficiency, >20%.

RDI: Men: 1.3 mg/day Women: 1.1 mg/day

Has a positive effect on energy, growth, normal appetite, and learning capacity.

Needed for muscle tone of intestines, stomach, and heart.

Acts as antioxidant, protecting body from degenerative effects of aging, alcohol consumption, and smoking.

Evaluate alcoholism impaired absorption, excess intravenous glucose infusion, in diets primarily of refined, unenhanced grain products

Cardiovascular (high-ouput congestive heart failure, low-output Shoshin disease)

Wernicke-Korsakoff syndrome (acute hemorrhagic polio-encephalitis)

Cerebral beriberi

Dependency states (thiamine-responsive megaloblastic anemia, lactic acidosis, ketoaciduria, subacute necrotizing encephalopathy, Leigh's disease).

Dextrose infusions (frequent, long-continued or highly concentrated)

Folate deficiency

High carbohydrate diet (mainly from milled [polished] rice)

Hyperthyroidism

Impaired absorption (ie, long-term diarrheas)

Impaired utilization (ie, severe liver disease)

Inadequate caloric or protein intake

Increase requirements (fever, lactation, pregnancy, strenuous physical exertion)

Poor memory

Renal dialysis

Long-term total parenteral nutrition

Unsupplemented

APPENDIX G

Minerals in Human Nutrition

Minerals are micronutrients needed in relatively small amounts. Unlike vitamins, the source for minerals comes from nonliving, naturally occurring elements, such as mineral salts in the soil that become a part of the chemical constituents of food or minerals that are dissolved in ocean water and ingested in seafoods. Mineral concentrations in blood, urine, and certain body tissues can be measured and reflect the nutritional status of the patient.

Normal Values

Dietary Reference Intakes (DRIs), the most recent approach adopted by the Food and Nutrition Board, Institute of Medicine, and National Academy of Sciences provide estimates of mineral intake. The DRIs look beyond deficiency disease and include the role of nutrients and food components in long-term health, prevention of chronic disease (ie, calcium balance and calcium retention). The DRIs consist of four reference intakes: RDAs, ULs, EARs, and AIs. See p. 1149 in the vitamin section. Recommended dietary allowances (RDAs) have been established, and Estimated Average Requirements (EAR) levels have been established for some minerals, including those with and without an assigned role in the human body.

Background

Minerals are either macronutrients (major) or micronutrients (trace or ultratrace). If the body requires a significant amount of the mineral (>100 mg/d) and an RDA has been established, it is a macronutrient; if the body requires less (a few milligrams per day) and an RDA or ESADDI has been established, it is a micronutrient trace mineral; if the body requires <1 mg/d and no RDA or ESADDI has been established, it is a micronutrient ultratrace mineral.

Macronutrients (*major minerals*) include calcium, chloride, magnesium, phosphorous, potassium, sodium, and sulfur. Macronutrients are not listed in this table; they are explained in Chapter 6.

Trace minerals include the micronutrients chromium, cobalt, copper, fluorine, iodine, iron, manganese, molybdenum, selenium, and zinc.

Ultratrace minerals include the micronutrients arsenic, boron, bromine, cadmium, lead, lithium, nickel, silicon, tin, and vanadium.

Minerals found in the body without an assigned metabolic role include aluminum, antimony, beryllium, bismuth, cyanide (an anion that forms a salt with minerals), gold, mercury, silver, thallium, and many others.

Explanation of Test

These measurements of minerals are used to assess occupational exposure and toxicity, monitor effectiveness of treatment, and evaluate mineral status along with other laboratory levels to verify deficiencies.

Procedure
Blood, urine, hair, or nail samples are examined for mineral levels by indirect and direct methods. The types of specimens required are listed in the table.

Clinical Implications
Increased and decreased levels and critical toxic ranges are found in the table.

Interfering Factors
Factors that affect mineral levels include genetic makeup, age or stage of life cycle, environmental factors drugs, intestinal malabsorption, stress, strenuous physical activity, smoking, and alcohol consumption, and dietary intake.

Patient Preparation
1. Evaluate overall nutritional status, dietary intake, and supplement usage to determine over consumption.
2. Evaluate signs and symptoms of occupational and environmental toxicity and mineral deficiencies that indicate the need for testing.
3. Explain the purpose of the test before collecting blood, urine, hair, or nail specimens.
4. Inform the patient that minerals are nutrients that can be detected in the blood and urine as an indication of toxicity or exposure and nutritional status. The amounts needed are determined by what is necessary for optimal function and health and to prevent disease.
5. See Chapter 1 guidelines for safe, effective, informed *pretest* and *intratest* care.

Patient Aftercare
1. Verify and report reference ranges (RR) and critical toxic ranges (CR). Take appropriate action when values are too high or too low.
2. Counsel the patient appropriately about abnormal results, follow-up testing, occupational and lifestyle changes, treatment, and diet. Reference ranges vary and are method dependent. Check with your laboratory. Notify employer, workplace, and physician about exposure results.
3. Follow Chapter 1 guidelines for safe, effective, informed *posttest* care.

Substance Tested (Specimen Needed), Reference Range (RR), Critical Toxic Range (CR), and RDIs if Available	Patient Preparation, Substance Function, and Indications for Test	Clinical Implications	
		Increase	Decrease
Aluminum (Al) (serum) RR: 0–6 ng/ml; <40 ng/ml dialysis patients (urine) RR: 0–32.0 µg/24 h	Collect urine in acid-washed polypropylene container. No metabolic role Metal used in other forms as an astringent (Burrow's solution) and as an antacid Access for occupational exposure, toxicity from antacids; monitor dialysis patients.	Aluminum absorption with citrate-containing drugs (effervescent or analgesics) Use of aluminum-containing astringents hydroxide gels, aluminum-containing phosphate binders Excessive occupational exposure. *Toxicity:* Aluminosis (lung disease) Aluminum-induced encephalopathy Hypophosphatemia Dialysis dementia Iron-resistant microcytic anemia Aluminum-related osteomalacia. In renal failure, when aluminum-containing antacids are used; long-term intermittent dialysis. *NOTE:* Aluminum is a neurotoxin. The primary symptom is motor dysfunction leading to dysarthria, myoclonus, or epilepsy. Aluminum	

(continued)

toxicity is not related to Alzheimer's disease. Aluminum can be found in laboratory solutions used with tissue samples and in laboratory dust. New testing methods are being adopted to rule out contamination.

Antimony (Sb)
(24-h urine)
RR: <50 μg/L
CR: >1 mg/L

No metabolic role.
Compounds used in alloys, medicines, poisons.

Assess for occupational exposure and toxicity.

Excessive occupational exposure (ore from mining, bronze ceramics)
Ingested compounds (drugs used in parasitic infections).

Toxicity: Acrid metallic taste, burning gastrointestinal pain (as in arsenic poisoning), throat constriction, dysphagia, pulmonary edema, liver and renal failure

Lethal dose: 5–50 mg/kg body weight

Arsenic (As)
(hair or nails)
<1.0 μg/g of hair or nails
(serum)
≥5 μg/ml
(24-h urine)

Ultratrace mineral; no function.
Found in pesticides and paints.
Used as a homicidal poison.
High selectivity

Dermatoses (hyperpigmentation, hyperkeratosis, desquamation, and hair loss); hematopoietic for hair and nails
Depression

(Continued)

Substance Tested (Specimen Needed), Reference Range (RR), Critical Toxic Range (CR), and RDIs if Available	Patient Preparation, Substance Function, and Indications for Test	Clinical Implications	
		Increase	Decrease
Normal concentration, <100 µg per specimen Toxic concentration, ≥5000 µg per specimen	Assess for occupational exposure, exposure from pesticides and herbicides, intentional poisoning.	Liver damage characterized by jaundice Peripheral neuropathy Accidental or intentional poisoning Excessive occupational exposure (ceramics, agriculture) *Toxicity:* Metallic taste and odor of garlic on breath, burning pain in gastrointestinal tract, shock syndrome, bloody diarrhea, pulmonary edema, liver failure. *Lethal dose:* 5–50 mg/kg body weight Arsenic trioxide (As/kg body weight): 0.35–0.91 µmol 10.2–26 nmol	
Beryllium (Be) (24-h urine) RR: 0.05 µg/d CR: >20 µg/L or 2.22 µmol/L	No metabolic role; a metallic element. Assess for occupational exposure and toxicity.	Acute beryllium disease (a chemical pneumonitis) Excessive occupational exposure (metal extraction, refinery, rocket base, nuclear plant, extensive coal burning); secondary polycythemia	

Bismuth (Bi)
(24-h urine)
RR: <20 µg/L,
<95.7 nmol/L (plasma)
RR: <1.0 µg/dl,
<47.9 mmol/L

Historical—beryllium mining, electronics, chemical plants, manufacture of fluorescent lights (inhalation, introduction into or under skin and/or conjunctiva): berylliosis or granulomatosis

NOTE: Almost impossible to distinguish from sarcoidosis.

Collect urine in metal-free container.

No metabolic role. Workers exposed in cosmetics, disinfectants, pigments, and solder industries. Used in some drugs; poisoning as a consequence of therapy for syphilis.

Assess for occupational exposure, toxicity, and medication levels.

Bismuth used as treatment for syphilis in a growing child when mother has been treated during pregnancy

Treatment of peptic ulcer with bismuth-containing drug (zolimidine, colloidal bismuth subcitrate)

Bismuth subcarbonate, subgallate, and subnitrate compounds (used as antiseptics, astringents, sedatives, and to treat diarrhea and inflamed skin)

Toxicity: Ulcerative stomatitis, anorexia, headache, rash, renal tubular damage, bluish line at gum margin, albuminuria;

(Continued)

Substance Tested (Specimen Needed), Reference Range (RR), Critical Toxic Range (CR), and RDIs if Available	Patient Preparation, Substance Function, and Indications for Test	Clinical Implications	
		Increase	*Decrease*
		resembles lead poisoning, without the blood changes and paralysis; rheumatic-like pain.	
Boron (Bo) (blood, 4-ml serum) total RR: 1 mg/dl CR: 10–20 mg/dl (plasma) RR: 200 ng/ml (24-h urine, 5 ml aliquot) RR: 0.3 μg/dl	Ultratrace mineral; a nonmetallic element, found as a compound such as boric acid or borox. Assess for exposure and toxicity, ingestion of boric acid, and unexpected absorption of boric acid from diapers or infant pacifier dipped in borax preparation and honey.	Increase in total plasma calcium concentrations and urinary excretions of calcium and magnesium *Toxicity:* Riboflavinuria; lethargy; gastrointestinal symptoms; bright, red rash; shock. *Infants:* reports of scanty hair; patchy, dry, erythema; anemia; seizure disorders. *Lethal dose* (adults): boric acid or borate salts, 50–500 mg/kg body weight	Decreased serum concentrations of 17β-estradiol, testosterone, and iodized calcium Depressed mental alertness

Substance	Description	Clinical Significance
Bromine (Br), Bromide (serum) RR: 1000–2000 µg/ml (plasma) RR: 3500 ng/dl	Ultratrace mineral; a central nervous system depressant. Bromine: liquid, nonmetallic element obtained from natural brines from wells and sea water. Compounds used in medicine and photography. Assess for occupational exposure to bromide in medicine or photography.	Bromide acne Neurologic disturbances Increased spinal fluid pressure *Toxicity:* Bromism or brominism *Lethal dose:* 500–5000 mg/kg body weight Recent findings support incidence of depressed growth, conception rate, milk fat production, and hemoglobin Central nervous system depressant
Cadmium (Cd) (blood) RR: 0–0.5 ng/ml urine preferred 0–5.0 µg/24h	Ultratrace mineral; a metallic element in zinc ores Used in electroplating and in atomic reactors. Its salts are poisonous. Assess for occupational exposure, environmental poisoning.	In tissue, in prostatic and renal cancer In urine, in hypertension, industrial exposure (electroplating, atomic reactors, zinc ores, cadmmium solder) In blood, poisoning from foods prepared in cadimum-lined vessels, inhalation of cadmium dust and fumes, softened drinking water, goods grown in soil heavily fertilized with superphosphate *Toxicity:* Severe gastroenteritis, mild liver damage, acute renal failure; pulmonary edema; cough; duck-like gait; brown urine *Lethal dose:* Several hundred mg/kg body weight

Substance Tested (Specimen Needed), Reference Range (RR), Critical Toxic Range (CR), and RDIs if Available	Patient Preparation, Substance Function, and Indications for Test	Clinical Implications	
		Increase	Decrease
Chromium (Cr) (plasma) RR: 0.3 µg/l; 0.5 ng/ml	Required for normal glucose metabolism; affects cholesterol synthesis. Assess for occupational exposure, poor diet, elderly at risk. Severe trauma and stress increase need.	Excessive industrial exposure (carcinogenic) Renal damage	Insulin resistance (hyperinsulinemia) Impaired glucose Increased risk for congestive heart disease Hypercholesterolemia Decreased fertility
Cobalt (Co) (part of the vitamin B_{12} molecule) (plasma) RR 0.007–6 µg/dl; 0.1–0.4 ng/ml	Essential element in vitamin B_{12}—stimulates production of red blood cells Assess for occupational exposure and monitor dialysis.	Cardiomyopathy after industrial exposure, during maintenance dialysis, and after drinking beer contaminated with cobalt during processing	Cobalamin (vitamin B_{12}) deficiency
Copper (Cu) (serum, 3 ml) RR (total): 85–150 µg/dl; (24-h urine) RR: 95–100 µg/d;	Required for hemoglobin synthesis; essential component of several enzyme systems; present in the liver and excreted by the kidneys and in bile.	T-cell proliferation Hepatic glutathione Wilson's disease (hepatolenticular degeneration) Ingestion of solutions of copper salts Contaminated water or dialysis fluids	Rheumatoid arthritis Menke's steely hair disease: lack of pigmentation of skin and hair Collagen abnormalities, osteoporosis

(plasma/500 RBC) RR: 0.47–0.067 mg/g Ceruloplasmin is an indirect test for copper: RR: 21–53 mg/dl, 210–530 mg/L (neonate: 5–18 mg/dl, 50–180 mg/L)	Assess for excessive antacid intake, nephronic malabsorptive disorder, hemodialysis, and consumption of water high in copper by infants	Indian childhood cirrhosis Female rheumatoid arthritis Oral contraceptive use Inflammatory conditions Cancer at injection sites or muscles *Toxicity:* Hepatic or renal failure *Lethal dose:* 50–500 mg/kg body weight	Ataxia Hypochromic anemia unresponsive to iron therapy Hypercholesterolemia Impaired cardiovascular system Over supplementation of zinc Altered interleukin-2 production Neutropenia, leukopenia Liver disease, kidney disease
Cyanide (Cn Radical) (blood, 5 ml) RR: <0.2 µg/ml Nonsmokers: toxic: ≥2 µg/ml	No metabolic role. The most common and most deadly poison—stops cellular respiration by inhibiting the actions of cytochrome oxidase, carbonic anhydrase, and other enzyme systems. Toxicity comes from inhalation or ingestion—a hazard to firefighters. Assess for industrial exposure, inhalation, or accidental poisoning from ingestion	Industrial exposure (pesticides, metallurgy) Inhalation of hydrocyanic acid and fumes from burning nitrogen- containing products Ingestion of salts and Laetrile (derived from broken seeds of apricots, peaches, jetberry bush, toyon, bitter almonds, and some apple seeds) *Toxicity:* Lethal dose is <5 mg/kg body weight (small child); fatal dose = 5–25 seeds. Death within 5 min of ingestion/inhalation. Adverse effects are dizziness, weakness, mental and motor impairment, and sudden death.	

Substance Tested (Specimen Needed), Reference Range (RR), Critical Toxic Range (CR), and RDIs if Available	Patient Preparation, Substance Function, and Indications for Test	Clinical Implications	
		Increase	**Decrease**
Fluorine (F) (plasma) RR: 0.01–0.2 μg/ml (urine) RR: 0.02–1.1 μg/ml RDI: men 4 mg/d women 3 mg/d	Gaseous chemical found in soil in combination with calcium. Used as a compound (fluoride) in toothpaste. Assess for excess ingestion; evaluate dental caries or mottling.	Fluorosis (excess fluorine use: >4 million ppm in water; treatment of osteoporosis, multiple myeloma, or Paget's disease) Osteosclerosis Exostoses of spine and genuvalgum Excess ingestion from swallowing fluoridated toothpaste. *Toxicity:* Peculiar taste with salivation and thirst (salty-soapy), hemorrhagic gastroenteritis; hypoglycemia; central nervous system depression; renal failure. *Lethal dose:* 50–500 mg/kg body weight; 5–10 g sodium fluoride	Marginal to deficient dietary intake from deficiencies in geochemical environments Dental caries Skeletal changes, especially in long bones

Element / Reference Range	Description	Clinical Significance
Gold (Au) (colloidal gold in cerebrospinal fluid) RR: minute amount (serum) RR: 0–0.1 mg/L; therapeutic, 1.0–2.0 mg/L	Collect in metal-free container. No metabolic role; a metallic element. Salts used in early rheumatoid arthritis and in nondisseminated lupus erythematosus. Detectable in serum 10 mo after cessation of treatment. Assess for toxicity in treatment of rheumatoid arthritis.	Rheumatoid arthritis if gold sodium thiomalate or gold thioglucose (aurothioglucose) is given parenterally; oral gold compound *Toxicity:* At least 35% of patients undergoing chrysotherapy develop some degree of toxicity Pruritus, dermatitis, stomatitis, albuminuria with or without nephrotic syndrome, agranulocytosis, thrombocytopenic purpura, and aplastic anemia *Adverse reactions:* Enterocolitis, intrahepatic cholestasis, skin hyperpigmentation, peripheral neuropathy, and pulmonary infiltrates
Iodine (I) (plasma) RR: 2–4 µg/dl, 60 ng/ml Deficiency: IDD (iodine deficiency disorders) (daily urine) Mild IDD, RR: 50–100 µg/d (median urine, 3.5–µg/dl) Moderate IDD, RR: 25–49 µg/d (median urine, 2–3.4 µg/dl)	Nonmetallic element belonging to the halogen group. Aids in the development and function of the thyroid gland, formation of thyroxine, and prevention of goiter. Assess for goiter.	Prolonged excessive intake of iodine leading to iodide-goiter and myxedema (common with pre-existing Hashimoto's thyroiditis) Excessive consumption of seaweed, kelp supplements; caffeine High dietary intake of known goitrogens (rutabagas, turnips, cabbages) Hypothyroidism in autoimmune Simple, endemic, colloid, or euthyroid goiter Endemic cretinism (neurologic and/or myxedematous) Fetus: abortions, stillbirths, congenital anomalies Child/teen: impaired mental function, retarded physical development

(Continued)

Substance Tested (Specimen Needed), Reference Range (RR), Critical Toxic Range (CR), and RDIs if Available	Patient Preparation, Substance Function, and Indications for Test	Clinical Implications	
		Increase	Decrease
Severe IDD, RR: <25 µg/d (median urine, 0–1.9 µg/dl) RDI: adults 150 µg/d		thyroid diseases, inhibition of thioamide drugs Dysgeusias Acne-like skin lesions	Adult: hypo- or hyper-thyroidism; impaired mental function
		Toxicity: Mucous membranes stained brown; burning pain in mouth and esophagus, laryngeal edema; shock, nephritis, circulatory collapse.	
		Lethal dose: 5–50 mg/kg body weight.	
Iron (Fe) (serum, 5 ml, diurnal; morning specimen shows higher values). RR: 35–140 µg/dl toxic: >300 µg/dl *Iron RR values:* Males: 50–160 µg/dl Females: 40–150 µg/dl Newborn: 100–250 µg/dl Child: 50–120 µg/dl *Total iron binding capacity (TIBC)* RR: RR 250–400 µg/dl	Essential to hemoglobin formation, transportation of oxygen and cellular respiration. Plays a role in the nutrition of epithelial tissues and the development of red blood cells. Assess for ingestion of iron pills or vitamin and mineral pills (toxicity). Populations at risk for deficiency are infants and children 0.5–4.0 y, early adolescents, and women	Diets high in heme iron or high in promoters of nonheme iron absorption Excessive iron absorption: hereditary hemochromatosis (African or "Bantu" siderosis); prolonged therapeutic administration of iron to subjects not iron deficient; chronic alcoholism or liver disease, pancreatic insufficiency potential; "shunt hemochromatosis;" severe anemia with ineffective	Iron deficiency anemia: inadequate diet (grossly iron deficient, high in cereals, low in animal protein and vitamin C) Koilonychia (spoon-shaped nails) Excessive menstrual loss Pregnancy, lactation Blood donors Premature infants; Intestinal

who are pregnant.

Transferrin RR values:
Adult: 250–425 mg/dl
Newborn: 130–275 mg/dl
Child: 203–360 mg/dl
RDI: Adults: 10–15 mg/d

erythropoiesis and increased
hemolysis; diabetes in 80% of
patients.
Transfusional hemosiderosis:
β-thalassemia major, some
chronic sideroblastic anemias,
hypoplastic or other refractory
anemias
Other: cancers (primary hepatic
carcinoma, acute leukemia, early
breast cancer); demyelinating
disease; Alzheimer's disease;
increased risk of congestive
heart disease, listeriosis
Also see Chapter 6

helminthiasis (especially
hookworm disease)
Malabsorption syndromes,
chronic diarrhea,
gastrectomy, patients with
atrophic gastritis and
achlorhydria, occult
gastrointestinal bleeding
Hereditary hemorrhagic
telangiectasia
Turner's syndrome
Angiodysplasia (vascular ectasis
or arteriovenous anomaly)
Blue rubber bleb nevi (hereditary cutaneous hemangiomas)
Menetrier's disease
Zollinger-Ellison syndrome,
pseudo-Zollinger-Ellison
syndrome (hypersecretion
of gastric HCl)
Drugs (aspirin, and ethanol),
adrenocortico-steroids or
non steroidal anti-
inflammatory agents
Sports anemia
Patterson-Kelly (Plummer-
Vinson) syndrome

Substance Tested (Specimen Needed), Reference Range (RR), Critical Toxic Range (CR), and RDIs if Available	Patient Preparation, Substance Function, and Indications for Test	Clinical Implications	
		Increase	Decrease
			Factitia iron deficiency anemia (Lasthenie de Ferjol syndrome—self-induced blood letting)
			Poor dietary intake
			Transferrin: severe protein-energy malnutrition
			Iron sequestration (idiopathic pulmonary hemosiderosis, paroxysmal nocturnal hemoglobinuria; chronic disease with inability to metabolize iron from reticuloendothelial cell deposits, congenital atransferrinemia [rare])
			Vitamin A deficiency—lack in developmental periods causes deficits in neural functioning and behavior

Lead (Pb)

(blood, preferred specimen 2 ml, collect with oxalate-fluoride mixture)
RR: 0–9 µg/dl in children and in most adults without occupational exposure
CR: >30 µg/dl in adults

(24-h urine)
RR: up to 500 µg/24h
CR: >400 µg/L

(hair)
RR: <5 µg/g
CR: >2 µg/g

Collect specimen in lead-free container and avoid airborne contaminants. For blood, use specifically monitored tubes for blood lead collection.

Ultratrace mineral; a metallic element—its compounds are poisonous, and any level of lead in blood is abnormal.

Lead oxides are used in paint pigment; lead additives in gasoline provide air pollutants.

Earthenware made of clay rich in lead salts; lead in some insecticides.

Assess for environmental or occupational contaminants and toxic exposure.

Children: irreversible cognitive deficits, acute encephalopathy
Adults: progressive, irreversible renal disease; toxic psychosis from inhalation of tetraethyl or tetramethyl-lead

Children and adults: hypochromic microcytic anemia.

Lead sources: Ingested or inhaled leaded paint (renovation dust); contaminated soil; contaminated water (lead pipes, lead solder on copper pipes, softened water); retention of a lead object in the stomach or joint (shot, curtain weight, fishing weight, bauble); contaminated acidic foods and beverages (storage in lead-glazed ceramics, leaded crystal, galvanized or nonstainless steel pots); inhalation (burning lead-painted wood or battery casings in home fireplaces or stoves); leaded gas fumes; occupational exposure

Lethal dose: 30 g/kg body weight

Depressed growth, altered iron metabolism

(Continued)

Substance Tested (Specimen Needed), Reference Range (RR), Critical Toxic Range (CR), and RDIs if Available	Patient Preparation, Substance Function, and Indications for Test	Clinical Implications	
		Increase	Decrease
Litbium (Li) (serum) RR: 0.0055 µg/ml (plasma) RR: 11 ng/ml Therapeutic range: Serum 0.6–1.5mmol/L or mEq/L Serum CR: >1.5 mEq/L, >1.5 mmol/L Lethal: >4.0mmol/L or mEq/L	Ultratrace mineral; a metallic element Lithium carbonate is used as drug to treat manic phase of manic-depressive illness. Decreased dietary sodium intake lowers the excretion rate of lithium. Assess psychotherapeutic drug monitoring.	Therapy for bipolar disorder. Diabetes insipidus Renal failure, weight gain Diminished taste perception High "hard water" levels	High dietary caffeine and/or sodium intake
Manganese (Mn) (serum) RR: 0.40–0.85 mg/ml CR: >100 ng/ml (24-h urine) RR: <0.3 µg per specimen CR: Urine: >10 µg per specimen	Essential for lipid and carbohydrate metabolism, bone and tissue formation, and reproductive processes. Assess for occupational exposure and evaluate certain diseases.	Chronic inhalation of airborne manganese (mines, steel mills, chemical industries) "Manganic madness," permanent crippling neurologic disorder of the extrapyramidal system (similar to lesions in Parkinson's disease)	High in nonheme iron; certain types of epilepsy; impaired bone metabolism, weak bone in association with low concentrations of copper and zinc; possibly in alcohol abuse

Increased urine levels in acute hepatitis, myocardial infarction and rheumatoid arthritis

Low tissue values in children with maple syrup disease and phenylketonuria.

Mercury (Hg)
(24-h urine)
RR: 0–50 µg/24 h
Whole blood—dark blue top container, refrigerate)
RR: 0–5 µg/dl

Use acid-washed, leakproof container; keep specimen on ice.

No metabolic role. Mercury is the only metal that is liquid at ordinary temperatures. Primarily absorbed by inhalation, but can also be absorbed through the skin and gastrointestinal tract. It is then distributed to the central nervous system and kidneys and excreted in the urine.

Evaluate for mercury toxicity, neurologic findings related to inorganic or organic mercurials, inhalation of mercury vapors.

Assess for occupational exposure, toxicity, and poisoning from contaminated fish.

Mercury poisoning; occupational activities (smelters, miners, gilders, hatters, and factory workers), hobbies (painting, ceramics, target shooting), home renovation, auto repair

Most common nonindustrial mercury poisoning is the consumption of methyl mercury contaminated fish.

Blood is recommended specimen for organic mercury, and urine is recommended specimen for inorganic mercury measurement

Iodine-containing drugs may cause false low levels

Organic mercury poisoning is more serious because it develops quickly

Inhalation of mercury vapors may lead to pneumonitis, cough, fever, and other pulmonary symptoms

Acute and chronic mercury

(Continued)

Substance Tested (Specimen Needed), Reference Range (RR), Critical Toxic Range (CR), and RDIs if Available	Patient Preparation, Substance Function, and Indications for Test	Clinical Implications	
		Increase	Decrease
		poisoning affects kidneys, central nervous system, and gastrointestinal tract.	
Molybdenum (Mo) (plasma) RR: 1.3 µg/dl (blood, mainly within red cells) RR: 2–6 ng/ml	A trace element, associated with the inborn error of molybdenum metabolism. Assess for genetic molybdenum deficiency and dietary.	Massive ingestion of tungsten (W) Occupational and high dietary intake (elevated uric acid blood concentration, gout) Sulfur amino acid toxicity Growth depression and anemia similar to copper deficiency	Sulfite oxidase deficiency (lethal inborn error of metabolism deranges cysteine metabolism) Prolonged total parenteral nutrition ("acquired molybdenum deficiency") Interference with copper metabolism
Nickel (Ni) (serum or plasma) RR: 1–2 ng/mL (urine) RR: 0.1–20 µg/dl	Ultratrace mineral; metallic element. Nickel carbonyl is an industrial chemical used in plating metals—toxic when inhaled, causes pulmonary edema Assess for occupational exposure.	Consistent in alcoholic liver disease Nickel dermatitis Inhalation of nickel carbonyl (promotes lung cancer)	Lack in diet, depressed iron absorption

Selenium (Se) (component of the enzyme glutathione peroxidase, isolated from human red blood cells) (plasma) RR: 100–300 ng/ml; RDI: men 50–70 µg/d women 50–55 µg/d	A chemical element resembling sulfur, found in soil. Has a role in the metabolism of enzymes. As a sulfide, used in treating dandruff and tinea versicolor (ie, Selsun Blue). Determine cause for loss of pigmentation of hair and skin.	Endemic selenosis. Nail and hair loss. Increased dietary intake owing to high soil concentrations (North Dakota, USA, China, Venezuela), excessive intake from "health store" tablets (skin lesions, polyneuritis). Hair and nail loss, changes in nail beds, inhibition of protein synthesis.	Keshan disease (endemic cardiomyopathy). Kashin-Beck disease (endemic osteoarthritis). Parenteral nutrition. Decreased dietary intake owing to low soil concentrations (New Zealand, China), aspermatogenesis. Long-term total parenteral nutrition (cardiomyopathy). Duchenne's muscular dystrophy, cataracts, tumor development. Whitening of nail beds, loss of pigmentation of hair and skin, muscle pain and weakness.
Silicon (Si)—silicic acid (H_2SiO_3) (plasma) RR: 500 µg/dl (serum or plasma) RR: 0.4–10.0 µg/ml	Ultratrace mineral; nonmetallic element in soil. Occurs in traces in skeletal structures (bones and teeth).	Long-term antacid therapy (magnesium trisilicate). Siliceous renal calculi.	

(Continued)

Substance Tested (Specimen Needed), Reference Range (RR), Critical Toxic Range (CR), and RDIs if Available	Patient Preparation, Substance Function, and Indications for Test	Clinical Implications Increase	Decrease
	Necessary for the formation of collagen, bones, and connective tissue; healthy nails, skin and hair; and calcium absorption in early stages of bone formation. Needed to maintain flexible arteries and major role in cardiovascular disease. Important in prevention of Alzheimer's disease and osteoporosis; inhibits aging process in tissues. Evaluate renal stone etiology.		
Silver (Ag) (serum) RR: 0.21 ± 0.15 ng/dl, 19.47 ± 13.90 nmol/L	Collect in metal-free container. No metabolic role. Salts used as antiseptic and bacteriostatic agents. In normal individuals, silver slowly accumulates in body tissue with age but causes no apparent harm.	Chemical conjunctivitis from silver nitrate Gastroenteritis (dose by mouth), grayish discoloration of mucous membranes Argyria (bluish gray skin discoloration from nose/eye drops over time or industrial exposure	

	Assess for occupational exposure or toxicity from medicinal uses of silver.	Silvadene topically for burns Silver picrate (antiseptic) *Lethal dose:* 3.5–35 g total dose.
Thallium (Tl) (blood) RR: 0–2.0 µg/dl CR: 10–800 µg/dl or 0.5–39.1 µmol/L (urine) RR: 0–2.0 µg/L/24h CR: 1.0–2.0 mg/L or 4.9–97.8 µmol/L	Collect in metal-free container. No metabolic role. Used in medications, cosmetics, and pesticides. Poisoning occurs from ingestion or from absorption through intact skin and mucous membranes; accumulates in liver, kidneys, bone, and muscle tissue. Assess for toxicity from either accidental ingestion or exposure.	Formerly used in ant, rat, and roach poisons. *Toxicity:* Thallitoxicosis or thallotoxicosis (ingestion of pesticides); vomiting, hair loss, delirium, coma, ataxia, pulmonary edema, paralysis, death Poisoning results in blindness, facial paralysis, paresthesias, peripheral neuropathy, liver and renal damage. *Lethal dose:* 5–50 mg
Tin (Sn) (plasma) RR: 23 ng/ml	Collect in metal-free container. Ultratrace mineral. Used in manufacturing of alloys, plating, food containers.	Diet high in canned fruits/juices Zinc balance negatively affected at 50 mg intakes, industrial exposure to organic tin compounds and dust.

(Continued)

Substance Tested (Specimen Needed), Reference Range (RR), Critical Toxic Range (CR), and RDIs if Available	Patient Preparation, Substance Function, and Indications for Test	Clinical Implications	
		Increase	Decrease
	Assess for industrial exposure.	Tin salts used in calico printing Organic compounds found in polyvinyl plastics, chlorinated rubber paints, fungicides, insecticides, and anthelmintics	
Vanadium (V) (plasma or serum) RR: 0.02–10 ng/ml (hair) RR: 0.01–2.2 μg/g (urine) RR: 0–10 μg/d	Collect in metal-free container. Ultratrace mineral. Used in the steel industry and to a lesser degree in photography and in the manufacturing of insecticides, dyes, inks, paints, and varnish. Assess for occupational exposure.	Occupational inhalation (fuel combustion for electricity): hemorrhagic endotheliotoxic with leukocytotactic and hematotoxic components. *Toxicity:* Industrial processes (sore eyes and bronchi), dermatitis, depletion of ascorbic acid, gastrointestinal distress; cardiac palpitation, kidney damage, central nervous system disturbances (lowers vanadium toxicity); green tongue and disturbances of mental function	
Zinc (Zn) (plasma) RR: 78–136 μg/ml	Fasting morning specimen. Plays a role in protein synthesis;	Zinc therapy for Wilson's disease Ingestion of food or beverage contaminated by storage in a	Decreased intake (chronic alcoholics, vegetarians, young women with

(serum) RR: 55–150 µg/ml (decreases with aging), 11–18 µmol/L (24-h urine) RR: 6–9 µmol/L (serum or plasma) RR: <70 µg/dl (deficiency) RDI: men 15 mg/d women 12 mg/d	critical for growth and sexual maturation. Important in wound healing and sensory perception (particularly taste and smell). Important in activating certain serum enzymes and in insulin and porphyrin metabolism. Assess population that may have increased needs for intake—alcoholism, chronic illness, stress, trauma, surgery, malabsorption, lactovegetarians, children consuming vegetarian diets, decubitus ulcers, anorexics.	galvanized container Long-term ingestion of excessive zinc supplements >150 mg/d (secondary copper deficiency) Low serum high-density lipoprotein Gastric erosion Depressed immune system Lethargy in dialysis patients Hyperzincuria increasing with the severity of diabetes Inhalation of zinc oxide fumes causing neurologic damage (metal fume fever, brass-founders' ague, zinc shakes), metallic taste, bloody diarrhea	anorexia nervosa), diarrhea Decreased circulatory and splenic T lymphocytes Prolonged bedrest Decrease in absorption of tetracycline Rheumatic diseases Infection Growth retardation Male hypogonadism and hypospermism Nyctalopia (night blindness) Hypogeusia Impaired wound healing, long-term total parenteral nutrition without zinc supplement Chronic liver disease Acrodermatitis enteropathica Dwarfism Parasitism (Egypt) Compromised immune function Low facteur thymique serique (FTS) Impaired embryogenesis Behavioral disturbances (impaired hedonic tone) Skeletal abnormalities, defective collagen synthesis, alopecia, impaired protein synthesis. Some cancers

APPENDIX H

Consent Form Examples

Informed consent, signifying agreement to testing, is required in many situations. For example, such agreement must be obtained before specimens are collected for human immunodeficiency virus (HIV) antibody testing or for witnessed urine drug screen testing.

Agency protocols, including legal codes, must be followed when obtaining an informed consent signed by the patient (or by the parent or guardian in the case of a minor). A properly executed informed consent form requires the date, consent signature, name of witness, and procedure type or test.

Before signing an informed consent form, the patient should be made aware of the difference between *confidential* and *anonymous* testing and the implications of each. Anonymous tests do not require the individual to give his or her name, whereas confidential tests do require names. As examples of implications, positive HIV test results may be reported to insurance companies or to local, state, or federal health agencies, and drug screening results may be reported to employers or law enforcement agencies.

It is important to document in the patient's record that the consent was obtained and to report anything out of the ordinary that occurred during the obtaining or witnessing of the consent.

Informed Consent and Agreement to HIV Testing

With my signature below I acknowledge that I have read (or have had read to me) and understand the following information:

Facts About HIV Testing

I HAVE BEEN TOLD THAT: (1) My blood will be tested for signs of an infection by the human immunodeficiency virus, the virus that causes AIDS; (2) My consent to have my blood tested for HIV should be FREELY given; and (3) Every attempt will be made to keep the results of this test confidential, but that confidentiality cannot be guaranteed.

What a NEGATIVE Result Means:

A negative test means that the laboratory has not found evidence of HIV infection in my blood sample.

What a POSITIVE Test Result Means:

A. A positive HIV test means that I have HIV infection and can spread the virus to others by having sex or by sharing needles;

B. A positive HIV test DOES NOT mean that I have AIDS – other tests are needed;

C. If my test result is positive, I may experience emotional discomfort and, if my test result becomes known to the community, I may experience discrimination in work, personal relationships, and insurance.

What Will Be Done for Me if My Test is Postiive:

A. I will be given a copy of the Department of Health and Mental Hygiene's publication, "Directory of Counseling and Referral Resources for HIV Seropositive Persons", which contains information about medical, social, psychological, and legal services that will be helpful to me;

B. I will be told how to keep from spreading my HIV infection by: (1) Avoiding sexual intercourse, or practicing SAFER sex; (2) Not sharing drug needles—better still, getting off drugs; (3) Not donating or selling my blood, plasma, organs, or sperm; (4) Avoiding pregnancy; and (5) Not breastfeeding, or donating breast milk;

C. Unless my test is performed at a designated anonymous test site approved by the Department of Health and Mental Hygiene, my unique patient identifying number will be given to the local health department and, if I have signs or symptoms of HIV infection, my name will be reported to the local health department to assist me in obtaining services and help the health department understand and control the AIDS problem;

D. I know that my local health department or doctor may assist me in notifying and referring my partners for medical services—without giving my name to my partners;

E. If I refuse to notify my partners, my doctor may either notify them, or have the local health department do so. In this case, my name will not be used. Maryland law requires that, when a local health department knows of my partners, it must refer them for care, support, and treatment; and

F. I have had a chance to have my questions about this test answered. My counselor has explained to me about the use of a portion of my Social Security number in the unique patient identifying number and I have indicated below whether or not a portion of my Social Security number can be used for this purpose.

☐ **YES,** I allow the use of a portion of my Social Security number.
☐ **NO, I DO NOT** allow the use of a portion of my Social Security number.

I hereby agree to have my blood drawn for an HIV test.

_____   _____
Name of Person Tested   Date

_____   _____
Signature of Patient or Authorized Substitute   Signature of Counselor

State of Maryland Health Department form for HIV testing.

Drug Screen Test Request (Chain of Custody)

CLIENT INFORMATION

Name

Address

Phone _____ Account Number

PATIENT DATA

PATIENT ID OR SOCIAL SECURITY NO.

CONTROL NUMBER **WD**

DATE COLLECTED

LOCATION IDENTIFIER

NAME (Last, First, Middle Initial)

COMMENTS

Comments Will Print on Report (Limit to 36 characters)

Please "X" Desired Profile

M50 **Drug Screen, Urine, for Drugs of Abuse (10-Drug Panel) with Confirmation of Positive Results**

Amphetamines, Barbiturates, Benzodiazepines, Cocaine, Marijuana, Methadone, Methaqualone, Opiates, Phencyclidine, Propoxyphene

44A **Drug Screen, Urine, for Drugs of Abuse (9-Drug Panel) with Confirmation of Positive Results**

Amphetamines, Barbiturates, Benzodiazepines, Cocaine, Marijuana, Methadone, Methaqualone, Opiates, Phencyclidine

M54 **Drug Screen, Urine, for Drugs of Abuse (7-Drug Panel) with Confirmation of Positive Results**

Amphetamines, Barbiturates, Benzodiazepines, Cocaine, Marijuana, Methaqualone, Opiates

M56 **Drug Screen, Urine, for Drugs of Abuse (6-Drug Panel) with Confirmation of Positive Results**

Amphetamines, Barbiturates, Benzodiazepines, Cocaine, Marijuana, Opiates

	Drug Screen, Urine, for Drugs of Abuse (5-Drug Panel) NIDA 5 Test Equivalent, with Confirmation of Positive Result
T24	Amphetamines, Cocaine, Marijuana, Opiates, Phencyclidine. **FOR NON-FEDERAL AGENCY USE ONLY.**
P29	Alcohol, Ethyl, Urine with Confirmation of Positive Results
M23	Alcohol, Ethyl, Blood with Confirmation of Positive Results
51A	Drug Screen, Urine, for Drugs of Abuse (5-Drug Panel + Alcohol) with Confirmation of Positive Results

Amphetamines, Cocaine, Marijuana, Opiates, Phencyclidine and Ethanol

For Laboratory Use Only

To be completed by collector. Read urine temperature within four minutes of collection

TEMPERATURE READ WITHIN 4 MINUTES	☐ YES	☐ NO

☐ Within Range	32.5–37.7 C 90.5–99.8 F	☐ Outside Range	Note Temperature (if outside range)

Donor Certification

I certify that I provided my specimen, (urine and / or blood) to the collector, that the specimen was sealed with a tamper-proof seal in my presence and that the information provided on this form is correct.

_____   _____
Donor Signature   Date

Collector Certification

I certify that the specimen, (urine and / or blood) identified on this form is the specimen presented to me by the donor providing the certification above, that it bears the same identification number as set forth above, and that is has been collected, labeled and sealed in accordance with MetPath Chain of Custody procedures.

_____   _____
Collector Signature   Date

_____   _____
Collection Site   Telephone No.

_____   _____
Lab Entry Signature   Date

Consent form used for witnessed urine drug testing in community, occupation, or clinic settings.

APPENDIX I

*Forms for Sleep Studies, Sleep Log,
Epworth Sleepiness Scale, and
Sleep Disorders Questionnaire*

As a part of the total assessment of sleep patterns, the patient may be required to complete charts or forms such as a sleep log, Epworth Sleepiness Scale, or Sleep Disorders Questionnaire. That information will be used in conjunction with the specific sleep study.

SLEEP LOG								
Name _____ Date _____							
Date of Birth _____ Sex M F Weight _____ Height _____							
Week #	S	M	T	W	TH	F	S
Date							
Time you went to bed							
Time lights out							
Time to fall asleep							
Time you awoke							
No. of times awake							
Time out of bed							
Medications							
Rate difficulty getting up 1 2 3 4 5 6 7 8 9 Not Very							
The following are for the preceding day							
Number of naps							
Total time of naps							
Total time outdoors							
Cups of coffee/soda							
Ounces of liquor							
Rate your fatigue 1 2 3 4 5 6 7 8 9 Not Very							

Typical sleep log, which is kept 1 or 2 weeks before sleep study.

EPWORTH SLEEPINESS SCALE

Name _____ Date _____

Date of birth _____ Sex   Male   Female

Please rate how likely you are to fall asleep in the following situations:

0 = never doze
1 = slight chance of dozing
2 = moderate chance of dozing
3 = high chance of dozing

Situation	Chance of dozing
Sitting and reading	_____
Watching TV	_____
Sitting inactive in a public place (meeting, theater, etc.)	_____
A passenger in a car for 1 hour without a break	_____
Lying down in the afternoon when circumstances permit	_____
Sitting and talking to someone	_____
Sitting quietly after lunch without alcohol	_____
In a car, while stopped for a few minutes in the traffic	_____

Total score <6 normal, scores >10 associated with mild sleep apnea, scores >16 associated with idiopathic hypersomnia, narcolepsy and moderate sleep apnea. Reference: Johns MW: A new method for measuring daytime sleepiness: The Epworth sleepiness scale. Sleep 14(6):540–545, 1991

SLEEP DISORDERS QUESTIONNAIRE

Name _____ Date _____

Date of birth _____ Sex M F Weight _____Height _____

Address _____

Doctor _____ Address _____

Describe your sleep problem _____

Current medications _____

Health problems _____

Allergies _____ Sinus problems _____

Breathing problems _____

Smoking history _____

1) Have you ever awakened with any of the following: (Circle)

Short of breath   Gasping or choking sensation   Headache

Burning sensation in chest or throat   Leg pain

2) Do you snore? Yes   No   3) Do you take naps? Yes   No

4) Do you fall asleep: (Circle)

Watching TV   Reading   Driving   Talking

5) What time do you go to bed?_____ Awaken?_____ Get up?_____

Do you drink alcohol?   Yes   No   Amount/Day _____

Do you drink coffee/soda?   Yes   No   Amount/Day _____

Typical questionnaire administered to a patient complaining of a sleeping problem.

APPENDIX J

*Drugs Affecting
Laboratory Test Values*

DRUGS AND LABORATORY TEST OUTCOMES

Many prescription medications, over-the-counter medications, vitamins, minerals, and herbal preparations can influence the results of laboratory tests. Mechanisms of drug effects are either pharmacologic (eg, furosemide usually increases the excretion of potassium, resulting in a low serum potassium level) or analytic (as when a drug in a patient's body fluid or tissue interferes with a chemical step in a laboratory test, resulting in an erroneous test result). The drug classes that cause the majority of analytic interferences include antibiotics, antihypertensives, anticonvulsants, hormones, and antidepressants.

Accurate and complete medication histories, including prescription medications, over-the-counter medications, vitamins, minerals, and herbal preparations, are essential to interpret laboratory test results that fall out of the normal range.

The following appendix is by no means exhaustive, and whenever laboratory results are suspected of being spurious, further research is necessary. There are many references available, including drug monographs in *AHFS Drug Information,* published by the American Society of Health System Pharmacists, and the *Physician's Desk Reference,* which contains official product information. Services that maintain this information include the Iowa Drug Information Service and Drugdex.

Drugs Affecting Laboratory Test Values for Selected Substances

Substance Determined	Drugs Causing Increased Values or False-Positive Values	Drugs Causing Decreased Values or False-Negative Values
EOSINOPHILS (BLOOD)	Aldesleukin, allopurinol, antibiotics (eg, cephalosporins, erythromycin, penicillins, quinolones, tetracyclines; anticonvulsants (eg, carbamazepine), antimalarials (eg, quinine), carisoprodol, chloral hydrate, chlorozoxazone, clofibrate, clozapine, dantrolene, dapsone, digitalis, enalapril,	Amphotericin B, aspirin, captopril, desipramine, glucocorticoids (eg, cortisone, hydrocortisone, prednisone), granulocyte colony-stimulating factor, indomethacin, interferon-α, niacin/niacinamide, procainamide

(continued)

Drugs Affecting Laboratory Test Values *(Continued)*

Substance Determined	Drugs Causing Increased Values or False-Positive Values	Drugs Causing Decreased Values or False-Negative Values
	epinephrine, etretinate, fluorides, fomepizole, glatiramer acetate, haloperidol, heparin, interleukin-3, iodides, isoniazide, ivermectin, levodopa, mefenamic acid, meprobamate, mercaptopurine, methyldopa, metyrosine, nonsteroidal antiinflammatory drugs (eg, aspirin), papaverine, paromomycin, penicillamine, phenothiazines (eg, promethazine), potassium iodide, probucol, procainamide, propafenone, ramipril, ranitidine, spironolactone, streptokinase, sulfonamides (eg, sulfasalazine), thiothixene, triamterene, tryptophan	
BASOPHILS		Procainamide, thiopental
MONOCYTES (BLOOD)	Ampicillin, carbenicillin, granulocyte colony-stimulating factor, griseofulvin, haloperidol, interleukin-3, methsuximide, phosphorus, pipercillin, prednisone, propylthiouracil, tumor necrosis factor	Glucocorticoids (eg, prednisone), granulocyte colony-stimulating factor
LYMPHOCYTES (BLOOD)	Aminosalicylic acid, chlorpropamide, dexamethasone, granulocyte colony-stimulating factors, griseofulvin, haloperidol, interleukin-3, levodopa, narcotics, niacinamide, propylthiouracil, spironolactone	Antineoplastics (eg, asparaginase, chlorambucil), cyclosporine A, folic acid, furosemide, glucocorticoids (eg, hydrocortisone, prednisone), ibuprofen lithium, niacin, phenytoin, pyridoxine, thiamine, tumor necrosis factor, x-ray therapy

(continued)

Drugs Affecting Laboratory Test Values *(Continued)*

Substance Determined	Drugs Causing Increased Values or False-Positive Values	Drugs Causing Decreased Values or False-Negative Values
RED CELL COUNT (BLOOD)	Antithyroid therapy (eg, propylthiouracil), cobalt, gentamicin, glucocorticoids, hydrochlorothiazide, methyldopa, pilocarpine, vitamin B_{12}	Acetaminophen, acyclovir, allopurinol, amphetamine, amyl nitrite, antibiotics (eg, ampicillin), anticonvulsants (eg, ethosuximide), antihistamines (eg, brompheniramine), antimalarials (eg, chloroquine), antineoplastics (eg, aminoglutethimide), antithyroid therapy (eg, propylthiouracil), arsenicals, auranofin, barbiturates (eg, phenobarbital), bismuth subsalicylate, captopril, carvedilol, chlordiazepoxide, chlorthalidone, cimetidine, clonazepam, corticosteroids, cyclosporine, dapsone, digitalis, dimercaprol, doxapram, etretinate, flucytosine, fluorides, furosemide, haloperidol, hydralazine, isoniazid, isotretinoin, levodopa/ methyldopa, lipomul, local anesthetics (eg, benzocaine), monoamine oxidase inhibitors, meprobamate, methazolamide, methylene blue, nitrites, nitrous oxide, nonsteroidal antiinflammatory drugs (eg, ibuprofen); oral contraceptives, penicillamine, pentoxifylline, phenothiazines (eg, chlorpromazine), phosphorus, probenecid, procainamide, quinidine,

Drugs Affecting Laboratory Test Values *(Continued)*

Substance Determined	Drugs Causing Increased Values or False-Positive Values	Drugs Causing Decreased Values or False-Negative Values
		radioactive compounds, sulfonamides (eg, sulfamethoxazole), sulfonylureas (eg, chlorpropamide), sulfasalazine, sulfinpyrazone, thiazides (eg, chlorothiazide), thiothixene, ticlopidine, tocainide, trazodone, tricyclic antidepressants (eg, amitriptyline), vitamin K, x-ray therapy, zidovudine
ERYTHROCYTE SEDIMENTATION RATE (BLOOD)	Anticonvulsants, aspirin, carbamazepine, cephalothin, clofazimine, cyclosporine A, dexamethasone, dextran, hydralazine, indomethacin, isotretinoin, methyldopa, nitrofurantoin, oral contraceptives, penicillamine, procainamide, propafenone, quinidine, sulfamethoxazole, theophylline, tretinoin, vitamin A	Adrenal steroids, aspirin, corticotropin, cortisone, cyclophosphamide, fluorides, gold, methotrexate, nonsteroidal antiinflammatory drugs, penicillamine, prednisone, quinine, salicylates, sulfasalazine, tamoxifen, trimethoprim
IRON (BLOOD)	Acetylsalicylic acid, blood transfusions, cefotaxime, chemotherapy, chloramphenicol, cisplatin, dextran, estrogens, ethanol, iron dextran, iron preparations, methicillin, methotrexate, methyldopa, oral contraceptives, rifampin	Adrenocorticotropic hormone, allopurinol, aspirin, cholestyramine, colchicine, cortisone, deferoxamine, metformin, methicillin, penicillamine, pyrazinamide, testosterone
FERRITIN (BLOOD)	Iron prepartions, oral contraceptives, theophylline, x-ray therapy	Antithyroid therapy, ascorbic acid, deferoxamine, methimazole

(continued)

Drugs Affecting Laboratory Test Values   *(Continued)*

Substance Determined	Drugs Causing Increased Values or False-Positive Values	Drugs Causing Decreased Values or False-Negative Values
METHEMOGLOBIN (BLOOD)	Aminosalicylic acid, amyl nitrite, analgesics (eg, acetaminophen), antimalarials (eg, primaquine), chloramphenicol, co-trimoxazole (SMX-TMP), dapsone, dimercaprol, furazolidone, isoniazid, isosorbide, local anesthetics (eg, benzocaine), methylene blue, metoclopramide, naphthalene, nitrates (eg, bismuth subnitrate), nitrofurantoin, nitroglycerin, phenazopyridine, phenytoin, potassium chloride, probenecid, quinidine, resorcinol, sulfonamide derivatives (eg, sulfacetamide)	
SULFHEMOGLOBIN (BLOOD)	Acetanilid, phenacetin, phenazopyridine, sulfanamides, sulfamethizole	
MYOGLOBIN (BLOOD)	Intramuscular injections, radioactive substances, simvastatin, streptokinase, succinylcholine	
VITAMIN B_{12} (SERUM)	Blood transfusion, chloral hydrate, granulocyte-macrophage colony-stimulating factor, Vitamin A, Vitamin C	Aminosalicylic acid, anticonvulsants, ascorbic acid, chlorpromazine, cholestyramine, colchicine, laxatives, metformin, neomycin, oral contraceptives, ranitidine
FOLIC ACID (SERUM)	Folic acid, metformin	Alcohol, aminoglutethimide, antacids, antibiotics (eg, ampicillin); anticonvulsants (eg, phenytoin), antimalarials (eg,

Drugs Affecting Laboratory Test Values *(Continued)*

Substance Determined	Drugs Causing Increased Values or False-Positive Values	Drugs Causing Decreased Values or False-Negative Values
		pyrimethamine), arsenicals, aspirin, barbiturates (eg, phenobarbital), cholestyramine, cycloserine, estrogens/oral contraceptives, iron, isoniazid, levodopa, metformin, methotrexate, sulfonamides (eg, sulfasalazine), triamterene
ERYTHROPOIETIN (SERUM)	Anabolic steroids, daunorubicin, fluoxymesterone, hydroxyurea, zidovudine	Amphotericin B, cisplatin, enalapril, theophylline
BLEEDING TIME (BLOOD)	Allopurinol, aminocaproic acid, antibiotics (eg, ampicillin), anticoagulants (eg, heparin), antithrombolitcs (eg, streptokinase), canola oil, dextran, ethanol, fluoxetine, mithramycin, nifedipine, nitroglycerin, nonsteroidal antiinflammatory drugs (eg, aspirin), radiographic contrast agents, propranolol, ticlopidine, valproic acid	Desmopressin
PLATELET COUNT (BLOOD)	Amoxapine, auranofin, clindamycin, danazol, dipyridamole, gemfibrozil, glucocorticoids, imipenem, interferon-α, interleukin-1β, interleukin-3, isotretinoin, lithium, metoprolol, miconazole, moxalactam, oral contraceptives, phosphorus, propranolol, tumor necrosis factor, zidovudine	Acetaminophen, acetazolamide, acetohexamide, albuterol, allopurinol, amiodaroine, amrinone, amphotericin B, antibiotics (eg, cephalosporins), anticonvulsants (eg, carbamazepine), antimalarials (eg, chloroquine), antineoplastics (eg, aminoglutethimide), arsenicals, aspirin, auranofin, barbiturates (eg, phenobarbital), betaxolol, bismuth

(continued)

Drugs Affecting Laboratory Test Values   *(Continued)*

Substance Determined	Drugs Causing Increased Values or False-Positive Values	Drugs Causing Decreased Values or False-Negative Values
		subsalicylate, captopril, carvedilol, chlorpheniramine, chlorthalidone, cimetidine, codeine, colchicine, dextroamphetamine, diazoxide, diethylstilbestrol, digitalis, enalapril, ethacrynic acid, fluconazole, flucytosine, fluorides, furosemide, granulocyte stimulating factors, hydralazine, immune globulin, interferon-α, interleukin-3, isoniazid, isotretinoin, itraconazole, levodopa/methyldopa, Lipomul, lovastatin, measles virus vaccine, meprobamate, metformin, methimazole, methylphenidate, mexiletine, miconazole, mumps virus vaccine, nitroglycerin, nonsteroidal antiinflammatory drugs (eg, fenoprofen), penicillamine, pentoxifylline, phenolphthalein, phenothiazines (eg, fluphenazine), poliovirus vaccine, potassium iodide, prednisone, probenecid, probucol, procainamide, propranolol, propylthiouracil, pyrazinamide, quinidine, ranitidine, reserpine, rubella virus vaccine, smallpox vaccine, spironolactone, sulfonamides, sulfonylureas (eg, chlorpropamide), tamoxifen, thiazide diuretics (eg, chlorothiazide, hydrochlorothiazide), thiothixene, ticlopidine, tocainide, tricyclic

Drugs Affecting Laboratory Test Values   *(Continued)*

Substance Determined	Drugs Causing Increased Values or False-Positive Values	Drugs Causing Decreased Values or False-Negative Values
		antidepressants (eg, amitriptyline), vitamin K, x-ray therapy, zidovudine
THROMBIN TIME (BLOOD)	Asparaginase, streptokinase, urokinase	Dextran, low-molecular-weight heparin
PARTIAL THROMBOPLASTIN TIME (BLOOD)	Antibiotics (eg, azlocillin), antihistamines, ascorbic acid, asparaginase, chlorpromazine, dextran, gold, heparin, naloxone, phenytoin, radiographic agents, salicylates (eg, aspirin), tolmetin	Low-molecular-weight heparin, oral contraceptives
COAGULATION TIME (BLOOD)	Anticoagulants, phosphorus, tetracycline	Aminophylline
PLASMINOGEN (BLOOD)	Anabolic steroids, danazol, fluoxymesterone, norethandrolone, oral contraceptives, oxymetholone, stanozolol	Alteplase, asparaginase, dextran, gemfibrozil, streptokinase
EUGLOBULIN CLOT LYSIS TIME (BLOOD)	Asparaginase, clofibrate, dextran, gemfibrozil, streptokinase	Adrenocorticotropic hormone, steroids
FIBRIN SPLIT PRODUCTS (PLASMA)	Barbiturates, heparin, streptokinase, urokinase	
FIBRINOGEN (PLASMA)	Aspirin, estrogens, gemfibrozil, norethandrolone, oral contraceptives, pyrazinamide	Anabolic steroids/androgens (eg, danazol), asparaginase, antithrombotics (eg, streptokinase), cefamandole, iron, kanamycin, lipid-lowering agents (eg, clofibrate), oral contraceptives, pentoxifylline, phenobarbital, phosphorus, ticlopidine, valproic acid

(continued)

Drugs Affecting Laboratory Test Values   *(Continued)*

Substance Determined	Drugs Causing Increased Values or False-Positive Values	Drugs Causing Decreased Values or False-Negative Values
GLUCOSE (CEREBROSPINAL FLUID)	Cefotaxime, dexamethasone	Cefotaxime
PROTEIN (CEREBROSPINAL FLUID)	Aminosalicylic acid, ascorbic acid, aspirin, cefotaxime, chloramphenicol, chlorpromazine, dextran, ibuprofen, imipramine, lidocaine, mannitol, methicillin, methotrexate	Acetaminophen, cefotaxime, cytarabine, dexamethasone
BLOOD IN STOOL	Anticoagulants, boric acid, bromides, colchicine, indomethacin, inorganic iron, iodine, iron, nonsteroidal antiinflammatory drugs, oxidizing agents, *Rauwolfia* derivatives, salicylates, steroids, vitamin C	Vitamin C
UROBILINOGEN (STOOL)	Amyl nitrite	Acetohexamide, aminosalicylic acid, antibiotics, chloramphenicol, chlorpromazine, chlorpropamide, erythromycin, methimazole, nalidixic acid, neomycin, oral contraceptives, prochlorperazine, promazine, sulfamethizole, sulfamethoxazole, sulfisoxazole, tetracycline, thiazides, tolazamide, tolbutamide, trifluoperazine
STOOL ELECTROLYTES *Sodium*	Neomycin	

Drugs Affecting Laboratory Test Values   *(Continued)*

Substance Determined	Drugs Causing Increased Values or False-Positive Values	Drugs Causing Decreased Values or False-Negative Values
Potassium		
	Neomycin	

DISCOLORATION OF STOOL

White or white speckling

Antacids,
aluminum
salts, barium

Black

Acetazolamide,
aminophylline,
amphetamine,
amphotericin,
bismuth
subsalicylate,
charcoal,
chlorpropamide,
clindamycin,
corticosteroids,
cyclophosphamide,
cytarabine,
digitalis,
ethacrynic acid,
fluorouracil,
hydralazine,
iodides, iron,
manganese,
melphalan,
methazolamide,
methotrexate,
phenylephrine,
potassium,
prednisolone,
procarbazine,
reserpine,
sulfonamides,
theophylline,
thiotepa,
warfarin

(continued)

Drugs Affecting Laboratory Test Values *(Continued)*

Substance Determined	Drugs Causing Increased Values or False-Positive Values	Drugs Causing Decreased Values or False-Negative Values
Black and white speckling Antibiotics		
Blue Chloramphenicol, methylene blue		
Red to black Anticoagulants, salicylates, tetracyclines (syrup)		
Orange Phenazopyridine, phenolphthalein, rifampin		
Green Indomethacin, medroxypro-gesterone		
CALCIUM (SERUM)	Anabolic steroids (eg, fluoxymesterone), androgens (eg, nandrolone), antacids (eg, aluminum hydroxide), cefotaxime, chlorpropamide, chlorthalidone, dihydrotachysterol, estrogens (eg, oral contraceptives), hydralazine, hypaque, lithium, magnesium salts, nisoldipine, parathyroid hormone, phenobarbital, potassium, prednisone, progestins, propranolol, secretin, tamoxifen, theophylline, thiazide diuretics (eg, chlorothiazide), vitamin D	Acetazolamide, aldesleukin, antibiotics (eg, genta-micin); anticonvulsants (eg, carbamazepine), antimalarials (eg, chloroquine), asparaginase, aspirin, calcitonin, cisplatin, citrates, corticosteroids (eg, prednisone), estrogens/oral contraceptives, etidronate, fluorides, foscarnet, heparin, indapamide, insulin, interferon, iron dextran complex, ketoconazole, laxatives, magnesium salts, methicillin, pamidronate, pentoxi-fylline, phenobarbital, phosphates, probucol, sodium acetate, sodium bicarbonate, sodium polystyrene sulfonate,

Drugs Affecting Laboratory Test Values *(Continued)*

Substance Determined	Drugs Causing Increased Values or False-Positive Values	Drugs Causing Decreased Values or False-Negative Values
		tamoxifen, thiazide diuretics (eg, quinethazone), trazodone, zalcitabine
CHLORIDE (SERUM)	Acetaminophen, acetazolamide, acetylcysteine, ammonium chloride, androgens, bromide, cannabis, carbamazepine, carvedilol, cefotaxime, chloride salts, chlorthalidone, cholestyramine, colestipol, corticosteroids (eg, hydrocortisone), cyclosporine, diazoxide, potassium-sparing diuretics (eg, amiloride, triamterene), estrogens, guanethidine, Hypaque, iodides, mafenide, methazolamide, methyldopa, neuromuscular blocking agents (eg, neostigmine), nifedipine, nonsteroidal antiinflammatory drugs (eg, ibuprofen), propantheline, sodium bromide, thiazide diuretics (eg, chlorothiazide)	Aldosterone, allopurinol, bicarbonate, cefotaxime, chlorpropamide, corticosteroids (eg, cortisone, hydrocortisone, prednisolone), dapsone, dirithromycin, diuretics (eg, bumetanide), fluorides, laxatives (eg, docusate), mannitol, polymyxin B, primidone, tolazoline, trimethoprim
PHOSPHATE (SERUM)	Aluminum hydroxide, aminosalicylic acid, anabolic steroids, antibiotics (eg, cefotaxime), ascorbic acid, β-blockers (eg, acebutolol, pindolol, timolol), colestipol, diuretics (eg, furosemide), etidronate disodium, foscarnet, lipids, mannitol, medroxyprogesterone, methotrexate, naproxen, nifedipine, oral contraceptives, phosphates, Phospho-Soda, potassium acid phosphate, theophylline, vitamin D	Acetazolamide, albuterol, amino acids, anesthetic agents, antacids (eg, aluminum hydroxide) antibiotics (eg, cefotaxime, plicamycin, tetracycline), anticonvulsants (eg, carbamazepine), calcitonin, citrates, foscarnet, gallium nitrate, insulin, isoniazid, levonorgestrel, lithium, mannitol, mestranol, mycophenolate, oral contraceptives, pamidronate, phenobarbital,

(continued)

Drugs Affecting Laboratory Test Values *(Continued)*

Substance Determined	Drugs Causing Increased Values or False-Positive Values	Drugs Causing Decreased Values or False-Negative Values
		phenothiazines (eg, promethazine), sucralfate, theophylline, vidarabine
MAGNESIUM (SERUM)	Aminoglycosides (eg, gentamicin), antacids, aspirin, calcifediol, calcitriol, cefotaxime, felodipine, foscarnet, indapamide, laxatives, lithium, loop diuretics (eg, furosemide), magnesium salts, nifedipine, potassium sparing diuretics (eg, amiloride), progesterones (eg, medroxyprogesterone), theophylline, thyroid medications	Albuterol, aldesleukin, aluminum hydroxide, amphotericin B, antibiotics (eg, cefotaxime), calcitriol, calcium gluconate, carboplatin, cisplatin, citrates, cyclosporin, digoxin, diuretics (eg, chlorothiazide), etidronate, haloperidol, indapamide, insulin, oral contraceptives, pamidronate, pentamidine, pentoxifylline, sodium polystyrene sulfonate, tacrolimus
POTASSIUM (SERUM)	Alprostadil, aminocaproic acid, amphotericin B, angiotensin-converting enzyme inhibitors (eg, captopril), antibiotics (eg, cefotaxime), antineoplastics (eg, aminoglutethimide), β-blockers (eg, atenolol), blood transfusions, cannabis, cyclosporine, danazol, dexamethasone, digitalis/digoxin, epinephrine, felodipine, fluorides, heparin, histamine, hydrochlorothiazide, iodides, isoniazid, ketoconazole, lipids, lithium, losartan, lovastatin, mannitol, mycophenolate, nifedipine, nonsteroidal anti-inflammatory drugs (eg, naproxen), pipercuronium, potassium-sparing diuretics (eg, spironolactone), potassium	Acetazolamide, albuterol, aldosterone, ammonium chloride, amphotericin B, antibiotics (eg, carbenicillin), betaxolol, captopril, carbamazepine, carboplatin, chloroquine, cidofovir, corticosteroids (eg, betamethasone), digoxin-specific Fab, disopyramide, diuretics (potassium-wasting) (eg, bumetanide), dobutamine, enalapril, epoprostenol, fludrocortisone, fluvoxamine, foscarnet, fosinopril, glucose, indapamide, insulin, isoetharine, itraconazole, laxatives (eg, bisacodyl), levodopa, lithium, magnesium salts, methazolamide, metoclopramide,

Drugs Affecting Laboratory Test Values   *(Continued)*

Substance Determined	Drugs Causing Increased Values or False-Positive Values	Drugs Causing Decreased Values or False-Negative Values
	supplements, procainamide, succinylcholine, terbutaline, theophylline, tromethamine, venlafaxine	nifedipine, phenolphthalein, phenothiazines (eg, promethazine), phosphates, salicylates (eg, aminosalicylic acid), sodium salts, sulfasalazine, sulfates, tacrolimus, terbutaline, vidarabine
SODIUM (SERUM)	Amiloride, amino acids, anabolic steroids (eg, danazol), antibiotics (eg, ampicillin), bicarbonate, calcium, cannabis, carbamazepine, chlorthalidone, cholestyramine, cisplatin, clonidine, corticosteroids (eg, betamethasone), diazoxide, estrogens/oral contraceptives, fluorides, fosphenytoin, isosorbide, lactulose, laxatives, mannitol, methyldopa, nonsteroidal antiinflammatory drugs (eg, fenoprofen); potassium, ramipril, reserpine, sodium salts (eg, sodium acetate), valproic acid	Acetaminophen, amphotericin B, angiotensin-converting enzyme inhibitors (eg, captopril), bicarbonate, calcium channel blockers (eg, nicardipine), carbamazepine, cisplatin, colestipol, cyclophosphamide, dapsone, desmopressin, diuretics (eg, amiloride), fluoxetine, foscarnet, gentamicin, glycerin, haloperidol, heparin, indapamide, itraconazole, ketoconazole, laxatives (eg, docusate), lithium, mannitol, methylprednisolone, miconazole, nonsteroidal anti-inflammatory drugs (eg, indomethacin), phenoxybenzamine, polymixin B, propafenone, somatostatin, sulfonylureas (eg, chlorpropamide), theophylline, tobramycin, vasopressin, vincristine, zalcitabine
C-PEPTIDE (SERUM)	Betamethasone, deferoxamine, glyburide, indapamide, isoproterenol, oral contraceptives, prednisone, rifampin, sulfonylureas, terbutaline	Atenolol, calcitonin, dexfenfluramine, enprostil

(continued)

Drugs Affecting Laboratory Test Values *(Continued)*

Substance Determined	Drugs Causing Increased Values or False-Positive Values	Drugs Causing Decreased Values or False-Negative Values
GLUCACON (PLASMA)	Amino acids, aspirin, calitonin, danazol, galactose, gastrin, glucocorticoids, guanabenz, hydrochlorothiazide, insulin, interferon-α, lipids, nifedipine, prednisolone, propranolol	Atenolol, insulin, metoprolol, octreotide, pindolol, propranolol, secretin, verapamil
INSULIN (PLASMA)	Acetohexamide, albuterol, amino acids, aspirin, calcium gluconate, cannabis, corticosteroids (eg, prednisone), deferoxamine, glucacon, hydrochlorothiazide, insulin, interferon-α, isoproterenol, levodopa, lisinopril, medroxyprogesterone, megestrol, niacin, oral contraceptives, perindopril, prazosin, quinine, rifampin, secretin, spironolactone, streptozocin, sulfonylureas (eg, chlorpropamide), terbutaline, trichlormethiazide, verapamil	Acarbose, acetohexamide, asparaginase, cimetidine, clofibrate, dexfenfluramine, diazoxide, diltiazem, diuretics (eg, ethacrynic acid), doxazosin, enalapril, metformin, midazolam, morphine, niacin, nifedipine, octreotide, phenytoin, prazosin, propranolol, psyllium, sulfonylureas (eg, chlorpropamide)
GLUCOSE TOLERANCE (SERUM)	Atenolol, caffeine, clofibrate, fenfluramine, glyburide, guanethidine, lisinopril, monoamine oxidase inhibitors, metformin, metoprolol, niacin, octreotide, phenytoin, prazosin, terazosin	Adrenoocorticotropic hormone, anabolic steroids (eg, danazol, mestranol), androgens, β-blockers (eg, acebutolol), calcitonin, cannabis, cimetidine, clofibrate, corticosteroids (eg, cortisone), diazoxide, diethylstilbestrol, diuretics (eg, chlorothiazide), estrogens/oral contraceptives, felodipine, glucagon, haloperidol, heparin, imipramine, interferon-α, iron, isoniazid, lithium, medroxyprogesterone, mefenamic acid, niacin/niacinamide, nicotine,

Drugs Affecting Laboratory Test Values *(Continued)*

Substance Determined	Drugs Causing Increased Values or False-Positive Values	Drugs Causing Decreased Values or False-Negative Values
		nifedipine, octreotide, phenolphthalein, phenothiazines (eg, perphenazine), phenytoin, progestins, thyroid hormone, verapamil
GLYCOSYLATED HEMOGLOBIN (BLOOD)	Aspirin, gemfibrozil, hydrochlorothiazide, indapamide, lovastatin, niacin, propranolol	Acarbose, deferoxamine, glyburide, insulin, lisinopril, metformin, ramipril, terazosin, verapamil
AMMONIA (PLASMA)	Acetaminophen, acetazolamide, alcohol, ammonium chloride, amobarbital, asparagine, baclofen, barbiturates, butabarbital sodium, chlorothiazide, chlorthalidone, diuretics (loop and thiazide), hydrochlorothiazide, mephobarbital, narcotics, parenteral nutrition, pentobarbital, polythiazide, trichlormethiazide, valproic acid derivatives	Broad-spectrum antibiotics, lactulose, *Lactobacillus,* levodopa, potassium salts
BILIRUBIN (SERUM)	Acetaminophen, acetazolimide, acetohexamide, acetophenazine, aldesleukin, allopurinol, amino acids, amiodarone, amphotericin B, amyl nitrite, anabolic steroids/androgens, antibiotics (eg, azithromycin), anticonvulsants (eg, carbamazepine), antifungal agents (eg, itraconazole), antihistamines (eg, cyproheptadine), antimalarials (eg, chloroquine), antineoplastics (eg, fluorouracil), arsenicals, ascorbic acid, barbiturates, benzodiaze-	Amikacin, amobarbital, anticonvulsants (eg, carbamazepine, phenytoin), ascorbic acid, barbiturates, caffeine, cyclosporine, hydroxyurea, isotretinoin, levodopa, mephobarbital, nitrofurantoin, penicillin, pentobarbital, phenobarbital, phenytoin, pindolol, prednisone, salicylates (eg, aspirin), sulfisoxazole, theophylline, thioridazine, ursodiol, valproic acid

(continued)

Drugs Affecting Laboratory Test Values *(Continued)*

Substance Determined	Drugs Causing Increased Values or False-Positive Values	Drugs Causing Decreased Values or False-Negative Values
	pines (eg, chlordiazepoxide), β-blockers (eg, carvedilol), bismuth subsalicylate, captopril, chloral hydrate, chloroform, cholestyramine, cholinergics (eg, bethanechol), cimetidine, clofibrate, clonidine, colchicine, cycloserine, dantrolene, dapsone, dextran, disopyramide, disulfiram, diuretics (eg, amiloride), estrogens/oral contraceptives, ethchlorvynol, ethionamide, factor IX complex (human), flucytosine, fluvastatin, glycopyrrolate, gold, haloperidol, hydralazine, indinavir, isoniazid, isoproterenol, levodopa/methyldopa, lamivudine, losartan, loxapine, monoamine oxidase inhibitors, megestrol acetate, meperidine, meprobamate, methacholine, methimazole, methoxsalen, morphine, niacin, nonsteroidal anti-inflammatory drugs (eg, indomethacin, sulindac), octreotide, ondansetron, papaverine, pegaspargase, pemoline, penicillamine, pentoxifylline, phenazo-pyridine, phenothiazines (eg, promethazine), phosphorus, probenecid, progesterones, propoxy-phene, propylthiouracil, pyrazinamide, quinidine, quinine, radiographic agents, reserpine, sorbitol, sulfadiazine, sulfamethox-azole, sulfasalazine, sulfisoxazole, sulfonylureas (eg, chlorpropamide, tolazamide, tolbutamide),	

Drugs Affecting Laboratory Test Values *(Continued)*

Substance Determined	Drugs Causing Increased Values or False-Positive Values	Drugs Causing Decreased Values or False-Negative Values
	tamoxifen, theophylline, thiothixene, ticlopidine, tricyclic antidepressants (eg, amitriptyline), warfarin	
BLOOD UREA NITROGEN	Acetaminophen, acetazolamide, acetohexamide, acyclovir, allopurinol, amantadine, amino acids, angiotensin-converting enzyme inhibitors (eg, captopril), antibiotics (eg, ampicillin/sulbactam), anticonvulsants (eg, carbamazepine), antineo-plastics (eg, asparaginase), aspirin, atovaquine, β-blockers (eg, atenolol, propranolol), bismuth subsalicylate, cefdinir, chloral hydrate, cimetidine, clonidine, codeine, danazol, dexamethasone, dextran, diuretics (eg, chlorthali-done), famotidine, flucyto-sine, fluorides, gold, griseofulvin, guanethidine, hydralazine, imipramine, immune globulin, interferon, iron, isosorbide, leuprolide, levodopa/methyldopa, losartan, methysergide, muromonab-CD3, nonsteroidal antiinflammatory drugs (eg, diclofenac), nifedipine, nizatidine, paromomycin, penicillamine, phenazopyridine, phosphorus, propylthiouracil, quinine, radiographic agents, streptokinase, tacrolimus, vasopressin, vitamin D	Amikacin, ascorbic acid, chloramphenicol, fluorides, levodopa, prednisone, streptomycin

(continued)

Drugs Affecting Laboratory Test Values *(Continued)*

Substance Determined	Drugs Causing Increased Values or False-Positive Values	Drugs Causing Decreased Values or False-Negative Values
CREATININE (SERUM)	Acetaminophen, acetohexamide, acyclovir, aldesleukin, alkaline antacids, amiodarone, amphotericin B, angiotensin-converting enzyme inhibitors (eg, captopil), antibiotics (eg, amikacin), antineoplastics (eg, methotrexate), arsenicals, ascorbic acid, atovaquone, barbiturates, β-blockers (eg, acebutolol), cefdinir, chlorpropamide, cidofovir, cimetidine, clofibrate, clonidine, cyclosprorine, danazol, dextran, dihydrotachysterol, diuretics (eg, bumetanide), dopamine, famotidine, flucytosine, foscarnet, ganciclovir, glycerin, griseofulvin, hydralazine, imipramine, interferon, lactulose, levodopa/methyldopa, lidocaine, Lipomul, lithium, losartan, mannitol, methylprednisolone, muromonab-CD3, nifedipine, nizatidine, nonsteroidal antiinflammatory drugs (eg, aspirin), paramomycin, penicillamine, phenytoin, prednisone, radiographic agents, ranitidine, streptokinase, sulfasalazine, tacrolimus, tretinoin, valsartan, vasopressin, vitamin D	Amikacin, ascorbic acid, cannabis, citrates, dopamine, ibuprofen, interferon, lisinopril, methyldopa, n-acetylcysteine, sulfonylureas (eg, chlorpropamide, glyburide), zidovudine
URIC ACID (SERUM)	Acetaminophen, acetazolamide, alcohol, anabolic steroids, antibiotics (eg, ampicillin), antineoplastics (eg, cisplatin), ascorbic acid, β-blockers (eg, atenolol), bismuth, blood transfusion,	Acetohexamide, acetophenazine, allopurinol, ascorbic acid, azathioprine, cannabis, canola oil, carbamazepine, cefotaxime, chloramphenicol,

Drugs Affecting Laboratory Test Values *(Continued)*

Substance Determined	Drugs Causing Increased Values or False-Positive Values	Drugs Causing Decreased Values or False-Negative Values
	caffeine, chloral hydrate, cimetidine, citrates, cyclosporine, dantrolene, dextran, diazoxide, didanosine, diuretics (eg, bumetanide), doxazosin, epinephrine, filgrastim, fluorides, hydralazine, indapamide, interferon, isoniazid, isotretinoin, levodopa/methyldopa, losartan, nelfinavir, niacin/ niacinamide, nonsteroidal antiinflammatory drugs (eg, ibuprofen), pancrelipase, phenothiazines (eg, promethazine), potassium, prednisone, probucol, propylthiouracil, radioactive compounds, salicylates (eg, aspirin), sulfinpyrazone, theophylline, thiamine, tretinoin, venlafaxine, warfarin, x-ray therapy	chlorine, clofibrate, corticosteroids (eg, cortisone), dicoumarol, diethylstilbestrol, diflunisal, doxazosin, enalapril, estrogens, ethacrynic acid, glucose infusion, griseofulvin, Guaifenesin, hydralazine, ibuprofen, indomethacin, levodopa/methyldopa, lisinopril, lithium, mannitol, mechlorethamine, mefenamic acid, mesoridazine, methotrexate, nifedipine, phenothiazines (eg, chlorpromazine), probenecid, radiographic agents, salicylates (eg, aspirin–high dose), sertraline, spironolactone, succimer, sulfamethox- azole, sulfinpyrazone, tetracycline, thiothixene, veapamil, vinblastine
ALDOSTERONE (PLASMA)	Amiloride, ammonium chloride, chlorthalidone, diazoxide, dobutamide, fenoldopam, hydralazine, hydrochlorothiazide, laxatives, metoclopramide, nifedipine, nitroprusside, opiates, potassium, pravastatin, spironolactone, triamterene, verapamil	Angiotensin-converting enzyme inhibitors (eg, captopril), calcium channel blockers (eg, nicardipine), clonidine, cyclosporine, dopamine, etomidate, fludro- cortisone, furosemide, guanfacine, ketoconazole, licorice, low-molecular-weight heparin, nonsteroidal antiinflammatory drugs (eg, ibuprofen), octreotide, propranolol, ranitidine, verapamil
ANTIDIURETIC HORMONE (PLASMA)	Acetaminophen, barbiturates, chlorthalidone, cholinergic agents (eg, bethanechol),	Alcohol, chlorpromazine, clonidine, guanfacine, phenytoin

(continued)

Drugs Affecting Laboratory Test Values *(Continued)*

Substance Determined	Drugs Causing Increased Values or False-Positive Values	Drugs Causing Decreased Values or False-Negative Values
	cisplatin, cyclophosphamide, estrogens, furosemide, lithium, narcotics, nicotine, oral hypoglycemic agents (eg, chlorpropamide), thiazide diuretics (eg, hydrochlorothiazide), tricyclic antidepressants (eg, amitriptyline)	
ATRIAL NATRIURETIC PEPTIDE (PLASMA)	Atenolol, captopril, carteolol, cyclosporin A, dopamine, doxorubicin, morphine, nifedipine, oral contraceptives, vasopressin, verapamil	Benazepril, chlorthalidone, clonidine, prazosin
CORTISOL (PLASMA)	Acetylsalicylic acid, amphetamines, anticonvulsants, atropine, clomipramine, corticosteroids (eg, cortisone), estrogen/oral contraceptives, fenfluramine, furosemide, glucagon, glyburide, insulin, interferon, interleukin, lithium, methadone, metoclopramide, naloxone, nonsteroidal antiinflammatory drugs (eg, diclofenac), octreotide, opiates, prostaglandin, ranitidine, spironolactone, tumor necrosis factor, vasopressin	Androgens (eg, danazol), barbiturates, clonidine, corticosteroids (eg, beclomethasone), dextroamphetamine, ephedrine, etomidate, ketoconazole, levodopa, lithium, magnesium sulfate, medroxyprogesterone, midazolam, morphine, nifedipine, nitrous oxide, oxazepam, phenytoin, pravastatin, ranitidine, trimipramine
CORTISOL SUPPRESSION	Carbamazepine, cortisol, estrogen, oral contraceptives, phenytoin, tetracycline	
CORTISOL STIMULATION	Corticosteroids, estrogens, spironolactone	
GROWTH HORMONE (PLASMA)	Amino acids, amphetamines, anabolic steroids, apomorphine, buspirone, clomipramine, clonidine, desipramine, dexametha-	Chlorpromazine, corticosteroids (eg, hydrocortisone), medroxyprogesterone, methyldopa, octreotide,

Drugs Affecting Laboratory Test Values *(Continued)*

Substance Determined	Drugs Causing Increased Values or False-Positive Values	Drugs Causing Decreased Values or False-Negative Values
	sone, diazepam, dopamine, estrogens/oral contraceptives, fenfluramine, glucagon, growth hormone–releasing hormone, indomethacin, interferon, levodopa/methyldopa, methamphetamine, metoclopramide, midazolam, niacin, nicotinic acid, pentagastrin, phenytoin, propranolol, prostaglandin $F_{2\alpha}$, pyridostigmine, tumor necrosis factor, vasopressin	phenothiazines (eg, promethazine), probucol, valproic acid
PARATHYROID HORMONE ASSAY (PLASMA)	Anticonvulsants, dopamine, estrogen/progestin therapy, foscarnet, furosemide, hydrocortisone (IV route), isoniazid, ketoconazole, lithium, octreotide, pamidronate, phenytoin, phosphates, prednisone, rifampin, steroids, tamoxifen, verapamil, vitamin D	Aluminum hydroxide, calcitrol, cimetidine, diltiazem, famotidine, gentamicin, pindolol, prednisone, propranolol, thiazides, vitamin A, vitamin D
SOMATOMEDIN C (INSULIN-LIKE GROWTH HORMONE) (PLASMA)	Aminoglutethimide, clonidine, dexamethasone, insulin-like growth factor-1, medroxyprogesterone, prednisolone, tamoxifen	Estrogens/oral contraceptives, methimazole, octreotide
CHORIONIC GONADOTROPIN (PLASMA)	Anticonvulsants, antiparkinsonian drugs, hypnotics, phenothiazines	Octreotide
FOLLICLE-STIMULATING HORMONE (PLASMA)	Anticonvulsants (eg, phenytoin), bromocriptine, cimetidine, gonadotropin-releasing hormone, growth hormone–releasing hormone, ketoconazole, levodopa, naloxone, phenytoin, pravastatin, spironolactone, tamoxifen	Anabolic steroids (eg, danazol), anticonvulsants (eg, carbamazepine), diethylstilbestrol, digoxin, estrogen/oral contraceptives, megestrol, octreotide, phenothiazines (eg, promethazine), pravastatin, tamoxifen, testosterone

(continued)

Drugs Affecting Laboratory Test Values *(Continued)*

Substance Determined	Drugs Causing Increased Values or False-Positive Values	Drugs Causing Decreased Values or False-Negative Values
LUTEINIZING HORMONE (PLASMA)	Anticonvulsants (eg, phenytoin), bromocriptine, clomiphene, finasteride, gonadotropin-releasing hormone, goserelin, growth hormone–releasing, hormone, ketoconazole mestranol, spironolactone	Anabolic steroids (eg, danazol), anticonvulsants (eg, carbamazepine), corticotropin-releasing hormone, diethylstilbestrol, digoxin, dopamine, estrogen/oral contraceptives, goserelin, megestrol, octreotide, phenothiazines (eg, thioridazine), pravastatin, progesterone, tamoxifen, testosterone
PROLACTIN (PLASMA)	Antihistamines, calcitonin, cimetidine, danazol, diethylstilbestrol, estrogens/oral contraceptives, fenfluramine, fenoldopam, furosemide, gonadotropin-releasing hormone, growth hormone–releasing hormone, haloperidol, histamine antagonists, insulin, interferon, labetalol, loxapine, megestrol, methyldopa, metoclopramide, monoamine oxidase inhibitors, molindone, morphine, nitrous oxide, opiates, parathyroid hormone, pentagastrin, phenothiazines (eg, chlorpromazine), phenytoin, ranitidine, reserpine, thiothixene, thyrotropin-releasing hormone, tumor necrosis factor, verapamil	Anticonvulsants (eg, carbamazepine), apomorphine, bromocriptine, calcitonin, clonidine, cyclosporin A, dexamethasone, dopamine, ergot alkaloid derivatives, levodopa, metoclopramide, morphine, nifedipine, octreotide, pergolide, ranitidine, rifampin, secretin, tamoxifen
PROGESTERONE (PLASMA)	Clomiphene, corticotropin, ketoconazole, progesterone, tamoxifen, valproic acid	Ampicillin, carbamazepine, danazol, goserelin, leuprolide, oral contraceptives, phenytoin, prostaglandin $F_{2\alpha}$, provastatin
TESTOSTERONE (SERUM)	Anabolic steroids (eg, danazol), anticonvulsants	Alcohol, androgens, carbamazepine,

Drugs Affecting Laboratory Test Values *(Continued)*

Substance Determined	Drugs Causing Increased Values or False-Positive Values	Drugs Causing Decreased Values or False-Negative Values
	(eg, phenytoin), barbiturates, bromocriptine, cimetidine, clomiphene, estrogens/oral contraceptives, finasteride, flutamide, gonadotropin, goserelin, pravastatin, rifampin, tamoxifen	cimetidine, corticosteroids (eg, dexamethasone), cyclophosphamide, diazoxide, diethylstil-bestrol, digoxin, fenoldopam, goserelin, ketoconazole, leuprolide, magnesium sulfate, medroxyprogesterone, octreotide, phenothiazines (thioridazine), pravastatin, spironolactone, stanozolol, tetracycline
ACID PHOSPHATASE (SERUM)	Androgens (in females), clofibrate, goserelin	Alcohol, fluorides, oxalates, phosphates
ALANINE AMINOTRANS-FERASE (SERUM)	Acetaminophen, acetohexamide, albendazole, allopurinol, aminosalicylic acid, amiodarone, amrinone, anabolic steroids, anesthetic agents (ketamine), anti-biotics (eg, amoxicillin, ampicillin), anticonvulsants (eg, carbamazepine), antifungals (eg, fluconazole), antineoplastic agents (eg, aminoglutethimide), ardeparin, arsenicals, aspirin, barbiturates (eg, phenobarbital), benzodiaze-pines (eg, alprazolam, chlordiazepoxide, diazepam, flurazepam, oxazepam), β-blockers (eg, betaxolol), bismuth subsalicylate, bromocriptine, buspirone, calcifediol, calcitriol, chenodiol, chloral hydrate, chlorzoxazone, cimetidine, clofibrate, clonidine, codeine, colchicine, cortisone, cycloserine, dantrolene, dapsone, delavirdine, diocumarol, dienestrol, diethylstilbestrol,	Acetylsalicylic acid, carvedilol, cyclosporine, ibuprofen, interferon, ketoprofen, metro-nidazole, phenothiazines, rifampin, ursodiol

(continued)

Drugs Affecting Laboratory Test Values *(Continued)*

Substance Determined	Drugs Causing Increased Values or False-Positive Values	Drugs Causing Decreased Values or False-Negative Values
	disopyramide, disulfiram, diuretics (eg, chlorothiazide), ethionamide, etretinate, famotidine, flucytosine, foscarnet, glycopyrrolate, gold, granulocyte colony-stimulating factors, halo-peridol, hydralazine, hydrocodone/homatropine, interferon, iron, isoniazid, isotretinoin, lamivudine, lavamisole, levodopa/methyldopa, levothyroxine, low-molecular-weight heparin, lovastatin, maprotiline, meperidine, meprobamate, methimazole, mexiletine, molindone, monoamine oxidase inhibitors, morphine, naltrexone, nedocromil, niacin, nizatidine, nonsteroidal antiinflam-matory drugs (eg, diclofenac), omeprazole, ondansetron, oral contra-ceptives, oxymetholone, papaverine, pegaspargase, pemoline, penicillamine, pentoxifylline, phenazo-pyridine, phenothiazines (eg, chlorpromazine), phosphorus, pravastatin, probenecid, procainamide, progesterone, propoxy-phene, propylthiouracil, pyrazinamide, quetiapine, quinidine, riluzole, saguinavir, simvastatin, streptokinase, succimer, sulfadiazine, sulfasalazine, sulfonylureas (eg, chlorpropamide), tacrine, thiabendazole, thiothixene, ticlopidine, tocainide, tretinoin, tricyclic antide-pressants (eg, amitriptyline), trioxsalen, ursodiol, verapamil, warfarin, zidovudine, zileuton	

Drugs Affecting Laboratory Test Values   *(Continued)*

Substance Determined	Drugs Causing Increased Values or False-Positive Values	Drugs Causing Decreased Values or False-Negative Values
ALAKLINE PHOSPHATASE (SERUM)	Albumin, aldesleukin, allopurinol, alprazolam, antibiotics (eg, cefamandole), anticonvulsants, antineoplastics, baclofen, chlorpropamide, colchicine, danazol, fluconazole, fluorides, fluvastatin, goserelin, indomethacin, isoniazid, mephobarbital, methyldopa, nicotinic acid, oral contraceptives, phenobarbital, phenothiazines, probenecid, succimer, verapamil	Arsenicals, calcifediol, calcitriol, clofibrate, cyanides, fluorides, nitrofurantoin, oxalates, zinc salts
ALDOLASE (SERUM)	Corticotropin, hepatotoxic agents, quinidine (IM), vasopressin	Phenothiazines, probucol
ANGIOTENSIN-CONVERTING ENZYME INHIBITORS (BLOOD)	Nicardipine, Triiodothyronine	Angiotensin-converting enzyme inhibitors, magnesium salts, steroids
AMYLASE (SERUM)	Adrenocorticotropic hormone, aminosalicylic acid, antibiotics (eg, nitrofurantoin), antineoplastics (eg, asparginase), aspirin, atovaquone, calcium salts, chloride salts, chlorpromazine, chlorthalidone, cholinergics (eg, bethanechol), cimetidine, codeine, cyproheptadine, didanosine, estrogens, ethycrynic acid, ethanol, fluorides, iodine-containing contrast media, lamivudine, meperidine, methylcholine, methyldopa, metoclopramide, metronidazole, pegaspargase, prochlorperazine, ranitidine, sulfonamides, sulindac, thiazide diuretics (eg, hydrochlorothiazide), triprolidine/pseudoephedrine, valproic acid	Citrates, dextrose (IV), oxalates, saquinavir

(continued)

Drugs Affecting Laboratory Test Values *(Continued)*

Substance Determined	Drugs Causing Increased Values or False-Positive Values	Drugs Causing Decreased Values or False-Negative Values
LIPASE (SERUM)	Adrenocorticotropic hormone, ardeparin, cholinergics (eg, bethanechol), didanosine, fat emulsions, furosemide, indomethacin, methacholine, methylprednisolone, metronidazole, narcotics (eg, codeine), oral contraceptives, pegaspargase, pentazocine, secretin, sulfisoxazole, thiazides (eg, hydrochlorothiazide), triprolidine/pseudoephedrine, valproic acid, x-ray therapy, zalcitabine	5-aminosalicylic acid, calcium ions, hydroxyurea, protamine, somatostatin
ASPARTATE TRANSAMINASE (SERUM)	Acetaminophen, acetohexamide, allopurinol, amantadine, aminocaproic acid, amiodarone, amrinone, anabolic steroids, anesthetic agents, antibiotics (eg, ampicillin), anticonvulsants (eg, carbamazepine), antifungal agents (eg, amphotericin), antineoplastic agents (eg, chlorambucil), ardeparin, ascorbic acid, baclofen, barbiturates, benzodiazepams (eg, alprazolam), β-blockers (eg, betaxolol), buspirone, captopril, chenodiol, chloral hydrate, chloroquine, chlorpropamide, chlorzoxazone, cholestyramine, chlolinergics (eg, bethanechol), cimetidine, clofibrate, clonidine, colchicine, dantrolene, dicoumarol, diethylstilbestrol, disopyramide, diuretics (eg, chlorthalidone), ethambutol, etretinate, famotidine, flucytosine, fluorides, flutamide,	Acetaminophen, allopurinol, ascorbic acid, cyclosporine, fluorides, ibuprofen, interferon, ketoprofen, metronidazole naltrexone, penicillamine, pindolol, prednisone, progesterone, rifampin, trifluoperazine, ursodiol

Drugs Affecting Laboratory Test Values *(Continued)*

Substance Determined	Drugs Causing Increased Values or False-Positive Values	Drugs Causing Decreased Values or False-Negative Values
	foscarnet, granulocyte colony-stimulating factor, gold, haloperidol, hydralazine, interferon, iron, isoniazid, isoproterenol, isotretinoin, lamivudine, levodopa, loracarbef, low-molecular-weight heparin, lovastatin, monoamine oxidase inhibitors, maprotiline, meprobamate, methacholine, *n*-acetylcysteine, naltrexone, narcotics (eg, meperidine), niacin, nizatidine, nonsteroidal antiinflammatory agents (eg, diclofenac), olsalazine, ondansetron, oral contraceptives, oxymetholone, papaverine, pemoline, penicillamine, pentoxifylline, phenazopyridine, phosphorus, pravastatin, probenecid, procainamide, progesterone, propafenone, propoxyphene, propylthiouracil, pyridoxine, quinidine, salicylates (eg, acetylsalicylic acid), simvastatin, streptokinase, sulfonamides, sulfonylureas, tacrine, tamoxifen, thiothixene, ticlopidine, tocainide, tretinoin, tricyclic antidepressants (eg, amitriptyline), venlafaxine, warfarin, zidovudine	
CREATINE PHOSPHOKINASE (SERUM)	Alcohol, aminocaproic acid, amphotericin, analgesics (IM injection) (eg, morphine), antibiotics (IM injection) (eg, ampicillin), anticoagulants, aspirin, bepridil, captopril, carteolol, cefotaxime, chlorthalidone, clonidine, colchicine,	Acetylsalicylic acid, amikacin, dantrolene, phenothiazines, pindolol, prednisone, sulfamethoxazole

(continued)

Drugs Affecting Laboratory Test Values   *(Continued)*

Substance Determined	Drugs Causing Increased Values or False-Positive Values	Drugs Causing Decreased Values or False-Negative Values
	danazol, dantrolene, dexamethasone, digoxin, dirithromycin, diuretics (IM route) (eg, chloro-thiazide), ethchlorvynol, hydrochlorothiazide, insulin, isotretinoin, labetalol, lithium, lidocaine, lipid-lowering agents (clofibrate), miconazole (IV), oral contraceptives, paraldehyde, penicillamine, phenothiazines (IM) (eg, chlorpromazine), phenytoin, pindolol, propranolol, quinidine (IM), strepto-kinase, succinylcholine, theophylline, trimethoprim, tubocurarine, vasopressin (IV), zidovudine	
LACTIC ACID DEHYDROGENASE (SERUM)	Acetaminophen, alcohol, amiodarone, amphotericin, anabolic steroids (eg, danazol), anesthetic agents, antibiotics (eg, carbenicillin), anticonvul-sants (eg, phenobarbital), antineoplastic agents (eg, estarmustine), bepridil, betaxolol, captopril, chlorpropamide, chlortha-lidone, cimetidine, clofibrate, dapsone, dicoumarol, etretinate, filgrastim, fluorides, furosemide, gold, hydralazine, imipramine, isotretinoin, itraconazole, levodopa/methyldopa, narcotics (eg, codeine), nonsteroidal antiinflam-matory agents, pemoline, penicillamine, phenobar-bital, phenothiazines (eg, chlorpromazine), procaina-mide, propoxyphene, propylthiouracil, quinidine, streptokinase, sulfasalazine, thiopental, vasopressin, verapamil	Acetylsalicylic acid, amikacin, ascorbic acid, cefotaxime, clofibrate, enalapril, fluorides, hydroxyurea, ketoprofen, methotrexate, naltrexone, theophylline

Drugs Affecting Laboratory Test Values   *(Continued)*

Substance Determined	Drugs Causing Increased Values or False-Positive Values	Drugs Causing Decreased Values or False-Negative Values
LACTATE DEHYDROGENASE ISOENZYMES (SERUM)	Bismuth subsalicylate, fluorides, morphine	Allopurinol
RENIN (PLASMA)	Captopril, furosemide	Oral contraceptives
γ-GLUTAMYL TRANSFERASE (SERUM)	Acetaminophen, alcohol, allopurinol, amiodarone, antibiotics (eg, chloramphenicol), anticonvulsants (eg, carbamazepine), antineoplastics (eg, aminoglutethimide), barbiturates (eg, phenobarbital), chlorpropamide, cimetidine, clomipramine, disulfiram, etretinate, haloperidol, hydrochloro-thiazide, isoniazid, isotretinoin, ketamine, levothyroxine, lovastatin, methyldopa, metoprololol, nonsteroidal antiinflam-matory drugs (eg, diclofenac), oral contraceptives, papaverine, phenothiazines (eg, chlorpromazine), propafenone, propoxy-phene, quinidine, strepto-kinase, sulfasalazine, warfarin, zidovudine	Cefotaxime, clofibrate, estrogens, ursodiol
α-ANTITRYPSIN (SERUM)	Aminocaproic acid, dextran, oral contraceptives, oxymetholone, streptokinase, tamoxifen, typhoid vaccine	
ETHANOL (BLOOD)	Cimetidine, ranitidine	
CHOLESTEROL (SERUM)	Acetohexamide, acetophenazine, acetylsalicylic acid (aspirin), amiodarone, amphotericin,	Acarbose, allopurinol, aluminum hydroxide, amiodarone, angiotensin-converting enzyme

(continued)

Drugs Affecting Laboratory Test Values *(Continued)*

Substance Determined	Drugs Causing Increased Values or False-Positive Values	Drugs Causing Decreased Values or False-Negative Values
	anabolic steroids, antibiotics (eg, cefotaxime), antineoplastic agents (eg, aminoglutethimide), arsenicals, ascorbic acid, β-blockers (eg, acebutolol), β-carotene, chlorpropamide, clonidine, corticosteroids (eg, prednisolone), cyclosporine, dantrolene, dapsone, dextran, disopyramide, disulfiram, diuretics (eg, chlorothiazide), epinephrine, etretinate, fat emulsion, fosinopril, glyburide, gold, imipramine, iodates, isotretinoin, levarterenol (norepinephrine), levodopa, lithium, meprobamate, methimazole, miconazole, moexipril, mycophenolate, oral contraceptives, oxymetholone, penicillamine, phenobarbital, phenothiazines (eg, chlorpromazine), phenytoin, quetiapine, sotalol, succimer, sulfonamides, tamoxifen, thiothixene, ticlopidine, venlafaxine, vitamin A, vitamin D	inhibitors (eg, captopril), antibiotics (eg, amikacin), ascorbic acid, aspirin, β-blockers (eg, acebutolol), bile salt–binding agents (eg, cholestyramine, colestipol), chlorpropamide, citrates, clomiphene, clonidine, coenzyme Q10, colchicine, diltiazem, diuretics (eg, amiloride, hydrochlorothiazide), doxazosin, fluorides, fluoxymesterone, glucagon, glyburide, granulocyte colony-stimulating factor, haloperidol, hydralazine, hydroxychloroquine, insulin, iodides, isoniazid, isotretinoin, isosorbide, ketoconazole, lipid-lowering agents (eg, niacin), low-molecular-weight heparin, monoamine oxidase inhibitors, medroxyprogesterone, metformin, methyldopa, metronidazole, nifedipine, nitrates, Norplant, oxymetholone, paromomycin, pectin, penicillamine, phenytoin, prazosin, progesterone, propofol, psyllium, pyridoxine, tamoxifen, terazosin, thyroid products, tolbutamide, ursodiol, verapamil
HIGH-DENSITY LIPOPROTEIN CHOLESTEROL (SERUM)	Albuterol, aminoglutethimide, angiotensin-converting enzyme inhibitor (eg, captopril), ascorbic acid, beclomethasone, β-blockers	Ascorbic acid, β-blockers (eg, acebutolol), chlorpropamide, clofibrate, danazol, diuretics (eg,

Drugs Affecting Laboratory Test Values *(Continued)*

Substance Determined	Drugs Causing Increased Values or False-Positive Values	Drugs Causing Decreased Values or False-Negative Values
	(eg, atenolol, carvedilol, pindolol), calcium channel blockers (eg, diltiazem), carbamazepine, cimetidine, diuretics (eg, furosemide, hydrochlorothiazide, indapamide), doxazosin, estrogen/oral contraceptives, glyburide, insulin, ketoconazole, lipid-lowering agents (eg, cholestyramine), metformin, minoxidil, phenobarbital, phenytoin, prazosin, prednisone, terbutaline	hydrochlorothiazide), ketoconazole, levothyroxine, medroxyprogesterone, methyldopa, oral contraceptives, prednisolone, stanozolol, tamoxifen
APOLIPOPROTEIN A (SERUM)	Carbamazepine, furosemide, gemfibrozil, phenobarbital, phenytoin, prednisolone	Estrogens, niacin, neomycin, stanozolol
APOLIPOPROTEIN B (SERUM)	Amiodarone, β-blockers (eg, metoprolol), cyclosporine, diuretics (eg, furosemide), etretinate, isotretinoin, oral contraceptives, phenobarbital, progestins, simvastatin, stanozolol	β-blockers (eg, bisoprolol), captopril, estrogens, interferon, ketoconazole, levothyroxine, lipid-lowering agents (eg, cholestyramine), low-molecular-weight heparin, medroxyprogesterone, neomycin, nifedipine, phenobarbital, phenytoin, prazosin, prednisolone, psyllium
TRIGLYCERIDES (SERUM)	Acetylsalicylic acid, amiodarone, ardeparin, asparaginase, β-blockers (eg, acebutolol) carbenicillin, chlordiazepoxide, cortico-steroids (eg, prednisolone), cyclosporine, danazol, diethylstilbesterol, disopyramide, diuretics (eg, chlorthalidone), enalapril, estrogens/oral contraceptives, ethylene glycol, etretinate, glycerin, isotretinoin,	Acarbose, acetylsalicylic acid, amiodarone, anabolic steroids, androgens, ascorbic acid, asparaginase, calcium channel–blocking agents (eg, diltiazem), chlorthalidone, citrates, dexfenfluramine, doxazosin, enalapril, fenfluramine, fosinopril, glucagon, guanfacine, hydroxychloroquine,

(continued)

Drugs Affecting Laboratory Test Values   *(Continued)*

Substance Determined	Drugs Causing Increased Values or False-Positive Values	Drugs Causing Decreased Values or False-Negative Values
	itraconazole, low-molecular-weight heparin, lovastatin, medroxyprogesterone, methadone, methicillin, methyldopa, miconazole, nitroglycerin, prazocin, ritonavir, sertraline, simvastatin, tamoxifen, warfarin	hydroxyurea, insulin, insulin-like growth factor, ketoconazole, levodopa/methyldopa, levothyroxine, lipid-lowering agents (eg, cholestyramine), low-molecular-weight heparin, medroxypro-gesterone, metformin, methimazole, methotrexate, metronidazole, naproxen, neomycin, Norplant, pentoxifylline, phenytoin, prazosin, prednisolone, psyllium, reserpine, rifampin, salicylates (high doses), sulfonylureas (eg, glyburide), terazosin
FATTY ACIDS, FREE (SERUM)	Aminophylline, amphetamine, chlorpromazine, desipramine, diazoxide, insulin-like growth factor, isoproterenol, levodopa, mescaline, molindone, oral contraceptives, prazocin, reserpine, somatostatin, terbutaline, theophylline, tolbutamide, valproic acid	Acebutolol, amino acids, asparaginase, aspirin, atenolol, clofibrate, glyburide, insulin, insulin-like growth factor, levothyroxine, metformin, metoprolol, neomycin, niacin, nifedipine, prazocin, propranolol, propylthiouracil, simvastatin, sotalol, streptozocin
CALCITONIN (PLASMA)	Estrogen/progestin, calcium, cholecystokinin, epinephrine, glucagon	Octreotide, phenytoin
THYROXINE T4 FREE (SERUM)	Amiodarine, aspirin, carbamazepine, danazol, furosemide, levothyroxine, phenytoin, probenecid, propranolol, radiographic agents, tamoxifen, thyroxine, valproic acid	Amiodarone, anabolic steroids, anticonvulsants (eg, carbamazepine), asparaginase, clofibrate, corticosteroids, furosemide, isotretinoin, levothyroxine, methadone, methimazole, octreotide, oral

Drugs Affecting Laboratory Test Values *(Continued)*

Substance Determined	Drugs Causing Increased Values or False-Positive Values	Drugs Causing Decreased Values or False-Negative Values
		contraceptives, phenobarbital, phenytoin, ranitidine
FREE TRIIODO-THYRONINE T3 (SERUM)	Amiodarone, aspirin, carbamazepine, fenoprofen, levothyroxine, phenytoin, ranitidine, thyroxine	Amiodarone, carbamazepine, corticosteroids, methimazole, phenytoin, propranolol, radiographic agents, somatostatin
FREE THYROXINE INDEX (SERUM)	Amiodarone, amphetamine, furosemide, oral contraceptives, propranolol	Aspirin, carbamazepine, clomiphene, corticosteroids, co-trimoxazole, ferrous sulfate, iodides, isotretinoin, lovastatin, methimazole, phenobarbital, phenytoin, primidone
NEONATAL THYROTROPIN-RELEASING HORMONE	Antithyroid drugs, aspirin, corticosteroids, estrogens, levodopa	
THYROGLOBULIN (SERUM)		Carbamazepine, neomycin, thyroxine
THYROID-STIMULATING HORMONE (SERUM)	Aminoglutethimide, amphetamine, calcitonin, carbamazepine, chlorpromazine, clomiphene, ethionamide, ferrous sulfates, furosemide, iodides, lithium, lovastatin, mercaptopurine, metoprolol, morphine, nitroprusside, phenytoin, potassium iodide, prazosin, prednisone, propranolol, radiographic agents, rifampin, sulfonamides, thyrotropin-releasing hormone	Amiodarone, anabolic steroids, antithyroid drugs, aspirin, carbamazepine, clofibrate, corticosteroids, danazol, dobutamide, dopamine, fenoldopam, growth hormone–releasing hormone, hydrocortisone, interferon, levodopa, levothyroxine, nifedipine, octreotide, phenytoin, pimozide, pyridoxine, somatostatin, thyroxine, troleandomycin
THYROXINE-BINDING GLOBULIN (SERUM)	Carbamazepine, clofibrate, diethylstilbestrol, estrogens, mestranol, oral contraceptives, perphenazine,	Anabolic steroids, asparaginase, aspirin, chlorpropamide, colestipol, corticosteroids,

(continued)

Drugs Affecting Laboratory Test Values *(Continued)*

Substance Determined	Drugs Causing Increased Values or False-Positive Values	Drugs Causing Decreased Values or False-Negative Values
	phenothiazines, progesterone, tamoxifen, thyroid agents, warfarin	cortisone, cytostatic therapy, phenytoin, propranolol, sulfonamides
TRIIODOTHYRONINE T3 TOTAL (SERUM)	Amiodarone, amphetamine, clofibrate, estrogens, fenoprofen, fluorouracil, insulin, levothyroxine, mestranol, methadone, opiates, phenothiazines, phenytoin, propylthiouracil, prostaglandins, ranitidine, rifampin, somatotropin, tamoxifen, terbutaline, thyrotropin-releasing hormone, valproic acid	Amiodarone, anabolic steroids, androgens, anticonvulsants (eg, phenytoin), asparaginase, aspirin, atenolol, cholestyramine, cimetidine, clomiphene, clomipramine, colestipol, corticosteroids, co-trimoxazole, furosemide, interferon, iodides, isotretinoin, lithium, methimazole, metoprolol, neomycin, netilmicin, oral contraceptives, penicillamine, phenobarbital, phenytoin, potassium iodide, propranolol, propylthiouracil, radiographic agents, reserpine, salicylates (eg, aspirin), somatostatin, sulfonylureas
TRIIODO-THYRONINE UPTAKE (BLOOD)	Anabolic steroids, androgens, aspirin, colestipol, corticosteroids, cytostatic therapy, dicoumarol, heparin, phenytoin, propranolol, salicylates, sulfonamides, thyroid agents, warfarin	Antiovulatory drugs, antithyroid drugs, carbamazepine, clofibrate, diethylstilbestrol, estrogens, heparin, heroin, mestranol, methadone, oral contraceptives, perphenazine, phenothiazines, progesterones, tamoxifen, thiazide diuretics (eg, hydrochlorothiazide), thyroid agents, warfarin
URINE SPECIFIC GRAVITY	Dextran, isotretinoin, penicillins, radiographic agents	Lithium

Drugs Affecting Laboratory Test Values   *(Continued)*

Substance Determined	Drugs Causing Increased Values or False-Positive Values	Drugs Causing Decreased Values or False-Negative Values
PROTEIN (URINE)	Acetaminophen, acetazolamide, aldesleukin, aminophylline, aminosalicylic acid, amphotericin, antibiotics (eg, bacitracin), arsenicals, ascorbic acid, asparaginase, auranofin, betaxolol, bicarbonate, bismuth subsalicylate, captopril, castor oil, chloral hydrate, chlorpromazine, chlorpropamide, cidofovir, cisplatin, codeine, corticosteroids, cyclosporine, dantrolene, dihydrotachysterol, diuretics (eg, chlorthalidone), doxapram, enalapril, ethosuximide, fenoprofen, fluorides, foscarnet, glyburide, glycerin, griseofulvin, hydralazine, interferon, iodine-containing drugs, iron-containing products, isoniazid, isotretinoin, lansoprazole, lithium, metahexamide, methenamine, methsuximide, mitomycin, mitotane, nifedipine, nizatidine, nonsteroidal antiinflammatory drugs (fenoprofen), penicillamine, phenazopyridine, phosphorus, probenecid, promazine, quinine, radiographic agents, ramipril, ranitidine, salicylates (eg, aspirin), sodium bicarbonate, streptokinase, streptozocin, theophylline, tolbutamide, trifluoperazine, vidarabine, vitamin D, vitamin K, x-ray therapy	Atenolol, captopril, clonidine, cyclophosphamide, diltiazem, enalapril, fosinopril, interferon, lisinopril, prednisolone, quinapril, ramipril
ALBUMIN (URINE)	Carbamazepine, cisplatin, gentamicin, nifedipine, oral contraceptives,	Angiotensin-converting enzyme inhibitors (eg, enalapril), atenolol,

(continued)

Drugs Affecting Laboratory Test Values   *(Continued)*

Substance Determined	Drugs Causing Increased Values or False-Positive Values	Drugs Causing Decreased Values or False-Negative Values
	radiographic agents, verapamil	diuretics (eg, furosemide), dypyridamole, ibuprofen
GLUCOSE (URINE)	Acetazolamide, aminosalicylic acid, antibiotics (eg, cephalosporins), ascorbic acid, aspirin, bismuth subsalicylate, captopril, carbamazepine, chloral hydrate, choline magnesium, trisalicylate, corticosteroids, dextroamphetamine, diazoxide, diuretics (eg, chlorthalidone), enalapril, ephedrine, estrogens, ethionamide, glucagon, glucose infusions, ifosfamide, indomethacin, isoniazid, levodopa, lithium, niacin, omeprazole, peroxide, phenazopyridine, phenothiazines, phenytoin, probenecid, reserpine, streptozocin, sulfonamides, theophylline, thiothixene	Antibiotics (eg, ampicillin), ascorbic acid, aspirin, bisacodyl, chloral hydrate, diazepam, digoxin, ferrous sulfate, flurazepam, furosemide, insulin, levodopa, phenazopyridine, phenobarbital, prednisone, propoxyphene, secrobarbital, vitamin preparations
KETONES (URINE)	Aspirin, captopril, cefixime, dimercaprol, etodolac, ifosfamide, insulin, isoniazid, levodopa, mesna, metformin, methyldopa, *n*-acetylcysteine, niacin, penicillamine, phenazopyridine, phenolphthalein, phenothiazines, pyrazinamide, streptozocin, succimer, valproic acid	Aspirin, phenazopyridine
BILIRUBIN (URINE)	Acetohexamide, acetophenazine, allopurinol, antibiotics, barbiturates, chlorpromazine, dapsone, etodolac, fluphenazine, imipramine, methyldopa,	Ascorbic acid, indomethicin

Drugs Affecting Laboratory Test Values   *(Continued)*

Substance Determined	Drugs Causing Increased Values or False-Positive Values	Drugs Causing Decreased Values or False-Negative Values
	norandrolone, oral contraceptives, perphenazine, phenothiazines, steroids, sulfonamides, tolmetin	
BLOOD CELLS AND RED CASTS (URINE)	Acetaminophen, acetazolamide, allopurinol, aminosalicylic acid, amphotericin, antibiotics, (eg, capreomycin), arsenicals, bismuth subsalicylate, carbamazepine, colchicine, colistin, cyclophosphamide, gold, hydralazine, ifosfamide, iron, levodopa, lipomul, mercaptopurine, methenamime, methocarbamol, mitotane, nonsteroidal antiinflammatory drugs (eg, aspirin), penicillamine, phenolphthalein, phosphorus, phytonadione, probenecid, propylthiouracil, radiographic agents, thiazide diuretics (eg, chlorothiazide), ticlopidine, warfarin	
POTASSIUM (URINE)	Acetazolamide, ammonium chloride, antibiotics (eg, gentamicin), atenolol, calcitonin, cathartics, citrates, corticosteroids, diuretics (eg, thiazide), dopamine, fenoldopam, isosorbide, levodopa, lithium, niacinamide, nifedipine, oral contraceptives, salicylates (eg, aspirin), sulfates	Amiloride, anesthetic agents, carbamazepine, cyclosporine, diazoxide, felodipine, ketoconazole, nicain, ramipril
SODIUM (URINE)	Acetazolamide, ammonium chloride, antibiotics (eg, tetracyclines, triamcinolone), aspirin, atenolol, calcitonin, captopril, carvedilol,	Anesthetic agents, carbamazepine, corticosteroids, cyclosporine, diazoxide, diuretics, enalapril,

(continued)

Drugs Affecting Laboratory Test Values *(Continued)*

Substance Determined	Drugs Causing Increased Values or False-Positive Values	Drugs Causing Decreased Values or False-Negative Values
	cisplatin, dexamethasone, digitalis, diuretics, (eg, ethacrynic acid), dopamine, enalapril, felodipine, fenoldopam, hydrocortisone, ifosfamide, insulin, isosorbide, laxatives, levodopa, lithium, mannitol, metoprolol, niacin, nicardipine, nifedipine, oral contraceptives, parathyroid extract, progesterones, secretin, sulfates, triamcinolone, verapamil, vincristine	etodolac, indomethacin, insulin, levarterenol, lithium, naproxen, octreotide, propranolol, ramipril
URIC ACID (URINE)	Acetaminophen, acetohexamide, ampicillin, ascorbic acid, asparaginase, clofibrate, cortisone, dicumarol, diethylstilbestrol, diuretics (eg, chlorothiazide), glycine, ifosfamide, levodopa/methyldopa, lithium, mannitol, mercaptopurine, methotrexate, niacinamide, nifedipine, phenothiazines, prednisolone, probenecid, salicylates (eg, aspirin), sulfamethoxazole, sulfinpyrazone, theophylline, verapamil, x-ray therapy	Acetazolamide, allopurinol, ascorbic acid, azathioprine, diazoxide, diuretics (eg, furosemide), ethambutol, hydralazine, niacin, probenecid, pyrazinamide, salicylates
CALCIUM (URINE)	Acetazolamide, aluminum hydroxide, ammonium chloride, anabolic steroids, androgens, antacids, anticonvulsants, ascorbic acid, asparaginase, calcitonin, calcitriol, calcium salts, cholestyramine, corticosteroids (eg, prednisolone), diltiazem, dimercaprol, diuretics (eg, amiloride), fenoldopam, mannitol, mithramycin, plicamycin, vitamin A, vitamin K	Antacids, bicarbonate, calcitonin, chlorthalidone, citrates, estrogens/oral contraceptives, ketoconazole, lithium, mestranol, neomycin, octreotide, pamidronate, phenytoin, phosphates, quinapril, spironolactone, thiazide diuretics, vitamin K

Drugs Affecting Laboratory Test Values *(Continued)*

Substance Determined	*Drugs Causing Increased Values or False-Positive Values*	*Drugs Causing Decreased Values or False-Negative Values*
MAGNESIUM (URINE)	Acetazolamide, ammonium chloride, amphotericin, calcitonin, cisplatin, corticosteroids, cyclosporine, diuretics (eg, bumetanide)	Acetazolamide, amiloride, calcium gluconate, diltiazem, glucuronic acid, interferon, oral contraceptives, parathyroid extract, phosphates
OXALATE (URINE)	Ascorbic acid, bumetanide, ethylene glycol, methoxyflurane	Ascorbic acid, calcium carbonate, pyridoxine
PREGNANEDIOL (URINE)	Adrenocorticotropic hormone/corticotropin, phenazopyridine, tamoxifen	Ampicillin, estrogens, medroxyprogesterone, oral contraceptives, phenothiazines, progesterones
URINE 5-HYDROXY-INDOLEACETIC ACID	Acetaminophen, benzodiazepines (eg, chlordiazepoxide, diazepam, flurazepam), cisplatin, ephedrine, fluorouracil, guaifenesin, heparin, melphalan, methamphetamine, methocarbamol, naproxen, phenobarbital, phentolamine, rauwolfia, reserpine, salicylates	Aspirin, ethyl alcohol, heparin, isoniazid, levodopa/methyldopa, monoamine oxidase inhibitors, methenamine, octreotide, phenothiazines, streptozocin, tricyclic antidepressants (eg, imipramine)
VANILLYMANDELIC ACID (URINE)	Aminosalicylic acid, caffeine, disulfiram, doxazosin, epinephrine, glucagon, griseofulvin, Guaifenesin, insulin, isoproterenol, labetalol, levodopa/methyldopa, lithium, methenamine, methocarbamol, nalidixic acid, nitroglycerin, oxytetracycline, penicillin, phenazopyridine, phenothiazines (eg, chlorpromazine, prochlorperazine), *Rauwolfia,* reserpine, salsalate, sulfonamides	Clofibrate, clonidine, disulfiram, guanethidine, guanfacine, levodopa/methyldopa, monoamine oxidase inhibitors, morphine, phenothiazines (eg, imipramine), radiographic agents, reserpine

(continued)

Drugs Affecting Laboratory Test Values   *(Continued)*

Substance Determined	Drugs Causing Increased Values or False-Positive Values	Drugs Causing Decreased Values or False-Negative Values
PORPHYRINE (URINE)	Aminoglutethimide, antibiotics (eg, ciprofloxacin), antipyretics, barbiturates, benzodiazepines (eg, chlordiazepoxide), chloral hydrate, chlorpropamide, ergot preparations, griseofulvin, hydroxychloroquine, meprobamate, methyldopa, pentazocine, phenazopyridine, phenytoin, progestin derivatives, vitamin K	Oral contraceptives
PORPHOBILINOGEN (URINE)	Aminoglutethimide, aminosalicylic acid, anticonvulsants (eg, phenytoin), barbiturates, cascara, chlordiazepoxide, chlorpropamide, griseofulvin, meprobamate, methyldopa, oral contraceptives, pentazocine, phenothiazines, procaine, tolbutamide	Actinomycin
PHENYLKETONURIA (URINE)	Antibiotics, phenols, phenothiazines, salicylates	Ascorbic acid
CREATININE (URINE)	Cefoxitin, cyclophosphamide, diuretics (eg, furosemide, torsemide), enalapril, fenoldopam, isosorbide, levodopa, mannitol, methylprednisolone, nifedipine, octreotide, oral contraceptives, prednisone, ramipril	Amphotericin, antibiotics (eg, cefoxitin, cephalothin, vancomycin), atenolol, cannabis, chlorpropamide, cimetidine, cisplatin, cyclosporine, diazoxide, diuretics (eg, chlorothiazide), ethambutol, etoposide, gold, griseofulvin, ketoconazole, lithium, mitomycin, nonsteroidal antiinflammatory drugs (eg, fenoprofen), octreotide, paromomycin, prednisone, probenecid
CYSTEINE (URINE)	Histidine, penicillamine	Ascorbic acid

Drugs Affecting Laboratory Test Values *(Continued)*

Substance Determined	Drugs Causing Increased Values or False-Positive Values	Drugs Causing Decreased Values or False-Negative Values
HYDROXYPROLINE (URINE)	Corticosteroids, danazol, parathyroid hormone, phenobarbital, phenytoin, thyroid, tolbutamide, vitamin D	Antineoplastic agents, ascorbic acid, aspirin, calcitonin, corticosteroids (eg, budesonide), estrogens/oral contraceptives, etidronate, gallium nitrate, pamidronate, plicamycin, propranolol, vitamin K
URINE AMINO ACIDS (TOTAL/ FRACTIONS)	Acetaminophen, aminocaproic acid, amphetamine, antibiotics (eg, amikacin), aspirin, bismuth subsalicylate, brompheniramine, cisplatin, colistin, dopamine, ephedrine, hydrocortisone, ifosfamide, insulin, levodopa/ methyldopa, methamphetamine, parathyroid extract, penicillamine, phenobarbital, phenylpropanolamine, primidone, pseudoephedrine, streptozocin, triamcinolone	Insulin
ANTINUCLEAR ANTIBODY TEST ANA (SERUM)	Acebutolol, anticonvulsants (eg, phenytoin), captopril, chlorpromazine, hydralazine, interferon, isoniazid, labetalol, methyldopa, mexiletine, nitrofurantoin, oral contraceptives, penicillamine, procainamide, propylthiouracil, quinidine, sulfasalazine, tocainide	
ANTI-DSDNA TSET (SERUM)	Chlorpromazine, valproic acid	
C3 COMPLEMENT (SERUM)	Cimetidine, cyclophosphamide, oral contraceptives	Danazol, hydralazine, methyldopa, phenytoin

(continued)

Drugs Affecting Laboratory Test Values *(Continued)*

Substance Determined	Drugs Causing Increased Values or False-Positive Values	Drugs Causing Decreased Values or False-Negative Values
C4 COMPLEMENT (SERUM)	Cyclophosphamide, danazol, oral contraceptives	Dextran, methyldopa, penicillamine
TOTAL HEMOLYTIC COMPLEMENT (CH50) (SERUM)	Chlorpropamide, cyclophosphamide, oral contraceptives	Hydralazine
RHEUMATOID FACTOR (SERUM)		Interferon α-2a; methotrexate, nonsteroidal antiinflammatory drugs
THYROID ANTIBODIES (SERUM)	Lithium	
ANTI–SMOOTH MUSCLE ANTIBODIES (SERUM)	Methyldopa, nitrofurantoin	
ANTIMITO-CHONDRIAL ANTIBODIES (SERUM)	Labetalol	Cyclosporine, ursodiol
ACETYLCHOLINE RECEPTOR ANTIBODIES (SERUM)	Penicillamine	
IMMUNOGLOBULIN E ANTIBODY (SERUM)	Aztreonam, penicillin G	Phenytoin
LATEX FIXATION (SERUM)	Procainamide	

Drugs Affecting Laboratory Test Values *(Continued)*

Substance Determined	Drugs Causing Increased Values or False-Positive Values	Drugs Causing Decreased Values or False-Negative Values
ANTICARDIOLIPIN ANTIBODIES (SERUM)	Chlorpromazine	
ANTICARDIOLIPIN-SPECIFIC IMMUNOGLOBULIN M ANTIBODIES (SERUM)	Chlorpromazine	
LEUKOAGGLUTININ TEST (SERUM)	Cephradine, methyldopa, sulfapyridine	
COOMBS' TEST (SERUM)	Aztreonam, cephalosporin antibiotics, ethosuximide, hydralazine, imipenem, isoniazid, levodopa, mefenamic acid, melphalan, moxalactam, penicillamine, phenytoin, procainamide, quinidine, quinine, streptomycin, sulfonylureas, tetracycline	
PLATELET ANTIBODY DETECTION TEST (BLOOD) *Drugs that may cause induction of antiplatelet antibodies*	Analgesics (eg, acetaminophen), antibiotics (eg, cephalosporins), diuretics, digoxin, disulfiram, heavy metals (eg, gold), heparin, hypoglycemics (oral) (eg, chlorpropamide), hypnotics (eg, phenobarbital), quinidine, propylthiouracil	

● INDEX

M

5198